Handbook of Practical Immunohistochemistry

Fan Lin • Jeffrey Prichard
Editors

Handbook of Practical Immunohistochemistry

Frequently Asked Questions

Haiyan Liu
Myra Wilkerson
Conrad Schuerch
Assoc. Editors

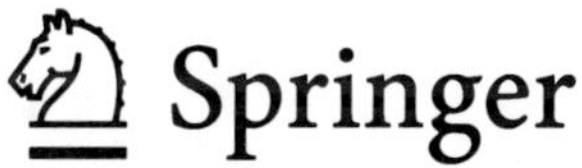

Editors
Fan Lin, MD, PhD
Department of Pathology and Laboratory Medicine
Geisinger Medical Center
Danville, PA 17822
USA
Flin1@geisinger.edu

Jeffrey Prichard, DO
Department of Pathology and Laboratory Medicine
Geisinger Medical Center
Danville, PA 17822
USA
jwprichard@geisinger.edu

ISBN 978-1-4419-8061-8 ISBN 978-1-4419-8062-5 (eBook)
DOI 10.1007/978-1-4419-8062-5
Springer New York Dordrecht Heidelberg London

Library of Congress Control Number: 2011928251

Printed on acid-free paper

Springer is part of Springer Science+Business Media (www.springer.com)

Preface and How to Use This Book

How Did Immunohistochemistry Evolve to Our Current Practices?

Over the past 20 years, four key discoveries can be viewed as the cornerstones in the continuing evolution of immunohistochemistry (IHC). They include (1) the development of monoclonal antibodies, significantly increasing diagnostic specificity; (2) the introduction of heat-induced and proteolytic enzyme antigen retrieval methods, providing a foundation for the utility of IHC on formalin-fixed paraffin-embedded surgical specimens; (3) the use of a highly sensitive secondary detection system, allowing detection of trace amounts of proteins in formalin-fixed tissue with little background staining; and (4) the invention of the automated immunohistochemical stainer, providing a device to run hundreds of IHC slides on the same day, in the same laboratory, with highly reproducible results. In the near future, digital pathology will certainly take IHC to a new level of practice.

Because of these advances, immunohistochemistry has been smoothly integrated into the practice of modern surgical pathology and cytopathology with regard to diagnosis, differential diagnosis, prognosis, and targeted therapy. However, there is a massive body of knowledge of IHC and new antibodies emerge continuously, challenging the general pathologist to keep current in all subspecialty areas.

What Is This Book For?

In much the same way that both positive and negative immunohistochemical results offer valuable insight into a disease process, we would like to describe for you both what this book is intended to be and what it is not. It is not an exhaustive reference work detailing the science and theory of immunohistochemistry to be read cover to cover. Many of us already own and treasure excellent volumes for this purpose. As these books have grown in size and scope, recording our expanding experience with the proteome of disease, our group felt a need for simplicity. This book is intended to be a practical, quick reference for information related to using immunohistochemistry in clinical diagnosis.

How Do I Use This Book to Find What I Am Looking For?

The concept of this book was derived from the Frequently Asked Questions (FAQs) portions of web sites, a format that has become an established and successful part of the Internet. The table of contents and chapters are organ-based and designed in a question-and-answer format.

Within each chapter, the questions are grouped and ordered by relationship to one another, so adjacent questions may provide additional information relevant to your search. The goal is to enable the reader to quickly find the specific information he or she is seeking and get back to work. The book is available in paper and electronic formats, reflecting the transitional and hybrid nature of our current information age. Some readers may find that the search function of the electronic version of the book serves them well in navigating the pages.

What Information Does the Book Contain and What Are the Unique Features of This Book?

We are all familiar with the daunting task faced as residents of learning the nuances of subspecialty diagnoses and the time-consuming reading involved in staying current as generalists while managing diverse caseloads. We all have collected stacks of notes and articles reminding us of useful antibody panels we want to remember next time. We offer this book as a "curbside consult" of practical knowledge shared by colleagues who work with these organ-specific diagnostic questions every day. The unique features of this book can be summarized as follows:

1. *Question-and-answer (Q&A) format with over 1,000 questions*: This Handbook is designed to be practical, concise, and credible. Most chapters are written in a Q&A (question-and-answer) format to recapitulate daily practice in surgical pathology and cytopathology, and how we think and work as pathologists.
2. *List of questions on first page of each chapter*: The first page of each chapter lists the FAQs about that particular organ, which provides easy access for a user. For organ-based chapters, each question is addressed in a table to provide the best answer.
3. *Suggested working antibody panels*: When you examine each individual table, you will notice that some of the antibodies in the table are highlighted by color. The color-highlighted set of antibodies is the suggested panel for an initial workup. Brief notes are provided for many tables, in order to reiterate the most important diagnostic applications and pitfalls that one may encounter.
4. *Color pictures from Geisinger Medical Laboratories (GML) IHC slides*: A fairly representative set of color pictures and diagrams, if available, is included in each chapter to illustrate some of the key antibodies used in that particular chapter. There are over 500 color pictures taken from GML IHC slides using the recommended staining protocols contained in the appendices of this book.
5. *GML data*: In many tables you will see a column containing data from GML in comparison to data from the literature. This is a unique feature of this book. The reproducibility of antibodies reported in the literature is sometimes in question; to improve the reproducibility, we have undertaken the daunting task of testing the antibodies listed in the appendices using more than 5,000 TMA slides (close to 100 TMA blocks) and 1,000 routine slides. These TMA sections contain thousands of tumors from various organs and normal tissues in the GML archives. If your laboratory follows the protocols in the appendices, you should obtain similar results to GML.
6. *IHC on normal tissues*: Immunophenotypes of many normal tissues, which receive little or no attention in other surgical pathology and IHC books, have been included in many chapters, such as normal breast, lung, pancreas, ampulla, colon, stomach, small intestine, and kidney.
7. *Antibody information*: The lack of detailed information about staining protocols in the literature is quite frustrating, especially when trying to reproduce published results;

therefore, we have included detailed antibody information in this book. Most antibodies mentioned in this book have been routinely used at GML, or have at least been optimized in both the Dako and Ventana systems. You will find the appendices (Appendix A, Antibodies Tested in the Dako System, and Appendix B, Antibodies Tested in the Ventana System) in the back of this book that provide detailed information for each antibody, including vendor, catalog number, clone, antigen retrieval method, antibody dilution, in vitro diagnostic use (IVD) vs. analyte-specific reagents (ASR) vs. research use only (RUO) class, staining pattern, positive control tissue, and the contact information for each vendor. No one in our group has a financial interest in any of these companies.

8. *Data interpretation*: To standardize on one manual scoring system, the following recording system is applied throughout this book, unless otherwise specified:
   (a) – = Usually less than 5% of cases are stained
   (b) + = Usually greater than 70% of cases are stained
   (c) + or – = Usually more than 50% but less than 70% of cases are stained
   (d) – or + = Usually less than 50% of cases are stained
   (e) v = Variable, or sometimes positive; data are somewhat inconsistent
   (f) ND = No data available
9. *Automated IHC – perspective from industry*: As an additional helpful note, we have included some brief chapters listing answers to questions regarding managing an immunohistochemistry laboratory. Topics include practical advice on choosing and optimizing antibody titers and retrieval methods, making choices regarding automated platforms, ways to monitor the quality of your processes and personnel, and regulatory issues related to running a clinical immunohistochemistry laboratory. We have also requested contributions from vendors to share their perspectives on where they perceive the industry to be and where the future of automating immunohistochemistry may take us.
10. *Expert contributions*: Last but not least, many chapters also include contributions from an expert in his or her field.

What Are the Points to Remember?

When you navigate through the chapters, you will notice (or you already have) that no single antibody is entirely specific and absolutely sensitive to a specific diagnosis. As a general rule, those initially reported as highly sensitive and specific "hot" antibodies may lose their popularity following extensive testing in various tumors and organs. Therefore, a few points should be emphasized here: (1) use of a single antibody to make a diagnosis is discouraged; instead, a small panel of antibodies should be considered; (2) if an unexpected positive or negative result occurs, proceed with caution and expand your panel; (3) one should focus on the whole picture, including clinical information, histopathology, radiological findings, and the IHC results; and (4) when things do not fit completely, go back to your H&E slides, because morphology is still the most crucial information available to us!

Since this is the first edition and the book was written within a relatively short period of time by the authors while still carrying our normal caseload, we fully expect to have some errors or even conflicting information. The editors sincerely ask for your understanding and also invite you to submit your feedback, suggestions, and comments to us (Flin1@geisinger.edu; Jwprichard@geisinger.edu; Hliu1@geisinger.edu; Mwilkerson@geisinger.edu; Cschuerch@geisinger.edu). With support from readers like you, we are confident that future editions will be even more complete and informative.

Fan Lin, MD, PhD
Jeffrey Prichard, DO
Haiyan Liu, MD
Myra Wilkerson, MD
Conrad Schuerch, MD

Acknowledgments

Producing this book was an enormous undertaking for our department and we wish to acknowledge the assistance and tremendous support we received from our staff. Therese Snyder, Vice President of Laboratory Operations, supported and encouraged this project from conception through completion. Sandy Mullay, Operations Director of Anatomic Pathology, always ensured we had the technical, secretarial, and clerical support needed for all phases of the project. Melissa Erb served as our project coordinator, keeping us organized and moving forward, doing whatever was needed from searching our archives for cases to editing references. Without her help and patience, this book would not exist. Tina Brosious, Histotechnologist, helped finalize, cut, and stain tissue microarrays. Kathy Fenstermacher was invaluable in editing and polishing book chapters, as well as in producing many of our diagrams. Glen Kauwell, Kris Bricker, and Laurie Kneller-Walter, Histotechnologists, helped stain tissue microarray sections. Mary Sejuit spent countless hours pulling and refiling slides and paraffin blocks, keeping everything well organized. Christy Attinger provided expert secretarial support. Bill Marple, Supervisor of Anatomic Pathology, helped with scheduling and coordination of technical staff. Jennifer Pettengill, CT(ASCP), Mayo Clinic, provided us with beautiful FISH images on urine samples, and Neogenomics provided us with additional FISH pictures. Finally, we need to thank our families and close friends for their understanding, especially during the final month of this project when we seemed to exist in a separate world. We are very fortunate to have your love and support.

Fan Lin, MD, PhD
Jeffrey Prichard, DO
Haiyan Liu, MD
Myra Wilkerson, MD
Conrad Schuerch, MD

Contents

Contributors

Nadine S. Aguilera, M.D.
Department of Hematopathology, Armed Forces Institute of Pathology,
Washington, DC 20306, USA

Angela Bitting, H.T.
Department of Pathology and Laboratory Medicine,
Geisinger Medical Center, Danville, PA 17822, USA
akbitting@geisinger.edu

Philip T. Cagle, M.D.
Department of Pathology and Laboratory Medicine, The Methodist Hospital
Physician Organization, Houston, TX 77030, USA
pcagle@tmhs.org

Ronald A. DeLellis, M.D.
Pathologist-in-Chief, Department of Pathology,
Rhode Island Hospital, Providence, RI 02903, USA
rdelellis@lifespan.org

R. Patrick Dorion, M.D.
Department of Pathology and Laboratory Medicine,
Geisinger Medical Center, Danville, PA 17822, USA
pdorion@geisinger.edu

Dirk M. Elston, M.D.
Department of Pathology and Laboratory Medicine,
Geisinger Medical Center, Danville, PA 17822, USA
dmelston@geisinger.edu

Tammie Ferringer, M.D.
Department of Pathology and Laboratory Medicine,
Geisinger Medical Center, Danville, PA 17822, USA
tferringer@geisinger.edu

Lawrence E. Gibson, M.D.
Professor, Department of Dermatology, Mayo Clinic College of Medicine,
Rochester, MN 55905, USA

Elizabeth Hammond, M.D.
Professor of Pathology, University of Utah School of Medicine Pathologist,
Intermountain Healthcare, LDS Hospital,
Dept of Pathology, 8th Ave and C Street, Salt Lake City, Utah 84143, USA
Elizabeth.Hammond@imail.ogr

David G. Hicks, M.D.
Professor of Pathology & Laboratory Medicine, Director of Surgical Pathology, University of Rochester, School of Medicine and Dentistry, 601 Elmwood Ave., Box 626, Rochester, NY 14642
David_Hicks@URMC.Rochester.edu

Hanna G. Kaspar, M.D.
Clinical Professor, Department of Pathology and Laboratory Medicine, Temple University School of Medicine, Philadelphia, PA, Staff Pathologist, Geisinger Wyoming Valley Medical Center, Wilkes-Barre, PA 18711, USA
hgkaspar@geisinger.edu

Heinz Kutzner, M.D.
Dermatopathologische, Gemeinschaftspraxis, Friedrichshafen, Germany

Jinhong Li, M.D., Ph.D.
Department of Pathology and Laboratory Medicine,
Assistant Professor, Pathology and Laboratory Medicine, Temple Univeristy, Geisinger Medical Center, Danville, PA 17822, USA
jli1@geisinger.edu

Fan Lin, M.D., Ph.D.
Department of Pathology and Laboratory Medicine,
Geisinger Medical Center, Danville, PA 17822, USA
flin1@geisinger.edu

Haiyan Liu, M.D., Ph.D.
Department of Pathology and Laboratory Medicine,
Geisinger Medical Center, Danville, PA 17822, USA
hliu1@geisinger.edu

Steven Meschter, M.D.
Department of Pathology and Laboratory Medicine,
Geisinger Medical Center, Danville, PA 17822, USA
smeschter@geisinger.edu

Markku Miettinen, M.D., Ph.D.
Department of Soft Tissue and Orthopedic Pathology,
Armed Forces Institute of Pathology, Washington, DC 20306-6000, USA

Douglas C. Miller, M.D., Ph.D.
Department of Pathology, 8 Anatomical Sciences, University of Missouri, School of Medicine, Columbia, MO 65212, USA

Barbara Paynton, Ph.D.
Department of Pathology and Laboratory Medicine,
Geisinger Medical Center, Danville, PA 17822, USA
bvpaynton@geisinger.edu

Erin Powell
Department of Pathology and Laboratory Medicine,
Geisinger Medical Center, Danville, PA 17822, USA
epowell1@geisinger.edu

Jeffrey Prichard, D.O.
Department of Pathology and Laboratory Medicine,
Geisinger Medical Center, Danville, PA 17822, USA
jwprichard@geisinger.edu

Ole F. Rasmussen, Ph.D.
Dako Denmark A/S, Glostrup, DK 2600, Denmark
ole.feldballe@dako.com

Angela Sattler
Ventana Medical System, Inc., Tucson, AZ 85755, USA
angi.sattler@ventana.roche.com

Andreas Schønau, M.S.
Dako Denmark A/S, Glostrup, Denmark

Conrad Schuerch, M.D.
Department of Pathology and Laboratory Medicine,
Geisinger Medical Center, Danville, PA 17822, USA
cschuerch@geisinger.edu

Jianhui Shi, M.D.
Department of Pathology and Laboratory Medicine,
Geisinger Medical Center, Danville, PA 17822, USA
jshi1@geisinger.edu

Jan F. Silverman, M.D.
Chairman, Department of Laboratory Medicine,
Allegheny General Hospital, Pittsburgh, PA 15212, USA;
Chairman, Department of Pathology, West Penn Hospital, Pittsburgh, PA, USA;
Chairman, Department of Pathology, West Penn Hospital Forbes Regional Campus, Pittsburgh, PA, USA;
Professor, Pathology and Laboratory Medicine, Drexel University College of Medicine, Philadelphia, PA, USA;
Professor, Pathology and Laboratory Medicine, Temple University, Philadelphia, PA, USA
jsilverm@wpahs.org

William B. Tyler, M.D.
Department of Pathology and Laboratory Medicine,
Geisinger Medical Center, Danville, PA 17822, USA
wtyler@geisinger.edu

Hanlin L. Wang, M.D., Ph.D.
Department of Pathology and Laboratory Medicine,
Cedars-Sinai Medical Center, Los Angeles, CA 90048, USA
Hanlin.wang@cshs.org

Myra Wilkerson, M.D.
Department of Pathology and Laboratory Medicine,
Geisinger Wyoming Valley Medical Center, PA 18711, USA
mwilkerson@geisinger.edu

Hueizhi (Hope) Wu, M.D., Ph.D.
Department of Pathology and Laboratory Medicine,
Geisinger Medical Center, Danville, PA 17822, USA
hwu1@geisinger.edu

Ximing J. Yang, M.D., Ph.D.
Professor, Department of Pathology, Robert H. Lurie Comprehensive
Cancer Center, Chicago, IL, USA;
Director, Pathology Core Facility, Robert H. Lurie Comprehensive
Cancer Center, Chicago, IL, USA;
Department of Surgical Pathology, Northwestern Memorial Hospital,
Northwestern University Feinberg School of Medicine, Chicago, IL 60611, USA
xyang@northwestern.edu

Hong Yin, M.D.
Department of Pathology and Laboratory Medicine,
Geisinger Medical Center, Danville, PA 17822, USA
hyin1@geisinger.edu

Qihui (Jim) Zhai, M.D.
Professor, Department of Pathology, University of Cincinnati,
Cincinnati, OH 45267, USA
qihui.zhai@uc.edu

Kai Zhang, M.D.
Department of Pathology and Laboratory Medicine,
Geisinger Medical Center, Danville, PA 17822, USA
kaizhang1@geisinger.edu

Xiaohong (Mary) Zhang, M.D.
Department of Pathology and Laboratory Medicine, Geisinger Wyoming
Valley Medical Center, Wilkes-Barre, PA 18711, USA
xmzhang1@geisinger.edu

Shaobo Zhu, M.D., Ph.D.
Department of Pathology and Laboratory Medicine, Geisinger Medical Center,
Danville, PA 17822, USA
szhu1@geisinger.edu

Chapter 1
Quality Management and Regulation

Jeffrey Prichard

Abstract Immunohistochemistry testing is highly complex with multiple steps. Assuring the optimum performance of your immunohistochemistry laboratory requires attention to numerous quality monitors. For testing performed on patient specimens, there are also additional regulatory requirements. This chapter answers questions about best practices in quality management in preanalytic, analytic, and postanalytic phases of the total immunohistochemistry test providing examples of possible quality improvement opportunities. It also provides information related to CLIA and FDA regulatory oversight medical devices, in vitro diagnostics (IVD), and analyte-specific reagents (ASR). With regard to immunohistochemistry laboratory accreditation, the final portion of this chapter draws attention to current best practice guidelines of the College of American Pathologists (CAP) relating to immunohistochemistry to prepare for inspection.

Keywords Quality • Regulation • CLIA • FDA • ASR • IVD • Controls • Validation • Inspection

FREQUENTLY ASKED QUESTIONS

IHC Quality Management

1. What should be the scope and significance of a quality management program for immunohistochemistry (IHC)? (p. 2)

Preanalytic Phase

2. How does specimen identification affect IHC quality? (p. 2)
3. How does specimen handling relate to IHC quality? (pp. 2–3)

Analytic Phase

4. How can I assure the qualifications of IHC testing personnel? (p. 3)
5. What role can research literature play in optimizing an IHC assay? (pp. 3–4)
6. How should RUO, ASR, and IVD designations be considered in selecting antibodies for optimizing an IHC assay? (p. 4)
7. How should I choose tissues for performing an optimization of an IHC assay? (p. 4)
8. What are the steps to vary in optimizing an IHC assay for a chosen antibody? (pp. 4–5)
9. What are the steps to validate an IHC assay for a chosen antibody? (p. 5)
10. What are the best control tissues for IHC assays? (pp. 5–6)
11. What are the parts of daily quality control in the IHC test? (p. 6)
12. What are the staining artifacts and failed control reactions to be aware of when interpreting IHC assay results? (p. 6)
13. What are some examples of quality assurance monitors for analytic phase of IHC testing? (p. 6)

Postanalytic Phase

14. What can be monitored in the postanalytic phase of IHC testing? (pp. 6–7)

Quality Improvement

15. What are some examples of possible quality improvement opportunities in IHC testing? (p. 7)

IHC Laboratory Regulation
CLIA and FDA Regulations

16. What is the law regulating IHC laboratory testing? (p. 7)
17. What is the concept of complexity with regard to laboratory testing regulation? (p. 7)
18. What are the agencies and organizations responsible for implementing CLIA regulations for clinical laboratories? (pp. 7–8)

J. Prichard (✉)
Department of Pathology and Laboratory Medicine,
Geisinger Medical Center, 100 North Academy Avenue, Danville, PA 17822, USA
e-mail: jwprichard@geisinger.edu

F. Lin and J. Prichard (eds.), *Handbook of Practical Immunohistochemistry: Frequently Asked Questions*,
DOI 10.1007/978-1-4419-8062-5_1, © Springer Science+Business Media, LLC 2011

19. What are the agencies and organizations responsible for implementing CLIA regulations for manufacturers of IHC reagents and instrumentation? (p. 8)
20. How does CLIA control the use of IHC testing through determination of laboratory and test complexity? (p. 8)
21. How does CLIA control the marketing and use of IHC testing through test class? (pp. 8–9)
22. What is the FDA's ASR rule? (p. 9)
23. What are the limitations placed on the information that a vendor can provide a laboratory for an ASR reagent? (p. 9)
24. How is the ASR rule related to in vitro diagnostic products labeled for research use only (RUO) or investigational use only (IUO)? (pp. 9–10)
25. What is the difference in FDA requirements for manufacturers of an ASR versus an RUO reagent? (p. 10)

CAP Regulations

26. What is the College of American Pathologists (CAP) Laboratory Accreditation Program (LAP)? (p. 10)
27. What are the CAP regulations for content of procedure manuals? (pp. 10–11)
28. What are the CAP regulations for instrument and reagents management? (p. 11)
29. What are the CAP regulations for microwaves used for IHC procedures? (p. 11)
30. What are the CAP regulations for formaldehyde and xylene use? (p. 11)
31. What are the CAP regulations for positive controls? (pp. 11–12)
32. What are the CAP regulations for negative controls? (p. 12)
33. What are the CAP regulations for endogenous biotin blocking? (p. 12)
34. What are the CAP regulations for new antibody validation? (pp. 12–13)
35. What are the CAP regulations for validation of new reagent lots? (p. 13)
36. What are the CAP regulations for reporting IHC results including ASRs? (p. 13)
37. What are the CAP regulations for slide or slide image retention? (p. 13)

1.1 What Should Be the Scope and Significance of a Quality Management Program for Immunohistochemistry?

Although immunohistochemistry (IHC) is a staining procedure, the factors that affect the quality of the results include events spanning from the identification of the specimen to the presentation in the report of the significance of the result to the submitting physician. So a program to manage the quality of IHC should address issues spanning the preanalytic, analytic, and postanalytic spectrum of the total testing process. Best practices should be implemented and processes monitored to detect and correct deficiencies to produce the best results. The need for quality results in IHC has only increased as the use of these tests has evolved from being markers of tumor differentiation to now include being predictive markers guiding the use of specific therapies. IHC stains are now, more than ever, an integral part of the practice of anatomic pathology. However, current and projected future healthcare economics make obvious the need for cost containment through comprehensive analysis and continuous quality improvements of workflow processes and appropriate utilization of IHC resources.

References: [1–11].

1.2 How Does Specimen Identification Affect IHC Quality?

The only way to provide a correct result for the correct patient is to ensure correct labeling of the specimen beginning from the initial acquisition of the specimen in the clinician's procedure room or operating room. To avoid confusion if specimen requisitions are separated from the specimen containers, both should be legibly labeled with at least two patient identifiers and the specimen type and location. This requirement for specimen identification should be monitored and enforced with submitting locations to emphasize the importance. Noncompliant specimen labels should be investigated to satisfactory resolution of identity with the submitting site or else rejected. The Joint Commission on Accreditation of Healthcare Organizations (JCAHO) has made the use of two patient identifiers, a National Patient Safety Goal applicable to laboratories. Modification of the requisition form may be necessary to help sites comply with specimen labeling requirements. Instances of problems with specimen labeling should be tracked and quantified to direct customer education resources to the most needed sites. Barcoding can be a major factor in reducing misidentification errors in anatomic pathology.

References: [11–17].

1.3 How Does Specimen Handling Relate to IHC Quality?

The topic of tissue handling and its effect on IHC testing has become common since the release in early 2007 of the American Society of Clinical Oncology (ASCO)/College of American Pathologists (CAP) guidelines for the Her-2 testing. The specifics of those guidelines will be discussed elsewhere in the book. But the inclusion of specific specimen handling recommendations in that report reinforces their importance.

The key issue in preanalytic specimen handling is to quickly get the tissue into standardized fixative to reduce the ischemic time until fixation and prepare the tissue for your validated antigen retrieval methods.

It is obvious that chemical breakdown resulting from ischemia would interfere in the detection of biomarkers in specimens. Whereas very stable markers such as DNA and intermediate filaments are able to be detected in necrotic tissue, other markers are far less resilient. Ischemic degradation is most noted with fragile mRNA molecules intended in vivo to be only fleetingly present to deliver their transcriptional messages. Breakdown of these molecules can be seen in a matter of minutes. CAP recommends limiting ischemic time for breast tissue specimens to be used for receptor studies to less than or equal to an hour.

Ischemic degradation of tissue is halted by the process of fixation by chemically stabilizing molecular structures, which creates linkages in the proteins. This has the effect of paralyzing tissue enzymes in addition to other proteins, which stops autolysis. Different fixative solutions have different times of tissue penetration and rates of fixation. Therefore, larger specimens should be refrigerated, if dissection is to be delayed. And when dissected, tissue sections should be thin enough so as not to be compressed by the cassette lid, which restricts fixative penetration. If breast tissue from a large resection is to be submitted for critical receptor studies, consideration should be given to either incising the tumor to expose the surface to fixative or submitting a single tissue section from the tumor prior to completing the full dissection.

Some biomarkers are affected differently by the use of different fixatives. An example of this is a loss of expression of S100 by IHC in tissue fixed in alcohol compared with the same tissue fixed in formalin. The effects of differences in fixation are not known for most biomarkers. And tissue fixation is probably the most out-of-control variable affecting the quality of IHC staining. So the best practice is to attempt to standardize the type and time of fixation used for tissues in your laboratory to optimize your antigen retrieval protocols to these fixation conditions. Methods recommended to standardize fixation in the preanalytic phase of testing include using only 10% neutral-buffered formalin (NBF). Formalin is not universally accepted to be the best fixative for all tissue types, but is the most commonly used fixative and provides for adequate histologic preparations for most antigens. Requiring formalin in your specimen submission requirements can help to achieve this goal. Of course alternative fixatives may be considered satisfactory, if the laboratory has performed validations of their IHC testing protocols using these alternative fixatives.

The other side of quickly placing tissues into fixative is controlling how long the tissues spend in the fixative solution. Tissues will be subjected to standardized antigen retrieval protocols designed to break down the bonds created by fixation. If tissue is inadequately fixed to withstand this retrieval process, target proteins may instead by destroyed, resulting in false-negative IHC results. This is known to occur with estrogen receptor protein testing performed on tissues fixed in formalin for less than 6 h. Tissues that are overfixed may also be falsely negative due to inadequacy of the standardized antigen retrieval protocol to reverse the effects of prolonged formalin fixation. In our experience, this is less commonly an issue with modern antigen retrieval methods. Each laboratory should have a procedure to control the minimum and maximum time tissues spend in fixative prior to processing and embedding. It is recommended that ischemic time and fixation type and time be recorded for tissues submitted for breast cancer receptor studies. Many laboratories have modified their specimen requisitions by providing an area of the form specifically for entering this data.

References: [18–39].

1.4 How Can I Assure the Qualifications of IHC Testing Personnel?

Histotechnologists (HTs) have the certification required to perform IHC testing, though the level of experience of histotechnologists with IHC varies greatly. The American Society of Clinical Pathology (ASCP) offers an additional certificate program for histotechnologists verifying advanced knowledge of the theory behind IHC testing as well as practical experience with optimization and performance of IHC. What is most critical is that staff have a familiarity with appropriate and inappropriate control reactions (nonspecific stromal staining, endogenous peroxide and biotin, staining artifacts, sub-cellular compartment of signal, and tissue pigments) and are able to recognize tissue artifacts before releasing slides to the pathologist. Competency testing of testing personnel should be performed and documented annually. Delays in the recognition of poor quality staining lead to delays in rerunning stains to produce adequate results. Such delays only serve to delay the final reports to the clinicians. The number of poor stains released should be monitored to direct re-education of staff. Providing images and descriptions of expected positive and negative staining patterns for each in-house stain can benefit histotechnologists as well as pathologists.

References: [4, 40–43].

1.5 What Role Can Research Literature Play in Optimizing an IHC Assay?

The first step to producing a clinically useful and valid IHC assays is by choosing clinically relevant and technically superior antibodies and reagents in your testing system. Our best advice is to review the literature to determine which antibody clones have associated clinical significance with reproducible protocols. Often requests for bringing on new antibodies are based on articles in the literature for a specific clinical application. In these cases, it would be advisable to acquire a copy of the article from the requesting pathologist or clinician to determine the clone and assay parameter used in the study to reproduce them as closely as possible in your laboratory. Even if the article does not provide sufficient information to reproduce the testing results, contacting the corresponding author is often fruitful. Otherwise, the article should, at least, indicate which tissue should produce positive and negative results so that these can be used to optimize the assay in your laboratory.

References: [2, 4, 44, 45].

1.6 How Should RUO, ASR, and IVD Designations Be Considered in Selecting Antibodies for Optimizing an IHC Assay?

Another consideration for choosing a clone is to determine which reagent class an antibody falls into. Antibodies developed in laboratories and not submitted to the FDA for approval are designated as research use only (RUO). As vendors pay for and accumulate research so that they are able to demonstrate increasingly reliable performance characteristics for their antibodies to the FDA, they received designations as either analyte-specific reagents (ASR) or, for the most fully characterized antibodies, there is a designation as an in vitro diagnostics (IVD). As vendors collect this research and obtain these higher class designations, they are able to supply more information. Datasheets for IVDs can contain more information regarding the expected performance of antibodies, often listing normal and abnormal tissue reactivities, indicating tissue types for optimization and control tissues. CAP-accredited laboratories have established rules for using RUO reagents. According to CAP guidelines, RUOs may only be used when no other class of antibody is available. RUOs purchased from commercial sources may be used in laboratory-developed tests, only if the laboratory has made a reasonable effort to search for IVD- or ASR-class reagents and the results of that failed search are documented by the laboratory director. If a CAP-accredited laboratory performs patient testing using Class I ASRs obtained or purchased from an outside vendor, federal regulations require that a disclaimer accompany the test result on the patient report stating, "This test was developed and its performance characteristics determined by (laboratory name). It has not been cleared or approved by the US Food and Drug Administration." CAP recommends adding an additional statement, "The FDA has determined that such clearance or approval is not necessary. This test is used for clinical purposes. It should not be regarded as investigational or for research. This laboratory is certified under the Clinical Laboratory Improvement Amendments (CLIA) as qualified to perform high complexity clinical laboratory testing." Attention to the class designation of antibodies is a Best Practice and CAP guideline.

References: [8, 46, 47].

1.7 How Should I Choose Tissues for Performing an Optimization of an IHC Assay?

Determining which choices to make for each of the steps of an IHC assay to achieve optimum performance is known as optimization. This process can be as simple as reproducing the vendor's recommended protocols with your equipment on your tissues. Unfortunately, it is the nature of reacting antibodies with fixed tissues that the optimization process is too often a long and confounding experience.

One of the most important keys to successful optimization is choosing the correct tissue. The first point to make is to choose tissues from your own paraffin archive of surgical specimens that were handled as typical specimens on which you would want to run the IHC test for diagnosis. Choosing tissues from autopsy cases can be a mistake, if the tissues were allowed to autolyze before fixation or were taken from tissues fixed for a much longer period of time. Autopsy tissues handled so differently from typical patient specimens are unlikely to react similarly or to serve as a good basis for test optimization. Similarly, tissues from other laboratories should not be used for optimization due to potential handling differences.

For markers intended to differentiate between two or more tumor types based on qualitatively positive or negative expression, the tissues chosen for optimization should reflect the positive and negative tissues types in that differential diagnosis. For assays designed to produce quantitative results or used to determine a certain threshold level of positive expression (such as Her-2), tissue used for optimization should be chosen to reflect the range of results on both sides of the diagnostic threshold for that marker.

References: [2, 6, 8, 44, 48].

1.8 What Are the Steps to Vary in Optimizing an IHC Assay for a Chosen Antibody?

Typically, researchers involved in optimizing newly developed primary antibodies or complex multi-antigen detection protocols will have years of experience with testing protocol variations with their open systems and will not be the people asking this question. In most instances, people new to optimizing IHC assays will be using well-characterized antibodies with dilutions recommended by the vendor on automated systems that have predefined detection protocols. In that setting, the choices to be considered in the beginning of an optimization process have been greatly simplified. For cases where the primary antibody has a recommended dilution from the vendor, attempting that dilution and dilutions at double and half that concentration are good starting points for testing. If the vendor has supplied a prediluted antibody, then the question of primary antibody dilution is moot, so choose a short, brief, and long antibody incubation time instead. In either case, attempt these antibody dilutions or incubation times on positive and negative control tissue sections (small sausage blocks are excellent for this purpose) with each of three different retrieval protocols: (1) heat-induced epitope retrieval (HIER) with pH 6 citrate buffer at 100°C for 20 min, (2) HIER with pH 8 EDTA buffer at 100°C for 20 min, and (3) a short 4-min protease digestion. Evaluate the results of these test protocols to determine the best combination of strong specific staining and minimize nonspecific background staining. The results of this initial set of tests should provide you with an indication of which direction to take your next optimization experiment. Additional blocking or amplification steps may be necessary to complete your optimization. For additional information related to stain optimization and troubleshooting, refer to Chap. 2.

References: [1–8, 44, 45, 48–54].

1.9 What Are the Steps to Validate an IHC Assay for a Chosen Antibody?

An optimization is a preliminary step to antibody validation during which the optimized protocol is tested to determine sensitivity and specificity of the IHC assay. To achieve this, numerous positive and negative control tissues representing typical specimen handling for your laboratory are obtained from your paraffin archive of cases. These positive and negative cases should reflect the types of tissues for which the test was developed to determine how the test will perform in the clinical setting. The NCCLS (CLSI) guideline requires IHC testing to undergo a validation, but most of the details of this validation are left to the discretion of the qualified laboratory director [6]. In its laboratory accreditation program guidelines, CAP has sited a commonly referenced article by Hsi [44] regarding the performance of IHC validation. This article suggests testing a minimum of ten positive and ten negative cases for well-established antibodies and at least 20 positive and 10 negative cases to determine the sensitivity and specificity of less well-characterized antibodies. An exception is made for very rare antigens such as ALK for which it may be more reasonable to collaborate with other institutions to aggregate enough cases for validation. Or alternatively, perform a prospective validation of your assay's performance in parallel to results obtained from an outside laboratory with an established, validated assay. In this way, the test can be introduced clinically based on the outside validation, while an internal validation is accumulated.

Newly announced guidelines regarding the validation of breast cancer receptor studies have far more specific requirements and will be addressed in their own chapter (see Chap. 9).

References: [1–8, 44, 45, 48].

1.10 What Are the Best Control Tissues for IHC Assays?

The best positive and negative control reactions are those present within the patient tissue sample. The best example of this is the presence of weak estrogen receptor (ER) protein expression in the normal breast ducts. If a section is chosen for ER testing to include normal benign duct structures along with tumor, then positive staining of the internal normal ducts is excellent confirmation of negative ER expression within the tumor on the same slide. Similarly, in a CD20 assay that is positive in B cells, the lack of staining of associated T cells is good evidence of the specificity of the positive CD20 reaction in the B cells. Of course, adequate control tissues are not always present on a slide to be tested. Fortunately, as a part of the process of a well-performed validation of an IHC assay's performance, positive and negative control tissues are identified and validated which can be used as controls in the clinical assays. If these are in sufficient supply, then these tissues are the ideal control tissue for the clinical assay. When ideal control tissues are scarce, often normal tissues that are in plentiful supply (e.g., tonsils, endomyometrium, and appendix) are substituted as control tissues. A drawback of this choice is that normal tissue often expresses characteristic proteins more strongly than tumor tissues, especially the very poorly differentiated tumors on which IHC assays are often ordered. There is a risk in using these strongly expressing tissues as positive control. In the event that the assay drops significantly in sensitivity, there may still be positive control staining, while the weakly expressing tumor tissue in the patient sample becomes falsely negative. For this reason, control tissues are best when they express at levels at the threshold level of detection for the patient tissues being tested.

Negative control studies lacking the primary antibody should be performed on sections cut from the patient block in parallel with the assay on the patient tissue to control for nonspecific staining. A negative control is required for each detection protocol used in the panel of assays performed on the patient tissue. If multiple types of antigen retrieval protocols are utilized, it is acceptable practice to perform the negative control assay using the retrieval protocol considered to be the most aggressive. Which is the most aggressive is not always clear, but as a general rule higher pH EDTA is considered more aggressive than pH 6 citrate HIER, and the addition of protease is even more aggressive.

References: [1–8, 55–58].

1.11 What Are the Parts of Daily Quality Control in the IHC Test?

The key to quality control in the performance of IHC staining is process standardization, which requires clear standard operating procedures and could benefit from automation (see Chaps. 3–5). Many additional techniques can aid in achieving quality control of the processes. Computer software and hardware utilizing barcode tracking of blocks, slides, and reagents can be leveraged to save time and reduce misidentification errors. Some barcoding systems can even offer real-time detection and correction of delays and bottlenecks in workflow due to staffing or equipment failure.

Attention needs to be paid to daily equipment calibration and maintenance. Reagent conditions also require attention with regard to storage and testing temperatures and expiration dates. Lot-to-lot comparisons of new reagents are required to assure equivalent performance to prior reagent lots.

Batch positive controls require review before release to the pathologist and must be made available to pathologists if needed. Other positive and negative controls performed along with patient cases should also be reviewed to detect assay failures prior to releasing to pathologists. Review of stain quality before releasing to pathologist detects and corrects staining errors sooner, avoiding delays in reordering and patient results. For this purpose, it is also essential to have established rejection criteria for slide acceptability for interpretation (e.g., control failure, mislabeling, background staining, cytoplasmic staining for a nuclear stain or vice versa, extensive edge artifact, lack of tissue adherence to slide, lack of coverslip, or insufficient mounting media).

There also needs to be a mechanism to permit feedback from the pathologist to the histotechnologists regarding the status of staining quality as another check on assay performance.

References: [1–8, 12].

1.12 What Are the Staining Artifacts and Failed Control Reactions to Be Aware of When Interpreting IHC Assay Results?

Quality control of the interpretation of an IHC slide should begin with the internal and external control reactions. Positive studies should always be confirmed by appropriate negative control reactions and vice versa. Even with appropriate external control reactions, the pathologist should be aware of staining pitfalls related to patient tissue conditions such as false-positive results related to edge artifact, crush artifact, necrosis, endogenous pigments, endogenous biotin or peroxidase, and detection of immunoglobulins in plasma cells. False-negative results may occur as a result of poor tissue preservation or nonstandard fixation. Uneven staining of patient tissue with appropriate controls should suggest poor tissue processing, and a different block from the case should be used if available.

Mistakes can also be avoided, if the pathologist is aware of the expected localization of the staining response and does not accept a positive cytoplasmic reaction as positive for a stain expected to be localized to the nucleus.

Failure of required control reactions should trigger a repeat of the assay, possibly on a different tissue block from the same case. The incidence of repeated stains should be monitored for evidence of a poorly performing assay. Repeated failure of the control study should trigger a thorough investigation of the parameters of the staining protocols and substitution of fresh reagents. Recalibration and maintenance of the equipment may be required to resolve the issue. When all these steps fail to correct the problem, a reoptimization and revalidation of the assay may be necessary.

References: [1–8, 36, 44, 45, 48, 53, 55–59].

1.13 What Are Some Examples of Quality Assurance Monitors for Analytic Phase of IHC Testing?

1. Monitor turnaround time for stain orders
2. Monitor trends in positive, equivocal, and negative results of predictive markers
3. Participation in external proficiency testing and laboratory accreditation inspections

References: [1–8, 38, 39, 60–63].

1.14 What Can Be Monitored in the Postanalytic Phase of IHC Testing?

Postsignout review of reports can be used to monitor the completeness of required documentation of stain and control results in the report and the accuracy of associated billing for IHC assays. The results of billed IHC testing are required to be documented for each antibody. Occurrences of duplicate billing when the same antibody is run multiple times on the same specimen part can be detected and credited. Identification of these types of mistakes can direct educational efforts and redesign of billing automatically triggered by laboratory information system processes.

References: [4, 5].

1.15 What Are Some Examples of Quality Improvement Opportunities in IHC Testing?

1. Identify root cause of infrequent, though critical zero-tolerance errors (lost or overly faced blocks, mislabeled slides, and tissue contaminants) for interventions.
2. Identify common issues causing inefficiencies in the IHC workflow (e.g., coordinate adequate staffing with timing of courier and processor runs, evaluate capacity of manual and automated staining processes for high slide volumes times, monitor IHC repeat orders as rework).
3. Update current equipment and antibody library to meet current clinical testing needs. This can be accomplished by monitoring the literature for newly available antibodies and equipment or new uses for existing antibodies and by following the migration of your existing antibodies from ASR to IVD status and polyclonal to monoclonal forms. With this information, proceed to validate assays for the use of the most clinically relevant antibody clones.
4. Monitor intradepartmental peer ordering patterns to target education for under or over utilization of testing.

Reference: [4].

1.16 What Is the Law Regulating IHC Laboratory Testing?

Congress passed the Clinical Laboratory Improvement Amendments (CLIA) in 1988, establishing quality standards for all laboratory testing to ensure the accuracy, reliability, and timeliness of patient test results regardless of where the test was performed. CLIA'88 establishes minimum performance standards for all clinical laboratories with regard to quality standards for proficiency testing (PT), patient test management, quality control, personnel qualifications, and quality assurance for laboratories performing moderate and/or high-complexity tests. Under CLIA, "A laboratory is any facility that does laboratory testing on specimens derived from humans to give information for the diagnosis, prevention, treatment of disease, or impairment of, or assessment of health." In total, CLIA covers approximately 200,000 laboratory entities. CLIA also regulates the manufacturers of commercially available reagents and instrumentation used for performing IHC and regards these as medical devices.

References: [64–69].

1.17 What Is the Concept of Complexity with Regard to Laboratory Testing Regulation?

Prior to CLIA'88, regulations regarding laboratory practices varied depending on the type of site (independent, hospital, or physician's office laboratory) with physician office laboratories loosely controlled. Under CLIA'88, laboratories in the USA are regulated based on the test complexity rather than by where the test is done. Laboratory tests categorized under CLIA as high complexity may only be performed in laboratories CLIA certified to perform high-complexity testing.

References: [65–69].

1.18 What Are the Agencies and Organizations Responsible for Implementing CLIA Regulations for Clinical Laboratories?

The Department of Health and Human Services (DHHS) is responsible for overseeing CLIA rules for all clinical laboratory testing (except research) performed on humans in the USA. The Centers for Medicare & Medicaid Services (CMS) under the DHHS assumes primary responsibility for financial management operations of the CLIA program. A laboratory must be CLIA certified to perform clinical laboratory testing and to receive Medicare payments for testing. The implementation of the CLIA Program regulations has fallen to the CMS Division of Laboratory Services, within the Survey and Certification Group, under the Center for Medicaid and State Operations (CMSO).

COLA, The Joint Commission on Healthcare Organizations (JCAHO), and the College of American Pathologists (CAP) are nongovernmental, professional organizations which have received deemed status from CMS to inspect and certify that laboratories meet the CLIA standards.

CAP's Laboratory Accreditation Program (LAP) is widely recognized as the "gold standard" and has served as a model for various federal, state, and private laboratory accreditation programs throughout the world. CAP accreditation is accepted for both CLIA and JCAHO certification. The CAP inspection program is internationally recognized and the only one of its kind that utilizes teams of practicing laboratory professionals as inspectors. Designed to go well beyond regulatory compliance, the program helps laboratories achieve the highest standards. There are more than 6,000 CAP-accredited laboratories nationwide.

Another nongovernmental organization related to laboratory standards, originally known as National Committee for

Clinical Laboratory (NCCLS), changed its name to the Clinical and Laboratory Standards Institute (CLSI) in January 2005. CLSI develops and publishes standards and guidelines through a consensus process that involves representatives from government, industry, and the patient-testing professions. CLSI has no regulatory authority of its own, so its standards and guidelines regarding the performance of IHC are only mandatory when they are referenced by other regulatory organizations such as CAP.

References: [38, 65–72].

1.19 What Are the Agencies and Organizations Responsible for Implementing CLIA Regulations for Manufacturers of IHC Reagents and Instrumentation?

In addition to regulating clinical laboratories, CLIA regulates the manufacturers of commercially available the reagents and instrumentation used for performing IHC and regards these as medical devices generically called In Vitro Diagnostics (IVD). Under CLIA'88, the Food and Drug Administration (FDA) Office of In Vitro Diagnostic Device Evaluation and Safety (OIVD) administers the CLIA test complexity program for medical devices. Within the OIVD are the Division of Immunology and Hematology Devices (DIHD), specifically responsible for tumor marker (cancer detection) tests, which is the most common use for IHC and ISH, and the Division of Microbiology Devices (DMD), responsible for any IHC or ISH tests for the detection of microorganisms (bacteria, fungi, mycobacteria, viruses).

References: [65–69].

1.20 How Does CLIA Control the Use of IHC Testing Through Determination of Laboratory and Test Complexity?

The Food and Drug Administration (FDA) Office of In Vitro Diagnostic Device Evaluation and Safety (OIVD) categorizes commercially marketed in vitro diagnostic (IVD) tests by level of complexity based on their potential for risk to public health as: (1) waived, (2) moderate or (3) high complexity. IHC testing is considered high-complexity testing. Therefore a laboratory must be accredited under CLIA to perform the level of complexity of the testing done in their facility.

References: [65–69].

1.21 How Does CLIA Control the Marketing and Use of IHC Testing Through Test Class?

Like other medical devices, IVDs are subject to premarket and postmarket controls to be determined by the FDA. Before a manufacturer can make an IHC testing reagent, test or instrument commercially available, it must determine the level of premarket documentation of performance characteristics and safety that will be required by the FDA. FDA classifies IVD products into Class I, II, or III according to the level of regulatory control that is necessary to assure safety and effectiveness. The classification of an IVD (or other medical device) determines the appropriate premarket process.

Class I – Class I devices are subject to the least regulatory control. They present minimal potential for harm to the user and are often simpler in design than Class II or Class III devices. Class I devices are subject to "General Controls," as are Class II and Class III devices. General controls include provisions that relate to adulteration; misbranding; device registration and listing; premarket notification; banned devices; notification, including repair, replacement, or refund; records and reports; restricted devices; and good manufacturing practices. The general use of IHC antibodies involved in determination of tumor differentiation is regarded as Class I or low risk and is almost always exempt from the premarket notification and approval requirements of Class II and Class III IHC antibodies.

Class II – Class II devices are those for which general controls alone are insufficient to assure safety and effectiveness, and existing methods are available to provide such assurances. In addition to complying with general controls, Class II devices are also subject to special controls also known as premarket notification or 510(k). Special controls placed on Class II devices may include special labeling requirements, mandatory performance standards and postmarket surveillance. IHC antibodies for estrogen and progesterone receptor proteins and Her-2 oncoprotein are used in testing to predict the use of hormone-based and trastuzumab therapy and are therefore considered of higher risk than general differentiation markers and fall into Class II requiring 510(k) premarket notification clearance. Automated microscopes for image analysis of IHC are also considered Class II by the FDA. Some vendors seek Class III premarket approval when it is not required to differentiate their product in the market.

Class III – Class III is the most stringent regulatory category for devices. Class III devices are those for which insufficient information exists to assure safety and effectiveness solely through general or special controls. Class III devices are usually those that support or sustain human life, are of substantial importance in preventing impairment of human health, or which present a potential, unreasonable risk of illness or injury. Premarket approval is the required process of scientific review to ensure the safety and effectiveness of Class III devices. Not all Class III devices require an approved premarket approval application to be marketed. Class III devices which are equivalent to devices legally marketed before May 28, 1976, may be marketed through the premarket notification [510(k)] process until the FDA has published a requirement for manufacturers of that generic type of device to submit premarket approval data. A 510(k) requires demonstration of substantial equivalence to another legally U.S. marketed device. A claim of substantial equivalence does not mean the new and predicate devices must be identical. Substantial equivalence means that the new device is at least as safe and effective as the predicate. A device is substantially equivalent if, in comparison to a predicate, it has the same intended use and technological characteristics as the predicate, or has the same intended use as the predicate but has different technological characteristics, and the information submitted to FDA does not raise new questions of safety and effectiveness and demonstrates that the device is at least as safe and effective as the legally marketed device. In IHC, testing for c-kit and epithelial growth factor receptor (EGFR) used to predict targeted therapies are considered Class III by the FDA and require the premarket approval process.

References: [65–69].

1.22 What is the FDA's ASR Rule?

ASR stands for analyte-specific reagent and is a designation created by the FDA for a special subset of IVD reagents that have fewer premarket requirements along with fewer premarket claims of testing performance. The ASR rule recognizes the difference between a general purpose reagent, such as buffers that lack specificity for an analyte, and antibodies or nucleic acid probes that by design have binding specificity for an analyte. It also recognizes the need for a difference between an in vitro diagnostic test (IVD) validated and marketed by a vendor and subject to premarket notification requirements [510(k)], and an antibody or probe sold to a CLIA-accredited laboratory used to develop an "in-house" assay to be validated by the laboratory itself, exempting the vendor from premarket notification requirements. The FDA created the ASR category as the least burdensome regulatory approach to foster cooperation between vendors and laboratories in developed tests. By accepting the ASR designation, vendors can make antibodies and probes available to laboratories sooner than if they were required to perform the premarket notification process for each antibody as an IVD. The ASR rule allows a description of the specific binding of an antibody or probe as long as there is no claim made for the clinical use which would change the antibody from the component of a test into a test itself. As such the FDA requires that clinical testing performed using ASRs provide documentation that the test has not been evaluated by the FDA and that the laboratory is certified to perform high-complexity testing and is responsible for and has validated the test that uses the ASR. An acceptable ASR disclaimer to satisfy the FDA would be, "This test was developed and its performance characteristics determined by (laboratory name). It has not been cleared or approved by the U.S. Food and Drug Administration."

References: [47, 65–69].

1.23 What Are the Limitations Placed on the Information that a Vendor Can Provide a Laboratory for an ASR Reagent?

Since ASRs are considered specific individual "building blocks" of laboratory-developed tests (LDT), a vendor is limited in the information that can be provided to a laboratory.

ASR labeling may indicate the affinity of the reagent to a molecular target, such as "anti-estrogen receptor antibody" or "CFTR nucleic acid probe" because it only describes the ligand to which the ASR is specific but does not claim to produce a particular clinical or analytical result. ASR manufacturers also should not promote, sell, or otherwise distribute other reagents, software or instrumentation that could imply that such packaging is needed to achieve a function of an ASR. Vendors should also not assist with the development or validation of an LDT using its specific ASR. Under the CLIA regulations, the laboratory must conduct validation and verification of test performance specification (42 CFR 493.1213). This validation by the laboratory is the minimum requirement under CLIA for the laboratory to generate clinical results for tests of high complexity. For ASRs the sole responsibility for how to use the ASR in testing lies with the performing laboratory.

References: [47, 65–69].

1.24 How Is the ASR Rule Related to In Vitro Diagnostic Products Labeled for RUO or IUO?

Products labeled for research use only (RUO) or investigational use only (IUO) are IVDs in different stages of development. The FDA considers RUO products to be products that are in the laboratory research phase of development; that is, either basic research or the initial search for potential clinical utility, and not represented as an effective in vitro diagnostic product. These products must be labeled, "For Research Use Only. Not for use in diagnostic procedures" as required under 21 CFR 809.10 (c)(2)(i).

FDA considers IUO products to be products that are in the clinical investigation phase of development. They may be classified with an investigational device exemption (IDE) from the requirements of 21 CFR Part 812 (21 CFR 812.2(c)), or may be regulated under 21 CFR Part 812 as either a non-significant risk device or a significant risk device. Diagnostic devices exempt from IDE requirements cannot be used for human clinical diagnosis unless the diagnosis is being confirmed by another, medically established diagnostic product or procedure [21 CFR 812.2(c)(3)(iv)]. This is a validation of the performance of the test using the RUO component performed by the laboratory CLIA certified to perform high-complexity testing. During this phase, the safety and effectiveness of the product are being studied (i.e., the clinical performance characteristics and expected values) are being determined in the intended patient population(s). These products must be labeled "For Investigational Use Only. The performance characteristics of this product have not been established" [21 CFR 809.10(c)(2)(ii)].

References: [47, 65–69].

1.25 What Is the Difference in FDA Requirements for Manufacturers of an ASR Versus an RUO Reagent?

Manufacturers establish and follow current good manufacturing practices (cGMPs), as established in the quality system regulation, to help ensure that their products are manufactured under controlled conditions that assure the devices meet consistent specifications across lots and over time (21 CFR Parts 808, 812, and 820. ASRs must be manufactured following cGMPs (21 CFR 809.20). FDA does not expect RUO reagents to be manufactured in compliance with cGMPs because products labeled as RUO reagents cannot be used as clinical diagnostic products [21 CFR 809.10(c)(2)(i)]. There is some controversy surrounding this and the fact that CAP regulations discourage but allow use of RUO reagents if ASR or IVD reagents are not available. CAP requires that assays developed using RUO reagents be validated by the performing laboratory and that there be documentation of at least annual attempts to identify appropriate ASR and IVD reagents to replace the RUO reagents as they become available. Some vendors in the IHC industry have expressed concern that this "RUO loophole" in CAP guidelines promotes the use of the RUO designation by industry rather than enduring the challenge of an ASR designation.

References: [47, 65–69].

1.26 What Is the College of American Pathologists (CAP) Laboratory Accreditation Program (LAP)?

The CAP Laboratory Accreditation Program (LAP) is an internationally recognized program and the only one of its kind that utilizes teams of practicing laboratory professionals as inspectors. Designed to go well beyond regulatory compliance, the program helps laboratories achieve the highest standards of excellence to positively impact patient care.

The program is based on rigorous accreditation standards that are translated into detailed and focused checklist requirements. The checklists, which provide a quality practice blueprint for laboratories to follow, are used by the inspection teams as a guide to assess the overall management and operation of the laboratory.

The Centers for Medicare and Medicaid Services (CMS) has granted the CAP LAP deeming authority acceptable for CLIA accreditation. It is also recognized by the Joint Commission on Accreditation of Healthcare Organizations (JCAHO), and can be used to meet many state certification requirements.

More than 6,000 laboratories worldwide are accredited through CAP LAP.

CAP guidelines are constantly being updated to address changes in technology and current best practices, so the laboratory should refer to materials provided by CAP for up-to-date guidelines. This chapter has included some specific requirements of the CAP LAP that relate specifically to IHC and ISH to help the section supervisor to prepare for CAP inspections, and in doing so, produce best laboratory practices (http://www.cap.org).

References: [8, 45, 73].

1.27 What Are the CAP Regulations for Content of Procedure Manuals?

Procedure manuals may be paper or electronic. Electronic manuals are easier to manage, especially in larger laboratories where the manual must be available at multiple benches, so making changes will not require updating multiple paper copies. If online manuals are used, backup copies on paper or CD must be available in the case of system downtime. Procedure manuals must include step-by-step instructions for performance of calibration and testing procedures for each method in current use and include access to any procedures retired in past 2 years. Manuals may include procedures provided by manufacturers if they describe the actual procedure employed in the lab. Any variations from manufacturer materials would require additional documentation so that the actual procedure is documented. Acceptable specimen conditions for testing must be defined in the manual, including fixation type and time, as well as conditions that may render a specimen unacceptable, such as hemorrhage, necrosis or autolysis. The location of batch control slides must be stated in the procedure manual to be available to all pathologists working with those stains. There must be annual documentation of review of the procedure manual by director or designee and testing personnel.

Reference: [8].

1.28 What Are the CAP Regulations for Instrument and Reagents Management?

All reagents must be properly labeled including expiration date. Dates may be recorded on the containers or in a paper or electronic log, providing that all containers are labeled to be traceable to the appropriate data in the log. If the manufacturer assigns an expiration date, it must be observed. If no expiration date is supplied by the manufacturer, the acceptable performance must be determined on an annual basis. All reagents must be stored as recommended by the manufacturer. There must be documentation of proper temperatures of refrigerators used for reagent storage. There must be documentation that the pH of the buffers used in IHC is tested when a new batch is prepared or received and routinely monitored. Maintenance records of automated IHC staining instruments and validation and calibration records of digital image analysis equipment should be kept.

Reference: [8].

1.29 What Are the CAP Regulations for Microwaves Used for IHC Procedures?

Microwave devices used for heat-induced epitope retrieval (HIER) must be monitored for consistency at least annually. Reproducibility may be evaluated by monitoring the temperatures of identical samples after microwave processing. Microwave devices used for hazardous or infection materials (excluding water, certain biological stains, paraffin tissue sections) should be placed in an appropriate ventilation hood or have an integral fume extractor that is certified by the manufacturer to contain airborne chemical contaminants and potentially infectious agents. The laboratory should consult the material safety data sheets (MSDS) received with reagents and stains to assist in determining proper handling requirements and safe use. Venting containers placed in microwave devices is necessary so that processing occurs at atmospheric pressure and to prevent explosion. For procedures above atmospheric pressure, specialized containers must be used strictly according to manufacturer instructions. The effectiveness of microwave ventilation should be monitored at least annually. The microwave device should be tested for radiation leakage if there is visible damage to the device.

References: [8, 74, 75].

1.30 What Are the CAP Regulations for Formaldehyde and Xylene Use?

The laboratory must have documentation of safe levels of formaldehyde and xylene vapors if used. Periodic measurements of formaldehyde and xylene vapors must be performed until results from two consecutive sampling periods taken at least 7 days apart show that employee exposure is below the action level and the short-term exposure limit (Table 1.1). Repeated measurement is required any time there is a change in production, equipment, process, personnel, or control measures, or when personnel report symptoms of respiratory or dermal conditions that may be associated with formaldehyde exposure.

Table 1.1 Formaldehyde and xylene exposure limits

	Formaldehyde (ppm)	Xylene (ppm)
Action level (8-h time-weighted exposure)	0.5	100
15 min Short-term average exposure limit (STEL)	2.0	150

References: [8, 76]

1.31 What Are the CAP Regulations for Positive Controls?

Positive controls should be performed in parallel to patient specimens and performed in the same manner and by the same personnel as patient samples. The laboratory director or designee must document the adequacy of controls, either in internal laboratory records or in the patient report each day of patient testing, and retain these records for 2 years. A statement such as, "All controls show appropriate reactivity" is sufficient. Ideal positive control tissue is present on the same slide and of the same tissue type as the patient tissue sample that possesses a low level of expression of the target antigen near the threshold of detection of the assay. Internal controls, such as normal breast ducts in hormone receptor assays, are often the best control for appropriate fixation and retrieval. Multi-tissue array blocks containing a variety of routinely processed tissue types known to both express and lack the target antigens may act as both positive and negative controls on the same slide.

An inventory of routinely processed formalin-fixed tissue samples can be used for patient specimens. These control tissues may be of different type from the patient specimen (decalcified tissues, alcohol fixed aspirate smears) if the laboratory has documented equivalent immunoreactivity by parallel testing a small panel of common markers. When batch controls are run, slides should be readily available to all pathologists working with those stains. For quantitative IHC testing, control materials at more than one level may be required to verify test performance at relevant decision points. Quantitative control results must be recorded and reviewed at least monthly to evaluate trends and detect problems. Control records must be readily available to the person performing the test. Immunofluorescence assays may utilize appropriate internal positive control reactions such as IgA-positive renal tubular casts, C3-positive arterial walls. For in situ hybridization (ISH) testing, internal or external control loci should be used during each hybridization. When available, a locus-specific probe at a different site on the same chromosome and/or a normal locus on the abnormal homolog should be used. For assays that may lack an internal control locus (e.g., a Y chromosome probe in a female), an external control that is known to have the probe target should be run in parallel with the patient sample.

References: [8, 38, 39, 77].

1.32 What Are the CAP Regulations for Negative Controls?

Negative control sections of the patient tissue sample should be performed in parallel to patient specimens for each block tested to assess nonspecific staining (specificity) related to intrinsic tissue elements (biotin or peroxidase), antigen retrieval conditions or the detection system. Appropriate staining of negative controls must be documented. The ideal negative control for monoclonal primary antibodies replaces the primary antibody with an unrelated antibody of the same isotype as the primary antibody. For polyclonal primary antibodies, an unrelated antibody from the same animal species as the primary antibody can be used. For staining kits, the negative control reagent specified by the vendor documentation and included in the kit should be used. Multi-tissue array blocks containing a variety of routinely processed tissue types known to both express and lack the target antigens may act as both positive and negative controls on the same slide. An acceptable negative control is a separate section of patient tissue processed using the same reagents and epitope retrieval protocol as the patient test slide, except that the primary antibody is omitted and replaced by diluent/buffer solution in which the primary antibody has been diluted. When performing panels of antibodies on sections from the same block employing varied antigen retrieval procedures, a reasonable negative control is to test the most aggressive retrieval procedure in the panel. Antigen retrieval aggressiveness (in decreasing order): pressure cooker, enzyme digestion, boiling, microwave, steamer, water bath. High pH retrieval is more aggressive than retrieval in buffer at pH 6.0. In the case of multiple blocks of similarly processed and stained sentinel lymph nodes, a single section from one of the blocks may be acceptable as the negative control reaction. Appropriate internal negative staining reactions can be considered adequate in lieu of separate negative control tissue sections. Immunofluorescence assays require separate sections of patient tissues omitting the primary antibody to act as negative control for autofluorescence.

References: [8, 38, 39, 56, 77].

1.33 What Are the CAP Regulations for Endogenous Biotin Blocking?

If the laboratory uses biotin in primary or dual-detection systems, there must be a policy that addresses nonspecific false-positive staining from endogenous biotin. Cell types with high metabolic activity tend to contain abundant mitochondria with the coenzyme biotin. Hepatocytes, renal tubules, gestational endometrium and many tumors are known to be rich in endogenous biotin. False-positive staining localized to metabolically active tumor cells may occur and be easily misinterpreted. Commercial and in-house (egg whites, milk) reagents should be used to block endogenous biotin before applying the biotin-based detection systems.

References: [8, 78].

1.34 What Are the CAP Regulations for New Antibody Validation?

Validation of all antibody assays must be performed prior to use in patient diagnosis to document the performance in its proposed differential diagnostic applications. The laboratory director or qualified designee must sign a statement documenting review of validation studies and approval of each test for clinical use. A statement such as "This validation study has been reviewed, and the performance of the method is considered acceptable for patient testing" should satisfy this requirement. With the exception of prescribed validation procedures for predictive markers Her-2/neu and hormone receptors (see Chap. 9), the specific parameters of IHC validation are left to the discretion of a qualified laboratory director. General guidance is given to require testing a sufficient number of cases to provide an idea of sensitivity and specificity of the assay and similarity of the assay to expected results. In general, a minimum of ten positive and ten negative tissues should be documented having appropriate results for well-established antibodies. More may be required for newer antibodies for which there is less experience in the literature. Antibodies FDA-designated as In Vitro Diagnostic (IVD) antibodies require demonstration of equivalence of staining reactions with expected results provided in the product literature supplied with the antibody from the vendor in order to validate performance in the laboratory. Vendors make no claims regarding expected performance of antibodies designated as analyte-specific reagents (ASR). Therefore, validation of ASR antibodies requires establishing the sensitivity and specificity of the assay in the laboratory. The laboratory must establish or verify the performance characteristics of tests using Class I ASRs in accordance with the Method Performance Specifications section of the Laboratory General Checklist. For testing to be performed on any specimens with significantly different handling (decalcification, frozen tissues, alternative fixatives, cytologic smears), additional validation of equivalent immunoreactivity with at least small panels of samples is needed.

References: [8, 38, 39, 44, 45, 77].

1.35 What Are the CAP Regulations for Validation of New Reagent Lots?

The performance of all types of new reagent lots (enzyme, antibody, detection system) must be validated prior to use on patient tissues. Documentation of equivalent staining of serial sections from a multi-tissue control tissue block, including positive and negative tissue reactions stained in parallel using old and new lots, will satisfy this requirement.

References: [6, 8, 77].

1.36 What Are the CAP Regulations for Reporting IHC Results Including ASRs?

If IHC or ISH is reported as an addendum or separate procedure, there must be a mechanism to reconcile morphologic diagnosis with potentially conflicting results of special studies such as immunohistochemistry.

If the laboratory employs antibodies or nucleic acid probes designated as an Analyte-Specific Reagent (ASR), federal regulations require that the following disclaimer accompany the test result on the patient report: "This test was developed and its performance characteristics determined by (laboratory name). It has not been cleared or approved by the U.S. Food and Drug Administration."

CAP recommends adding the following statement to the ASR disclaimer: "The FDA has determined that such clearance or approval is not necessary. This test is used for clinical purposes. It should not be regarded as investigational or for research. This laboratory is certified under the Clinical Laboratory Improvement Amendments (CLIA) as qualified to perform high complexity clinical laboratory testing."

There is no specific guidance from CAP regarding the use of a disclaimer for "research use only" (RUO). But the laboratory may put a single ASR disclaimer on the pathology report to address all IHC and ISH studies used in a particular case. Separately tracking each reagent used for a case and selectively applying the disclaimer to only the Class I ASRs is unnecessary.

CAP has additional requirements for reporting results of predictive marker studies for breast cancer which are addressed in Chap. 9.

References: [8, 46].

1.37 What Are the CAP Regulations for Slide or Slide Image Retention?

IHC slides, including the control slides, must be readable and retained for 10 years. Fluorescence slides will fade over time, so a diagnostic image of the fluorescent slide findings should be included on the report or maintained separately for 10 years to meet the requirement of being readable for 10 years. Representative images of FISH assays with at least one cell for normal results, and at least two cells for each abnormal result must be retained for 10 years' documentation.

References: [8, 34, 79].

References

1. Taylor CR, Cote RJ. Immunomicroscopy, a diagnostic tool for the surgical pathologist. 3rd ed. Philadelphia, PA: Elsevier; 2006.
2. Dabbs DJ. Diagnostic immunohistochemistry. New York: Churchill Livingstone; 2002.
3. Leong AS-Y, Cooper K, Leong FJW-M. Manual of diagnostic antibodies for immunohistology. 2nd ed. London: Greenwich Medical Media; 2003.

4. Brown RW. Quality management in immunohistochemistry. In: Nakleh RE, Fitzgibbons PL, editors. Quality management in anatomic pathology: promoting patient safety through systems improvement and error reduction. Northfield, IL: CAP; 2005. p. 93–110.
5. Taylor CR. The total test approach to standardization of immunohistochemistry. Arch Pathol Lab Med. 2000;124(7):945–51.
6. National Committee on Clinical Laboratory Standards (NCCLS) MM4-A. Quality assurance for immunocytochemistry; approved guideline. Wayne, PA: National Committee on Clinical and Laboratory Standards; 1999.
7. O'Leary TJ. Standardization in immunohistochemistry. Appl Immunohistochem Mol Morphol. 2001;9(1):3–8.
8. Laboratory Accreditation Program. College of American Pathologists. Northfield, IL.
9. Novis DA. Detecting and preventing the occurrence of errors in the practices of laboratory medicine and anatomic pathology: 15 years' experience with the College of American Pathologists' Q-PROBES and Q-TRACKS programs. Clin Lab Med. 2004;24(4):965–78.
10. Condel JL, Sharbaugh DT, Raab SS. Error-free pathology: applying lean production methods to anatomic pathology. Clin Lab Med. 2004;24(4):865–99. Review.
11. Muirhead D, Aoun P, Powell M, Juncker F, Mollerup J. Pathology economic model tool: a novel approach to workflow and budget cost analysis in an anatomic pathology laboratory. Arch Pathol Lab Med. 2010;134(8):1164–9.
12. Zarbo RJ, Tuthill JM, D'Angelo R, et al. The Henry Ford production system: reduction of surgical pathology in-process misidentification defects by bar code-specified work process standardization. Am J Clin Pathol. 2009;131(4):468–77.
13. Valenstein PN, Sirota RL. Identification errors in pathology and laboratory medicine. Clin Lab Med. 2004;24(4):979–96. vii.
14. Makary MA, Epstein J, Pronovost PJ, Millman EA, Hartmann EC, Freischlag JA. Surgical specimen identification errors: a new measure of quality in surgical care. Surgery. 2007;141(4):450–5.
15. Nakhleh RE, Zarbo RJ. Surgical pathology specimen identification and accessioning: a College of American Pathologists Q-probes study of 1 004 115 cases from 417 institutions. Arch Pathol Lab Med. 1996;120(3):227–33.
16. Nakhleh RE, Zarbo RJ. Amended reports in surgical pathology and implications for diagnostic error detection and avoidance: a College of American Pathologists Q-probes study of 1,667,547 accessioned cases in 359 laboratories. Arch Pathol Lab Med. 1998;122(4):303–9.
17. Nakhleh RE, Gephardt G, Zarbo RJ. Necessity of clinical information in surgical. Arch Pathol Lab Med. 1999;123(7):615–9.
18. Barnes RO, Parisien M, Murphy LC, Watson PH. Influence of evolution in tumor biobanking on the interpretation of translational research. Cancer Epidemiol Biomarkers Prev. 2008;17(12):3344–50.
19. Mazumder A, Wang Y. Gene-expression signatures in oncology diagnostics. Pharmacogenomics. 2006;7(8):1167–73.
20. De Cecco L, Musella V, Veneroni S, et al. Impact of biospecimens handling on biomarker research in breast cancer. BMC Cancer. 2009;9:409.
21. Dumur CI, Sana S, Ladd AC, et al. Assessing the impact of tissue devitalization time on genome-wide gene expression analysis in ovarian tumor samples. Diagn Mol Pathol. 2008;17(4):200–6.
22. Hopwood D. Fixatives and fixation: a review. Histochem J. 1969;1(4):323–60.
23. Mason JT, O'Leary TJ. Effects of formaldehyde fixation on protein secondary structure: a calorimetric and infrared spectroscopic investigation. J Histochem Cytochem. 1991;39(2):225–9.
24. Medawar PB. The rate of penetration of fixatives. J R Microsc Soc. 1941;61:46–57.
25. Ostrowski K, Komender J, Kwarecki K. Quantitative investigations on the solubility of proteins extracted from tissues fixed by different chemical and physical methods. Ann Histochim. 1961;6:501–6.
26. Petsko GA, Ringe D. Protein structure and function. Sunderland, MA: Sinauer; 2004.
27. Burnett MG. The mechanism of the formaldehyde clock reaction: methylene glycol dehydration. J Chem Educ. 1982;59(2):160.
28. Fox CH, Johnson FB, Whiting J, Roller PP. Formaldehyde fixation. J Histochem Cytochem. 1985;33(8):845–53.
29. Goldstein NS, Ferkowicz M, Odish E, Mani A, Hastah F. Minimum formalin fixation time for consistent estrogen receptor immunohistochemical staining of invasive breast carcinoma. Am J Clin Pathol. 2003;120(1):86–92.
30. Gown AM. Unmasking the mysteries of antigen or epitope retrieval and formalin fixation. Am J Clin Pathol. 2004;121(2):172–4.
31. Helander KG. Kinetic studies of formaldehyde binding in tissue. Biotech Histochem. 1994;69(3):177–9.
32. Helander KG. Formaldehyde binding in brain and kidney: a kinetic study of fixation. J Histotechnol. 1999;22(4):317–8.
33. Hewlett BR. Penetration rates of formaldehyde. Microsc Today. 2002;10(6):30.
34. National Committee on Clinical Laboratory Standards MM7-A. Fluorescence in situ hybridization (FISH) methods for medical genetics; approved guideline. Wayne, PA: National Committee on Clinical and Laboratory Standards; 2004.
35. Williams JH, Mepham BL, Wright DH. Tissue preparation for immunocytochemistry. J Clin Pathol. 1997;50(5):422–8.
36. Yaziji H, Taylor CR. Begin at the beginning, with the tissue! The key message underlying the ASCO/CAP task-force guideline recommendations for HER2 testing. Appl Immunohistochem Mol Morphol. 2007;15(3):239–41.
37. Leake R, Barnes D, Pinder S, et al. Immunohistochemical detection of steroid receptors in breast cancer: a working protocol. UK Receptor Group, UK NEQAS, The Scottish Breast Cancer Pathology Group, and The Receptor and Biomarker Study Group of the EORTC. J Clin Pathol. 2000;53(8):634–45.
38. Wolff AC, Hammond ME, Schwartz JN, et al. American Society of Clinical Oncology/College of American pathologists guideline recommendations for human epidermal growth factor receptor 2 testing in breast cancer. Arch Pathol Lab Med. 2007;131(1):18–43.
39. Hammond ME, Hayes DF, Dowsett M, et al. American Society of Clinical Oncology/College of American Pathologists guideline recommendations for immunohistochemical testing of estrogen and progesterone receptors in breast cancer. Arch Pathol Lab Med. 2010;134(6):907–22.
40. Enterline HT. Pathologist and histotechnologist: a marriage in need of counseling. Pathol Annu. 1975;10:205–11.
41. Buesa RJ. Histology aging workforce and what to do about it. Ann Diagn Pathol. 2009;13(3):176–84.
42. Buesa RJ. Staffing benchmarks for histology laboratories. Ann Diagn Pathol. 2010;14(3):182–93.
43. Buesa RJ. Productivity standards for histology laboratories. Ann Diagn Pathol. 2010;14(2):107–24.
44. Hsi ED. A practical approach for evaluating new antibodies in the clinical immunohistochemistry laboratory. Arch Pathol Lab Med. 2001;125(2):289–94.
45. College of American Pathologists. 2010 CAP LAP audioconference: test validation: a brave new world for anatomic pathology. May 19, 2010.
46. Brown RW, Sharkey FE. Standards and guidelines for clinical genetics laboratories. 2nd ed. Bethesda, MD: American College of Medical Genetics; 1999.
47. Graziano C. Disclaimer now needed for analyte-specific reagents. CAP Today. 1998;12(11):5–11.
48. U.S. Department of Health and Human Services, Food and Drug Administration. Guidance for industry and fda staff – commercially distributed analyte specific reagents (ASRs): frequently asked questions. http://www.fda.gov/MedicalDevices/DeviceRegulationandGuidance/GuidanceDocuments/ucm078423.htm. Published 14 Sep 2007. Accessed 30 Jul 2010.
49. Clinical and Laboratory Standards Institute (CLSI) GP2-A5. Laboratory documents: development and control; approved

guideline – fifth edition. Wayne, PA: Clinical and Laboratory Standards Institute; 2006.

50. Rhodes A, Jasani B, Balaton AJ, et al. Study of interlaboratory reliability and reproducibility of estrogen and progesterone receptor assays in Europe. Documentation of poor reliability and identification of insufficient microwave antigen retrieval time as a major contributory element of unreliable assays. Am J Clin Pathol. 2001;115(1):44–58.
51. Larsson LI. Section pre-treatment, epitope demasking, and methods for dealing with unwanted staining. In: Larson LI, editor. Immunocytochemistry: theory and practice. Boca Raton: CRC; 1988. p. 147–70.
52. Shi SR, Gu J, Taylor CR, editors. Antigen retrieval techniques: immunohistochemistry and molecular morphology. Natick, MA: Eaton; 2000.
53. Sompuram SR, Vani K, Messana E, Bogen SA. A molecular mechanism of formalin fixation and antigen retrieval. Am J Clin Pathol. 2004;121(2):190–9.
54. Werner M, Chott A, Fabiano A, Battifora H. Effect of formalin fixation and processing on immunohistochemistry. Am J Surg Pathol. 2000;24(7):1016–9.
55. Fitzgibbons PL, Murphy DA, Hammond ME, Allred DC, Valenstein PN. Recommendations for validating estrogen and progesterone receptor immunohistochemistry assays. Arch Pathol Lab Med. 2010;134(6):930–5.
56. Miller RT, Groothuis CL. Multitumor "sausage" blocks in immunohistochemistry. Simplified method of preparation, practical uses, and roles in quality assurance. Am J Clin Pathol. 1991;96(2):228–32.
57. Chan JK, Wong CS, Ku WT, Kwan MY. Reflections on the use of controls in immunohistochemistry and proposal for application of a multitissue spring-roll control block. Ann Diagn Pathol. 2000;4(5):329–36.
58. Burry RW. Specificity controls for immunocytochemical methods. J Histochem Cytochem. 2000;48(2):163–6.
59. Weirauch M. Multitissue control block for immunohistochemistry. Lab Med. 1999;30(7):448–9.
60. Clinical Laboratory Standards Institute GP28-A. Microwave device use in the histology laboratory; approved guideline. Wayne, PA: Clinical and Laboratory Standards Institute; 2005.
61. Vyberg M, Torlakovic E, Seidal T, Risberg B, Helin H, Nielsen S. Nordic immunohistochemical quality control. Croat Med J. 2005;46(3):368–71.
62. United Kingdom National External Quality Assessment Service. http://www.ukneqas.org.uk/content/Pageserver.asp. Accessed 30 Jul 2010.
63. Nordic Immunohistochemistry Quality Control. http://www.nordiqc.org/. Accessed 30 Jul 2010.
64. Joint Commission on Accreditation of Healthcare Organizations. Accreditation manual for pathology and clinical laboratory services. Oakbrook Terrace, IL: Joint Commission on Accreditation of Healthcare Organizations (JCAHO); 1996.
65. Goris JA, Ang S, Navarro C. Minimizing the toxic effects of formaldehyde. Lab Med. 1997;29(1):39–42.
66. Clinical Laboratory Improvement Amendments (CLIA). http://www.fda.gov/MedicalDevices/DeviceRegulationandGuidance/IVDRegulatoryAssistance/ucm124105.htm. Accessed.
67. Sliva CA. FDA's CLIA complexity process. IVD roundtable 510(k) workshop. 23 April 2002. http://www.fda.gov/MedicalDevices/DeviceRegulationandGuidance/IVDRegulatoryAssistance/ucm124269.htm. Accessed 30 Jul 2010.
68. U.S. Department of Health and Human Services, U.S. Food and Drug Administration. Overview of IVD regulation. http://www.fda.gov/MedicalDevices/DeviceRegulationandGuidance/IVDRegulatoryAssistance/ucm123682.htm. Accessed 30 Jul 2010.
69. U.S. Department of Health and Human Services, U.S. Food and Drug Administration. Medical device databases. http://www.fda.gov/MedicalDevices/DeviceRegulationandGuidance/Databases/default.htm. Accessed 30 Jul 2010.
70. U.S. Department of Health and Human Services. Medicare, medicaid and CLIA programs: regulations implementing the clinical laboratory improvement amendments of 1988 (CLIA '88). Final rule. Federal Reg. 1992;57:7002–186.
71. COLA. COLA laboratory accreditation manual. Columbia, MD: Commission on Office Laboratory Accreditation; 1996.
72. National Committee on Clinical and Laboratory Standards GP2-A3. Clinical laboratory technical procedure manuals – third edition. approved guideline. Wayne, PA: National Committee on Clinical Laboratory Standards; 1996.
73. CAP accreditation and laboratory improvement: about the CAP accreditation program. http://www.cap.org/. Accessed 30 Jul 2010.
74. Arber DA. Effect of prolonged formalin fixation on the immunohistochemical reactivity of breast markers. Appl Immunohistochem Mol Morphol. 2002;10(2):183–6.
75. U. S. Department of Labor, Occupational Safety and Health Administration. 29CFR part 19 standards 10.1048 and 10.1450, revised 1 Jul 1998.
76. National Committee on Clinical and Laboratory Standards C24A2. Statistical quality control for quantitative measurements: principles and definitions – second edition; approved guideline. Wayne, PA: National Committee on Clinical and Laboratory Standards; 1998.
77. Miller RT, Swanson PE, Wick MR. Fixation and epitope retrieval in diagnostic immunohistochemistry: a concise review with practical considerations. Appl Immunohistochem Mol Morphol. 2000;8(3):228–35.
78. Miller RT, Kubier P, Reynolds B, Henry T. Blocking of endogenous avidin-binding activity in immunohistochemistry: the use of skim milk as an economical and effective substitute for commercial biotin solutions. Appl Immunohistochem Mol Morphol. 1999;7(1):63–5.
79. College of American Pathologists. Retention of laboratory records and materials. http://www.cap.org/apps/cap.portal?_nfpb=true&cntvwrPtlt_actionOverride=%2Fportlets%2FcontentViewer%2Fshow&_windowLabel=cntvwrPtlt&cntvwrPtlt%7BactionForm.contentReference%7D=policies%2Fpolicy_appPP.html&_state=maximized&_pageLabel=cntvwr. Accessed 30 Jul 2010.

Chapter 2
Technique and Troubleshooting of Antibody Testing

Fan Lin and Jianhui Shi

Abstract This chapter provides a practical overview of common problems encountered when testing a new antibody and how to approach and solve these problems in a simple way.

Keywords Antigen retrieval • Heat-induced • Proteolytic-induced • Staining signal • Staining background

FREQUENTLY ASKED QUESTIONS

2.1 What Are the Results and Common Problems Encountered When Testing a New Antibody?

Troubleshooting problems encountered in an immunohistochemical staining procedure can be straightforward or a very complicated task. Many articles and book chapters have addressed these potential issues in great detail; therefore, this chapter is not intended to be comprehensive or to substitute for published literature. Instead, it attempts to reemphasize the key points one should remember when working on these problems. The nine most likely immunostaining results and potential problems one may encounter when testing and optimizing a new antibody in a positive control tissue block are summarized in the following table. The possible causes and solutions for each specific problem will be addressed in Question #3 [1–5].

F. Lin (✉)
Department of Pathology and Laboratory Medicine, Geisinger Medical Center, 100 N. Academy Avenue, Danville, PA 17822, USA
e-mail: flin1@geisinger.edu

Table 2.1 Summary of possible staining results when testing a new antibody

	Staining signal		
Background	Strong staining signal	Weak staining signal	No staining signal
No background	A	D	G
Weak background	B	E	H
Strong background	C	F	I

2.2 What Are the General Approaches Before Getting into a Demanding Technical Issue?

As a general rule, before getting into the demanding technical issues as listed in Table 2.1, the best approach is to follow this simple checklist:

- Follow all steps and instructions in the manufacturer's protocol.
- Consult the data sheet for general recommendation such as positive control tissue, antigen retrieval technique, antibody dilution, blocking reagent, etc.
- Confirm the compatibility of a secondary antibody to the species and subclass immunoglobulin of a primary antibody (such as rabbit monoclonal antibody or mouse monoclonal antibody).
- Be sure to use the "right" tissue or tumor as a positive control, which should contain abundant and well-preserved antigen to be tested.
- Use a positive control block (such as tissue microarray block) containing multiple tissue sections, if it is available.
- Ensure the water bath and oven temperatures do not exceed 60°C.

F. Lin and J. Prichard (eds.), *Handbook of Practical Immunohistochemistry: Frequently Asked Questions*,
DOI 10.1007/978-1-4419-8062-5_2,

- Perform all relevant blocking steps to eliminate background staining, including endogenous peroxidases and phosphatases.
- Check all reagents for appropriate preparation, expiration date, and storage condition.
- Be aware that inadequate fixation (under-fixation), inappropriate fixative (other than 10% neutral-buffered formalin), and high acidity or prolonged decalcification may result in a false-negative result for many antibodies [1–5].

2.3 What are the Possible Solutions for Each Specific Technical Problem in Table 2.1?

2.3.1 A. If Strong Staining Signal and No Background Staining Is Obtained

- The next step is to test the primary antibody in multiple dilutions, to obtain the highest dilution with the optimal result, to save the primary antibody and cut down the cost.

2.3.2 B. If Strong Staining Signal and Weak Background Staining Is Obtained

- Reduce the primary antibody concentration.
- Shorten the primary antibody incubation time.
- Shorten the second antibody incubation time.
- Further block the background staining.

2.3.3 C. If Strong Staining Signal and Strong Background Staining Is Obtained

- Reduce the primary antibody concentration.
- Shorten the primary antibody incubation time.
- Shorten the second antibody incubation time.
- Further block the background staining.
- Try different antigen retrieval methods.

2.3.4 D. If Weak Staining Signal and No Background Staining Is Obtained

- Increase the primary antibody concentration.
- Increase the incubation time for the primary antibody.
- Increase the incubation time for the second antibody.
- Switch to a more sensitive secondary detecting system.
- Try different antigen retrieval methods.

2.3.5 E. If Weak Staining Signal and Weak Background Staining Is Obtained

- Increase the primary antibody concentration and reduce the incubation time.
- Further block background staining.
- Increase the incubation time for the second antibody.
- Switch to a more sensitive secondary detecting system.
- Try different antigen retrieval methods.
- Use a different primary antibody.

2.3.6 F. If Weak Staining Signal and Strong Background Staining Is Obtained

- Further block background staining.
- Switch to a more sensitive secondary detecting system.
- Try different antigen retrieval methods.
- Use a different primary antibody.

2.3.7 G. If No Staining Signal and No Background Staining Is Obtained

- Follow the general approaches step-by-step.
- Increase the primary antibody concentration and incubation time.
- Try different antigen retrieval methods.
- Switch to a more sensitive secondary detecting system.
- Contact the technical department of the primary antibody supplier for assistance.
- Use a different primary antibody.

2.3.8 H. If No Staining Signal and Weak Background Staining Is Obtained

- Follow the general approaches step-by-step.
- Increase the primary antibody concentration and incubation time.
- Try different antigen retrieval methods.
- Switch to a more sensitive secondary detecting system.
- Contact the technical department of the primary antibody supplier for assistance.
- Use a different primary antibody.

2.3.9 *I. If No Staining Signal and Strong Background Staining Is Obtained*

- Follow the general approaches step-by step.
- Try different antigen retrieval methods.
- Switch to a more sensitive secondary detecting system.
- Contact the technical department of the primary antibody supplier for assistance.
- Use a different primary antibody.

2.4 How To Determine Whether or Not a Primary Antibody Works? Table/Diagram 2.2

The following diagram will give you a quick idea whether or not a primary antibody works on positive control tissue. If the testing result appears in the zones I–III, the primary antibody will work well after fine-tuning. If the testing result falls into zones IV–VI, after additional testing and adjustments of the staining condition, the primary antibody is most likely working. If the testing result ends up in the zones VII–IX, the primary antibody is unlikely to work; therefore, to save time, a new antibody from a different vendor should be considered (Table Diagram 2.2).

Table 2.2 Summary of possible staining results

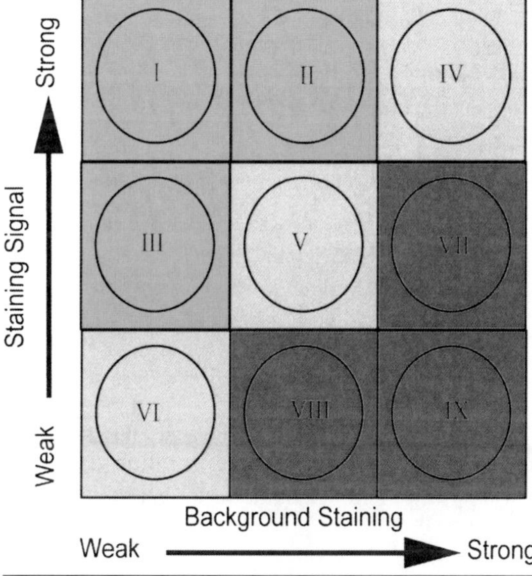

2.5 What Are the Commonly Used Antigen Retrieval Methods?

Antigen retrieval (AR) technique is a process to unmask an antibody-binding site for a specific antibody on formalin-fixed, paraffin-embedded tissue sections. It can significantly enhance the immunohistochemical staining signal. There are two main AR techniques. One is called heat-induced epitope retrieval (HIER). Another method uses enzymatic digestion and is called proteolytic-induced epitope retrieval (PIER).

Many enzymes can be used in PIER, such as trypsin, proteinase K, pepsin A, and pronase. The key factors to obtain an optimal result include enzyme concentration, time of digestion, temperature, and pH. Proteinase K will provide an effective enzymatic digestion for membrane antigens such as VHL, CD31, and vWF. Over-digestion may result in poor tissue morphology and even a false-positive staining; in contrast, under-digestion may cause a false-negative result.

Microwave oven and water bath are the most commonly used heating devices for HIER in our lab. Other devices may include microwave pressure cooker, vegetable steamer, and decloaker device. A heating and cooling time of 20 min each appears to be adequate for many antibodies. EDTA at pH 8.0 is the most frequently used retrieval solution in our practice; citrate buffer at pH 6.0, target retrieval solution pH 6.1, and target retrieval solution pH 8.0 (HipH) are also suitable for some antibodies.

A combination of HIER and PIER is an alternative approach to unmask so-called difficult antigens when other methods fail to work. It is especially useful when performing double or triple labeling for two or more antigens simultaneously. However, special attention should be paid because two retrieval methods may cause a false-negative staining result for one of the two antibodies, and sometimes a tissue section may fall off the slide due to the prolonged retrieval time.

2.6 What Are the Commonly Used Antigen Retrieval Protocols?

2.6.1 *Protocol #1: Citrate Buffer Antigen Retrieval Method*

2.6.1.1 Solutions and Reagents

Citric acid monohydrate (Fisher Scientific, Cat #A104-500)

10.505 g, Dilute in 500 mL of distilled water, mix to dissolve (0.1 M)

Sodium citrate (Fisher Scientific, Cat #S93364)

14.704 g, Dilute in 500 mL of distilled water, mix to dissolve (0.1 M)

Store the solutions at 4°C refrigeration for longer storage.

Fresh preparation of citrate buffer before use:

9 mL of 0.1 M citric acid
41 mL of 0.1 M sodium citrate } Dilute in 500 mL of distilled water, mix to dissolve

Adjust pH to 6.0 with 1 N NaOH and 1 N HCl and mix well.

Formalin or other aldehyde fixation forms protein cross-linking that masks the antigenic sites in tissue specimens, which in turns gives weak or false-negative staining for immunohistochemical detection of certain proteins. The citrate-based solution is designed to break the protein cross-linking; thereby, unmasking the antigens and epitopes in formalin-fixed and paraffin-embedded tissue sections, then enhancing staining intensity of antibodies.

2.6.1.2 Procedure

1. Dewax paraffin-embedded tissue sections with two changes of Histoclear solution or xylene, 5 min each.
2. Rehydrate the sections in two changes of 100 and 95% ethanol for 30 s each, and 70% ethanol for 30 s; then rinse in distilled water.
3. Inserted the slides in a slide holder and immerse the slides into the microwave dish containing 500 mL of citrate buffer. Set the lid loosely on top of the microwave dish.
4. Heat the dish for 5 min at high power (level 10) and 15 min at medium power (level 5).
5. Transfer the dish to room temperature and allow the slides to cool for 20 min. Rinse sections in a cool running tap water; then put the slides into Tris-buffered saline with 0.05% Tween (TBST) solution.
6. Continue with an appropriate antibody staining protocol.

2.6.2 Protocol #2: EDTA Buffer Antigen Retrieval Protocol

2.6.2.1 Solutions and Reagents

EDTA buffer (1 mM EDTA, pH 8.0):

EDTA (Fisher Scientific, Cat #BP120-500)	0.372 g
Distilled water	1,000 mL

Mix to dissolve. Adjust pH to 8.0 using 1 N NaOH. Store at room temperature for up to 3 months or at 4°C for longer storage.

This buffer works well for many antibodies, but sometime it gives high background staining; therefore, a primary antibody can often be diluted in a lower concentration. It is very useful for low-affinity antibodies or when tissue antigens are not abundant.

The EDTA solution is also designed to break the protein cross-links; thereby, unmask the antigens and epitopes in formalin-fixed and paraffin-embedded tissue sections, thus enhancing the staining intensity of the antibodies.

2.6.2.2 Procedure

1. Dewax the sections in two changes of xylene, 5 min each.
2. Rehydrate the slides in two changes of 100 and 95% ethanol for 30 s each and 70% ethanol for 30 s; then rinse in distilled water.
3. Place the slides in a slide holder and immerse slides inserted in the microwave dish containing 500 mL of EDTA buffer. Set the lid loosely on top of the microwave dish.
4. Heat the dish for 5 min at high power (level 10) and 15 min at medium power (level 5).
5. Transfer the dish to room temperature and allow the slides to cool for 20 min.
6. Rinse sections in a running cool tap water; then put the slides into Tris-buffered saline with 0.05% Tween (TBST) solution.
7. Ready for an appropriate antibody staining protocol.

2.6.3 Protocol #3: Target Retrieval Solution Buffer Antigen Retrieval Protocol

2.6.3.1 Solutions and Reagents

Target retrieval solution, pH 6.1	(DAKO Cat #S1700)
Target retrieval solution, pH 8.0	(DAKO Cat #S3308)
Target retrieval solution, pH 9.0	(DAKO Cat #S2368)

These products are to be used on formalin-fixed, paraffin-embedded tissue sections mounted on glass slides for target retrieval prior to IHC procedures.

The retrieval procedure involves incubating the sections in preheated target retrieval solution in a water bath for 20 min. The treatment of target retrieval solution prior to IHC procedures results in an increase in staining intensity with many primary antibodies.

2.6.3.2 Procedure

1. Fill Coplin staining jar or other suitable container with a sufficient quantity of target retrieval solution. Place the container in a water bath. Heat the water bath to 95–99°C (do not boil).
2. Dewax the sections in two changes of xylene, 5 min each.
3. Rehydrate the slides in two changes of 100 and 95% ethanol for 30 s each and 70% ethanol for 30 s; then rinse in distilled water.
4. Incubate the sections in preheated target retrieval solution in a water bath for 20 min.
5. Transfer the entire container with slides from the water bath. Allow it to cool for 20 min at room temperature.

6. Rinse the sections in a running cool tap water; then put the slides into Tris-buffered saline with 0.05% Tween (TBST) solution.
7. Ready for an appropriate antibody staining protocol.

2.6.4 Protocol #4: Retrieve-All Antigen Unmasking System Retrieval Protocol

2.6.4.1 Solutions and Reagents

Universal, 1× (SIGNET) catalog number: SIG-31912.

Retrieve-All is an antigen unmasking solution available in the following three pH formulas for use in heat-induced unmasking. Retrieve-All 1 (universal pH 8) is the most frequently used in our immunohistochemical laboratory in all the Retrieve-All solutions.

Retrieve-All 1 (universal pH 8).
Retrieve-All 2 (basic pH 10).
Retrieve-All 3 (acidic pH 4.8).

2.6.4.2 Procedure

1. Fill Coplin staining jar or other suitable container with a sufficient quantity of Retrieve-All 1 solution. Place the container in a water bath. Heat the water bath to 95–99°C (do not boil).
2. Dewax the sections in two changes of xylene solution, 5 min each.
3. Rehydrate the sections in two changes of 100 and 95% ethanol for 30 s each and 70% ethanol for 30 s; then rinse in distilled water.
4. Incubate the sections in preheated Retrieve-All 1 solution in a water bath for 10 min.
5. Remove the entire jar or container with slides from the water bath. Allow it to cool down for 10 min at room temperature.
6. Rinse sections in running cool tap water; then put the slides into Tris-buffered saline with 0.05% Tween (TBST) solution.

2.6.5 Protocol #5: Proteinase K Antigen Retrieval Protocol

2.6.5.1 Solutions and Reagents

Proteinase K solution (DAKO Cat #S3020).

Proteolytic enzyme solution diluted in 0.05 mol/L Tris–HCl, 0.015 mol/L sodium azide, pH 7.5.

Proteinase K is used for the proteolytic digestion of formalin-fixed, paraffin-embedded tissue sections prior to an immunohistochemical staining protocol. Enzymatic digestion unmasks certain epitopes/sites which have been masked during formalin-fixation process; therefore, unmasking the antigens and epitopes in formalin-fixed and paraffin-embedded tissue sections will enhance staining intensity of antibodies. This method may cause tissue damage, if the tissue sections are under-fixed. It is crucial to select the appropriate incubation time (5–20 min) and temperature of incubation (20–60°C) for a specific application and try to avoid over-digestion of the tissue sections' tissues. Proteinase K is a very useful antigen unmasking solution to some cell membrane antigens.

2.6.5.2 Procedure

1. Dewax the sections in two changes of Histoclear or xylene solution, 5 min each.
2. Rehydrate in two changes of 100 and 95% ethanol for 30 s each and 70% ethanol for 30 s; then rinse in distilled water.
3. Transfer the sections into Proteinase K working solution and incubate for 5–15 min at room temperature in a humidified chamber (optimal incubation time may vary depending on tissue type and degree of fixation).
4. If you use DAKO Autostainer, after performing avidin/biotin blocking such as peroxidase block (DAKO Cat #K4007) processing, you can set up a step for Proteinase K incubation before primary antibody incubation. Certainly, a polymer detecting system is more favorable choice.
5. Ready for an appropriate antibody staining protocol.

References

1. Chu PG, Weiss LM, editors. Modern immunohistochemistry. New York, NY: Cambridge University Press; 2009.
2. Dabbs DJ. Diagnostic immunohistochemistry: theranostic and genomic applications. 3rd ed. Philadelphia, PA: Saunders Elsevier; 2010.
3. Taylor C, Cote R, editors. Major problems in pathology, Immunomicroscopy: a diagnostic tool for the surgical pathologist, vol. 19. 3rd ed. Philadelphia, PA: Saunders Elsevier; 2006.
4. Renshaw S, editor. Immunohistochemistry: methods express. Oxfordshire, England: Scion; 2007.
5. Haytt MA. Microscopy, immunohistochemistry and antigen retrieval methods: for light and electron microscopy. New York, NY: Kluwer Academic/Plenum; 2002.

Chapter 3
Overview of Automated Immunohistochemistry

Jeffrey Prichard, Angela Bitting, and Joe Myers

Abstract The past decade has produced major innovations and a great variety of features available in automated staining instruments. This chapter is a "buyer's guide" for automated IHC instruments. For those new to the topic of automated staining, it begins with discussions of the advantages and disadvantages of automated versus manual staining techniques to help you decide if automation is the right choice for your laboratory. The basics of the general types of mechanics that differentiate the platforms are illustrated. Industry jargon about "open" and "closed" systems are better defined. To help with creating a thoughtful business plan to justify the budget expense of automation, the considerations that include the cost and potential savings of operating the equipment over and above the purchase price are presented. The different strategies for slide capacity and continuous processing that affect overall test throughput are described. A comprehensive feature comparison table is included to reveal how the current clinical instruments stack up side by side. With the information in this chapter you will know how to evaluate whether an instrument is right for you and understand the value of technological advancements as they arrive in the future.

Keywords Automation • Instrument • Cost • Slide capacity • Waste • Predilute • Barcode

FREQUENTLY ASKED QUESTIONS

1. What are the advantages of automating immunohistochemistry when compared to manual staining? (pp. 23–24)
2. What are the disadvantages of automating immunohistochemistry when compared to manual staining? (p. 24)
3. What are "Open" and "Closed" staining systems? (p. 24)
4. What is the purpose of automation that includes the ability to heat slides? (pp. 24–25)
5. What are Matrix and Rotary platforms? (pp. 25–26)
6. What should be considered when evaluating the cost of an automated staining system? (p. 26)
7. How do slide capacity and batch size affect the speed of stain production? (p. 26)
8. What other system features effect the speed of the staining? (p. 26)
9. What are the advantages and disadvantages of using prediluted antibodies and other reagents? (p. 26)
10. What are the consideration surrounding waste disposal strategies? (p. 27)
11. What should be considered when comparing automated staining platforms? (pp. 27–29)

3.1 What Are the Advantages of Automating Immunohistochemistry When Compared to Manual Staining?

There are several reasons that people begin to consider adding automated immunohistochemistry. The main advantages of automating your staining protocols involve standardization and labor savings. In both of these cases, the greatest benefits of automation lay in addressing higher volume workloads. The higher the volume at a laboratory, the more likely testing will involve multiple histotechnologists on multiple shifts, each with individual tendencies and variable interruptions that could benefit from the standardization provided by automation. Additionally, many of us are experiencing shortages of qualified histotechnologists throughout the laboratory, and need the personnel we have working at cutting and embedding stations that lack a reasonable option for automation. Automating the immunohistochemistry section of your laboratory will free up technologist's time to perform these essential tasks. And although optimizing and troubleshooting staining and reviewing control tissue reactions require extensive knowledge and experience with the science and theory of IHC, performing the prepared protocols on the automated instruments is less demanding. With automation, you may consider sharing the responsibility for performing IHC stains with a larger number of your staff. Many instruments offer assistance to staff with

J. Prichard and A. Bitting (✉)
Department of Pathology and Laboratory Medicine, Geisinger Medical Center, 100 N. Academy Avenue, Danville, PA 17822, USA

F. Lin and J. Prichard (eds.), *Handbook of Practical Immunohistochemistry: Frequently Asked Questions*,
DOI 10.1007/978-1-4419-8062-5_3,

additional process monitoring for errors in the form of alarms for such events as inappropriate temperatures, inadequate reagent volumes, or even incorrectly selected reagents identified through barcode tracking. These systems may also employ computerized software capable of tracking reagent stock and expiration dates, aiding reagent inventory management [1].

3.2 What Are the Disadvantages of Automating Immunohistochemistry When Compared to Manual Staining?

We consider machines to be tirelessly reproducible engines of productivity. But in reality, we must keep in mind that any machine periodically requires maintenance or repair. And the more moving parts an instrument has, the more opportunities there are for parts to malfunction. More complex systems are not necessarily better systems. Laboratories dependent on automation are at the mercy of their instrumentation. Sufficient redundancy should be considered to accommodate instrument downtime, scheduled, or otherwise.

Another disadvantage of automation noted by many is its effect on the working knowledge of staff. A decade or more ago, immunohistochemistry was only performed by a small number of staff highly knowledgeable about the IHC staining processes from spending endless hours of trial and error attempting to optimize manual stains. These people are particularly valuable to have in your laboratory when trying to troubleshoot poorly performing stains because of their hands-on experience with each of the steps of the staining process. In much of current practice, automation separates us from the staining process through mechanization. Because of this, less experienced personnel are able to participate in the IHC section of the laboratory. But this comes with the increasing likelihood that the person running the IHC instrumentation does not have sufficient knowledge to troubleshoot the staining process when a control reaction is suboptimal. Implementation of an automated system does not assure that high-quality results will be produced. Whether assays are manual or automated, they are subject to (a) the effects of specimen fixation and processing, (b) the effects of specimen pretreatments – e.g., heat/enzyme-induced retrieval, endogenous enzyme, protein/immunoglobulin, and/or biotin blocking, (c) detection system reagent compatibility, and (d) selection of positive and negative control specimens and methods. Any laboratory performing IHC needs to have some personnel overseeing the IHC section with specialized knowledge adequate to assure proper function of the assays.

The greatest advantages of manual staining come in the almost infinite flexibility in choosing reagents, retrieval methods, and in the ability to attempt subtle variation in technique when optimizing a staining protocol. In the transition from manual to automated staining, many note frustrations related to lack of control or awareness of the processes going on within the instrument. There is reason to believe that flexibility is sacrificed to greater or lesser degrees depending on how open or closed an instrument is with regard to variables permitted at each of the staining steps. This is discussed further in the next question.

3.3 What Are "Open" and "Closed" Staining Systems?

When compared to the flexibility of "open" manual staining options, the standardization of automation is achieved by "closing" the instrument to opportunities for variations introduced by human participation. Although it is not necessary to limit open optimization options in an instrument, in order to have it capable of closed reproducible production of assays, it is often the case in the IHC automation offerings that standardization is increased at the expense of flexibility.

This has resulted in automated systems being designed and described as "open" meaning that they offer similar flexibility to manual staining in diverse reagent choices and timing of staining steps. In fact, open automated systems are the easiest to migrate to from manual protocols with the least need for alterations. The term open is also used to refer to systems that do not perform onboard heat-induced epitope retrieval (HIER), in contrast to "closed" systems that perform onboard HIER under the "closed" lids of the system. Open automated systems are often preferred in research settings where the main concern may be developing new staining protocols for an ever-growing number of target biomarkers, requiring flexibility in protocol options.

In contrast, in the clinical setting where priority is given to reproducing established protocols in greater volumes performed by a greater number of testing personnel, assays can benefit from the reproducibility of "closed" standardized processes. Automated systems are described as increasingly "closed," the more they limit protocols to the use of proprietary antibodies and reagents, and restrict the options available in the software to vary the steps of the protocol. Closed systems can be perceived as easier to operate because of the fewer options, but there is also a perception of the testing being done in a "black box" out of sight and understanding of the operator. Obviously, there are strengths and weaknesses to both open and closed system and the appropriate balance of function should be sought for the laboratory's purpose [2].

3.4 What Is the Purpose of Automation that Includes the Ability to Heat Slides?

Heat can be used for several purposes in the staining process. The most well known is the use of slide heating for HIER. A great emphasis is placed on this because HIER is necessary in the vast majority of staining protocols, and when not performed onboard, these procedures must be performed manually prior to loading the slides on the staining instrument. Heating is also one of the necessary steps in denaturing DNA targets for DNA in situ hybridization procedures such as those to detect Human Papilloma Virus (HPV). Heat is not required, however, for in situ hybridization to detect RNA such as in the case of Epstein Barr virus (EBV) which can be performed on nonheated platforms as long as there is a detection system from in situ hybridization available for the instrument.

Both Dako Autostainers™ and Thermo Autostainer 2D™ have adopted the strategy of creating pretreatment (PT) modules separate from their staining instruments. This provides automation for pretreatment in a single module that may supply retrieved slides for multiple staining instruments in the laboratory.

Other instruments, such as the Ventana Benchmarks™, Leica Bond™ series, and the Celerus WAVE RPD™· have incorporated onboard HIER into their staining instruments. An advantage for systems that incorporating the slide heating function into the staining instrumentation is the ability to apply heat during incubation of reagents to accelerate reaction times [3].

3.5 What Are Matrix and Rotary Platforms?

Matrix and rotary are terms used to describe the motion of the robotic mechanisms that bring the reagents to the microscopic slides in automated IHC systems. The vast majority of automated systems utilize the matrix architecture, also known as array architecture (Fig. 3.1). In these matrix systems, the slides and reagents are each arranged in rows and/or columns and robotic arms move back and forth across the array of slides, dispensing reagents, and return to the matrix of reagent vials to rinse and refill with the next reagent to dispense. In the rotary systems, the slides and reagents are each placed around rotating circular racks (Fig. 3.2). The reagent platter

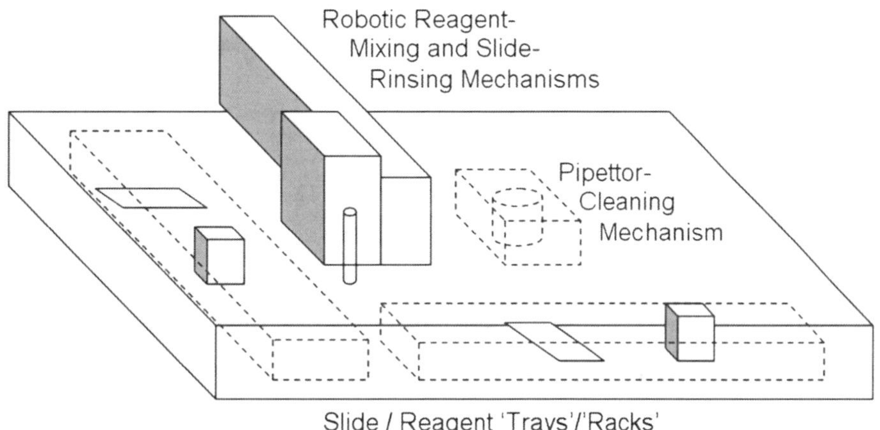

Fig. 3.1 Matrix system "layout"

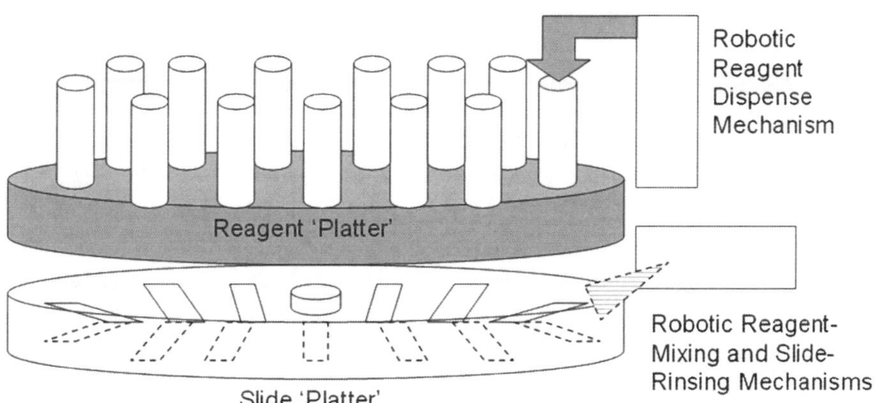

Fig. 3.2 Rotary system "layout"

is located above the slide platter. Rotation of the platters brings the reagent containers into position over slides to directly dispense their fluids onto the slides. In this way, each reagent container acts as its own dispenser eliminating possibility for cross contamination. There is no need to rinse the aspiration probes or exchange disposable pipette tips between uses on different reagents as is done in the matrix systems.

3.6 What Should Be Considered When Evaluating the Cost of an Automated Staining System?

One of the obvious issues to be addressed in acquiring staining automation equipment is the topic of cost. And consideration should be given to the ongoing operating costs in addition to the initial purchase price of a system. Costs may come in the form of consumables (proprietary reagents, containers, pipette tips), service contracts, waste disposal, and even interfacing costs to connect to laboratory information systems. If chosen correctly to match the demands of your testing volumes, turn-around time, and needs for standardization and labor savings, automation can actually save money compared to the manual alternative. But there will most likely still be the need to show consideration of these factors in a cost justification to someone responsible for purchasing equipment in this price range [4].

3.7 How Do Slide Capacity and Batch Size Affect the Speed of Stain Production?

The overall throughput that a system is capable of is a result of how many slides can be loaded on the system and how quickly the steps of staining can be performed. For most systems, the rate-limiting steps are the lengths of the staining protocols and the total number of slides that can be placed on the system at a time is called the instrument slide capacity. The rate of reagent delivery rarely is the bottleneck in the process, because the robotic components that distribute reagents to the slides only work intermittently in between periods of reagent incubation. In this sense, having a large slide capacity can improve throughput by having more slides staining at a time. But of course it is not as simple as just slide capacity and protocol length.

Consider that there can be great variation in the time required for different slides in a batch to complete their staining cycle. In fact different staining protocols may vary from minutes for some direct immunofluorescence assays to several hours for multiplexed stains or in situ hybridization. If a staining system requires all of the stains in a batch to remain while the slide with the longest protocol finishes, all of the slides and the slots they are occupying could be held hostage for hours. Because of this variation in protocol lengths, we would ideally want batch sizes to be singular and be able to load and unload individual slides independently. With single slide batches, each of the slots in a platform achieves the fastest throughput. Systems representing all points on the spectrum of slide capacity and batch size can be found in the market. Most vendors offer a compromise of large instrument capacity systems divided into multiple, smaller, independently operated racks or drawers. Finding the correct balance of capacity and batch size for your volume and protocol mix will provide you the best slide throughput [5].

3.8 What Other System Features Effect the Speed of the Staining?

Incubations can be accelerated by introducing energy into the reaction in the form of either heat or mixing techniques. Systems that contain slide heating plates utilized during HIER may also employ heat to expedite reagent incubation periods. There are some quite unique instruments on the market that use mixing methods to hasten reagent reactions. Air vortex mixing and dynamic capillary mixing are two examples of this.

3.9 What Are the Advantages and Disadvantages of Using Prediluted Antibodies and Other Reagents?

Prediluted reagents, particularly antibodies, provide significant convenience over reagents that must be prepared from concentrate, then optimized/validated as needed; it should be noted that detection reagents are almost always available in "ready-to-use" format, regardless of vendor/system. Prediluted primary antibodies limit optimization steps to adapting the retrieval method and primary antibody incubation times, since the antibody dilution cannot be altered.

3.10 What Are the Consideration Surrounding Waste Disposal Strategies?

Waste separation – diaminobenzidine (DAB) is the most common chromogen used in IHC assays. Unfortunately, DAB is hazardous with special, more expensive handling requirement as a waste product. If kept separate from nonhazardous waste, less volume needs the expensive handling or neutralization. But if mixed into the nonhazardous waste, all of the waste must be processed as hazardous waste.

Limiting waste – several vendors use strategies that limit the initial volumes of reagents required. Examples include employing small, walled off reaction chambers on the slides, or permitting control of the amount of reagent that is dispensed. Rinsed probe systems are considered better at being able to dispense small amounts of concentrated reagents when compared to disposable pipettes or disposable dispensers. The Celerus Wave RPD™ employs a very unique waste strategy that produces no liquid waste since all waste is collected in an absorbant material within the waste cartridge and disposed as solid waste. In the end, limiting the amount of reagents used saves both the reagent costs and costs for the disposal of waste produced.

3.11 What Should Be Considered When Comparing Automated Staining Platforms?

The first thing to understand is that there is no best system on the market for all purposes. In fact the existence of so many diverse staining technologies argues that each has an audience with diverse needs and wants. If you are considering adopting an automated staining system, the best approach is to start with the understanding of your proposed use. Consider the following:

- Size of the platform and required reagents compared to the size of your laboratory space
- Capacity, speed, and flexibility of batches for continuous processing compared to your needs for volumes and turnaround time
- Flexibility and openness of the reagent choices and protocol options compared to the number and difficulty of optimizations you will be performing
- Flexibility and precision for dispensing small amounts of expensive reagents or those in low supply in customized protocols
- The value of automated heating to perform onboard retrieval protocols and DNA target denaturation
- Ability of the permitted detection systems to produce dual color staining and in situ hybridization compared to your testing needs
- Utility of reagent chilling for preservation of unstable chromogen substrates useful in dual antigen staining procedures
- Ease of use of the software and the computer capabilities of your testing personnel
- Whether LIS interfacing for automated stain ordering and label printing will benefit your workflow
- The time-saving and quality control benefits of systems supporting bar-coding or other technologies to track slides and reagents
- Degree to which the software aids you in providing quality control and quality assurance functionality, including operator alerts of suboptimal heating or insufficient or incorrect reagents, workload reports, stain utilization, lot to lot validations, and reagent inventory management
- Overall operating costs of the testing system and the potential to better utilize limited staff for other manual tasks

The following tables summarize many features of the variety of automated staining platforms currently available (Table 3.1). The following chapters (4 and 5) also offer perspectives and insights on the past, present, and future of automated staining systems from industry leading experts whose business is to develop the instruments that we will use.

Table 3.1 Feature comparison of automated IHC slide staining systems

	Capacities and capabilities	Biocare Medical intelliPath FLX®	BioGenex Laboratories Xmatrx Diagnostics®	BioGenex Laboratories i6000 Diagnostics™	Celerus Diagnostics Wave RPD™
Onboard automated staining functions	Slide baking	No	Yes	No	Yes
	Dewaxing capability	No	Yes	No	Yes
	Heat-induced retrieval	No	Yes	No	Yes
	On board ISH	RNA	DNA/RNA	RNA	DNA/RNA[a]
	Counterstaining	Yes	Yes	Yes	Yes
	Dehydration and clearing	No	Yes	No	No
	Coverslipping	No	Yes	No	No
Space	System space requirements	Benchtop	Floor	Benchtop	Benchtop
	Weight	145 lbs	400 lbs	124 lbs	125 lbs
	Size ($W \times D \times H$) (inches)	40×25×24"	46×29×59	38.5×24×18"	43×27.5×23.5"
Slide	Slide capacity/ batch size	50	40	60	16
	Bar-code labeled slides	Yes	Yes	Yes	Yes
	Continuous-processing/ batch size	Yes	Yes	Yes	No
	Slide-placement format	5 drawers of 10 slides	4 racks of 10 slides	5 drawers of 12 slides	16 (1 rack of 8 paired slides)
Antibodies/reagents/ protocols	Robotic movement	Matrix/array	Matrix/array	Matrix/array	Clamshell
	Reagent container capacity	48	49	60	8
	Bar-code labeled reagents	Yes	Yes	Yes	Memory chip
	Any protocol, any position	Yes	Yes	Yes	Yes
	Manage two buffers in same run[c]	Yes	No	No	No
	Accepts other vendor's reagents	All types	Primary antibodies	Primary antibodies	Primary antibodies
	Dual color stain capable	Yes	Yes	Yes	No
	Reagent chilling capability	Yes	No	No	No
	Reagent application method	Rinsed probe tip	Disposable pipette tips	Disposable pipette tips	Disposable cartridge
	Adjustable dispense volume	Yes	Yes	Yes	No
	Reagent incubation/mixing method	Open slide	Microchamber	Open slide	Dynamic capillary mix
	Waste separation	Yes	No	No	No
IT	LIS-interface capability	Yes	Yes	Yes	Yes
	Qty. units controlled by one PC	4	1	1	Unlimited
Proprietary issues	Special (required) accessories	Reagent vials	Pipette tips	Pipette tips	Reagent and waste cartridges
	Unique features	Simultaneous multiplexed stains, reagent chilling chamber	Total automation with onboard coverslipping	IHC, ISH and special stains	Plug and Play Reagents® Rapid IHC® (1 h)

[a]DNA/RNA expected by 2011

[b]Optical characters

[c]Helpful for combining runs of stains with a standard buffer with Dako's FDA approved Her-2 stain and proprietatry buffer [6–11]

Green shading indicates the onboard presence of a feature. Red shading indicates absence of a feature. Yellow shading indicates partial conformity or off-board automation of a feature

Dako		Leica Microsystems		Thermo-Lab Vision	Roche – Ventana	
Autostainer Plus™	Autostainer Link 48™	Bond-III™	Bond-Max™	Autostainer 2D™ 360/720	Benchmark XT™	Benchmark ULTRA™
No	No	Yes	Yes	No	Yes	Yes
Separate module	Separate module	Yes	Yes	Separate module	Yes	Yes
Separate module	Separate module	Yes	Yes	Separate module	Yes	Yes
Separate module DNA/RNA	Separate module DNA/RNA	RNA	RNA	RNA	DNA/RNA	DNA/RNA
Yes	Yes	Yes	Yes	Yes	Yes	Yes
No	No	No	No	No	No	No
No	No	No	No	No	No	No
Benchtop	Benchtop	Floor	Benchtop	Benchtop	Floor	Floor
140 lbs	147 lbs	543 lbs	265 lbs	119/174 lbs	385 lbs	650 lbs
40×27×24"	34×26×18"?	53.5×31×31"	30×30.5 ×28"	30/50×26 ×23 cm	35×26×60"	44×33×62"
48	48	30	30	36/84	30	30
No	Yes	Yes[b]	Yes[b]	Yes	Yes	Yes
No	No	Yes	Yes	Yes	No	Yes
4 racks of 12 slides	4 racks of 12 slides	3 racks of 10 slides	3 racks of 10 slides	3/7 racks of 12	1 wheel of 30 slides	30 random access slides
Matrix/array	Matrix/array	Matrix/array	Matrix/array	Matrix/array	Rotary	Rotary
64	42	36	36	40/84	35	35
No	Yes	Yes	Yes	Yes	Yes	Yes
Yes	Yes	No	No	Yes	Yes	Yes
No	Yes	No	No	No	No	No
All types	All types	All types	All types	All types	Primary antibodies	Primary antibodies
Yes	Yes	Yes	Yes	Yes	Yes	Yes
No	No	No	No	No	No	No
Rinsed probe tip	Rinsed probe tip	Rinsed probe tip	Rinsed probe tip	Rinsed probe tip	Disposable dispensers	Disposable dispensers
Yes	Yes	No	Yes	Yes	No	No
Open slide	Open slide	Covertiles™	Covertiles™	Open slide	Liquid coverslip, vortex mix	Liquid coverslip, vortex mix
Yes	Yes	Yes	Yes	Yes	No	No
No	Yes	Yes	Yes	Yes	Yes	Yes
1	3	5	5	4	4	8
Reagent vials	Reagent vials	Covertiles™	Covertiles™	Reagent vials	Reagent dispensers	Reagent dispensers
Open platform	Open platform with connectivity of multiple modules and LAN/LIS	3 Bulk reagent dispensing arms, Covertile™ microchambers	Covertile™ microchambers	Open platforms of in small and large sizes	Liquid coverslip chamber	Individual random access slide drawers

References

1. Myers J. Automated slide stainers for special stains, immunohistochemistry, and in situ hybridization. Med Lab Obs. 2004;36(1):28–30.
2. Myers J. Primer for selecting lab equipment. Med Lab Obs. 2007;39(1):26–7.
3. Myers J. Antigen retrieval: a review of commonly used, methods and commercially available devices. Med Lab Obs. 2006;38(6):10–5.
4. Myers J. Reducing immunohistochemistry expense – Part 2. Adv Admin Lab. 2004;13(10):18–22.
5. Myers J. The technical, clinical, and financial benefits of multi-antigen immuno-staining (MAIS) procedures. HistoLogic. 2006;4(2):25–9.
6. http://www.biocare.net.
7. http://www.biogenex.com.
8. http://www.dako.com.
9. http://www.leica.com.
10. http://www.thermoscientific.com.
11. http://www.ventanamed.com.

Chapter 4
Automated Staining: Dako Perspective

Ole F. Rasmussen and Andreas Schønau

Abstract Dako has been an industry leader developing automated staining instruments for decades. We have invited Dako to offer perspectives and insights on the past, present, and future of automated staining systems. Experts from Dako answer questions regarding what automation can and cannot provide, how automation can improve workflow and secure high staining quality, gains from connection to laboratory information systems, automated in situ hybridization assays, and the next steps in automation of staining and other processes in the pathology laboratory.

Keywords Dako • Automation • Quality • Reagents • Connectivity • CISH • Future • Immunohistochemistry

FREQUENTLY ASKED QUESTIONS

4.1 What Is Automation in Immunohistochemistry?

A simple definition of automation of immunohistochemistry (IHC) slide staining is automation of each step of the manual procedure conducted at the laboratory bench from baking to coverslipping. Over the past years we have also seen that automation facilitates new ways of handling single steps or unit operations or even combination of unit operations. A good example of this is the three-in-one pre-treatment procedure that is carried out in the Dako PT Link instrument where deparaffinization, target retrieval, and rehydration are combined into one step reducing the overall time and manual handling.

Another example is the reagent mixing carried out during the staining process on Celerus' Wave RPD System that helps reduce the incubation time. In future instrument generations, we will surely see new features where automation introduces new technologies that improve IHC staining parameters over existing systems. These improvements are likely to be made within the areas of robustness, turn-around-time (TAT), performance, new test types, and reduced environmental impact to solve green issues.

4.2 How Do You Differentiate Between Automation and Workflow?

A simple explanation of the difference between automation and workflow is that automation describes WHAT is being done, whereas workflow describes HOW things are being done.

O.F. Rasmussen (✉)
Dako Denmark A/S, Produktionsvej 42,
DK-2600 Glostrup, Denmark
e-mail: ole.feldballe@dako.com

F. Lin and J. Prichard (eds.), *Handbook of Practical Immunohistochemistry: Frequently Asked Questions*,
DOI 10.1007/978-1-4419-8062-5_4, © Springer Science+Business Media, LLC 2011

Thus, automation is one of several vehicles for an effective workflow in the laboratory. For the anatomic pathology laboratory, the workflow covers the process from sample receipt to the final delivery of the diagnostic report. The workflow is complex and it changes with the sample load, sample type, and staffing levels; thus metrics within the laboratory on their performance are never exact, and there is much variation from laboratory to laboratory.

4.3 What Are the Prime Benefits of Automation?

In a paper on automation from 1998, Moreau et al. [1] describe the tedious process of manual IHC: "before beginning the staining process the specimens should be circled with a delimiting pen that serves as a guide when wiping away excess liquid to prevent the specimen from being accidentally wiped off; that to avoid evaporation of solution, the slides should be laid flat with the specimen facing upward in a humidity chamber; that during buffer wash excess liquid should be wiped off using an absorbent tissue and consequently that when processing a large number of specimens, only three to five slides should be wiped at one time before applying the appropriate solution."

While many today take automation of IHC staining for granted, the 12 year old paper puts some of the benefits of automation nicely into perspective:

(a) Freeing up of resources by reducing hands-on time and by that overcoming the issue of labor shortages and the fact that laboratories, irrespective of geography, experience increasing difficulties in recruiting skilled staff.
(b) Standardization, facilitating similar procedures to be aligned and carried out in the same way and not depend on differences in personal skills or preferences.
(c) Reproducibility, ensuring that any given step always is carried out in the same way.
(d) Optimized use of reagents.

In addition, with increased focus on the user interface of the software, tracking capabilities, and data management, automation now provides further freeing up of resources and a long range of possibilities for reduction of (manual) errors and controls.

4.4 Can Automation Give Basis for Improved Workflow?

Within the pathology laboratory, the best example on impact the new automation can have on the workflow is probably the rapid processing instruments that have emerged over the past few years allowing significant reduction in time to result and also significantly impacting how specimen handling is organized in the laboratory.

In general, automation can give basis for improved workflow if it is able to do one or more of the following:

- Reduce the amount of manual handling
- Reduce the amount of data entry and log book entry
- Reduce the amount of checking and rechecking that is a very frequent process with ALL laboratory actions between unit operations (stop and start, send and receive)
- Reduce the defect level
- Reduce the risk of errors, and is as "error free" and "easy to use" as possible

To give some specific examples, within IHC staining, the introduction of the PT Link for three-in-one pre-treatment has made parallel processing of pre-treatment and staining highly efficient and ensures optimal utilization of the instrumentation. Furthermore, the use of the same slide rack both in the PT Link and the Autostainer ensures an easy and efficient work process. Other IHC staining instruments have random access features facilitating a different type of workflow based on smaller batches of slides and/or arrangement into a patient case-oriented handling.

4.5 How Can Automation Help in Reducing Hands-On Time?

The move from manual handling to automation of IHC staining has significantly reduced the hands-on time per slide, not only directly via the use of the instruments but also indirectly via reduction of errors. There will continuously be focus on developing automation to make the IHC staining process even more efficient, and this will include not only automation of more steps but also software with a more intuitive user interface and software allowing for reuse of patient data already available from the laboratory information system (LIS).

In general, automation will reduce hands-on-time if it can do any of the following:

- Replace manual steps and facilitate easy interfaces between adjacent steps in the workflow.
- Reduce the number of protocols so that in the best case there is just one, as this will reduce, e.g., reagent preparation.
- Accept slide requests either via LAN or LIS connection, thus reducing the need for data entry.
- Facilitate work planning by providing an easy and manageable automated work list.
- Predict end time to ensure the user has predictable "hands-off time" while the instrument is running enabling the user to do other things during "machine-time."

One interesting aspect is the relation between flexible workflow and hands-on time. Whereas instruments with random access allow for flexible workflow, this also introduces more user interactions with the instrument, and thus relatively more hands-on time per slide compared to staining on a high slide capacity instrument in a batch-mode. Here, the laboratory must choose what best suits their primary needs.

4.6 What Is the Difference Between an Open and a Closed System?

In an open IHC staining system such as the Autostainer Classic, the users can select any reagent and design any protocol they prefer, including buffers and visualization systems, number of steps and incubation times, and wash steps. In closed systems at least the visualization system is locked, and it has also been seen that, e.g., the target retrieval buffers are locked. In most cases, today, the protocols are also locked with the exception of primary antibody incubation time. There will always be flexibility for the antibodies as it is not realistic that one supplier will be able to offer all antibodies that a laboratory needs.

There are no completely strict lines between open and closed systems, as a closed system may be "un-locked" and an open system may be used fully or primarily as a closed system. An example of the latter is the Autostainer Link system used with the EnVision™ FLEX/FLEX+ visualization system and the full package of more than 100 ready-to-use (RTU) antibodies. An important benefit of closed systems is the high level of standardization, whereas open systems allows a high degree of flexibility.

4.7 How Does Automation Help Secure High Staining Quality?

Automation as such does not ensure high staining quality, but it must provide the basis for obtaining a high quality by securing an optimal process basis, e.g., adequate reagent application and correct incubation times. In addition, it ensures that the instrument processes are carried out in a reproducible manner.

The key point here is that high staining quality is first and only obtained when the instrument is combined with high quality reagents and protocols optimized for the reagents on the specific type of instrument. On top of that – to consistently maintain high staining quality – the personnel operating the instrument must be properly instructed in operation of the full system and that they do not deviate from protocol or take risks with the system. Furthermore, the instruments must be well maintained according to the manufacturer's instructions.

4.8 What Can Automation Not Provide?

While automation of IHC staining has facilitated significant progress in quality, standardization, and reproducibility, the dependency on prefixation handling, tissue fixation, and processing is high, and it can be argued that the computer-related adage, "garbage-in, garbage-out" applies to IHC staining as well. The importance of fixation on staining quality has been discussed considerably in the literature [2, 3], and insufficient fixation – typically below 12 h when using formalin- can result in a mixture of formalin-based and alcohol-based fixation and result in easily recognizable patchy staining.

Another parameter of importance that has had much less attention is baking of sectioned tissue. In a study by Williams et al. [4], the temperature and duration of baking and drying were found to have significant impact on staining quality. With baking at 60°C for 1 h as reference, baking at 30 min on a 70°C hot plate negatively affected staining of 4 out of 12 antibodies: L26, UCHL1, PC10, and Desmin.

Finally, but not least, automation cannot replace the users, the instruments need the users to function, and it will NEVER replace the pathologist's staining interpretation or give the full diagnosis. However, automation is likely eventually to cover some of the diagnostic work as we have seen with liquid-based cytology screening.

4.9 How Do You See Automation Help in Quality Control?

Today's visual control of stained control slides is still a highly manual process; however, if improper staining is indicated, the automation of the staining process offers a range of possibilities for investigating the cause of improper staining by investigating the instrument operations including protocol and reagent used, actual incubation times, and potential instrument process irregularities.

In addition to this, automation provides quality "proactively" by controlling a range of parameters prior to start of the staining run, e.g., only approved protocols are run, only reagents with proper remaining shelf life are used, only approved users initiate a run and required instrument maintenance is flagged.

However, in order to secure proper quality control, it is advisable to follow "the Dutch model" of having positive control material on every single slide. This may seem as double work, but will ensure that staining quality can be assessed for every single slide stained.

4.10 What Role Do Reagents Play in Relation to Automation?

You cannot have one without the other; thus you need high quality reagents that work optimally together on an instrument in a specified protocol. Important reagent parameters include conditions providing efficient target retrieval, high sensitivity and specificity of the antibodies, and high sensitivity visualization systems with a low background. The "garbage-in, garbage-out" also definitely apply to reagents.

The market has accepted that the closed systems are the way to go. With the EnVision™ FLEX/FLEX+ visualization system, the concomitantly developed FLEX RTU primary antibodies and well-defined set of protocols for the Autostainer Link platform Dako has made a solution that consistently provides exceptional staining results, and the staining quality for each of the antibodies has been endorsed by expert pathologists from the Unites States, Europe, and Japan.

4.11 What Can We Gain from Connection to LISs?

Integration of the IHC staining instruments with LIS enables seamless flow of patient and sample data bi-directionally to and from the instruments. This ensures patient data integrity and a significant reduction of the possibility to introduce errors. Furthermore, this frees up technologist time from the time-consuming task of (re-)entering test requests into the instruments. Connectivity to LIS and/or Local Area Network allows for easy access to data wherever and whenever needed facilitating efficient information flow for everyone in the pathology laboratory.

4.12 How Do We Get the Most out of Our Instruments or Systems?

When you get a new cell phone, you can easily find out how to make and receive telephone calls, but for most people it takes a long time to figure out all the features – and learn to use those you benefit from in your daily life. You may parallelize this to an IHC staining system, the point being that in order to be able to use the system in an efficient way; you need to understand your IHC stainer system sufficiently well to take advantage of the features that are important for your specific tasks in your laboratory. This may relate to a number of parameters, e.g., software features, standardization of protocols, or organization of the system in relation to workflow. It is likewise important to understand how new features in instrument, software, and/or reagent updates may or may not be utilized in the laboratory and that new personnel are trained sufficiently.

It should also be considered how the IHC stainer features can be best aligned with other instruments and processes in the laboratory, the goal being to establish the overall most efficient work processes or workflow to fulfill the laboratory needs.

4.13 How Do We Get the Most out of CISH Staining?

Chromogenic in situ hybridization (CISH) is a powerful tool for the detection of gene amplification, gene deletion, or genomic translocations. While flourescence in situ hybridization (FISH) is a very accurate and sensitive method, and today it is regarded as a "reference test" with respect to HER2 testing [5], the method does have some limitations. The evaluation of FISH stains requires a fluorescence microscope, and the evaluation of tissue and tumor morphology through FISH may be difficult and time-consuming. Fluorescence signals are also known to fade relatively quickly making inspection of FISH signals impossible after a few months of storage. These limitations can be overcome by CISH which allows for interpretation by bright field microscopy with the morphology of the tissue visible at the same time.

Converting the fluorescent signals of well-established FISH probes directly to chromogenic signals, while maintaining high signal resolution and distinct signals allows for a direct dot-to-dot conversion of signals. This is important for high concordance between FISH and CISH assays, which has been demonstrated in several publications [6–8].

To get the most out of CISH, all required information should be present at the same slide, including the gene signal and the reference signal, eliminating the need for combining information from multiple slides. A dual-color CISH technique hence makes it easier to distinguish true gene amplifications from chromosomal aneuploidy [9].

4.14 What Does the Laboratory Need to Do to Keep the Instrument at Speed?

It is important that the instruments are properly installed and that daily as well as periodic maintenance is followed according to manufacturer's instructions. Furthermore, if instruments are moved or major repair done, be sure to subsequently control that the instruments are working correctly.

As an example, several reports on improper staining have been shown to have incorrect instrument leveling as the root-cause.

4.15 What Do You See as the Next Steps in Automation of IHC Staining?

The next steps in automation will be driven by impact on time of the process, reduction of hands-on time, and cost reduction – without compromising staining quality. Automated baking on H&E or IHC stainers is a good example of the complexity of the combination of improvements. Some of today's stainers have the capability of automated baking, yet many laboratories do not use this capability because it takes too long time and reduces the efficiency of the system and/or process.

If we were to point to some specific steps or other improvements in automation this would include an efficient baking, efficient target retrieval, and coverslipping as this would allow true patient case handling from cutting of slides to microscopy and diagnosis by the pathologist. Looking at the question in a little wider perspective, improvements in instrument capability will allow the systems – with new reagents and software – to be able to address diagnostic questions requiring a much higher sensitivity than we see today, perhaps even allowing detection of single point mutations. There will definitely also be a move toward systems facilitating increased load of information on one slide, including both more methods (IHC/ISH) and more colors on the same slide – and this of course in combination with image analysis.

4.16 What Will Be the Next Steps for Automation Within Pathology?

There will in general be much focus directed toward reducing today's 3–5 day response time down to a response that can be given within an 8 h shift, allowing the oncologist to talk with the patients while still in the hospital, and potentially to initiate therapy. Another general trend will be to continue with standardization initiatives, and to have the anatomic pathology laboratory more and more to mimic the clinical pathology laboratory in the level of automation.

If we look beyond slide-based staining we will surely see a significant increase of nonslide-based technologies entering the pathology laboratory, and these will all be in at least a semi-automated form. There is a great potential in combining the tissue and slide-based technologies with a range of solution-based assays such as PCR which is already in use some places today.

What we hope to see one day would be automated tissue cutting, as this would give significant workflow benefits, reduce repeating work procedures, and decrease hands-on time dramatically. This will, however, require significant developments for the process itself, and it would also require optimization of the interface between the tissue cutting instrument and the staining instrument to have a fully automated procedure. We will probably have to wait some years for that to come.

References

1. Moreau A, Neel TE, Joubert M. Approach to automation in immunohistochemistry. J Clin Chim Acta. 1998;278:177–84.
2. Boenisch T. Effect of heat-induced antigen retrieval following inconsistent formalin fixation. Appl Immunol Mol Morphol. 2005;13(3):283–6.
3. Shi S-R, Liu C, Taylor CR. Standardization of immunohistochemistry for formalin-fixed, paraffin-embedded tissue sections based on the antigen-retrieval technique: from experiments to hypothesis. J Histochem Cytochem. 2007;55(2):105–9.
4. Williams JH, Mapham BL, Wright DH. Tissue preparation for immunocytochemistry. J Clin Pathol. 1997;50:422–8.
5. Wolff AC, Hammond ME, Schwartz JN, et al. American Society of Clinical Oncology/College of American Pathologists guideline recommendations for human epidermal growth factor receptor 2 testing in breast cancer. J Clin Oncol. 2007;25(1):118–45.
6. García-Caballero T, Grabau D, Green AR, et al. Determination of HER2 amplification in primary breast cancer using dual-color chromogenic in situ hybridization is comparable to fluorescence in situ hybridization: a European multicenter study involving 168 specimens. Histopathology. 2010;56(4):472–80.
7. Hoff K, Jørgensen JT, Müller S, et al. Visualization of FISH Probes by dual-color chromogenic in situ hybridization. Am J Clin Pathol. 2009;133(2):205–11.
8. Pedersen M, Rasmussen BB. The correlation between dual-color chromogenic in situ hybridization and fluorescence in situ hybridization in assessing HER2 gene amplification in breast cancer. Diagn Mol Pathol. 2009;18(2):96–102.
9. Tanner M, Gancberg D, Di Leo A, et al. Chromogenic in situ hybridization: a practical alternative for fluorescence in situ hybridization to detect HER-2/neu oncogene amplification in archival breast cancer samples. Am J Pathol. 2000;157(5):1467–72.

Chapter 5
Automated Staining: Ventana Perspective

Angela Sattler

Abstract Ventana has risen to its current position in the industry by offering some of the most integrated automation solutions. We have invited Ventana to offer perspectives and insights on the role of automation in immunohistochemistry. Ventana experts answer questions regarding the types of technology available and how these technologies address challenges in automating the staining process. They also discuss the process of transferring assays from manual to automated techniques, the role of automation in quality control, connectivity with computer infrastructures, image analysis, the function of automated retrieval methods, and the changing portfolio of antibodies for testing and the new role of multicolor staining protocols.

Keywords Ventana • Automation • Capillary gap • Quality • Connectivity • Multiplex assay • Retrieval • Image analysis

FREQUENTLY ASKED QUESTIONS

5.1 What Is the State of Immunohistochemistry? How Far Have We Come?

The question of whether immunohistochemistry (IHC) is a volume production tool invaluable to modern pathology or just an esoteric technique suited only to obtaining supporting diagnostic information has certainly moved toward the former opinion in recent years. Original methods, using directly labeled fluorescent antibodies, provided limited information to the general pathology world. From there, indirect techniques and their utilization of enzyme labels, followed by the

A. Sattler (✉)
Ventana Medical System, Inc., 1910 E. Innovation Park Dr., Tucson, AZ 85755, USA
e-mail: angi.sattler@ventana.roche.com

F. Lin and J. Prichard (eds.), *Handbook of Practical Immunohistochemistry: Frequently Asked Questions*, DOI 10.1007/978-1-4419-8062-5_5, © Springer Science+Business Media, LLC 2011

various avidin biotin systems, were developed. Now, the widespread use of polymer and other nonavidin biotin detection systems has elevated the role of IHC to one of a central diagnostic tool in most fields of histopathology.

IHC was originally developed using manual techniques requiring extensive input from skilled personnel. Automation was seen as a way of improving throughput without requiring legions of technicians to cope with huge numbers of tests. Once a laboratory is performing a hundred or so tests a day, reproducibility and quality can suffer due to the increased pressure on the technician to ensure that they can stain each slide correctly, every time, to the highest level. One of the key demands on any system designed to provide large volumes of specific types of information is reproducibility. It is of no use being able to demonstrate a diagnostically valuable cellular component, present only in minute concentrations, if you can only do this on a Thursday when technician X is at work. There are also other requirements of any IHC service that favor some form of automation. These include:

1. Increased output to cope with demand
2. Improvement in reproducibility and therefore quality
3. Reduction in costs – both labor and consumables can be affected
4. Increased standardization allowing better interlaboratory comparisons

One of the potential negative consequences of increased automation is the perceived "dumbing-down" of what is an intricate series of chemical and biological reactions. One perception could be that technicians are merely becoming "button pushers," in reality this is not the case. Automated IHC provides both pathologists and technicians with a tool which can free up their time to be productive in other areas of the laboratory; work up new antibodies which require manual first steps, or develop new services which the laboratory can then offer to their customers.

5.2 What Types of Technology Are Being Used to Automate Immunohistochemistry?

There are three main types of technology currently used in most automated IHC instrumentation:

Capillary Gap Technology – Instruments utilizing this type of technology use variations of a common theme that being the production of a narrow gap between two surfaces which then draws fluid into that space by capillary action.

Liquid Overlay Technology – This places a layer of inert fluid over the whole slide. Reagents, including pretreatments, antibodies, and detection reagents can be overlaid with, or introduced into, this fluid where they are mixed thoroughly, allowing elevated temperatures to quickly equilibrate throughout the reagents without any potential harm from drying out.

Open System Technology – These instruments often closely mimic manual techniques. Slides are held in a rack, often horizontally, and reagents are applied by a dispensing mechanism in a similar way to a manual application via a pipette. In many cases, open systems can be quickly established using the same reagents and protocols utilized in manual procedures. In some cases, "open" systems are used to develop a particular procedure which is then moved over to a more "hands off" or closed type of instrumentation. One of the main advantages of an open system is that the user-defined reagents can be used rather than having to rely on the manufacturer's recommendations.

5.3 How Is the Space Between Slides Maintained as It Is So Small in Capillary Gap Systems?

Two slides (or one slide and a reuseable cover plate) can be placed face to face with each other, test sections on the inside, held apart by the thickness of painted surfaces at the top and bottom corners of the slide. When placed in a solution the gap allows solutions to be drawn up into the gap covering the sections, typically 150–200 μl. Fluid is drawn out of the gap by blotting, and rinsing can take place by flowing fluid through the gap during this blotting procedure.

5.4 Do All Capillary Gap Systems Work in the Same Way as I Do Not Want to Have to Use "Special Slides"?

Another version of the system has test slides placed horizontally as in conventional manual staining. The slide is overlaid by a replaceable cover slide which can be moved back and forth by the instrument. The cover slide can be retracted for the application of reagent and then moved back into place to produce a pseudo-capillary gap. Fluid contained therein spreads to cover the entire area. Again, volumes of 150–200 μl are typical.

5.5 Why Is It a Problem If Slides Dry Out?

One way to increase throughput or decrease processing time for an IHC test is to increase the temperature of the system. The inherent danger of elevated temperatures is that the sections are prone to drying out; something to be avoided at all cost during any IHC procedure.

Slide drying can not only ruin a run, but can also preclude that slide from being restained. Background chromogen deposition often makes even a seemingly completed run unreadable. To avoid this possibility, and to keep the slide covered with fluid at all times, some systems use what is known as a liquid coverslip system. This places a layer of inert fluid over the whole slide. Reagents, including pretreatments, antibodies, and detection reagents can be overlaid with, or introduced into, this fluid where they are mixed thoroughly, allowing elevated temperatures to quickly equilibrate throughout the reagents without any potential harm from drying out.

5.6 What Are the Advantages of Having "User-Defined" Reagents?

User-defined reagents enable the user to choose exactly what type of reagent to use, at what concentration, and from which vendor. This can also be a disadvantage, especially to the smaller more inexperienced laboratory that does not have the resources (both personnel and budgetary) or desire to work up entire IHC procedures and thus would prefer essentially a "plug and play" type system.

Most new systems that are being developed are trending toward a more integrated approach. A variety of systems are now becoming incorporated onto one instrument, these include on-line deparaffinization and antigen retrieval, reagent and slide monitoring, and interfacing to a Laboratory Information System (LIS). Many of these newer innovations are important not only for inventory control and budgetary management, but also for quality control and statistical analysis of workload.

5.7 What Things Should I Consider When Transferring an Assay from Manual to Automation?

When transferring to automation from a manual assay, there are many aspects that you need to keep in mind in order to be successful. Key factors that play an important role in the automation of an assay, may seem like common sense, are often overlooked.

Concentration of the antibody, diluents, and incubation times are some of the biggest factors that should be considered. Time can increase or decrease depending upon the platform that you are moving to and how your manual incubations were performed. You will find that the dilution will change dramatically once the assay is automated. Initially, a higher concentration of the antibody may be needed to allow for adequate signal intensity. Subsequently, you may be able to further dilute the antibody depending on the platform's features and your ability to adapt incubation times to meet your workflow.

Specific automation effects and their features will play an important part in transferring your assay. On-board heating, humidity control, mixing/agitation, and slide volumes all play an important role during automation and many times are not considered to be as significant as they are. The kinetics of the platform are key to shortening assay times and increasing turn around. Conversely, the very attributes that make automation desirable can produce unexpected results if you attempt to transfer your assay directly from the manual protocol steps. An example of this is automating an antibody that is directed against estrogen receptor (ER). Automation allows you to increase the temperature of the reaction and thus shorten run time. However, this can produce an overly intense result if the manual times and steps are directly applied.

5.8 How Do These Integrated Instruments Help Maintain or Improve Quality and Productivity?

On-Line Procedures – By removing the need for user involvement, reproducibility and hence quality should increase. There are inevitable variations in technique of any laboratory staff and IHC has always been sensitive to minute alterations in time, concentration of reagents, pH, etc. The use of on-line procedures removes this variability as the instrument should do the same thing every single time. Obviously, careful preventive maintenance is called for to ensure that any instrument is performing up to manufacturer's specifications.

The main aim of introducing any automated operation is standardization; being able to produce the same result consistently, regardless of who is performing the test. This is a must for any laboratory that wishes to produce quality work which will have a positive outcome on patient care.

5.9 How Can an Automated System Help When Things Go Wrong?

Reagent and Slide Management – It is important to know what reagents were used in which particular procedure because if a stain fails, the whole procedure can be reexamined. This provides the user with the ability to ensure that the correct reagents were used, that lot numbers were not mixed up, and that expiry dates were not passed. The ability to know exactly which position on a machine a particular slide was run can help pinpoint peculiar machine errors, for example, inappropriate volume dispenses, heating errors, etc.

Inventory control is very important, especially for the larger laboratory. On-line reagent management takes away some of the need to manually check reagent stocks. Re-order levels can be assigned and when a reagent nears that level an automatic notification to re-order is generated. Some facilities will be able to interface this to their ordering system to enable automated orders to be placed. Security is built into the system to ensure that only authorized orders are placed.

The demand for this type of application has led several instrument manufacturers to develop extensive yet user friendly systems to enable accurate monitoring of all reagents and slides used for each test in a run.

5.10 Many Hospitals Have Extensive IT Infrastructures; Can Automated IHC Be Accommodated and Integrated Within Those Organizations?

LIS Interface – As workload increases the need to maximize the amount of technician output has also increased. This places demands on the efficiency of any system. The ability to enter data into a laboratory LIS once and have that data automatically be interpreted by any instrument can improve this efficiency by avoiding duplication of tasks. Most, if not all, instruments being used or developed today are designed to have multiple interfaces which can be readily connected to a facility's existing IT system

The traditional model has the case or specimen entered into an accessioning system which captures patient demographics, billing information, and tests ordered. A technician then interprets the request and performs the tests, either entering them on to some form of work sheet or programming those tests into an automated instrument.

By interfacing automated IHC instruments to an LIS all the test data can be immediately accessed by that instrument once entered thus avoiding the duplication of data entry and its attendant human error of entering incorrect tests. It also frees up some time for technicians to perform other associated tasks such as preparing machines for that day's runs. There are quality issues and business rules to be taken into consideration, there must be appropriate quality checks that the correct tests have been entered before an instrument run is started.

5.11 How Is the Portfolio of Antibodies Available for Testing Changing?

Antibody Developments – When IHC first started it was always reassuring to see the color development at the end of the procedure. From there the reliability of IHC increased and procedures became more robust and achieved sufficient sensitivity to identify very low levels of target antigen within tissue even if that tissue was not optimally fixed and processed. The notion of an IHC stain not working was less of an issue.

The idea of being able to perform two antibodies on one slide to test for two different components was mooted by several workers. As technology improved, what once a novel research was only tool moved into the mainstream. Several combinations of antibody and chromogen are being used in conjunction to provide valuable diagnostic information. Today, not only are double stains being offered by large reference laboratories but also triple and quadruple stains. Many of these use straightforward procedures which can be readily adopted by smaller routine laboratories.

5.12 Multiple Stains on One Slide Sounds Complex and Time Consuming, I Am Not Sure Our Facility Has the Skills to Accomplish This While Maintaining Good Quality and an Adequate Turnaround Time. Can Automation Help?

Several companies have made it even easier to perform multiple staining to the point where they have become routine. Many of these multiple stain procedures employ a cocktail of primary antibodies, each component of which is raised in a different species thus avoiding cross reactions. Cocktails of secondary antibodies and chromogens of different color provide excellent definition of each tissue element under investigation. A novel example of the way multiple stains are developing can be explained as follows: a stain needs to be developed to identify three separate components in a particular tissue, one of these components is cytoplasmic and two are nuclear. Two solutions for specific identification arise:

1. Use three different color chromogens to identify each component.
2. Use two different color chromogens, one to identify one of the nuclear and one of the cytoplasmic components and another to identify the other nuclear marker. There can be no confusion as long as there is no co-expression (and even this can be sorted by modern image analysis).

The procedure can be kept to a manageable length of time due to only using essentially two procedures rather than three.

5.13 What Are the Next Steps with These Multiplex Assays?

This type of thinking does take something of a mind shift away from the traditional approach of each marker being specifically identified by individual colors to that of identifying by location essentially regardless of color. This approach also offers the opportunity of using three or four colors to potentially identify five, six, or more markers in one slide. When combined with tissue microarrays we have the capability to produce an enormous amount of information on one slide instead of having to rely on a whole battery of tests and a multitude of slides. This not only saves technician time but also, and possibly of more value, pathologists time in having to scan a tray full of slides as opposed to one or two.

The following examples highlight the usefulness of multiple stains

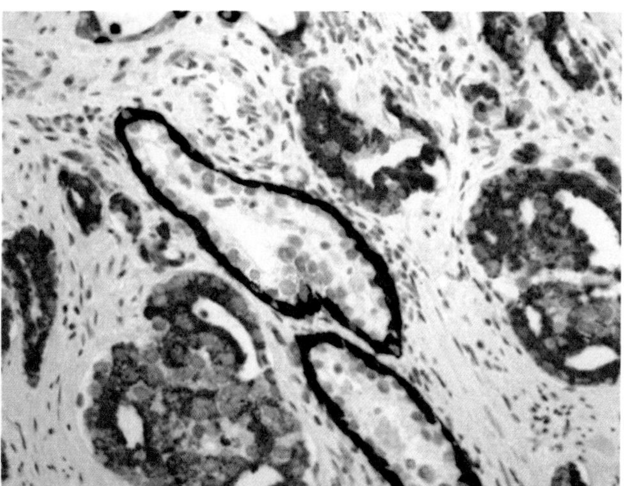

Fig. 5.1 Dual color stain of prostate cancer. Red chromogen labels cytoplasmic P504s in cancer glands lacking in benign central glands. Brown DAB chromogen highlights the basal layer of the central benign glands with nuclear p63 and cytoplasmic high molecular weight cytokeratin lacking in the surrounding cancer glands

5.14 What Is PIN 4 Cocktail (P504s, p63, and HMW-CK)?

Expression of P504s protein is found in prostatic adenocarcinoma, but not in benign prostatic tissue. It has also been found to stain premalignant high-grade prostatic intraepithelial neoplasia (PIN) and atypical adenomatous hyperplasia. In combination with antibodies to p63 and high molecular weight cytokeratin (HMW-CK), a very useful cocktail is available for diagnosing PIN (see Fig. 5.1). Anti-P504s stains cytoplasm in prostate adenocarcinoma and atypical hyperplasia and the anti-p63 and anti-HMW-CK stain normal and benign prostate glands respectively. By using a DAB chromogen for p63 and HMW-CK antibodies strong basal staining is produced highlighting glandular structures. Anti-P504s is labeled with red chromogen and any malignancy is immediately highlighted due to the contrast between the brown and red chromogens.

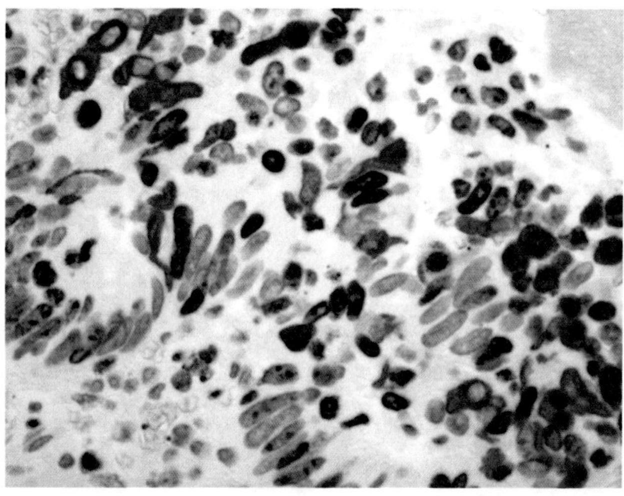

Fig. 5.2 Dual color stain of in situ and invasive breast cancer. Anti-CK 8/18 (red cytoplasmic staining) labels all ductal or lobular epithelial cells. Anti-CK 5/6 (cytoplasmic brown staining) and anti-p63 (nuclear brown staining) identify myoepithelial cells surrounding the duct carcinoma in situ (*lower left*). The invasive tumor glands (*upper right*) lack myoepithelial staining

5.15 What Is Breast Microinvasion Cocktail (Cytokeratin 5/6 + p63 + Cytokeratin 8/18)?

Antibodies to CK 5/6 + p63 + CK 8/18 have been combined to form a Microinvasion cocktail (see Fig. 5.2). This set of markers can be extremely useful for distinguishing ductal carcinoma in situ from microinvasive breast carcinoma. This cocktail is also excellent at deciphering other diagnostic challenges, for example, radial scar and infiltrating carcinoma. Anti-CK 5/6 (cytoplasmic brown staining) and anti-p63 (nuclear brown staining) combine to produce intense staining of myoepithelial cells. Anti-CK 8/18 (red cytoplasmic staining) labels all ductal or lobular epithelia. CK 8/18 has been shown to be useful for identifying adenocarcinoma. Therefore, the combination of these three markers should distinguish invasive from noninvasive breast lesions with the presence or absence of myoepithelium (CK 5/6 and/or p63 brown) and glandular staining of breast carcinoma with CK 8/18 (red).

5.16 What Is M30 (Apoptotic CK 18) and Ki 67 Cocktail?

M30 antibody recognizes a neo-epitope formed early in the apoptotic cascade by caspase cleavage of cytokeratin 18. Apoptosis is a process, in which cells activate an intrinsic suicide mechanism that destroys themselves. The Ki-67 nuclear antigen is associated with cell proliferation. It is found throughout the cell cycle that includes the G1, S, G2, and M phases; but not the (GO) phase. This antibody cocktail was designed to provide information on cell death (apoptosis) (CK 18 – red) versus cell proliferation (Ki 67 – brown) (see Fig. 5.3). By establishing a base line of the amount of cells undergoing proliferation against those undergoing apoptosis, a true measure of actual tumor growth or decay can be ascertained.

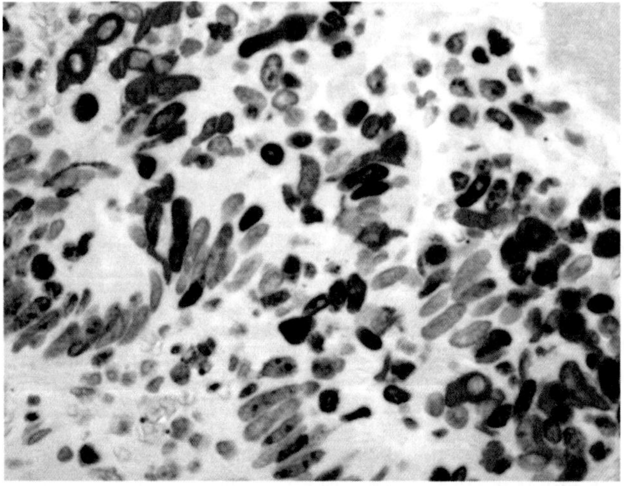

Fig. 5.3 This antibody cocktail was designed to provide information on cell death (apoptotic CK 18 – *red*) versus cell proliferation (Ki 67 – *brown*)

5.17 As Stains Become More Complex How Do We Manage to Extract All the Information They Provide?

Image Analysis – Over the years many attempts have been made to overcome the subjectivity of the human eye in the analysis of histological preparations, no more so than in IHC and specifically with breast markers. A "new breed" of imaging and image analysis equipment has been developed in recent years and is widely used across the world. The approach was to move away from the traditional "total solution in one box." A more open system was developed utilizing a specifically designed image capture instrument allied to highly intuitive and customizable analysis software. This system allows objective algorithms to be developed to analyze any particular stain of interest. The system is actually taught what tumor cells look like and the algorithms are designed to only analyze those cells. In older instruments, a simple colorimetric analysis was made between blue and brown staining relying on user expertise to determine if the cells were of tumor origin or not. With the new system, all the imaging is done in house and is then transmitted over high speed internet lines to the client facility where they can perform their own analysis, using supplied software. Images and analyses can be produced in the host laboratory and be made available to their clients almost immediately after the stains are completed, over the high speed lines. Security and access are obviously closely scrutinized to ensure patient privacy at all times.

This so-called "Virtual Image" technology expands the possibilities of the use of IHC. Not only can the system be used as an analysis tool but also as an educational and teaching aid. Real-time telepathology is eminently simple with a system of this design and anyone wishing to partake of the service gets the benefit of expert pathology opinions from the host laboratory that they may not have in their own facility. Images can be viewed by multiple users and manipulated to examine a test result just as if you were looking down a multiheaded microscope. Conference telephone calls can be established and peer review of cases becomes a simple task

The future for IHC is looking ever more promising; automation and virtual technology are taking us to previously unthought of solutions to technical and diagnostic challenges. It will be interesting, perhaps, to look back in 10 years at the technology available today and wonder how we coped with such archaic and outdated designs. After all what do the designers of the Space Shuttle think of Wilbur and Orville Wright's Flyer? Where we go is only limited by our own abilities. Let us embrace the new technology and take our whole science to new heights.

5.18 What Are the Benefits of Automated Immunohistochemistry in a Small-Sized Pathology Laboratory?

Automation in small-sized pathology laboratories has flourished in recent times due to the chronic shortage of histotechnologists, increased financial benefits, and readily available, state-of-the-art technology. Small laboratories have proven that automating immunohistochemistry can improve not only the bottom line, but also the quality, patient safety, and workflow.

Even in small laboratories, the cost of histotechs can be put to better use by dedicating their expertise to skilled tasks, while automated technology handles the less-skilled, routine functions. Not only is this more cost-effective, but it also allows room for growth with expanding antibody menus and improves quality and patient safety.

One must consider that people make mistakes and repetitive tasks become inconsistent. Automating immunohistochemistry removes the variables and produces consistent, reproducible results. At the same time, when fewer people handle patient tissue, the fewer number of errors will occur. Therefore, when managed correctly, automating immunohistochemistry can be extremely beneficial in a small-sized pathology laboratory.

5.19 What Are the Benefits of Automated Epitope Unmasking vs. Traditional Methods?

Epitope unmasking is the science of using a buffered solution with a specific pH combined with heat to undo the effects of a cross-linking fixative on an antigen of interest. Epitope unmasking is critical to providing the sensitivity and specificity required of many diagnostically valuable antibodies.

Traditionally, manual methods of epitope unmasking utilized pressure cookers, steamers, and microwave ovens to heat slides immersed in buffer to perform the unmasking. These procedures are fundamentally unreliable because it is extremely difficult to regulate the local temperature of a single slide for a desired length of time. Variations in local temperature and "hot spots" make this technique challenging to consistently reproduce manually.

Automated epitope unmasking methods use a combination of volumetrically delivered buffers, mixing, and precise heat control to very reliably manage the precision and duration of the reaction. Independent slide heating also allows for a slide having epitope unmasking performed at 95°C or to be sitting directly next to a slide that does not need unmasking and is being incubated at a 37°C. This protocol flexibility provides the increased efficiency which is required in today's anatomic pathology laboratory.

Chapter 6
Tissue Microarray

Myra Wilkerson and Erin Powell

Abstract Tissue microarray (TMA) is a powerful tool for performing population level studies using tissues routinely processed in surgical pathology. They are used for a variety of applications including validation of cDNA array data; validation of the sensitivity and specificity of antibodies; quality assurance in immunohistochemistry; translation of data from cell line, xenograft, and animal models to human cancer; collaborative studies, especially for aggregation and preservation of rare tumor tissues; molecular profiling of large series of tumors or diseased tissue and correlation with clinical endpoints; and evaluation of diagnostic, prognostic, and therapeutic potential of newly discovered genes and molecules. Most standard histologic and molecular techniques can be applied to TMA sections. Image analysis and data management are crucial issues, but many tools are available.

Keywords Tissue microarray • Tissue cores • Population studies • Virtual microscopy • Data exchange standards • Validation studies • Quality assurance

Abbreviations

FFPE	Formalin fixed, paraffin embedded
IHC	Immunohistochemistry
mAB	Monoclonal antibody
TMA	Tissue microarray

FREQUENTLY ASKED QUESTIONS

6.1 What Is a Tissue Microarray?

A tissue microarray (TMA) consists of up to 1,000 cores of formalin-fixed paraffin-embedded tissue obtained from donor blocks that are placed into a single recipient paraffin block.

M. Wilkerson (✉)
Department of Pathology and Laboratory Medicine, Geisinger Wyoming Valley Medical Center, PA 18711, USA
e-mail: mwilkerson@geisinger.edu

F. Lin and J. Prichard (eds.), *Handbook of Practical Immunohistochemistry: Frequently Asked Questions*,
DOI 10.1007/978-1-4419-8062-5_6, © Springer Science+Business Media, LLC 2011

This recipient block can subsequently be sectioned and the sections placed on glass slides. Depending on the length of the cores, as many as 300 slides can be produced from one array [1].

6.2 What Is the Scalability of TMAs?

TMAs are population level research tools. Each slide produced from a TMA can be used for a single experiment to probe for a DNA, RNA, or protein target on as many as 1,000 tissues at one time [1–4].

6.3 What Are the Applications of TMAs?

Validation of cDNA array data: A single cDNA array experiment can generate data about the gene expression patterns of up to 50,000 genes in a single tissue. These genes can be expressed in multiple cell types; however, most molecular methods have a common problem, that the tissues must be disintegrated prior to testing. TMA experiments can identify the specific cellular type and compartmental localization of the gene products of interest. This is particularly helpful as candidate genes may be expressed in many tissue types other than diseased tissue, so validating protein expression of potential markers using TMA experiments as a screening tool eliminates the time and labor associated with using full tissue sections [1, 3, 5–7].

Validation of the sensitivity and specificity of a newly discovered antibody: Using TMAs containing a variety of tumors and normal tissues is a very efficient and cost-effective way to validate the sensitivity and specificity of new antibodies, as well as to optimize the appropriate staining protocol.

Utilization of TMAs with cytologic specimens: Biopsies obtained through radiologic procedures in many cases result in a very limited amount of material available for pathologic diagnosis. Often, no surgical resection specimens are taken if the initial cytology specimen is diagnostic. TMAs can be constructed from cell block material, although it may be necessary to add another one or two cores to insure adequate cellularity on array sections.

Quality assurance in immunohistochemistry (IHC): Performing IHC on TMA sections offers a way to quickly assess the performance characteristics of antibodies, including comparison of different mABs that may be directed at different epitopes of a target protein antigen; optimization of staining conditions; interlab comparison of IHC staining results; and standardization of morphologic interpretation. Using TMA sections to test new antibodies is especially useful to quickly optimize staining conditions, such as antigen retrieval, reagent concentrations or antibody titers, incubation times with primary and secondary antibodies, temperatures, and wash conditions. This eliminates the variation between batches that use full size tissue sections [1, 6, 8, 9].

Translation of data from cell line, xenograft, and animal models to human cancer: TMAs can be constructed from experimental tissues and cell lines. An array of cell lines makes it possible to screen for amplification of a gene of interest [4, 5, 10].

Collaborative studies: TMAs require little tissue from individual cases and therefore provide a means of making tissue available for study in a compact form (one slide) that is easily shared. This is a convenient way to share tissue resources in a large collaborative study such as a multicenter clinical trial, while also preserving archived tissues from rare tumors or diseases for additional future studies. This also allows multiple laboratories to standardize and optimize protocols and use of various probes, as well as to validate the data generated from multiple centers [4, 9].

Molecular profiling of large series of tumors or diseased tissue and correlation with clinical endpoints: Clinical data accompanying each core may be crucial for discovery of significant patterns or alterations in tissue when compared to profiles of nondiseased tissue. This is an important consideration when designing an array and choosing appropriate cases for inclusion. This correlation may result in more refined molecular classifications of tumors and other disease states than was possible in the past, especially if materials are drawn from, and evaluated by, multiple institutions [4, 10].

Evaluation of diagnostic, prognostic, and therapeutic potential of newly discovered genes and molecules: TMAs provide an easy and quick means to evaluate new markers and alterations or responsiveness of tissues to new candidate drugs in a large number of tissues simultaneously [4, 10].

6.4 What Are the Types of TMAs Designed?

Multitumor TMAs: These TMAs contain samples of several different tumor types in order to screen for the prevalence of a molecular alteration across many different tumor types, or to test the specificity of a new mAB [4].

Progression TMAs: These TMAs contain samples of one tumor type at different stages in order to study the changes or similarities in gene amplification or protein expression at different stages in a particular tumor type [4, 5].

Prognosis TMAs: These TMAs contain samples of tumors with associated long-term follow-up clinical data in order to identify and evaluate prognostic markers and alterations for the prediction of clinical response to therapeutic interventions such as chemotherapeutic drugs or radiation therapy [4, 5].

Normal tissue TMAs: These TMAs contain sample of normal tissues in order to evaluate the expression of candidate genes in multiple tissues for their potential as therapeutic targets [6].

Rare tumors or unusual diseases: In order to preserve as much tissue as possible for future studies of rare malignancies or diseases, TMAs provide the means to utilize a small sample that can be arrayed with tissue cores obtained from multiple institutions, preserving very limited resources.

6.5 What Types of Assays Can Be Applied to TMAs and Are There Special Considerations?

Immunohistochemistry: IHC is the technique most commonly applied to TMA sections. It is a multiparameter assay involving many variables that need to be optimized. The most important step is choosing a primary antibody that is specific for the protein of interest. Ideally, the antibody should usually only produce one detectable band on a Western blot, but often there are multiple bands. When applied to tissue, it needs to produce a staining pattern in the appropriate cellular compartment of the expected cell types. IHC in TMAs faces the same difficulties as full size tissue sections; however, TMA sections are particularly susceptible to tissue loss during deparaffinization and antigen retrieval steps. They are susceptible to edge staining effect. These can be avoided by using replicate cores placed in different locations within the array. Some laboratories also place a rim of cores around the edge of the array of other tissue types, and find that more fibrous tissue is helpful. There are two categories of proteins that are challenging for IHC, transcription factors because there are very few copies per cell that may not be visibly detectable and cytokines which may diffuse throughout the tissue and produce nonspecific staining [8, 11].

Chromogenic in situ hybridization (CISH): CISH requires intact cells to probe for the nucleic acid sequence of interest. Formalin fixation and tissue processing preserve tissue morphology, but also cause conformational changes that affect probe attachment. The chromogenic signal is usually localized to the nucleus and cytoplasm, and interpreted similarly to IHC [11, 12].

Fluorescent in situ hybridization (FISH): FISH is a method used to detect translocations, gene deletions, and gene amplifications in tumors. Formalin fixation preserves the structure of tissue by forming crosslinking methylene bridges, but this has the disadvantage of reducing the accessibility of the hybridization target. Pretreatment steps, such as use of sodium thiocyanate and pepsin digestion to unmask the target DNA, need to be optimized for each tissue type. Since multitumor TMA sections contain many different tissue types that may require different pretreatment conditions, this needs to be considered when designing the appropriate array for an experiment. For more information on problems encountered in FISH assays in TMAs and possible solutions, see [13].

Quantum dots (QDs): QDs are nanoscale semiconductor crystals with several properties that offer advantages over conventional organic and fluorescent dyes. Their broad excitation spectra and narrow emission spectra allow for simultaneous excitation and quantifiable observation of up to ten QDs in the same sample. QDs are highly resistant to photobleaching, unlike both organic and fluorescent dyes. They have been used in imaging tumor vasculature, studying apoptosis, and gene expression analysis. They have been applied to TMA sections as multiplex assays to distinguish renal carcinoma from normal tissue by detecting MDM-2 and beta-actin protein targets, as well as examining simultaneous antigen expression of EGFR, E-cadherin, and CK in xenograft lung cancer specimens [14, 15].

Multiplex immunoblotting: Proteins can be transferred from a single TMA section to a stack of up to ten replicate membranes. These membranes can be probed using conventional immunoblotting techniques, increasing the number of antibodies that can be utilized in an experiment. The advantage is that this method works with phosphor-specific antibodies, as well as many antibodies that do not work well in FFPE tissue samples [16–18].

6.6 What Instruments Are Available to Construct TMAs?

Beecher Instruments (Sun Prairie, WI) manufactures both the manual and automated tissue arrayer. Other manufacturers include Veridian (Poway, CA) and Unitma (Seoul, Korea). All work similarly and employ hollow needles with slightly different diameters – a larger bore needle to remove a core of tissue from a recipient block and a slightly smaller bore needle to remove the tissue from a donor block for insertion into the hollow cylinder created in the recipient block. Since most of the costs of constructing a TMA are associated with the time spent in the selection of tissues to be arrayed, there is little advantage in using the more expensive automated arrayer, unless the laboratory is a core facility that will be making arrays daily. The punching needles on the automated arrayers wear out more quickly. Manually producing an array is tedious, but when compared to an automated arrayer, it is easier to get all cores level, it is simpler to repair, and the cores can be punched out more precisely within a localized area. It is also not recommended to use the automated arrayer on calcified tissue or bone [5, 19].

6.7 How Is a TMA Designed?

Selecting tissue: The most important consideration is the availability of clinical data that can be compiled and associated with each sample in an array. Even though a TMA may be initially designed for a specific set of experiments, the remaining sections may be used for future experiments and the value of those sections may depend on the accompanying annotated data. Donor blocks of FFPE tissues should be selected for thickness. Ideally, the tissue should be 3–4-mm thick. The tissue should not be necrotic or contain heavily calcified or bony areas that have not been decalcified. In situ lesions or thin epithelial cancers can be difficult to obtain representative cores. It is also difficult to array certain micro-anatomical structures, such as an entire hepatic lobule or the full thickness of an epithelium [1, 5, 20, 21].

Selecting controls: The inclusion of normal tissue on all arrays is essential. If a biotinylated detection system is used, either liver or kidney should be included to demonstrate false background staining due to endogenous biotin in the tissue [21].

6.8 How Is a Paraffin-Based TMA Constructed?

1. Search databases for appropriate cases.
2. Examine H&E-stained slides to select appropriate blocks and mark areas to be sampled. Use different colors of markers on the slide to indicate different areas to be cored and arrayed, such as black for tumor, green for normal benign tissue, and blue for inflammatory changes.
3. Acquire paraffin blocks that correspond to the slides selected and marked. Examine to check for block integrity (our laboratory actually had a fungus colonize several years' worth of paraffin blocks in storage) and to see if adequate tissue remains for sampling.
4. Design the TMA block in a diagram. We designed three templates in MS Excel that show a grid with the coordinates of each core based on the core diameter to be used. The case number, paraffin block, and color of the sample area on the H&E slide for each core are indicated in individual cells on the spreadsheet. This map is crucial for the person constructing the array and for data collection after the TMA is sectioned. This also lets the array designer know how many spaces are available to be filled.
5. Prepare recipient blocks. The manual arrayer from Beecher Instruments allows four replicate blocks to be produced simultaneously. The recipient blocks should be formed from low melting point paraffin. Standard metal pans used for tissue blocking in histology can be used, although many laboratories prefer to make blocks of double thickness so that longer cores can be arrayed. A tissue cassette should be placed on one side of the block so that it can be cut in a fashion similar to routine histology blocks.
6. Set coordinates on the arrayer and remove the first core of paraffin from the recipient block.
7. Remove a core from the donor block by aligning the marked slide over the block face to find the region of interest.
8. Place the donor core into the hollow cylinder in the recipient block. If the tissue in the donor block is thin, multiple cores can be removed, the excess paraffin trimmed from the cores, and the shorter tissue cores can be stacked inside the hollow cylinder.
9. Repeat steps 6–8 until the array is completed. This process will cause the paraffin to buckle, so that occasional rows should be left empty in order to maintain alignment. Designing and building the array in sectors with empty spaces also make the location of specific cores easier when scoring staining patterns. See Fig. 6.1 [5, 6, 19, 21, 22].

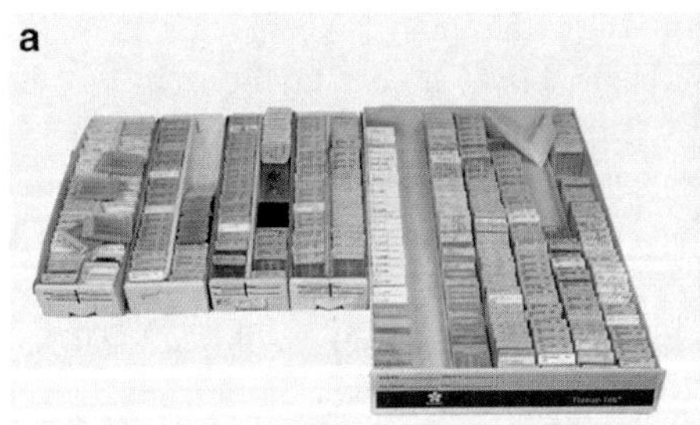

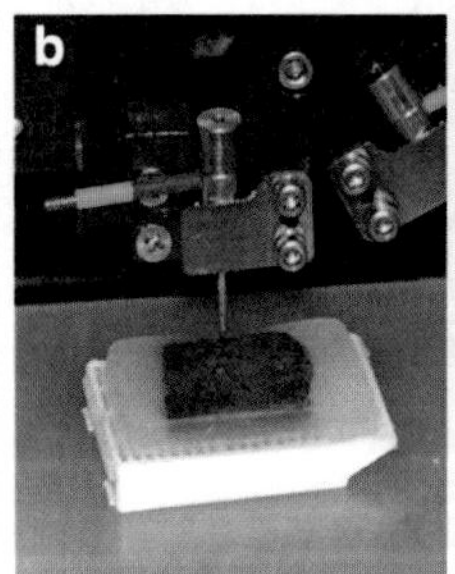

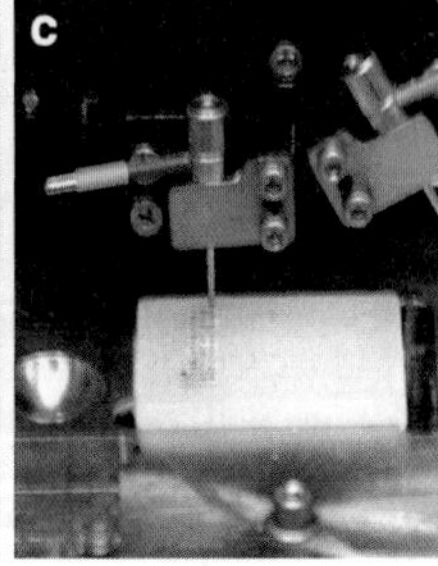

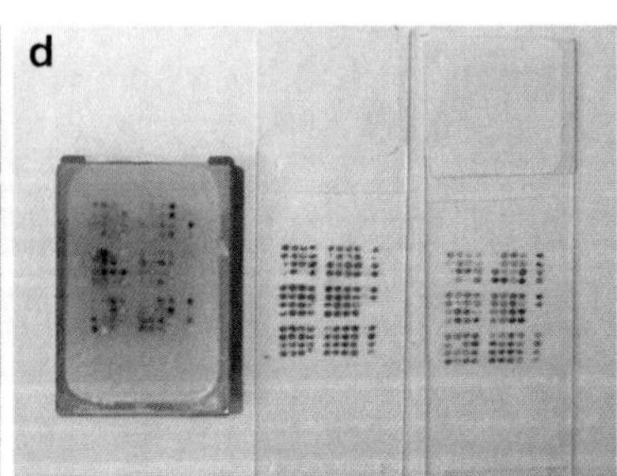

Fig. 6.1 Workflow for constructing TMAs. (**a**) The most time-consuming step in building a TMA is selecting appropriate cases and the most representative FFPE blocks containing adequate tissue from those cases for inclusion in the array. (**b**) The areas to be cored from a donor block are usually marked on an H&E stained slide that can be overlaid on the donor block, then the core of tissue in the selected area can be removed from the donor block. (**c**) The donor core is then placed into a predetermined hollow cylinder that was previously removed from the recipient block with a hollow needle that is slightly larger in diameter than the donor core. (**d**) The completed TMA should be tempered to let the donor cores anneal to the recipient block paraffin, then the TMA can be sectioned and the resulting slides stained similarly to routine histology practices

6.9 Can TMAs Be Constructed from Material Other Than Paraffin Embedded Tissue?

Frozen tissues in gel: Recipient blocks can be formed from a gel made of formalin, gelatin, sucrose, agarose, and PBS. Arrays of frozen tissue can be arrayed in this block at room temperature or at −5 to −10°C. This helps to preserve RNA and protein quality [23].

Frozen TMAs using OCT: Recipient blocks can be formed by freezing OCT. The advantage is preservation of DNA, RNA, and proteins; however, morphology may be distorted as compared to paraffin or gel arrays. Lipids will also be preserved, another advantage over FFPE tissues. Fewer cores of tissue can be arrayed due to the brittle nature of frozen OCT and the completed TMA must be stored in the frozen state. Antibodies that do not work well on formalin-fixed tissue may work better on frozen tissues. In situ hybridization assays also work well on frozen tissues [11, 12, 24–26].

Cell line microarrays: Drug development studies often require use of cell lines rather than FFPE archival tissues. Methods have been developed for cell culture lines to be fixed, paraffin embedded, and arrayed [21, 24, 27].

Xenograft tumor arrays: TMAs can be constructed using tissues from xenograft models or from transgenic or knockout mice. These TMAs provide a means for rapid assessment of gene expression and drug responsiveness [24, 28].

Cutting edge matrix assembly (CEMA): Tissues can be shaved from paraffin blocks, trimmed into rectangular primary plates, then stacked and bonded either by heat that anneals the paraffin together, or with cyanoacrylate glue that will dissolve during processing. Stacks of bonded primary plates are then transversely cut and bonded edge-to-edge, forming high-density arrays lacking an intervening matrix between the tissue samples. This has several advantages over TMAs in that up to 12,000 pieces of tissue can be arrayed in a block, and those pieces of tissue are much longer than the cores used in TMAs, so more slides can be produced from a CEMA. Because the tissue samples are bonded together and of the same length, less tissue is lost when the array is sectioned and floated on a water bath for placement on a glass slide. CEMA solves the problem of creating arrays of thin-walled structures such as blood vessels or ducts, full-thickness representation of layered epithelia, or larger micro-anatomical structures, such as hepatic lobules [29–31].

Tissue immunoblotting: TMA sections on a glass slide can be treated with enzymes and the proteins subsequently transferred to a stack of nitrocellulose membranes, producing up to ten replicate protein array membranes. These protein arrays can then be probed with antibodies for quantitative protein analysis [16, 24].

6.10 How Are Sections Cut from an Array Block?

The array block should be tempered prior to cutting. Place the block in a 37°C incubator for 10 min, then gently press the surface with a glass slide to flatten the cores. Place the block back in the incubator for 1 h, then cool on an ice block or in a −4°C freezer for 15 min and repeat incubation and cooling two more times. This helps the paraffin in the recipient block adhere to the cores so that the cores do not pop out and tissue spots are not lost during sectioning. The tissue spots on the slides will have fewer defects if this is done correctly. This is why recipient blocks should be molded from low melting point (58–65°C) paraffin [21].

Sections may be cut from the block on a microtome and floated on a water bath for placement onto a positively charged slide. Some tissue spots may be lost in this process and to prevent this, many laboratories employ a tape sectioning aid (Instrumedics Inc., Hackensack, NJ). This system includes adhesive coated slides, adhesive tape for section transfer, and a UV lamp. In our experience, a competent histotechnologist does not require such an aid. It is difficult to clear all adhesive residues from the slide and this residue may interfere with ISH, FISH, and phosphorylated antibodies in IHC. This residue can also make automated image analysis more difficult. It has also been reported that IHC using the capillary gap method will not work with the tape transfer system. In addition, the oil coverslip of some automated stainers seems to interfere with the staining process on the adhesive coated slides [5, 7, 12, 27, 32].

We recommend performing an H&E stain on the first section and every 50 sections thereafter for quality assurance. If an array has not been sectioned and stained for some time, it may also be beneficial to perform stains to check the viability of antigens. Examples would be vimentin or pancytokeratin for IHC, or a probe for housekeeping genes, such as glyceraldehyde-3-phosphate dehydrogenase, beta-actin, or histone H3 for in situ hybridization methods [21].

6.11 How Many Cores of Tissue Are Considered Representative of a Tumor?

Many studies comparing IHC findings in core samples from TMA blocks to large section histology have been conducted in several tumor types for a variety of markers. The concern is whether tumor heterogeneity can be accounted for in such small samples and what size and number of cores are optimal. The overall consensus is that three 0.6 mm diameter cores provides adequate representation and most researchers are assuming that one of the three tissue spots will be lost during transfer to a glass slide or during staining so that two cores will be available for scoring. Similarly, two 1.0 or 1.5 mm cores are also considered representative. Use of 2.0 mm cores may allow one to demonstrate larger structures, such as a hepatic lobule, but they are more difficult to array in the recipient blocks due to fractures created in the paraffin when removing cores. Taking the cores from different tissue blocks may help account for tissue heterogeneity, especially in diseases like lymphoma or when looking at markers of hypoxia. Adding more than four or five core samples does not appear to improve concordance with large sections. These studies have included prognostic markers such as estrogen and progesterone receptors and Her-2/neu, as well as proliferation markers such as Ki-67, and all have shown excellent concordance (most were between 94 and 100%) with large tissue sections. TMA cores may actually be more representative than larger sections in necrotic tumors because the best areas are sampled and much of the background staining associated with necrosis is eliminated. Some studies have also shown that fixation differences between central and peripheral regions of tumors do not impact the concordance between TMA cores and large sections. One important fact to remember is that these studies are based on the assumption that standard tissue sampling practice is actually the gold standard and representative of an entire tumor. Consider that a tumor measuring 3 × 2 × 3 cm has a volume of about 18 cm^3, one large tissue section represents about 1/7,500 of the tumor volume. A 0.6-mm core represents about 1/1,600 of the volume of a standard large tissue section, so the greater problem is not the correlation between TMA cores and large tissue sections, but between large tissue sections and large volume tumors [1, 3, 5, 7, 10, 20, 32–38].

6.12 How Do TMA IHC Results Compare to Large Tissue Slide Results in Various Tumors?

TMA IHC results have been reported in many cancers including (but not limited to) nonsmall cell lung carcinoma, breast carcinoma (both invasive and in situ), Hodgkin lymphoma, non-Hodgkin lymphoma, acute myelogenous leukemia in bone marrow trephine biopsies, endometrial carcinoma, ovarian carcinoma, kidney carcinoma, urinary bladder carcinoma, sarcomas, thyroid carcinoma, and cell blocks from effusions. All studies looked at multiple markers and concordance of phenotypic expression patterns ranged from 80 to 100%. All studies were able to reproduce known associations between phenotypic expression patterns or molecular changes and clinical endpoints. One advantage of TMA studies compared to large tissue section studies is the degree of consistency and standardization of staining on a single TMA slide vs. the corresponding large tissue sections. Scoring of large tissue sections is also more subjective as one chooses what is most representative, whereas a TMA tissue spot is usually scored in its entirety [3, 20, 33–44].

6.13 How Long Do FFPE Tissues Retain Their Antigenicity?

Tissue oxidation starts when a block is sectioned; however, some proteins will retain their antigenicity for greater than 60 years if they were originally fixed in neutral-buffered formalin. Antigens in a cytoplasmic or nuclear distribution may be less susceptible to long-term storage degradation than those with a membranous distribution [35, 45].

6.14 How Should TMA Blocks and Slides Be Stored?

There is no consensus on the best method of storage. Some laboratories section the entire TMA block all at once, whereas others cut 20 sections at a time and then coat the surface of the block with a thin layer of paraffin. Cold storage appears to slow antigen degradation, but does not stop it entirely. Some store cut slides in a refrigerator inside a sealed container with a dessicant. Other laboratories coat freshly cut slides in paraffin and may store them at room temperature, in a refrigerator (some in a nitrogen dessicator), or in a freezer; however, adequate deparaffinization prior to staining may be problematic and freezer storage may introduce ice crystal artifact [12, 35, 46].

6.15 Do Standards Exist for TMA Data Exchange?

An open source TMA data exchange specification was developed by the Association for Pathology Informatics to facilitate data sharing between laboratories that employ a variety of information systems containing source data for tissue, experimental protocols, imaging modalities, data capture, and data storage. It consists of an XML document that defines 80 common data elements and six semantic rules. The data exchange specification has been evaluated and validated with files from AIDS and Cancer Specimen Resource TMA data [47, 48].

6.16 What Features Should TMA Data Management Software Offer?

1. Registration of patients and specimens
2. Means to catalog and manage paraffin block and frozen tissue archives
3. Management of common data element sets for general and organ-specific clinical information
4. Management of common data elements for TMA construction and studies
5. De-identification of data for HIPAA compliance
6. Data mining tools
7. Web accessibility
8. Experimental results scoring, both quantitative and qualitative
9. Data exporting functions to other database and spreadsheet programs
10. Data importing functions from other database and spreadsheet programs
11. Security features including audit trails
12. Access for collaborators

6.17 What Software Is Currently Available for TMA Data Management?

Open access software: Stanford University currently offers TMAD for designing, viewing, scoring, and analyzing TMAs [49]. Another set of open source software tools for managing TMA data and images is TMAJ [8].

Commercial software: There are numerous commercial software packages available with a wide range of features. Many are associated with whole slide imaging equipment. For a partial list, please see "Resources for TMA" at the end of this chapter.

6.18 What Statistical Methods Have Been Utilized to Handle the Large Data Sets Associated with TMAs?

The statistics utilized depend on the study design and questions to be answered. The following is a brief summary of a few of the more complex mathematical models that have been employed. For open access software related to these models, please refer to the "Resources for TMA" listed at the end of this chapter.

Hierarchical clustering analysis: This technique has been applied previously to gene expression microarray studies to detect patterns of expression and can be similarly applied to TMA data. In this model, relatedness is independent of clinical or histological parameters and is therefore considered unsupervised. IHC scoring has a much more narrow range than that of cDNA array results and clustering of data may therefore be less defined in IHC. The cluster analysis process groups similar IHC profiles together into columns in a clustergram. The relationships between cases and IHC profiles can then be depicted as a dendrogram [11, 50–52].

Hierarchical naïve Bayes model: This is a population level model that takes sample heterogeneity into account where replicate measurements are available for the same sample [53].

Tissue microarray object model: This is a data model that attempts to manage different sets of clinical and histopathologic information, as well as integrate that data with other biological data such as gene expression or proteomics data [48].

Random forest clustering: Unlike other clustering models, this one does not depend on dissimilarity measures between tumor samples. It is not dependent on other covariates, but does look at relatedness between covariates. The model will also accommodate missing values [54].

6.19 What Are the Advantages and Limitations of Manual Analysis of TMA IHC Slides?

A pathologist can manually score approximately 1,000 TMA tissue spots over a 1–2-h period using a standard microscope if a single antibody marker is used, normal cells are easily distinguished from neoplastic cells, and artifacts are easily identified.

Sources of variability in TMA IHC manual analysis include:

Orientation: The greatest difficulty is keeping track of which tissue spot you are examining and scoring when the slide contains several hundred spots, making it easy to lose orientation. This is further complicated when arrays have misaligned cores, or when tissue spots are lost during transfer from the microtome to a water bath to a glass slide. It helps to have distinctly different control tissues scattered throughout the array.

Classification protocol: A well-defined system of classifiers will help reduce interobserver variability. It should address attributes of both the tumor and the antibody used such as expected staining patterns and grading of staining intensity.

Sequence of review: Most pathologists can easily recognize cores taken from the same tumor. Scattering cores from the same tumor into different sectors in the same array may help to insure that each core is scored independently, especially with regard to staining intensity.

Workload: Prolonged visual study results in eye fatigue and it becomes more difficult to reliably distinguish color changes.

Quantitative vs. qualitative scoring: The number and complexity of categories used for scoring affects inter- and intra-observer agreement. Qualitative scoring (present vs. absent, or + vs. −) is simple but does not indicate intensity. Quantitative scoring is usually a numeric scale (e.g., 0, 1, 2, 3, 4) that accounts for staining intensity, but the intermediate categories tend to be overused because the human eye cannot always reliably discriminate between subtle differences in staining color or intensity. When scoring tissue samples, we recommend the following parameters be used for consistency and ease of comparison between studies or institutions:

Indicate a semiquantitative scale for staining:

Negative = no staining

1+ = <25% of appropriate cells stain

2+ = 26–50% of appropriate cells stain

3+ = 51–75% of appropriate cells stain

4+ = >75% of appropriate cells stain

Indicate intensity of staining:

Strong, intermediate, or weakIndicate compartmental localization:

Nuclear, cytoplasmic, membranous, or combinations*Illumination*: The typical light bulbs used in microscopes usually have a yellow tint that may influence the perception of staining intensity. The contrast introduced by filters and condenser settings will also influence the amount of light transmitted and can change the observer's perceptions.

Human vision: Vision is highly variable and every person views objects and colors slightly differently. Vision is very subjective and IHC observations will be affected by the amount of tumor present, background staining, and stromal staining. Contrast, or the average brightness of the tissue vs. the background brightness, is especially important when assessing membranous staining patterns. If no cytoplasmic staining is present, membranous staining is perceived as more intense than if cytoplasmic staining were present. This effect is called conditional contrast [5, 8, 54, 55].

6.20 What Are the Advantages and Limitations of Automated Analysis (Virtual Microscopy) of TMA IHC Slides?

Virtual microscopy via a slide scanner helps overcome some of the limitations of human vision as subtle differences in staining intensity and color can be detected and scored on a continuous scale with highly reproducible results. Slide scanners are not subject to eye fatigue and illumination is standardized. However, virtual microscopes and their associated software programs have difficulty accounting for daily variability in slide staining and other artifacts such as edge effect in IHC and tissue folds that pathologists recognize easily.

Several types of scanners are available. There are three basic types: field of view devices that capture a digital image of a field and use software to stitch the images together; linear array devices that scan a slide in strips that are stitched together by software; and area array scanners that have several fiber optic cameras to take an image of a slide simultaneously and the software stitches the images together. The area array scanners are the fastest (about 1 min/slide) but they are much more expensive. Important features to look for in a scanner include scanning time, image resolution, *z*-stacking capability of the software (equivalent to focusing up and down on a microscope), file formats (many are proprietary) and types of compression for images, and usability of software for slide viewing. Commercially available scanners offer brightfield microscopy, but some are starting to offer fluorescence capabilities. For a list of vendors, please see "Resources for TMA" section at the end of this chapter.

Another limitation of automated systems is image storage requirements. The image size depends on the scanning resolution and area scanned in two dimensions. Images for research will probably need to be maintained for several years and should have a backup system. Indexing of images for easy retrieval is essential [8].

6.21 Resources for TMA

Tissue arrayer instrument vendors:

http://www.beecherinstruments.com

http://www.veridiamTissueArrayer.com

http://www.unitma.com

TMA supplies (manual punches and molds):

http://www.ihcworld.com/tissuearray.htm*Open source software TMA tools:*

http://tma.stanford.edu

http://bioinformatics.mdanderson.org/tad.html

http://tmaj.pathology.jhmi.edu/

Commercial software TMA tools:

http://www.premierbiosoft.com/tissue-microarray/index.html

http://www.slidepath.com/

http://www.alphelys.com/site/us/pIMG_Spotbrowser3.htm

http://www.definiens.com/

Slide scanners with TMA management software:

http://www.aperio.com

http://sales.hamamatsu.com

http://www.bioimagene.com

http://www.3dhistech.com/

http://www.dakousa.com/prod_productrelatedinformation?url=acis_iii_-_index.htm

http://www.historx.com/launch/technology/software_instrumentation.html

http://www.genetix.com/en/systems/ariol/introduction/index.html

Other slide scanners:

http://www.demetrix.net

http://www.olympusamerica.com/seg_section/seg_vm.asp

http://www.bioptonics.com/Home.htm

Open source statistical software:

http://www.r-project.org/

http://www.genetics.ucla.edu/labs/horvath/kidneypaper/RCC.htm

http://rana.lbl.gov/EisenSoftware.htm

Tape section transfer system:

http://www.Instrumedics.com

References

1. Kallioniemi OP, Wagner U, Kononen J, Sauter G. Tissue microarray technology for high-throughput molecular profiling of cancer. Hum Mol Genet. 2001;10(7):657–62.
2. Nocito A, Kononen J, Kallioniemi OP, Sauter G. Tissue microarrays (TMAs) for high-throughput molecular pathology research. Int J Cancer. 2001;94(1):1–5.
3. Torhorst J, Bucher C, Kononen J, et al. Tissue microarrays for rapid linking of molecular changes to clinical endpoints. Am J Pathol. 2001;159(6):2249–56.
4. Bubendorf L. High-throughput microarray technologies: from genomics to clinics. Eur Urol. 2001;40(2):231–8.
5. Simon R, Mirlacher M, Sauter G. Tissue microarrays in cancer diagnosis. Expert Rev Mol Diagn. 2003;3(4):421–30.
6. Simon R, Sauter G. Tissue microarrays for miniaturized high-throughput molecular profiling of tumors. Exp Hematol. 2002;30(12):1365–72.
7. Skacel M, Skilton B, Pettay JD, Tubbs RR. Tissue microarrays: a powerful tool for high-throughput analysis of clinical specimens: a review of the method with validation data. Appl Immunohistochem Mol Morphol. 2002;10(1):1–6 [see comment].
8. Conway C, Dobson L, O'Grady A, Kay E, Costello S, O'Shea D. Virtual microscopy as an enabler of automated/quantitative assessment of protein expression in TMAs. Histochem Cell Biol. 2008;130(3):447–63.
9. Moch H, Kononen T, Kallioniemi OP, Sauter G. Tissue microarrays: what will they bring to molecular and anatomic pathology? Adv Anat Pathol. 2001;8(1):14–20.
10. Al Kuraya K, Simon R, Sauter G. Tissue microarrays for high-throughput molecular pathology. Ann Saudi Med. 2004;24(3):169–74.
11. Hewitt SM. The application of tissue microarrays in the validation of microarray results. Methods Enzymol. 2006;410:400–15.
12. Watanabe A, Cornelison R, Hostetter G. Tissue microarrays: applications in genomic research. Expert Rev Mol Diagn. 2005;5(2):171–81.
13. Brown LA, Huntsman D. Fluorescent in situ hybridization on tissue microarrays: challenges and solutions. J Mol Histol. 2007;38(2):151–7.
14. Caldwell ML, Moffitt RA, Liu J, Parry RM, Sharma Y, Wang MD. Simple quantification of multiplexed quantum dot staining in clinical tissue samples. Conf Proc IEEE Eng Med Biol Soc. 2008;2008:1907–10.
15. Ghazani AA, Lee JA, Klostranec J, et al. High throughput quantification of protein expression of cancer antigens in tissue microarray using quantum dot nanocrystals. Nano Lett. 2006;6(12):2881–6.
16. Takikita M, Chung JY, Hewitt SM. Tissue microarrays enabling high-throughput molecular pathology. Curr Opin Biotechnol. 2007;18(4):318–25.
17. Chung JY, Braunschweig T, Baibakov G, et al. Transfer and multiplex immunoblotting of a paraffin embedded tissue. Proteomics. 2006;6(3):767–74.
18. Chung JY, Braunschweig T, Tuttle K, Hewitt SM. Tissue microarrays as a platform for proteomic investigation. J Mol Histol. 2007;38(2):123–8.
19. Schweizer MS, Schumacher L, Rubin MA. Constructing tissue microarrays for research use. Curr Protoc Hum Genet. 2004. Chapter 10:Unit 10.7.
20. Zimpfer A, Schonberg S, Lugli A, et al. Construction and validation of a bone marrow tissue microarray. J Clin Pathol. 2007;60(1):57–61.
21. Hewitt SM. Design, construction, and use of tissue microarrays. Methods Mol Biol. 2004;264:61–72.
22. Kramer MW, Merseburger AS, Hennenlotter J, Kuczyk M. Tissue microarrays in clinical urology – technical considerations. Scand J Urol Nephrol. 2007;41(6):478–84.
23. Zhou L, Hodeib M, Abad JD, Mendoza L, Kore AR, Hu Z. New tissue microarray technology for analyses of gene expression in frozen pathological samples. BioTechniques. 2007;43(1):101–5.
24. Avninder S, Ylaya K, Hewitt SM. Tissue microarray: a simple technology that has revolutionized research in pathology. J Postgrad Med. 2008;54(2):158–62.
25. Schoenberg Fejzo M, Slamon DJ. Frozen tumor tissue microarray technology for analysis of tumor RNA, DNA, and proteins. Am J Pathol. 2001;159(5):1645–50.
26. Hoos A, Cordon-Cardo C. Tissue microarray profiling of cancer specimens and cell lines: opportunities and limitations. Lab Invest. 2001;81(10):1331–8.
27. Fedor HL, De Marzo AM. Practical methods for tissue microarray construction. Methods Mol Med. 2005;103:89–101.
28. Henshall S. Tissue microarrays. J Mammary Gland Biol Neoplasia. 2003;8(3):347–58.
29. Cutting edge matrix assembly: a new high density tissue microarray technology. Cancer Biol Ther. 2005;4(8):ii.
30. Rimm DL. Tissue microarrays without cores. Nat Methods. 2005;2(7):492–3. doi:10.1038/nmeth0705-492.
31. Rui H, LeBaron MJ. Creating tissue microarrays by cutting-edge matrix assembly. Expert Rev Med Devices. 2005;2(6):673–80.
32. Packeisen J, Korsching E, Herbst H, Boecker W, Buerger H. Demystified...tissue microarray technology. Mol Pathol. 2003;56(4):198–204.
33. de Jong D, Xie W, Rosenwald A, et al. Immunohistochemical prognostic markers in diffuse large B-cell lymphoma: validation of tissue microarray as a prerequisite for broad clinical applications (a study from the Lunenburg Lymphoma Biomarker Consortium). J Clin Pathol. 2009;62(2):128–38.
34. Fons G, Hasibuan SM, van der Velden J, ten Kate FJ. Validation of tissue microarray technology in endometrioid cancer of the endometrium. J Clin Pathol. 2007;60(5):500–3.
35. Camp RL, Neumeister V, Rimm DL. A decade of tissue microarrays: progress in the discovery and validation of cancer biomarkers. J Clin Oncol. 2008;26(34):5630–7.
36. Warnberg F, Amini RM, Goldman M, Jirstrom K. Quality aspects of the tissue microarray technique in a population-based cohort with ductal carcinoma in situ of the breast. Histopathology. 2008;53(6):642–9.

37. Kyndi M, Sorensen FB, Knudsen H, et al. Tissue microarrays compared with whole sections and biochemical analyses. A subgroup analysis of DBCG 82 b&c. Acta Oncol. 2008;47(4):591–9.
38. Hecht JL, Kotsopoulos J, Gates MA, Hankinson SE, Tworoger SS. Validation of tissue microarray technology in ovarian cancer: results from the Nurses' Health Study. Cancer Epidemiol Biomarkers Prev. 2008;17(11):3043–50.
39. Linderoth J, Ehinger M, Akerman M, et al. Tissue microarray is inappropriate for analysis of BCL6 expression in diffuse large B-cell lymphoma. Eur J Haematol. 2007;79(2):146–9.
40. Schmidt LH, Biesterfeld S, Kummel A, et al. Tissue microarrays are reliable tools for the clinicopathological characterization of lung cancer tissue. Anticancer Res. 2009;29(1):201–9.
41. Henriksen KL, Rasmussen BB, Lykkesfeldt AE, Moller S, Ejlertsen B, Mouridsen HT. Semi-quantitative scoring of potentially predictive markers for endocrine treatment of breast cancer: a comparison between whole sections and tissue microarrays. J Clin Pathol. 2007;60(4):397–404.
42. Pu RT, Giordano TJ, Michael CW. Utility of cytology microarray constructed from effusion cell blocks for immunomarker validation. Cancer. 2008;114(5):300–6.
43. Simon R, Mirlacher M, Sauter G. Tissue microarrays. BioTechniques. 2004;36(1):98–105.
44. Tzankov A, Went P, Zimpfer A, Dirnhofer S. Tissue microarray technology: principles, pitfalls and perspectives–lessons learned from hematological malignancies. Exp Gerontol. 2005;40(8–9):737–44.
45. Eguiluz C, Viguera E, Millan L, Perez J. Multitissue array review: a chronological description of tissue array techniques, applications and procedures. Pathol Res Pract. 2006;202(8):561–8.
46. Fergenbaum JH, Garcia-Closas M, Hewitt SM, Lissowska J, Sakoda LC, Sherman ME. Loss of antigenicity in stored sections of breast cancer tissue microarrays. Cancer Epidemiol Biomarkers Prev. 2004;13(4):667–72.
47. Berman JJ, Edgerton ME, Friedman BA. The tissue microarray data exchange specification: a community-based, open source tool for sharing tissue microarray data. BMC Med Inform Decis Mak. 2003;3:5.
48. Lee HW, Park YR, Sim J, Park RW, Kim WH, Kim JH. The tissue microarray object model: a data model for storage, analysis, and exchange of tissue microarray experimental data. Arch Pathol Lab Med. 2006;130(7):1004–13.
49. Marinelli RJ, Montgomery K, Liu CL, et al. The Stanford tissue microarray database. Nucleic Acids Res. 2008;36(Database issue):871–7.
50. Au NH, Cheang M, Huntsman DG, et al. Evaluation of immunohistochemical markers in non-small cell lung cancer by unsupervised hierarchical clustering analysis: a tissue microarray study of 284 cases and 18 markers. J Pathol. 2004;204(1):101–9.
51. Hsu FD, Nielsen TO, Alkushi A, et al. Tissue microarrays are an effective quality assurance tool for diagnostic immunohistochemistry. Mod Pathol. 2002;15(12):1374–80.
52. Makretsov NA, Huntsman DG, Nielsen TO, et al. Hierarchical clustering analysis of tissue microarray immunostaining data identifies prognostically significant groups of breast carcinoma. Clin Cancer Res. 2004;10(18 Pt 1):6143–51.
53. Demichelis F, Magni P, Piergiorgi P, Rubin MA, Bellazzi R. A hierarchical Naive Bayes Model for handling sample heterogeneity in classification problems: an application to tissue microarrays. BMC Bioinform. 2006;7:514.
54. Breiman L. Random forests. Mach Learn. 2001;45:5–32.
55. Conway CM, O'Shea D, O'Brien S, et al. The development and validation of the virtual tissue matrix, a software application that facilitates the review of tissue microarrays on line. BMC Bioinform. 2006;7:256.
56. Simon R, Sauter G. Tissue microarray (TMA) applications: implications for molecular medicine. Expert Rev Mol Med. 2003;5(26): 1–12.

Chapter 7
Unknown Primary/Undifferentiated Neosplasms in Surgical and Cytologic Specimens

Fan Lin and Haiyan Liu

Abstract This chapter provides a practical overview of frequently used markers in the diagnosis and differential diagnosis of both common and rare metastatic tumors and undifferentiated neoplasms with a specific focus on epithelial/epithelioid neoplasms and their mimickers. The chapter contains 89 questions; each question is addressed with a table, a concise note, and representative pictures if applicable. In addition to the literature review, the authors have included their own experience and tested numerous antibodies reported in the literature for a wide range of entities from various organs on both TMA sections and routine sections. The most effective differential diagnostic panels of antibodies have been recommended for many entities, such as TTF1, MOC-31, CEA, calretinin, WT1, and CK5/6 being suggested as the best diagnostic panel for the distinction of pulmonary adenocarcinoma from mesothelioma. In addition, frequently asked questions on differential diagnosis of fine needle aspiration biopsy specimens have been included. Application and potential pitfalls of some important markers have been emphasized.

Keywords Unknown primary • Undifferentiated neoplasm • Carcinoma • Sarcoma • Melanoma • Germ cell tumor • Lymphoma • Mesothelioma

FREQUENTLY ASKED QUESTIONS

F. Lin (✉)
Department of Pathology and Laboratory Medicine, Geisinger Medical Center, 100 N. Academy Ave, Danville, PA 17822, USA
e-mail: flin1@geisinger.edu

F. Lin and J. Prichard (eds.), *Handbook of Practical Immunohistochemistry: Frequently Asked Questions*,
DOI 10.1007/978-1-4419-8062-5_7,

27. VHL-positive and negative tumors (Table 7.26, Fig. 7.8) (pp. 68, 69)
28. RCCMa-positive tumors (Table 7.27) (p. 69)
29. P504S-positive tumors (Table 7.28) (p. 69)
30. OCT4-positive tumors (Table 7.29) (p. 69)

Diagnostic Panels for Common Histomorphologies:

31. Markers for malignant melanoma (see Table 30.2) (pp. 523–524)
32. Markers for lymphomas and other hematopoietic neoplasms (see Chap. 27) (p. 461)
33. Markers for germ cell tumors (Table 7.30; also see Table 21.3) (p. 70, 357)
34. Markers for small round cell tumors (Table 7.31) (p. 70)
35. Markers for spindle cell tumors (Table 7.32) (p. 70)
36. Markers for pleomorphic tumors (Table 7.33) (p. 70)
37. Markers for epithelioid tumors (Table 7.34) (p. 71)

Differential Diagnosis:

Lung vs. Other Primaries:

38. Lung adenocarcinoma vs. mesothelioma (Table 7.35) (p. 71)
39. Lung adenocarcinoma vs. breast carcinoma (Table 7.36) (p. 71)
40. Lung adenocarcinoma vs. pancreatic adenocarcinoma (Table 7.37) (p. 71)
41. Lung adenocarcinoma vs. gastric adenocarcinoma (Table 7.38) (p. 72)
42. Lung adenocarcinoma vs. endometrial carcinoma (Table 7.39) (p. 72)
43. Lung adenocarcinoma vs. ovarian serous carcinoma (Table 7.40) (p. 72)
44. Lung adenocarcinoma vs. colorectal adenocarcinoma (Table 7.41) (p. 72)
45. Lung adenocarcinoma vs. esophageal adenocarcinoma (Table 7.42) (p. 72)
46. Lung adenocarcinoma vs. papillary thyroid carcinoma (Table 7.43) (p. 72)
47. Lung poorly differentiated non-small cell carcinoma vs. anaplastic thyroid carcinoma (Table 7.44) (p. 72)
48. Lung adenocarcinoma vs. renal cell carcinoma (Table 7.45) (p. 73)
49. Lung adenocarcinoma vs. adrenal cortical neoplasm (Table 7.46) (p. 73)

Breast vs. Other Primary Sites:

50. Lung adenocarcinoma vs. breast carcinoma (see Table 7.36) (p. 71)
51. Breast carcinoma vs. pancreatic adenocarcinoma (Table 7.47) (p. 73)
52. Breast carcinoma vs. ovarian serous carcinoma (Table 7.48) (p. 73)
53. Breast carcinoma vs. endometrial carcinoma (Table 7.49) (p. 73)
54. Breast carcinoma vs. gastric carcinoma (Table 7.50) (p. 73)

Renal Cell Carcinoma vs. Other Primaries:

55. Lung adenocarcinoma vs. renal cell carcinoma (see Table 7.45) (p. 73)
56. Clear cell renal cell carcinoma vs. adrenal cortical neoplasm (Table 7.51) (p. 73)
57. Renal cell carcinoma/clear cell vs. ovarian clear cell carcinoma (Table 7.52) (p. 74)
58. Renal cell carcinoma/clear cell vs. brain hemangioblastoma (Table 7.53) (p. 74)
59. Renal cell carcinoma/clear cell vs. hepatocellular carcinoma (Table 7.54) (p. 74)
60. Papillary renal cell carcinoma vs. papillary urothelial carcinoma (Table 7.55) (p. 74)
61. Collecting duct carcinoma vs. urothelial carcinoma (Table 7.56) (p. 74)

Colorectal Adenocarcinoma vs. Other Primaries:

62. Lung adenocarcinoma vs. colorectal adenocarcinoma (see Table 7.41) (p. 72)
63. Colorectal adenocarcinoma vs. breast ductal carcinoma (Table 7.57) (p. 74)
64. Colorectal adenocarcinoma vs. bladder adenocarcinoma (Table 7.58) (p. 75)
65. Colorectal adenocarcinoma vs. pancreatic adenocarcinoma (Table 7.59) (p. 75)
66. Colorectal adenocarcinoma vs. intrahepatic cholangiocarcinoma (Table 7.60) (p. 75)
67. Colorectal adenocarcinoma vs. gastric adenocarcinoma (Table 7.61) (p. 75)
68. Colorectal adenocarcinoma vs. small intestinal adenocarcinoma (Table 7.62) (p. 75)

Pancreas/Biliary Tract Adenocarcinoma vs. Other Primaries:

69. Pancreatic/biliary adenocarcinoma vs. lung adenocarcinoma (see Table 7.37); vs. breast (see Table 7.47); vs. colorectal (see Table 7.59) (pp. 71, 73, 75)
70. Pancreatic adenocarcinoma vs. ovarian serous carcinoma (Table 7.63) (p. 75)
71. Pancreatic adenocarcinoma vs. urothelial carcinoma (Table 7.64) (p. 75)
72. Pancreatic adenocarcinoma vs. gastric adenocarcinoma (Table 7.65) (p. 76)

Other Differential Diagnoses:

73. Small cell carcinoma vs. Merkel cell carcinoma (Table 7.66) (p. 76)

74. Prostatic adenocarcinoma vs. urothelial carcinoma (Table 7.67) (p. 76)
75. Ovarian mucinous carcinoma vs. other mucinous tumors (Table 7.68, Fig. 7.9) (pp. 76, 77)

Fine Needle Aspiration Specimens on Cellblock Preparation:

76. Salivary gland oncocytoma vs. acinar cell carcinoma (Table 7.69, Fig. 7.10) (pp. 77, 78)
77. Mucoepidermoid carcinoma vs. salivary duct carcinoma (Table 7.70) (p. 78)
78. Adenoid cystic carcinoma vs. benign mixed tumor (Table 7.71) (p. 78)
79. Diagnostic panels for common thyroid neoplasms (Table 7.72) (p. 79)
80. Diagnostic panel for lung small cell carcinoma, adenocarcinoma, and squamous cell carcinoma (Table 7.73) (p. 79)
81. Thymic carcinoma vs. lung adenocarcinoma (Table 7.74) (p. 79)
82. Pancreatic adenocarcinoma vs. chronic pancreatitis (Table 7.75, Fig. 7.11) (pp. 79, 80)
83. Diagnostic panel for pancreatic cystic lesions (Table 7.76) (p. 81)
84. Differential diagnosis of pancreatic endocrine neoplasm (Table 7.77) (p. 81)
85. Anaplastic thyroid carcinoma vs. a lung metastasis (see Table 7.44) (p. 72)
86. Hepatocellular carcinoma vs. cholangiocarcinoma and common metastatic carcinomas (see Chap. 23)
87. Diagnostic panel for GIST and mimickers (see Table 24.18)
88. Diagnostic panel for small round cell tumors (see Table 7.31) (p. 70)
89. Diagnostic panels for soft tissue tumors (see Tables 7.21–7.24 and Chap. 26) (p. 68)

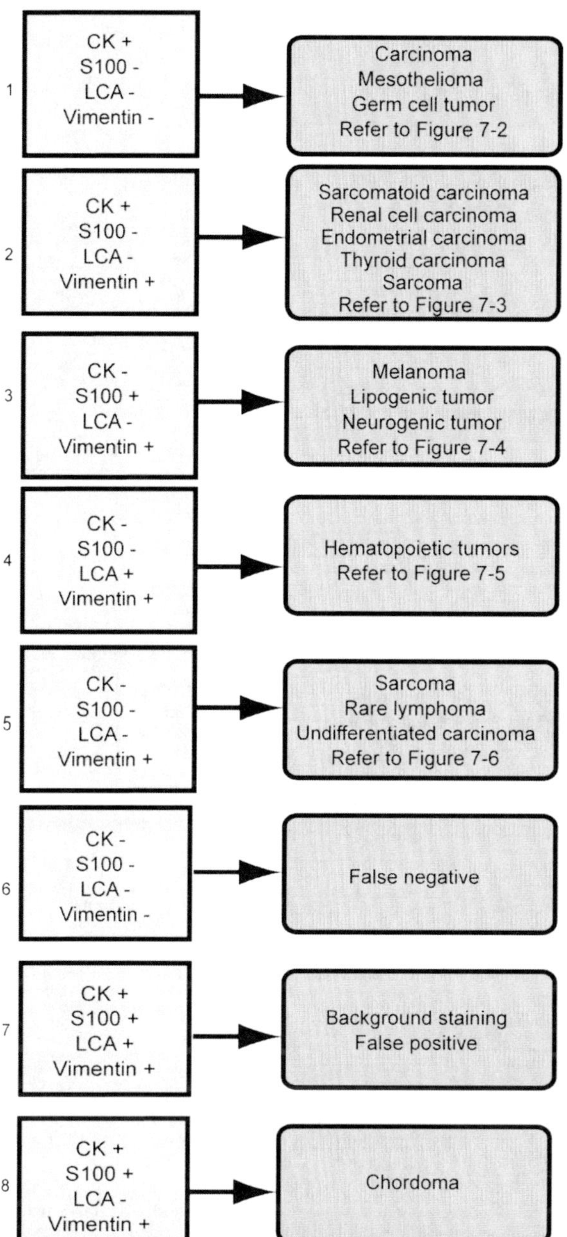

Fig. 7.1 A diagram showing how to approach an unknown primary/undifferentiated neoplasm by using CK (both AE1/AE3 and CAM 5.2), S100, LCA, and vimentin as a start-up panel

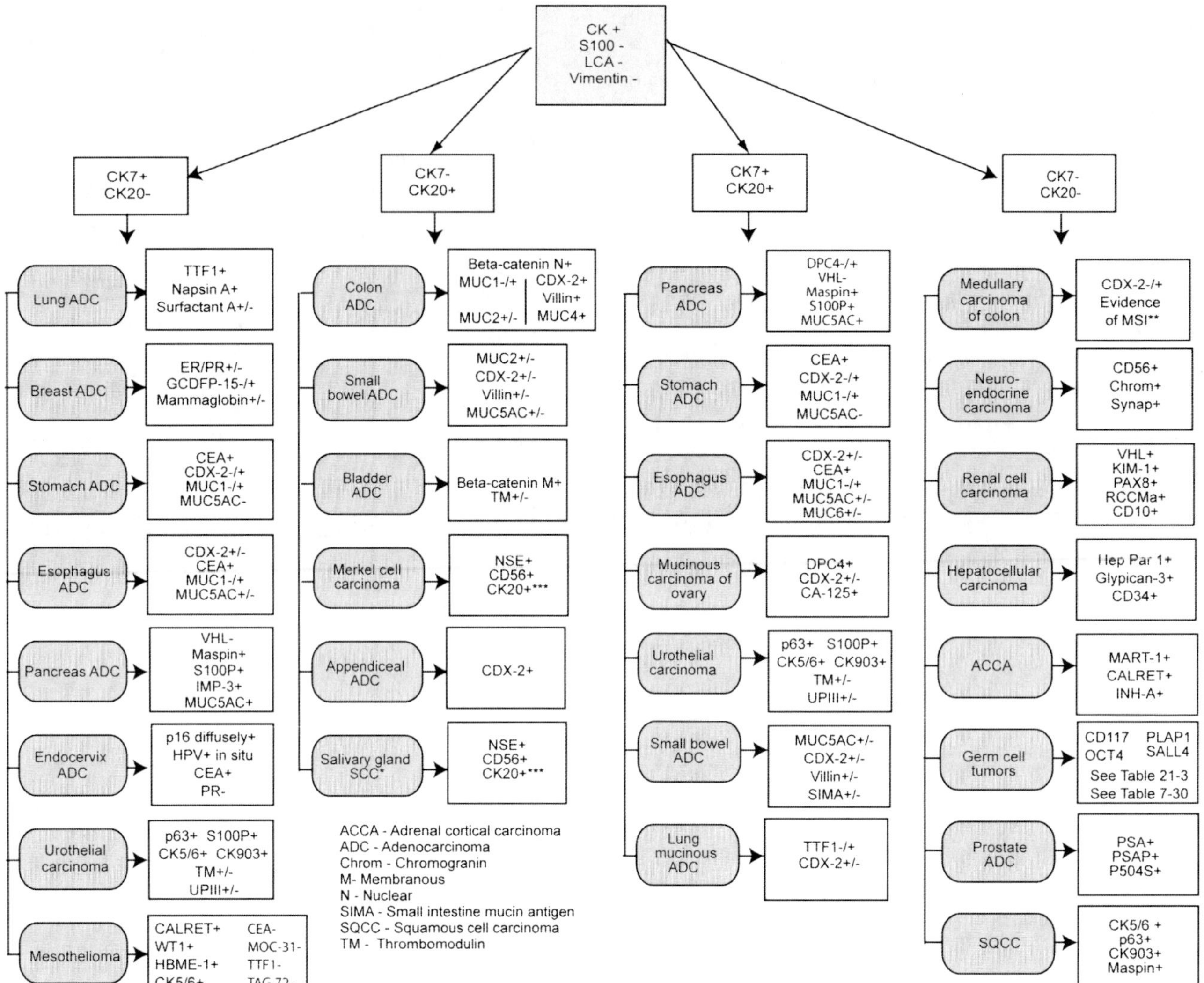

Fig. 7.2 A diagram showing the use of CK7 and CK20 to further classify CK+ and S100–/LCA–/vimentin– neoplasms. Endometrial ADC and ovarian serous carcinoma See Table 7.3

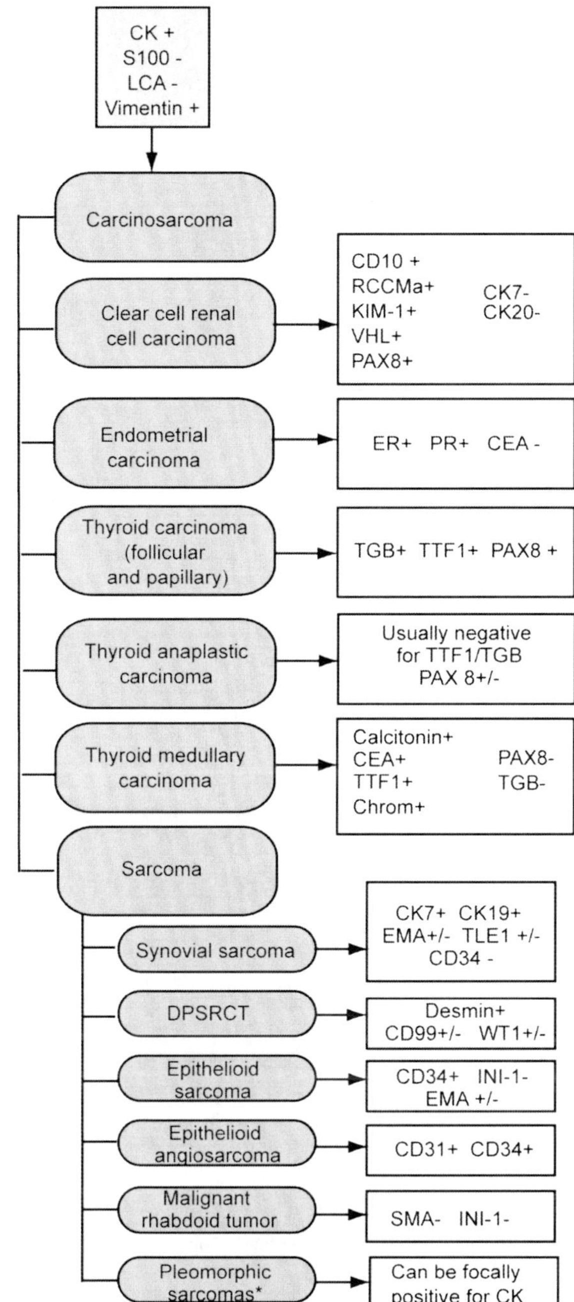

Fig. 7.3 A diagram showing the neoplasms that are likely to demonstrate CK+/vimentin+ and LCA–/S100– and how to perform a further workup

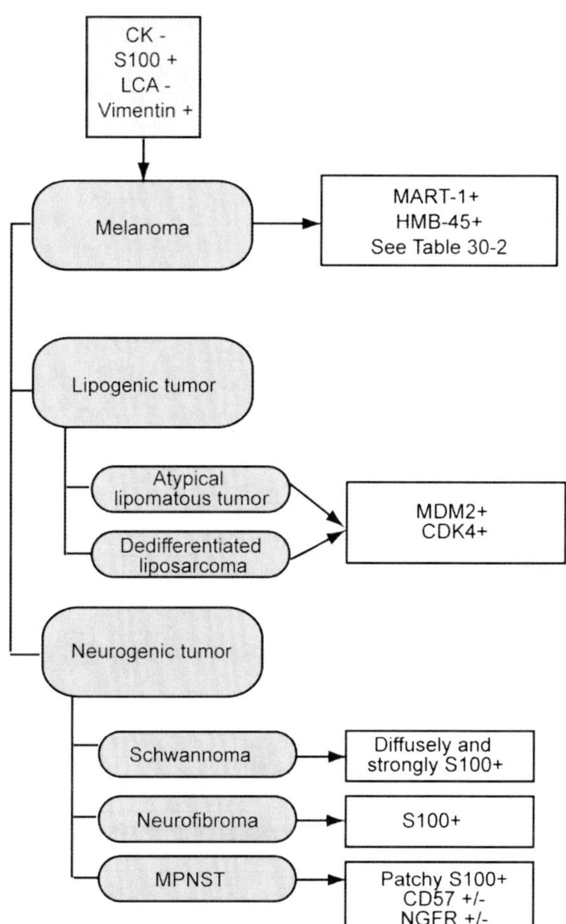

Fig. 7.4 A diagram showing the neoplasms that are likely to demonstrate S100+/vimentin+ and LCA–/CK– and how to perform a further workup

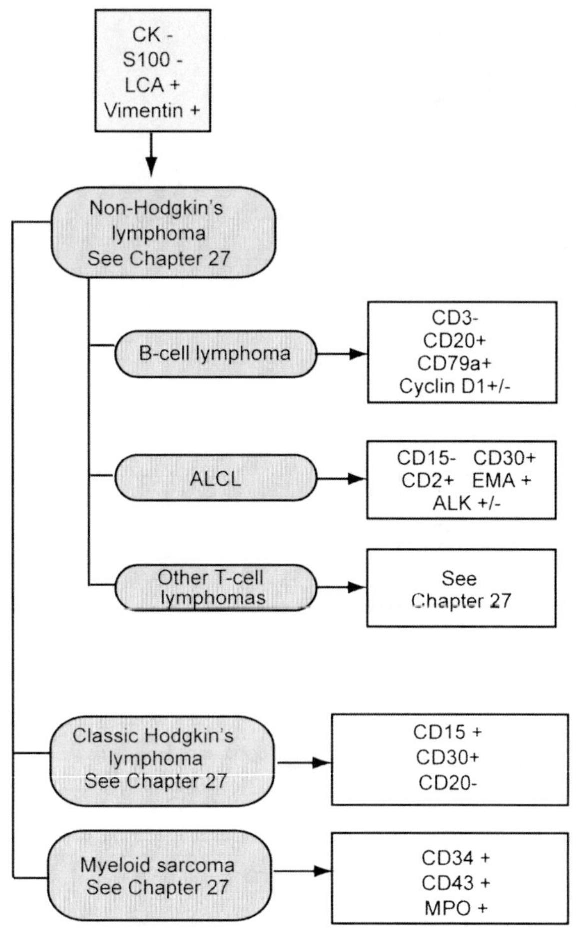

Fig. 7.5 A diagram showing the neoplasms that are likely to demonstrate LCA+/vimentin+ and CK–/S100– and how to perform a further workup

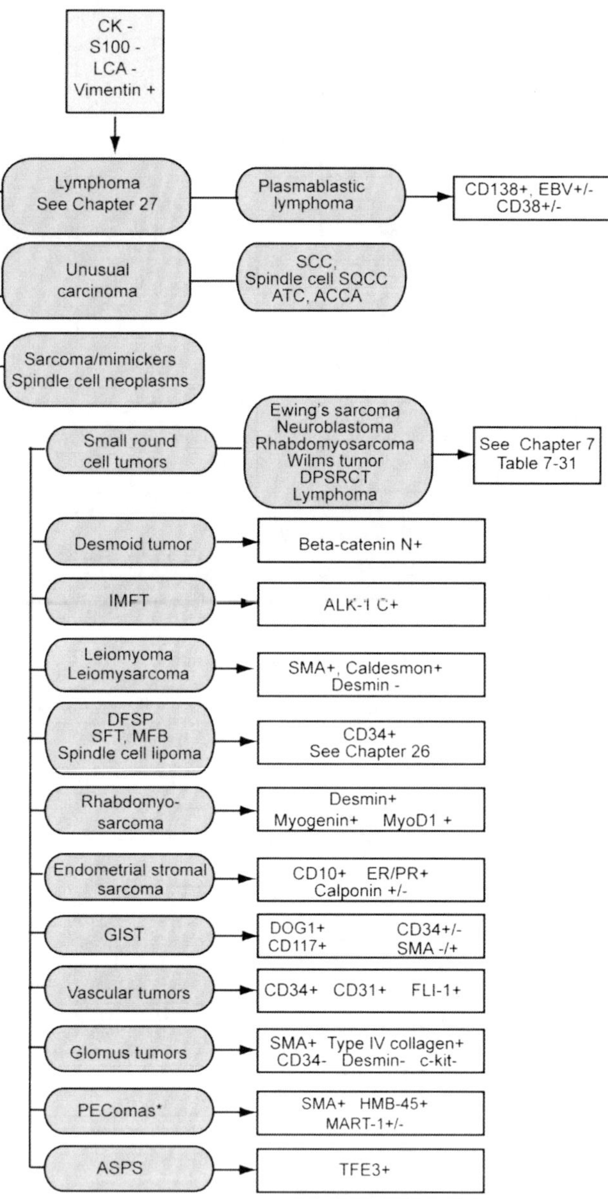

Fig. 7.6 A diagram showing the neoplasms that are likely to demonstrate vimentin+ and CK–/LCA–/S100– and how to perform a further workup

Table 7.1 Markers useful in the diagnosis of undifferentiated neoplasms/unknown primaries

A. Epithelial markers:
AE1/AE3, CAM 5.2, CK7, CK20, CK5/6, CK903, CK17, CK19, EMA

B. Myoepithelial markers:
p63, S100, calponin, SMA, SMMH-1, CK14, maspin

C. Mesenchymal markers:
Vimentin, SMA, MSA, desmin, MyoD1, myogenin, NF, S100, p63, CD10, calponin, myoglobin, MDM2, CDK4, FLI-1, CD117, DOG1, CD31, CD34, Factor XIIIa, CD99

D. Melanocytic markers:
S100, HMB-45, MART-1, tyrosinase, MiTF

E. Mesothelial markers:
Calretinin, CK5/6, WT1, D2-40, HBME-1, mesothelin, thrombomodulin

F. Neuroendocrine markers:
Chromogranin, synaptophysin, CD56, PGP 9.5, NSE, insulin, PTH, calcitonin, thyroglobulin, prolactin

G. Germ cell tumor markers:
PLAP, OCT4, CD117 (c-kit), SALL4, CD30, alpha-fetoprotein, beta-hCG, glypican-3, inhibin-alpha, calretinin, EMA, CAM 5.2

H. Transcription factors, receptors, and nuclear staining markers:
TTF1, CDX-2, Ki-67 (MIB1), MSI markers (MLH1, MSH2, MSH6, PMS2), ARP, ER, PR, INI-1, FLI-1, TFE3, MDM2, CDK4, p53, p63, beta-catenin, WT1, DPC4, OCT4, myogenin, p16

I. Tumor-associated markers:
MUC1, MUC2, MUC4, MUC5AC, MUC6, CEA, Ber-EP4, MOC-31, TAG72 (B72.3), CA19-9, CA125, GCDFP-15, mammaglobin, PSA, PSAP, P504S, Hep Par1, glypican-3, PAX8, PLAP, OCT4, SALL4, CD117 (c-kit), IMP-3, maspin, VHL, S100P, RCC marker, inhibin-alpha, napsin A, CD30, KIM-1, uroplakin III, S100A6, S100A1, GFAP

J. Hematopoietic markers:
CD2, CD3, CD5, CD10, CD20, CD38, CD21, CD35, CD15, CD30, CD79a, CD43, CD138, Bcl-2, Bcl-6, cyclin D1, MUM1, CD68, CD1a, S100, MPO

K. Markers for infectious agents:
EBV, HHV-8

Note: Numerous antibodies are used in diagnosis and differential diagnosis of undifferentiated neoplasms or tumors of unknown origin. A complete list of antibodies with detailed information is summarized in the Appendices. The function, applications, and potential pitfalls of each antibody can be found in the first table of many chapters throughout this book

In general, however, the most useful antibodies in the diagnosis of undifferentiated neoplasms/unknown primaries can be divided into 11 categories as summarized above. The above list of antibodies provides good coverage for a wide spectrum of diagnostic entities, which is suitable for the initial setup of an immunohistochemical laboratory

Table 7.2 Useful markers for identifying tumor origin

Marker	Tumor/organ	Comment
Calcitonin, CEA	Medullary carcinoma of the thyroid	CEA is a highly sensitive marker for medullary carcinoma; up to 5% of calcitonin-negative medullary carcinomas have been reported
Insulin, glucagon, somatostatin	Pancreatic endocrine neoplasms	Some of the functioning pancreatic endocrine tumors
CK20	Merkel cell carcinoma	Perinuclear dot staining
HMB-45, MART-1, SMA	Angiomyolipoma	Positivity can be very focal; negative for S100
S100, HMB-45, MART-1, vimentin	Melanoma	Only 1–2% of melanomas are negative for S100
CD117 (c-kit), DOG1	GI and extra-GI stromal tumors	5–10% of GISTs may be negative for CD117 by IHC but show mutation of PDGFR at the molecular level
CD5, p63	Thymic carcinoma	Thymoma is also positive for p63
CK20, CDX-2, beta-catenin, villin	Colorectal carcinoma	Medullary carcinoma of the colon may be negative for both CDX-2 and CK20 but show MSI (loss of one or more MSI markers such as MLH1, MSH2, MSH6, and PMS2)
Androgen receptor protein (ARP), GCDFP-15	Salivary duct carcinoma	ARP and GCDFP-15 are frequently positive in this entity. Both GCDFP-15 and ARP can be positive in a high-grade mucoepidermoid carcinoma
GCDFP-15, ER, PR, mammaglobin	Breast	High-grade breast carcinoma tends to exhibit loss of ER and PR expression

(continued)

Table 7.2 (continued)

Marker	Tumor/organ	Comment
TTF1, napsin A, surfactant A	Lung adenocarcinoma	TTF1 is also positive in thyroid carcinoma and can be positive in small cell carcinoma of the bladder and prostate; it is rarely positive in endometrial ADC or other carcinomas
TTF1, thyroglobulin, PAX8	Thyroid papillary and follicular carcinomas	Anaplastic carcinoma of the thyroid is usually negative for both TTF1 and thyroglobulin. PAX8 can be positive.
CD1a, S100	Langerhans cell histiocytosis	CD1a is a specific marker
PSA, PSAP, P504S	Prostatic adenocarcinoma	P504S is also positive in many other tumors, such as papillary RCC, clear cell RCC, colorectal adenocarcinoma, and some urothelial carcinomas
CK, EMA, S100	Chordoma	
P504S/KIM-1/RCCMa	Papillary RCC	Expression of these markers tends to be stronger in type II PRCC than in type I PRCC
RCCMa, KIM-1, PAX8, pVHL	Clear cell RCC	PAX8 is also positive in thyroid carcinoma and ovarian serous carcinoma; KIM-1 is also positive in ovarian and uterine clear cell carcinoma and rarely in high-grade urothelial carcinoma
MIB1 (Ki-67)	Hyalinizing trabecular adenoma of the thyroid	Unique membranous staining pattern
OCT4/CD117/PLAP/D2-40	Seminoma	Usually negative for AE1/AE3, CK7, and CK20
CK+ desmin	Desmoplastic small round cell tumor (DPSRCT)	Frequently positive for CD99 and WT1 as well
Glypican-3, Hep Par1	Hepatocellular carcinoma	Hep Par1 expressed in normal liver and hepatocellular adenoma
Alpha-fetoprotein/glypican-3/PLAP/SALL4	Yolk sac carcinoma	Only a small percentage of HCC is positive for AFP
OCT4/CD30/SOX2/SALL4/PLAP	Embryonal carcinoma	Negative for D2-40 and CD117
MDM2, CDK4	Adipose tissue/liposarcoma	Atypical lipomatous tumor and pleomorphic liposarcoma
Myogenin, desmin, MyoD1	Rhabdomyosarcoma	Myogenin tends to have a stronger signal than MyoD1
SMA, MSA, desmin	Leiomyosarcoma/smooth muscle tumor	
p16, HPV in situ	Cervical and endocervical carcinoma	Serous carcinoma is usually diffusely positive for p16 as well; endometrioid carcinoma tends to be patchy positive
ER, WT1, PAX8	Ovarian serous carcinoma	PAX8 is also positive in clear cell RCC and thyroid carcinoma
CD10, ER	Endometrial stromal sarcoma	Loss of or reduced expression in high-grade endometrial stromal sarcoma
Maspin, VHL	Pancreatic ductal adenocarcinoma (PDA)	Loss of expression of VHL is seen in pancreatic, common bile duct, and gallbladder adenocarcinoma, but expression of VHL is retained in intrahepatic cholangioCA
CD2, CD3	T-cells	A high percentage of anaplastic large cell lymphoma is negative for CD3
CD20, PAX5, CD79a	B-cells	Plasmablastic lymphoma is usually negative for these markers but positive for CD138 and EBV in situ
CD43, CD34, CD33, MPO	Myeloid cells	Myeloid sarcoma
CD117 (c-kit), tryptase	Mast cells	Tryptase is the most sensitive and specific marker for mast cells
CD21, CD35	Follicular dendritic cells	Follicular dendritic cell tumor

References: [1–52]

Table 7.3 Summary of common immunostaining markers in adenocarcinomas, mesothelioma, melanoma, and germ cell tumors

Marker	Lung	Pancreas	Breast	Stomach	Ovary	Uterus	Cervix	Colon	Kidney	Bladder	Prostate	Liver	Meso	Mel	GCT
CK7	+	+	+	+	+	+	+	–	–	+	–	–	+	–	– or +
CK20	–	– or +	–	– or +	–	–	–	+	–	+ or –	–	–	–	–	–
CK5/6	–	–	–	–	–	–	–	–	–	+	–	–	+	–	–
p63	–	–	–	–	–	–	–	–	–	+	–	–	–	–	–
TTF1	+	–	–	–	–	–	–	–	–	–	–	C+	–	–	–
CDX-2	–	– or +	–	+ or –	–	–	– or +	+	–	–	–	–	–	–	–
ER	–	–	+	–	+	+	– or +	–	–	–	–	–	–	–	–
CD10	–	–	–	–	–	–	–	–	+	– or +	–	+	–	– or +	– or +
RCCMa	–	–	–	–	–	–	–	–	+	–	–	–	–	–	–
VHL	–	–	–	–	–	–	–	–	+	–	–	–	–	–	–
PAX8	–	–	–	–	+	–	–	–	+	–	–	–	–	–	–
S100	– or +	–	+ or –	–	–	–	–	–	+ or –	–	–	–	–	+	–
S100P	+ or –	+	– or +	–	–	–	–	+ or –	–	+	–	–	–	–	–
Vimentin	–	–	–	–	–	+ or –	–	–	+	–	–	–	– or +	+	–
PSA	–	–	–	–	–	–	–	–	–	–	+	–	–	–	–
Hep Par1	–	–	–	–	–	–	–	–	–	–	–	+	–	–	–
Glypican-3	–	–	–	–	–	–	–	–	–	–	–	+	–	–	– or +
HMB-45	–	–	–	–	–	–	–	–	–	–	–	–	–	+	–
SALL4	–	–	–	–	–	–	–	–	–	–	–	–	–	–	+

Note: *Meso* mesothelioma; *Mel* melanoma; *GCT* germ cell tumors (includes seminoma and non-seminomatous tumors)

Lung mucinous adenocarcinoma with BAC features tends to be negative for TTF1 and can be positive for CDX-2

Typical seminoma tends to be negative for cytokeratin (such as AE1/AE3, CK7, and CK20) and can be positive for CAM 5.2. In contrast, non-seminomatous tumors are usually positive for AE1/AE3. Seminoma is usually positive for PLAP, CD117, OCT4, D2-40, and SALL4

Embryonal carcinoma is usually positive for OCT4 and SALL4 and often positive for CD30; yolk sac tumor is frequently positive for AFP, SALL4, and glypican-3, and negative for OCT4; choriocarcinoma is positive for beta-hCG and CD10

Colon: Medullary carcinoma of the colon tends to be negative or only very focally positive for CK20 and CDX-2; to complicate the matter further, some can be focally positive for CK7 but usually present with MSI (loss of expression of MLH1 and PMS2, or MSH2 and MSH6). Therefore, caution should be taken because negativity for both CK20 and CDX-2 does not automatically exclude the possibility of a colorectal origin

Kidney: The staining profile shown in this table is for clear cell RCC. Type I papillary RCC is usually positive for CK7, P504S, KIM-1, and CD10 with the exception of the type II PRCC, which is frequently negative for CK7, strongly positive for P504S and CD10, and can be focally positive for CK20. KIM-1, RCCMa, PAX8, and VHL are the most effective panel of markers to identify a metastatic renal cell carcinoma

Endocervical adenocarcinoma: It is usually diffusely and strongly positive for p16 and positive for HPV by in situ hybridization. In contrast, endometrial adenocarcinoma tends to be only focally positive for p16 and also positive for ER/PR and vimentin, but negative for CEA

References: [1–52]

Table 7.4 Markers for the determination of a broad category of neoplasms

Marker/tumor	Carcinoma	Sarcoma	Melanoma	Lymphoma	GCT	Mesothelioma
CK	+	–	–	–	+ or –	+
Vimentin	–	+	+	+	–	–
S100	– or +	–	+	–	–	–
LCA	–	–	–	+	–	–
SALL4	–	–	–	–	+	–

Note: *GCT* germ cell tumor

A combination of AE1/AE3 and CAM 5.2 or EMA is the effective panel of markers for identifying the epithelial lineage. AE1/AE3 by itself is insufficient to exclude an epithelial lineage

References: [1, 32–35]

Table 7.5 Expression of high and low molecular weight cytokeratins in various tumors

LMWCK+HMWCK	LMWCK (CAM 5.2)	HMWCK (34betaE12)
Breast	HCC	SQCC
Urothelial CA	RCC	
Ovarian CA	Colorectal ADC	
Pulmonary ADC	Endometrial ADC	
Pancreatic ADC	Prostatic ADC	
Mesothelioma	Neuroendocrine CA	
Thymoma		

Note: *LMWCK* low molecular weight cytokeratin, *HMWCK* high molecular weight cytokeratin; *ADC* adenocarcinoma, *CA* carcinoma, *HCC* hepatocellular carcinoma, *RCC* renal cell carcinoma, *SQCC* squamous cell carcinoma

References: [1, 32–35, 53]

Table 7.6 Expression of CK7 and CK20 in various tumors

CK7+/CK20–	CK7–/CK20+	CK7+/CK20+	CK7–/CK20–
Lung	Colorectal ADC	Urothelial CA	CRCC
Breast	Bladder ADC	Pancreatic/biliary CA	HCC
Mesothelioma	Merkel cell carcinoma	Ovarian mucinous CA	Prostatic ADC
Endometrial ADC	Appendiceal CA	Small bowel CA	ACCA
Endocervical ADC	Small bowel CA	Cholangiocarcinoma	SCC
Ovarian serous CA		Gastric CA	SQCC
Thymoma		Bladder ADC	Mesothelioma
Pancreatic/biliary ADC			

Note: *ADC* adenocarcinoma, *CA* carcinoma, *CRCC* clear cell renal cell carcinoma, *HCC* hepatocellular carcinoma, *SCC* small cell carcinoma, *SQCC* squamous cell carcinoma, *ACCA* adrenal cortical carcinoma

References: [1, 32–35]

Table 7.7 Expression of MUC1, MUC2, MUC5AC, and MUC6 in adenocarcinomas of various organs

Organ/marker	MUC1	MUC2	MUC5AC	MUC6
Breast	+	–	–	– or +
Lung	+	–	+ or –	– or +
Esophagus	+	–	+ or –	ND
Stomach	+[a]	– or +	+ or –	+ or –
Pancreas	+	–	+	– or +
Endometrium	+	–	–	–
Ovary	+	– or +	+ or –	ND
Colon	– or +	+	– or +	–

Note: Mucinous adenocarcinomas from various organs are positive for MUC2, such as colloid carcinoma of the pancreas and breast

References: [1, 32–35, 49]

[a]Our data ($N = 22$) showed only 13% of gastric adenocarcinomas are positive for MUC1

Table 7.8 Markers for neuroendocrine carcinomas of various organs

Markers	Tumors/organ
Calcitonin	Medullary carcinoma of the thyroid
TTF1	Small cell carcinoma of the lung, bladder, and prostate
CDX-2	GI tract
CK20 perinuclear dot-like stain	Merkel cell carcinoma
Insulin, glucagon, PAX8	Pancreatic endocrine neoplasms
PTH	Parathyroid gland
Prolactin	Pituitary gland

References: [1, 32–35]

Table 7.9 Tumors that frequently and rarely express both cytokeratin and vimentin

Carcinomas that frequently express both	Sarcomas that frequently express both	Carcinomas that rarely express both
Renal cell carcinoma	Synovial sarcoma	Breast carcinoma
Anaplastic thyroid carcinoma	DPSRCT	Ovarian carcinoma
Endometrial carcinoma	Epithelioid sarcoma	GI carcinoma
Thyroid carcinomas	Epithelioid angiosarcoma	Lung small cell carcinoma
Sarcomatoid carcinoma	Malignant rhabdoid tumor	Lung non-small cell carcinoma
	Leiomyosarcoma	Prostatic carcinoma

Note: Follicular, papillary, and medullary thyroid carcinomas are nearly 100% positive for vimentin. Metaplastic breast carcinoma usually expresses both cytokeratin and vimentin in addition to high molecular weight cytokeratins and myoepithelial markers

References: [1, 32–35]

Table 7.10 Expression of epithelial markers in non-epithelial neoplasms

Marker	Tumors
EMA	Plasmacytoma
CK7, CK19, EMA	Synovial sarcoma
AE1/AE3, CAM 5.2	Epithelioid sarcoma, angiosarcoma
AE1/AE3, CAM 5.2	DPSRCT
AE1/AE3, CAM 5.2	Malignant rhabdoid tumor
EMA	Anaplastic large cell lymphoma

Note: *DPSRCT* desmoplastic small round cell tumor

References: [1, 32–35]

Table 7.11 Expression of hematopoietic markers in nonhematopoietic neoplasms

Marker	Tumor
CD5	Thymic carcinoma, CC
CD30	Embryonal carcinoma
CD138	Carcinoma of the lung, CC, UC
CD10	RCC, HCC, ESS, chorioCA
CD15	Carcinoma of the lung and other organs; renal oncocytoma
CD56	Neuroendocrine carcinomas and thyroid carcinomas

Note: *RCC* renal cell carcinoma, *HCC* hepatocellular carcinoma, *ESS* endometrial stromal sarcoma; *UC* urothelial carcinoma; *CC* cholangiocarcinoma, *chorioCA* choriocarcinoma

CD5 has been reported in breast carcinoma, colonic carcinoma, pancreatic carcinoma, and lung carcinoma. CD138 is also frequently positive in squamous cell carcinoma, and can be positive in breast carcinoma, ovarian carcinoma, adrenal cortical carcinoma, and renal cell carcinoma

CD56 is the most sensitive, but not an entirely specific marker for neuroendocrine neoplasms, including some small cell carcinomas, which may lose expression of cytokeratins and other neuroendocrine markers, but still show expression of CD56. A significant percentage of thyroid carcinomas are immunoreactive for CD56 as well in the literature. Our experience showed positivity for CD56 in thyroid tissue and tumor 100% (20/20), 27% (12/45), 90% (47/52), 44% (16/36), and 100% (10/10) for normal thyroid follicular cells, papillary thyroid carcinoma, follicular adenoma, follicular carcinoma, and medullary carcinoma, respectively

References: [1, 32–35, 38, 51, 54]

Table 7.12 Carcinomas with markedly reduced expression or loss of cytokeratins

Tumors	Comment
Small cell carcinoma	Can be negative for AE1/AE3, CAM 5.2, EMA, and other cytokeratins, but CD56 is usually still positive
Anaplastic thyroid carcinoma	Can be only patchy positive for CAM 5.2 and negative for other cytokeratins
Medullary carcinoma of the colon	Can be negative for AE1/AE3, CK20, CK7, and other cytokeratins
Adrenal cortical carcinoma	Usually negative for AE1/AE3, CK7, and CK20
Renal cell carcinoma (Clear cell)	Up to 10% of cases can be negative for AE1/AE3, CK7, CK20, EMA, and other cytokeratins

References: [1, 32–35]

Table 7.13 TTF1-positive and negative tumors

TTF1-positive tumors	TTF1-negative tumors
Lung adenocarcinoma	Breast carcinoma
Carcinoma of the thyroid (follicular, papillary, and medullary carcinoma)	Adrenal cortical carcinoma
Small cell carcinoma of the lung	Mesothelioma
Small cell carcinoma of the bladder	Urothelial carcinoma
Small cell carcinoma of the prostate	Prostatic adenocarcinoma
	Pancreatic adenocarcinoma
	Colon carcinoma
	Renal cell carcinoma

Note: Anaplastic thyroid carcinoma is usually negative for TTF1; medullary carcinoma of the thyroid tends to be weakly positive. Approximately 75% of pulmonary adenocarcinomas, 90% of small cell carcinomas of the lung and 40% of small cell carcinomas of the bladder or prostate are positive for TTF1. TTF1 immunoreactivity has been reported in a small percentage of carcinomas from various organs such as endometrial adenocarcinoma, endocervical adenocarcinoma, and ovarian carcinoma. The TTF1-negative tumors may also rarely demonstrate TTF1 positivity

References: [1, 32–35, 52]

Table 7.14 Napsin A-positive and negative tumors

Tumor	Literature	GML% (*N*)
Lung ADC	+	93% (54)
Papillary RCC	+	69% (26)
Clear cell RCC	– or +	38% (53)
LCCA of the lung	– or +	ND
SQCC	–	5% (42), focal
Mesothelioma	–	ND
Pancreas ADC	–	5% (56), focal
Breast ADC	–	0 (62)
Colon ADC	–	29% (38)
Esophageal ADC	–	17% (30)
Urothelial CA	–	2.5% (40), focal
PTC	–	18% (45)

Note: *RCC* renal cell carcinoma; *ADC* adenocarcinoma; *CA* carcinoma; *LCCA* large cell carcinoma of the lung; *PTC* papillary thyroid carcinoma; *SQCC* squamous cell carcinoma of the lung; *ND* no data

Napsin A is useful marker for confirming the diagnosis of adenocarcinoma of the lung and helpful in differentiating a lung primary from other sites. However, caution should be taken since many other tumors can be positive for napsin A. Examples of the expression of napsin A in papillary renal cell carcinoma and esophageal adenocarcinoma are shown in Fig. 7.7a, b

References: [1, 32–37]

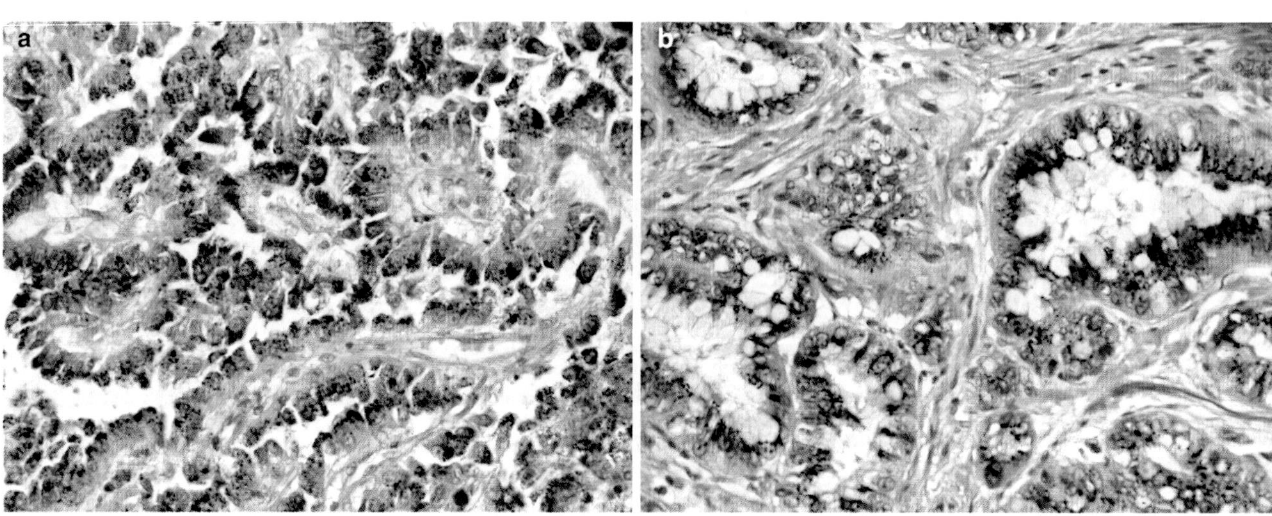

Fig. 7.7 (**a**, **b**) In addition to lung adenocarcinoma, napsin A can be positive in other carcinomas, such as papillary renal cell carcinoma (**a**) and esophageal adenocarcinoma (**b**)

Table 7.15 CEA-positive and negative tumors

CEA-positive tumors	CEA-negative tumors
Lung adenocarcinoma	Endometrial carcinoma
Colorectal carcinoma	Ovarian serous carcinoma
Gastric carcinoma	Renal cell carcinoma
Pancreatic carcinoma	Prostatic adenocarcinoma
Breast carcinoma	Mesothelioma
Urothelial carcinoma	Adrenal cortical carcinoma
Medullary carcinoma of the thyroid	
Endocervical carcinoma	

References: [1, 32–35]

Table 7.16 CDX-2-positive and negative tumors

Tumors	CDX-2
Colorectal ADC	+
Small intestinal ADC	+
Neuroendocrine neoplasm of the GI tract	+ or –
Upper GI ADC	+ or –
Ovarian mucinous ADC	+ or –
Pancreas/biliary ADC	– or +
Breast ADC	–
Lung ADC	–
Urothelial CA	–
RCC	–

References: [1, 32–35]

Table 7.17 ER- and PR-positive and negative tumors

ER-positive tumors	PR-positive tumors	ER-negative tumors
Breast carcinoma	Breast carcinoma	Colorectal adenocarcinoma
Ovarian carcinoma	Ovarian carcinoma	Gastric adenocarcinoma
Endometrial carcinoma	Endometrial carcinoma	Hepatocellular carcinoma
Ovarian-like stroma of MCN	Ovarian-like stroma of MCN	Endocervical carcinoma
Endometrial stromal sarcoma	Endometrial stromal sarcoma	Pancreatic adenocarcinoma
	SPT	Renal cell carcinoma
	Meningioma (I and II)	

Note: *MCN* mucinous cystic neoplasm of the pancreas, *SPT* solid and pseudopapillary neoplasm of the pancreas

ER positivity has been reported in up to 5% of pulmonary adenocarcinomas. However, we have not encountered a single case of clinically proven pulmonary adenocarcinoma with an unequivocal ER immunoreactivity

References: [1, 32–35]

Table 7.18 CD10-positive nonhematopoietic tumors

Tumor	CD10
RCC	+
HCC	+
SPT	+
ChorioCA	+
ESS	+

Note: *RCC* renal cell carcinoma, *HCC* hepatocellular carcinoma, *SPT* solid and pseudopapillary neoplasm of the pancreas, *chorioCA* choriocarcinoma, *ESS* endometrial stromal sarcoma

CD10 is a relatively nonspecific marker; many other carcinomas have been reported to be focally or diffusely positive for CD10. Caution should be taken when using CD10 as a diagnostic marker

References: [1, 22, 32–35]

Table 7.19 CD34-positive tumors

Tumors	Comment
Hematopoietic progenitor cells	Also positive for CD33 and MPO
Vascular tumors	Also positive for CD31 and Factor VIII
DFSP	Negative for Factor XIII
Solitary fibrous tumor	Also positive for CD99 and Bcl-2
GI and extra-GI stromal tumors	50% of cases positive for CD34; also positive for CD117 and DOG1
Epithelioid sarcoma	Also positive for cytokeratin/EMA and loss of INI-1 expression
PHAT of soft part	Negative for S100 and HMB-45
Spindle cell lipoma	Spindle cells are negative for S100

Note: *DFSP* dermatofibrosarcoma protuberans, *PHAT* pleomorphic hyalinizing angiectatic tumor of soft part

References: [1, 32–35]

Table 7.20 CD117 (c-kit)-positive tumors

Tumors	Comment
GIST	Approximately 10% of GISTs can be negative
CML	
Seminoma	Also positive for PLAP, OCT4, and SALL4
Chromophobe RCC	Positive for CK7 and Ep-CAM (Ber-EP4), and negative for S100A1
Oncocytoma	Positive for S100A1 and PAX2, and negative or focally positive for CK7
Mastocytosis	Tryptase is the best diagnostic marker

Note: *CML* chronic myelogenous leukemia, *GIST* gastrointestinal stromal tumor

References: [1, 32–35]

Table 7.21 S100-positive tumors

S100-positive tumors	Comment
Malignant melanoma	Very sensitive marker, including for spindle cell melanoma
Schwannoma	Diffuse and strong positivity
Neurofibroma	The intensity of the positive staining tends to be weaker than in schwannoma
Granular cell tumor	
Clear cell renal cell carcinoma	Very similar to S100A1; it is also positive in oncocytoma, but negative in ChRCC
Langerhans' cell histiocytosis	CD1a is more specific marker
Chordoma	Coexpression of cytokeratin
Carcinomas from various organs	Carcinomas from the lung, breast, and kidney
Lipogenic tumor	Usually negative in spindle cell lipoma, which is positive for CD34
MPNST	Only focally and weakly positive

Note: *MPNST* malignant peripheral nerve sheath tumor, *ChRCC* chromophobe renal cell carcinoma

References: [1, 32–35]

Table 7.22 HMB-45-positive tumors

HMB-45-positive tumors	Comment
Melanoma	S100+, MART-1+
Clear cell (sugar) tumor of the lung	Focal S100+
Clear cell sarcoma of soft part	Also S100+ and MART-1+
Angiomyolipoma	SMA+ and S100–
Lymphangioleiomyomatosis	S100–
Cardiac rhabdomyoma	S100–
Renal translocation carcinoma	TFE3+

Note: It is important to know that HMB-45 can be positive in non-melanocytic tumors. In addition, other melanocytic marker such as MART-1 can be positive in adrenal cortical neoplasm or other PEComas (perivascular epithelioid cell tumors)

References: [1, 32–35]

Table 7.23 CD99 (MIC-2)-positive and negative tumors

CD99-positive tumors	CD99-negative tumors
Ewing's sarcoma/PENT	Neuroblastoma
Lymphoblastic lymphoma	Rhabdomyosarcoma
Thymoma	Embryonal carcinoma
Poorly differentiated synovial sarcoma	Esthesioneuroblastoma
Solitary fibrous tumor	Wilms' tumor
Granular cell tumor	
Proximal-type epithelioid sarcoma	
DPSRCT	

Note: *DPSRCT* desmoplastic small round cell tumor

References: [1, 32–35]

Table 7.24 Myogenin-positive and negative tumors

Tumor	Myogenin
Embryonal RHMS	+
Alveolar RHMS	+
Pleomorphic RHMS	+ or –
Synovial sarcoma	– or + (<10%)

Note: *RHMS* rhabdomyosarcoma, *MPNST* malignant peripheral nerve sheath tumor

Epithelioid sarcoma, Ewing's sarcoma/PNET, MPNST, neuroblastoma, leiomyosarcoma, and pleomorphic sarcoma (MFH) are usually negative for myogenin

References: [1, 31–35]

Table 7.25 PAX8-positive and negative tumors

PAX8-positive tumors	PAX8-negative tumors
Thyroid carcinomas (follicular and papillary)	Lung small cell and non-small cell carcinomas
Renal cell carcinomas	Pancreatic/biliary carcinomas
Ovarian serous carcinoma	GI carcinomas
Ovarian clear cell carcinoma	Breast DAC
Nephrogenic adenoma	Urothelial CA

Note: Medullary carcinoma of the thyroid is negative for PAX8, and data on the expression of PAX8 in poorly differentiated and anaplastic thyroid carcinomas are inconsistent. Our data also demonstrated 53% ($N = 17$) cases of the endocervical adenocarcinoma and 3% cases of colorectal adenocarcinoma ($N = 68$) are positive for PAX8

References: [1, 10–12, 32–35]

Table 7.26 VHL-positive and negative tumors

VHL-positive tumors	VHL-negative tumors
Renal cell carcinomas	Pancreatic ADC
Intrahepatic cholangiocarcinoma	Gallbladder ADC
Salivary oncocytoma	Salivary acinar cell carcinoma
Clear cell carcinoma of the ovary	Breast ADC
Clear cell carcinoma of the uterus	Lung ADC
Renal oncocytoma	Common bile duct ADC

Note: *ADC* adenocarcinoma

Normal/reactive pancreatic ducts, acini, gallbladder mucosa, common bile ducts, and hepatic bile ducts are positive for VHL. The expression VHL in intrahepatic cholangiocarcinoma can be potentially used as a diagnostic marker in differentiating it from other pancreatic/biliary tract carcinomas. Our study also demonstrated VHL was focally positive (<25% of the tumor cells) in 16% of colorectal ADCs ($N = 38$) and 13% of esophageal ADCs ($N = 30$). Examples of the expression of VHL in ovarian clear cell carcinoma and intrahepatic cholangiocarcinoma are demonstrated in Fig. 7.8a–c

References: [41–43]

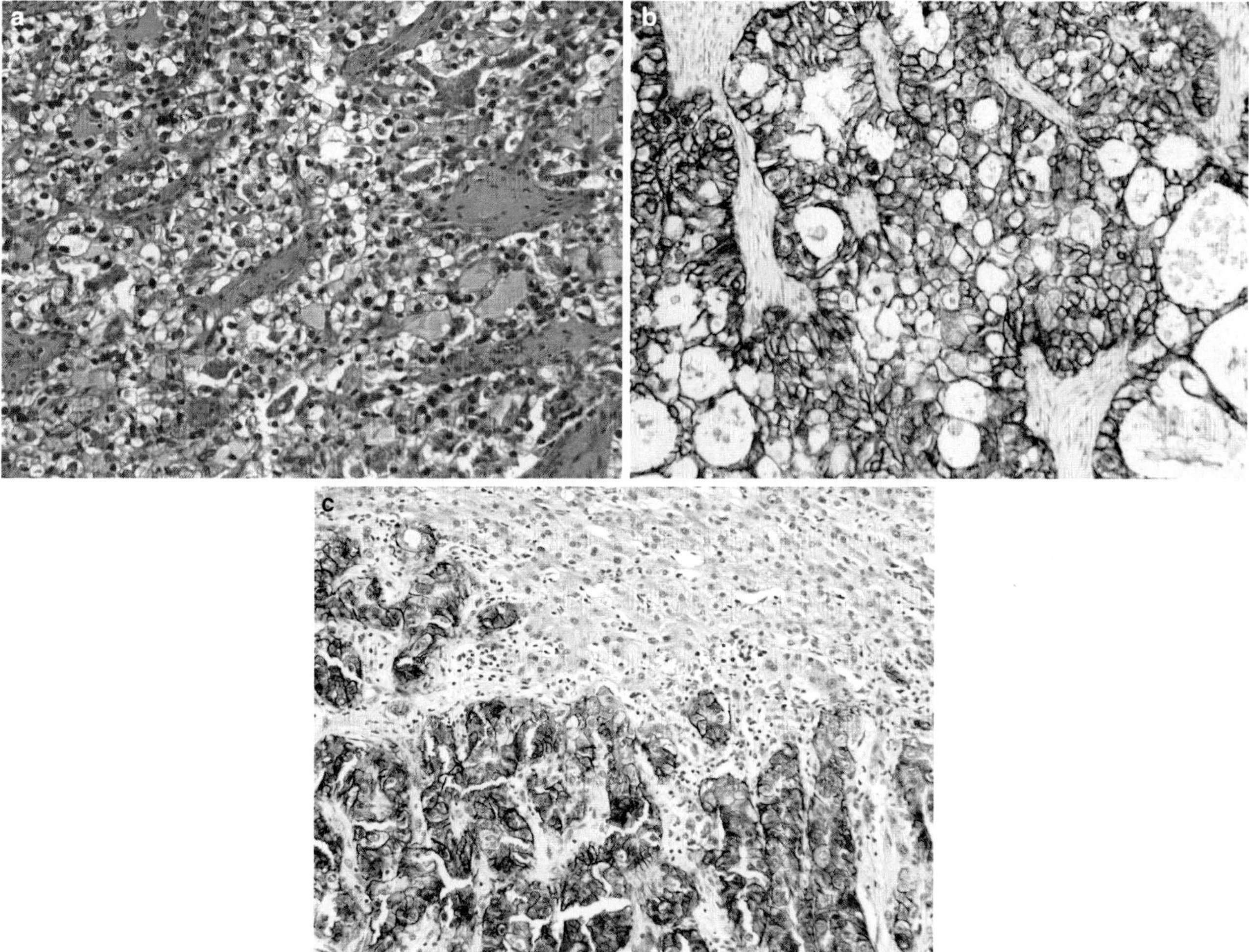

Fig. 7.8 Ovarian clear cell carcinoma, H & E (**a**) VHL can be a useful marker for ovarian clear cell carcinoma (**b**) and intrahepatic cholangiocarcinoma (**c**)

Table 7.27 RCCMa-positive tumors

Tumors	RCCMa
CRCC	+
PRCC	+
Renal oncocytoma	–
ChRCC	–
TFC	+ or –
PTC	– or +

Note: *CRCC* clear cell re nal cell carcinoma, *PRCC* papillary renal cell carcinoma, *ChRCC* chromophobe renal cell carcinoma, *TFC* thyroid follicular carcinoma, *PTC* papillary thyroid carcinoma

Our study demonstrates that the immunoreactivity for RCCMa is present in 96% (50/52), 27% (12/45), and 72% (26/36) of follicular adenomas, PTCs, and TFCs, respectively. Therefore, RCCMa is not a good marker to identify a metastatic renal cell carcinoma in the thyroid

References: [1, 32–35]

Table 7.28 P504S-positive tumors

Tumors	P504S
Prostatic ADC	+
PRCC	+
Colorectal ADC	+
NGA	+
CRCC	+ or –
UC	– or +

Note: *ADC* adenocarcinoma, *NGA* nephrogenic adenoma, *CRCC* clear cell renal cell carcinoma, *PRCC* papillary renal cell carcinoma, *UC* urothelial carcinoma

References: [1, 32–35, 39, 40]

Table 7.29 OCT4-positive tumors

Tumors	OCT4
Seminoma	+
Embryonal carcinoma	+
Yolk sac tumor	–
Teratoma	–
Choriocarcinoma	–

References: [1, 29, 32–35]

Table 7.30 Markers for germ cell tumors

Markers	Seminoma	EBC	YST	ChorioCA	Teratoma
AE1/AE3	–	+	+	+	+
CK7					
PLAP	+	+	+	+	–
CD117 (c-kit)	+	–	+ or –	–	–
OCT4	+	+	–	–	–
SALL4	+	+	+	+	–
CD30	–	+	–	–	–
Alpha-fetoprotein	–	–	+	–	–
Glypican-3	–	–	+	+ or –	–
Beta-hCG	–	–	–	+	–

Note: *EBC* embryonal carcinoma, *YST* yolk sac tumor, *ChorioCA* choriocarcinoma

References: [1, 2, 29, 32–35, 50, 55]

Table 7.31 Markers for small round cell tumors

Marker/diagnosis	NB	ES/PNET	RHMS	LYM	DPSRCT	SCC
Desmin	–	–	+	–	+	–
Myogenin	–	–	+	–	–	–
CD99	–	+	– or +	+ or –	+ or –	–
NSE	+	+	–	–	– or +	+ or –
LCA	–	–	–	+	–	–
S100	–	–	–	–	–	–
Vimentin	+	+	+	+	+	–
CK	–	–	–	–	+	+
WT1	–	–	–	–	+ or –	–
FLI-1	–	+	–	–	–	–

Note: *NB* neuroblastoma, *ES/PNET* Ewing's sarcoma, *RHMS* rhabdomyosarcoma, *LYM* lymphoma, *DPSRCT* desmoplastic small round cell tumor, *SCC* small cell carcinoma

References: [2, 31, 56]

Table 7.32 Markers for spindle cell tumors

Diagnosis/markers	CK	S100	Vimentin	SMA	Desmin	CD34	CD117
Spindle cell carcinoma	+	–	+ or –	–	–	–	–
Spindle cell melanoma	–	+	+	–	–	–	–
Neurogenic tumor	–	+	+	–	–	–	–
GIST	–	–	+	– or +	–	+ or –	+
Smooth muscle tumor	–	–	+	+	+	–	–
Fibrosarcoma	–	–	+	–	–	–	–
DFSP	–	–	+	–	–	+	–
SFT	–	–	+	–	–	+	–
Synovial sarcoma	+	–	+	–	–	–	–
Kaposi sarcoma	–	–	+	–	–	+ or –	–

Note: *GIST* gastrointestinal stromal tumor, *DFSP* dermatofibrosarcoma protuberans, *SFP* solitary fibrous tumor

References: [1, 32–35]

Table 7.33 Markers for pleomorphic tumors

Diagnosis/markers	CK	Vimentin	S100	Desmin	Myogenin	SMA
Carcinoma	+	– or +	–	–	–	–
Pleomorphic sarcoma (MFH)	–	+	–	–	–	–
Liposarcoma	–	+	Focal +	–	–	–
Rhabdomyosarcoma	–	+	–	+ or –	+ or –	+ or –
Leiomyosarcoma	–	+	–	– or focal +	–	+
Melanoma	–	+	+	–	–	–

References: [1, 32–35]

Table 7.34 Markers for epithelioid tumors

Diagnosis/markers	CK	S100	Myogenin	CD117	SMA	CD34	CD31
Carcinoma	+	–	–	–	–	–	–
Mesothelioma	+	–	–	–	–	–	–
Epithelioid sarcoma	+	–	–	–	–	+ or –	–
Epithelioid angiosarcoma	– or focal +	–	–	–	–	+	+
Clear cell sarcoma	–	+	–	–	–	–	–
Epithelioid GIST	–	–	–	+	– or +	+ or –	–
Epithelioid MPNST	– or focal +	Focal +	–	–	–	–	–
Alveolar soft part sarcoma	–	–	–	–	–	–	–
*PEComas	–	–	–	–	+	–	–
Chordoma	+	+	–	–	–	–	–

Note: Alveolar soft part sarcoma may be positive for TFE3. Epithelioid sarcoma frequently shows loss of INI-1 expression. PEComas (Perivascular epithelioid cell tumors) can be patchy positive for S100 and usually positive for HMB-45 and MART-1 as well

References: [1, 17, 18, 32–35]

Table 7.35 Lung adenocarcinoma vs. mesothelioma

Antibody	LADC (literature)	LADC (GML%, *N* = 54)	Mesothelioma (literature)
Calretinin	–	2%	+
WT1	–	0	+
CK5/6	–	4%	+
D2-40	–	0	+
Mesothelin	–	33%	+
CEA	+	100%	–
MOC-31	+	100%	–
Ber-EP4	+	87%	–
TTF1	+	89%	–
Napsin A	+	93%	–

Note: *LADC* lung adenocarcinoma

References: [1, 23, 32–35]

Table 7.36 Lung adenocarcinoma vs. breast carcinoma

	LADC		BCA	
Markers	Literature	GML% (*N* = 54)	Literature	GML% (*N*)
Napsin A	+	93%	–	0 (62)
TTF1	+	89%	–	0 (88)
ER	–	0	+	60% (88)
GCDFP-15	–	2%	– or +	30% (88)
Mammaglobin	–	0	+ or –	41% (88)

Note: *LADC* lung adenocarcinoma, *BCA* breast carcinoma

References: [1, 32–35]

Table 7.37 Lung adenocarcinoma vs. pancreatic adenocarcinoma

	LADC		PADC	
Markers	Literature	GML% (*N*)	Literature	GML% (*N*)
CK17	ND	13% (54)	+	60% (70)
TTF1	+	78% (54)	–	0 (70)
Napsin A	+	93% (54)	–	5% (56)
DPC4	+	95% (55)	– or +	41% (70)
Maspin	+	51% (55)	+	100% (70)
CA19-9	– or +	28% (55)	+	84% (70)
MUC4	– or +	28% (55)	+ or –	50% (70)
MUC5AC	– or +	16% (55)	+	67% (70)
Mesothelin	– or +	33% (54)	+	60% (70)

Note: *LADC* lung adenocarcinoma, *PADC* pancreatic adenocarcinoma

References: [1, 32–35]

Table 7.38 Lung adenocarcinoma vs. gastric adenocarcinoma

	LADC		GADC	
Markers	Literature	GML% (*N* = 54)	Literature	GML% (*N*)
TTF1	+	89%	–	0 (18)
Napsin A	+	93%	–	6% (18)
CK20	–	4%	– or +	61% (18)
CDX-2	–	0	+ or –	39% (18)
MUC1	+	100%	+	13% (22)

Note: *ND* no data, *LADC* lung adenocarcinoma, *GADC* gastric adenocarcinoma

Other markers including CK7, CK17, maspin, IMP-3, MUC4, MUC5AC, MUC2, and MUC6 are not very useful

References: [1, 32–35]

Table 7.39 Lung adenocarcinoma vs. endometrial carcinoma

	LADC		
Antibodies	Literature	GML% (*N* = 54)	ECA (literature)
TTF1	+	89%	–
Napsin A	+	93%	–
ER	–	0	+
Vimentin	–	4%	+
CEA	+ or –	100%	–

Note: *LADC* lung adenocarcinoma, *ECA* endometrial carcinoma

References: [1, 32–35]

Table 7.40 Lung adenocarcinoma vs. ovarian serous carcinoma

	LADC		OSCA	
Antibodies	Literature	GML% (*N* = 54)	Literature	GML% (*N* = 15)
TTF1	+	89%	–	0
Napsin A	+	93%	–	0
PAX8	–	0	+	100%
WT1	–	0	+	73%
CA125	– or +	39%	+	87%
ER	–	0	+	80%
CEA	+	100%	–	7%
CD15	+	85%	–	7%

Note: *ND* no data, *LADC* lung adenocarcinoma, *OSCA* ovarian serous carcinoma

References: [1, 32–35]

Table 7.41 Lung adenocarcinoma vs. colorectal adenocarcinoma

	LADC		CRADC	
Markers	Literature	GML% (*N* = 54)	Literature	GML% (*N* = 38)
CK7	+	96%	–	3%
CK20	–	4%	+	97%
CDX-2	–	0	+	95%
TTF1	+	89%	–	0
Napsin A	+	93%	–	29%
Villin	–	6%	+	82%
MUC1	+	100%	–	16%

Note: *LADC* lung adenocarcinoma, *CRADC* colorectal adenocarcinoma

References: [1, 32–35]

Table 7.42 Lung adenocarcinoma vs. esophageal adenocarcinoma

	LADC		EADC	
Markers	Literature	GML% (*N* = 54)	Literature	GML% (*N* = 30)
TTF1	+	89%	–	0
Napsin A	+	93%	–	17%
CDX-2	–	0	+ or –	43%
CK20	–	4%	+ or –	37%
MUC1	+	100%	– or +	27%
MUC5AC	– or +	16%	+	43%
Villin	– or +	6%	+	17%

Note: *LADC* lung adenocarcinoma, *EADC* esophageal adenocarcinoma

References: [1, 32–35]

Table 7.43 Lung adenocarcinoma vs. papillary thyroid carcinoma

	LADC		PTC	
Markers	Literature	GML% (*N* = 54)	Literature	GML% (*N* = 45)
TTF1	+	89%	+	100%
Napsin A	+	93%	–	0
PAX8	–	0	+	93%
Thyroglobulin	–	0	+	100%
Vimentin	–	4%	+	100%
CEA	+ or –	100%	–	7%

Note: *LADC* lung adenocarcinoma, *PTC* papillary thyroid carcinoma

References: [1, 32–35]

Table 7.44 Lung poorly differentiated non-small cell carcinoma vs. anaplastic thyroid carcinoma

Antibody	LPNSCC	ATC
TTF1	+ or –	–
PAX8	–	+ or –
CK7	+ or –	– of focal +
p63	+ or –	– or focal +
CK5/6	+ or –	– or focal +

Note: *LPNSCC* lung poorly differentiated non-small cell carcinoma, *ATC* anaplastic thyroid carcinoma

References: [1, 24, 32–35]

Table 7.45 Lung adenocarcinoma vs. renal cell carcinoma

	LADC		RCC	
Markers	Literature	GML% (*N* = 54)	Literature	GML% (*N*)
TTF1	+	89%	–	0 (76)
PAX8	–	0	+	95% (94)
KIM-1	+	0	+	75%
VHL	–	0	+	99% (77)
CK7	+	96%	–	11% (79)
CD10	– or +	13%	+	90% (82)
Vimentin	–	4%	+	86% (88)
CEA	+ or –	100%	–	ND

Note: *LADC* lung adenocarcinoma, *RCC* renal cell carcinoma, *ND* no data. KIM-1 – based on our previously published data

References: [1, 11, 12, 32–35, 42, 44]

Table 7.46 Lung adenocarcinoma vs. adrenal cortical neoplasm

	LADC		ACN	
Markers	Literature	GML% (*N* = 54)	Literature	GML% (*N*)
TTF1	+	89%	–	0 (29)
Napsin A	+	93%	–	0 (29)
MART-1	–	ND	+	97% (29)
Calretinin	–	2%	+	100% (24)
CK7	–	96%	–	0 (29)
Inhibin-alpha	–	6%	+	41% (29)

Note: *ND* no data, *LADC* lung adenocarcinoma, *ACN* adrenal cortical neoplasm

Inhibin-alpha staining tends to be weak in our laboratory

References: [1, 32–35]

Table 7.47 Breast carcinoma vs. pancreatic adenocarcinoma

	BCA		PADC	
Markers	Literature	GML% (*N* = 88)	Literature	GML% (*N* = 70)
IMP-3	N/D	6%	+	95%
ER	+	60%	–	0
MUC5AC	–	0	+	67%
CK17	–	8.4%	+	60%
MUC4	–	0	+ or –	50%
DPC4	+	90%	– or +	41%
Maspin	N/D	24%	+	100%
CA19-9	– or +	16%	+	84%
GCDFP-15	– or +	30%	–	0
Mammaglobin	+ or –	41%	–	0

Note: *BCA* breast carcinoma, *PADC* pancreatic adenocarcinoma, *ND* no data

References: [1, 32–35, 57]

Table 7.48 Breast carcinoma vs. ovarian serous carcinoma

	Breast carcinoma		OSCA	
Markers	Literature	GML% (*N*)	Literature	GML% (*N* = 15)
PAX8	–	0 (62)	+	100%
WT1	–	8% (62)	+	73%
GCDFP-15	– or +	30% (88)	–	0
Mammaglobin	+ or –	41% (88)	–	ND
CA125	– or +	3% (62)	+	87%

Note: *ND* no data, *OSCA* ovarian serous carcinoma

References: [1, 12, 32–35]

Table 7.49 Breast carcinoma vs. endometrial carcinoma

	Breast carcinoma		Endometrial carcinoma
Antibody	Literature	GML% (*N*)	Literature
Mammaglobin	+ or –	41% (70)	–
GCDFP-15	– or +	30% (70)	–
Vimentin	–	0 (70)	+
CEA	+	40% (62)	–

References: [1, 32–35]

Table 7.50 Breast carcinoma vs. gastric carcinoma

	Breast carcinoma		Gastric carcinoma	
Markers	Literature	GML% (*N*)	Literature	GML% (*N* = 18)
ER	+	60% (88)	–	0 (18)
CXD2	–	0 (62)	+ or –	39% (18)
CK20	–	0 (88)	+ or –	61% (18)
GCDFP-15	– or +	30% (88)	–	0 (18)
Mammaglobin	+ or –	40% (88)	–	0 (18)
MUC1	+	96% (88)	– or +	13% (22)

Note: *ND* no data

References: [1, 32–35]

Table 7.51 Clear cell renal cell carcinoma vs. adrenal cortical neoplasm

	ACN		CRCC	
Markers	Literature	GML% (*N*)	Literature	GML% (*N*)
CD10	–	7% (29)	+	90% (80)
RCC marker	–	0 (20)	+	89% (80)
VHL	–	0 (29)	+	98% (80)
PAX8	–	0 (24)	+	95% (80)
MART-1	+	97% (29)	–	0 (36)
Inhibin-alpha	+	41% (29)	–	0 (36)
Calretinin	+	100% (24)	–	0 (36)
EMA	–	3% (29)	+	85% (80)
NSE	+	93% (29)	–	92% (36)

Note: *CRCC* clear cell renal cell carcinoma, *ACN* adrenal cortical neoplasm

GML data of 29 adrenal cortical neoplasms included 5 cases of adrenal cortical adenoma and 24 cases of adrenal cortical carcinoma

References: [1, 22, 32–35, 42]

Table 7.52 Renal cell carcinoma/clear cell vs. ovarian clear cell carcinoma

Antibody	CRCC (literature)	CRCC (GML% N = 80)	OCCC (literature)
CK7	–	11%	+
RCCMa	+	89%	–
Vimentin	+	86%	–
CD10	+	90%	–

Note: *CRCC* renal cell carcinoma/clear cell, *OCCC* ovarian clear cell carcinoma

Both tumors are usually positive for PAX8, KIM-1, and VHL

References: [1, 32–35, 42, 44]

Table 7.53 Renal cell carcinoma/clear cell vs. brain hemangioblastoma

Antibody	CRCC (literature)	CRCC (GML%, *N*)	BHB (literature)
EMA	+	85% (80)	–
RCCMa	+	89% (80)	–
PAX8	+	95% (80)	–
VHL	+	99% (80)	–
Inhibin-alpha	–	0 (80)	+
NSE	ND	92% (36)	+

Note: *CRCC* renal cell carcinoma/clear cell, *BHB* brain hemangioblastoma, *ND* no data

References: [1, 32–35, 42, 43]

Table 7.54 Renal cell carcinoma/clear cell vs. hepatocellular carcinoma

	CRCC		HCC	
Markers	Literature	GML% (*N*)	Literature	GML% (*N* = 18)
EMA	+	85% (80)	–	0
Vimentin	+	86% (80)	–	0
RCC marker	+	89% (80)	–	0
Glypican-3	–	0 (36)	+	72%
Hep Par1	–	0 (36)	+	94%
PAX8	+	95% (80)	–	0
VHL	+	98% (80)	ND	0

Note: *CRCC* renal cell carcinoma/clear cell, *HCC* hepatocellular carcinoma

References: [1, 32–35]

Table 7.55 Papillary renal cell carcinoma vs. papillary urothelial carcinoma

	PRCC		PUC	
Markers	Literature	GML% (*N* = 24)	Literature	GML% (*N* = 40)
CK7	+	91%	+	98%
CK20	–	0	+	58%
CK903	–	ND	+	93%
p63	–	0	+	98%
S100P	ND	0	+	68%
VHL	+	100%	ND	0
P504S	+	96%	– or +	20%
RCCMa	+	88%	–	0

Note: *PRCC* papillary renal cell carcinoma, *PUC* papillary urothelial carcinoma, *ND* no data

Type II PRCC shows a different immunophenotype, which is frequently negative for CK7, focally positive for CK20, and diffusely and strongly positive for P504S and KIM-1. MUC1 is usually negative

References: [1, 32–35, 40, 42]

Table 7.56 Collecting duct carcinoma vs. urothelial carcinoma

Antibody	CDC (literature)	UC (literature)	UC (GML%, *N* = 40)
PAX8	+	–	0
p63	–	+	98%
CK20	–	+ or –	58%
CD10	+	– or +	35%
CA IX	+	– or +	30%

CDC collecting duct carcinoma, *UC* urothelial carcinoma

References: [1, 10, 32–35]

Table 7.57 Colorectal adenocarcinoma vs. breast ductal carcinoma

	CRADC		BDCA	
Markers	Literature	GML% (*N* = 38)	Literature	GML% (*N* = 88)
CK7	–	3%	+	91%
CK20	+	97%	–	0
CDX-2	+	95%	–	0
ER	–	0	+	60%
Mammaglobin	–	ND	+ or –	41%
GCDFP-15	–	0	– or +	30%
MUC1	– or +	16%	+	96%
MUC2	+	55%	–	0

Note: *CRADC* colorectal adenocarcinoma, *BDCA* breast ductal carcinoma, *ND* no data

References: [1, 32–35]

Table 7.58 Colorectal adenocarcinoma vs. bladder adenocarcinoma

	CRADC		BADC
Antibody	Literature	GML% (*N* = 38)	Literature
CK7	–	3%	+ or –
CK20	+	97%	+ or –
CDX-2	+	95%	– or +
Beta-catenin	+, N	63%, M + N	+, M
TM	–	ND	+ or –

Note: *N* nuclear, *M* membranous, *CRADC* colorectal adenocarcinoma, *BADC* primary bladder adenocarcinoma

References: [1, 27, 32–35]

Table 7.59 Colorectal adenocarcinoma vs. pancreatic adenocarcinoma

	CRADC		PADC	
Markers	11.596 pt	GML% (*N* = 38)	Literature	GML% (*N* = 70)
CK7	–	3%	+	96%
CK20	+	97%	– or +	15%
CDX-2	+	95%	– or +	5%
MUC5AC	–	26%	+	67%
MUC2	+	55%	–	4%
Beta-catenin	+, M + N	63%, M + N	+, M	100%

Note: *M* membranous, *N* nuclear, *CRADC* colorectal adenocarcinoma, *PADC* pancreatic adenocarcinoma

References: [1, 27, 32–35]

Table 7.60 Colorectal adenocarcinoma vs. intrahepatic cholangiocarcinoma

	CRADC		ICC	
Markers	Literature	GML% (*N* = 38)	Literature	GML% (*N* = 11)
CK7	–	3%	+	100%
CK20	+	97%	+ or –	20%
CDX-2	+	95%	– or +	0
MUC2	+	55%	–	0
Beta-catenin	+, M + N	63%, M + N	+, M	100%, M
VHL	ND	16%	ND	80%

Note: *M* membranous, *N* nuclear, *CRADC* colorectal adenocarcinoma, *ICC* intrahepatic cholangiocarcinoma

References: [1, 32–35]

Table 7.61 Colorectal adenocarcinoma vs. gastric adenocarcinoma

	CRADC		GADC	
Markers	Literature	GML% (*N* = 38)	Literature	GML% (*N* = 18)
CK7	–	3%	+	83%
CK20	+	97%	+ or –	61%
CDX-2	+	95%	+ or –	39%
MUC2	+	55%	– or +	17%
Beta-catenin	+, M + N	63%	+, M	6%, M + N
P504S	+	90%	–	39%

Note: *ND* no data, *CRADC* colorectal adenocarcinoma, *GADC* gastric adenocarcinoma

References: [1, 32–35]

Table 7.62 Colorectal adenocarcinoma vs. small intestinal adenocarcinoma

Antibody	CRADC	SIADC
CK7	–	+
P504S (AMACR)	+	–
Beta-catenin	N+	N+ or –
CK20	+	+ or –
CDX-2	+	+ or –
Villin	+	+ or –
MUC2	+	+ or –
MUC5AC	+ or –	+ or –
Hep Par1	– or +	– or +

Note: *N* nuclear, *CRADC* colorectal adenocarcinoma, *SIADC* small intestinal adenocarcinoma

All the 24 reported SIADC (non-ampullary) showed CK7 immunoreactivity with a diffuse staining in 54% cases. Only 1 of the 24 SIADC demonstrated focal P504S positivity, whereas 62% (41/66) of CRADC exhibited a variable degree of P504S positivity. Nuclear localization beta-catenin was observed in 71% of CRADC and only in 19% of SIADC. Hep Par1 was expressed in 23% SIADC (9 of 39) and 10% of CRADC. Hep Par1 is usually expressed in normal small intestinal mucosa, but not in normal colonic mucosa

References: [58–62]

Table 7.63 Pancreatic adenocarcinoma vs. ovarian serous carcinoma

	PADC		OSCA	
Markers	Literature	GML% (*N* = 70)	Literature	GML% (*N* = 15)
CK17	+	60%	ND	0
MUC5AC	+	67%	–	0
DPC4/SMAD4	– or +	41%	+	ND
WT1	–	0	+	73%
PAX8	–	0	+	100%

Note: *ND* no data, *PACD* pancreatic adenocarcinoma, *OSCA* ovarian serous carcinoma

References: [1, 12, 32–35]

Table 7.64 Pancreatic adenocarcinoma vs. urothelial carcinoma

	PADC		UC	
Markers	Literature	GML% (*N* = 70)	Literature	GML% (*N* = 40)
p63	–	0	+	98%
CK903	– or +	0	+	93%
Uroplakin III	– or +	0	–	40%
MUC1	+	95%	+ or –	55%
MUC5AC	+	67%	–	5%

Note: *PADC* pancreatic adenocarcinoma; *UC* urothelial carcinoma

References: [1, 32–35]

Table 7.65 Pancreatic adenocarcinoma vs. gastric adenocarcinoma

	PADC		GADC	
Markers	Literature	GML% (N = 70)	Literature	GML% (N)
CK7	+	96%	+	83% (18)
CK20	+ or −	15%	+ or −	61% (18)
CK17	+	60%	−	0 (18)
MUC1	+	95%	+ or −	13% (22)
MUC5AC	+	67%	−	0 (18)
CDX-2	− or +	5%	+ or −	39% (18)

Note: *PADC* pancreatic adenocarcinoma, *GADC* gastric adenocarcinoma

References: [1, 32–35]

Table 7.66 Small cell carcinoma (SCC) vs. Merkel cell carcinoma (MCCA)

Antibody	SCC	MCCA
CK20	−	+
TTF1	+	−
Chromogranin	+ or −	+
NF	−	+ or −

Note: *SCC* small cell carcinoma, *MCCA* Merkel cell carcinoma

References: [1, 32–35]

Table 7.67 Prostatic adenocarcinoma vs. urothelial carcinoma

	PADC		UC	
Markers	Literature	GML% (N = 100)	Literature	GML% (N = 40)
CK7	−	3%	+	98%
CK20	−	1%	+ or −	58%
S100P	−	1%	+	68%
PSA	+	100%	−	0
P504S	+	97%	− or +	20%
*UPIII	−	ND	+	40%

Note: *PADC* prostatic adenocarcinoma, *UC* urothelial carcinoma

The staining signal for UPIII in our system tends to be weak

References: [1, 32–35]

Table 7.68 Ovarian mucinous carcinoma vs. other mucinous tumors

Antibody	OMC	CRADC	AADC	PADC	EADC	BDCA	LADC
CK7	+	−	− or +	+	+	+	+
CK20	+, p	+	+	− or +	−	−	−
CDX-2	+ or −	+	+	− or + (10%)	−	−	−
MUC1	ND	− or +	−	+	+ or −	+	+
MUC5AC	+	+ or −	+	+	−	−	−
p16	−	−	−	−	+, D	−	−
HPV	−	−	−	−	+	−	−

Note: *OMC* ovarian mucinous carcinoma, *CRADC* colorectal adenocarcinoma, *AADC* appendical adenocarcinoma, *PADC* pancreatic adenocarcinoma, *EADC* endocervical adenocarcinoma, *BDCA* breast ductal carcinoma, *LADC* lung adenocarcinoma, *D* diffuse

An example of metastatic adenocarcinoma of the endocervix mimicking the primary ovarian adenocarcinoma is shown in Fig. 7.9a–c, in which the tumor is diffusely positive for p16 and positive for HPV in situ

References: [1, 32–35]

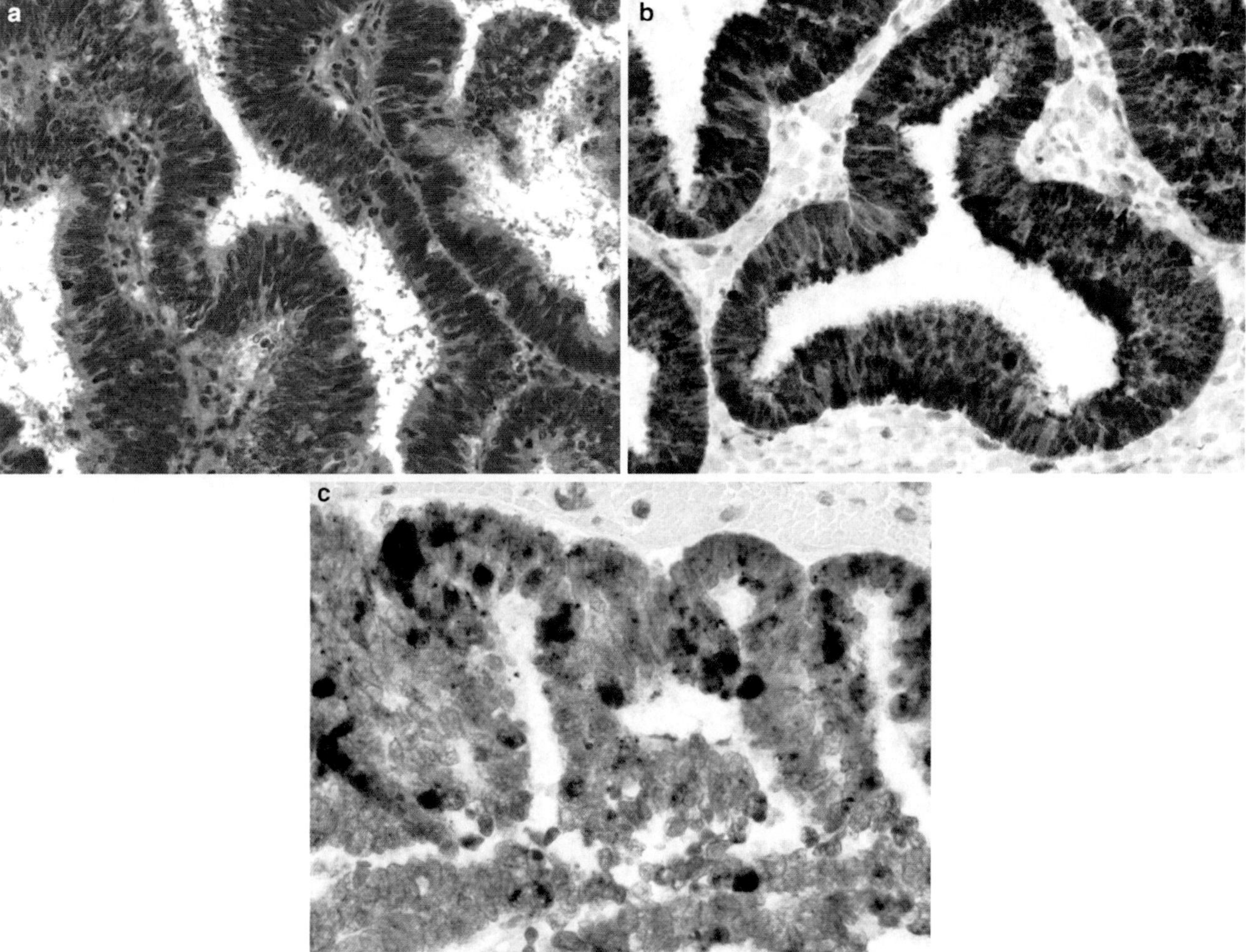

Fig. 7.9 (**a**–**c**) Metastatic endocervical adenocarcinoma in the ovary H & E section (a). The tumor is diffusely positive for p16 (**b**) and positive for HPV by in situ hybridization (**c**)

Table 7.69 Salivary gland oncocytoma vs. acinar cell carcinoma

Antibody	Acinar cell carcinoma	Oncocytoma
VHL	–	+
p63	–	+ or –
CEA	+ or –	–
PAS-D	+	–

Note: Differential diagnosis of oncocytoma from acinar cell carcinoma of the salivary gland on cytological specimens can be difficult. Our study demonstrates that VHL is a useful marker in distinction of these two entities. Examples on both fine needle aspiration biopsy and the follow-up surgical specimens are shown in Fig. 7.10a–d. Caution should be taken both acinar cell carcinoma and normal acini are negative for VHL

References: [1, 32, 33, 57]

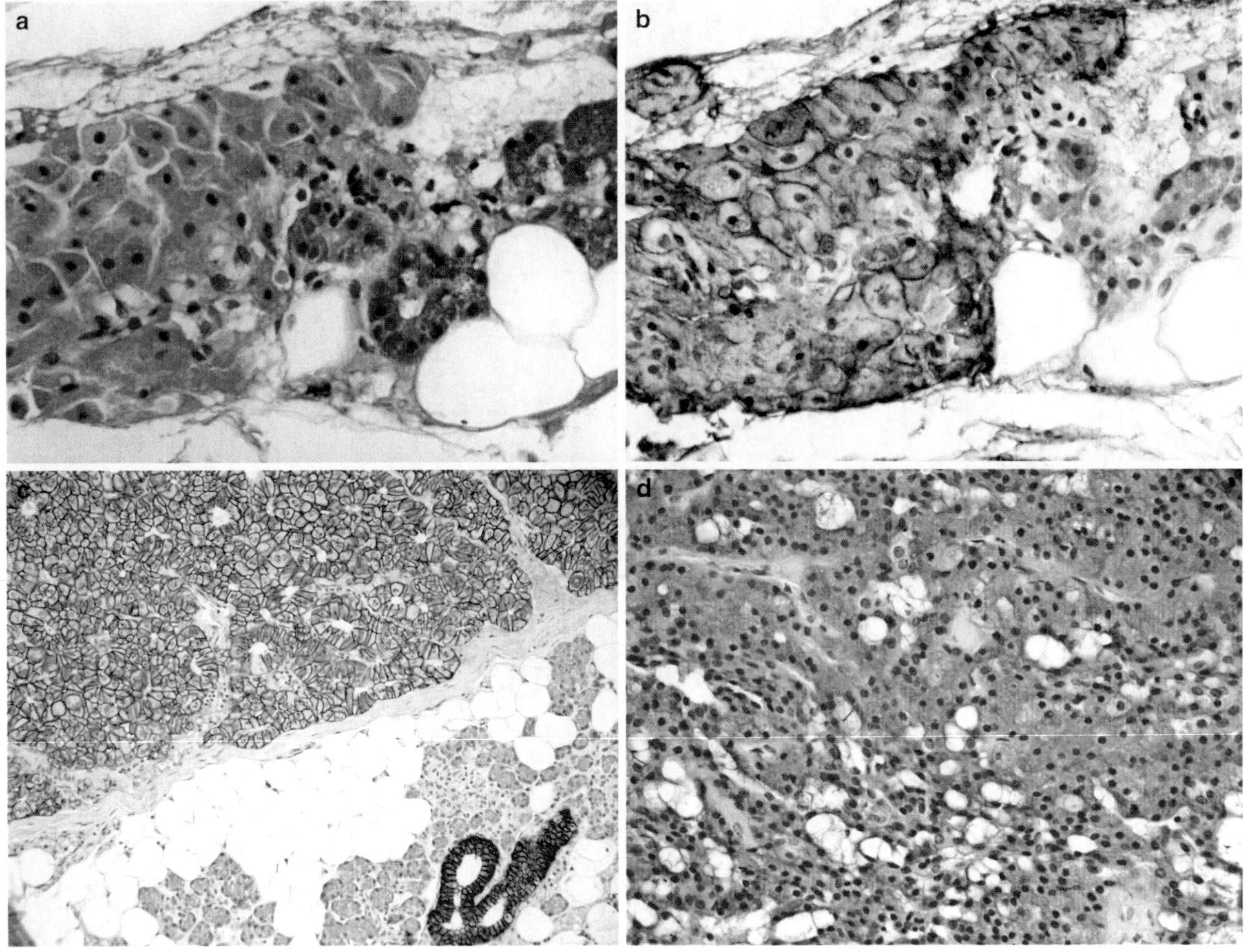

Fig. 7.10 (**a–d**) Expression of VHL in salivary oncocytoma, but not in acinar cell carcinoma. Note that the cell block section demonstrates oncocytic neoplasm and normal acini (**a**), expression of VHL in the tumor, but not in normal acini on the cytology specimen (**b**) and follow-up surgical specimen (**c**), and no immunoreactivity in acinar cell carcinoma (**d**)

Table 7.70 Mucoepidermoid carcinoma vs. salivary duct carcinoma

Antibody	MEC	SDC
ARP	–	+
GCDFP-15	– or +	+ or –
S100	–	+ or –
Mucin	+	–
CK7	+	+

Note: *MEC* mucoepidermoid carcinoma, *SDC* salivary duct carcinoma, *ARP* androgen receptor protein

References: [1, 32–35]

Table 7.71 Adenoid cystic carcinoma vs. benign mixed tumor

Antibody	ACCA	BMT
CD117	+	–
GFAP	–	+ or –
MIB1 (Ki-67)	*4%	Usually <2%

Note: *ACCA* adenoid cystic carcinoma, *BMT* benign mixed tumor

A mean of 4% has been reported

References: [1, 32–35]

Table 7.72 Diagnostic panels for common thyroid neoplasms

Antibody	PTC	TFN	TMC	HTA	ATC
CK7	+	+	+	+	– or +
CK19	+	– or +	–	– or +	–
HBME-1	+	– or +	–	– or +	–
Galectin-3	+	– or +	– or +	– or +	+ or –
Calcitonin	–	–	+	–	–
CEA	–	–	+	–	–
Chromogranin	–	–	+	–	–
MIB1 (Ki-67)	N	N	N	M	N
PAX8	+	+	–	+	+ or –
TTF1	+	+	+, weak	+	–
Thyroglobulin	+	+	–	+	–

Note: *N* nuclear, *M* membranous, *PTC* papillary thyroid carcinoma, *TFN* thyroid follicular neoplasm, *TMC* thyroid medullary carcinoma, *HTA* hyalinizing trabecular adenoma, *ATC* anaplastic thyroid carcinoma

References: [1, 32–35]

Table 7.73 Diagnostic panel for lung small cell carcinoma, adenocarcinoma, and squamous cell carcinoma

Antibody	SCC	ADC	SQCC
CAM 5.2	+	+	+
CK7	– or +	+	– or patchy +
CK5/6	–	–	+
p63	– or +	– or patchy +	+
CD56	+	–	– or +
Synaptophysin	+	–	–
Chromogranin	Patchy + or –	–	–
TTF1	+	+	–
Napsin A	–	+	–
MIB1 (Ki-67)	Usually >30%	High	High

Note: *SCC* small cell carcinoma, *ADC* adenocarcinoma, *SQCC* squamous cell carcinoma

It has been reported in the literature that a small percentage of SQCCs may be positive for TTF1; however, our study ($N = 41$) demonstrated only one case with focal (5% of the tumor cells) positivity

References: [1, 32–35]

Table 7.74 Thymic carcinoma vs. lung adenocarcinoma

Antibody	Thymic carcinoma	LADC
TTF1	–	+
Napsin A	–	+
CD5	+	–
p63	+	–
CK7	+ or –	+

Note: *LADC* lung adenocarcinoma

References: [1, 32–35, 51, 54]

Table 7.75 Pancreatic adenocarcinoma vs. chronic pancreatitis

Antibody	PADC	CP
VHL	–	+
Maspin	+	–
S100P	+	–
IMP-3	+	–
CEA	+	–
MUC5AC	+	–

Note: *PADC* pancreatic adenocarcinoma, *CP* chronic pancreatitis

Our experience shows that the above panel is the most effective working panel to differentiate PADC from CP/reactive/benign pancreatic ducts. Caution should be taken as intrahepatic cholangiocarcinoma tends to demonstrate a reverse staining pattern for VHL and maspin (positive for VHL and negative or patchy positive for maspin). Ampullary adenocarcinoma may show a similar staining pattern as that of intrahepatic cholangiocarcinoma. An example of PADC on cellblock preparation with the positive staining for maspin, IMP-3 (KOC), and S100P, and loss of VHL expression is demonstrated in Fig. 7.11a–e

References: [1, 32–35, 43, 63]

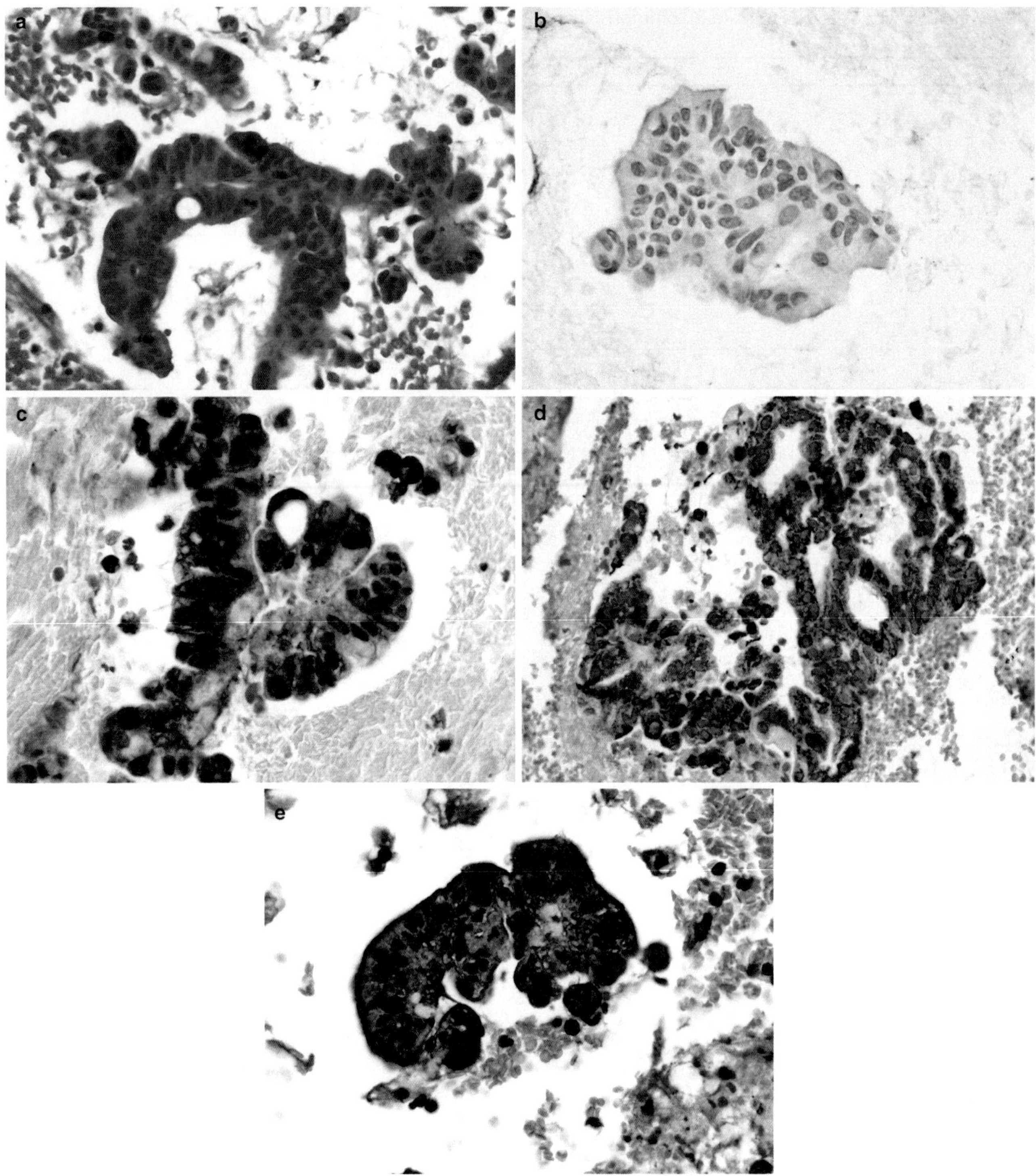

Fig. 7.11 (**a**–**e**) Expression of VHL, maspin, IMP-3, and S100P in a case of pancreatic adenocarcinoma on the cytology specimen. Note the loss of expression of VHL (**b**), and overexpression of maspin (**c**), IMP-3 (**d**), and S100P (**e**) in the tumor cells

Table 7.76 Diagnostic panel for pancreatic cystic lesions

Antibodies	MCN	SMA	GC	SIC
pVHL	–	+	–	–
NSE	–	+	–	–
MUC6	–	+	–	–
Inhibin-alpha	–	+	–	–
Maspin	+	–	+	–
Hep Par1	–	–	–	+
CK20	+ or –	–	+	+
CDX-2	+ or –	–	–	+
MUC5AC	+ or –	–	+	–

Note: *MCN* mucinous cystic neoplasm, *SMA* serous microcystic adenoma, *GC* gastric contaminants, *SIC* small intestinal contaminants

References: [1, 32–35, 64]

Table 7.77 Differential diagnosis of pancreatic endocrine neoplasm

Antibodies	PEN	DAC	ACC	SPN
CAM 5.2	+	+	+	– or patchy +
CK7	– or patchy +	+	– or patchy +	–
Maspin	–	+	–	–
Beta-catenin	M	M	M or N	N and M
Chromogranin	+	–	–	–
CD10	–	–	–	+
Trypsin	–	–	+	–
Vimentin	–	–	–	+

Note: *PEN* pancreatic endocrine neoplasm, *DAC* ductal adenocarcinoma, *ACC* acinar cell carcinoma, *SPN* solid–pseudopapillary neoplasm

References: [1, 32–35]

Note for All Tables

Note: "+" – usually greater than 70% of cases are positive; "–" – less than 5% of cases are positive; "+ or –" – usually more than 50% of cases are positive; "– or +" – less than 50% of cases are positive.

References

1. Dabbs DJ. Diagnostic immunohistochemistry. 3rd ed. Philadelphia, PA: Churchill Livingstone Elsevier; 2010.
2. Cheng L, Zhang S, Talerman A, Roth LM. Morphologic, immunohistochemical, and fluorescence in situ hybridization study of ovarian embryonal carcinoma with comparison to solid variant of yolk sac tumor and immature teratoma. Hum Pathol. 2010;41(5):716–23.
3. Kandil D, Leiman G, Allegretta M, Evans M. Glypican-3 protein expression in primary and metastatic melanoma: a combined immunohistochemistry and immunocytochemistry study. Cancer Cytopathol. 2009;117(4):271–8.
4. Maeda D, Ota S, Takazawa Y, et al. Glypican-3 expression in clear cell adenocarcinoma of the ovary. Mod Pathol. 2009;22(6):824–32.
5. Wang HL, Anatelli F, Zhai QJ, Adley B, Chuang ST, Yang XJ. Glypican-3 as a useful diagnostic marker that distinguishes hepatocellular carcinoma from benign hepatocellular mass lesions. Arch Pathol Lab Med. 2008;132(11):1723–8.
6. Baumhoer D, Tornillo L, Stadlmann S, Roncalli M, Diamantis EK, Terracciano LM. Glypican 3 expression in human nonneoplastic, preneoplastic, and neoplastic tissues: a tissue microarray analysis of 4,387 tissue samples. Am J Clin Pathol. 2008;129(6):899–906.
7. Herawi M, Drew PA, Pan CC, Epstein JI. Clear cell adenocarcinoma of the bladder and urethra: cases diffusely mimicking nephrogenic adenoma. Hum Pathol. 2010;41(4):594–601.
8. Chivukula M, Dabbs DJ, O'Connor S, Bhargava R. PAX2: a novel Mullerian marker for serous papillary carcinomas to differentiate from micropapillary breast carcinoma. Int J Gynecol Pathol. 2009;28(6):570–8.
9. Ozcan A, Zhai J, Hamilton C, et al. PAX-2 in the diagnosis of primary renal tumors: immunohistochemical comparison with renal cell carcinoma marker antigen and kidney-specific cadherin. Am J Clin Pathol. 2009;131(3):393–404.
10. Albadine R, Schultz L, Illei P, et al. PAX8 (+)/p63 (–) immunostaining pattern in renal collecting duct carcinoma (CDC): a useful immunoprofile in the differential diagnosis of CDC versus urothelial carcinoma of upper urinary tract. Am J Surg Pathol. 2010;34(7):965–9.
11. Long KB, Srivastava A, Hirsch MS, Hornick JL. PAX8 Expression in well-differentiated pancreatic endocrine tumors: correlation with clinicopathologic features and comparison with gastrointestinal and pulmonary carcinoid tumors. Am J Surg Pathol. 2010;34(5):723–9.
12. Laury AR, Hornick JL, Perets R, et al. PAX8 reliably distinguishes ovarian serous tumors from malignant mesothelioma. Am J Surg Pathol. 2010;34(5):627–35.
13. Cao D, Guo S, Allan RW, Molberg KH, Peng Y. SALL4 is a novel sensitive and specific marker of ovarian primitive germ cell tumors and is particularly useful in distinguishing yolk sac tumor from clear cell carcinoma. Am J Surg Pathol. 2009;33(6):894–904.
14. Miettinen M. Keratin 20: immunohistochemical marker for gastrointestinal, urothelial, and Merkel cell carcinomas. Mod Pathol. 1995;8(4):384–8.
15. Chu PG, Weiss LM. Expression of cytokeratin 5/6 in epithelial neoplasms: an immunohistochemical study of 509 cases. Mod Pathol. 2002;15(1):6–10.
16. Armah HB, Parwani AV. Xp11.2 translocation renal cell carcinoma. Arch Pathol Lab Med. 2010;134(1):124–9.
17. Hornick JL, Dal Cin P, Fletcher CD. Loss of INI1 expression is characteristic of both conventional and proximal-type epithelioid sarcoma. Am J Surg Pathol. 2009;33(4):542–50.
18. Cheng JX, Tretiakova M, Gong C, Mandal S, Krausz T, Taxy JB. Renal medullary carcinoma: rhabdoid features and the absence of INI1 expression as markers of aggressive behavior. Mod Pathol. 2008;21(6):647–52.
19. Vollmer RT. Primary lung cancer vs metastatic breast cancer: a probabilistic approach. Am J Clin Pathol. 2009;132(3):391–5.
20. Parker DC, Folpe AL, Bell J, et al. Potential utility of uroplakin III, thrombomodulin, high molecular weight cytokeratin, and cytokeratin 20 in noninvasive, invasive, and metastatic urothelial (transitional cell) carcinomas. Am J Surg Pathol. 2003;27(1):1–10.
21. Erickson LA, Papouchado B, Dimashkieh H, Zhang S, Nakamura N, Lloyd RV. Cdx2 as a marker for neuroendocrine tumors of unknown primary sites. Endocr Pathol. 2004;15(3):247–52.
22. Chu P, Arber DA. Paraffin-section detection of CD10 in 505 nonhematopoietic neoplasms. Frequent expression in renal cell carcinoma and endometrial stromal sarcoma. Am J Clin Pathol. 2000;113(3):374–82.

23. Miettinen M, Sarlomo-Rikala M. Expression of calretinin, thrombomodulin, keratin 5, and mesothelin in lung carcinomas of different types: an immunohistochemical analysis of 596 tumors in comparison with epithelioid mesotheliomas of the pleura. Am J Surg Pathol. 2003;27(2):150–8.
24. Miettinen M, Franssila KO. Variable expression of keratins and nearly uniform lack of thyroid transcription factor 1 in thyroid anaplastic carcinoma. Hum Pathol. 2000;31(9):1139–45.
25. Wennerberg AE, Nalesnik MA, Coleman WB. Hepatocyte paraffin 1: a monoclonal antibody that reacts with hepatocytes and can be used for differential diagnosis of hepatic tumors. Am J Pathol. 1993;143(4):1050–4.
26. Chu PG, Ishizawa S, Wu E, Weiss LM. Hepatocyte antigen as a marker of hepatocellular carcinoma: an immunohistochemical comparison to carcinoembryonic antigen, CD10, and alpha-fetoprotein. Am J Surg Pathol. 2002;26(8):978–88.
27. Wang HL, Lu DW, Yerian LM, et al. Immunohistochemical distinction between primary adenocarcinoma of the bladder and secondary colorectal adenocarcinoma. Am J Surg Pathol. 2001;25(11):1380–7.
28. Hishima T, Fukayama M, Fujisawa M, et al. CD5 expression in thymic carcinoma. Am J Pathol. 1994;145(2):268–75.
29. Jones TD, Ulbright TM, Eble JN, Baldridge LA, Cheng L. OCT4 staining in testicular tumors: a sensitive and specific marker for seminoma and embryonal carcinoma. Am J Surg Pathol. 2004;28(7):935–40.
30. Binh MB, Sastre-Garau X, Guillou L, et al. MDM2 and CDK4 immunostainings are useful adjuncts in diagnosing well-differentiated and dedifferentiated liposarcoma subtypes: a comparative analysis of 559 soft tissue neoplasms with genetic data. Am J Surg Pathol. 2005;29(10):1340–7.
31. Kumar S, Perlman E, Harris CA, Raffeld M, Tsokos M. Myogenin is a specific marker for rhabdomyosarcoma: an immunohistochemical study in paraffin-embedded tissues. Mod Pathol. 2000;13(9):988–93.
32. Taylor C, Cote R, editors. Immunomicroscopy: a diagnostic tool for the surgical pathologist. Major problems in pathology, vol. 19. 3rd ed. Philadelphia, PA: Saunders Elsevier; 2006.
33. Chu PG, Weiss LM. Modern immunohistochemistry. New York, NY: Cambridge University Press; 2009.
34. Bahrami A, Truong LD, Ro JY. Undifferentiated tumor: true identity by immunohistochemistry. Arch Pathol Lab Med. 2008;132(3): 326–48.
35. Krishna M. Diagnosis of metastatic neoplasms: an immunohistochemical approach. Arch Pathol Lab Med. 2010;134(2): 207–15.
36. Bishop JA, Sharma R, Illei PB. Napsin A and thyroid transcription factor-1 expression in carcinomas of the lung, breast, pancreas, colon, kidney, thyroid, and malignant mesothelioma. Hum Pathol. 2010;41(1):20–5.
37. Dejmek A, Naucler P, Smedjeback A, et al. Napsin A (TA02) is a useful alternative to thyroid transcription factor-1 (TTF-1) for the identification of pulmonary adenocarcinoma cells in pleural effusions. Diagn Cytopathol. 2007;35(8):493–7.
38. Pallesen G, Hamilton-Dutoit SJ. Ki-1 (CD30) antigen is regularly expressed by tumor cells of embryonal carcinoma. Am J Pathol. 1988;133(3):446–50.
39. Jiang Z, Fanger GR, Woda BA, et al. Expression of alpha-methylacyl-CoA racemase (P504s) in various malignant neoplasms and normal tissues: a study of 761 cases. Hum Pathol. 2003;34(8):792–6.
40. Tretiakova MS, Sahoo S, Takahashi M, et al. Expression of alpha-methylacyl-CoA racemase in papillary renal cell carcinoma. Am J Surg Pathol. 2004;28(1):69–76.
41. Levy M, Lin F, Xu H, Dhall D, Spaulding BO, Wang HL. S100P, von Hippel-Lindau gene product, and IMP3 serve as a useful immunohistochemical panel in the diagnosis of adenocarcinoma of endoscopic bile duct biopsy. Hum Pathol. 2010;41:1210–9.
42. Lin F, Shi J, Liu H, et al. Immunohistochemical detection of the von Hippel-Lindau gene product (pVHL) in human tissues and tumors: a useful marker for metastatic renal cell carcinoma and clear cell carcinoma of the ovary and uterus. Am J Clin Pathol. 2008; 129(4):592–605.
43. Lin F, Shi J, Liu H, et al. Diagnostic utility of S100P and von Hippel-Lindau gene product (pVHL) in pancreatic adenocarcinoma-with implication of their roles in early tumorigenesis. Am J Surg Pathol. 2008;32(1):78–91.
44. Lin F, Zhang PL, Yang XJ, et al. Human kidney injury molecule-1 (hKIM-1): a useful immunohistochemical marker for diagnosing renal cell carcinoma and ovarian clear cell carcinoma. Am J Surg Pathol. 2007;31(3):371–81.
45. Adley BP, Gupta A, Lin F, Luan C, Teh BT, Yang XJ. Expression of kidney-specific cadherin in chromophobe renal cell carcinoma and renal oncocytoma. Am J Clin Pathol. 2006;126(1):79–85.
46. Lin F, Yang W, Betten M, Teh BT, Yang XJ, French Kidney Cancer Study Group. Expression of S-100 protein in renal cell neoplasms. Hum Pathol. 2006;37(4):462–70.
47. Coston WM, Loera S, Lau SK, et al. Distinction of hepatocellular carcinoma from benign hepatic mimickers using Glypican-3 and CD34 immunohistochemistry. Am J Surg Pathol. 2008;32(3):433–44.
48. Lau SK, Weiss LM, Chu PG. D2-40 immunohistochemistry in the differential diagnosis of seminoma and embryonal carcinoma: a comparative immunohistochemical study with KIT (CD117) and CD30. Mod Pathol. 2007;20(3):320–5.
49. Lau SK, Weiss LM, Chu PG. Differential expression of MUC1, MUC2, and MUC5AC in carcinomas of various sites: an immunohistochemical study. Am J Clin Pathol. 2004;122(1):61–9.
50. Ushiku T, Shinozaki A, Shibahara J, et al. SALL4 represents fetal gut differentiation of gastric cancer, and is diagnostically useful in distinguishing hepatoid gastric carcinoma from hepatocellular carcinoma. Am J Surg Pathol. 2010;34(4):533–40.
51. Tateyama H, Eimoto T, Tada T, Hattori H, Murase T, Takino H. Immunoreactivity of a new CD5 antibody with normal epithelium and malignant tumors including thymic carcinoma. Am J Clin Pathol. 1999;111(2):235–40.
52. Cheuk W, Kwan MY, Suster S, Chan JK. Immunostaining for thyroid transcription factor 1 and cytokeratin 20 aids the distinction of small cell carcinoma from Merkel cell carcinoma, but not pulmonary from extrapulmonary small cell carcinomas. Arch Pathol Lab Med. 2001;125(2):228–31.
53. Miettinen M. Keratin immunohistochemistry: update of applications and pitfalls. Pathol Annu. 1993;28(Pt 2):113–43.
54. Chu PG, Arber DA, Weiss LM. Expression of T/NK-cell and plasma cell antigens in nonhematopoietic epithelioid neoplasms. An immunohistochemical study of 447 cases. Am J Clin Pathol. 2003; 120(1):64–70.
55. Kandil DH, Cooper K. Glypican-3: a novel diagnostic marker for hepatocellular carcinoma and more. Adv Anat Pathol. 2009;16(2):125–9.
56. Folpe AL, Hill CE, Parham DM, O'Shea PA, Weiss SW. Immunohistochemical detection of FLI-1 protein expression: a study of 132 round cell tumors with emphasis on CD99-positive mimics of Ewing's sarcoma/primitive neuroectodermal tumor. Am J Surg Pathol. 2000;24(12):1657–62.
57. Liu H, Shi J, Liang K, Meschter S, Lin F. Loss of or reduced expression of the von Hipple-Linadu gene product (pVHL) in malignant salivary epithelial neoplasms – with an implication of its role in tumorigenesis [USACP abstract 1089]. Mod Pathol. 2008;21(Suppl 1s):238A.
58. Chen ZM, Wang HL. Alteration of cytokeratin 7 and cytokeratin 20 expression profile is uniquely associated with tumorigenesis of

primary adenocarcinoma of the small intestine. Am J Surg Pathol. 2004;28(10):1352–9.

59. Chen ZM, Ritter JH, Wang HL. Differential expression of alpha-methylacyl coenzyme A racemase in adenocarcinomas of the small and large intestines. Am J Surg Pathol. 2005;29(7):890–6.
60. Zhang MQ, Chen ZM, Wang HL. Immunohistochemical investigation of tumorigenic pathways in small intestinal adenocarcinoma: a comparison with colorectal adenocarcinoma. Mod Pathol. 2006;19(4):573–80.
61. Zhang MQ, Lin F, Hui P, Chen ZM, Ritter JH, Wang HL. Expression of mucins, SIMA, villin, and CDX2 in small-intestinal adenocarcinoma. Am J Clin Pathol. 2007;128(5):808–16.
62. Mac MT, Chung F, Lin F, Hui P, Balzer BL, Wang HL. Expression of hepatocyte antigen in small intestinal epithelium and adenocarcinoma. Am J Clin Pathol. 2009;132(1):80–5.
63. Anandan V, Shi J, Liu H, Meschter S, Lin F. Identification of an effective antibody panel in the diagnosis of pancreatic ductal adenocarcinoma on fine needle aspiration biopsy specimens [USACP abstract 381]. Mod Pathol. 2010;23(Suppl 1s):87A.
64. Lin F, Shi J, Liu H, Wilkerson M, Meschter S. S100P, pVHL, CDX2 and mucicarmine are a panel of useful markers in distinguishing mucin-producing neoplasms of the pancreas from gastrointestinal contaminants [American Society of Cytopathology Platform Presentation PF08]. Cancer Cytopathol. 2008;114(Suppl S5):347.

Chapter 8
Exfoliative Cytopathology

Steven Meschter and Jan F. Silverman

Abstract Exfoliative cytology is often challenging. Correct diagnosis can be significantly enhanced by the use of cellblocks and immunocytochemical assays. This chapter offers panels of immunocytochemical assays that are designed to assist in differentiating commonly encountered processes in effusions. For example, adenocarcinomas of the lung or breast can be difficult to distinguish from reactive mesothelial cells or from epithelioid mesotheliomas using morphology alone. Other commonly encountered dilemmas include classifying malignant cells of undetermined primary sites. Undifferentiated tumor cells may also be tricky and panels to initiate classification are provided. Details for producing an adequate cellblock are discussed.

Keywords Effusion • Adenocarcinoma • Epithelioid mesothelioma • Reactive mesothelial cells • Lymphoma • Calretinin • TTF-1 • MOC-31

FREQUENTLY ASKED QUESTIONS

Diagnosis Question List

1. Antibody list (Table 8.1) (pp. 86–87)
2. What is the immunohistochemical phenotype for malignant epithelioid mesothelioma in an effusion? (Fig. 8.1, Table 8.2) (p. 88)
3. What is the immunohistochemical phenotype for lung carcinoma in effusions? (Fig. 8.2, Table 8.3) (pp. 88–89)
4. What is the immunohistochemical phenotype for small cell carcinoma in effusions? (Figs. 8.3 and 8.4, Table 8.4) (pp. 89–90)
5. What is the immunohistochemical phenotype for melanoma in effusions? (Table 8.5) (p. 90)
6. What is the immunohistochemical phenotype for breast carcinoma in effusions? (Female effusions: Table 8.6) (p. 90)
7. What is the immunohistochemical phenotype for clear cell renal cell carcinoma in effusions? (Effusions: Table 8.7) (p. 90)
8. What is the immunohistochemical phenotype for urothelial carcinoma in effusions? (Effusions: Table 8.8) (p. 90)
9. What immunophenotype can resolve reactive mesothelium vs. epithelioid malignant mesothelioma? (Pleural/pericardial effusions: Table 8.9) (p. 91)
10. What is the immunohistochemical phenotype for epithelioid mesothelioma vs. lung adenocarcinoma in effusions? (Pleural/pericardial effusions: Table 8.10) (p. 91)
11. What is the immunohistochemical phenotype for epithelioid mesothelioma vs. breast carcinoma in female pleural/pericardial effusions? (Pleural/pericardial effusions: Table 8.11) (p. 91)
12. What immunophenotype would help distinguish lung carcinoma vs. breast carcinoma in a female pleural/pericardial effusion? (Pleural/pericardial effusion: Table 8.12) (p. 91)
13. What is a good screening panel for classifying poorly differentiated malignant cells in an effusion? (Effusion screening panel: triage of malignant effusion cell type: Table 8.13) (p. 92)
14. What is the immunohistochemical phenotype for epithelioid mesothelioma vs. squamous cell carcinoma in effusions? (Pleural/pericardial effusions: Table 8.14) (p. 93)
15. What is the immunohistochemical phenotype for clear cell variant of mesothelioma vs. clear cell renal cell carcinoma in effusions? (Pleural/pericardial effusions, peritoneal: Table 8.15) (p. 93)
16. What is the immunohistochemical phenotype for sarcomatoid carcinoma vs. sarcomatoid mesothelioma in effusions? (Pleural/pericardial effusions: Table 8.16) (p. 93)
17. What is the immunohistochemical phenotype for mesothelioma vs. nongynecologic adenocarcinoma (colonic carcinoma, gastric carcinoma, pancreatic carcinoma, and bile duct carcinoma) in peritoneal effusions in males? (Peritoneal effusions, male: Fig. 8.5, Table 8.17) (pp. 93–94)

S. Meschter (✉)
Department of Pathology and Laboratory Medicine, Geisinger Medical Center, 100 North Academy Avenue, Danville, PA 17822, USA
e-mail: smeschter@geisinger.edu

F. Lin and J. Prichard (eds.), *Handbook of Practical Immunohistochemistry: Frequently Asked Questions*,
DOI 10.1007/978-1-4419-8062-5_8,

18. What is the immunohistochemical phenotype for peritoneal malignant mesothelioma (PMM) vs. papillary serous carcinoma (PSC) in female peritoneal effusions? (Peritoneal effusions, female: Table 8.18) (p. 94)
19. What is the immunohistochemical phenotype for ovary (mucinous and endometrioid) vs. colon in female peritoneal effusions? (Female peritoneal effusions: Table 8.19) (p. 94)
20. What is the immunohistochemical phenotype for ovary vs. breast vs. colon in female peritoneal effusions? (Female peritoneal effusions: Table 8.20) (p. 95)
21. What immunophenotype might help to resolve ovarian adenocarcinoma vs. metastatic pancreatic/bile duct carcinoma in female peritoneal effusions? (Peritoneal effusions, female: Table 8.21) (p. 95)
22. What is the immunohistochemical phenotype for selected lymphomas/leukemias in effusions? (Effusions: Figs. 8.6 and 8.7, Table 8.22) (pp. 95–96)
23. What is the immunohistochemical phenotype for small round cell tumors in adult effusions? (Pleural/pericardial/peritoneal: Table 8.23) (p. 97)
24. What is the immunohistochemical phenotype for small round cell tumors in pediatric effusions? (Pleural/pericardial/peritoneal: Table 8.24) (p. 98)
25. What is the immunohistochemical phenotype for seminoma vs. nonseminomatous germ cell tumors (NSGCT) in effusions? (Effusions: Table 8.25) (p. 98)
26. What are the advantages of using cellblocks for immunohistochemical analysis in exfoliative cytopathology? (p. 92)
27. How is the cellblock prepared? (p. 92)

Table 8.1 Antibody list

Antibody	Staining pattern	Comment
MOC31	M	In effusions, stains adenocarcinoma
BerEP4	M	Lung adenocarcinoma, breast carcinoma
Calretinin	C/N	Mesothelium and epithelioid mesothelioma
WT-1 protein	C/N	Expressed in mesothelioma, serous ovarian carcinoma, and primary peritoneal serous carcinoma
Podoplanin (D2-40)	M	Reactive mesothelium and mesothelioma
CK5/6	C[a]	Mesothelium and mesothelioma, poorly differentiated squamous carcinoma
B72.3	C	Tumor-associated glycoprotein, adenocarcinoma
ER (estrogen receptor)	N	Breast carcinoma, endometrium, ovary
GCDFP-15	C	Marker of breast carcinoma
TTF-1	N	Marker for lung carcinomas and thyroid carcinoma. Helpful in distinguishing pulmonary adenocarcinoma from epithelioid mesothelioma
CK7	C	Breast, lung, ovary, and urothelial carcinoma
CK20	C	Cytokeratin associated with colon carcinoma. Also shows a specific paranuclear dot pattern in small cell carcinomas of the skin (Merkel cell carcinoma)
CKAE1,3	C	Broad spectrum cytokeratin cocktail useful for identifying epithelial tumors
CAM5.2	C	When combined with CKAE1,3, this low molecular weight cytokeratin (detects CK18) provides a broad spectrum of keratins for the purpose of identifying epithelial tumors
P63	N	Marker useful in identifying poorly differentiated squamous cell carcinoma
CEA	C	Lung, colon, and breast carcinoma
BG8 (Lewis Y antigen)	M/C	Blood group-related antigen lung, adenocarcinoma, breast carcinoma
CD15 (Leu-M1)	M/C	Granulocyte-associated antigen positive in various carcinomas including lung, breast, colon, pancreas, and prostate
CA19-9	M/C[b]	Marker for pancreatic carcinoma
EMA	M	Glandular and ductal epithelial differentiation. Expressed by adenocarcinomas and mesotheliomas
HMFG-2	M/C	Human milk fat globulin protein-2 useful in resolving carcinoma vs. reactive mesothelium
Thrombomodulin	M/C	Marker for mesothelial cells. Also can be used in a panel to identify urothelial carcinoma
E-cadherin	M	Transmembrane epithelial protein associated with cellular adhesion
CD45 (LCA)	M/C	Useful for identifying tumor cells of lymphoid origin
CD20	M	Lymphocytes of B-cell linage
CD3	M	T-cell lymphocyte marker
TdT	N	Marker for acute lymphoblastic lymphoma/leukemia
Desmin	C	In serous effusions, useful in identifying reactive mesothelium
CD30	M	Anaplastic large cell lymphoma and Hodgkins lymphoma (Reed–Sternberg cells), primary effusion lymphoma
CD138	M	Plasma cell marker
HMB-45	C	Used to confirm melanoma
Mart-1	C	Marker for melanoma

(continued)

Table 8.1 (continued)

Antibody	Staining pattern	Comment
Vimentin	C	Good screening assay for poorly differentiated tumors where melanoma is suspected. Can be used in conjunction with other cytokeratin to identify epithelial tumors that coexpress vimentin and cytokeratin
S100	C/N (both must be positive)	Good screening assay for poorly differentiated tumors where melanoma is suspected
HBME-1	C/M	Human mesothelial cell antibody, for identifying mesothelial differentiation
CD56	M	Marker for poorly differentiated small cell carcinoma and other neuroendocrine carcinomas. Also found on NK cells and NK lymphomas
Neuron-specific enolase	C	Marker of neuroendocrine differentiation
Synaptophysin	C	Marker of neuroendocrine differentiation
Chromogranin	C	Marker of neuroendocrine differentiation
CD79a	M	Marker of B-cell lymphocytes
Pax-5	N	Marker for B-cell linage lymphomas
ALK-1	C/N	Marker for anaplastic large cell lymphoma
CD45rb	M/C	Marker for nucleated cells of hematopoietic origin
HHV-8		Marker associated with primary effusion lymphoma
CD117	M	Marker in acute myelogenous leukemia and in plasma cell tumors. Also can be used to identify seminomas
Myeloperoxidase	C	Marker for acute myelogenous leukemia and granulocytic cell sarcomas
CD31	M (not cytoplasmic)	Confirms vascular origin of tumors
CD34	M	Useful in identifying an epithelioid angiosarcoma or hemangioendothelioma. Also may be used to identify acute leukemic blasts
PR (progesterone receptor)	N	Breast carcinoma, endometrium, ovary
Androgen receptor	N	Useful as a breast marker
Mammaglobin	C	Useful as a breast marker
Napsin A	C	Marker for adenocarcinoma of the lung
ES-1	C	Marker for adenocarcinoma of the lung
PLAP	C	Marker for germ cell tumors, useful with seminoma
OCT-4	N	Marker for germ cell tumor, useful for seminoma and embryonal cell carcinoma
CD117	M	Can be used to identify seminoma
Alpha feto protein	C	Marker for distinguishing germ cell tumors (yolk-sac tumor)
Beta-HCG	C	Marker for germ cell tumor (choriocarcinoma)
HLA-G	M	Marker for germ cell tumor (choriocarcinoma)
Inhibin	C	Marker for germ cell tumor (choriocarcinoma). Also positive in adrenal cortical carcinoma
GCP-3	M	Marker for germ cell tumors
CD99	M	Marker for Ewing's sarcoma/PNET, lymphoblastic lymphoma/leukemia, myelogenous leukemia, granulocytic sarcoma, and desmoplastic small round cell tumor
Myo-D1	N	Marker for myoblasts in developing skeletal muscle
H-caldesmon	N/C	Marker for mesothelioma
Mesothelin	M[b]	Marker of mesothelioma
Glut-1	M/C	Reactive mesothelium vs. mesothelioma
Pax-2	N	Marker for clear cell variant of renal cell carcinoma
CD10	M/C	Marker for glomerular epithelial cells and brush border of proximal convoluted tubules (kidney marker)
MUC5AC	C and extracellular	Mucin in mucinous ovarian carcinoma
Beta-catenin	M/C	Marker for colon carcinoma
RCC	M/C	Marker for primary renal cell carcinoma clear cell type
CDX-2	N	Marker for colonic carcinoma
MITF	N	Marker for melanoma
Tyrosinase	C	Marker for melanoma
Uroplakin	M	Marker for urothelial carcinoma
CA-125	M/C	Marker for ovarian carcinoma
P53	N	Is useful in discriminating reactive mesothelium from epithelioid mesothelioma

[a]Cytoplasmic staining with perinuclear enhancement

[b]Apical

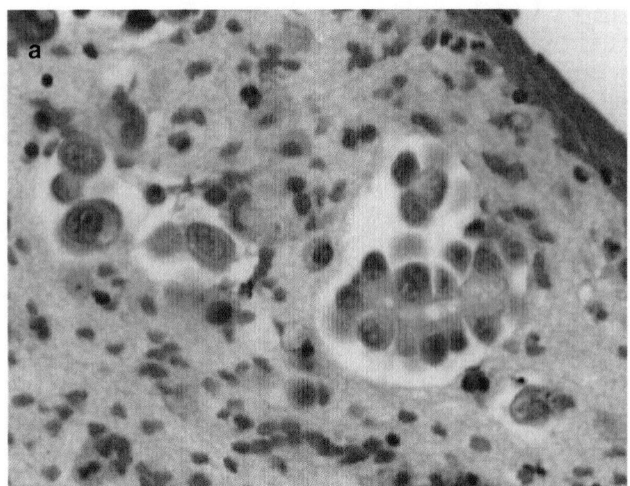

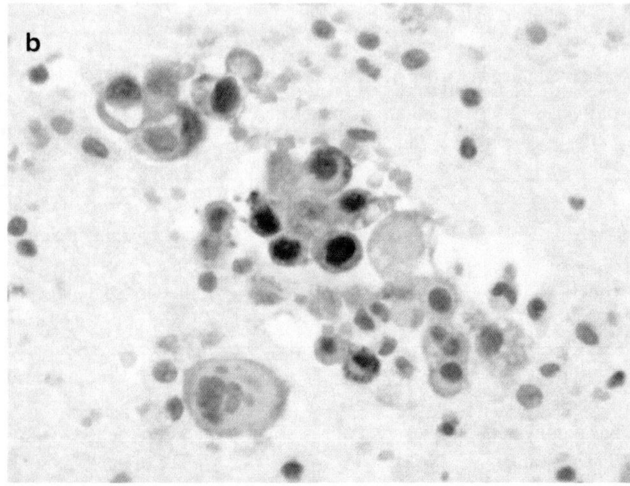

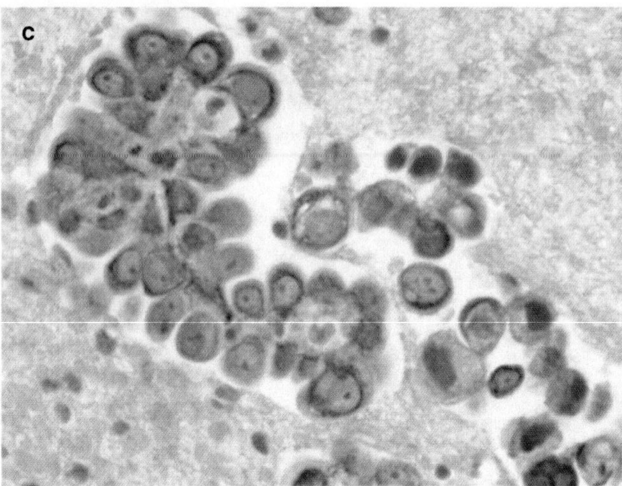

Fig. 8.1 Epithelioid mesothelioma: (**a**) H&E, (**b**) calretinin, (**c**) CK5/6, (×450)

Table 8.2 Effusions: epithelioid mesothelioma

Antibody	Mesothelioma
Calretinin	+
CK5/6	+
WT-1	+
Podoplanin (D2-40)	+
MOC-31	−
B72.3	−
BerEp4	−
TTF-1	−
mCEA[a]	−
BG8 (Lewis Y antigen)	−
CD15	−
Pancytokeratin	+
CKAE1,3	+

A minimal panel includes pancytokeratin, two mesothelial markers, and two adenocarcinoma markers as recommended by the International Mesothelioma Panel

WT-1 shows strong nuclear staining in mesothelioma

Positive staining with TTF-1, even if only focally, is very strong evidence that the tumor is not a mesothelioma. There is no reported case of a confirmed mesothelioma that is positive with TTF-1

[a]**Note**: mCEA is monoclonal. pCEA, or polyclonal CEA will stain histiocytes.

References: [1, 2]

Table 8.3 Effusions: lung carcinoma

Antibody	Reaction
Thyroid transcription factor-1 (TTF-1)	+/−
CK7	+/−
P63	−/+
CK5/6	−/+
ES1	+
Napsin A	+

Note: While not specific for the purpose of diagnosis, immunocytochemical markers can be helpful in classifying poorly differentiated nonsmall cell carcinomas of the lung. A panel of four markers is useful: CK7, TTF-1 (positive in adenocarcinomas, and negative in squamous cell carcinoma), and p63, CK5/6 (positive in squamous cell carcinomas and negative in adenocarcinomas). These results are helpful in directing the selection of chemotherapy agents for these patients.

References: [3–5]

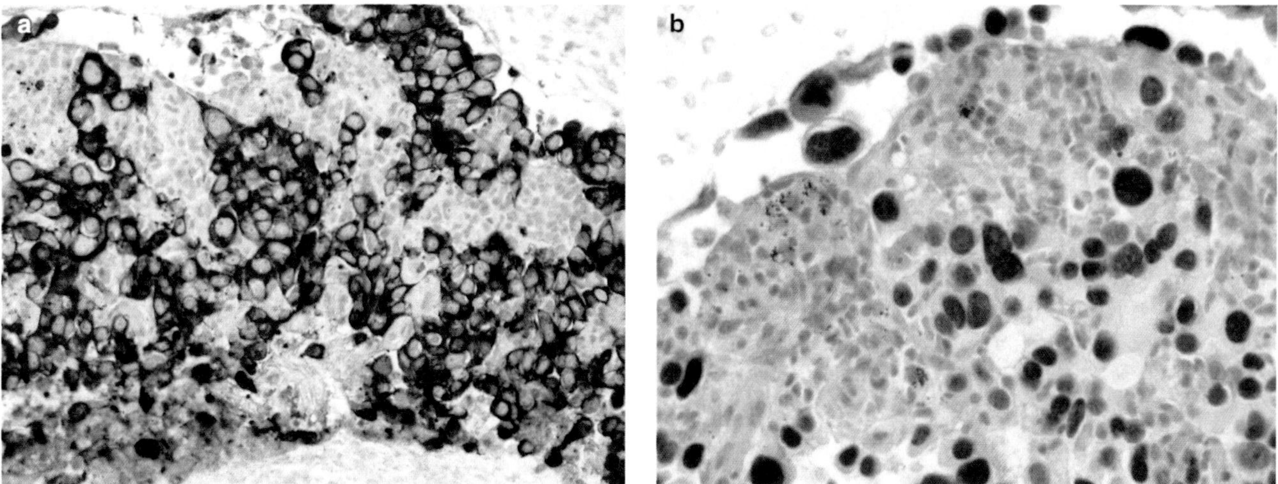

Fig. 8.2 Non-small cell carcinoma of lung, favor adenocarcinoma: (**a**) CK7 (**b**) TTF-1 (×450)

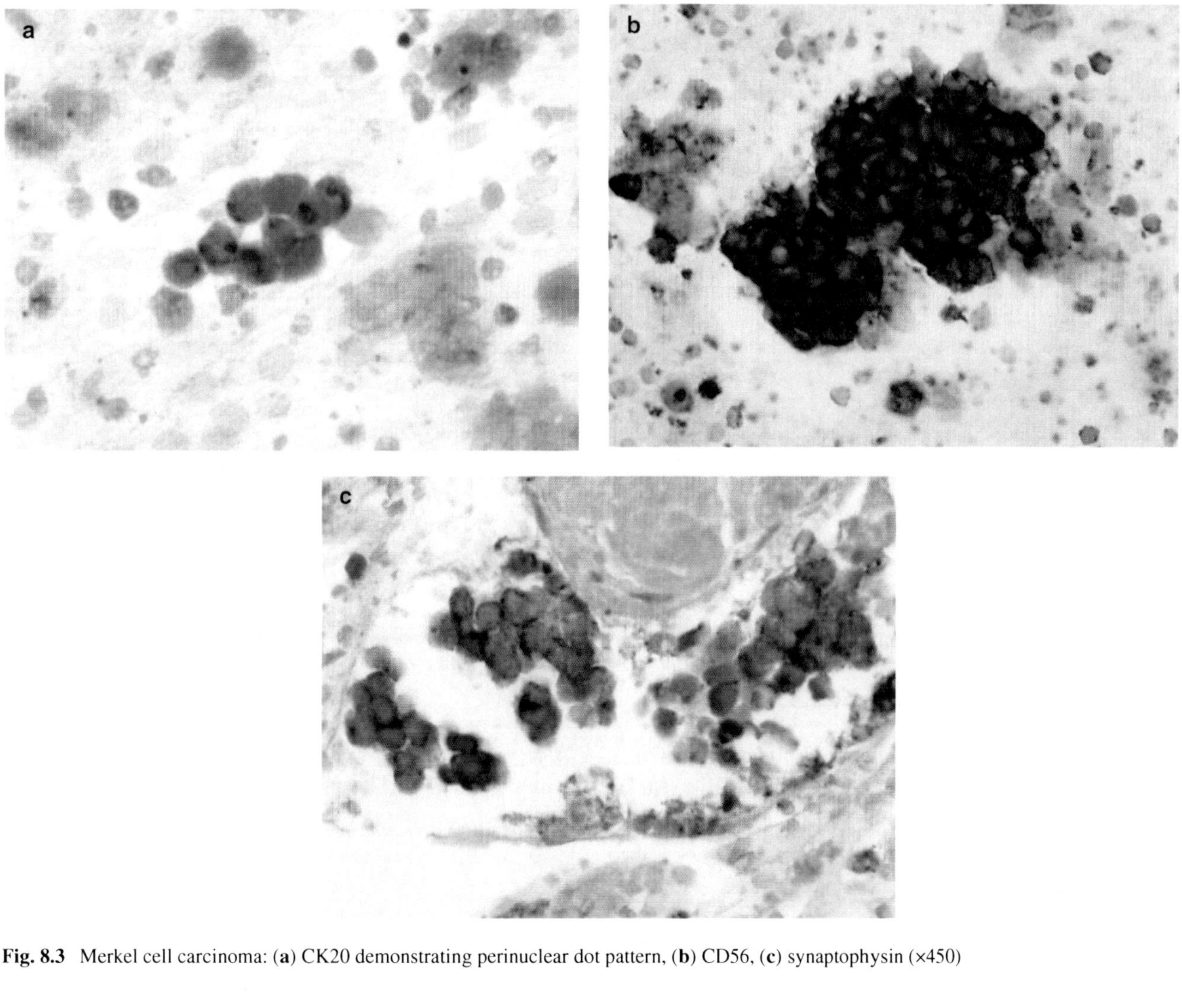

Fig. 8.3 Merkel cell carcinoma: (**a**) CK20 demonstrating perinuclear dot pattern, (**b**) CD56, (**c**) synaptophysin (×450)

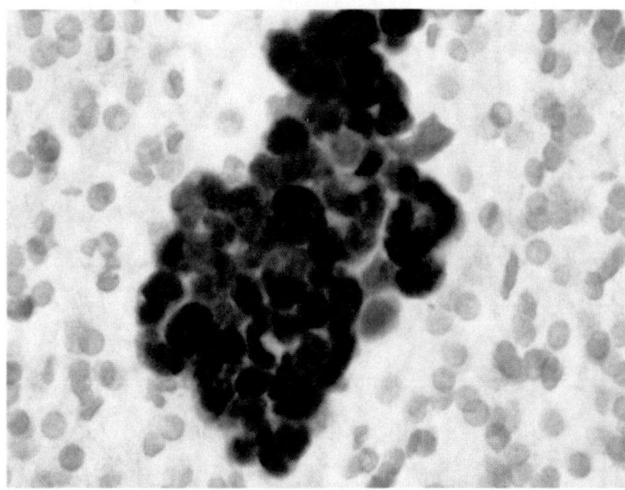

Fig. 8.4 Small cell carcinoma of lung: TTF-1 (×450)

Table 8.4 Effusions: small cell carcinoma

Antibody	Primary site
Cam 5.2	+/– (All sites)
CKAE1,3	+/– (All sites)
NSE	+ (All sites)
CD56	+ (All sites)
Synaptophysin	+/– (All sites)
Chromogranin	–/+ (All sites)
CK20 paranuclear punctate pattern	+ (Merkel cell, SCC of skin)
TTF-1	+ (Lung)
Estrogen receptor/progesterone receptor	–/+ (Breast)
CDX-2	+/– (Colon/small intestine)

References: [3,6]

Table 8.5 Effusions: melanoma

Antibody	Reaction
S100	+[a]
HMB-45	+
Melan A/MART 1	+
Vimentin	+
MITF (microphthalmia transcription factor)	+/–
Tyrosinase	+

[a]**Note**: S100 is the only of these markers that is reliably positive in desmoplastic variants of malignant melanoma. These tumors are frequently negative with HMB45, Melan A/MART-1, MITF, and tyrosinase

Reference: [6]

Table 8.6 Effusions, female: breast carcinoma

Antibody	Reaction
Estrogen	+
Progesterone	+/–
Androgen receptor	+/–[a]
Gross cystic disease fluid protein-15 (GCDFP-15)	+/–[b]
CK7	+
Mammaglobin	+/–[c]

[a]High-grade breast carcinomas, particularly as a metastasis show a high percentage of staining with androgen (82%)

[b]GCDFP-15 will decorate some skin adnexal tumors with apocrine differentiation

[c]Mammaglobulin is not very specific and will be positive in salivary gland carcinomas and endometrial carcinomas

References: [3, 7–9]

Table 8.7 Effusions: clear cell renal cell carcinoma

Antibody	Renal cell carcinoma clear cell type
CK7	–
CK20	–
Vimentin	+
RCC	+
CD10	+
CEA	–
CAM 5.2	+
Pax-2	+

References: [10, 11]

Table 8.8 Effusions: urothelial carcinoma

Antibody	Urothelial carcinoma
CK7	+
CK20	+
Uroplakin	+
Thrombomodulin	+
P63	+
CK5/6	–/+
EMA	+

References: [10, 12, 13]

Table 8.9 Pleural/pericardial effusions: benign/reactive mesothelium vs. epithelioid mesothelioma

Antibody	Benign mesothelium	Malignant mesothelioma
Desmin	+	−/+
EMA	−/+	+
P53	−	−/+
GLUT-1	−	+

References: [1, 14–18]

Table 8.10 Pleural/pericardial effusions: lung adenocarcinoma vs. epithelioid mesothelioma

Antibody	Adenocarcinoma	Mesothelioma
Calretinin	−/+	+
CK5/6	−/+	+
WT-1	−	+[a]
Podoplanin (D2-40)	−	+
H-caldesmon	−	+
MOC-31	+	−/+
B72.3	+	−
BerEp4	+	−/+
TTF-1	+	−[b]
CEA	+	−
BG8	+	−
CD15	+	−
CKAE1,3	+	+

Note: A minimal panel for establishing the diagnosis of epithelioid mesothelioma includes CKAE1,3 (pancytokeratin), two mesothelial markers, and two adenocarcinoma markers as recommended by the International Mesothelioma Panel

[a] WT-1 shows strong nuclear staining in mesothelioma, but may show granular cytoplasmic staining in adenocarcinoma of the lung and endothelial cells

[b] Positive staining with TTF-1, even if only focally, is very strong evidence that the tumor is not a mesothelioma. There is no reported case of a confirmed mesothelioma that is positive with TTF-1

References: [1, 19–33]

Table 8.11 Pleural effusion/pericardial, effusions, female: breast carcinoma vs. epithelioid mesothelioma

Antibody	Breast carcinoma	Mesothelioma
Calretinin	−/+	+
CK5/6	−/+	+
WT-1	−	+
Podoplanin (D2-40)	−	+
Estrogen receptor	+	−
Progesterone receptor	+	−
Gross cystic disease fluid protein (GCDFP)	+	−
BG8	+	−
MOC-31	+	−/+
CKAE1,3	+	+
CEA	+	−

Note: A minimal panel for the diagnosis of mesothelioma includes CKAE1,3 (pancytokeratin), two mesothelial markers, and two breast markers as recommended by the International Mesothelioma Panel

References: [1, 20–23, 28, 34]

Table 8.12 Pleural effusion/pericardial, effusions, female: primary lung carcinoma vs. breast carcinoma

Antibody	Lung carcinoma	Breast carcinoma
TTF-1	+	−
GCDFP-15	−	+/−
Estrogen receptor (ER)	−	+
Progesterone receptor (PR)	−	+/−
Mammaglobulin	−/+	+
CK7	+	+
Androgen	−	+
Napsin A	+[a]	−

Note: Some well-differentiated adenocarcinomas of the lung may show some estrogen receptor positivity with the Ventana antibody. Similar tumors are usually negative with the Dako estrogen antibody

[a] Napsin A is specific for adenocarcinomas of the lung

References: [35–37]

8.1 Discussion

8.1.1 Why Use Cellblock Preparations for Immunohistochemical Analysis?

There are a number of technical challenges implicit in performing immunohistochemistry on cytologic preparations. Although there are published procedures available for performing immunohistochemistry on direct smears and other intact cellular preparations (cytospins, thin-layer preparations, etc.), these are limited by significant short comings. Standard immunohistochemical procedures intended for histologic tissue sections need to be separately tested, adjusted, and validated on cytologic preparations due to the variety of fixation methods (alcohol based), the fact that the cells remain intact, and the variations in cellular volume/thickness in these preparations. Control materials, whether cytologic or histologic are also a challenge. A very valuable alternative for establishing a standardized series of protocols is the use of cellblock preparations.

Cellblock preparations using fresh cellular materials are fixed in formalin and processed via the identical procedures utilized for paraffin-embedded tissues. These can generate multiple sections (ten or more depending on cellularity), which are then subjected to validated immunohistochemical procedures. The cellular materials are sectioned via a microtome and internal cellular antigens are readily exposed to the antibody solutions. Control tissues prepared for standard tissue sections are suitable as controls for the cellblock sections and the results are equivalent to other paraffin-embedded tissues. The basic shortcoming of this procedure is in cases of cytologic preparations with very limited cellularity (such as cerebral spinal fluid). This circumstance is fortunately infrequently encountered in the case of most effusions or other exfoliative cytologic specimens.

8.1.2 How Is the Cellblock Prepared?

Procedure: Plasma-thrombin cell block technique for use with fresh fluids not containing natural clot. Clotted specimens can be fixed in formalin directly (proceed to step 8):

1. Label 50 ml falcon tubes and Histology cassette with Accession #.
2. Spin down specimen in labeled 50 ml falcon tubes for 10 min at 2,000 rpm in preset centrifuge.
3. Remove falcon tubes from centrifuge, pour off supernatant, taking care to preserve cell button.
4. Add approximately five drops of Plasma[1] to cell button and resuspend as appropriate.
5. Add approximately five drops of Thrombin[2] and let stand for 10 min.
6. Add 10–20 ml formalin to tube and fix for 1 h.

[1] Screened plasma is obtained from Blood Bank, divided into 20–50 ml aliquots in Falcon tubes and frozen. Tubes are thawed for use as needed. Once thawed the plasma expires in 2 days and must be discarded.
[2] Bovine thrombin is obtained through Fisher Scientific Item #23-306291, reconstituted as directed on package, and frozen in glass tubes in 1–2 ml aliquots. Thrombin is thawed as needed and must be used the same day.

Table 8.13 Effusions: effusion screening panel for poorly differentiated tumor cells

Antibody	Mesothelioma	Adeno-carcinoma	Melanoma	Sarcoma Epithelioid hemangioendothelioma	Sarcoma Angiosarcoma	Lymphoma
CD45	–	–	–	–	–	+
CD20	–	–	–	–	–	+
CD30	–	–	–	–	–	+
S100	–	–	+	–	–	–
HMB-45	–	–	+	–	–	–
CD31	–	–	–	+	+	–
CD34	–	–	–	+	+	–
CKAE1,3	+	+	–	–	–	–
Cam 5.2	+	+	–	–	–	–
EMA	+	+	–	–	–	–/+
Vimentin	+/–	+/–	+	+	+	–/+

Note: Almost all mesotheliomas are positive with a pancytokeratin, CKAE1,3. Tumors that are negative with these broad-spectrum keratins are likely not mesotheliomas or carcinomas and other tumor types as outlined above should be considered. A screening panel is very useful in this context

Note: Epithelioid angiosarcomas can be cytokeratin positive. Vascular markers (CD 31, CD34) need to be done to identify these rare tumors

Reference: [1]

7. Transfer the cellblock material into a biopsy bag by pouring the contents of the falcon tube into a biopsy bag over a funnel and beaker.
8. Place cell block/biopsy bag into Histology cassette labeled with the Cytology Accession # on front of cassette and patient's name on the side of the cassette.
9. Add cassette to tissue processor with other tissues for paraffin processing and embedding.

Table 8.14 Pleural/pericardial effusions: squamous cell carcinoma (scc) of the lung vs. epithelioid mesothelioma

Antibody	Squamous cell carcinoma	Mesothelioma
WT-1	–	+a
Calretinin	+/–	+
P63	+	–
MOC-31	+	–
BG8 (Lewis)	+	–/+
BerEp4	+	+/–

[a]WT-1 shows strong nuclear staining in mesothelioma, but may show granular cytoplasmic staining in adenocarcinoma of the lung and endothelial cells

Note: CK5/6 is not helpful in this differential as 100% of squamous cell carcinomas are positive and 75–100% of mesotheliomas are positive

Note: Podoplanin (D2-40) is not useful in this panel due to significant staining in both squamous cell carcinoma and mesothelioma

References: [1, 20, 22, 38]

Table 8.15 Pleural/pericardial effusions: clear cell renal cell carcinoma vs. epithelioid clear cell mesothelioma

Antibody	Renal cell carcinoma	Mesothelioma
Calretinin	–	+
CK5/6	–	+
WT-1	–/+	+a
Podoplanin (D2-40)	–	+
CD15	+	–
RCC	+	–/+
MOC-31	+	–/+
Mesothelin	–	+b
PAX2	+	–

[a]WT-1 shows strong nuclear staining in mesothelioma, but may show granular cytoplasmic staining in adenocarcinoma of the lung and endothelial cells

[b]Mesothelin is a sensitive marker for mesothelioma; however, it lacks specificity. It appears that it is not frequently positive in renal cell carcinoma, and thus has some utility in this specific panel

References: [1, 11, 20–22, 38, 39]

Table 8.16 Pleural/pericardial/peritoneal effusion: sarcomatoid carcinoma vs. sarcomatoid mesothelioma

Antibody	Sarcomatoid carcinoma	Sarcomatoid mesothelioma
Calretinin	–	+
D2-40	–	+
CKAE1,3	+	+
Cam5.2	+	+
CK18	+	+
CK7	+	+

Note: Pleomorphic, malignant cells with sarcomatoid features rarely occur in pleural effusions. However, when they are identified the most common differential remains between sarcomatoid variant of carcinoma (lung or renal) and sarcomatoid mesothelioma

Note: WT-1, CK5/6, BerEp4,CEA, and MOC-31 do not provide significant additional information in this differential

Note: This differential is usually only resolved in situations where the calretinin and D2-40 are positive, in addition to cytokeratin. Calretinin and D2-40 positivity alone should be regarded as insufficient evidence of mesothelial differentiation. Positive cytokeratins are seen in both of these entities and do not adequately distinguish them. However, in the absence of cytokeratin staining, the tumor may not be a carcinoma, or mesothelioma but some other spindled tumor such as melanoma or angiosarcoma. Thus, it is important to start by establishing positive cytokeratin staining. Because the expression of these can be limited in both sarcomatoid carcinomas and sarcomatoid mesotheliomas, a more extensive panel of cytokeratins may be necessary

Reference: [1]

Table 8.17 Peritoneal effusion, male: nongynecologic adenocarcinoma vs. peritoneal malignant mesothelioma

Antibody	Nongynecologic adenocarcinoma (AdCa)	Peritoneal malignant mesothelioma (PMM)
Calretinin	–/+ (Pancreatic AdCa)	+
WT-1	– (Gastric AdCa)	+/–
D2-40	– (Negative in pancreatic and gastric AdCa)	+
MOC-31	+ (AdCa)	–
BG8	+ (AdCa)	–/+
CEA	+ (AdCa)	–
B72.3	+ (Pancreas AdCa)+ (Bile duct AdCa) + (Colonic AdCa)	–
BerEp4	+ (Pancreas AdCa)+ (Gastric AdCa)	–/+

Note: CK5/6 is not useful as a marker for PMM in this panel as it is positive in 38% of pancreatic AdCa

References: [1, 20, 21, 40]

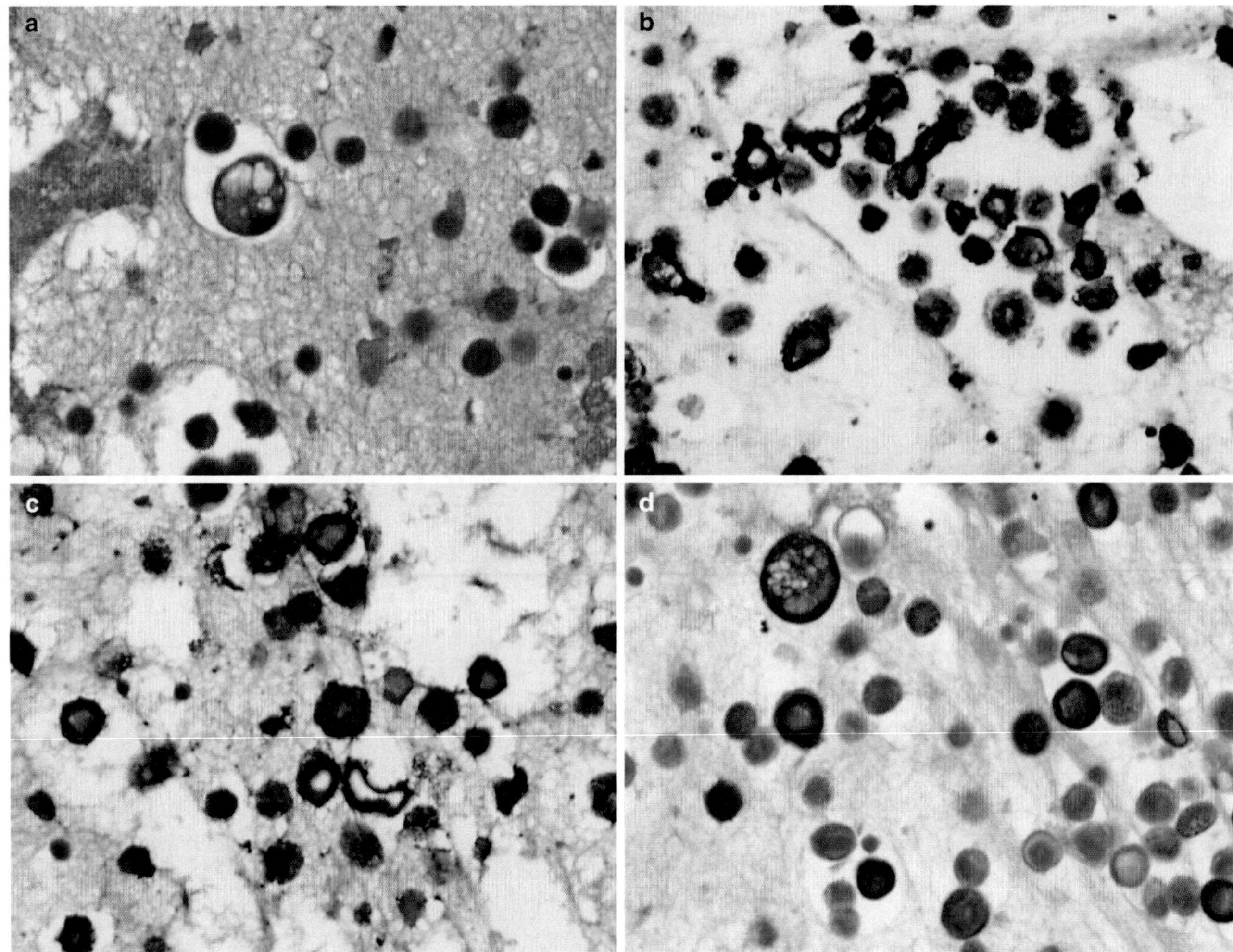

Fig. 8.5 Gastric carcinoma: (**a**) H&E, (**b**) BerEp-4, (**c**) MOC31, and (**d**) CK20 (×450)

Table 8.18 Peritoneal effusion, female: papillary serous carcinoma (PSC) vs. peritoneal malignant mesothelioma (PMM)

Antibody	PSC	PMM
Calretinin	−/+	+
D2-40	−/+	+
MOC-31	+	−
BG8 (Lewis)	+	−/+
BerEp4	+	−/+
Estrogen receptor	+	−
Progesterone receptor	+/−	−
H-caldesmon	−	+

Note: This panel is specific for female patients in whom PSC is a differential consideration

Note: WT-1 is not useful in this panel as it is usually positive in both PSC and PMM

Note: CK5/6 is not useful in this panel as it is positive in 53–100% PMM and 22–35% PSC

Note: CEA is not useful, 0–45% in PSC and 0% in PMM

References: [1, 20, 21, 33, 41]

Table 8.19 Peritoneal effusion, female: ovary (mucinous and endometrioid) vs. colon

Antibody	Mucinous adenocarcinoma of ovary	Endometrioid adenocarcinoma of the ovary	Colon adenocarcinoma
CK7	+	+	−
CK20	+	−	+
Estrogen receptor (ER)	+/−	+/−	−
Progesterone receptor (PR)	+/−	+/−	−
Beta catenin	−	−	+
MUC5AC	+	−	−
CDX2	+/−	−	+
CA-125	+	+	−
Vimentin	−	+	−

References: [42–47]

Table 8.20 Peritoneal effusion, female: ovary (mucinous and endometrioid) vs. breast vs. colon

Antibody	Adenocarcinoma of ovary	Breast carcinoma	Colon adenocarcinoma
CK7	+	+	–
CK20	+	–	+
Estrogen receptor (ER)	+/–	+/–	–
Progesterone receptor (PR)	+/–	+/–	–
GCDFP-15	–	+/–	–
Beta catenin	–	–	+
MUC5AC	+	–	–
CDX2	+/–	–	+
CA-125	+	–	–
Vimentin	+/–	–	–

References: [42, 46]

Table 8.21 Peritoneal effusion, female: mucinous adenocarcinoma of the ovary vs. pancreatic/bile duct adenocarcinoma

Antibody	Mucinous adenocarcinoma of ovary	Pancreatic adenocarcinoma	Bile duct adenocarcinoma
CK7	+	+	+
CK20	+	+	+/–
Estrogen receptor (ER)	+/–	–	–
Progesterone receptor (PR)	+/–	–	–
MUC5AC	+	+	+
CDX2	+/–	–/+	–/+
CA-125	+	–	–
CA 19-9	–	+	+

References: [6, 42, 48]

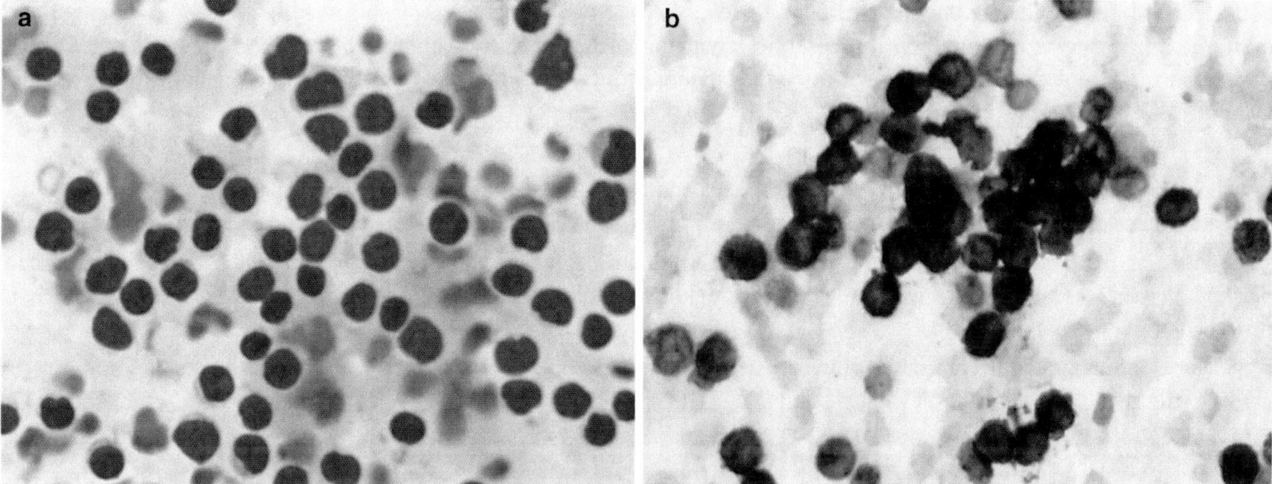

Fig. 8.6 Reactive pleural effusion lymphocytes (**a**) Diff-Quick and (**b**) CD3 (×450)

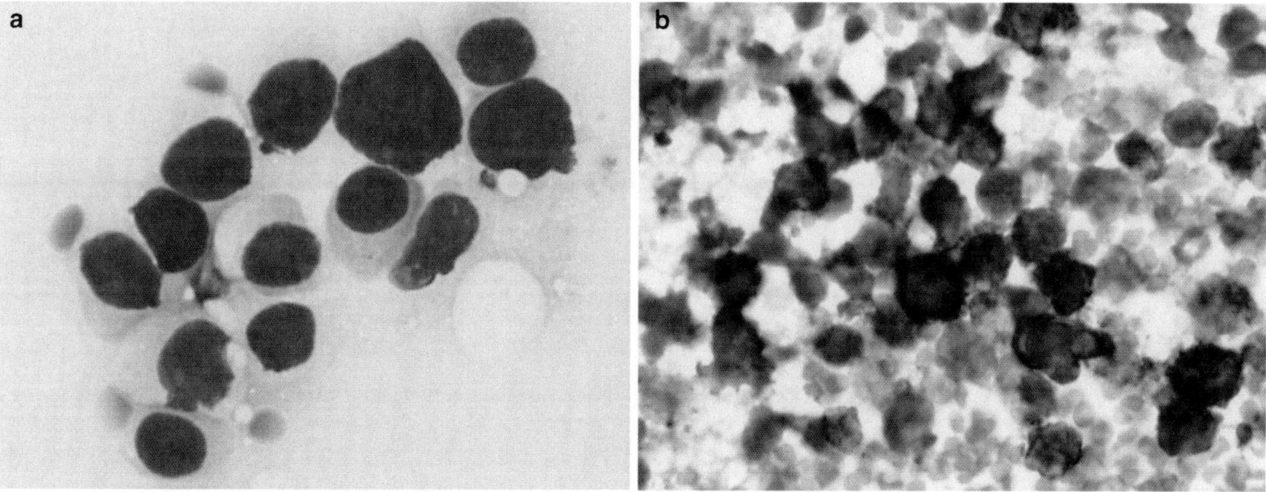

Fig. 8.7 Myeloma (**a**) Diff quick and (**b**) CD138 (×450)

Table 8.22 Effusions: selected lymphomas/leukemias in pediatric and adult effusions

Antibody	B-SLL	DLBCL	PL	PEL	BL	ALCL	BALL	TALL	AML	CHL
CD3	−	−	−	−	−	+	−	+[a]	−	−
CD20	−/+[b]	+	+	−	+	−	−/+	−	−	−
CD79a	+	+	+	+	+	−	+	−	−	−
PAX5	+	+	−	+/−	+	−	+	−	+	−
CD45rb	+	+	−/+[c]	+	+	−[c]	−/+[c]	−/+[c]	+[c]	−[c]
CD15	−	−	−	−	−	−	+/−	+/−	+/−	+
CD30	−	−	+	+	−	+	−	−	−	+
ALK-1	−	−/+	−	−	−	+	−	−	−	−
CD138	−	−/+	+	+	−	−	−	−	−	−
CD56	−	−	+	−	−	−/+	−	−	+/−	−
Ig	+[d]	+/−[d]	+	−	+/−	−	−	−	−	−
HHV8	−	−	−	+	−	−	−	−	−	−
EMA	−	−/+	+	+	−	−	−	−	−	+
TdT	−	−	−		−	−	+	+	−/+	−
CD34	−	−	−	−	−	−	+	+		−
CD117	−	−	+	−	−	−	−	−	+	−
MPO	−	−	−	−	−	−	−	−	+	−

SLL small lymphocytic lymphoma, *DLBCL* diffuse large B-cell lymphoma, *PL* plasmacytoid and plasmablastic lymphomas, *PEL* primary effusion lymphoma, *BL* Burkitt's lymphoma, *ALCL T-cell* anaplastic large cell lymphoma, *BALL* B-cell lymphoblastic lymphoma/leukemia, *TALL* T-cell lymphoblastic lymphoma/leukemia, *AML* acute myelogenous leukemia, *CHL* classic Hodgkin's lymphoma

[a]CD3 staining is cytoplasmic in immature T-cells

[b]CD20 may be very weak or negative in SLL. CD79a and Pax-5 usually are positive in these cases

[c]CD45 is usually strongly positive in non-Hodgkin lymphomas and weakly positive in acute leukemias (ALL, and AML), some cases of B-LBL and all cases of AML with erythroid and megakaryocytic differentiation. Other hematopoietic neoplasms that can be CD45rb negative are classical Hodgkin's lymphoma (Reed–Sternberg cells), anaplastic large cell lymphoma, and plasma cell tumors

[d]Surface immunoglobulins are not well demonstrated with paraffin-embedded, cellblock tissues. These are more readily evident with flow cytometric studies

References: [49–54]

Table 8.23 Effusions, adult: small round cell tumors in adults

Antibody	SmCC [a]	PDSS	DSRCT [b]	EWS/PNET	Lymphoma/leukemia [c]	Melanoma [d]
CKAE1,3	+	+[e]	+	–/+	–	–
CAM5.2	+	+[e]	+	–/+	–	–
CD45	–	–	–	–	+[f]	–
S100	–	–/+	–	–	–	+
CD99[g]	–	+	–/+	+	–/+[c,f]	–/+[h]
Desmin	–	–	+[i]	–	–	–
CD56	+	+	–/+	–/+	–	–/+[j]
WT-1	–	–	+	–	–	–/+

Note: *SmCC* small cell carcinoma (poorly differentiated neuroendocrine carcinoma, including Merkel cell carcinoma, small cell carcinoma of the breast, small cell carcinoma of the prostate, small cell carcinoma of the colon, and small cell carcinoma of the salivary gland) *PDSS* poorly differentiated synovial sarcoma, round cell type, *DSRCT* desmoplastic small round cell tumor, *EWS/PNET* Ewing's sarcoma, primitive neuroectodermal tumor

[a]SmCC shows simultaneous epithelial and neuroendocrine differentiation, with CK expression, particularly low molecular weight cytokeratin CK8, and CK18. Neuroendocrine differentiation is identified by NSE, CD56, synaptophysin, chromogranin, in order of increasing specificity. SmCC arises in many sites. Some of these can be identified by additional phenotyping: CK20 is positive in >97% of Merkel cell carcinoma (SmCC from skin); CK20 is positive in 60% of salivary gland SmCC; ER/PR is positive in 66% of breast SmCC; TTF-1 is positive in 80–100% of lung SmCC; and CDX-2 is positive in 20% of SmCC of colon

[b]Frequently desmoplastic small round cell tumor coexpresses cytokeratin and vimentin. However, the coexpression of cytokeratin and desmin is unique and the most specific means of identifying this tumor

[c]Granulocytic sarcoma (myeloid sarcoma) is usually positive with CD45 (75%) and frequently expresses CD99. It is also positive with CD43 (100%). Myeloperoxidase and lysozyme can also be helpful

[d]Nasopharyngeal melanomas can present as a small round cell morphology and thus are included in this differential. These tumors would be only very rarely encountered in effusions

[e]EMA staining is 100% in poorly differentiated synovial sarcomas, round cell type

[f]Lymphoblastic lymphoma/leukemia may negative for CD45 but is usually positive with CD99. If lymphoblastic lymphoma is suspected, an additional panel of TdT, CD43, and CD79a should be used

[g]CD99 shows strong membranous staining in Ewing's sarcoma/primitive neuroectodermal tumors. It is also strongly positive in lymphoblastic lymphoma/leukemia (>90%), myelogenous leukemia, granulocytic sarcoma, small cell variant of poorly differentiated synovial sarcoma, and desmoplastic small round cell tumors. When lymphoblastic lymphoma is a differential consideration TdT and CD79a should be evaluated as they are positive in lymphoblastic lymphoma. FLI1 protein overexpression is seen in 70% of Ewing's sarcoma. It can be detected immunohistochemically but does not exclude lymphoblastic lymphoma which is 88% positive for FLI1 protein

[h]CD99 can be positive in up to 60% of small cell variants of malignant melanoma

[i]A paranuclear dot-like pattern is seen with desmin staining of desmoplastic small round cell tumors

[j]Small cell variants of malignant melanoma may be positive with CD56 (13%)

References: [3, 6, 55–61]

Table 8.24 Effusions, pediatric: small round cell tumors in children

Antibody	WT	NB	DSRCT [a]	EWS/PNET	Lymphoma/leukemia [b]	RMS
CKAE1,3	–/+	–/+	+	–/+	–	–
CAM5.2	–/+	–	+	–/+	–	–
CD45	–	–	–	–	– [c]	–
S100	–	–	–	–	–	–
CD99 [d]	–/+	–	–/+	+	–/+ [b,c]	–/+
Desmin	+	–	+ [e]	–	–	+
Myogenin [f]	–/+ [g]	–	+	–	–	+
CD56	+	+ [h]	–/+	–/+	–	+
WT-1	+	–	+	–	–	+ [i]

WT Wilms tumor, *NB* Neuroblastoma, *DSRCT* desmoplastic small round cell tumor, *EWS/PNET* Ewing's sarcoma, primitive neuroectodermal tumor, *RMS* rhabdomyosarcoma

[a] Frequently desmoplastic small round cell tumor coexpresses cytokeratin and vimentin. However, the coexpression of cytokeratin and desmin is unique and the most specific means of identifying this tumor

[b] Granulocytic sarcoma (myeloid sarcoma) is usually positive with CD45 (75%) and frequently expresses CD99. It is also positive with CD43 (100%). Myeloperoxidase and lysozyme can also be helpful

[c] Lymphoblastic lymphoma/leukemia may negative for CD45 but is usually positive with CD99. If lymphoblastic lymphoma is suspected, an additional panel of TdT, CD43, and CD79a should be used

[d] CD99 shows strong membranous staining in Ewing's sarcoma/primitive neuroectodermal tumors. It is also strongly positive in lymphoblastic lymphoma/leukemia (>90%), myelogenous leukemia, granulocytic sarcoma, small cell variant of poorly differentiated synovial sarcoma, and desmoplastic small round cell tumors. When lymphoblastic lymphoma is a differential consideration TdT and CD79a should be evaluated as they are positive in lymphoblastic lymphoma. FLI-1 protein overexpression is seen in 70% of Ewing sarcoma's. It can be detected immunohistochemically but does not exclude lymphoblastic lymphoma. Lymphoblastic lymphoma is 88% positive for FLI-1 protein

[e] A paranuclear dot-like pattern is seen with desmin staining of desmoplastic small round cell tumors

[f] Nuclear staining for myogenin or Myo-D1 is considered specific. Cytoplasmic staining is nonspecific and should not be considered evidence of skeletal muscle differentiation. Myo-D1 is prone to background and cytoplasmic staining. Myogenin is technically preferable

[g] Rhabdomyomatous Wilms tumors are positive with MyoD-1

[h] Neuroblastomas are positive with CD56 (100%). Other neuronal phenotypic markers include NSE (38–95%), neurofilament protein (65–85%), synaptophysin (65–85%), and chromogranin (60–80%). Synaptophysin and chromogranin are the most specific

[i] WT-1 demonstrates a cytoplasmic staining pattern in rhabdomyosarcoma

References: [6, 55, 56, 62–73]

Table 8.25 Effusions, adult and pediatric: seminoma vs. nonseminomatous germ cell tumors (NSGCT)

Antibody	Seminoma	Embryonal carcinoma	Yolk sac tumor	Choriocarcinoma
Cam 5.2	–	+	+	+
CKAE1,3	–	+	+	+
CK7	–	–	–	–
CK20	–	–	–	–
PLAP	+	+	+/–	+
OCT4	+	+	–	–
Podoplanin D2-40	+	–	–	–
Alpha feto protein	–	–	+	–
Beta HCG	–	–	–	+
CD30	–	+	–	–
CD117	+	–	–	–
HLA-G	–	–	–	+
Inhibin	–	–	–	+
GCP-3	–	–	+	+

References: [10, 74–77]

Note for All Tables

Note: "+" – usually greater than 70% of cases are positive; "–" – less than 5% of cases are positive; "+ or –" – usually more than 50% of cases are positive; "– or +" – less than 50% of cases are positive.

References

1. Husain AN, Colby TV, Ordonez NG, et al. Guidelines for pathologic diagnosis of malignant mesothelioma: a consensus statement from the International Mesothelioma Interest Group. Arch Pathol Lab Med. 2009;133(8):1317–31.
2. Yaziji H, Battifora H, Barry TS, et al. Evaluation of 12 antibodies for distinguishing epithelioid mesothelioma from adenocarcinoma: identification of a three-antibody immunohistochemical panel with maximal sensitivity and specificity. Mod Pathol. 2006;19(4):514–23.
3. Jagirdar J. Application of immunohistochemistry to the diagnosis of primary and metastatic carcinoma to the lung. Arch Pathol Lab Med. 2008;132(3):384–96.
4. Mai KT, Perkins DG, Zhang J, Mackenzie CR. ES1, a new lung carcinoma antibody – an immunohistochemical study. Histopathology. 2006;49(5):515–22.
5. Ueno T, Linder S, Elmberger G. Aspartic proteinase napsin is a useful marker for diagnosis of primary lung adenocarcinoma. Br J Cancer. 2003;88(8):1229–33.
6. Bahrami A, Truong LD, Ro JY. Undifferentiated tumor: true identity by immunohistochemistry. Arch Pathol Lab Med. 2008;132(3):326–48.
7. Bhargava R, Beriwal S, Dabbs DJ. Mammaglobin vs GCDFP-15: an immunohistologic validation survey for sensitivity and specificity. Am J Clin Pathol. 2007;127(1):103–13.
8. Han JH, Kang Y, Shin HC, et al. Mammaglobin expression in lymph nodes is an important marker of metastatic breast carcinoma. Arch Pathol Lab Med. 2003;127(10):1330–4.
9. Sasaki E, Tsunoda N, Hatanaka Y, Mori N, Iwata H, Yatabe Y. Breast-specific expression of MGB1/mammaglobin: an examination of 480 tumors from various organs and clinicopathological analysis of MGB1-positive breast cancers. Mod Pathol. 2007;20(2):208–14.
10. Hammerich KH, Ayala GE, Wheeler TM. Application of immunohistochemistry to the genitourinary system (prostate, urinary bladder, testis, and kidney). Arch Pathol Lab Med. 2008;132(3):432–40.
11. Gokden N, Gokden M, Phan DC, McKenney JK. The utility of PAX-2 in distinguishing metastatic clear cell renal cell carcinoma from its morphologic mimics: an immunohistochemical study with comparison to renal cell carcinoma marker. Am J Surg Pathol. 2008;32(10):1462–7.
12. Kaufmann O, Volmerig J, Dietel M. Uroplakin III is a highly specific and moderately sensitive immunohistochemical marker for primary and metastatic urothelial carcinomas. Am J Clin Pathol. 2000;113(5):683–7.
13. Wang HL, Lu DW, Yerian LM, et al. Immunohistochemical distinction between primary adenocarcinoma of the bladder and secondary colorectal adenocarcinoma. Am J Surg Pathol. 2001;25(11): 1380–7.
14. Attanoos RL, Griffin A, Gibbs AR. The use of immunohistochemistry in distinguishing reactive from neoplastic mesothelium. A novel use for desmin and comparative evaluation with epithelial membrane antigen, p53, platelet-derived growth factor-receptor, P-glycoprotein and Bcl-2. Histopathology. 2003;43(3):231–8.
15. Krismann M, Muller KM, Jaworska M, Johnen G. Pathological anatomy and molecular pathology. Lung Cancer. 2004;45 Suppl 1:S29–33.
16. Kato Y, Tsuta K, Seki K, et al. Immunohistochemical detection of GLUT-1 can discriminate between reactive mesothelium and malignant mesothelioma. Mod Pathol. 2007;20(2):215–20.
17. Acurio A, Arif Q, Gattuso P, et al. Value of immunohistochemical markers in differentiating benign from malignant mesothelial lesions: United States and Canadian Academy of Pathology annual meeting. Mod Pathol. 2008;21:334A.
18. Davidson B, Nielsen S, Christensen J, et al. The role of desmin and N-cadherin in effusion cytology: a comparative study using established markers of mesothelial and epithelial cells. Am J Surg Pathol. 2001;25(11):1405–12.
19. Galateau-Salle F, Brambilla E, Cagle PT, et al. Classification and histologic features of epithelioid mesotheliomas. In: Galateau-Salle F, editor. Pathology of malignant mesothelioma. London, England: Springer-Verlag; 2006. Accessed 5 Mar 2010.
20. Trupiano JK, Geisinger KR, Willingham MC, et al. Diffuse malignant mesothelioma of the peritoneum and pleura, analysis of markers. Mod Pathol. 2004;17(4):476–81.
21. Chu AY, Litzky LA, Pasha TL, Acs G, Zhang PJ. Utility of D2-40, a novel mesothelial marker, in the diagnosis of malignant mesothelioma. Mod Pathol. 2005;18(1):105–10.
22. Ordonez NG. D2-40 and podoplanin are highly specific and sensitive immunohistochemical markers of epithelioid malignant mesothelioma. Hum Pathol. 2005;36(4):372–80.
23. Hammar SP. Macroscopic, histologic, histochemical, immunohistochemical, and ultrastructural features of mesothelioma. Ultrastruct Pathol. 2006;30(1):3–17.
24. Carella R, Deleonardi G, D'Errico A, et al. Immunohistochemical panels for differentiating epithelial malignant mesothelioma from lung adenocarcinoma: a study with logistic regression analysis. Am J Surg Pathol. 2001;25(1):43–50.
25. Johnston WW. Applications of monoclonal antibodies in clinical cytology as exemplified by studies with monoclonal antibody B72.3. The George N. Papanicolaou award lecture. Acta Cytol. 1987;31(5):537–56.
26. Sun Y, Wu GP, Fang CQ, Liu SL. Diagnostic utility of MOC-31, HBME-1 and MOC-31 mRNA in distinguishing between carcinoma cells and reactive mesothelial cells in pleural effusions. Acta Cytol. 2009;53(6):619–24.
27. Dejmek A, Hjerpe A. Reactivity of six antibodies in effusions of mesothelioma, adenocarcinoma and mesotheliosis: stepwise logistic regression analysis. Cytopathology. 2000;11(1):8–17.
28. Miedouge M, Rouzaud P, Salama G, et al. Evaluation of seven tumour markers in pleural fluid for the diagnosis of malignant effusions. Br J Cancer. 1999;81(6):1059–65.
29. Ichihara T, Nagura H, Nakao A, Sakamoto J, Watanabe T, Takagi H. Immunohistochemcial localization of CA 19-9 and CEA in pancreatic carcinoma and associated diseases. Cancer. 1987;61(2):324–33.
30. Deniz H, Kibar Y, Guldur ME, Bakir K. Is D2-40 a useful marker for distinguishing malignant mesothelioma from pulmonary adenocarcinoma and benign mesothelial proliferations? Pathol Res Pract. 2009;205(11):749–52.
31. King JE, Thatcher N, Pickering CA, Hasleton PS. Sensitivity and specificity of immunohistochemical markers used in the diagnosis of epithelioid mesothelioma: a detailed systematic analysis using published data. Histopathology. 2006;48(3):223–32.
32. Ordonez NG. The immunohistochemical diagnosis of mesothelioma: a comparative study of epithelioid mesothelioma and lung adenocarcinoma. Am J Surg Pathol. 2003;27(8):1031–51.
33. Comin CE, Saieva C, Messerini L. h-Caldesmon, calretinin, estrogen receptor, and Ber-EP4: a useful combination of

immunohistochemical markers for differentiating epithelioid peritoneal mesothelioma from serous papillary carcinoma of the ovary. Am J Surg Pathol. 2007;31(8):1139–48.

34. Epenetos AA, Canti G, Taylor-Papadimitriou J, Curling M, Bodmer WF. Use of two epithelium-specific monoclonal antibodies for diagnosis of malignancy in serous effusions. Lancet. 1982;320(8306):1004–6.
35. Fabian CB, Dabbs DJ. Breast Carcinoma versus lung adenocarcinoma: the immunohistochemical discrimination of breast carcinoma metastatic in lung. Breast J. 2007;3(3):135–41.
36. Yang MC, Bannan M, Chiriboga L, et al. Immunohistochemical differential expression in lung and breast cancers. Mod Pathol. 2007;1:334A.
37. Yang M, Nonaka D. A study of immunohistochemical differential expression in pulmonary and mammary carcinomas. Mod Pathol. 2010;23(5):654–61.
38. Ordonez NG. The diagnostic utility of immunohistochemistry in distinguishing between epithelioid mesotheliomas and squamous carcinomas of the lung: a comparative study. Mod Pathol. 2006;19(3):417–28.
39. Ordonez N. Value of mesothelin immunostaining in the diagnosis of mesothelioma. Mod Pathol. 2003;16(3):192–7.
40. Sadeghi B, Arvieux C, Glehen O, et al. Peritoneal carcinomatosis from non-gynecologic malignancies: results of the EVOCAPE 1 multicentric prospective study. Cancer. 2000;88(2):358–63.
41. Baker PM, Clement PB, Young RH. Malignant peritoneal mesothelioma in women: a study of 75 cases with emphasis on their morphologic spectrum and differential diagnosis. Am J Clin Pathol. 2005;123(5):724–37.
42. Mittal K, Soslow R, McCluggage WG. Application of immunohistochemistry to gynecologic pathology. Arch Pathol Lab Med. 2008;132(3):402–23.
43. Lagendijk JH, Mullink H, Van Diest PJ, Meijer GA, Meijer CJ. Tracing the origin of adenocarcinomas with unknown primary using immunohistochemistry: differential diagnosis between colonic and ovarian carcinomas as primary sites. Hum Pathol. 1998;29(5):491–7.
44. Chou YY, Jeng YM, Kao HL, Chen T, Mao TL, Lin MC. Differentiation of ovarian mucinous carcinoma and metastatic colorectal adenocarcinoma by immunostaining with beta-catenin. Histopathology. 2003;43(2):151–6.
45. Groisman GM, Meir A, Sabo E. The value of Cdx2 immunostaining in differentiating primary ovarian carcinomas from colonic carcinomas metastatic to the ovaries. Int J Gynecol Pathol. 2004;23(1):52–7.
46. Lagendijk JH, Mullink H, van Diest PJ, Meijer GA, Meijer CJ. Immunohistochemical differentiation between primary adenocarcinomas of the ovary and ovarian metastases of colonic and breast origin. Comparison between a statistical and an intuitive approach. J Clin Pathol. 1999;52(4):283–90.
47. Albarracin CT, Jafri J, Montag AG, Hart J, Kuan SF. Diffe-rential expression of MUC2 and MUC5AC mucin genes in primary ovarian and metastatic colonic carcinoma. Hum Pathol. 2000;31(6):672–7.
48. Zapata M, Cohen C, Siddiqui MT. Immunohistochemical expression of SMAD4, CK19 and CA19-9 in fine needle aspiration samples of pancreatic adenocarcinoma: utility and potential role. Cytojournal. 2007;4:13.
49. Chen CC, Raikow RB, Sonmez-Alpan E, Swerdlow SH. Classification of small B-cell lymphoid neoplasms using a paraffin section immunohistochemical panel. Appl Immunohistochem Mol Morphol. 2000;8(1):1–11.
50. Torlakovic E, Torlakovic G, Nguyen PL, Brunning RD, Delabie J. The value of anti-pax-5 immunostaining in routinely fixed and paraffin-embedded sections: a novel pan pre-B and B-cell marker. Am J Surg Pathol. 2002;26(10):1343–50.
51. Lewis RE, Cruse JM, Sanders CM, et al. The immunophenotype of pre-TALL/LBL revisited. Exp Mol Pathol. 2006;81(2):162–5.
52. Nador RG, Cesarman E, Chadburn A, et al. Primary effusion lymphoma: a distinct clinicopathologic entity associated with the Kaposi's sarcoma-associated herpes virus. Blood.1996;88(2):645–56.
53. Ely SA, Knowles DM. Expression of CD56/neural cell adhesion molecule correlates with the presence of lytic bone lesions in multiple myeloma and distinguishes myeloma from monoclonal gammopathy of undetermined significance and lymphomas with plasmacytoid differentiation. Am J Pathol. 2002;160(4):1293–9.
54. Drexler HG, Uphoff CC, Gaidano G, Carbone A. Lymphoma cell lines: in vitro models for the study of HHV-8+ primary effusion lymphomas (body cavity-based lymphomas). Leukemia. 1998;12(10):1507–17.
55. Ozdemirli M, Fanburg-Smith JC, Hartmann DP, et al. Precursor B-lymphoblastic lymphoma presenting as a solitary bone tumor and mimicking Ewing's sarcoma: a report of four cases and review of the literature. Am J Surg Pathol. 1998;22(7):795–804.
56. Zhang PJ, Goldblum JR, Pawel BR, Fisher C, Pasha TL, Barr FG. Immunophenotype of desmoplastic small round cell tumors as detected in cases with EWS-WT1 gene fusion product. Mod Pathol. 2003;16(3):229–35.
57. Shipley WR, Hammer RD, Lennington WJ, Macon WR. Paraffin immunohistochemical detection of CD56, a useful maker for neural cell adhesion molecule (NCAM), in normal and neoplastic fixed tissues. Appl Immunohistochem. 1997;5:87.
58. Shin SJ, DeLellis RA, Ying L, Rosen PP. Small cell carcinoma of the breast: a clinicopathologic and immunohistochemical study of nine patients. Am J Surg Pathol. 2000;24(9):1231–8.
59. Ordonez NG. Value of thyroid transcription factor-1 immunostaining in distinguishing small cell lung carcinomas from other small cell carcinomas. Am J Surg Pathol. 2000;24(9):1217–23.
60. Erickson LA, Papouchado B, Dimashkieh H, Zhang S, Nakamura N, Lloyd RV. Cdx2 as a marker for neuroendocrine tumors of unknown primary sites. Endocr Pathol. 2004;15(3):247–52.
61. Thompson LD, Wieneke JA, Miettinen M. Sinonasal tract and nasopharyngeal melanomas: a clinicopathologic study of 115 cases with a proposed staging system. Am J Surg Pathol. 2003;27(5):594–611.
62. Folpe AL, Hill CE, Parham DM, O'Shea PA, Weiss SW. Immunohistochemical detection of FLI-1 protein expression: a study of 132 round cell tumors with emphasis on CD99-positive mimics of Ewing's sarcoma/primitive neuroectodermal tumor. Am J Surg Pathol. 2000;24(12):1657–62.
63. Riopel M, Dickman PS, Link MP, Perlman EJ. MIC2 analysis in pediatric lymphomas and leukemias. Hum Pathol. 1994;25(4):396–9.
64. Zhang PJ, Barcos M, Stewart CC, Block AW, Sait S, Brooks JJ. Immunoreactivity of MIC2 (CD99) in acute myelogenous leukemia and related diseases. Mod Pathol. 2000;13(4):452–8.
65. Garin-Chesa P, Fellinger EJ, Huvos AG, et al. Immunohistochemical analysis of neural cell adhesion molecules. Differential expression in small round cell tumors of childhood and adolescence. Am J Pathol. 1991;139(2):275–86.
66. Khanlari B, Buser A, Lugli A, Tichelli A, Dirnhofer S. The expression pattern of CD56 (N-CAM) in human bone marrow biopsies infiltrated by acute leukemia. Leuk Lymphoma. 2003;44(12):2055–9.
67. Rossi S, Orvieto E, Furlanetto A, Laurino L, Ninfo V, Dei Tos AP. Utility of the immunohistochemical detection of FLI-1 expression in round cell and vascular neoplasm using a monoclonal antibody. Mod Pathol. 2004;17(5):547–52.
68. Kumar S, Perlman E, Harris CA, Raffeld M, Tsokos M. Myogenin is a specific marker for rhabdomyosarcoma: an immunohistochemical study in paraffin-embedded tissues. Mod Pathol. 2000;13(9):988–93.
69. Wirnsberger GH, Becker H, Ziervogel K, Hofler H. Diagnostic immunohistochemistry of neuroblastic tumors. Am J Surg Pathol. 1992;16(1):49–57.

70. Sebire NJ, Malone M. Myogenin and MyoD1 expression in paediatric rhabdomyosarcomas. J Clin Pathol. 2003;56(6):412–6.
71. Wang NP, Marx J, McNutt MA, Rutledge JC, Gown AM. Expression of myogenic regulatory proteins (myogenin and MyoD1) in small blue round cell tumors of childhood. Am J Pathol. 1995;147(6):1799–810.
72. Cessna MH, Zhou H, Perkins SL, et al. Are myogenin and myoD1 expression specific for rhabdomyosarcoma? A study of 150 cases, with emphasis on spindle cell mimics. Am J Surg Pathol. 2001;25(9):1150–7.
73. Carpentieri DF, Nichols K, Chou PM, Matthews M, Pawel B, Huff D. The expression of WT1 in the differentiation of rhabdomyosarcoma from other pediatric small round blue cell tumors. Mod Pathol. 2002;15(10):1080–6.
74. Hattab EM, Tu PH, Wilson JD, Cheng L. OCT4 immunohistochemistry is superior to placental alkaline phosphatase (PLAP) in the diagnosis of central nervous system germinoma. Am J Surg Pathol. 2005;29(3):368–71.
75. Lau SK, Weiss LM, Chu PG. D2-40 immunohistochemistry in the differential diagnosis of seminoma and embryonal carcinoma: a comparative immunohistochemical study with KIT (CD117) and CD30. Mod Pathol. 2007;20(3):320–5.
76. Mao TL, Kurman RJ, Huang CC, Lin MC, Shih I. Immunohistochemistry of choriocarcinoma: an aid in differential diagnosis and in elucidating pathogenesis. Am J Surg Pathol. 2007;31(11):1726–32.
77. Shih IM, Kurman RJ. Immunohistochemical localization of inhibin-alpha in the placenta and gestational trophoblastic lesions. IntJ Gynecol Pathol. 1999;18(2):144–50.

Chapter 9
Predictive Markers of Breast Cancer: ER, PR, and HER2

Jeffrey Prichard, David Hicks, and Elizabeth Hammond

Abstract With the new role of immunohistochemistry as a test to guide the use of specific therapies, new demands for quantitative accuracy and reproducibility have been placed on laboratories. In response to this need increased quality of IHC testing, the College of American Pathologists (CAP) has released guidelines for the validation, performance, and ongoing quality management of receptor testing in breast cancer cases. This chapter reviews the new requirements of these testing guidelines to help laboratories adopt these best practices. Information is offered on the FDA approval of current antibodies for this testing. Diagrams illustrate the recommended testing algorithm combining results of immunohistochemical and in situ hybridization testing for HER2. Photomicrographs of positive, negative, and equivocal staining reactions are provided to aid in the interpretation of immunohistochemical and in situ hybridization assays. Figures demonstrating the use of appropriate and inappropriate internal control reactions serve to help decide, if results are valid and can be reported or should be rejected.

Keywords Estrogen • Progesterone • Receptor • HER2 • Predictive • Hybridization • Guidelines • Breast

FREQUENTLY ASKED QUESTIONS

Breast Cancer Receptor Studies Overview

HER2 Testing

ER/PR Testing

J. Prichard (✉)
Department of Pathology and Laboratory Medicine, Geisinger Medical Center, Danville, PA 17822, USA
e-mail: jwprichard@geisinger.edu

F. Lin and J. Prichard (eds.), *Handbook of Practical Immunohistochemistry: Frequently Asked Questions*, DOI 10.1007/978-1-4419-8062-5_9,

9.1 Why Have Specific Guidelines Been Created for Performing Estrogen Receptor (ER), Progesterone Receptor (PR), and HER2 Testing?

In 1998, when the FDA approved the use of Trastuzumab for treating breast cancer patients with a positive IHC result for overexpression of the HER2 receptor oncoprotein, a new demand for accuracy in IHC testing was created. In the past, IHC was mainly a binary test of tumor differentiation with positive or negative results. With the arrival of the Dako Herceptest™ in 1998, pathologists were now being asked to differentiate moderately positive from strongly positive intensity and distribution of IHC staining. And that single interpretation would be the sole basis for determining whether a patient would receive Trastuzumab therapy. As patients entered clinical trials, their semiquantitative HER2 IHC results from laboratories across the country were frequently different from results obtained at centralized laboratories for the clinical trials. Over the following years, greater emphasis was placed on the accuracy of interpreting HER2 IHC. Fluorescence in situ hybridization (FISH) testing for gene amplification touted as the gold standard in HER2 testing was not widely available and also showed unacceptable reproducibility outside the setting of large centralized laboratories. Digital image analysis systems were created to standardize the interpretation. But the accuracy and reproducibility of HER2 IHC testing was still unacceptable, largely due to other uncontrolled factors in the specimen handling. Issues of variable formalin fixation affecting the accuracy of ER IHC testing also became apparent. It became clear to pathologists and oncologists that standardized best practices for receptor testing that had not existed previously would need to be developed to address this problem. In response, a team of experts reviewed all available research regarding best practices for all the steps in receptor testing. The result was the joint publications from the American Society of Clinical Oncology (ASCO) and the College of American Pathologist (CAP) in 2007 and 2010 establishing standards for performing ER, PR, and HER2 testing [1, 2]. There has been abundant attention paid to these guidelines at national meetings and they have been integrated into the CAP laboratory accreditation program (LAP) guidelines. CAP has produced excellent material to better explain the many requirements of these guidelines and changes they demand from laboratory practices. Many of these materials are available on the CAP website (www.cap.org) including a clear and authoritative Frequently Asked Questions (FAQ) document in the style of this book that we will not attempt to replicate here. But since there are so many questions asked about these receptor testing guidelines, and we believe in the importance of disseminating these best practices to the IHC community, we will attempt to answer a few of them.

References: [1–9]

9.2 What Are the Optimal Tissue Handling Requirements of Breast Specimens Used for ER, PR, and HER2 Receptor Testing?

The time from tissue acquisition to fixation should be as short as possible. Prolonged cold ischemia time can lead to preferential loss of HER2 probe signals in FISH testing that may lead to false negative results. The greatest challenge in this respect usually involves needle localization specimens that require specimen radiography prior to fixation. It is almost always possible to be able to get even these specimens into formalin within the hour that is recommended to minimize cold ischemic changes. Recommended fixation is in 10% neutral-buffered formalin (NBF) for a minimum of 6 hours for both biopsies and resection specimens. Recommended maximum fixation HER2 testing is 48 hours, while maximum fixation for ER/PR testing is to 72 hours. Use of alternative fixatives or longer fixation times requires a separate validation of the immunoreactivity of these specimens. To facilitate good penetration of the resection tissues by the formalin, samples should be sliced at 5-mm intervals after appropriate gross inspection and margins designation and placed in at least 10-fold the volume of NBF as the volume of the specimen to allow adequate tissue penetration. Sections should be thin enough so as not to be compressed when placed in the cassette for processing as this will impede the infiltration of the tissue during processing. If complete dissection of a tumor in a resection specimen is delayed due to overnight storage or transportation from a remote site, consideration should be given to formalin fixation of a sample of the tumor for predictive marker studies within the first hour of ischemia. This can be achieved by bisecting the specimen to expose the tumor surface directly to formalin or dissecting a small tumor sample into a cassette prior to any storage or transportation delay. Time tissue is removed from patient, time tissue is placed in fixative, duration of fixation, and fixative type must be recorded and noted on accession slip or in report. Storage of slides for more than 6 weeks before analysis is not recommended.

References: [1–9, 36, 37]

9.3 What Is HER2 and Does It Have Other Names?

HER2 is an oncogene on the long arm of chromosome 17 and there is usually one copy on each of the copies of chromosome 17. HER2 is also the name for the associated

185-kDa oncoprotein product. The HER2 oncoprotein is a glycoprotein and one of many tyrosine kinase receptors found in epithelial cell membranes directing cell growth from the outside of the cell to the nucleus inside the cell. In fact, it belongs to a family of human epidermal growth factor receptors from which "HER" originates. Another closely related and well-known member of this receptor family is HER1 also known as epidermal growth factor receptor (EGFR). This HER family of receptors is also known as the ErbB family named after the avian erythroblastosis tumor virus, which encodes an aberrant form of the receptor. This family gives HER2, its other name is c-erbB2. Other variations on these themes are used such as ErbB2 and her-2/neu, CD340, and p185. In normal tissues, HER2 does not have a known ligand to trigger its signaling but instead is triggered by dimerization with other members of its receptor family. In tumors with HER2 overexpression, HER2 also homodimerizes with itself causing activation. Activation of the HER2 signally pathway leads to cell growth and differentiation. *HER2* gene amplification is the mechanism of the HER2 protein overexpression in almost all HER2 positive breast cancers. Because of this close association between gene amplification and protein overexpression, a breast cancer is considered positive for HER2, if it exhibits either gene amplification or strong protein overexpression.

References: [1, 2, 4–6, 11, 12]

9.4 What Is the Prognostic and Predictive Significance of a Positive HER2 Result?

Prognostically, HER2 positivity in invasive breast cancer is associated with higher rates of recurrence and mortality without adjuvant therapy. HER2 positivity, as a surrogate for topoisomerase II coamplification, is predictive of better response from anthracycline therapy. HER2 overexpression, in both primary and metastatic breast cancer, predicts response from therapies that targets HER2 oncoprotein (trastuzumab and lapatinib), reducing recurrence and mortality. HER2 overexpression also predicts resistance to selective estrogen receptor modulator therapy (tamoxifen). A falsely positive HER2 result would not just unnecessarily incur the significant cost of trastuzumab therapy. It may also misdirect treatment choices denying the patient of the benefits of alternative treatment in addition to subjecting the patient to a 1–8% increased risk of cardiac toxicity. A falsely negative HER2 result would deny the potential benefit of targeted therapy and subject the patient to the potential harm of alternative therapies.

References: [1, 2, 4–6, 10, 13–15]

9.5 What Tests Are FDA Approved for Performing HER2 Testing?

There are several of polyclonal and monoclonal antibodies available for use in HER2 IHC assays. The original Dako Herceptest™ with its polyclonal primary antibody, the older Ventana Pathway® with its mouse monoclonal CB11, and now the newer Ventana Pathway® with its rabbit monoclonal 4B5 primary antibody all have achieved premarket approval (PMA) from the Food and Drug Administration (FDA) as IHC assays for testing HER2. (Table 9.1).

Both FISH and Chromogen In Situ Hybridization (CISH) assays have been FDA approved for *HER2* testing. Abbott PathVysion® and Dako *HER2* FISH pharmDX™ are both FDA-approved FISH assays for *HER2* testing of gene amplification. More recently, the FDA has approved a CISH brightfield assay called SPOT-Light® *HER2* CISH made by Invitrogen and marketed by BioCare Medical. There is a Silver In Situ Hybridization (SISH) assay available from Ventana that has yet to receive FDA approval. Ventana and Dako have both developed highly anticipated brightfield two-color in situ hybridization assays that can co-visualize *HER2* and a *CEP17* control probe on a single slide, but these assays have not yet been approved by the FDA (Table 9.2).

Table 9.1 FDA-approved (PMA) and FDA-cleared [510(k)] antibodies for *HER2*

HER2 IHC				
Company	Clonality	Antibody/kit	FDA process	FDA date
Biogenex	Monoclonal mouse	InSite CB11	PMA	12/22/2004
Cell Marque	Monoclonal mouse	CB11	PMA	11/27/2002
Dako	Polyclonal	Herceptest kit	PMA	9/25/1998
Ventana	Monoclonal rabbit	Pathway 4B5	PMA	11/28/2000

Table 9.2 FDA-approved (PMA) and FDA-cleared [510(k)] ISH probes for *HER2*

HER2 ISH, *HER2:CEP17*				
Company	Test type	Kit	FDA process	FDA date
Abbott	FISH	PathVysion FISH	PMA	12/31/2001
Dako	FISH	pharmDx FISH	PMA	5/3/2005
Invitrogen	CISH (2 slide)	Spot-Light CISH	PMA	7/1/2008

9.6 What Are the Differences Between FISH, CISH, and SISH?

The vast majority of *HER2* gene testing is performed by FISH. It is an older, established technology with FDA-approved assays available. FISH, of course, required fluorescence microscopy which is performed with limited ability to visualize tissue and cell morphology to locate appropriate cells to examine. Another drawback is that fluorescence signals fade over time. The frustrations with "working in the dark" performing FISH assays has lead to the newer brightfield CISH where the signals are labeled with chromogens similar to IHC and can be seen with a conventional microscope. In addition, there is the advantage of being able to see more conventional histology with counterstains that make the process of identifying the appropriate areas to count much easier. SISH is Silver In Situ Hybridization which has the same advantages of CISH, because they share the use of brightfield technology. SISH may have the advantage of producing sharper and better contrasted signals than those produced by conventional chromogens with a more rapid protocol. The factors, which are holding back widespread adoption of CISH and SISH, are that the FDA-approved methods available in the USA require two separate slides to view two signals to count both the *HER2* and the chromosome 17 control signal, which can be done on the same slide by two-color FISH. At least two dual-color *HER2* CISH/SISH assays have been developed, and once FDA-approved, it is very likely to become the new standard for *HER2* testing.

References: [1, 2, 4–6, 16–20, 23–25]

9.7 What Are the Requirements for the Initial HER2 Validation Study?

The initial validation must be completed before assay can be placed into clinical service. Although clinical validation is formally required in the ER guideline, this is not specifically required for HER2. The HER2 guideline states that laboratories should use FDA approved antibodies or those used in FDA approved kits to imply clinical validation. Validation for a new HER2 IHC or FISH assay may be performed against a clinically validated IHC or FISH assay by demonstrating 95% concordance with the validated assay. The HER2 guideline requires between 25 and 100 cases, but the validation paper by Fitzgibbons et al says the initial validation should include 80 cases. The next update of the HER2 guidelines is expected to reflect this minimum of 80 cases. Image analysis improves the consistency of interpretation of IHC. But if image analysis is used clinically, the method must be validated and thresholds positive, equivocal, and negative determined for 100% correlation with FISH results for positive and negative categories. The HER2 guideline that the laboratory director must assure competency of the Pathologists performing HER2 testing to include periodic or continuous peer comparisons among reviewing pathologists. No specific interval is specified.

Reference: [1, 35]

9.8 What Are the Requirements for Assuring Ongoing of HER2 Testing Quality?

If image analysis is used, annual rechecking of IHC samples results (11–26) against FISH is required to assure that thresholds are valid according to Appendix G of the HER2 guideline. Competency testing of technical personnel at regular intervals is required. Perform periodic or continuous trend analysis of HER2 positive, equivocal, and negative rates by pathologists compared with intradepartmental peers. Participation in external proficiency testing program with at least two testing events per year is mandatory. Use standardized, well-defined, negative, equivocal, and positive control materials with each run. If pathologists use several different microscopes to read assays, a system of calibration of these instruments should be implemented to ensure consistent interpretation. Validated image analysis procedures that are calibrated and subjected to regular maintenance are recommended as an effective tool aiding the pathologists for achieving consistent interpretation. Pathologist must confirm if the correct tissue is evaluated and the image analysis result. Consideration should be given to minimizing the number of Pathologists interpreting HER2 testing or referring to a central laboratory so pathologist will interpret a greater number of cases. A new initial validation study should be performed whenever a significant change is made to the test system such as use of a new primary antibody, antigen retrieval method or detection system, or when results of ongoing quality monitoring demonstrate the need.

Reference: [1]

Fig. 9.2 *HER2* FISH assay rejection criteria. (**a**, **d**) *CEP17* filter image, (**b**, **e**) *HER2* filter image, (**c**, **f**) multibandpass filter images for both *HER2* and *CEP17* signals. DAPI staining shows some blue tumor nuclei. *CEP17* is a centromere enumeration probe for chromosome 17 and is labeled with a green fluorescent signal. *HER2* is labeled with orange fluorescent signals. (**a–c**) Decalcification: The tissue in images A/B/C has been decalcified in strong acid resulting in complete loss of all ISH probe signals with all filters. (**d–f**) Weak nonuniform signals: The tissue in images D/E/F does contain faint blue DAPI-labeled nuclei containing few, nonuniform green and red-orange probe signals, but these are of insufficient quality to use for an adequate *HER2* FISH study and should be rejected

9.9 What Are the Criteria for Rejection of Results of IHC and ISH Testing of HER2?

Tissues submitted in alternative, unvalidated fixative should be rejected. Sample with prolonged cold ischemia time or formalin fixation duration <6 h or >72 h should call into question a negative results and this should be documented in the report. Specimens that have been decalcified using strong acids producing poor signals should be rejected. Anytime internal or external controls are not as expected, the test should be repeated. Many laboratories will not perform receptor HER2 studies on microinvasive cancer because foci are often gone on subsequent sections used for the studies and microinvasive foci can be very difficult to identify with FISH. IHC with strong membrane staining of internal normal duct epithelium (Fig. 9.1) or edge, crush or retraction artifacts involving most of a sample should be rejected. FISH with nonuniform signals, poor signal quality, poor nuclear resolution, obscuring background, or autofluorescence should be rejected (Fig. 9.2). When an IHC assay fails, the study could be switched to FISH testing as alternative, or vice versa.

Reference: [1]

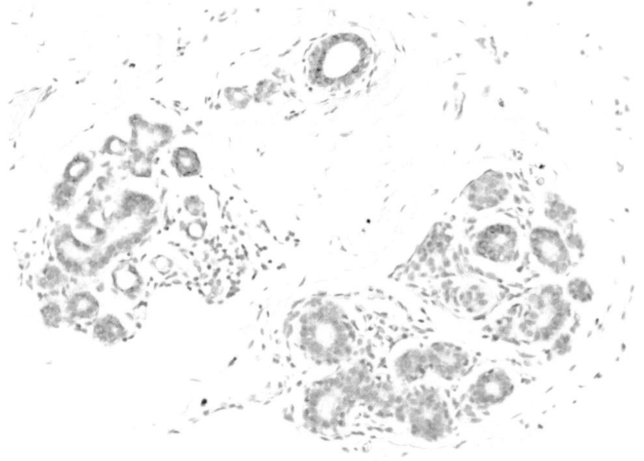

Fig. 9.1 Internal control for HER2 IHC. When available, blocks that include both tumor and normal duct epithelium should be chosen for performing receptor studies. Normal breast ducts can serve as internal control reactions for the appropriateness if the IHC staining. For HER2 IHC, there should be no strong membrane staining of internal normal duct epithelium except for areas of apocrine metaplasia When normal duct staining is present in a HER2 IHC study where tumor is also positive, consider a false-positive reaction and reject the study

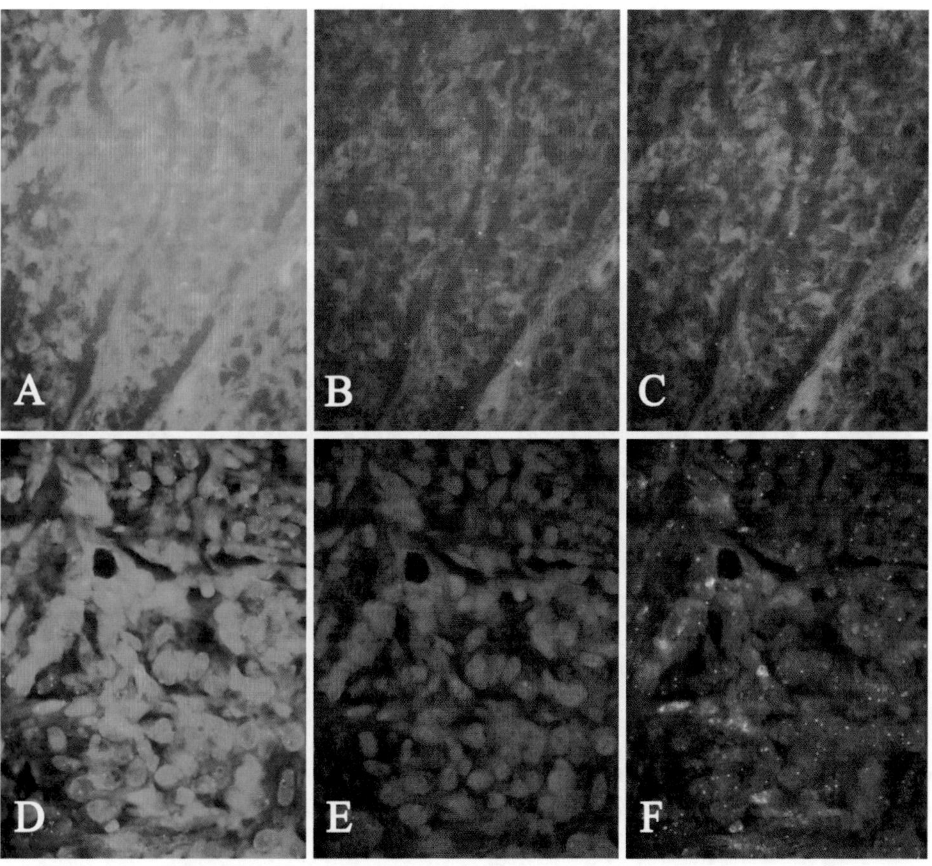

9.10 What Are the Criteria for Scoring HER2 IHC Stains?

First determine whether the slide passes the rejection criteria for testing. If the assay is adequate, proceed with scoring invasive tumor cells by assessing the extent, intensity, and completeness of circumferential staining of cell membranes. There are four results that fall into three categories for adequate HER2 IHC results. 0 or 1+ are negative, 2+ is equivocal, and 3+ is positive.

Negative for HER2 IHC is no (0) (Fig. 9.3a) or weak (1+) (Fig. 9.3b) circumferential cell membrane staining in less than 10% of tumor cells.

Equivocal for HER2 IHC is weak or nonuniform (2+) complete circumferential cell membrane staining in at least 10% of tumor cells (Fig. 9.3c).

Positive for *HER2* IHC is intense, uniform (3+) complete circumferential cell membrane staining in greater than 30% of tumor cells (Fig. 9.3d).

Reference: [1]

9.11 What Are the Criteria for Scoring *HER2* ISH Assays Stains?

First determine whether the slide passes the rejection criteria for testing. If the assay is adequate, proceed with scoring invasive tumor nuclei by counting the number of *HER2*, or *HER2* and *CEP17* signals per cell if using a dual-signal test. There are three categories for adequate *HER2* ISH assay results: negative, equivocal, and positive based on the

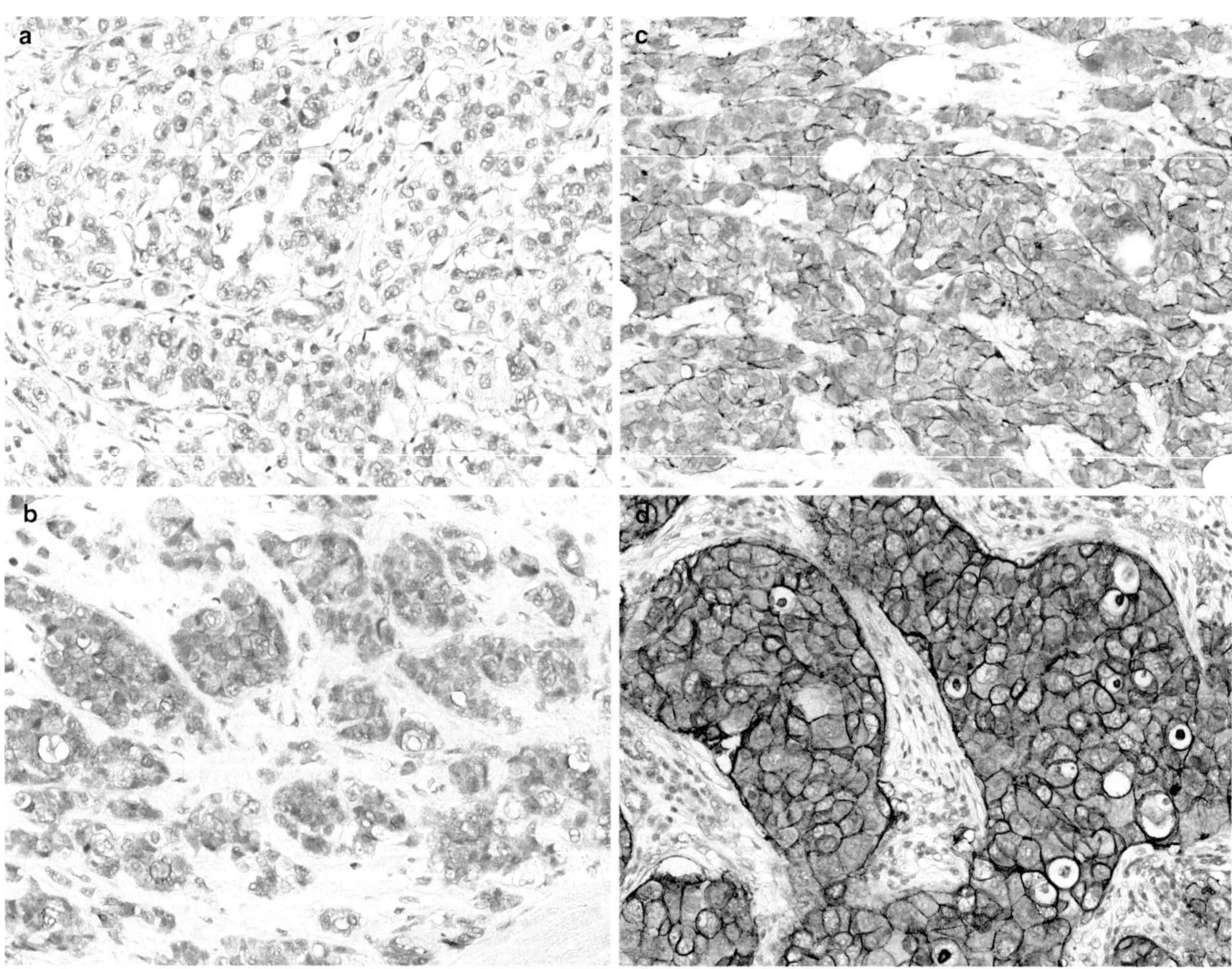

Fig. 9.3 HER2 IHC assay scoring. (**a**) HER2 IHC Negative (0) result with no complete circumferential membrane staining. (**b**) HER2 IHC Negative (1+) result with weak circumferential membrane staining in less than 10% of tumor cells. (**c**) HER2 IHC Equivocal (2+) result with moderate nonuniform complete circumferential membrane staining in at least 10% of tumor cells. (**d**) HER2 IHC Positive (3+) result with intense, uniform complete circumferential membrane staining in at least 30% of tumor cells

average signals per invasive tumor cell nucleus or total number of *HER2* signals, if no control probe is used for these counts.

Negative for *HER2* ISH is an average ratio of <1.8 of *HER2* to *CEP17* signals per nucleus or <4 signals per nucleus for tests without a *CEP17* internal control probe (Fig. 9.4a–c). Equivocal for *HER2* ISH is an average ratio that falls between 1.8 and 2.2 *HER2* to *CEP17* signals per nucleus or between 4 and 6 signals per nucleus for tests without a *CEP17* internal control probe (Fig. 9.4d–f).

Positive for *HER2* ISH is an average ratio of >2.2 of *HER2* to *CEP17* signals per nucleus or >6 signals per nucleus for tests without a *CEP17* internal control probe (Fig. 9.4g–i).

When the number of *HER2* signals is greater than 2 and the number of CEP17 control probe signals is proportionally amplified, this is an indication that the entire chromosome 17 is replicated rather than simply amplification of the area of the long arm with the *HER2* gene. This result of proportional increase of *HER2* and *CEP17* is called polysomy and does not qualify for a *HER2*-amplified result, because the average ratio of *HER2* to *CEP17* is not increased above 2.2. Polysomy is not infrequently seen associated with low level increases in *HER2* protein expression in ISH testing referred from 2+ equivocal IHC testing (Fig. 9.4j–l).

Of course, it requires two probes to measure the ratio of *HER2* to *CEP17* and diagnose polysomy. Single probe assays cannot determine if an increase in *HER2* signal is due to amplification or polysomy so two probe assays are most often used. To allow for the use of single probe *HER2* ISH testing by CISH, the CAP guidelines use a cutoff of >6 average *HER2* signals per nucleus to qualify as amplified, since most all cases of polysomy have *HER2* signal counts below 6.

References: [1, 17–22]

9.12 What Is the Recommended Algorithm for HER2 Test Interpretation?

HER2 testing may be performed initially by either ISH or IHC testing to produce a negative or positive result. First determine whether the slide passes the rejection criteria for testing. If the assay is adequate, the slide may be interpreted. If results are equivocal for the either assay initially, the test can be repeated with the other technique to attempt to clarify the result. If the second result is positive, then the patient result is positive. If the second result is negative, then the result is negative. If the results of both IHC and ISH testing are equivocal, then the oncologist can consider that prior to these guidelines, patients with *HER2* FISH scores of at least 2.0 were eligible for adjuvant Trastuzumab clinical trials (Fig. 9.5).

References: [1, 2]

9.13 What Are the Required Reporting Elements for HER2 IHC?

The HER2 guideline requires standardization of reporting elements for HER2 testing. Some of these elements may be documented in laboratory records rather than the patient report. The reporting elements for a HER2 IHC result report are:

- Patient identification information
- Submitting physician information
- Date of Service
- Specimen identification (case and block number)
- Specimen site and type
- Time to fixation (if available)
- Type and duration of fixation (if available)
- Antibody clone/vendor
- Method used (test/vendor and if FDA approved)
- Image analysis method (if used)
- Controls (high, low, and negative protein expression levels and internal control if present)
- Adequacy of the sample for evaluation
- Results including percentage of tumor cells exhibiting complete membrane staining
- Uniformity of staining
- Homogenous, dark circumferential pattern (present or absent)
- Interpretation: Positive, Equivocal, Negative or not interpretable
- Comment whether an FDA method is used, modified, or not used it should be stated in the report. The report should also state that the test has been validated and that the laboratory takes responsibility for the quality of the test performance.

Reference: [1]

9.14 What Are the Required Reporting Elements for *HER2* ISH?

The HER2 guideline requires standardization of reporting elements for HER2 testing. Some of these elements may be documented in laboratory records rather than the patient report. The reporting elements for a *HER2* ISH result report are:

- Patient identification information
- Submitting physician information
- Date of Service
- Specimen identification (case and block number)
- Specimen site and type
- Time to fixation (if available)

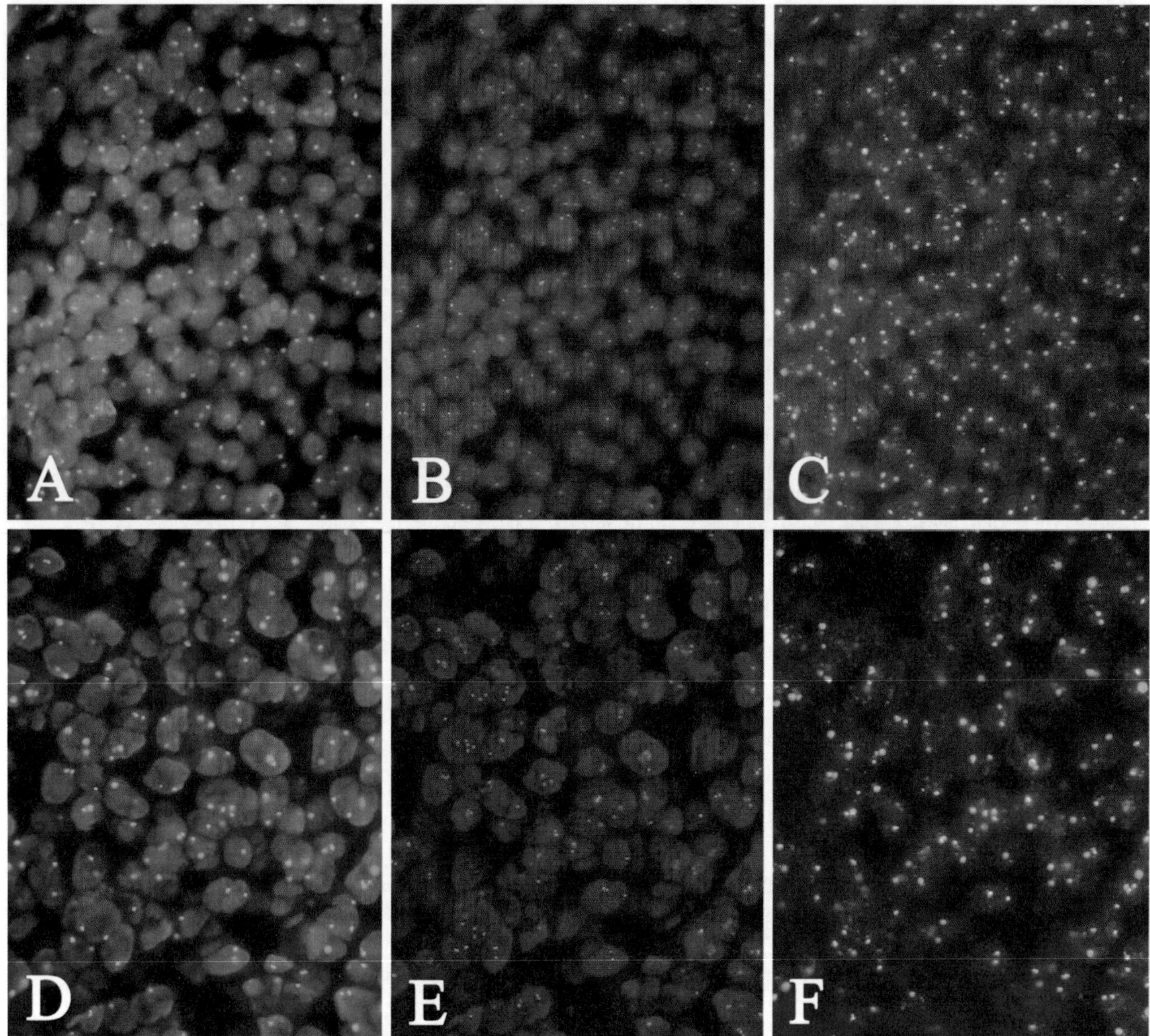

Fig. 9.4 *HER2* FISH assay. (**a**, **d**, **g**, **j**) CEP17 filter image, (**b**, **e**, **h**, **k**) *HER2* filter image, (**c**, **f**, **i**, **l**) multibandpass filter images combining both *HER2* and CEP17 signals. DAPI stains nuclei blue. CEP17 is a centromere enumeration probe for chromosome 17 and is labeled with a green fluorescent signal. *HER2* is labeled with orange fluorescent signals. (**a–c**) Normal gene number: The tissue in images (**a–c**) shows normal gene signals in each blue DAPI nucleus with an average of two green in (**a**) and (**c**) and two orange in (**b**) and (**c**). (**d–f**) Equivocal *HER2* gene amplification: The tissue in images (**d–f**) shows an equivocal level of *HER2* amplification. (**d**) An average of two green CEP17 signals per blue DAPI nucleus, but (**e**) and (**f**) both show an average of four orange HER2 signals per nucleus. This average *HER2*:CEP17 ratio of 2.0:1 falls in the equivocal range for *HER2* FISH results.

- Type and duration of fixation (if available)
- Probe(s) identification
- Method used (test/vendor and if FDA approved)
- Image analysis method (if used)
- Controls (amplified, equivocal, and not amplified levels and internal control)
- Adequacy of the sample for evaluation (adequate number of invasive tumor cells present with adequate signal quality)
- Results including number of tumor cells counted, number of observers, average number of *HER2* signals/nucleus or tile, average number of *CEP17* chromosome signals/nucleus or tile if performed, average ratio of *HER2*/*CEP17* probe signals if *CEP17* performed
- Interpretation: Amplified, Equivocal, Not Amplified or Not Interpretable
- Comment whether an FDA method is used, modified, or not used it should be stated in the report. The report should also state that the test has been validated and that the laboratory takes responsibility for the quality of the test performance.

Reference: [1]

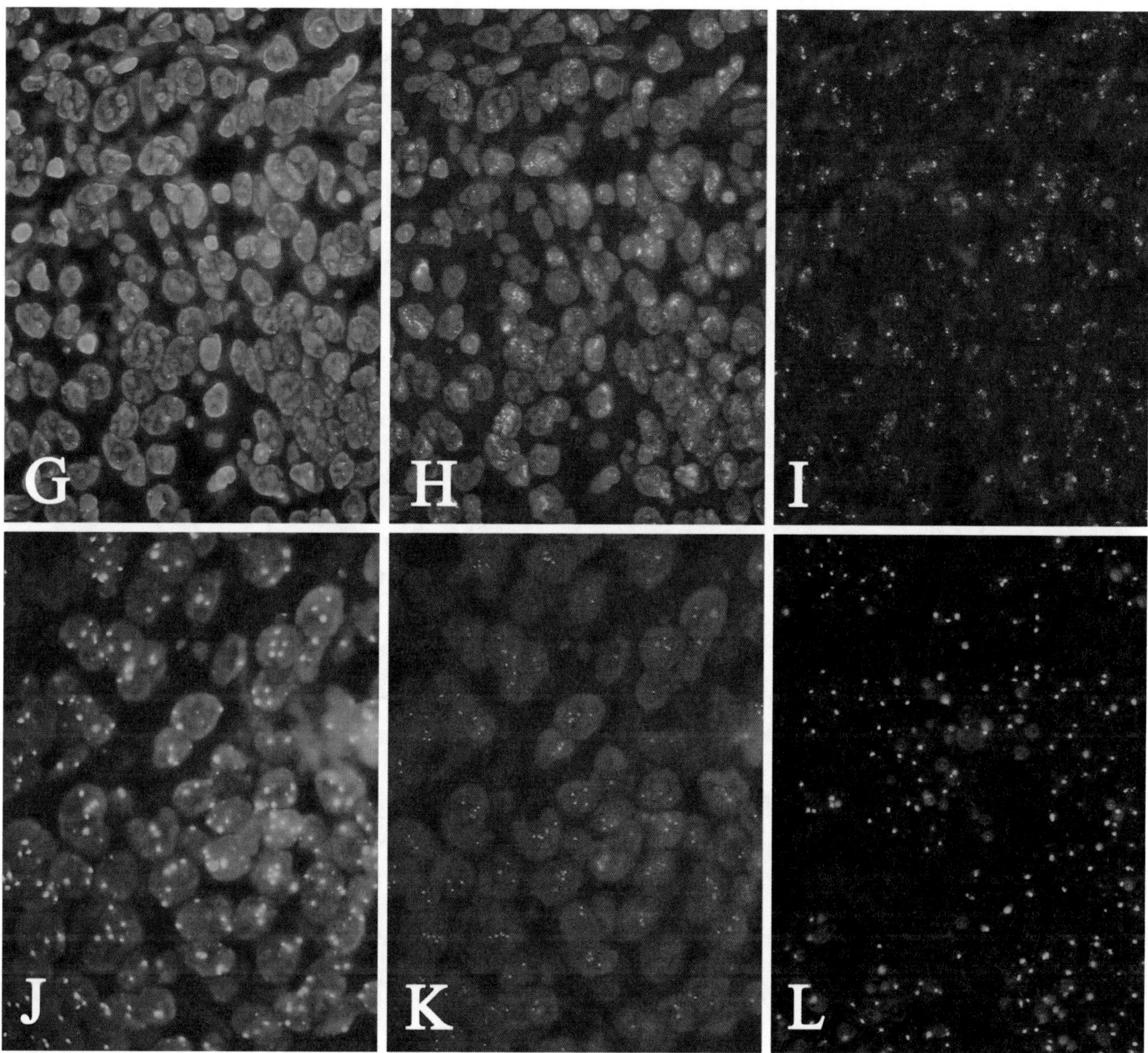

(**g–i**) Positive for *HER2* gene amplification: The tissue in images (**g–i**) shows a normal average of two green *CEP17* signals per nucleus and amplified orange *HER2* signal that are >20 per nucleus. The resulting *HER2*:*CEP17* ratio is markedly greater than 2.2:1 and qualifies as Positive for *HER2* gene amplification. (**j–l**) Polysomy/Negative for *HER2* gene amplification: The tissue in images (**j–l**) shows proportionally increased *CEP17* green signals and *HER2* orange signals indicating an increase in the total number of chromosomes rather than simply an amplification of the *HER2* gene on the long arm of chromosome 17. Although the total number of signals is increased for both *CEP17* and *HER2*, the average ratio of *HER2*: *CEP17* is less than 1.8 and qualifies a Negative for *HER2* gene amplification

9.15 What Are Estrogen Receptor (ER) and Progesterone Receptor (PR)?

What we refer to as estrogen receptor relating to IHC testing is actually a family of intracellular receptors that are all activated by estrogen hormones. There are two different forms of the estrogen receptor designated as alpha and beta and are encoded by two genes ESR1 and ESR2. ER alpha is the form associated with breast cancer and is also known as NR3A1. Once activated by estrogen, the estrogen receptor dimerizes with itself. In its active form, its main function is as nuclear transcription factor. One of the many results of the activation of ER in normal tissues is the production of the progesterone receptor. It is because of this relationship between ER and PR that ER is required to be present whenever PR is detected. Progesterone receptor, also known as NR3C3, is also a hormone receptor, but activated instead by its ligand, the progesterone hormone. When activated, PR also dimerizes and functions as a nuclear transcription factor causes the production of proteins. There are two

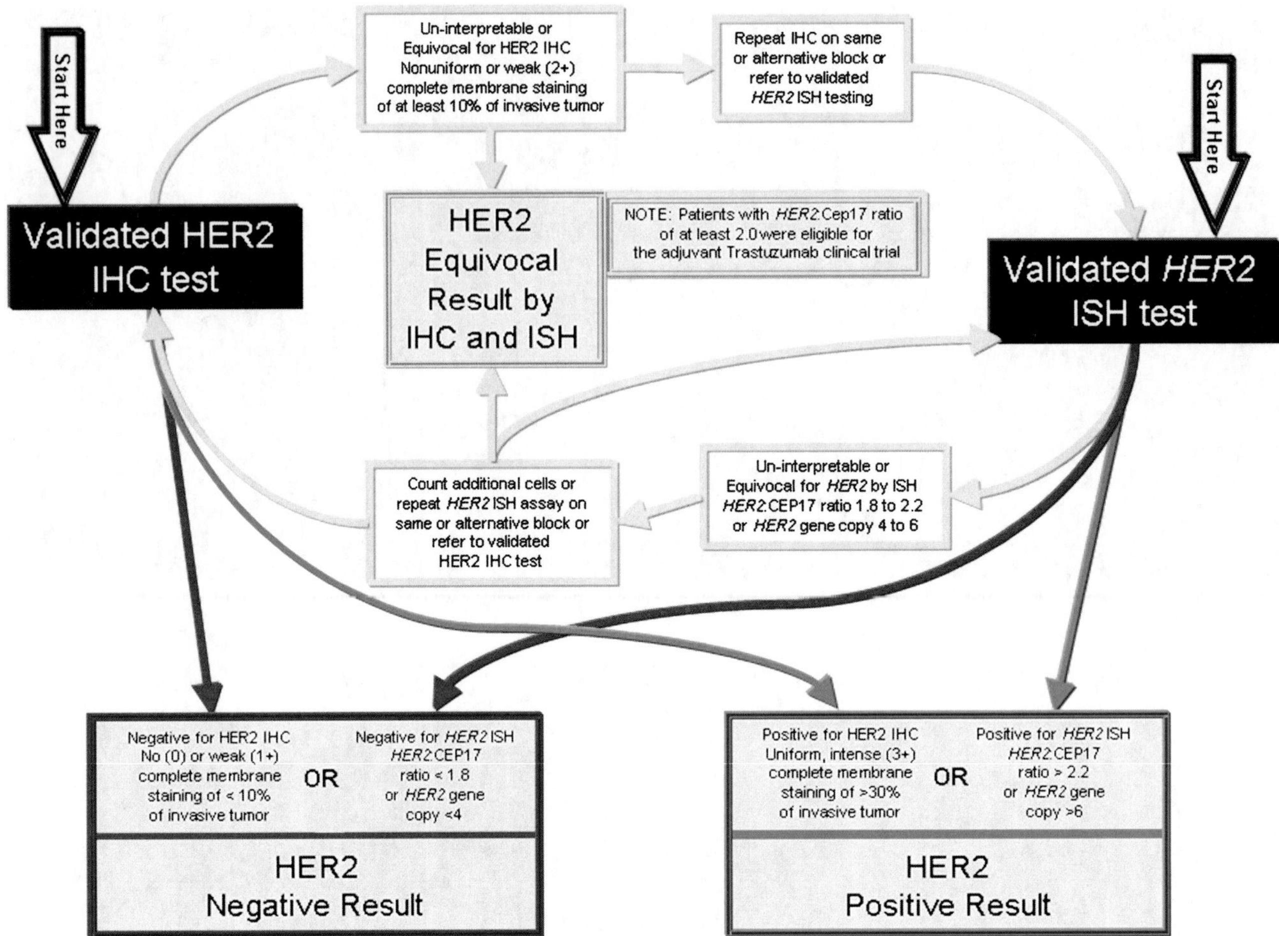

Fig. 9.5 HER2 testing algorithm. Testing for HER2 can benign with either IHC or ISH indicated by the *black starting arrows*. Either of initial tests can produce a positive or negative result directly if criteria are met. If either assay results in an equivocal or uninterpretable, it may be repeated or referred to the other testing method. If an assay is equivocal by both IHC and ISH methods, the clinician may consider patients with at least 2.0:1 ratio for *HER2*:CEP17 were eligible for the adjuvant Trastuzumab clinical trial

forms of the progesterone receptor that induce the production of different groups of proteins that have both proliferation and inhibition effects on cell growth. A breast cancer is considered positive for hormone receptors, if either ER or PR is positive by IHC.

References: [3, 7, 8, 26–30]

9.16 What Is the Prognostic and Predictive Significance of a Positive ER/PR Result?

Several studies have demonstrated substantial benefit from endocrine-based therapies for patients with ER-positive and no benefit for patients with ER-negative tumors. Endocrine therapies reduce morbidity and mortality in patients with ER-positive breast cancer and can also an effective chemopreventive strategy. Progesterone receptor assay is performed along with the estrogen receptor assay for a couple of reasons. First is that patients with ER-positive and PR-negative breast cancers have a worse prognosis than patients who have PR-positive tumors. However, studies have not shown that ER-positive/PR-negative patients response differently from ER-positive/PR-positive patients in terms of predicting benefit from antiestrogen therapies. Performing the PR assay alongside the ER assay also serves as a quality control measure to detect false-negative ER results since it is believed that ER must be present in order for PR to be present and detectable by IHC. Falsely positive hormone receptor studies are unusual, but could subject a patient to endocrine-based therapies that would offer no benefit and subject the patient to an increased risk for possibly fatal thromboembolic events and uterine cancer. False-negative hormone receptor results are thought to be too common and deny patients the substantial benefits of endocrine therapy while simultaneously misdirecting therapy to potentially toxic alternatives.

References: [3, 7, 8, 30–33]

9.17 What Tests Are FDA Cleared for Performing ER/PR Testing?

Numerous antibodies have been cleared by the FDA as Class II In Vitro Diagnostics (IVD) Devices for ER and PR IHC testing. There are no ER or PR antibodies that have completed an FDA PMA as was done for HER2 antibodies. Each hormone receptor antibody has been cleared through the less stringent premarket notification process of the FDA [510(k)] by establishing equivalence with either a dextran-coated charcoal technique established prior to 1976 or a different previously cleared antibody (Table 9.3).

9.18 What Are the Requirements for the Initial ER/PR Validation Study?

The initial validation must be completed before assay can be placed into clinical service unless laboratory has the documentation of existing clinically validated FDA-cleared or FDA-approved ER or PR assay used on at least 200 clinical specimens. This existing validation may be used to satisfy this requirement for validation if the study conformed to the manufacturer's FDA-cleared recommendation or with the current guidelines. If image analysis is used clinically, then it must be incorporated in the validation study. The initial validation studies must include at least 40 positive (^{3}1% cells staining) and 40 negative specimens (<1% cells staining). At least 10 of the 40 positive cases should be weakly positive (1–10% of cells staining). Staining should be performed in at least two batches and by multiple testing personnel so that it parallels clinical practice. Results should be either directly clinically validated or compared with results of assay performed on same specimens validated through any of the following:

- Clinical outcomes
- Previously validated ligand binding assay
- Assay from laboratory providing written attestation of conformance with CAP/ASCO guidelines and its own validation meeting the guidelines
- Alternative clinically validated method for measuring hormone receptor expression such as gene expression array
- Formal proficiency testing program including at least 50 laboratories and the PT vendor
- Technically validated tissues provided by organization such as CAP or NIST
- Concordance with clinically validated assay should be ^{3}90% for positive results and ^{3}95% for negative results. Each pathologist who interprets ER/PR results must perform a skill validation (competency testing) on at least 20 positive and 20 negative specimens, including some weakly negative specimens. Slides from the initial validation may be used for skill validations. Acceptable performance for a skill validation is no more than 2 of 40 incorrect results (95% concordance).

References: [3, 35]

Table 9.3 FDA-approved (PMA) and FDA-cleared [510(k)] ER and PR antibodies

	Company	Clonality	Antibody	FDA process	FDA date
Estrogen receptor	Biogenex	Monoclonal mouse	ER88	510(k)	2/28/2002
	Dako	Monoclonal rabbit	SP1	510(k)	5/8/2009
	Dako	Monoclonal mouse	1D5	510(k)	3/3/2000
	Labvision	Monoclonal rabbit	SP1	510(k)	6/27/2006
	Ventana	Monoclonal mouse	6F11	510(k)	8/12/1999
	Vision Biosystems	Monoclonal mouse	6F11	510(k)	5/25/2006
Progesterone receptor	Biogenex	Monoclonal mouse	PR88	510(k)	3/8/2002
	Dako	Monoclonal mouse	PgR 636	510(k)	2/28/2002
	Dako	Monoclonal mouse	PgR 1294	510(k)	2/15/2005
	Vision Biosystems	Monoclonal mouse	PgR 16	510(k)	1/29/2007
	Labvision	Monoclonal rabbit	Sp2	510(k)	4/24/2006
	Ventana	Monoclonal mouse	1A6	510(k)	7/23/1999
	Ventana	Monoclonal rabbit	1E2	510(k)	Pending

Notes: Dako received clearance to market its ER 1D5 and PR PgR1294 clones together as an ER/PR PharmDx kit on 2/15/2005. Ventana has submitted its 1E2 rabbit monoclonal on its Ultra platform for FDA clearance still pending at press time.

9.19 What Are the Requirements for Assuring Ongoing of ER/PR Testing Quality?

Following the initial test validation, there should be ongoing quality control and equipment maintenance. The use of standardized operating procedures including routine use of external control materials with each batch of testing and routine evaluation of internal normal epithelial elements, or the inclusion of normal breast sections on each tested slide is best practice wherever possible. There needs to be ongoing training and competency assessment of both technical staff and pathologists. Ongoing assay reassessment should be done at least semiannually. ER-positive and -negative rates should be trended by pathologist, by patient age and by tumor grade. Positive and negative rates of the overall assay and those interpreted by each pathologist should be evaluated at least semiannually. Overall ER-negative rate should be less than 30%. In women over 65, ER-negative rate for invasive tumor should be £20%. Low-grade tumor ER-negative rate should be £5%. For cases with available gene expression analyses for ER and PR such as through OncotypeDX®, concordance with IHC results should be at least 95%. Participation in external proficiency testing program for ER and PR with at least two testing events (mailings) per year is mandatory. Satisfactory performance requires at least 90% correct responses on graded challenges for both tests. Unsuccessful performance results in suspension of laboratory testing for ER or PR. A new initial validation study must be performed whenever a significant change is made to the test system such as use of a new primary antibody, antigen retrieval method or detection system, or when results of ongoing quality monitoring demonstrate the need. CAP on-site inspection is to be performed every other year with annual self-inspections to review laboratory validation, procedures, QA results and processes, and reports. Unsatisfactory performance will require laboratory to respond according to accreditation agency program requirements.

References: [3, 35]

9.20 What Are the Criteria for Rejection of Result of IHC Testing of ER and PR?

Tissues submitted in alternative, unvalidated fixative should be rejected. Sample with prolonged cold ischemia time or formalin fixation duration <6 h or >72 h should call into question a negative results and this should be documented in the report. Specimens that have been decalcified using strong acids producing poor staining should be rejected. Anytime internal or external controls are not as expected, the test should be repeated. When internal normal epithelial elements and/or normal positive control on same slide show no staining, negative staining in the patient tumor cells should be rejected (Fig. 9.6). Reject the sample if excessive cytoplasmic staining occurs. The ER and PR results should fit the clinical profile of the patient being evaluated: Consider the type of invasive cancer and the grade of the cancer in interpretation; some cancer types such as lobular, mucinous, and tubular carcinoma are almost always strongly ER-positive and only rarely ER-negative. Specimens exhibiting the unlikely immunophenotype of ER-negative and PR-positive, most likely indicates a false-negative ER assay or a false-positive PR assay. Tissue specimens where a microinvasive tumor cannot be clearly identified should be rejected. A Ductal Carcinoma In Situ (DCIS) score may be provided if made clear in the report that the scoping was performed on DCIS rather than invasive tumor. Cytology specimens with limited or weak staining must contain at least 100 cells. For rejected studies, a separate tumor block can be chosen to repeat the study or the test can be deferred to IHC studies on a previous or subsequent additional specimen of the tumor.

Reference: [3]

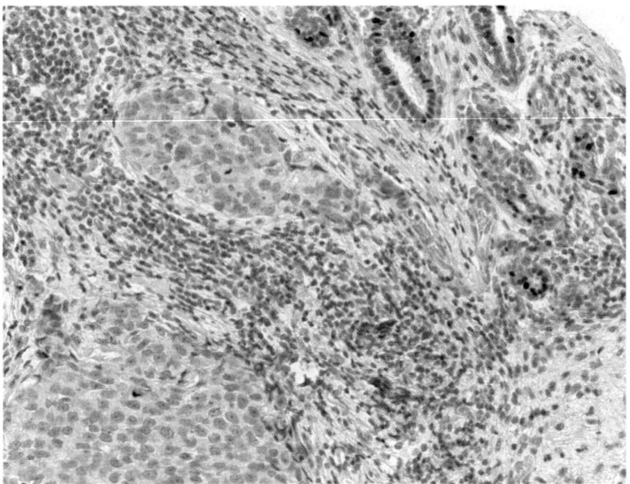

Fig. 9.6 Internal control for ER and PR IHC. The image shows invasive breast cancer in the *lower left* contrasted with appropriately positive staining internal control normal duct epithelium in the *upper right*. When available, blocks that include both tumor and normal duct epithelium should be chosen for performing receptor studies. Normal breast ducts can serve as internal control reactions for the appropriateness if the IHC staining. For ER and PR IHC, there should be some nuclear staining of internal normal duct epithelium. When normal duct staining is not present in an ER or PR IHC study where tumor is also negative, consider a false-negative reaction and reject the study

9.21 What Are the Criteria for Scoring the Results of IHC Testing of ER and PR?

First determine whether the slide passes the rejection criteria for testing. If the assay is adequate, proceed with scoring invasive tumor nuclei by counting for percentage positivity and average intensity. There are only two categories for adequate ER or PR IHC results: negative or positive. An ER or PR study is negative when <1% of tumor cells with ER or PR staining (Fig. 9.7a). For an ER or PR assay to have a positive result, ^{3}1% of tumor cells are immunoreactive (Fig. 9.7b, c). Reporting the results of ER and PR studies should include scores for both average intensity and percentage of nuclei staining included in the report. A combined percentage and intensity score such as H score, Allred score, or Quick score may be provided in addition to individual percentage and intensity scores. Positive staining for either ER or PR is considered a positive result for hormone receptor status of breast cancer, though a result that is ER-negative and PR-positive should call into question to result and hormone receptor studies should be repeated on a different block or specimen if available. Quantitative image analysis is encouraged for samples with low percentages of nuclear staining or in cases with multiple observers in the same institution. It is also a valuable way to quantify intensity and assure day-to-day consistency of control tissue reactivity.

References: [3, 30–32]

9.22 What Are the Required Reporting Elements for ER and PR IHC?

The items to be included in an ER/PR IHC result report are:

- Patient identification information
- Submitting physician information
- Date of Service
- Specimen identification (case and block number)
- Specimen site and type
- Results including percentage and average intensity (weak, moderate, strong) of invasive tumor cells exhibiting nuclear staining (DCIS resulting is optional), scores combining intensity and percentage positivity are optional
- Interpretation: Positive, Equivocal, Negative or not interpretable for ER or PR protein expression
- Internal and external controls: positive, negative, or not present
- Standard assay condition net/not met/unknown (ischemia/fixation)
- Comment should explain reason for an uninterpretable result or any other unusual condition, if applicable
- The following items must be documented on the accession slip or in internal laboratory records if not included in an ER/PR IHC result report:
- Cold ischemia time (time to fixation)
- Type and duration of fixation (if available)
- Staining method (details of the primary antibody/test kit/vendor and if FDA approved, and method of test validation)

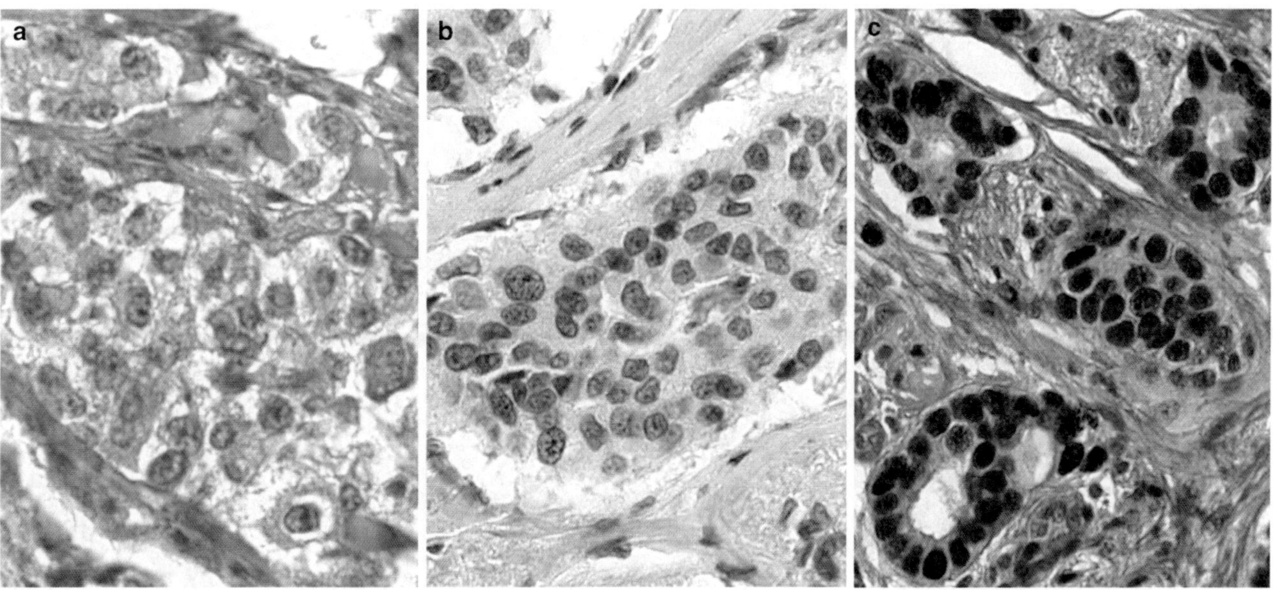

Fig. 9.7 ER and PR IHC assay scoring. (**a**) ER/PR IHC Negative result with less 1% positive tumor nuclei staining. (**b**) ER/PR IHC Weakly Positive result with weak staining in 1–10% of tumor nuclei staining in at least 10% of tumor cells. (**c**) ER/PR IHC Strongly Positive result with intense, uniform staining of all tumor nuclei

- Controls (high protein expression, low-level protein expression, negative protein expression, internal elements or from normal breast tissue included with sample)
  Image analysis method (if used)

Reference: [3]

References

1. Wolff AC, Hammond ME, Schwartz JN, Hagerty KL, Allred DC, Cote RJ, et al. American Society of Clinical Oncology/College of American Pathologists guideline recommendations for human epidermal growth factor receptor 2 testing in breast cancer. Arch Pathol Lab Med. 2007;131(1):18–43.
2. Carlson RW, Moench SJ, Hammond ME, Perez EA, Burstein HJ, Allred DC, et al. HER2 testing in breast cancer: NCCN Task Force report and recommendations. J Natl Compr Canc Netw. 2006;4 Suppl 3:S1 22.
3. Hammond ME, Hayes DF, Dowsett M, et al. American Society of Clinical Oncology/College of American Pathologists guideline recommendations for immunohistochemical testing of estrogen and progesterone receptors in breast cancer. Arch Pathol Lab Med. 2010;134(6):907–22.
4. Paik S, Bryant J, Tan-Chiu E, Romond E, Hiller W, Park K, et al. Real-world performance of HER2 testing–National Surgical Adjuvant Breast and Bowel Project experience. J Natl Cancer Inst. 2002;94(11):852–4.
5. Roche PC, Suman VJ, Jenkins RB, Davidson NE, Martino S, Kaufman PA, et al. Concordance between local and central laboratory HER2 testing in the breast intergroup trial N9831. J Natl Cancer Inst. 2002;94(11):855–7.
6. Perez EA, Suman VJ, Davidson NE, Martino S, Kaufman PA, Lingle WL, et al. HER2 testing by local, central, and reference laboratories in specimens from the North Central Cancer Treatment Group N9831 intergroup adjuvant trial. J Clin Oncol. 2006;24(19):3032–8.
7. Badve SS, Baehner FL, Gray RP, Childs BH, Maddala T, Liu ML, et al. Estrogen- and progesterone-receptor status in ECOG 2197: comparison of immunohistochemistry by local and central laboratories and quantitative reverse transcription polymerase chain reaction by central laboratory. J Clin Oncol. 2008;26:2473–81.
8. Viale G, Regan MM, Maiorano E, Mastropasqua MG, Dell'Orto P, Rasmussen BB, et al. Prognostic and predictive value of centrally reviewed expression of estrogen and progesterone receptors in a randomized trial comparing letrozole and tamoxifen adjuvant therapy for postmenopausal early breast cancer: BIG 1–98. J Clin Oncol. 2007;25:3846–52.
9. Bloom K, Harrington D. Enhanced accuracy and reliability of HER-2/neu immunohistochemical scoring using digital microscopy. Am J Clin Pathol. 2004;121(5):620–30.
10. Munro AF, Cameron DA, Bartlett JM. Targeting anthracyclines in early breast cancer: new candidate predictive biomarkers emerge. Oncogene. 2010;29(38):5231–40.
11. Olayioye MA. Update on HER-2 as a target for cancer therapy: intracellular signaling pathways of ErbB2/HER-2 and family members. Breast Cancer Res. 2001;3(6):385–9. doi:10.1186/bcr327. PMID 11737890.
12. Libermann TA et al. Tyrosine kinase receptor with extensive homology to EGF receptor shares chromosomal location with neu oncogene. Science. 1985;230(4730):1132–9.
13. Idirisinghe PK, Thike AA, Cheok PY, Tse GM, Lui PC, Fook-Chong S, et al. Hormone receptor and c-ERBB2 status in distant metastatic and locally recurrent breast cancer. Pathologic correlations and clinical significance. Am J Clin Pathol. 2010;133(3):416–29.
14. Ross JS, Slodkowska EA, Symmans WF, Pusztai L, Ravdin PM, Hortobagyi GN. The HER-2 receptor and breast cancer: ten years of targeted anti-HER-2 therapy and personalized medicine. Oncologist. 2009;14(4):320–68.
15. Mohsin SK. HER2 testing: state of the laboratories. Arch Pathol Lab Med. 2010;134(5):660–6. Online publication date: 1 May 2010.
16. Downey L, Livingston RB, Koehler M, Arbushites M, Williams L, Santiago A, et al. Chromosome 17 polysomy without human epidermal growth factor receptor 2 amplification does not predict response to lapatinib plus paclitaxel compared with paclitaxel in metastatic breast cancer. Clin Cancer Res. 2010;16(4):1281–8.
17. Penault-Llorca F, Bilous M, Dowsett M, Hanna W, Osamura RY, Rüschoff J, et al. Emerging technologies for assessing HER2 amplification. Am J Clin Pathol. 2009;132(4):539–48.
18. Francis GD, Jones MA, Beadle GF, Stein SR. Bright-field in situ hybridization for HER2 gene amplification in breast cancer using tissue microarrays: correlation between chromogenic (CISH) and automated silver-enhanced (SISH) methods with patient outcome. Diagn Mol Pathol. 2009;18(2):88–95.
19. Papouchado BG, Myles J, Lloyd RV, Stoler M, Oliveira AM, Downs-Kelly E, et al. Silver in situ hybridization (SISH) for determination of HER2 gene status in breast carcinoma: comparison with FISH and assessment of interobserver reproducibility. Am J Surg Pathol. 2010;34(6):767–76.
20. Zhao J, Wu R, Au A, Marquez A, Yu Y, Shi Z. Determination of HER2 gene amplification by chromogenic in situ hybridization (CISH) in archival breast carcinoma. Mod Pathol. 2002;15(6):657–65.
21. Krishnamurti U, Hammers JL, Atem FD, Storto PD, Silverman JF. Poor prognostic significance of unamplified chromosome 17 polysomy in invasive breast carcinoma. Mod Pathol. 2009;22(8):1044–8.
22. Vanden Bempt I, Van Loo P, Drijkoningen M, Neven P, Smeets A, Christiaens MR, et al. Polysomy 17 in breast cancer: clinicopathologic significance and impact on HER-2 testing. J Clin Oncol. 2008;26(30):4869–74.
23. Gruver AM, Peerwani Z, Tubbs RR. Out of the darkness and into the light: bright field in situ hybridisation for delineation of ERBB2 (HER2) status in breast carcinoma. J Clin Pathol. 2010;63(3):210–9.
24. Mayr D, Heim S, Weyrauch K, Zeindl-Eberhart E, Kunz A, Engel J, et al. Chromogenic in situ hybridization for Her-2/neu-oncogene in breast cancer: comparison of a new dual-colour chromogenic in situ hybridization with immunohistochemistry and fluorescence in situ hybridization. Histopathology. 2009;55(6):716–23.
25. Kato N, Itoh H, Serizawa A, Hatanaka Y, Umemura S, Osamura RY. Evaluation of HER2 gene amplification in invasive breast cancer using a dual-color chromogenic in situ hybridization (dual CISH). Pathol Int. 2010;60(7):510–5.
26. Coussens L, Yang-Feng TL, Liao YC, Chen E, Gray A, McGrath J, et al. International Union of Pharmacology. LXIV. Estrogen receptors. Pharmacol Rev. 2006;58(4):773–81.
27. Levin ER. Integration of the extranuclear and nuclear actions of estrogen. Mol Endocrinol. 2005;19(8):1951–9.
28. Gadkar-Sable S, Shah C, Rosario G, Sachdeva G, Puri C. Progesterone receptors: various forms and functions in reproductive tissues. Front Biosci. 2005;10:2118–30.
29. Kastner P, Krust A, Turcotte B, Stropp U, Tora L, Gronemeyer H, et al. Two distinct estrogen-regulated promoters generate transcripts encoding the two functionally different human progesterone receptor forms A and B. EMBO J. 1990;9(5):1603–14.
30. Fisher ER, Anderson S, Dean S, Dabbs D, Fisher B, Siderits R, et al. Solving the dilemma of the immunohistochemical and other

methods used for scoring estrogen receptor and progesterone receptor in patients with invasive breast carcinoma. Cancer. 2005;103(1): 164–73.
31. Harvey JM, Clark GM, Osborne CK, Allred DC. Estrogen receptor status by immunohistochemistry is superior to the ligand-binding assay for predicting response to adjuvant endocrine therapy in breast cancer. J Clin Oncol. 1999;17:1474–81.
32. Mohsin SK, Weiss H, Havighurst T, Clark GM, Berardo M, le Roanh D, et al. Progesterone receptor by immunohistochemistry and clinical outcome in breast cancer: a validation study. Mod Pathol. 2004;17:1545–54.
33. Visvanathan K, Lippman SM, Hurley P, Temin S. American Society of Clinical Oncology clinical practice guideline update on the use of pharmacologic interventions including tamoxifen, raloxifene, and aromatase inhibition for breast cancer risk reduction. J Clin Oncol. 2009;27(19):3235–58.
34. Yamashita H, Yando Y, Nishio M, Zhang Z, Hamaguchi M, Mita K, et al. Immunohistochemical evaluation of hormone receptor status for predicting response to endocrine therapy in metastatic breast cancer. Breast Cancer. 2006;13:74–83.
35. Fitzgibbons PL, Murphy DA, Hammond MEH, et al. Recommendations for validating estrogen and progesterone receptor immunohistochemistry assays. Arch Pathol Lab Med. 2010; 134(6):930–5.
36. Goldstein NS, Ferkowicz M, Odish E, Mani A, Hastah F. Minimum formalin fixation time for consistent estrogen receptor immunohistochemical staining of invasive breast carcinoma. Am J Clin Pathol. 2003;120:86–92.

Chapter 10
Central and Peripheral Nerve System Tumors

Hueizhi (Hope) Wu, Conrad Schuerch, and Douglas C. Miller

Abstract This chapter addresses frequently asked practical questions about the application of immunohistochemistry to the central nervous system (CNS). The first table, Table 10.1, is a summary table of frequently used antibodies in the CNS. The markers for individual tumor types in the CNS are given in Tables 10.2–10.20. Tables 10.21–10.34 list markers useful in differential diagnosis of CNS tumors. The last four tables, Tables 10.35–10.38, are markers for non-neoplastic lesions in the CNS, listing the markers for neurodegenerative disorders (Table 10.35), virus and parasite infections (Table 10.36), epilepsy (Table 10.37), and histiocytic disorders (Table 10.38).

Keywords Central nervous system • Tumors • Immunohistochemistry • Antibodies • Neurodegenerative disease

FREQUENTLY ASKED QUESTIONS

Antibodies Frequently Used in the CNS:

Tumor: Markers for Tumors in the CNS:

Tumor: Markers for Differential Diagnosis in the CNS:

H. (Hope) Wu (✉)
Department of Pathology and Laboratory Medicine, Geisinger Medical Center, 100 N. Academy Ave, Danville, PA 17822, USA
e-mail: hwu1@geisinger.edu

F. Lin and J. Prichard (eds.), *Handbook of Practical Immunohistochemistry: Frequently Asked Questions*,
DOI 10.1007/978-1-4419-8062-5_10,

31. Markers for tumors with chordoid pattern: chordoid glioma vs. chordoid meningioma vs. chordoma (Table 10.31) (p. 131)
32. Markers for tumors with giant cell pattern (Table 10.32) (p. 131)
33. Markers for tumors with spindle cell pattern (Table 10.33) (p. 131)
34. Markers for metastases in CNS (Table 10.34) (p. 132)

Markers for Non-neoplastic Lesions in the CNS:

35. Markers for neurodegenerative disorders (Table 10.35) (p. 133)
36. Markers for virus and parasite infections of the CNS (Table 10.36) (p. 133)
37. Markers for epilepsy (Table 10.37) (p. 133)
38. Markers for histiocytic disorders in CNS (Table 10.38) (p. 134)

Table 10.1 Frequently used antibodies in the CNS

Antibodies	Staining pattern	Function	Key applications and pitfalls
Alpha-B-crystallin	C	Neurons, major protein component of Rosenthal fibers	Swollen neurons, neurons in degenerative disorders, Rosenthal fibers
Alpha-beta-amyloid	Extracellular	Amyloid	Cerebral amyloid angiopathy
			Amyloid plaques of Alzheimer's disease
Alpha-subunit/C	C		Pituitary adenoma
Alpha-synuclein		Lewy bodies	Lewy bodies and Lewy neurites in Parkinson's disease and diffuse Lewy body disease
BAF47/SNF5 (INI-1)	N	Regulator of chromatin structure	*Positive*:
			Mosaic pattern in familial schwannomatosis
			Rhabdoid cells in rhabdoid glioblastoma (GBM)
			Rhabdoid meningiomas
			Absent expression in: Atypical teratoid/rhabdoid tumor
Beta-amyloid precursor protein	C, Extracellular	Axonal spheroids	Damaged axons, cell bodies; senile plaques of Alzheimer's disease
			Hypoxic–ischemic encephalopathy
CAM5.2	C	Low molecular weight cytokeratin	Epithelial neoplasms[a]
			Sparsely positive in growth hormone and ACTH producing pituitary adenomas
Carbonic anhydrase isoenzyme II	C	Cytosolic enzyme	Widely distributed enzyme, in the brain principally in oligodendroglial cells. Present in glial tumors, myxopapillary ependymoma and others
CD1a	M	Langerhans cells	Langerhans cell histiocytosis[b]
C-Kit/CD117	M, C	Transmembrane tyrosine kinase receptor	Glial cells, glial tumors, reactive glial cells
			Germinomas
CD3	M + C	T cells	Pan T cell marker–T cells
CD4	M	T cells	T cell subset
CD8	M	T cells	T cell subset
CD20	M	B cells	B cells
CD31	M	Vascular endothelium	Vascular hyperplasia in Hypoxic–ischemic encephalopathy
CD34	M	Vascular endothelium	Endothelial neoplasms
			Solitary fibrous tumor of dura
			Ganglioglioma neurons
			Neurofibroma
			Epithelioid sarcoma
CD45	M	All differentiated hematopoietic cells except erythrocytes and plasma cells. Also known as leukocyte common antigen (LCA)	Macrophages and microglia in demyelination, infection, infarcts
CD56	C	NK cells, activated T cells, the brain and cerebellum, and neuroendocrine tissues. Also called neural cell adhesion molecule (NCAM)	Neuroendocrine tumors
			Adult neuroblastoma
			Metastatic small cell lung carcinoma
			Primitive neuroectodermal tumor (PNET)
CD68	M	Macrophages and microglial cells	Infarcts
			Demyelinating processes
			Necrotic neoplasms
			Wallerian (White matter tract) degeneration

(continued)

Table 10.1 (continued)

Antibodies	Staining pattern	Function	Key applications and pitfalls
Chromogranin	C	Present in the cores of amine and peptide hormone and neurotransmitter dense-core secretory vesicles in endocrine and neuroendocrine cells	Positive in neuroendocrine tumors including pituitary adenomas, paragangliomas, and some cells in some neuronal tumors
CK7	M + C	54-kDa type II keratin	Epithelial marker, positive in metastatic carcinomas (e.g., in most lung cancers and most breast cancers, and in some gastric cancers), but it is usually negative in colon and rectal adenocarcinomas
CK20	M + C	46-kDa low-molecular-weight keratin	Epithelial marker, positive in choroid plexus tumors, metastatic carcinomas (e.g., Positive in the large majority of colon and rectal adenocarcinomas)
Claudin 6	M + C	Key component for tight junction	Positive in atypical teratoid/rhabdoid tumor
Cytokeratin AE1/AE3	C	Pankeratin cocktail containing high and low molecular weight keratins	Marker of most carcinomas and epithelial neoplasms. Stains some glial tumors[c]
Cytomegalovirus (CMV)	C + M	Cytomegalovirus	CMV-infected cells
Desmin	C	Intermediate filament of skeletal, smooth, and cardiac muscle	Myogenic differentiation in neoplasms Rhabdomyoma/sarcoma; leiomyoma/sarcoma
EMA (Epithelial membrane antigen)	M + C	Normal and neoplastic epithelia; notochord; perineural cells; arachnoidal cells; plasma cells	Carcinoma Meningioma Synovial sarcoma Epithelioid sarcoma Perineurioma Chordoma Atypical teratoid/rhabdoid tumor Some plasmacytomas Dot-like cytoplasmic positivity in ependymomas and angiocentric glioma
Factor XIIIa	M	Clotting factor	Positive in endoneurial fibroblasts, neurofibroma
GFAP	C	Astrocytes; ependymal cells; immature oligodendrocytes. GFAP-like protein expressed by nonmyelinating Schwann cells	Reactive fibrillary astrocytes Astrocytoma, except sarcomatous elements in gliosarcoma Ependymoma Gliofibrillary oligodendrocytes and oligodendroglial minigemistocytes Some schwannomas
HMB45	C	Melanoma extract antigen	Melanocytic tumors, especially to distinguish metastatic melanoma from other S100+ brain tumors
HSV	N + C	Herpes simplex virus	Infected cells in Herpes encephalitis
Kappa and lambda light chains	M + C	Immunoglobulin components	Clonal vs. mixed plasma cell or lymphocytic proliferations[d]
Leu7 (CD57)	M	Transmembrane adhesion molecule	Natural killer cells, neuroglial progenitor cells
MAP2	C	Microtubule-associated protein of brain tissue	Axons
Mart-1/Melan-A	C	Glycoproteinaceous antigenetic group	Melanocytic tumors, especially to distinguish metastatic melanoma from other S100+ brain tumors
Melan-A	C	Melanoma antigen	Some melanomas are HMB-negative and Melan-A helps identify these cases
MIB1	N	Ki67 nuclear antigen associated with cell proliferation during all active phases of the cell cycle (G1, S, G2, and mitosis); absent from resting cells (G0)	Proliferation index Important for CNS tumor grading
MSA	C	Muscle-specific actin, a contractile protein	Smooth muscle cells
NeuN	N	Neuronal nuclei; not in Purkinje cells, neurons of the internal nuclear layer of the retina, and sympathetic chain ganglia	Neuronal and glioneural tumors; also very useful for the examination of cortical architecture in specimens from epilepsy surgery
Neurofilament protein	C	Neuronal characteristic intermediate filament; nonphosphorylated in perikaryon, phosphorylated in neurites	Neuronal and glioneuronal tumors. Accumulation in neurons and axons swollen due to injury[e]
OCT4 (POU5T-1)	N	18-kDa Pou-domain transcription factor in embryonic stem cells and primordial germ cells	Germinoma

(continued)

Table 10.1 (continued)

Antibodies	Staining pattern	Function	Key applications and pitfalls
p53	N	Transcription factor and TP53 tumor suppressor gene product	Increased staining is an indirect marker of a mutant TP53 gene or of wild-type TP53 inactivation from hypoxia or DNA damage Immunopositive in some WHO Grade II–IV astrocytomas but not in pilocytic astrocytoma Atypical pituitary adenoma and pituitary carcinoma Seen in reactive changes status post radiation therapy[f]
PGP9.5	C	Ubiquitin C-terminal hydrolase	Swollen neuron
Progesterone receptor (PR)	N	Receptor for progesterone	Meningioma, absence indicates increased risk of recurrence
pVHL	M	Von Hippel–Lindau gene product, a tumor suppressor protein	Positive in renal cell carcinoma, oncocytoma
RMDO20	C	Antibody to neurofilament protein, intermediate molecular weight	Neuronal and glioneuronal tumors[e]
S100	N + C	Calcium-binding proteins	Cells derived from the neural crest (Schwann cells, melanocytes, and glial cells), chondrocytes, adipocytes, myoepithelial cells, macrophages, Langerhans cells, dendritic cells, and keratinocytes Chordoma, gliomas, melanomas, schwannomas, neurofibromas, and chondrosarcomas
Smooth muscle actin	C	Myogenic differentiation, including myofibroblastic and myoepithelial tissues	Myogenic differentiation in neoplasms Highlights vascular hyperplasia
SV40		Simian virus 40, a polyomavirus	Surrogate for immunolabeling of JC virus-infected cells in progressive multifocal leukoencephalopathy (PML)
Synaptophysin	C	Synaptic vesicle protein	Neuronal, pineal, and choroid plexus tumors Pituitary adenoma Paraganglioma Gray matter neuropil (synapses)[g]
TDP43	C	TAR-DNA binding protein, altered form of a transcription regulator protein	Pathologic protein in types of frontotemporal dementia and amyotrophic lateral sclerosis
Thyroid transcription factor-1 (TTF1)	N	Protein that regulates transcription of genes specific for the thyroid, lung, and diencephalon	Metastatic lung or thyroid carcinoma Ependymoma of the 3rd ventricle
Transthyretin (TTR)	C	CSF protein carrier of thyroxine	Choroid plexus tumors
Ubiquitin	C	Ubiquitin protein	Swollen neurons; inclusions of a variety of neurodegenerative diseases (tangles, Lewy bodies, others)
Vimentin	C	Intermediate filament	Mesenchymal cells, myoepithelial cells, spindled carcinoma cells, melanocytes, endocrine cells, endothelial cells, and many others Tumor of these cell types, including most gliomas

Note: *N* nuclear staining, *M* membranous staining, *C* cytoplasmic staining

[a] CAM5.2 is positive in metastatic carcinomas, primary choroid plexus papillomas, and most choroid plexus carcinomas. It is not positive in endothelial tumors such as angiosarcoma

[b] Primary CNS Langerhans Cell Histiocytosis is, for some reason, often CD1a negative

[c] There is well-known cross-reactivity with the AE1/AE3 cocktail and GFAP, which should not be misinterpreted as evidence of epithelial differentiation in glial tumors

[d] Immunostains for Kappa and Lambda light chains are often not very clean; kappa and lambda in situ hybridization provides better visualization

[e] NFP comes in three molecular weights: low (NF-L), intermediate (NF-M), and high (NF-H). Antibody cocktails to all three are often most useful for tumor diagnosis, and NF-M antibodies are the next best choice

[f] A few pilocytic tumors have been shown to be p53 positive

[g] The patterns of synaptophysin immunopositivity are important as these are often difficult for general pathologists. In Ganglioglioma and related ganglion cell tumors, the diagnostic pattern is a coarse granular surface immunopositivity on the cell body of the neoplastic ganglion cell: "perikaryal surface immunopositivity." An example for Synaptophysin immunostain to demonstrate "perikaryal surface immunopositivity" in dysembryoplastic neuroepithelial tumor is shown in Fig. 10.10

In neurocytic tumors, sometimes the cell body's cytoplasm is positive, but more often the neuropil between the tumor cells has a granular immunopositivity. This must be differentiated from normal granular immunopositivity of gray matter and can be recognized by finding it in white matter or subarachnoid space

References: [1–10, 16, 64–66]

Table 10.2 Markers for astrocytoma

Antibodies	Literature
GFAP	+
S100	+
Vimentin	+
Synaptophysin	–
NeuN	–
CAM5.2	–
MIB1	+[a]
CD117/C-kit	+ or –[b]

Notes:

[a]Low-grade astrocytomas generally have less than 4% MIB labeling index. Higher indices are generally associated with more aggressive tumors. Anaplastic astrocytomas mostly have indices between 5 and 10%

[b]CD117 expression has been reported strongest in higher-grade astrocytomas

References: [1–7, 62]

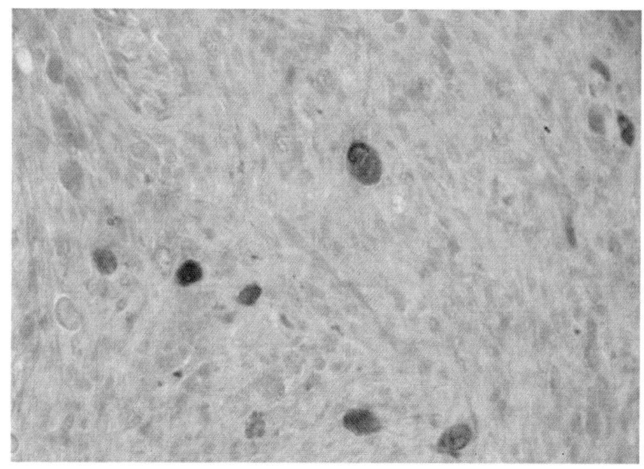

Fig. 10.2 Synaptophysin demonstrates positivity in pleomorphic xanthoastrocytoma tumor cells

Table 10.3 Markers for pleomorphic xanthoastrocytoma

Antibodies	Literature
GFAP	+
S100	+
Vimentin	+
Synaptophysin	+
NeuN	+
CAM5.2	–
MIB1	+ (<1%)

Note: Representative markers for pleomorphic xanthoastrocytoma are shown in Figs. 10.1–10.4

References: [1–7]

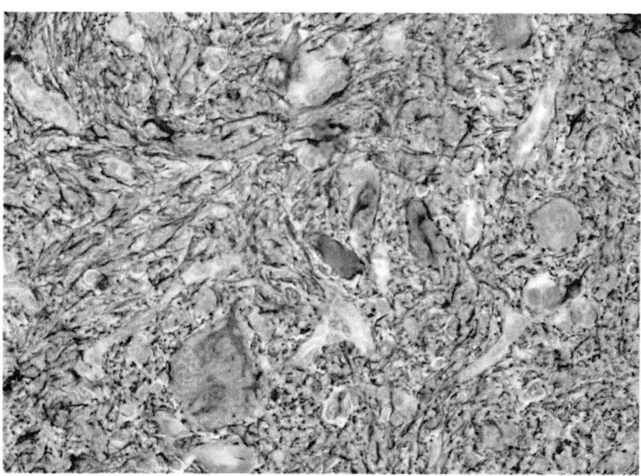

Fig. 10.3 GFAP demonstrates positivity in pleomorphic xanthoastrocytoma tumor cells

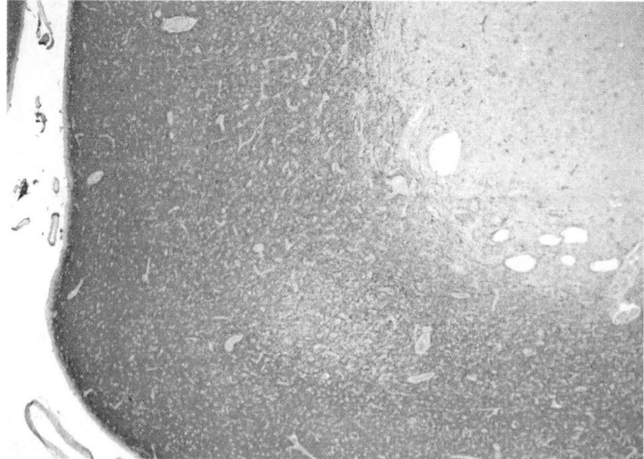

Fig. 10.1 Synaptophysin demonstrates strong diffuse neuropil staining in gray matter, and negative staining in white matter. The normal staining pattern is disrupted by pleomorphic xanthoastrocytoma

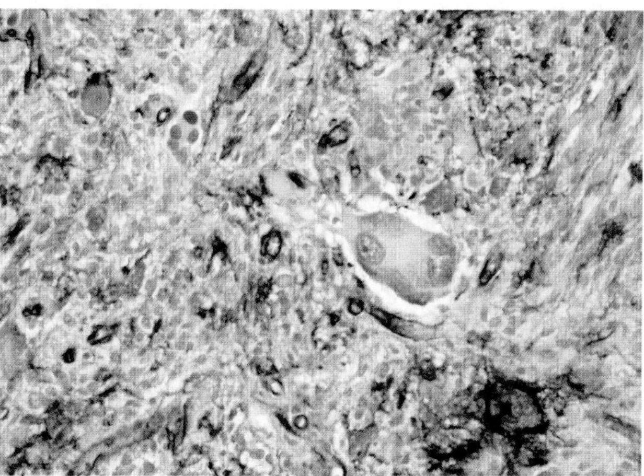

Fig. 10.4 CD34 demonstrates positivity in pleomorphic xanthoastrocytoma tumor cells

Table 10.4 Markers for oligodendroglioma

Antibodies	Literature
GFAP[a]	– or +
Vimentin[b]	– or +
NFP[c]	–
Synaptophysin[c]	–
NeuN[c]	–
Leu7 (CD57)	+ or –
MIBI	+ (<6%)

Notes:

[a]GFAP is positive in minigemistocytes and neoplastic astrocytic cells in oligodendroglioma. An example of GFAP positivity in the astrocytic component in anaplastic oligoastrocytoma is shown in Fig. 10.5

[b]Vimentin is positive in neoplastic astrocytic cells in oligodendroglioma

[c]Neuronal markers highlight entrapped neurons or they indicate that the "oligodendroglioma" is actually a neurocytoma. However, occasional reports of neuronal-associated antigens, including synaptophysin, NFP, and NeuN positivity in so-called oligodendrogliomas raise questions about cytogenesis, producing confusion in the classification of these tumors. Please see Table 10.28 for differential diagnosis in neurocytoma vs. oligodendroglioma

An example for GFAP immunostain positivity in astrocytic component in anaplastic oligoastrocytoma is shown in Fig. 10.5

References: [1–7, 11, 12]

Table 10.5 Markers for ependymal tumors

Antibodies	Literature
GFAP	+
EMA	+
CD99	+
MIB1/Ki 67	+[a]
Vimentin	+
S100	+
CKAE1/3	+
CAM5.2	– or +
CK7	– or +

[a]**Note**: MIB1 proliferation rates 5% or greater have been associated with shorter survival time

A perivascular positive pattern for GFAP and positivity in pseudorosettes are strong evidence of ependymoma

A "dot-like" pattern of EMA, tiny dot-like positivity, or small rings of positivity are indicative of intracellular lumina

A Ki67 labeling index <4% is associated with longer survival times

An example of GFAP immunostain positivity in myxopapillary ependymoma is shown in Fig. 10.6

References: [1–7, 13–15, 61, 67]

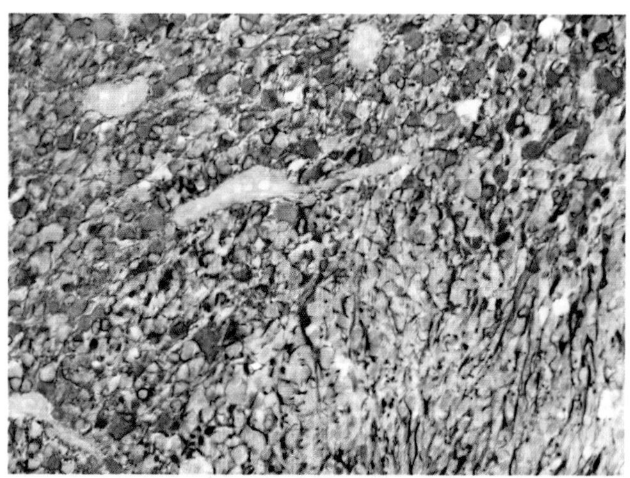

Fig. 10.5 GFAP demonstrates positivity in the astrocytic component in anaplastic oligoastrocytoma (on the *left side*). The oligodendroglioma component is GFAP negative (on the *right side*)

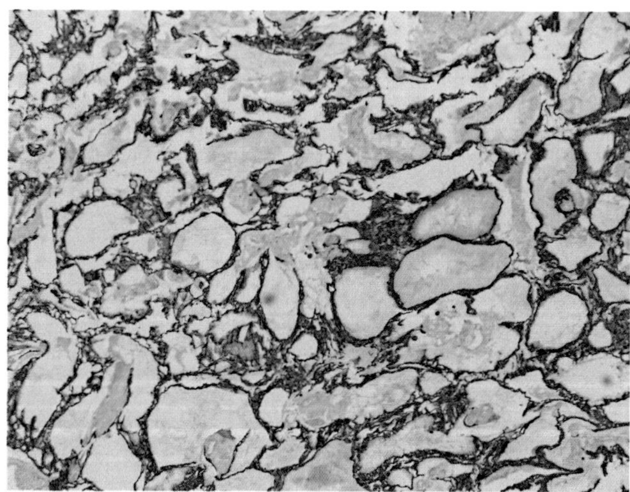

Fig. 10.6 GFAP demonstrates positivity in myxopapillary ependymoma. CAM5.2 and EMA immunostains were negative (data not shown)

Table 10.6 Markers for choroid plexus tumor

Antibody	Literature
CAM5.2	+
Transthyretin (TTR)	+[b]
GFAP	+
CK7	+ or −
CK20	+ or −
Synaptophysin	+ or −
ECad	+
S100	+[b]
AE1/AE3	+
MAP2	− or +
MIB1	+[a]

Notes:

[a]MIB proliferation index for choroid plexus papilloma is generally reported from 0.2 to 6% and for choroid plexus carcinoma in the range of 7.3–60%

[b]A number of markers usually described for choroid plexus papilloma and so-called atypical papilloma may be negative in choroid plexus carcinoma

References: [1–7]

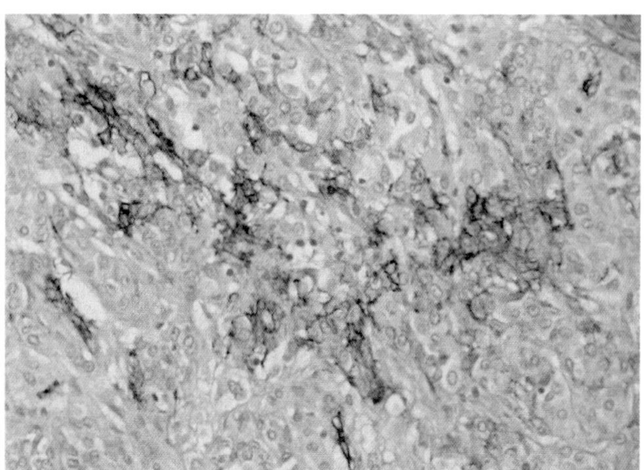

Fig. 10.8 CD34 demonstrates positivity in chordoid glioma

Table 10.7 Markers for chordoid glioma

Antibodies	Literature
GFAP	+
Keratin	− or +[a]
Synaptophysin	−
S100	+
NFP	+
MIB1	+ (5%)
CD34	+
Vimentin	+
P53	−
EGF	+
EMA	+

[a]**Note**: Focal or variable staining with various keratin antibodies have been reported in case reports of these tumors

Representative markers for chordoid glioma are shown in Figs. 10.7–10.9

References: [1–7, 17–20]

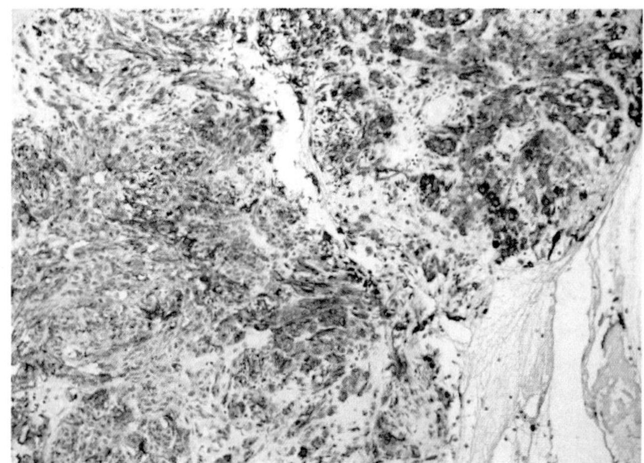

Fig. 10.9 CK7 demonstrates positivity in chordoid glioma

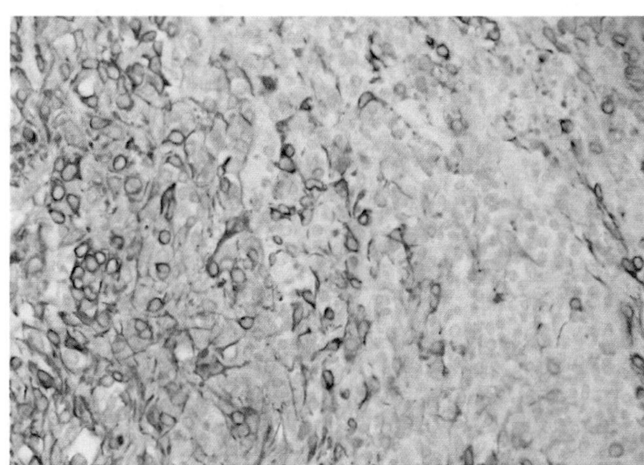

Fig. 10.7 GFAP demonstrates positivity in chordoid glioma

Table 10.8 Markers for mixed neuronal–glial tumors

Antibodies	Literature
GFAP	+
NeuN	+
Synaptophysin	+
NF-M (RMDO20)	+
NFP	+[a]
MIB1	+ (0–8%)

[a]**Note**: NFP positivity is for NF-M (middle molecular weight neurofilament protein) and NF cocktails, not for NFH (high molecular weight)

Representative markers for dysembryoplastic neuroepithelial tumor are shown in Figs. 10.10 (Synaptophysin) and 10.11 (GFAP)

References: [1–7, 21]

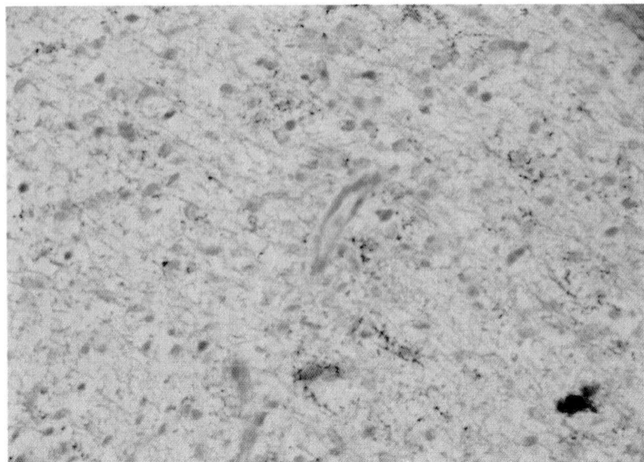

Fig. 10.10 Synaptophysin demonstrates "perikaryal surface immunopositivity" in dysembryoplastic neuroepithelial tumor

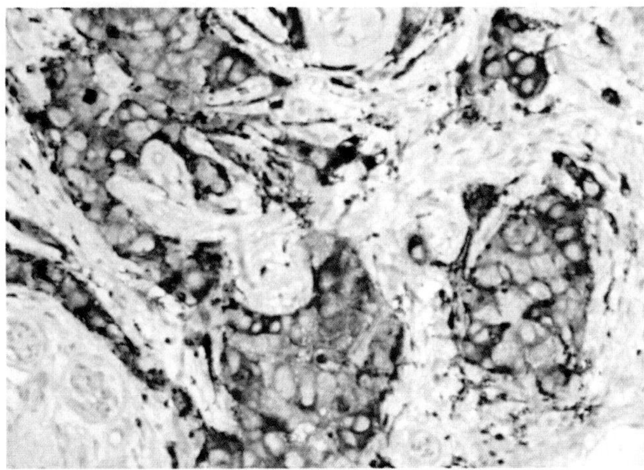

Fig. 10.12 Synaptophysin demonstrates positivity in spinal paraganglioma

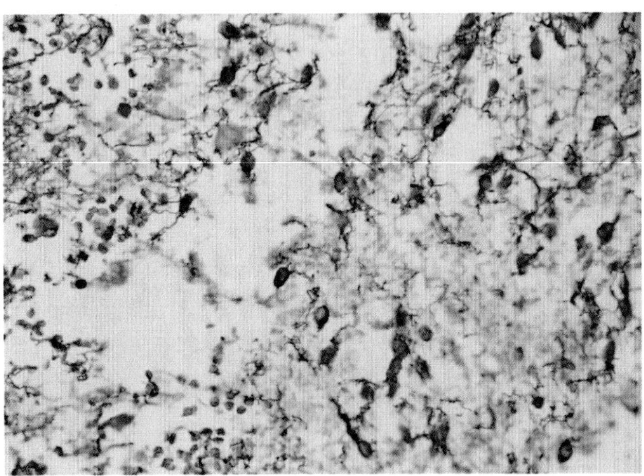

Fig. 10.11 GFAP demonstrates positivity in dysembryoplastic neuroepithelial tumor

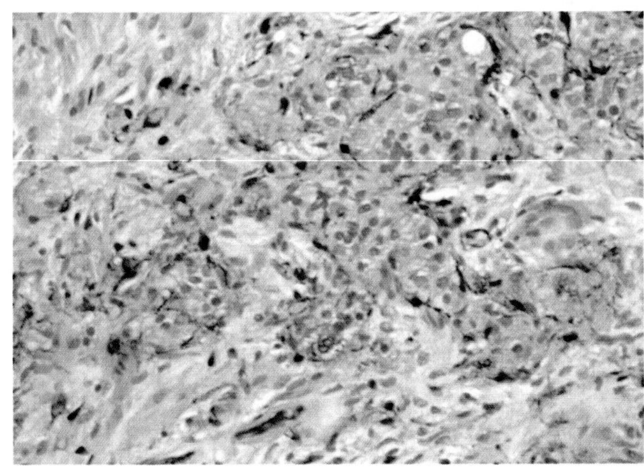

Fig. 10.13 S-100 demonstrates positivity in spinal paraganglioma, highlighting the sustentacular cells

Table 10.9 Markers for spinal paraganglioma

Antibodies	Literature
Synaptophysin	+
S100	+
Chromogranin	+
CAM5.2	+
NFP	+
EMA	–
GFAP	+

Note: S100 highlights the sustentacular cells. GFAP usually shows positivity for the sustentacular cells as well. NFP can be positive in the paraganglion cells ("chief cells")

Representative markers for spinal paraganglioma are shown in Figs. 10.12–10.14

References: [1–7, 22]

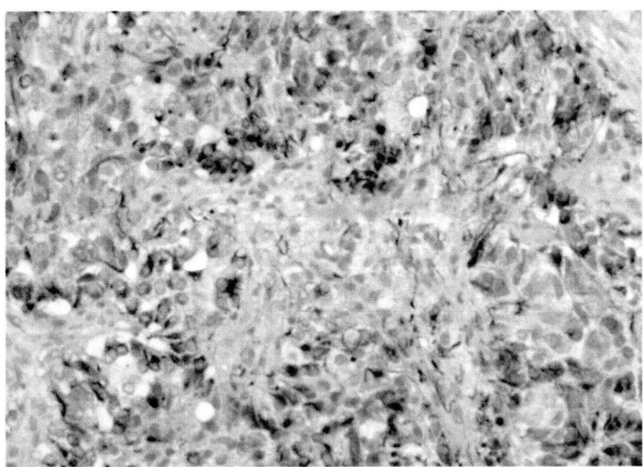

Fig. 10.14 CAM5.2 demonstrates positivity in spinal paraganglioma

Table 10.10 Markers for pineal parenchymal tumors

Antibodies	Literature
NeuN	+
Synaptophysin	+
NSE	+
NFP	+

Note: These markers typically label pineocytomas and pineal parenchymal tumors of intermediate differentiation. Pineoblastomas are PNETs and show more variable labeling with these and other antibodies

References: [1–7, 23–25]

Table 10.11 Markers for medulloblastoma

Antibodies	Literature
GFAP	– or +
NeuN	+ or –
Synaptophysin	+
CAM5.2	–
NFP	– or +
MIB1	+ (50%)
LCA	–
P53	+

Note: Medulloblastoma may exhibit differentiation along myogenic or melanocytic lines or show areas of desmoplastic/nodular growth pattern. Desmoplastic/nodular Medulloblastoma is composed of nodules with strong neuropil granular positivity for NeuN and NFP. MIB1 labeling index is low in nodules. Medulloblastoma with myogenic differentiation has immunopositivity for anti-fast-myosin and myoglobulin. Medulloblastoma with melanotic differentiation has immunopositivity for S100

References: [1–7, 26–28]

Table 10.12 Markers for primitive neuroectodermal tumors (PNET)

Antibodies	Literature
NSE	+
CD99[a]	–
CD57	– or +
Synaptophysin	+ or – (focal)
S100	+ or –
Vimentin	+
Cytokeratin	– or +
GFAP	– or +
NFP[b]	– or +
Carbonic anhydrase isoenzyme II	– or +

Notes:

[a]In contrast to peripheral Ewing Sarcoma/PNET, central nervous system PNET is negative for CD99, evidence that peripheral and central PNETs are different pathologic entities

[b]The WHO classification of central nervous system primitive neuroectodermal tumors includes tumors which are purely primitive and those which show differentiation along the lines of neuroblasts, neuroepithelial elements, and ependymal elements (central neuroblastomas, medulloepitheliomas, and ependymoblastomas). Neural markers are most prevalent in neuroblastoma, while cytokeratin is expressed in neuroepithelial elements and ependymal elements

References: [1–7, 30–31, 63]

Table 10.13 Markers for atypical teratoid/rhabdoid tumor

Antibodies	Literature
GFAP	– or +
NeuN	+ or –
Synaptophysin	+
Claudin 6	+
NFP	– or +
MIB1	+
BAF47/SNF5 (INI-1)	–
EMA	+ or –
MSA	+ or –
Vimentin	+ or –

References: [1–10, 32]

Table 10.14 Markers for tumors of the cranial and paraspinal nerves

Antibodies	Schwannoma	Neurofibroma	MPNST
Desmin	–	–	(Triton+)
MSA	–	–	(Triton+)
GFAP	– or +	–	Rare
S100	+ (strong)	+	+ or –
Leu7 (CD57)	+ or –	+	– or +
Myelin basic protein	+ or –	–	– or +
HMB45	(Melanotic+)	–	–
INI-1	+[a]	+	+
MIB1	+	– or +	+
CD34	–	+ (focal)	+ (focal)
Calretinin	+	– or +	N/A
Factor XIIIa	– or +	+	N/A
CD56	+	– or +	N/A
NFP	–	+[b]	N/A

Notes:

[a]INI-1: May be a mosaic pattern in tumor from patients with schwannomatosis

[b]NFP: Used to demonstrate entrapped neuronal processes, which are found within neurofibromas, but not generally within schwannomas

N/A not available

References: [1–7, 33, 65, 66]

Table 10.15 Markers for meningioma

Antibodies	Literature
GFAP	–
CAM5.2	–
Synaptophysin	–
Vimentin	+
EMA	+
PR	+
MIB1	+ or –[a]
S100	– or +

[a]**Note**: MIB1 proliferation index is significantly associated with WHO grade in meningiomas. However, there is some overlap among grades. Grade I meningiomas are associated with average MIB1 index of 0.08 ± 0.05%, grade II 4.8 ± 0.9%, and grade III 19 ± 4.7%

References: [1–7]

Table 10.16 Markers for lymphoma in CNS

Markers	B-Cell lymphomas	T-Cell lymphomas	Anaplastic lymphoma	NK/T-Cell lymphoma
CD3	–	+	– or +	+ or –
CD20	+	–	–	–
CD10	+ or –	–	–	–
Bcl2	+ or –	+ or –		
Bcl6	+ or –	–	–	–
PAX5	+[a]	–	–	–
CD4	–	– or +	– or +	–
CD5	–	+ or –	– or +	– or +
CD8	–	– or +	– or +	+ or –
EBV	– or +[b]	–	–	+

Notes:

[a]PAX5 is a very useful B-cell marker. CD4 and CD8 are useful in T-cell lymphoma, when restricted to all CD4 or all CD8. CD5 can be useful in some T-cell lymphomas as they can be CD3 negative, but CD5 positive (antigenic aberrency)

[b]Angiocentric and plasmablastic lymphomas are EBV positive

An example of markers for diffuse large B-cell malignant lymphoma is shown in Figs. 10.15 (CD20) and 10.16 (BCL-6)

References: [1–7, 29]

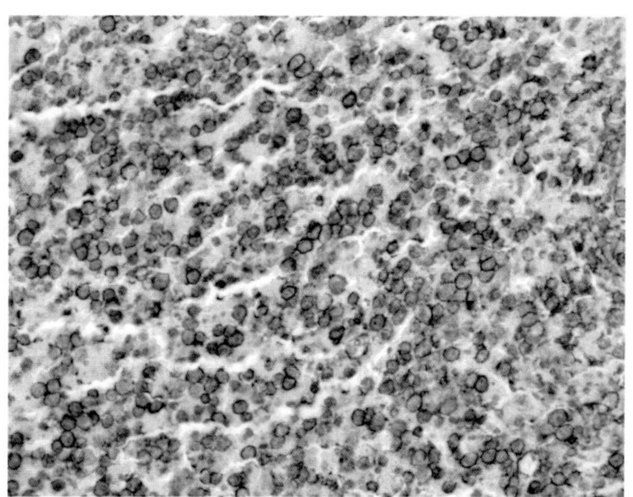

Fig. 10.15 CD20 demonstrates positivity in diffuse large B-cell malignant lymphoma

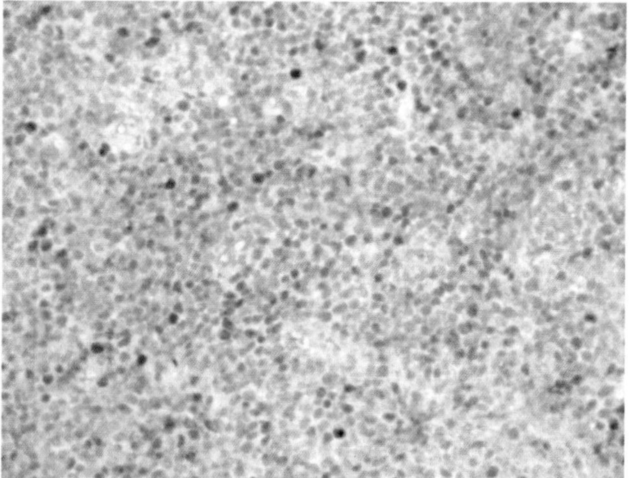

Fig. 10.16 BCL-6 demonstrates positivity in diffuse large B-cell malignant lymphoma

Table 10.17 Markers for germ cell tumors

Antibodies	Germinoma	Teratoma	Yolk-sac tumor	Embryonal carcinoma	Chori CA
AFP	–	+[a]	+	–	–
HCG	– or + (focal)[b]	–	–	–	+
HPL	– or +	–	–	–	+
PLAP	+	–	+ or –	+	+ or –
CAM5.2[c]	–	+	+	+	+
C-kit/CD117[d]	+	+ or –	–	–	+ or –
OCT4	+	–	–	+	–
CD30	–	–	–	+	–
EMA	–	+ or –	–	+ or –	+

Notes:

[a]Alpha-fetoprotein is usually restricted to enteric-type glandular components

[b]Many germinomas contain HCG positive syncytiotrophoblastic giant cells. Syncytiotrophoblastic giant cells that may be found in otherwise pure germinomas (or in any of the other CNS GCT types) will be immunoreactive for human chorionic gonadotropin (HCG) and human placental lactogen (HPL)

[c]A minority of germinomas exhibit cytokeratin reactivity that is usually distributed in patchy fashion. Cytokeratin reactivity is a feature of epithelial components. Cytokeratin immunoreactivity is a regular feature of syncytiotrophoblastic giant cells, while cytotrophoblastic *cells are* often negative

[d]C-kit has been reported to have immunoexpression limited to some mesenchymal and epithelial components

Representative markers for germinoma are shown in Figs. 10.17 (C-kit/CD117) and 10.18 (OCT-4)

References: [1–7, 10]

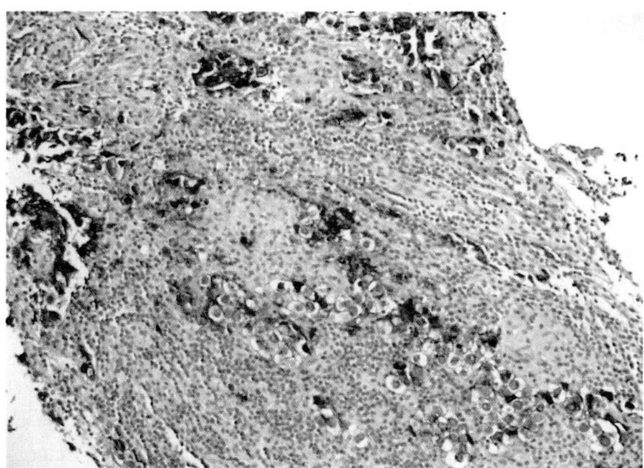

Fig. 10.17 C-kit/CD117 demonstrates cytoplasmic positivity and membranous positivity in germinoma

Fig. 10.18 OCT-4 demonstrates nuclear positivity in germinoma

Table 10.18 Markers for hemangioblastoma

Antibodies	Literature
GFAP	– or +[a]
CAM5.2	–
Synaptophysin	–
pVHL	+ (stromal cells)
Alpha-inhibin	+ (stromal cells)
NSE	+ (stromal cells)
CD10	–
Cytokeratin	–
EMA	–
CD56	+ (stromal cells)
CD34	+ (vascular)
CD31	+ (vascular)
S100	+ or – (stromal cells)
PR	+

[a]**Note**: The expression of glial fibrillary acidic protein (GFAP) in hemangioblastomas is controversial. Some studies report a frequent positive immunoreactivity, whereas others observe only occasional positive cells in hemangioblastomas. One study finds GFAP to be consistently negative in hemangioblastoma stromal cells. It is also unclear whether scattered GFAP positive cells represent entrapped reactive astrocytes, stromal cells with glial differentiation, or stromal cells with intracytoplasmic GFAP from phagocytic activity

References: [1–7, 34–40]

Table 10.19 Markers for craniopharyngioma

Antibodies	Adamantinomatous	Squamous papillary
CAM5.2	+	+
CK7	+[a]	+
Beta-catenin	+[b]	+

Notes:

[a]Adamantinomatous craniopharyngioma demonstrates full thickness staining for CK7. Squamous papillary craniopharyngioma demonstrates surface epithelial staining

[b]Adamantinomatous craniopharyngioma demonstrates diffuse staining for Beta-catenin. Squamous papillary craniopharyngioma demonstrates focal staining

References: [1–7, 42, 58, 59]

Table 10.20 Markers for pituitary adenoma

Antibodies	Literature	Tumor type
GH	+	GH cell adenoma
PRL	+	PRL cell adenoma
ACTH	+	ACTH cell adenoma
TSH[a]	+	TSH cell adenoma
FSH	+	FSH cell adenoma
LH	+	LH cell adenoma
Alpha-subunit (Alpha-SU)	+	GH, FSH, LH, TSH cell adenomas
Chromogranin	+	All adenomas[b]
Synaptophysin	+	All adenomas[b]

Notes:

[a]TSH cell adenomas are very rare

[b]Chromogranin and synaptophysin are positive in all adenomas including null cell adenoma, which is negative for all the other pituitary hormone antibodies

References: [1–7]

Table 10.21 Markers for hemangiopericytoma vs. solitary fibrous tumor

Antibodies	Hemangiopericytoma	Solitary fibrous tumor
CD34	+ or –	+
GFAP	–	–
CAM5.2	–	–
Synaptophysin	–	–
SMA	– or +	–
Desmin	–	–
Vimentin	– or +	+
MSA	+	–
Bcl2	–	+

Note: CD34 immunoreactivity in HPC tumor cells and endothelial cells. SFT has a diffusely positive pattern

References: [1–7, 41, 43–49]

Table 10.22 Markers for astrocytic tumor vs. oligodendroglioma

Antibodies	Astrocytic tumor	Oligodendroglioma
GFAP	+	– or +
Vimentin	+	– or +
MBP	–	– or +
Leu7 (CD57)	+	+
NeuN	–	–

Note: GFAP is positive in minigemistocytes in oligodendroglioma

No immunohistochemical reagent consistently and specifically identifies neoplastic cells as oligodendroglial

References: [1–7, 50]

Table 10.23 Markers for astrocytic tumor vs. neuronal tumor

Antibodies	Astrocytic tumor	Neuronal tumor
GFAP	+	– or +
CAM5.2	–	–
Synaptophysin	–	+
Vimentin	+	–
NeuN	–	+

Note: Many "neuronal tumors" are mixed, containing stromal/glial elements so they will also have GFAP and vimentin positive cells

References: [1–7]

Table 10.24 Markers for astrocytic tumor vs. demyelinating disease

Antibodies	Astrocytic tumor	Demyelinating disease
GFAP	+	+
CD68	–	+
CD4	–	+
MBP	–	+
CD8	–	+
LCA	–	+

Note: GFAP-positive cells in astrocytic tumor are crowded, with atypical nuclei; in demyelinating disease, the reactive cells are predominantly CD68-positive foamy macrophages which contain luxol fast blue (LFB)-positive phagocytosed myelin. In astrocytic tumors, reactive histiocytes and activated microglial cells are present. Therefore, CD68 positive cells may be of little help to distinguish a neoplastic from a reactive condition. LCA, a lymphocytic marker, is negative in tumor cells but will be positive in perivascular infiltrates in either condition. The lymphoid infiltrates in demyelinating disease are primarily T-cells, whereas the majority of lymphomas are B-cell. The use of NFP is not helpful in distinguishing infiltrating astrocytoma vs. demyelination, as neurofilaments will be preserved. However, in areas of infarction, the loss of NFP can be a helpful observation

References: [1–7]

Table 10.25 Markers for glioblastoma vs. metastatic carcinoma

Antibodies	Glioblastoma	Metastatic carcinoma
GFAP	+	–
CAM5.2	–	+
Vimentin	+	–
AE1/AE3	– or +	+
Pan keratin	– or +	+
EMA	– or +	+

Note: AE1/AE3 can react with glial cells. For this reason, CAM5.2 is preferred. See Table 10.34 for specific markers for metastatic tumor types

References: [1–7]

Table 10.26 Markers for perivascular lymphocytic infiltration

Antibodies	Lymphoma	Glioma	Infection
CD3	+ or –	+	+
CD20	+	+	+
GFAP	– or + (in gliosis)	+	+ or –
CD68	–	–	+

Note: Lymphoma cells are negative for GFAP. However, there is almost always a marked gliosis in or around primary CNS lymphomas, as can be demonstrated with a GFAP stain. CD68 positive macrophages are common in CNS lymphomas and not uncommon in astrocytomas

References: [1–7]

Table 10.27 Markers for ependymoma vs. choroid plexus tumor

Antibodies	Classic ependymoma	Supratentorial papillary ependymoma	Choroid plexus papilloma	Spinal papillary ependymoma
GFAP	+	– or +	– or +	+
EMA	+ or –	– or +	– or +	+
TTR	– or +	+	+	+
CD99	+	–	– or +	+
NCAM	+	+	–	+
ECad	–	–	+	+
MAP2	– or +	+	– or +	+
Cytokeratin	– or +	N/A	+	–

Note: *N/A* not available, *TTR* transthyretin

References: [51, 61]

Table 10.28 Markers for neurocytoma and dysembryoplastic neuroepithelial tumor (DNET) vs. oligodendroglioma

Antibodies	Neurocytoma	DNET	Oligodendroglioma
GFAP	–	+	– or + (focal)
NeuN	+	+ (focal)	–
Synaptophysin	+ (diffuse)	+ (focal)	–
Carbonic anhydrase isoenzyme II	–	–	+

References: [30, 52–56]

Table 10.29 Markers for selected tumors with epithelioid pattern: Glioblastoma vs. meningioma vs. atypical teratoid/rhabdoid tumor (AT/RT)

Antibodies	Glioblastoma	Meningioma	AT/RT
GFAP	+	–	– or +
INI-1	+	+	–
CAM5.2	–	–	–
S100	+	–	– or +
EMA	–	+	+
Claudin 6	–	NA	+
PR	–	+	–

Note: *N/A* not available

References: [1–8]

Table 10.30 Markers for tumors with clear cell pattern: hemangioblastoma vs. clear cell renal carcinoma (CRCC) vs. clear cell meningioma

Antibodies	Hemangioblastoma	CRCC	Clear cell meningioma
pVHL	+	+	N/A
PAX2	–	+	N/A
AE1/3	–	+	–
S100	–	–	– or +
EMA	–	– or +	+
Vimentin	–	+	+
PR	–	–	+
CD10	–	+	–
RCC	–	+	–
InhibinA	+	–	–

Note: *N/A* not available

References: [1–7, 57]

Table 10.31 Markers for tumors with chordoid pattern: chordoid glioma vs. chordoid meningioma vs. chordoma

Antibodies	Chordoid glioma	Chordoid meningioma	Chordoma
GFAP	+	–	–
D2-40	+	+	–
S100	+	– or +	+
EMA	+	+	+
Brachyury	–	–	+
PR	–	+	–

References: [1–7, 17]

Table 10.32 Markers for tumors with giant cell pattern

Antibodies	Giant cell glioblastoma	Pleomorphic xanthoastrocytoma (PXA)
GFAP	+	+ or –
Vimentin	+	–
Synaptophysin	–	+
S100	+	+
P53	+	+ or –
CD68	–	+

References: [1–7]

Table 10.33 Markers for tumors with spindle cell pattern

Antibodies	Meningioma	Schwannoma	Hemangiopericytoma
Vimentin	+	+	+
EMA	+	–	–
PR	+	–	–
S100	– or +	+	–
CD34	–	–	– or +
NFP	+	+	–
MSA	–	–	+

References: [1–7]

Table 10.34 Markers for metastases in CNS

Markers	Kidney	SCC	Lung-A	Mel.	Stomach	Lung-S	Colon	Breast
CK5/6	–	+	–	–	–	–	–	–
CK7	–	+ or –	+	–	+	– or +	–	+
CK20	–	–	–	–	+ or –	–	+	–
CK903	–	+ or –	–	–	–	–	–	–
S100	+ or –	–	–	+	–	–	–	– or +
HMB45	–	–	–	+	–	–	–	–
Mart1	–	–	–	+	–	–	–	–
p63	–	+	–	–	–	–	–	–
MOC31	– or +	–	+	–	+	– or +	+	+
TTF1	–	–	+	–	–	+	–	–
NapsinA	– or +	–	+	–	–	–	–	–
CDX2	–	–	–	–	– or +	–	+	–
KIM1	+	–	–	–	–	–	–	–
CD10	+	–	–	+ or –	–	–	–	–
ER	–	–	–	–	–	–	–	+
Synap	–	–	–	–	–	+	–	–

SCC squamous cell carcinoma, *Lung-A* lung adenocarcinoma, *Mel*-melanoma *Lung-S* lung small cell carcinoma. Mucinous adenocarcinomas of the lung are occasionally positive for CDX2 and negative for TTF1; in addition, a small percentage of lung adenocarcinomas can be positive for ER

S100 is a highly sensitive (98%) but not specific marker for screening melanoma. Caution should be taken if the sample is fixed in alcohol, since the S100 antigen is not preserved well after alcohol fixation. If melanoma is suspected, then other markers, including Mart1 and HMB45, should be done

Some metastatic small cell carcinomas of the lung can be negative for both synaptophysin and chromogranin, but they are very infrequently negative for CD56. MIB1 (Ki67) proliferative index tends to be very high (>50%); it would be extremely unusual to have a small cell carcinoma with a low-MIB1 index

The majority (>90%) of the metastatic colonic adenocarcinomas are positive for both CK20 and CDX2; however, it should be noted that medullary carcinoma of the colon with microsatellite instability (MSI) frequently shows the loss of expression of both CDX2 and CK20. In this case, the tumor cells would demonstrate the loss of expression of either MLH1/PMS2 or MSH2/MSH6

Representative markers for brain with metastatic adenocarcinoma of the lung are shown in Figs. 10.19 (TTF-1) and 10.20 (Napsin)

References: [1–7]

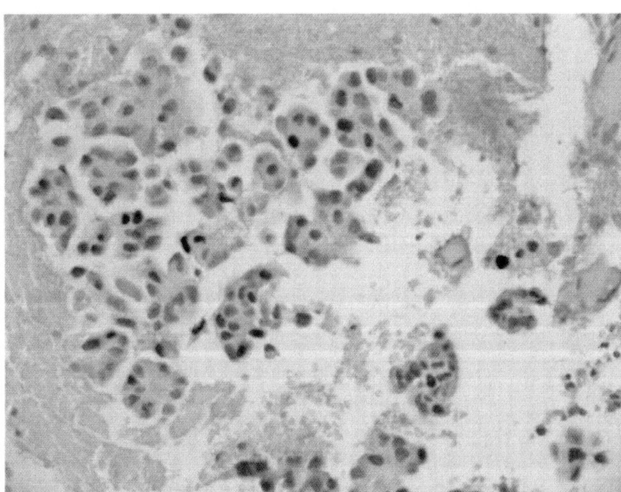

Fig. 10.19 TTF-1 demonstrates nuclear positivity in metastatic adenocarcinoma of the lung

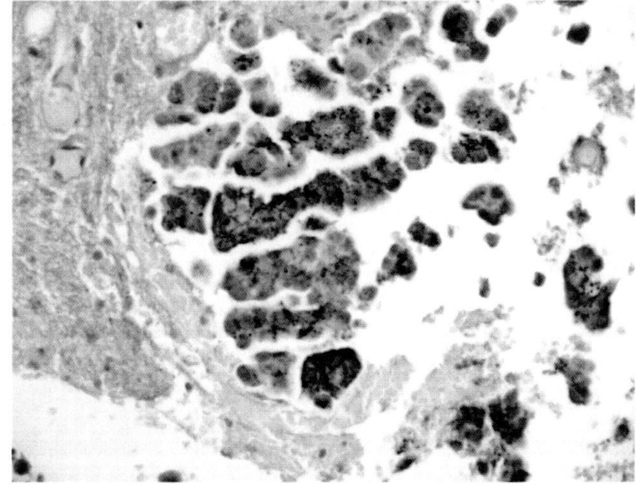

Fig. 10.20 Napsin-A demonstrates cytoplasmic positivity in metastatic adenocarcinoma of the lung

Table 10.35 Markers for neurodegenerative disorders

Antibodies	Key application	Location
Phosphorylated tau	Major component of neurofibrillary tangles in Alzheimer disease and frontotemporal lobar degeneration. Present in inclusions, in Pick disease and progressive supranuclear palsy (PSP), also in Corticobasal Degeneration (CBD)	In Pick disease neuronal inclusions in outer cortical layers of frontal and temporal lobes. In PSP neuronal and glial inclusions in globus pallidus, subthalamic nucleus substantia nigra, colliculi, periaqueductal gray matter, and dentate nucleus. In CBD present in glial cells and neurons
Amyloid precursor protein (APP) or peptides (A-Beta)	Alzheimer disease, cerebral amyloid angiopathy (CAA)	Plaques and vessels
Ubiquitin	Dementia with diffuse Lewy body disease, idiopathic Parkinson's disease, multiple system atrophy (MSA), frontotemporal labor degeneration (FLD), Pick disease	In Lewy bodies especially in substantia nigra and locus ceruleus in Parkinson's disease. In MSA, neuronal inclusions are in the cerebellar peduncles, pons, medulla substantia nigra, and striatum. In FLD, inclusions are in the outer cortical layers of the temporal and frontal and the dentate gyrus. Pick bodies
Alpha-synuclein	Dementia with diffuse Lewy body disease, idiopathic Parkinson's disease, multiple system atrophy, frontotemporal lobar degeneration. Absent in Pick disease	In Lewy bodies especially in substantia nigra and locus ceruleus in Parkinson's disease. In MSA, neuronal inclusions are in the cerebellar peduncles, pons, medulla substantia nigra, and striatum. In FLD, inclusions are in the outer cortical layers of the temporal and frontal and the dentate gyrus
Human prion protein	Creutzfeldt–Jakob disease and other prion diseases	Extracellular in Kuru plaques, mainly in gray matter. Also diffuse granular staining of neuropil and of occasional neurons
TDP43	Frontotemporal lobar degeneration with ubiquitinated inclusions Amyotrophic lateral sclerosis	Cytoplasmic and nuclear inclusions

References: [1–7, 60, 68–71]

Table 10.36 Markers for virus and parasite infection of the CNS

Antibodies	Key application	Location
HSV Herpes I/II	Herpes simplex encephalitis	Encephalitis; Cowdry A amphophilic nuclear inclusions of 90–100 nm target capsids
Toxoplasma	Toxoplasmosis	Necrosis containing 3–5 μm tachyzoites; (cysts); (inflammation)
JCV/SV40	Progressive multifocal leukoencephalopathy	Demyelinated areas; bizarre glia; amphophilic nuclear inclusions of 15–25 or 30–40 nm diameter filaments or spheres
CMV	CMV	Cytoplasmic and nuclear inclusions in endothelial cells and ependymal cells
PrP	Dementia/Creutzfeldt–Jakob disease	Extracellular in Kuru plaques, mainly in gray matter. Also diffuse granular staining of neuropil and of occasional neurons

References: [1–7, 68]

Table 10.37 Markers for epilepsy

Antibodies	Key application	Location
GFAP	Highlights gliosis, focal or diffuse, secondary to chronic seizure disorder	Superficial, subpial (Chaslin type), or diffuse fibrillary, in cortex and white matter
Synaptophysin	Highlights cortex, positive marker for neurons. Helpful for the identification of cortical dysplasia	Cortical neuron loss, neurons in white matter (neuronal migration failure, neuronal heterotopia)
NeuN	Identifies neurons. Helpful for the identification of cortical dysplasia	Cortical neuron loss and neurons in white matter (neuronal migration failure, neuronal heterotopia)
NFP	Identifies neurons. Helpful for the identification of cortical dysplasia	Cortical neuron loss and neurons in white matter (neuronal migration failure, neuronal heterotopia)
Vimentin	Identification of areas of scar/fibrosis	Any cerebral location
CD45/LCA	Highlights inflammatory focus (presumed secondary to placement of monitoring device)	Meninges, cortex
CD68	Highlights inflammatory focus, microglial activation (presumed secondary to the placement of monitoring device)	Meninges, cortex

References: [2–6]

Table 10.38 Markers for histiocytic disorders in CNS

Antibodies	Langerhans cell histiocytosis	Rosai–Dorfman disease	Juvenile xanthogranuloma	Xanthomatous inflammation
CD1a	+	–	–	–
S100	+	+	+ or –	–
Factor XIIIa	–	–	+	– or + (focal)
CD68	+	–	+	+

References: [1–7]

References

1. Louis DN, Ohgaki H, Wiestler OD, Cavenee WK. WHO classification of tumours of the central nervous system. 4th ed. Lyon: IARC (International Agency for Research on Cancer); 2007.
2. Miller DC. Modern surgical neuropathology. Cambridge: Cambridge University Press; 2009.
3. Ellison D, Love S, Chimelli L, et al. Neuropathology. Amsterdam: Elsevier; 2003.
4. Dabbs DJ. Diagnostic immunohistochemistry. 3rd ed. Philadelphia: Churchill Livingstone Elsevier; 2010.
5. Perry A, Brat DJ. Practical surgical neuropathology: a diagnostic approach. Philadelphia: Churchill Livingstone Elsevier; 2010.
6. Vogel H. Nervous system. Cambridge: Cambridge University Press; 2009.
7. Burger PC, Scheithauer BW. Tumors of the central nervous system, vol. Fascicle 7. 4th ed. Washington: American Registry of Pathology; 2007.
8. Kleinschmidt-DeMasters BK, Alassiri AH, Birks DK, Newell KL, Moore W, Lillehei KO. Epithelioid versus rhabdoid glioblastomas are distinguished by monosomy 22 and immunohistochemical expression of INI-1 but not claudin 6. Am J Surg Pathol. 2010; 34(3):341–54.
9. Birks DK, Kleinschmidt-DeMasters BK, Donson AM, et al. Claudin 6 is a positive marker for atypical teratoid/rhabdoid tumors. Brain Pathol. 2010;20(1):140–50.
10. Edgar MA, Rosenblum MK. The differential diagnosis of central nervous system tumors: a critical examination of some recent immunohistochemical applications. Arch Pathol Lab Med. 2008;132(3):500–9.
11. Perry A, Scheithauer BW, Macaulay RJ, Raffel C, Roth KA, Kros JM. Oligodendrogliomas with neurocytic differentiation. A report of 4 cases with diagnostic and histogenetic implications. J Neuropathol Exp Neurol. 2002;61(11):947–55.
12. Wharton SB, Chan KK, Hamilton FA, Anderson JR. Expression of neuronal markers in oligodendrogliomas: an immunohistochemical study. Neuropathol Appl Neurobiol. 1998;24(4):302–8.
13. Vege KD, Giannini C, Scheithauer BW. The immunophenotype of ependymomas. Appl Immunohistochem Mol Morphol. 2000;8(1): 25–31.
14. Vaishali SS, Tatke M, Daljit S, Ajay S. Histological spectrum of ependymomas and correlation of p53 and Ki-67 expression with ependymoma grade and subtype. Indian J Cancer. 2004;41(2):66–71.
15. Wolfsberger S, Fischer I, Hoftberger R, et al. Ki-67 immunolabeling index is an accurate predictor of outcome in patients with intracranial ependymoma. Am J Surg Pathol. 2004;28(7):914–20.
16. Preusser M, Laggner U, Haberler C, Heinzl H, Budka H, Hainfellner JA. Comparative analysis of NeuN immunoreactivity in primary brain tumours: conclusions for rational use in diagnostic histopathology. Histopathology. 2006;48(4):438–44.
17. Sangoi AR, Dulai MS, Beck AH, Brat DJ, Vogel H. Distinguishing chordoid meningiomas from their histologic mimics: an immunohistochemical evaluation. Am J Surg Pathol. 2009;33(5):669–81.
18. Reifenberger G, Weber T, Weber RG, et al. Chordoid glioma of the third ventricle: immunohistochemical and molecular genetic characterization of a novel tumor entity. Brain Pathol. 1999;9(4):617–26.
19. Horbinski C, Dacic S, McLendon RE, et al. Chordoid glioma: a case report and molecular characterization of five cases. Brain Pathol. 2008;19(3):439–48.
20. Sugita Y, Ohshima K, Shigemori M, Arakawa M, Kuramoto T, Nakayama K. The tumor of the third ventricle. Neuropathology. 2010;30(1):97–100.
21. McLendon RE, Bentley RC, Parisi JE, et al. Malignant supratentorial glial-neuronal neoplasms: report of two cases and review of the literature. Arch Pathol Lab Med. 1997;121(5):485–92.
22. Moran CA, Rush W, Mena H. Primary spinal paragangliomas: a clinicopathological and immunohistochemical study of 30 cases. Histopathology. 1997;31(2):167–73.
23. Fevre-Montange M, Jouvet A, Privat K, et al. Immunohistochemical, ultrastructural, biochemical and in vitro studies of a pineocytoma. Acta Neuropathol (Berl). 1998;95(5):532–9.
24. Okuda Y, Taomoto K, Saya H, et al. Pineoblastoma with neuronal differentiation – immunohistochemical and immunocytochemical studies. J Neurooncol. 1988;6(2):193–8.
25. Mena H, Rushing EJ, Ribas JL, Delahunt B, McCarthy WF. Tumors of pineal parenchymal cells: a correlation of histological features, including nucleolar organizer regions, with survival in 35 cases. Hum Pathol. 1995;26(1):20–30.
26. Badiali M, Iolascon A, Loda M, et al. p53 gene mutations in medulloblastoma. Immunohistochemistry, gel shift analysis, and sequencing. Diagn Mol Pathol. 1993;2(1):23–8.
27. McLendon RE, Friedman HS, Fuchs HE, Kun LE, Bigner SH. Diagnostic markers in paediatric medulloblastoma: a Paediatric Oncology Group Study. Histopathology. 2001;34(2):154–62.
28. Giordana MT, Mauro A, Migheli A, Schiffer D. Contributions of immunohistochemistry to the problem of differentiation in medulloblastoma. Ital J Neurol Sci. 1983;4(4):411–5.
29. Jaffee ES, Harris NL, Stein H, et al. WHO classification of tumours: pathology and genetics of tumors of haematopoietic and lymphoid tissues. Lyon: IARC Press; 2001.
30. Parkkila AK, Herva R, Parkkila S, Rajaniemi H. Immunohistochemical demonstration of human carbonic anhydrase isoenzyme II in brain tumours. Histochem J. 1995;27(12):974–82.
31. Cruz-Sanchez FF, Haustein J, Rossi ML, Cervos-Navarro J, Hughes JT. Ependymoblastoma: a histological, immunohistological and ultrastructural study of five cases. Histopathology. 1988;12(1): 17–27.
32. Ertan Y, Sezak M, Turhan T, et al. Atypical teratoid/rhabdoid tumor of the central nervous system: clinicopathologic and immunohistochemical features of four cases. Childs Nerv Syst. 2009;25(6): 707–11.
33. Weiss SW, Goldblum JR. Enzinger and Weiss's soft tissue tumors. 5th ed. St Louis: Mosby Elsevier; 2008.
34. Jung SM, Kuo TT. Immunoreactivity of CD10 and inhibin alpha in differentiating hemangioblastoma of central nervous system from metastatic clear cell renal cell carcinoma. Mod Pathol. 2005;18(6):788–94.

35. Glasker S, Li J, Xia JB, et al. Hemangioblastomas share protein expression with embryonal hemangioblast progenitor cell. Cancer Res. 2006;66(8):4167–72.
36. Lach B, Gregor A, Rippstein P, Omulecka A. Angiogenic histogenesis of stromal cells in hemangioblastoma: ultrastructural and immunohistochemical study. Ultrastruct Pathol. 1999;23(5):299–310.
37. Bohling T, Plate KH, Haltia MJ, Alitalo K, Neumann HPH. Von Hippel-Lindau disease and capillary hemangioblastoma. In: Kleihues P, Cavenee WK, editors. World Health Organization classification of tumours, Pathology and genetics-tumours of the nervous system. Lyon: IARC Press; 2000.
38. Becker I, Paulus W, Roggendorf W. Histogenesis of stromal cells in cerebellar hemangioblastomas. An immunohistochemical study. Am J Pathol. 1989;134(2):271–5.
39. Hufnagel TJ, Kim JH, True LD, Manuelidis EE. Immunohistochemistry of capillary hemangioblastoma. Immunoperoxidase-labeled antibody staining resolves the differential diagnosis with metastatic renal cell carcinoma, but does not explain the histogenesis of the capillary hemangioblastoma. Am J Surg Pathol. 1989;13(3):207–16.
40. Hoang MP, Amirkhan RH. Inhibin alpha distinguishes hemangioblastoma from clear cell renal cell carcinoma. Am J Surg Pathol. 2003;27(8):1152–6.
41. Vuorinen V, Sallinen P, Haapasalo H, Visakorpi T, Kallio M, Jaaskelainen J. Outcome of 31 intracranial haemangiopericytomas: poor predictive value of cell proliferation indices. Acta Neurochir. 1996;138(12):1399–408.
42. Kurosaki M, Saeger W, Ludecke DK. Immunohistochemical localisation of cytokeratins in craniopharyngioma. Acta Neurochir (Wien). 2001;143(2):147–51.
43. Veltrini VC, Etges A, Magalhaes MH, de Araujo NS, de Araujo VC. Solitary fibrous tumor of the oral mucosa – morphological and immunohistochemical profile in the differential diagnosis with hemangiopericytoma. Oral Oncol. 2003;39(4):420–6.
44. Thompson LD, Miettinen M, Wenig BM. Sinonasal-type hemangiopericytoma: a clinicopathologic and immunophenotypic analysis of 104 cases showing perivascular myoid differentiation. Am J Surg Pathol. 2003;27(6):737–49.
45. Hori E, Kurimoto M, Fukuda O, et al. Recurrent intracranial solitary fibrous tumor initially diagnosed as hemangiopericytoma. Brain Tumor Pathol. 2007;24(1):31–4.
46. Shidham VB, Chivukula M, Gupta D, Rao RN, Komorowski R. Immunohistochemical comparison of gastrointestinal stromal tumor and solitary fibrous tumor. Arch Pathol Lab Med. 2002;126(10):1189–92.
47. Rodriguez F, Scheithauer BW, Ockner DM, Giannini C. Solitary fibrous tumor of the cerebellopontine angle with salivary gland heterotopia: a unique presentation. Am J Surg Pathol. 2004;28(1):139–42.
48. Wang J, Arber DA, Frankel K, Weiss LM. Large solitary fibrous tumor of the kidney: report of two cases and review of the literature. Am J Surg Pathol. 2001;25(9):1194–9.
49. Suzuki SO, Fukui M, Nishio S, Iwaki T. Clinicopathological features of solitary fibrous tumor of the meninges: an immunohistochemical reappraisal of cases previously diagnosed to be fibrous meningioma or hemangiopericytoma. Pathol Int. 2000;50(10):808–17.
50. Nakagawa Y, Perentes E, Rubinstein LJ. Immunohistochemical characterization of oligodendrogliomas: an analysis of multiple markers. Acta Neuropathol (Berl). 1986;72(1):15–22.
51. Dulai MS, Caccamo DV, Briley AL, Edwards MS, Fisher PG, Lehman NL. Intramedullary papillary ependymoma with choroid plexus differentiation and cerebrospinal fluid dissemination to the brain. J Neurosurg Pediatr. 2010;5(5):511–7.
52. Fujisawa H, Marukawa K, Hasegawa M, et al. Genetic differences between neurocytoma and dysembryoplastic neuroepithelial tumor and oligodendroglial tumors. J Neurosurg. 2002;97(6):1350–5.
53. Yuen ST, Fung CF, Ng TH, Leung SY. Central neurocytoma: its differentiation from intraventricular oligodendroglioma. Childs Nerv Syst. 1992;8(7):383–8.
54. McKeever PE. The brain, spinal cord, and meninges. In: Mills SE, Carter D, Greenson JK, et al., editors. Sternsburg's diagnostic surgical pathology. 5th ed. Philadelphia: Lippincott Williams & Wilkins; 2010; p. 351–448.
55. Kubota T, Hayashi M, Kawano H, et al. Central neurocytoma: immunohistochemical and ultrastructural study. Acta Neuropathol. 1991;81(4):418–27.
56. Giangaspero F, Cenacchi G, Losi L, Cerasoli S, Bisceglia M, Burger PC. Extraventricular neoplasms with neurocytoma features. A clinicopathological study of 11 cases. Am J Surg Pathol. 1997;21(2):206–12.
57. Lin F, Shi J, Liu H, et al. Immunohistochemical detection of the von Hippel-Lindau gene product (pVHL) in human tissues and tumors: a useful marker for metastatic renal cell carcinoma and clear cell carcinoma of the ovary and uterus. Am J Clin Pathol. 2008;129(4):592–605.
58. Hofmann BM, Kreutzer J, Saeger W, et al. Nuclear beta-catenin accumulation as reliable marker for the differentiation between cystic craniopharyngiomas and rathke cleft cysts: a clinico-pathologic approach. Am J Surg Pathol. 2006;30(12):1595–603.
59. Xin W, Rubin MA, McKeever PE. Differential expression of cytokeratins 8 and 20 distinguishes craniopharyngioma from rathke cleft cyst. Arch Pathol Lab Med. 2002;126(10):1174–8.
60. Dickson DW. Review article: neuropathology of non-Alzheimer degenerative disorders. Int J Clin Exp Pathol. 2010;3(1):1–23.
61. Mahfouz S, Aziz AA, Gabal SM, el-Sheikh S. Immunohistochemical study of CD99 and EMA expression in ependymomas. Medscape J Med. 2008;10(2):41.
62. Cetin N, Dienel G, Gokden M. CD117 expression in glial tumors. J Neurooncol. 2005;75(2):195–202.
63. Gyure KA, Prayson RA, Estes ML. Extracerebellar primitive neuroectodermal tumors: a clinicopathologic study with bcl-2 and CD99 immunohistochemistry. Ann Diagn Pathol. 1999;3(5):276–80.
64. Matsuda R, Takahashi T, Nakamura S, et al. Expression of the c-kit protein in human solid tumors and in corresponding fetal and adult normal tissues. Am J Pathol. 1993;142(1):339–46.
65. Akiyama H, Kondo H, Ikeda K, Arai T, Kato M, McGleer PL. Immunohistochemical detection of coagulation factor XIIIa in postmortem human brain tissue. Neurosci Lett. 1995;202(1–2):29–32.
66. Takata M, Imai T, Hirone T. Factor-XIIIa-positive cells in normal peripheral nerves and cutaneous neurofibromas of type-1 neurofibromatosis. Am J Dermatopathol. 1994;16(1):37–43.
67. Choi YL, Chi JG, Suh YL. CD99 immunoreactivity in ependymoma. Appl Immunohistochem Mol Morphol. 2001;9(2):125–9.
68. Kovacs GG, Head MW, Hegyi I, et al. Immunohistochemistry for the prion protein: comparison of different monoclonal antibodies in human prion disease subtypes. Brain Pathol. 2002;12(1):1–11.
69. Neumann M, Kwong LK, Sampathu DM, Trojanowski JQ, Lee VM. TDP-43 proteinopathy in frontotemporal lobar degeneration and amyotrophic lateral sclerosis: protein misfolding diseases without amyloidosis. Arch Neurol. 2007;64(10):1388–94.
70. Hasegawa M, Arai T, Nonaka T, et al. Phosphorylated TDP-43 in frontotemporal lobar degeneration and amyotrophic lateral sclerosis. Ann Neurol. 2008;64(1):60–70.
71. Freeman SH, Spires-Jones T, Hyman BT, Growdon JH, Frosch MP. TAR-DNA binding protein 43 in Pick disease. J Neuropathol Exp Neurol. 2008;67(1):62–7.

Chapter 11
Thyroid and Parathyroid Gland

Haiyan Liu, Fan Lin, and Ronald A. DeLellis

Abstract This chapter provides a practical overview of frequently used markers in the diagnosis and differential diagnosis of both common and rare neoplasms of the thyroid and parathyroid glands, with a specific focus on papillary thyroid carcinoma and its mimickers. The chapter contains 28 questions; each question is addressed with a table, concise note, and representative pictures if applicable. In addition to the literature review, the authors have included their own experience and tested numerous antibodies reported in the literature. The most effective diagnostic panels of antibodies have been recommended for many entities, such as CK19, HBME-1, and galectin-3 being suggested as the best diagnostic panel for identifying papillary thyroid carcinoma. Furthermore, immunophenotypes of normal thyroid tissue have been described, which tends to be neglected in literature.

Keywords Papillary thyroid carcinoma • Medullary carcinoma • Follicular carcinoma • Anaplastic carcinoma • PAX8 • HBME-1 • CK19 • Galectin-3

FREQUENTLY ASKED QUESTIONS

Thyroid Gland

Differential Diagnosis

H. Liu (✉)
Department of Pathology and Laboratory Medicine, Geisinger Medical Center, 100 N. Academy Ave, Danville, PA 17822, USA
e-mail:hliu1@geisinger.edu

F. Lin and J. Prichard (eds.), *Handbook of Practical Immunohistochemistry: Frequently Asked Questions*,
DOI 10.1007/978-1-4419-8062-5_11,

Parathyroid Gland

26. Summary of useful markers in the evaluation of the parathyroid gland (Table 11.26) (p. 150)
27. Markers for normal parathyroid gland (Table 11.27) (p. 150)
28. Markers for parathyroid neoplasms (Table 11.28 and Fig. 11.20) (p. 150)

Table 11.1 Summary of applications and limitations of useful markers

Antibodies	Staining pattern	Function	Key applications and pitfalls
TTF1	N	A nuclear transcription factor	Both follicular cells and C cells are positive Anaplastic carcinomas are usually nonreactive
Thyroglobulin (TGB)	C	The primary product of thyroid, representing the macromolecular precursor of iodinated thyroid hormones: thyroxine (T4) and triiodothyroxine (T3)	A follicular cell-specific marker, but anaplastic carcinomas are nonreactive False positive: due to the tendency to diffuse through adjacent tissue
PAX8	N	A family of developmental control genes that encode transcription factors	Similar to TTF1 as a sensitive marker for thyroid tumors; anaplastic carcinomas are frequently positive as well
CK19	M + C	Cytokeratin expressed by simple and glandular epithelium	Usually strong and diffuse stain in PTC; less intense and more focal stain in FA and FC; negative in normal thyroid follicles
HBME-1	C	A monoclonal antibody generated against the microvillous surface of mesothelial cells	A useful marker of malignancy in thyroid nodules
Galectin-3	C, N	A member of the non-integrin beta-galactoside-binding lectin family that plays an important role in cell–cell adhesion and in cell–matrix interaction	Overexpressed in thyroid malignant tumors. Also expressed in macrophages, neutrophils, mast cells, and Langerhans cells
FN-1	C, M	Multifunctional adhesive glycoproteins found in the extracellular matrix and body fluids	Oncofetal FNs are highly expressed in fetal and neoplastic tissues, including thyroid follicular cell-derived tumors
IMP-3	C	A member of the insulin-like growth factor II mRNA binding protein (IMP) family	Reported high expression in thyroid follicular cell-derived carcinomas, correlating with the differentiation of the tumor
HMGA2	N	A member of nonhistone nuclear proteins that orchestrate the assembly of nucleoprotein complexes	Upregulated in several malignant neoplasms including thyroid tumors
CLDN 1	M	A multi-pass membrane protein, as an important structural and functional component of tight junction mediated in paracellular transport	Increased claudin-1 mRNA levels have been observed in PTC. IHC studies claim expression in PTC, FC, and FA
NIS	M, C	An integral plasma membrane glycoprotein that mediates active iodine transport	Reduced expression in general in thyroid carcinomas; not detected immunohistochemically in ACs
RET/PTC	C	A somatic rearrangement of RET proto-oncogene; plays a key role in the pathogenesis of PTC	Molecular testing appears superior to IHC methods in detecting those rearrangements currently
Beta-catenin	C/N	A 94-kDa protein, as part of a membrane-bound cell growth-signaling complex, plays a role in cell adhesion, as well as in the promotion of growth through activation of the Wnt signaling pathway	Malignant thyroid tumors: the loss of M staining with C and N staining, associated with progressive loss of tumor differentiation Cribriform-morular variant PTC (frequently associated with familial adenomatous polyposis) with aberrant nuclear localization
DPPIV (CD26)	M	An exopeptidase involved in T-cell activation	Absent from normal thyroid tissue but highly expressed in malignant thyroid cells
TPO	C	A thyroid-specific enzyme expressed by differentiated thyroid cells	Studies of TPO expression by ISH and IHC show reduced or lost expression of TPO in malignant tissue compared with normal and benign neoplastic tissue
CD44v6	M	A member of immunologically related integral membrane glycoproteins mediating cell–cell and cell–matrix interactions through its affinity for hyaluronic acid	Intense membrane stain had been detected in benign (~40%) and malignant thyroid tumors, with highest in well-differentiated PTC (75–90%) and FC (90–100%)
CK7	M + C	Epithelial marker	Thyroid tumors are positive
CK20	M + C	Epithelial marker	Differentiated thyroid carcinoma is nonreactive
p63	N	A transcription factor belonging to the p53 gene family	Diffusely positive in SCN, CASTLE, MEC, SMEC, and nearly half of AC
CDX-2	N	Intestine-specific transcription factor directing intestinal development, differentiation, proliferation, and maintenance of the intestinal phenotype	Rarely being reported positive in PTCs. A recent single study of three cases of columnar cell variant PTC shows diffuse nuclear stain for CDX-2

(continued)

Table 11.1 (continued)

Antibodies	Staining pattern	Function	Key applications and pitfalls
COX-2	C	Important enzymes involved in the arachidonic acid pathway and synthesis of prostaglandins	Higher expression in PTCs and FCs than in normal follicular epithelium and follicular adenomas
Calcitonin	C	A secreted protein produced by parafollicular C cells	Rare cases of MC are negative for calcitonin
CGRP	C	A widely distributed vasodilatory peptide, encoded by calcitonin gene (CALCA)	Useful marker for the diagnosis of MCs
mCEA	C, M	Carcinoembryonic antigens	Very sensitive marker for MC and hyperplastic or neoplastic C-cells
E-cadherin	M	An adhesion molecule of the integrin and cadherin family, involving the induction and maintenance of a functional organization of polarized epithelia	Reduced or lost expression in differentiated thyroid carcinomas; lost expression in PDCs and ACs

Note: *N* nuclear staining, *M* membranous staining, *C* cytoplasmic staining

TGB thyroglobulin, *PAX8* peroxidase proliferative-activated receptor gamma, *CGRP (CALCA)* calcitonin gene-related peptide (calcitonin-related polypeptide alpha), *HBME-1* Hector Battifora mesothelial cell 1, *FN-1* fibronectin-1, *IMP-3* insulin-like growth factor mRNA-binding protein 3, *CLDN 1* claudin protein 1, *NIS* Na^{+}/I^{+} symporter, *COX-2* cyclooxygenase-2, *HMGA2* high-mobility group A2, *DPPIV* dipeptidyl aminopeptidase IV, *LCA* leukocyte common antigen, *PTH* parathyroid hormone, *Gcm2* Glial cells missing homolog 2, also known as chorion-specific transcription factor GCMb, *PTC* papillary thyroid carcinoma, *FA* follicular adenomam, *FC* follicular carcinoma, *MC* medullary carcinoma, *HCC* Hurthle cell carcinoma, *PDC* poorly differentiated carcinoma, *ATC* anaplastic thyroid carcinoma, *CASTLE* carcinomas showing thymus-like differentiation of the thyroid, *SMECE* Primary sclerosing mucoepidermoid carcinoma with eosinophilia, *MEC* primary mucoepidermoid carcinoma

TTF1 is expressed both in follicular epithelial cells and C-cells; however, the intensity of staining in the follicular cells is stronger than in the C-cells. In tumors, PTCs and follicular adenomas are strongly positive; in contrast, medullary carcinoma tends to be weakly or focally positive. A significant portion of follicular carcinomas demonstrate weak reactivity to TTF1 as well. In our study, 16 of 36 cases of follicular carcinoma showed only weak positivity for TTF1. In general, poorly differentiated carcinomas are less intensely positive than differentiated carcinomas. Anaplastic carcinoma of the thyroid is usually negative for TTF1. Examples of the expression of TTF1 on normal thyroid tissue and various thyroid tumors are shown in Fig. 11.1a–d

PAX8 is more often expressed in FC (reported 53–100%), less often in PTC (reported 0–49% in early studies and 100% in one recent study with 17 cases) and FA (8–62% in early studies and 100% in one recent study with 18 cases); PDCs are reported non-expressed in early studies and positive in a recent study with seven cases. PAX8 was reported to be positive in 79% of ATCs. Our study shows PAX8 is positive in 96, 93, and 80% of follicular adenomas, PTCs and follicular carcinomas, respectively. The expression of PAX8 tends to be weaker in follicular carcinomas than in PTCs and follicular adenomas. A small number of medullary carcinomas ($N = 10$) are negative for PAX8, and two of five anaplastic thyroid carcinomas are focally positive for PAX8. Examples of the expression of PAX8 in various tumors are shown in Fig. 11.2a–d

Galectin-3 represents one of the most studied molecules for thyroid cancer diagnosis, especially for PTC. Galectin-3 is highly expressed in thyroid cancer but not in normal thyroid tissue and infrequently in benign thyroid lesions. In classic PTC, galectin-3 expression was reported in 58–100% of cases, with the majority of reports within the range of 90–100%. However, the expression of galectin-3 is usually lower in follicular variant PTC than in classic PTC. Variable expression was identified in MTC, HCC, and PDTC. In ATC, galectin-3 expression was identified in 75–100% of reported cases. Galectin-3 expression was reported in 0–45% of cases of FA. In NG, no galectin-3 was identified, with few exceptions. Normal thyroid tissue is generally negative for galectin-3

Fibronectin was reported to be upregulated in thyroid carcinoma compared with normal and benign thyroid tissue. An immunohistochemical panel consisting of FN-1, galectin-3, and HBME-1 has been reported to be effective in the diagnosis of follicular cell-derived thyroid tumors. Fibroblasts were detected containing a high number of copies of oncofetal FN mRNA, which may cause false-positive results in molecular-based diagnosis of thyroid carcinomas in FNA biopsy specimens

IMP-3 expression was reported highest in undifferentiated carcinomas (95%), and not detected in benign thyroid tissue (normal or benign neoplastic tissue)

Thyroid carcinomas, in general, have reduced the expression of NIS when compared with normal thyroid tissue. Normal thyroid tissue shows more of the basolateral membranous staining. Apical staining was not noted in normal thyroid tissue, which has been noted in a proportion of thyroid carcinomas. NIS protein redistribution (cytoplasmic instead of basolateral membranous staining by immunostain) has been reported in several studies

Immunohistochemical studies for CD26/DPPIV show all PTCs and the majority of FCs are strongly positive. It is rare in FA and AC and nonreactive in MC, normal and goiters

References: [1–8, 10–92]

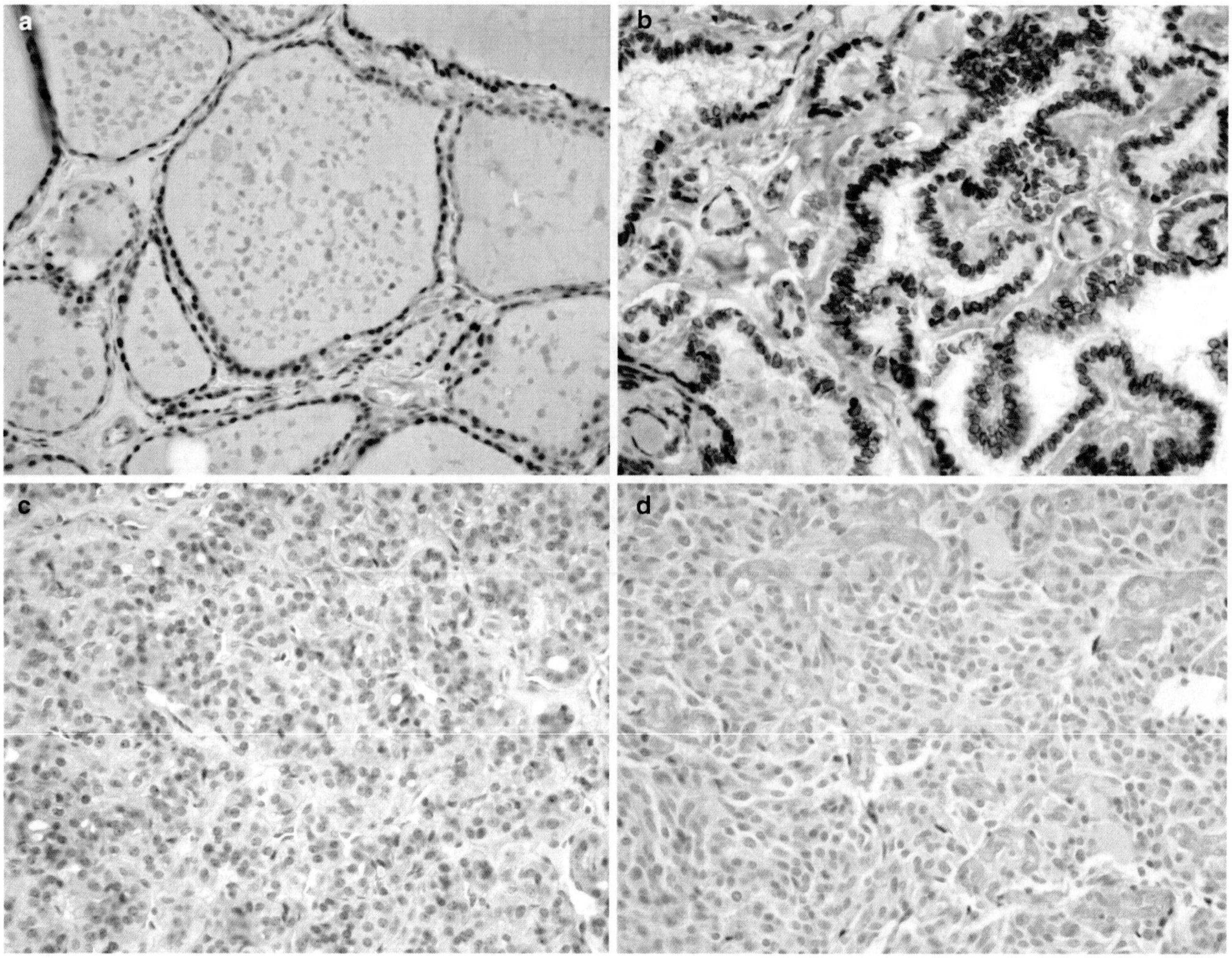

Fig. 11.1 Expression of TTF1 in normal thyroid tissue (**a**), papillary carcinoma (**b**), follicular carcinoma (**c**), and medullary carcinoma (**d**). Note that the weak staining in both follicular carcinoma and medullary carcinoma

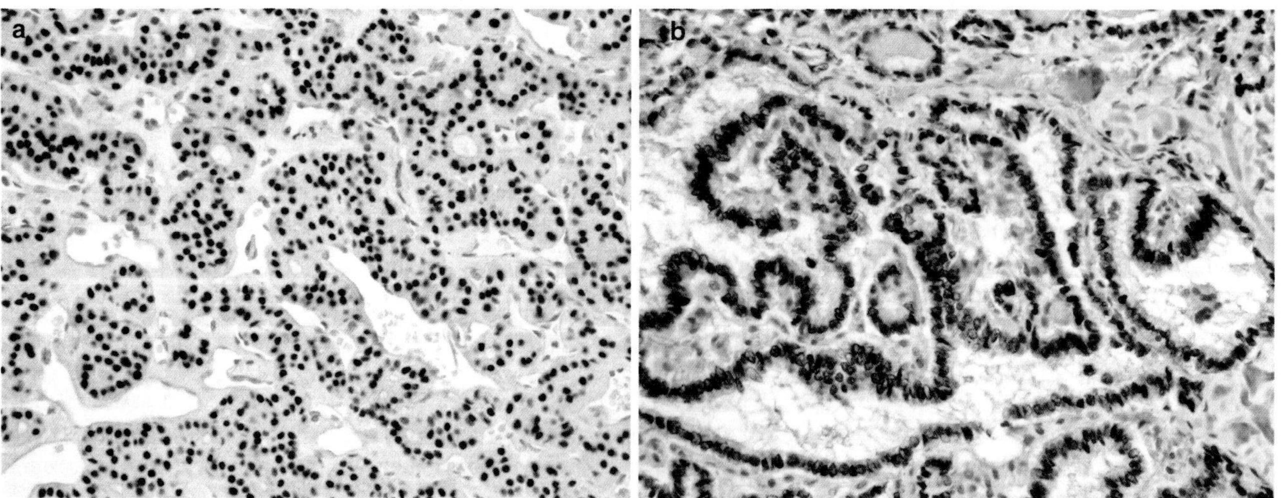

Fig. 11.2 Expression of PAX8 in follicular adenoma (**a**), papillary carcinoma (**b**), follicular carcinoma (**c**), and medullary carcinoma (**d**). Note that the weak staining in follicular carcinoma and the absence of staining in medullary carcinoma

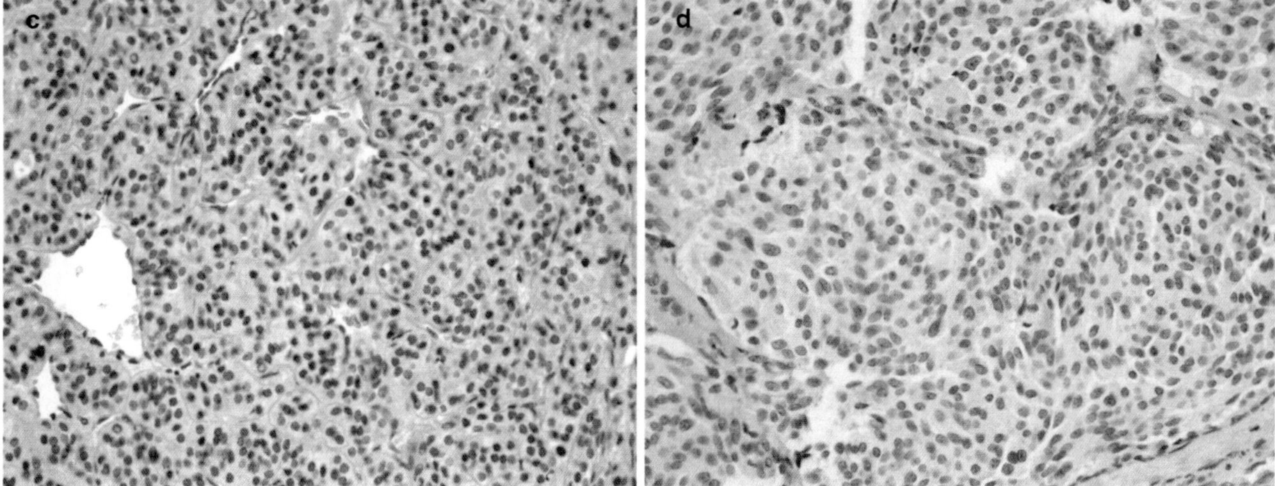

Fig. 11.2 (continued)

Table 11.2 Markers for normal thyroid follicles

	Follicular cells	
Antibodies	Literature	GML data (*N* = 14)
Thyroglobulin	+	100%
TTF1	+	100%
PAX8	–	100%
Calcitonin	–	0
PTH	–	0
CEA	–	0
CK19	–	0
HBME-1	–	14%
FN-1	–	ND
Galectin-3	–	14%
AE1/AE3	+	100%
CK7	+	100%
EMA	+	0
Chromogranin	–	0
Synaptophysin	–	0

Note: *ND* no data

References: [1, 12–17, 67, 93–97]

Table 11.3 Summary of useful markers in common tumors of the thyroid gland

Antibodies	PTC	FC	MC	PDTC	ATC
CK7	+	+	+	+ or –	+ or –
CK20	–	–	–	–	–
CK19	+	– or +	– or +	– or +	–
HBME-1	+	– or +	– or +	– or +	– or +
Galectin-3	+	– or +	– or +	–	+ or –
Calcitonin	–	–	+	–	–
CEA	–	–	+	ND	–
PAX8	+	+/–	–	+/–	+
TGB	+	+	–	+ or –	–
TTF1	+	+	+	+ or –	–
Synaptophysin	+ or –	+/–	+	ND	–
Chromogranin	–	–	+	ND	–

Note: *PTC* papillary thyroid carcinoma, *FC* follicular carcinoma, *MC* medullary thyroid carcinoma, *PDC* poorly differentiated thyroid carcinoma, *ATC* anaplastic thyroid carcinoma, *ND* no data

The intensity of PAX8 and TTF1 is stronger in PTC than in follicular carcinoma. TTF1 tends to be weakly expressed in medullary carcinoma and negative in anaplastic carcinoma. PAX8 is negative in medullary carcinoma. CEA is a more sensitive marker for medullary carcinoma than calcitonin; up to 5% of medullary carcinomas can be negative for calcitonin, and nearly all cases are positive for CEA

CK19, HBME-1, and galectin-3 is the best panel of marker to confirm a diagnosis of PTC with over 90% sensitivity; however, the percentage tends to be lower in follicular variant PTC

References: [1, 4, 10, 13–15, 30, 60, 66, 67, 97–116]

Table 11.4 Markers for solid cell nests

Antibodies	Literature
p63	+
CEA	+
TGB	–
TTF1	– or W+
Calcitonin	–
CGRP	–
Chromogranin	–
Galectin-3	+
AE1/AE3	+
HBME-1	–

Note: *W* weak

Solid cell nests demonstrate diffuse p63 staining. p63-positive foci are often present in PTC and Hashimoto's thyroiditis but usually absent in normal, nodular goiter, oncocytic follicular adenoma, and FC. Solid cell nests are usually positive for CAM 5.2, AE1/AE3, 34betaE12, and CK7 and negative for CK20

References: [1, 32, 82, 117–128]

Table 11.5 Markers for hyalinizing trabecular adenoma

Antibodies	Literature
MIB-1, monoclonal	M and C+
TGB	+
TTF1	+
Calcitonin	–
HBME-1	–
CK7	+
p63	–
Galectin-3	– or +
RET/PTC	– or +
CK19	– or +
CK20	–

Note: Distinct membranous and cytoplasmic staining for monoclonal antibody to MIB-1 is shown in Figs. 11.3 and 11.4. Type IV collagen and PAS demonstrate reactivity around tumor cells and nuclear pseudoinclusion

References: [1, 29, 78, 93, 129–140]

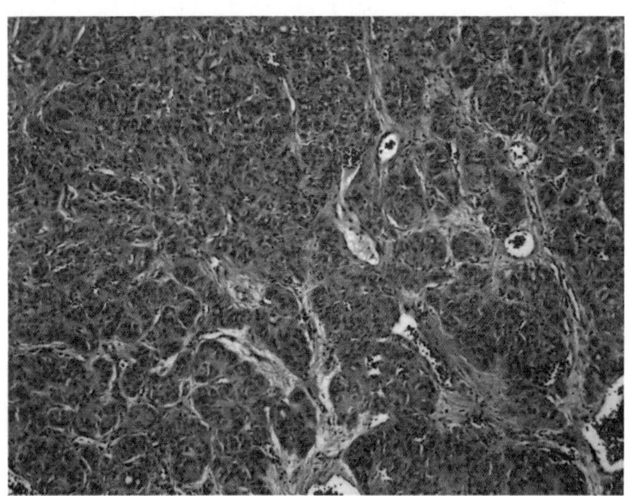

Fig. 11.3 Hyalinizing trabecular adenoma on H&E section

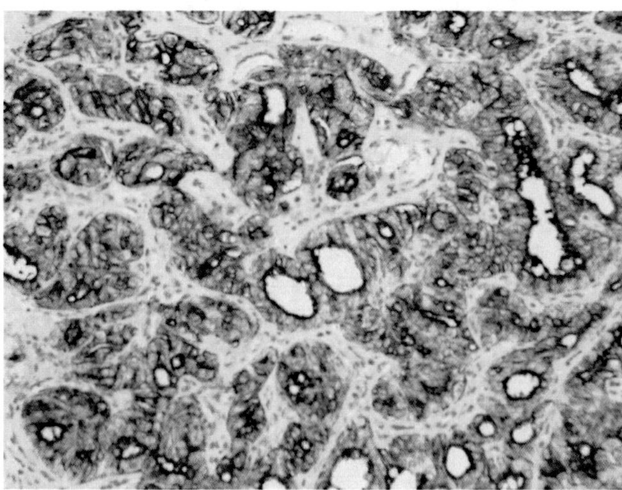

Fig. 11.4 Hyalinizing trabecular adenoma showing membranous and cytoplasmic staining pattern for Ki-67 (MIB-1)

Table 11.6 Markers for paraganglioma

Antibodies	Literature
Cytokeratins	–
Chromogranin	+
Synaptophysin	+
S100 protein	–

Note: Immunostain for S100 protein is negative in paraganglioma, except in the sustentacular cells, which are positive for S100 protein

Immunohistochemical studies for CEA, calcitonin, thyroglobulin, EMA, and vimentin are usually negative

References: [1, 141–149]

Table 11.7 Markers for Hurthle cell neoplasm

Antibodies	Literature
TTF1	+
Thyroglobulin	+
AE1/AE3	+
CK7	+
S100A1 and S100A6	+

References: [1, 36, 94, 111, 150–156]

Table 11.8 Markers for follicular thyroid carcinoma

Antibodies	Literature	GML data (*N* = 36)
Thyroglobulin	+	100%
TTF1	+	94%
Galectin-3	– or +	25%
CK17	–	0
CK19	– or +	17%
HBME-1	+	38%
FN-1	+	N/D
AE1/AE3	+	81%
CK7	+	97%
Vimentin	+	100%
Cyclin D1	+	94%

(continued)

Table 11.8 (continued)

Antibodies	Literature	GML data (*N* = 36)
S100A1	+	94%
Chromogranin	–	0
COX-2	–/+	N/D
CD56	–/+	44%
p53	–/+	44%
Calcitonin	Usually negative	0
mCEA	–	0

Note: Our data (unpublished) reveal that approximately 20% cases of follicular carcinoma are nonreactive to AE1/AE3, but nearly all of those cases are positive for CK7 (97%). RCC marker is very frequently expressed in follicular carcinoma and follicular adenoma and less frequently in PTC (27%). The staining signal of cyclin D1 is weaker in FC than in PTC. CEA and chromogranin are usually negative, but CD56 is detected in 44% of cases in our study. An example of FC negative for AE1/AE3 and positive for RCC is shown in Fig. 11.5a, b

Some follicular carcinomas can be positive for CK19, HBME-1, and galectin-3

References: [1, 7, 9, 49]

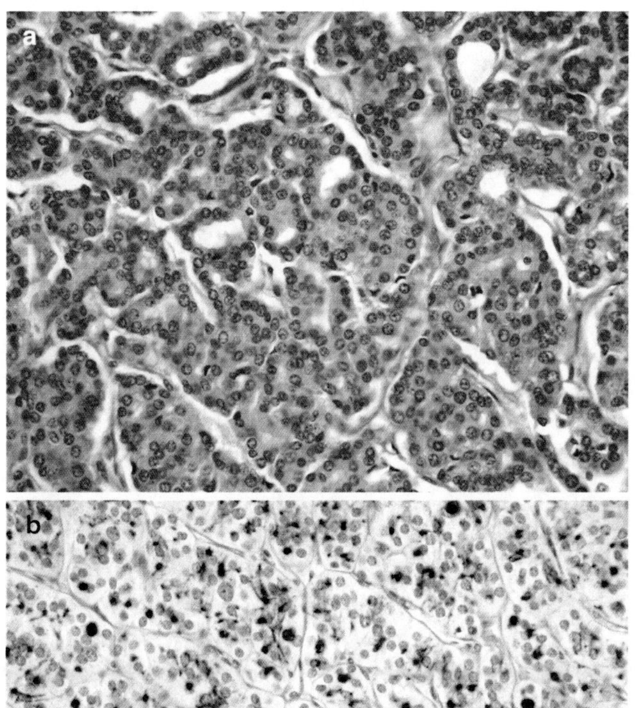

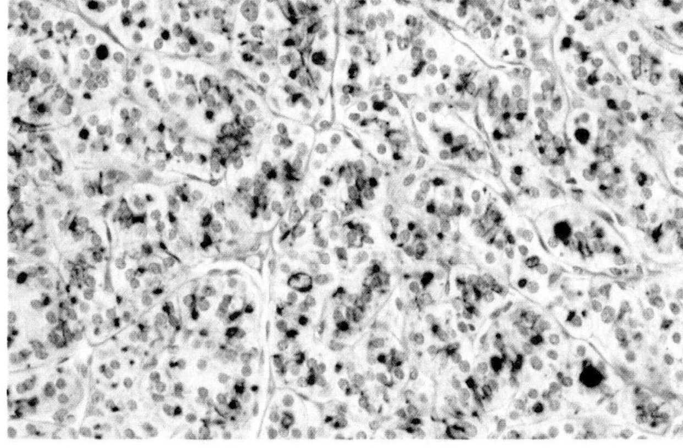

Fig. 11.5 Follicular carcinoma can be negative for AE1/AE3 (**a**) and positive for RCC (**b**)

Table 11.9 Markers for papillary thyroid carcinoma

Antibodies	Literature	GML data (*N* = 45)
TTF1	+	100%
TGB	+	100%
Galectin-3	+	93%
CK 19	+	91%
FN-1	+	ND
CITED1	+	ND
HBME-1	+	93%
Calcitonin	–	0
Chromogranin	–	0
mCEA	–	9% Focal +
RET/PTC	+	ND
S100A1	+	100%
S100A6	+	100%
RCC	ND	27%
CDX-2	ND	2%
Beta-catenin	–/+	100%
CK7	+	100%
AE1/AE3	+	100%
Vimentin	+	100%
p53	–/+	9%
CD56	–/+	27%
CD57	+	ND
PAX8	+	100%

Note: *ND* no data

Galectin-3 is overexpressed in malignant tumors of thyroid gland and usually absent in hyperplastic nodules, NG, and normal follicular epithelium. PTC characteristically demonstrates intense and diffuse cytoplasmic staining for CK19, HBME-1, galectin-3, cyclin D1, S100A1, and vimentin as shown in Figs. 11.6–11.13. Rare cases may express CDX-2 in addition to TTF1 as shown in Fig. 11.14a–c. Papillary carcinoma, cribriform-morular variant, poorly differentiated and anaplastic carcinomas show aberrant nuclear stain for beta-catenin in contrast to the membranous staining in other thyroid carcinomas. TTF1 and TGB are usually negative in areas of squamous differentiation

Although galectin-3, HBME-1, and CK19 are not entirely sensitive and specific for the diagnosis of PTC, at the present time it is considered the most effective panel of markers in confirming a diagnosis of PTC, including papillary microcarcinomas

Both S100A1 and S100A6 are usually positive in papillary carcinomas; however, normal thyroid follicles are positive as well. Our experience showed S100 is usually negative in both normal thyroid follicles and PTC

RT/PTC and NIS have been tested in the Dako system with various antigen retrieval methods. The results are suboptimal, and they are not recommended as routine diagnostic markers based on our experience

References: [1, 12, 15, 22, 23, 81, 86, 99, 100, 157–168]

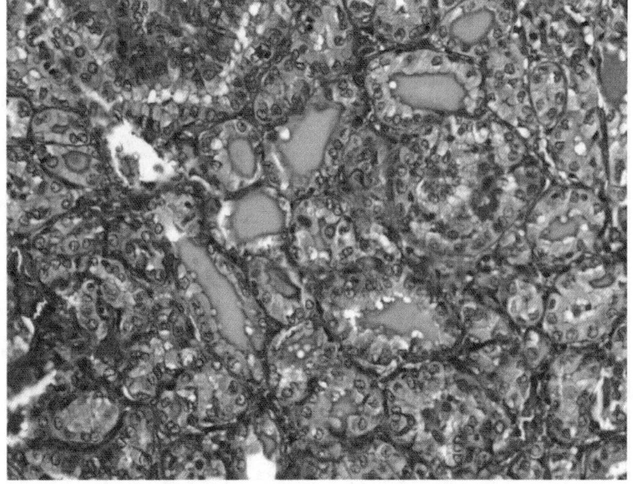

Fig. 11.6 A typical immunostaining profile for a PTC: the H&E-stained section

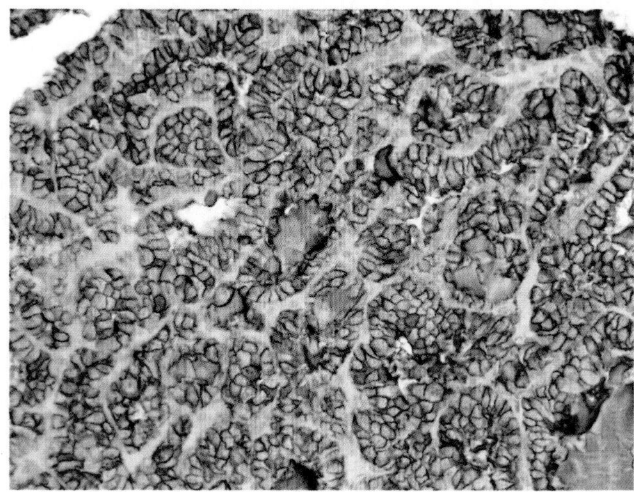

Fig. 11.9 A typical immunostaining profile for a PTC: HBME-1

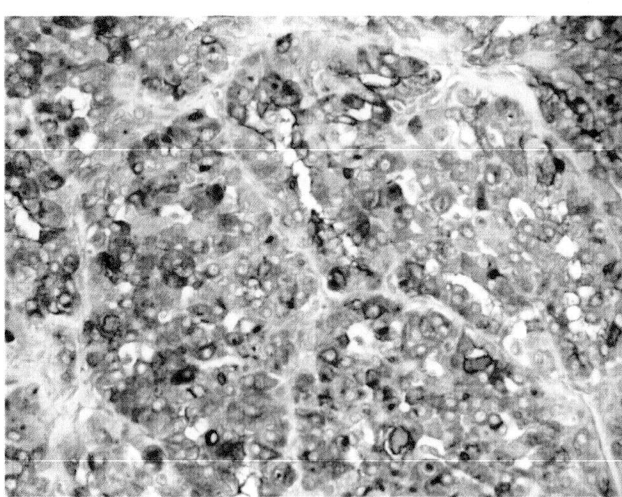

Fig. 11.7 A typical immunostaining profile for a PTC: thyroglobulin

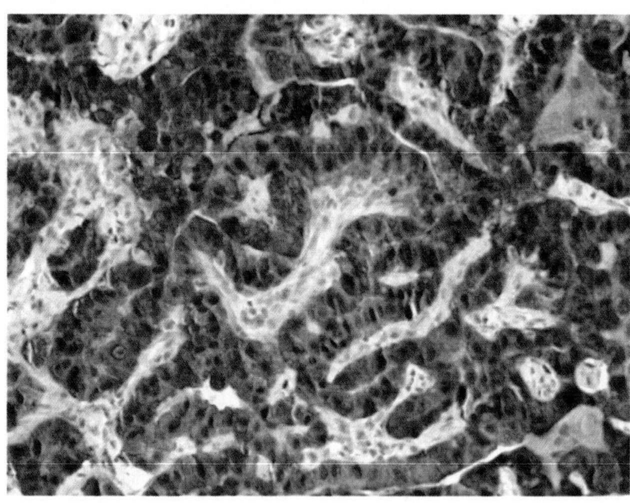

Fig. 11.10 A typical immunostaining profile for a PTC: galectin-3

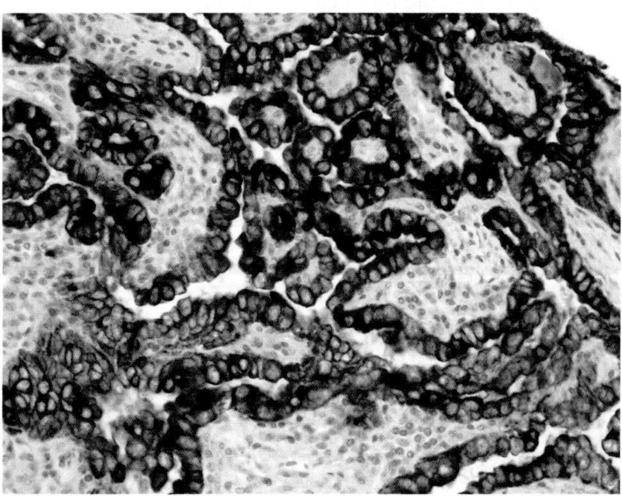

Fig. 11.8 A typical immunostaining profile for a PTC: CK19

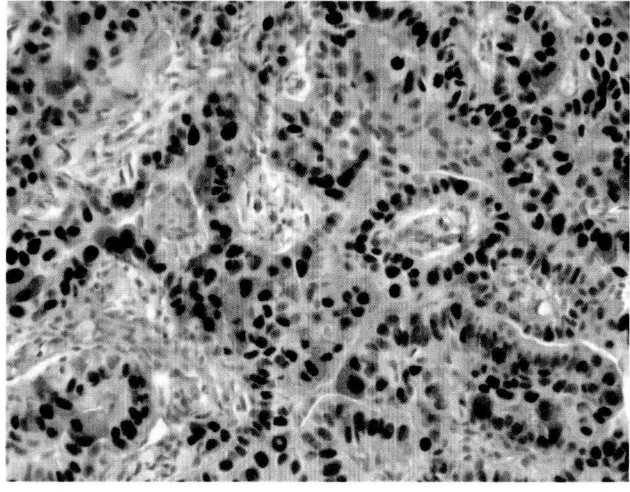

Fig. 11.11 A typical immunostaining profile for a PTC: cyclin D1

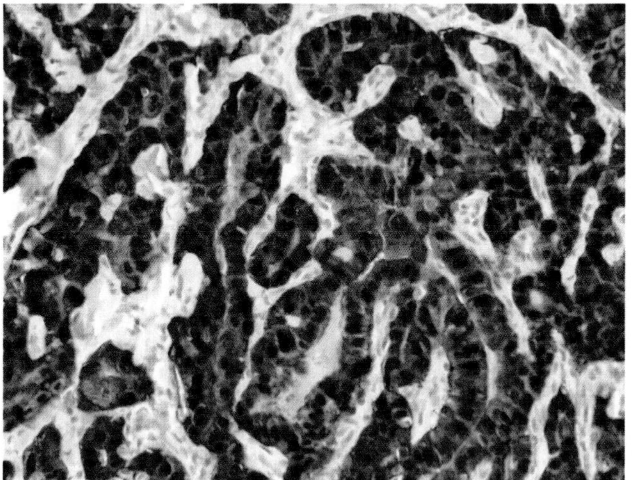

Fig. 11.12 A typical immunostaining profile for a PTC: S100A1

Fig. 11.13 A typical immunostaining profile for a PTC: vimentin

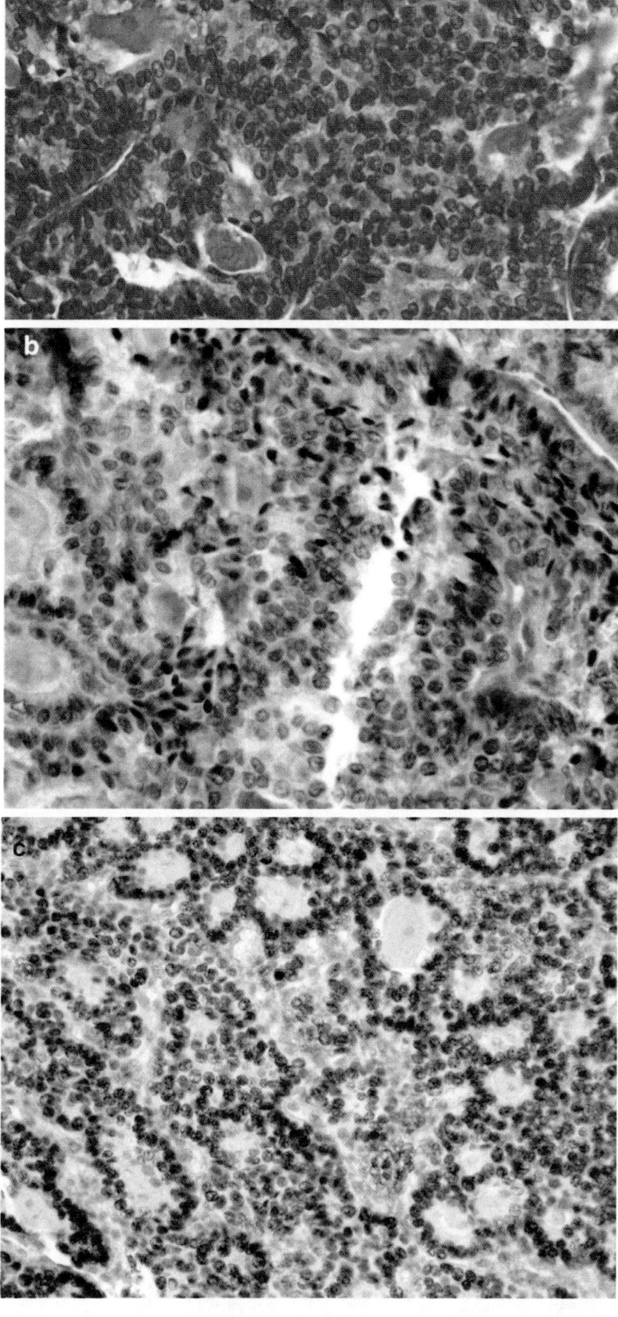

Fig. 11.14 CDX-2 is expressed in a rare case of papillary thyroid carcinoma. Note that papillary carcinoma on H&E section (**a**), and positive for TTF1 (**b**) and CDX-2 (**c**)

Table 11.10 Markers for medullary thyroid carcinoma

Antibodies	Literature	GML data (N = 10)
Calcitonin	+	100%
Thyroglobulin	–	0
TTF1	+	100%, w+
CEA	+	100%
Chromogranin	+	100%
Synaptophysin	+	100%
CGRP	+	ND
NFP	+	ND
AE1/AE3	+	100%
CK7	+	100%
CK20	–	0
CK5/6	–	0
Vimentin	+ or –	100%
COX-2	+	ND
Galectin-3	– or +	0
S100A1	ND	10%
S100A6	ND	100%

Note: Typical phenotype of MC is positive for calcitonin, CGRP, TTF1, mCEA, and neuroendocrine markers and negative for TGB (with focal stain in entrapped follicles or deposits). Rare cases of MC are negative for calcitonin (reported in up to 5% of cases); and the calcitonin-negative MC cases are usually positive for mCEA. It has been reported that 85% of cases of MC are positive for NFP, whereas normal C-cells are usually negative

Our data also showed MC is usually positive for Ber-EP4 and S100A6 but negative for TAG 72 and S100A1. An example of MC positive for calcitonin, CEA, and S100A6 and negative for S100A1 is shown in Figs. 11.15–11.19

References: [1, 31, 60, 62–66, 68, 104, 108, 109, 169–177]

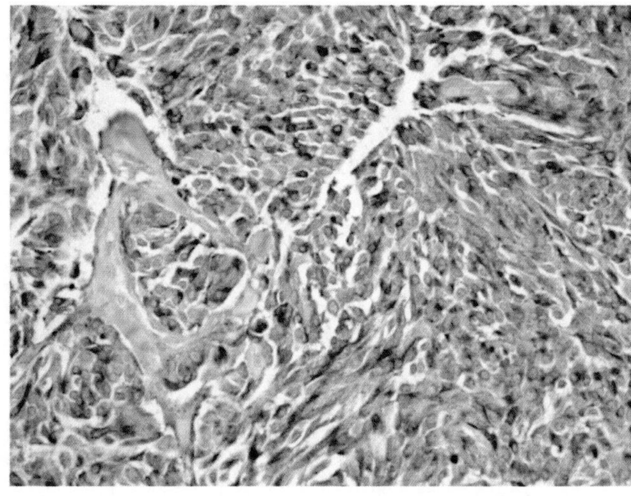

Fig. 11.16 Medullary carcinoma positive for calcitonin

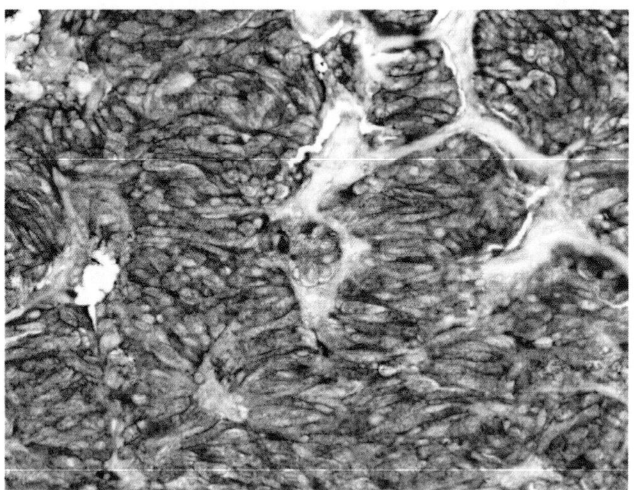

Fig. 11.17 Medullary carcinoma: CEA

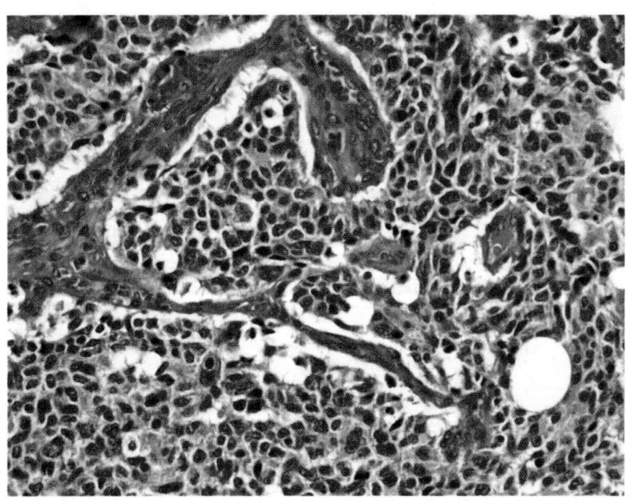

Fig. 11.15 Medullary carcinoma on H&E section

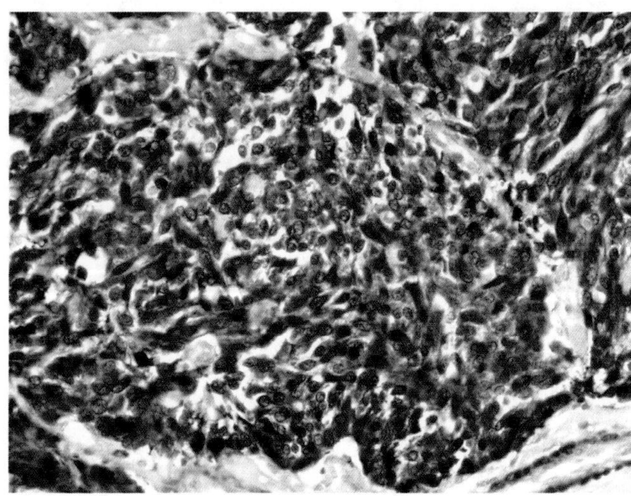

Fig. 11.18 Medullary carcinoma: S100A6

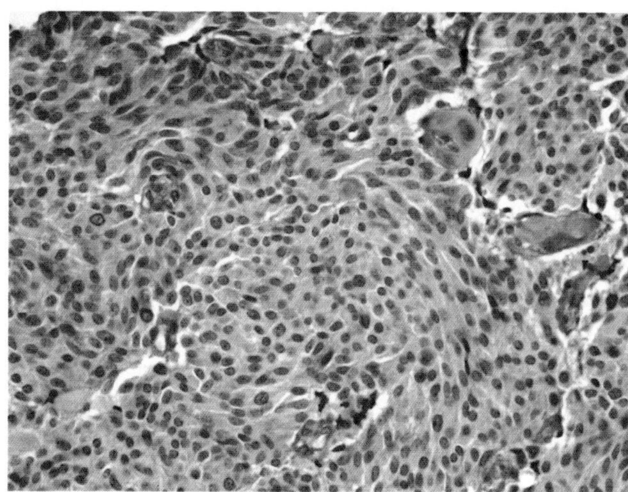

Fig. 11.19 Medullary carcinoma negative for S100A1

Table 11.11 Markers for insular carcinoma

Antibodies	Literature
Thyroglobulin	+
TTF1	+
CEA	–
AE1/AE3	+
Cyclin D1	+, N
HBME-1	+ or –
CK19	+ or –
RET/PTC	+ or –
Galectin-3	–
PAX2	–
p53	–

Note: TGB stain is often weak and focal, showing a peculiar pattern of dot-like paranuclear staining which is not specific and may be observed in other benign or malignant lesions with a predominantly solid/trabecular pattern of growth

References: [1, 4, 110, 111, 178–188]

Table 11.12 Markers for anaplastic thyroid carcinoma

Antibodies	Literature
AE1/AE3	+
Pan-CK	+
Vimentin	+
PAX8	+ or –
Thyroglobulin	–
TTF1	–
Galectin-3	+
p53	+
mCEA	–
Calcitonin	–
HBME-1	– or +
CK19	– or +
EMA/MUC1	– or +
CD56	–

Note: The most useful epithelial markers for ATC are cytokeratins, with a reported positivity rate of 50–100%. By using AE1/AE3 or Pan-CK, about 80% of cases demonstrate cytokeratin expression. Thyroglobulin is negative in ATC. When present, it is most likely the result of diffusion from entrapped or adjacent non-neoplastic thyroid tissue or from residual well-differentiated neoplastic components. TTF1 is usually nonreactive in ATC. Few studies show rare cases of ATC demonstrating isolated TTF1-reactive tumor cells, which may be due to the presence of a differentiated thyroid carcinoma component. ATCs typically show strong reactivity to p53. PAX8 is positive in about 79% of ATCs and is negative in normal and neoplastic lung tissue. Therefore, PAX8 can be a useful marker in the differential diagnosis of ATC from poorly differentiated pulmonary adenocarcinoma. In our study, only two of five cases of ATC were positive for PAX8

References: [1, 10, 11, 16, 23, 25, 30, 34, 38, 112, 189–199]

Table 11.13 Markers for mucoepidermoid carcinoma of thyroid

Antibody	Pattern
CKs (AE1/AE3, CAM 5.2)	+
Thyroglobulin	+
Calcitonin	–
NSE	+
Vimentin	+
P-cadherin	+
CGRP	–
Chrom, Synap	–
TTF1	+ or –
CEA	+ or –

Note: There are only small numbers of case report in the literature. Immunohistochemically, most of these cases are reported positive for cytokeratin (AE1/AE3, CAM 5.2), thyroglobulin (at least focally), and NSE and negative for calcitonin and neuroendocrine markers (chromogranin and synaptophysin). The immunoprofile for CEA (polyclonal or monoclonal) is variable

References: [1, 200–214]

Table 11.14 Sclerosing mucoepidermoid carcinoma with eosinophilia of thyroid

Antibody	Literature
CKs (AE1/AE3, CAM 5.2)	+
Thyroglobulin	–
Calcitonin	–
TTF1	+ or –
CEA	+ or –

Note: There are only few cases reported in the literature. Immunohistochemically, most of these cases are reported positive for cytokeratin (AE1/AE3, CAM 5.2) and negative for thyroglobulin and calcitonin

References: [1, 200–214]

Table 11.15 Solid cell nests (SCN) vs. nodular C-cell hyperplasia (CCH)

Antibody	SCN	Nodular CCH
p63	+	–
Calcitonin	–	+
Galectin-3	+	–
Chromogranin	–	+
Synaptophysin	–	+
TTF1	–	+, focal
Thyroglobulin	–	–
AE1/AE3	+	+
CEA	+	+

References: [1, 29, 78, 129–140, 215–219]

Table 11.16 Solid cell nest (SCN) vs. papillary microcarcinoma (PTmC)

Antibody	SCN	PTmC
CEA	+	–
Thyroglobulin	–	+
p63	+, diffuse	–/+, focal, variable
TTF1	– or focal w+	+, diffuse and strong
HBME-1	–	+
CGRP	–	–
AE1/AE3	+	+
CK19	+	+
Galectin-3	+	+
Chromogranin	–	– or +
Synaptophysin	–	– or +
Calcitonin	–	–

References: [1, 32, 82, 117–128]

Table 11.17 Hyalinizing trabecular adenoma (HTA) vs. paraganglioma (PG)

Antibody	HTA	PG
Thyroglobulin	+	–
TTF1	+	–
CK7	+	–
AE1/AE3	+	–
MIB-1 (Ki-67)	+, M, C	–
Chromogranin	– or +	+
S100	–	Scattered SC +
Vimentin	+	–
Calcitonin	–	–

Note: *SC* Sustentacular cell

References: [1, 29, 78, 93, 129–149]

Table 11.18 Hyalinizing trabecular tumor (HTA) vs. papillary carcinoma (PC)

Antibody	HTA	PC
MIB-1	+, M, C	+, N
HBME-1	– or +	+
34betaE12	–	+
CK19	– or +	+
Galectin-3	– or +	+
Thyroglobulin	+	+
TTF1	+	+
Calcitonin	–	–
CK7	+	+

Note: MIB-1 is a marker labeling nuclei in general, but demonstrating membranous and cytoplasmic staining pattern in HTA

References: [1, 12, 15, 22, 23, 29, 78, 81, 86, 93, 99, 100, 129–140, 157–168]

Table 11.19 Hyalinizing trabecular tumor (HTA) vs. medullary carcinoma (MC)

Antibody	HTA	MC
Calcitonin	–	+
MIB-1 (Ki-67)	+, M, C	+, N
TGB	+	–
mCEA	N/A	+
Chromogranin	– or focal +	+
TTF1	+	Weakly +
CK7	+	+

References: [1, 29, 31, 60, 62–66, 68, 78, 93, 104, 108, 109, 129–140, 169–177]

Table 11.20 Follicular adenoma vs. follicular carcinoma

Antibody	FA	FC
FN-1	– or +	+
HBME-1	– or +	+ or –
CITED1	– or +	+ or –
Galectin-3	– or +	+ or –
CK19	– or +	– or +
RET/PTC	–	+ or –
CD44v6	– or +	+

References: [1, 19, 21, 23, 25, 29, 34, 36, 49, 53, 167, 220–231]

Table 11.21 Differentiation of follicular adenoma with clear cell changes

Antibody	FA with clear cell changes	Met. renal cell carcinoma	Parathyroid adenoma
Chromogranin	–	–	+
TTF1	+	–	–
Thyroglobulin	+	–	–
PTH	–	–	+
KIM-1	–	+	–
VHL	–	+	–
RCC	– or +	+	+
CD10	–	+	N/A
CK7	+	– or +	N/A
Vimentin	+	+	N/A

Note: Our experience shows that VHL and KIM-1 (kidney injury molecule-1) are usually positive in metastatic RCC and negative in follicular adenoma and parathyroid adenoma or carcinoma. RCC marker is not very useful, since the positive staining is frequently observed in normal thyroid follicular epithelium and neoplasms

References: [1, 232–234]

Table 11.22 Follicular variant of PTC (FVPTC) vs. follicular neoplasm (FN)

Antibody	FVPTC	FN
CK19	+	– or +
FN-1	+	–
HBME-1	+	– or +
Galectin-3	+	– or +
CD57	+	– or +

References: [1, 12, 15, 20, 21, 95, 165, 168, 225, 235–239]

Table 11.23 Differential diagnosis of anaplastic carcinoma

Antibody	Anaplastic carcinoma	Rhabdomyo-sarcoma	Leiomyo-sarcoma	Angio-sarcoma	Malignant melanoma
PAX8	+ or –	–	–	–	–
AE1/AE3	+	–	–	– or +	–
MSA	–	+	+	– or +	–
Desmin	–	+	+	–	–
Myogenin	–	+	–	–	–
MyoD1	–	+	–	–	–
Factor VIII	–	–	–	+	–
CD31	– or +	–	–	+	–
CD34	– or +	– or +	– or +	+	–
S100	– or +	–	–	–	+
HMB-45	N/A	–	– or +	–	+
MART-1	–	–	–	–	+
Vimentin	+	+	+	+	+

References: [1, 111, 189, 240–261]

Table 11.24 Cystic metastatic papillary carcinoma (Met. PTC) vs. metastatic cystic squamous cell carcinoma (Met. SCC)

Antibody	Met. PTC	Met SCC
CD57	+	–
CK5/6	–	+
Rb	–	+
TTF1	+	Usually –
CK14	– or +	+
CK7	+	– or +
Vimentin	+	– or +
p63	– or +	+
CK19	+	+

Reference: [1]

Table 11.25 Proliferative, prognostic, and cell cycling markers in normal follicular epithelium and thyroid carcinomas

Antibody	NL	WDTC	PDTC	UDTC
MIB-1 (Ki-67)	Very low (<5%)	Low (<10%)	Intermediate (10–30%)	High (>30%)
Bcl-2	+	+	Usually +	–
Cyclin D1	–	Low	Intermediate	High
p27	+	High	Intermediate	Low

Note: Bcl-2 has been reported a prognostic marker for worse survival. Some groups found low levels of expression of p27 in PTCs. Studies show variably reduced E-cadherin expression in well-differentiated thyroid carcinomas, and it is frequently absent in poorly differentiated and anaplastic carcinomas. Loss of E-cadherin expression is an adverse prognostic factor in differentiated thyroid carcinomas. Studies reveal that the loss of membrane beta-catenin immunostaining is an indicator of loss of differentiation and adverse prognosis. Aberrant nuclear immunoreactivity of beta-catenin is associated with stabilizing CTNNB1 exon 3 mutations that are found almost exclusively in PDCs and ATCs. The cribriform-morular variant of PTC has been reported to demonstrate cytoplasmic and nuclear accumulation of beta-catenin and CTNNB1 exon 3 mutation

References: [1, 22, 181, 240, 262–268]

Table 11.26 Summary of useful markers in the evaluation of the parathyroid gland

Antibodies	Staining pattern	Function	Key applications and pitfalls
PTH	C	An 84-amino acid peptide secreted by parathyroid chief cells, regulating calcium metabolism	Parathyroid gland specific; staining is more intense in normal than in hyperplastic or neoplastic tissue
Chromogranin A	C	A member of a family of acidic glycoproteins that localize within secretory granules of endocrine, neuroendocrine, and neuronal tissue	Positive in normal, hyperplastic, and neoplastic parathyroid tissue, more intense in normal than in hyperplastic or neoplastic tissue
Gcm2	N	The key transcription factor that acts as an essential regulator of parathyroid gland development	Highly specific for parathyroid tissue
CK8/18	C	Members of the keratin family, expressed in simple epithelia, not in stratified epithelial cells	Positive in adenomatous and normal parathyroid tissue
CK19	C	A member of the keratin family of intermediate filament proteins	Positive in adenomatous and normal parathyroid tissue
Parafibromin (HRPT2)	N, C	The 531-amino acid protein product of HRPT2 gene responsible for hyperthyroidism-jaw tumor syndrome	Loss of expression has been suggested to be of value in making the diagnosis of parathyroid carcinoma

Note: *Gcm2* glial cells missing homolog 2 also known as chorion-specific transcription factor GCMb

References: [1, 269–292]

Table 11.27 Markers for normal parathyroid gland

Antibodies	Chief cells
Parathyroid hormone (PTH)	+, C
Gcm2	+, N
Chromogranin A	+, C
p53	–

Note: *C* cytoplasmic, *N* nuclear

References: [1, 269, 270, 272, 278–284, 287–291]

Table 11.28 Markers for parathyroid neoplasms

Antibodies	Parathyroid adenoma	Parathyroid carcinoma
Parathyroid hormone (PTH)	+	+
Chromogranin A	+	+
Parafibromin (HRPT2)	+	–
Galectin-3	–	+
MIB-1 (Ki-67)	Low	High
p27, Bcl-2, MDM2	+	– or +
Thyroglobulin	–	–
TTF1	–	–
CK8, 18, 19	+	+
Rb protein	+	+ or –
RCC	+	+ or –

Note: *Rb protein* retinoblastoma protein

Immunohistochemical studies may be helpful in supporting a diagnosis of carcinoma or adenoma, but none is discriminant. Many studies (molecular and/or immunohistochemical analyses) reveal that the overexpression of p27, Bcl-2, and MDM2 is a more frequent finding among parathyroid adenoma than carcinoma, but this finding is not consistent among studies. High Ki-67 proliferative index is more often seen in parathyroid carcinoma. An example of expression of parafibromin in parathyroid adenoma and carcinoma is shown in Fig. 11.20a, b

References: [1, 250, 293–296]

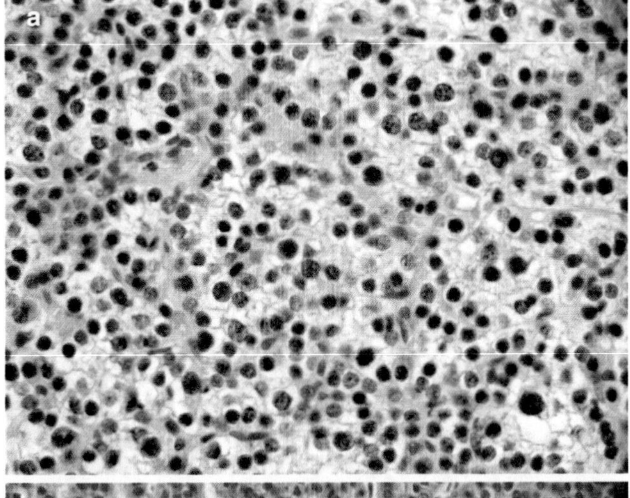

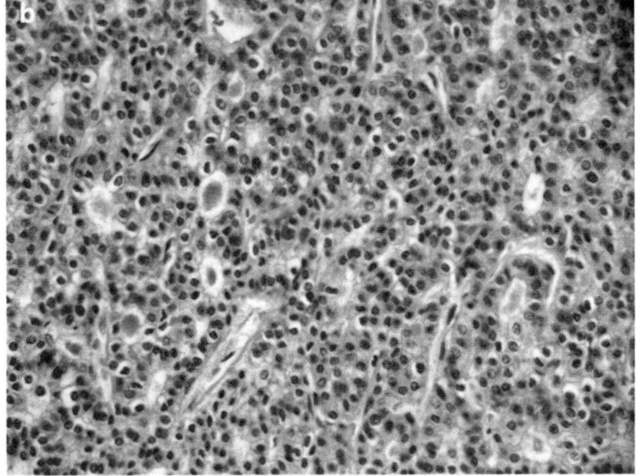

Fig. 11.20 Expression of parafibromin is more frequently positive in parathyroid adenoma (**a**) and negative in parathyroid carcinoma (**b**)

References

1. Dabbs DJ. Diagnostic immunohistochemistry. 3rd ed. Philadelphia: Churchill Livingstone Elsevier; 2010.
2. Fischer S, Asa SL. Application of immunohistochemistry to thyroid neoplasms. Arch Pathol Lab Med. 2008;132(3):359–72.
3. Civitareale D, Lonigro R, Sinclair AJ, Di Lauro R. A thyroid-specific nuclear protein essential for tissue-specific expression of the thyroglobulin promoter. EMBO J. 1989;8(9):2537–42.
4. Bejarano PA, Nikiforov YE, Swenson ES, Biddinger PW. Thyroid transcription factor-1, thyroglobulin, cytokeratin 7, and cytokeratin 20 in thyroid neoplasms. Appl Immunohistochem Mol Morphol. 2000;8(3):189–94.
5. Fabbro D, Di Loreto C, Beltrami CA, Belfiore A, Di Lauro R, Damante G. Expression of thyroid-specific transcription factors TTF-1 and PAX-8 in human thyroid neoplasms. Cancer Res. 1994;54(17):4744–9.
6. Liles N, Hamilton G, Shen SS, Krishnan B, Truong LD. PAX-8 is a sensitive marker for thyroid differentiation. Comparison with PAX-2, TTF-1 and thyroglobulin [USCAP abstract 573]. Mod Pathol. 2010;23(Suppl ls):130A.
7. Marques AR, Espadinha C, Frias MJ, et al. Underexpression of peroxisome proliferator-activated receptor (PPAR)gamma in PAX8/PPARgamma-negative thyroid tumours. Br J Cancer. 2004;91(4):732–8.
8. Marques AR, Espadinha C, Catarino AL, et al. Expression of PAX8-PPAR gamma 1 rearrangements in both follicular thyroid carcinomas and adenomas. J Clin Endocrinol Metab. 2002;87(8): 3947–52.
9. Gustafson KS, LiVolsi VA, Furth EE, Pasha TL, Putt ME, Baloch ZW. Peroxisome proliferator-activated receptor gamma expression in follicular-patterned thyroid lesions. Caveats for the use of immunohistochemical studies. Am J Clin Pathol. 2003;120(2): 175–81.
10. Nonaka D, Tang Y, Chiriboga L, Rivera M, Ghossein R. Diagnostic utility of thyroid transcription factors Pax8 and TTF-2 (FoxE1) in thyroid epithelial neoplasms. Mod Pathol. 2008;21(2):192–200.
11. Nikiforova MN, Biddinger PW, Caudill CM, Kroll TG, Nikiforov YE. PAX8-PPARgamma rearrangement in thyroid tumors: RT-PCR and immunohistochemical analyses. Am J Surg Pathol. 2002;26(8):1016–23.
12. Cheung CC, Ezzat S, Freeman JL, Rosen IB, Asa SL. Immunohistochemical diagnosis of papillary thyroid carcinoma. Mod Pathol. 2001;14(4):338–42.
13. Lam KY, Lui MC, Lo CY. Cytokeratin expression profiles in thyroid carcinomas. Eur J Surg Oncol. 2001;27(7):631–5.
14. Choi YL, Kim MK, Suh JW, et al. Immunoexpression of HBME-1, high molecular weight cytokeratin, cytokeratin 19, thyroid transcription factor-1, and E-cadherin in thyroid carcinomas. J Korean Med Sci. 2005;20(5):853–9.
15. Baloch ZW, Abraham S, Roberts S, LiVolsi VA. Differential expression of cytokeratins in follicular variant of papillary carcinoma: an immunohistochemical study and its diagnostic utility. Hum Pathol. 1999;30(10):1166–71.
16. Miettinen M, Franssila KO. Variable expression of keratins and nearly uniform lack of thyroid transcription factor 1 in thyroid anaplastic carcinoma. Hum Pathol. 2000;31(9):1139–45.
17. Sahoo S, Hoda SA, Rosai J, DeLellis RA. Cytokeratin 19 immunoreactivity in the diagnosis of papillary thyroid carcinoma: a note of caution. Am J Clin Pathol. 2001;116(5):696–702.
18. Asa SL, Cheung CC. The mind's eye. Am J Clin Pathol. 2001;116(5):635–6.
19. Mase T, Funahashi H, Koshikawa T, et al. HBME-1 immunostaining in thyroid tumors especially in follicular neoplasm. Endocr J. 2003;50(2):173–7.
20. de Matos PS, Ferreira AP, de Oliveira Facuri F, Assumpcao LV, Metze K, Ward LS. Usefulness of HBME-1, cytokeratin 19 and galectin-3 immunostaining in the diagnosis of thyroid malignancy. Histopathology. 2005;47(4):391–401.
21. Liu YY, Morreau H, Kievit J, Romijn JA, Carrasco N, Smit JW. Combined immunostaining with galectin-3, fibronectin-1, CITED-1, Hector Battifora mesothelial-1, cytokeratin-19, peroxisome proliferator-activated receptor-{gamma}, and sodium/iodide symporter antibodies for the differential diagnosis of non-medullary thyroid carcinoma. Eur J Endocrinol. 2008;158(3):375–84.
22. Papotti M, Rodriguez J, De Pompa R, Bartolazzi A, Rosai J. Galectin-3 and HBME-1 expression in well-differentiated thyroid tumors with follicular architecture of uncertain malignant potential. Mod Pathol. 2005;18(4):541–6.
23. Prasad ML, Pellegata NS, Huang Y, Nagaraja HN, de la Chapelle A, Kloos RT. Galectin-3, fibronectin-1, CITED-1, HBME1 and cytokeratin-19 immunohistochemistry is useful for the differential diagnosis of thyroid tumors. Mod Pathol. 2005;18(1):48–57.
24. Coli A, Bigotti G, Zucchetti F, Negro F, Massi G. Galectin-3, a marker of well-differentiated thyroid carcinoma, is expressed in thyroid nodules with cytological atypia. Histopathology. 2002;40(1):80–7.
25. Herrmann ME, LiVolsi VA, Pasha TL, Roberts SA, Wojcik EM, Baloch ZW. Immunohistochemical expression of galectin-3 in benign and malignant thyroid lesions. Arch Pathol Lab Med. 2002;126(6):710–3.
26. Tanaka T, Umeki K, Yamamoto I, Sakamoto F, Noguchi S, Ohtaki S. CD26 (dipeptidyl peptidase IV/DPP IV) as a novel molecular marker for differentiated thyroid carcinoma. Int J Cancer. 1995;64(5):326–31.
27. Savin S, Cvejic D, Isic T, et al. Thyroid peroxidase immunohistochemistry in differential diagnosis of thyroid tumors. Endocr Pathol. 2006;17(1):53–60.
28. Savin S, Cvejic D, Isic T, Paunovic I, Tatic S, Havelka M. Thyroid peroxidase and galectin-3 immunostaining in differentiated thyroid carcinoma with clinicopathologic correlation. Hum Pathol. 2008;39(11):1656–63.
29. Gaffney RL, Carney JA, Sebo TJ, et al. Galectin-3 expression in hyalinizing trabecular tumors of the thyroid gland. Am J Surg Pathol. 2003;27(4):494–8.
30. Katoh R, Kawaoi A, Miyagi E, et al. Thyroid transcription factor-1 in normal, hyperplastic, and neoplastic follicular thyroid cells examined by immunohistochemistry and nonradioactive in situ hybridization. Mod Pathol. 2000;13(5):570–6.
31. Cvejic D, Savin S, Golubovic S, Paunovic I, Tatic S, Havelka M. Galectin-3 and carcinoembryonic antigen expression in medullary thyroid carcinoma: possible relation to tumour progression. Histopathology. 2000;37(6):530–5.
32. Faggiano A, Talbot M, Baudin E, Bidart JM, Schlumberger M, Caillou B. Differential expression of galectin 3 in solid cell nests and C cells of human thyroid. J Clin Pathol. 2003;56(2):142–3.
33. Chiu CG, Strugnell SS, Griffith OL, et al. Diagnostic utility of galectin-3 in thyroid carcinoma. Am J Pathol. 2010;176(5): 2067–81.
34. Gasbarri A, Martegani MP, Del Prete F, Lucante T, Natali PG, Bartolazzi A. Galectin-3 and CD44v6 isoforms in the preoperative evaluation of thyroid nodules. J Clin Oncol. 1999;17(11): 3494–502.
35. Bartolazzi A, Gasbarri A, Papotti M, et al. Application of an immunodiagnostic method for improving preoperative diagnosis of nodular thyroid lesions. Lancet. 2001;357(9269):1644–50.
36. Nascimento MC, Bisi H, Alves VA, Longatto-Filho A, Kanamura CT, Medeiros-Neto G. Differential reactivity for galectin-3 in Hurthle cell adenomas and carcinomas. Endocr Pathol. 2001;12(3):275–9.
37. Casey MB, Lohse CM, Lloyd RV. Distinction between papillary thyroid hyperplasia and papillary thyroid carcinoma by immuno-

histochemical staining for cytokeratin 19, galectin-3, and HBME-1. Endocr Pathol. 2003;14(1):55–60.
38. Feilchenfeldt J, Totsch M, Sheu SY, et al. Expression of galectin-3 in normal and malignant thyroid tissue by quantitative PCR and immunohistochemistry. Mod Pathol. 2003;16(11):1117–23.
39. Mehrotra P, Okpokam A, Bouhaidar R, et al. Galectin-3 does not reliably distinguish benign from malignant thyroid neoplasms. Histopathology. 2004;45(5):493–500.
40. Hesse E, Musholt PB, Potter E, et al. Oncofoetal fibronectin – a tumour-specific marker in detecting minimal residual disease in differentiated thyroid carcinoma. Br J Cancer. 2005;93(5):565–70.
41. Castellone MD, De Falco V, Rao DM, et al. The beta-catenin axis integrates multiple signals downstream from RET/papillary thyroid carcinoma leading to cell proliferation. Cancer Res. 2009;69(5):1867–76.
42. Lantsov D, Meirmanov S, Nakashima M, et al. Cyclin D1 overexpression in thyroid papillary microcarcinoma: its association with tumour size and aberrant beta-catenin expression. Histopathology. 2005;47(3):248–56.
43. Meirmanov S, Nakashima M, Kondo H, et al. Correlation of cytoplasmic beta-catenin and cyclin D1 overexpression during thyroid carcinogenesis around Semipalatinsk nuclear test site. Thyroid. 2003;13(6):537–45.
44. Hirokawa M, Maekawa M, Kuma S, Miyauchi A. Cribriform-morular variant of papillary thyroid carcinoma – cytological and immunocytochemical findings of 18 cases. Diagn Cytopathol. 2010;38(12):890–6. doi:10.1002/dc.21309.
45. Ando M, Nakanishi Y, Asai M, Maeshima A, Matsuno Y. Mucoepidermoid carcinoma of the thyroid gland showing marked ciliation suggestive of its pathogenesis. Pathol Int. 2008;58(11):741–4.
46. Garcia-Rostan G, Camp RL, Herrero A, Carcangiu ML, Rimm DL, Tallini G. Beta-catenin dysregulation in thyroid neoplasms: down-regulation, aberrant nuclear expression, and CTNNB1 exon 3 mutations are markers for aggressive tumor phenotypes and poor prognosis. Am J Pathol. 2001;158(3):987–96.
47. Xu B, Yoshimoto K, Miyauchi A, et al. Cribriform-morular variant of papillary thyroid carcinoma: a pathological and molecular genetic study with evidence of frequent somatic mutations in exon 3 of the beta-catenin gene. J Pathol. 2003;199(1):58–67.
48. Sugenoya A, Usuda N, Adachi W, Oohashi M, Nagata T, Iida F. Immunohistochemical studies on the localization of fibronectin in human thyroid neoplastic tissues. Endocrinol Jpn. 1988;35(1):111–20.
49. Prasad ML, Pellegata NS, Kloos RT, Barbacioru C, Huang Y, de la Chapelle A. CITED1 protein expression suggests papillary thyroid carcinoma in high throughput tissue microarray-based study. Thyroid. 2004;14(3):169–75.
50. Slosar M, Vohra P, Prasad M, Fischer A, Quinlan R, Khan A. Insulin-like growth factor mRNA binding protein 3 (IMP3) is differentially expressed in benign and malignant follicular patterned thyroid tumors. Endocr Pathol. 2009;20(3):149–57.
51. Huang WC, Jeng YM. IMP3 expression in thyroid carcinomas [USCAP abstract 564]. Mod Pathol. 2010;23(Suppl 1s):127A.
52. Lu D, Vohra P, Chu PG, Woda B, Rock KL, Jiang Z. An oncofetal protein IMP3: a new molecular marker for the detection of esophageal adenocarcinoma and high-grade dysplasia. Am J Surg Pathol. 2009;33(4):521–5.
53. Belge G, Meyer A, Klemke M, et al. Upregulation of HMGA2 in thyroid carcinomas: a novel molecular marker to distinguish between benign and malignant follicular neoplasias. Genes Chromosomes Cancer. 2008;47(1):56–63.
54. Kanehira K, Merzianu M. HMGA2 nuclear expression in thyroid tissue is restricted to neoplastic lesions and is associated with a malignant phenotype [USCAP abstract 566]. Mod Pathol. 2010;23(Suppl 1s):128A.
55. Kajita S, Ruebel KH, Casey MB, Nakamura N, Lloyd RV. Role of COX-2, thromboxane A2 synthase, and prostaglandin I2 synthase in papillary thyroid carcinoma growth. Mod Pathol. 2005;18(2):221–7.
56. Lo CY, Lam KY, Leung PP, Luk JM. High prevalence of cyclooxygenase 2 expression in papillary thyroid carcinoma. Eur J Endocrinol. 2005;152(4):545–50.
57. Casey MB, Zhang S, Jin L, Kajita S, Lloyd RV. Expression of cyclooxygenase-2 and thromboxane synthase in non-neoplastic and neoplastic thyroid lesions. Endocr Pathol. 2004;15(2):107–16.
58. Ito Y, Yoshida H, Nakano K, et al. Cyclooxygenase-2 expression in thyroid neoplasms. Histopathology. 2003;42(5):492–7.
59. Haynik DM, Prayson RA. Immunohistochemical expression of cyclooxygenase 2 in follicular carcinomas of the thyroid. Arch Pathol Lab Med. 2005;129(6):736–41.
60. Katoh R, Miyagi E, Nakamura N, et al. Expression of thyroid transcription factor-1 (TTF-1) in human C cells and medullary thyroid carcinomas. Hum Pathol. 2000;31(3):386–93.
61. Erickson LA, Lloyd RV. Practical markers used in the diagnosis of endocrine tumors. Adv Anat Pathol. 2004;11(4):175–89.
62. Baloch ZW, LiVolsi VA. Neuroendocrine tumors of the thyroid gland. Am J Clin Pathol. 2001;115(Suppl):S56–67.
63. Saad MF, Fritsche Jr HA, Samaan NA. Diagnostic and prognostic values of carcinoembryonic antigen in medullary carcinoma of the thyroid. J Clin Endocrinol Metab. 1984;58(5):889–94.
64. Talerman A, Lindeman J, Kievit-Tyson PA, Droge-Droppert C. Demonstration of calcitonin and carcinoembryonic antigen (CEA) in medullary carcinoma of the thyroid (MCT) by immunoperoxidase technique. Histopathology. 1979;3(6):503–10.
65. Lloyd RV, Sisson JC, Marangos PJ. Calcitonin, carcinoembryonic antigen and neuron-specific enolase in medullary thyroid carcinoma. Cancer. 1983;51(12):2234–9.
66. Dasovic-Knezevic M, Bormer O, Holm R, Hoie J, Sobrinho-Simoes M, Nesland JM. Carcinoembryonic antigen in medullary thyroid carcinoma: an immunohistochemical study applying six novel monoclonal antibodies. Mod Pathol. 1989;2(6):610–7.
67. Wilson NW, Pambakian H, Richardson TC, Stokoe MR, Makin CA, Heyderman E. Epithelial markers in thyroid carcinoma: an immunoperoxidase study. Histopathology. 1986;10(8):815–29.
68. Uribe M, Fenoglio-Preiser CM, Grimes M, Feind C. Medullary carcinoma of the thyroid gland. Clinical, pathological, and immunohistochemical features with review of the literature. Am J Surg Pathol. 1985;9(8):577–94.
69. Rocha AS, Soares P, Seruca R, et al. Abnormalities of the E-cadherin/catenin adhesion complex in classical papillary thyroid carcinoma and in its diffuse sclerosing variant. J Pathol. 2001;194(3):358–66.
70. Rocha AS, Soares P, Fonseca E, Cameselle-Teijeiro J, Oliveira MC, Sobrinho-Simoes M. E-cadherin loss rather than beta-catenin alterations is a common feature of poorly differentiated thyroid carcinomas. Histopathology. 2003;42(6):580–7.
71. Aratake Y, Umeki K, Kiyoyama K, et al. Diagnostic utility of galectin-3 and CD26/DPPIV as preoperative diagnostic markers for thyroid nodules. Diagn Cytopathol. 2002;26(6):366–72.
72. Salvatore G, Giannini R, Faviana P, et al. Analysis of BRAF point mutation and RET/PTC rearrangement refines the fine-needle aspiration diagnosis of papillary thyroid carcinoma. J Clin Endocrinol Metab. 2004;89(10):5175–80.
73. Tallini G, Asa SL. RET oncogene activation in papillary thyroid carcinoma. Adv Anat Pathol. 2001;8(6):345–54.
74. Fenton CL, Lukes Y, Nicholson D, Dinauer CA, Francis GL, Tuttle RM. The ret/PTC mutations are common in sporadic papillary thyroid carcinoma of children and young adults. J Clin Endocrinol Metab. 2000;85(3):1170–5.
75. Bounacer A, Wicker R, Caillou B, et al. High prevalence of activating ret proto-oncogene rearrangements, in thyroid tumors from

patients who had received external radiation. Oncogene. 1997;15(11):1263–73.

76. Fischer AH, Bond JA, Taysavang P, Battles OE, Wynford-Thomas D. Papillary thyroid carcinoma oncogene (RET/PTC) alters the nuclear envelope and chromatin structure. Am J Pathol. 1998;153(5):1443–50.
77. Fusco A, Chiappetta G, Hui P, et al. Assessment of RET/PTC oncogene activation and clonality in thyroid nodules with incomplete morphological evidence of papillary carcinoma: a search for the early precursors of papillary cancer. Am J Pathol. 2002;160(6):2157–67.
78. Cheung CC, Boerner SL, MacMillan CM, Ramyar L, Asa SL. Hyalinizing trabecular tumor of the thyroid: a variant of papillary carcinoma proved by molecular genetics. Am J Surg Pathol. 2000;24(12):1622–6.
79. Lloyd RV. Hyalinizing trabecular tumors of the thyroid: a variant of papillary carcinoma? Adv Anat Pathol. 2002;9(1):7–11.
80. Cerilli LA, Mills SE, Rumpel CA, Dudley TH, Moskaluk CA. Interpretation of RET immunostaining in follicular lesions of the thyroid. Am J Clin Pathol. 2002;118(2):186–93.
81. Enriquez ML, Ende LB, Zhang PJ, Montone KT, LiVolsi VA. CDX2 expression in columnar cell variant of papillary thyroid carcinoma [USCAP abstract 561]. Mod Pathol. 2010;23(Suppl 1s):127A.
82. Reimann JD, Dorfman DM, Nose V. Carcinoma showing thymus-like differentiation of the thyroid (CASTLE): a comparative study: evidence of thymic differentiation and solid cell nest origin. Am J Surg Pathol. 2006;30(8):994–1001.
83. Bishop JA, Sharma R, Illei PB. Napsin A and thyroid transcription factor-1 expression in carcinomas of the lung, breast, pancreas, colon, kidney, thyroid, and malignant mesothelioma. Hum Pathol. 2010;41(1):20–5.
84. Colato C, Ambrosetti MC, et al. Claudin proteins, PAX8 and NIS immunohistochemical evaluation in human fetal thyroid development [USCAP abstract 558]. Mod Pathol. 2010;23(Suppl 1s):126A.
85. Asioli S, Erickson LA, Sebo TJ, et al. Papillary thyroid carcinoma with prominent hobnail features: a new aggressive variant of moderately differentiated papillary carcinoma. A clinicopathologic, immunohistochemical, and molecular study of eight cases. Am J Surg Pathol. 2010;34(1):44–52.
86. Ishigaki K, Namba H, Nakashima M, et al. Aberrant localization of beta-catenin correlates with overexpression of its target gene in human papillary thyroid cancer. J Clin Endocrinol Metab. 2002;87(7):3433–40.
87. Umeki K, Tanaka T, Yamamoto I, et al. Differential expression of dipeptidyl peptidase IV (CD26) and thyroid peroxidase in neoplastic thyroid tissues. Endocr J. 1996;43(1):53–60.
88. Umeki K, Yamamoto I, Maruta J, et al. CD26/dipeptidyl peptidase IV and thyroid peroxidase as molecular markers for differentiated thyroid carcinoma [in Japanese]. Rinsho Byori. 1996;44(1):42–50.
89. Mishra A, Pal L, Mishra SK. Distribution of Na^{+}/I^{-} symporter in thyroid cancers in an iodine-deficient population: an immunohistochemical study. World J Surg. 2007;31(9):1737–42.
90. Filetti S, Bidart JM, Arturi F, Caillou B, Russo D, Schlumberger M. Sodium/iodide symporter: a key transport system in thyroid cancer cell metabolism. Eur J Endocrinol. 1999;141(5):443–57.
91. Ajjan RA, Kamaruddin NA, Crisp M, Watson PF, Ludgate M, Weetman AP. Regulation and tissue distribution of the human sodium iodide symporter gene. Clin Endocrinol (Oxf). 1998;49(4):517–23.
92. Castro MR, Bergert ER, Goellner JR, Hay ID, Morris JC. Immunohistochemical analysis of sodium iodide symporter expression in metastatic differentiated thyroid cancer: correlation with radioiodine uptake. J Clin Endocrinol Metab. 2001;86(11):5627–32.
93. Hirokawa M, Shimizu M, Manabe T, Kuroda M, Mizoguchi Y. Hyalinizing trabecular adenoma of the thyroid: its unusual cytoplasmic immunopositivity for MIB1. Pathol Int. 1995;45(5):399–401.
94. Asa SL. My approach to oncocytic tumours of the thyroid. J Clin Pathol. 2004;57(3):225–32.
95. Cameron BR, Berean KW. Cytokeratin subtypes in thyroid tumours: immunohistochemical study with emphasis on the follicular variant of papillary carcinoma. J Otolaryngol. 2003;32(5):319–22.
96. Miettinen M, Kovatich AJ, Karkkainen P. Keratin subsets in papillary and follicular thyroid lesions. A paraffin section analysis with diagnostic implications. Virchows Arch. 1997;431(6):407–13.
97. Fonseca E, Nesland JM, Hoie J, Sobrinho-Simoes M. Pattern of expression of intermediate cytokeratin filaments in the thyroid gland: an immunohistochemical study of simple and stratified epithelial-type cytokeratins. Virchows Arch. 1997;430(3):239–45.
98. Kaserer K, Scheuba C, Neuhold N, et al. C-cell hyperplasia and medullary thyroid carcinoma in patients routinely screened for serum calcitonin. Am J Surg Pathol. 1998;22(6):722–8.
99. Ferreiro JA, Hay ID, Lloyd RV. Columnar cell carcinoma of the thyroid: report of three additional cases. Hum Pathol. 1996;27(11):1156–60.
100. Wenig BM, Thompson LD, Adair CF, Shmookler B, Heffess CS. Thyroid papillary carcinoma of columnar cell type: a clinicopathologic study of 16 cases. Cancer. 1998;82(4):740–53.
101. Putti TC, Bhuiya TA. Mixed columnar cell and tall cell variant of papillary carcinoma of thyroid: a case report and review of the literature. Pathology. 2000;32(4):286–9.
102. Gaertner EM, Davidson M, Wenig BM. The columnar cell variant of thyroid papillary carcinoma. Case report and discussion of an unusually aggressive thyroid papillary carcinoma. Am J Surg Pathol. 1995;19(8):940–7.
103. Komminoth P, Roth J, Saremaslani P, Matias-Guiu X, Wolfe HJ, Heitz PU. Polysialic acid of the neural cell adhesion molecule in the human thyroid: a marker for medullary thyroid carcinoma and primary C-cell hyperplasia. An immunohistochemical study on 79 thyroid lesions. Am J Surg Pathol. 1994;18(4):399–411.
104. Schroder S, Kloppel G. Carcinoembryonic antigen and nonspecific cross-reacting antigen in thyroid cancer. An immunocytochemical study using polyclonal and monoclonal antibodies. Am J Surg Pathol. 1987;11(2):100–8.
105. Matsuki Y, Tanimoto A, Hamada T, Sasaguri Y. Histidine decarboxylase expression as a new sensitive and specific marker for small cell lung carcinoma. Mod Pathol. 2003;16(1):72–8.
106. Satoh F, Umemura S, Yasuda M, Osamura RY. Neuroendocrine marker expression in thyroid epithelial tumors. Endocr Pathol. 2001;12(3):291–9.
107. Hirsch MS, Faquin WC, Krane JF. Thyroid transcription factor-1, but not p53, is helpful in distinguishing moderately differentiated neuroendocrine carcinoma of the larynx from medullary carcinoma of the thyroid. Mod Pathol. 2004;17(6):631–6.
108. Osamura RY, Yasuda O, Kawakami T, Itoh Y, Inada K, Kakudo K. Immunoelectron microscopic demonstration of regulated pathway for calcitonin and constitutive pathway for carcinoembryonic antigen in the same cells of human medullary carcinomas of thyroid glands. Mod Pathol. 1997;10(1):7–11.
109. Kargi A, Yorukoglu, Aktas S, Cakalagaoglu, Ermete M. Neuroendocrine differentiation in non-neuroendocrine thyroid carcinoma. Thyroid. 1996;6(3):207–10
110. Volante M, Collini P, Nikiforov YE, et al. Poorly differentiated thyroid carcinoma: the Turin proposal for the use of uniform diagnostic criteria and an algorithmic diagnostic approach. Am J Surg Pathol. 2007;31(8):1256–64.
111. Judkins AR, Roberts SA, Livolsi VA. Utility of immunohistochemistry in the evaluation of necrotic thyroid tumors. Hum Pathol. 1999;30(11):1373–6.
112. Pilotti S, Collini P, Del Bo R, Cattoretti G, Pierotti MA, Rilke F. A novel panel of antibodies that segregates immunocytochemically

poorly differentiated carcinoma from undifferentiated carcinoma of the thyroid gland. Am J Surg Pathol. 1994;18(10):1054–64.
113. Huss LJ, Mendelsohn G. Medullary carcinoma of the thyroid gland: an encapsulated variant resembling the hyalinizing trabecular (paraganglioma-like) adenoma of thyroid. Mod Pathol. 1990;3(5):581–5.
114. Zhang PJ, Genega EM, Tomaszewski JE, Pasha TL, LiVolsi VA. The role of calretinin, inhibin, melan-A, BCL-2, and C-kit in differentiating adrenal cortical and medullary tumors: an immunohistochemical study. Mod Pathol. 2003;16(6):591–7.
115. Arber DA, Tamayo R, Weiss LM. Paraffin section detection of the c-kit gene product (CD117) in human tissues: value in the diagnosis of mast cell disorders. Hum Pathol. 1998;29(5):498–504.
116. Fonseca E, Nesland JM, Sobrinho-Simoes M. Expression of stratified epithelial-type cytokeratins in hyalinizing trabecular adenomas supports their relationship with papillary carcinomas of the thyroid. Histopathology. 1997;31(4):330–5.
117. Faggiano A, Talbot M, Lacroix L, et al. Differential expression of galectin-3 in medullary thyroid carcinoma and C-cell hyperplasia. Clin Endocrinol (Oxf). 2002;57(6):813–9.
118. Reis-Filho JS, Preto A, Soares P, Ricardo S, Cameselle-Teijeiro J, Sobrinho-Simoes M. p63 expression in solid cell nests of the thyroid: further evidence for a stem cell origin. Mod Pathol. 2003;16(1):43–8.
119. Cameselle-Teijeiro J, Varela-Duran J, Sambade C, Villanueva JP, Varela-Nunez R, Sobrinho-Simoes M. Solid cell nests of the thyroid: light microscopy and immunohistochemical profile. Hum Pathol. 1994;25(7):684–93.
120. Mizukami Y, Nonomura A, Michigishi T, et al. Solid cell nests of the thyroid. A histologic and immunohistochemical study. Am J Clin Pathol. 1994;101(2):186–91.
121. Martin V, Martin L, Viennet G, Challier B, Carbillet J, Fellmann D. Solid cell nests and thyroid pathologies. Retrospective study of 1,390 thyroids [in French]. Ann Pathol. 2000;20(3):196–201.
122. Burstein DE, Nagi C, Wang BY, Unger P. Immunohistochemical detection of p53 homolog p63 in solid cell nests, papillary thyroid carcinoma, and Hashimoto's thyroiditis: a stem cell hypothesis of papillary carcinoma oncogenesis. Hum Pathol. 2004;35(4):465–73.
123. Burstein DE, Unger P, Nagi C, Wang BY. Thinking "out of the nest" – a reply to "a stem-cell role for thyroid solid cell nests [letter]". Hum Pathol. 2005;36(5):591–2.
124. Cameselle-Teijeiro J, Preto A, Soares P, Sobrinho-Simoes M. A stem cell role for thyroid solid cell nests. Hum Pathol. 2005;36(5):590–1.
125. Asioli S, Erickson LA, Lloyd RV. Solid cell nests in Hashimoto's thyroiditis sharing features with papillary thyroid microcarcinoma. Endocr Pathol. 2009;20(4):197–203.
126. Unger P, Ewart M, Wang BY, Gan L, Kohtz DS, Burstein DE. Expression of p63 in papillary thyroid carcinoma and in Hashimoto's thyroiditis: a pathobiologic link? Hum Pathol. 2003;34(8):764–9.
127. Vollenweider I, Hedinger C. Solid cell nests (SCN) in Hashimoto's thyroiditis. Virchows Arch A Pathol Anat Histopathol. 1988;412(4):357–63.
128. Preto A, Cameselle-Teijeiro J, Moldes-Boullosa J, et al. Telomerase expression and proliferative activity suggest a stem cell role for thyroid solid cell nests. Mod Pathol. 2004;17(7):819–26.
129. Hirokawa M, Carney JA. Cell membrane and cytoplasmic staining for MIB-1 in hyalinizing trabecular adenoma of the thyroid gland. Am J Surg Pathol. 2000;24(4):575–8.
130. Ohtsuki Y, Watanabe R, Kimura M, et al. Immunohistochemical and electron microscopic studies of a case of duodenal gangliocytic paraganglioma. Med Mol Morphol. 2009;42(4):245–9.
131. Galgano MT, Mills SE, Stelow EB. Hyalinizing trabecular adenoma of the thyroid revisited: a histologic and immunohistochemical study of thyroid lesions with prominent trabecular architecture and sclerosis. Am J Surg Pathol. 2006;30(10):1269–73.
132. Carney JA. Hyalinizing trabecular tumors of the thyroid gland: quadruply described but not by the discoverer. Am J Surg Pathol. 2008;32(4):622–34.
133. Casey MB, Sebo TJ, Carney JA. Hyalinizing trabecular adenoma of the thyroid gland identification through MIB-1 staining of fine-needle aspiration biopsy smears. Am J Clin Pathol. 2004;122(4):506–10.
134. Hirokawa M, Carney JA, Ohtsuki Y. Hyalinizing trabecular adenoma and papillary carcinoma of the thyroid gland express different cytokeratin patterns. Am J Surg Pathol. 2000;24(6):877–81.
135. Papotti M, Volante M, Giuliano A, et al. RET/PTC activation in hyalinizing trabecular tumors of the thyroid. Am J Surg Pathol. 2000;24(12):1615–21.
136. LiVolsi VA. Hyalinizing trabecular tumor of the thyroid: adenoma, carcinoma, or neoplasm of uncertain malignant potential? Am J Surg Pathol. 2000;24(12):1683–4.
137. Nose V, Volante M, Papotti M. Hyalinizing trabecular tumor of the thyroid: an update. Endocr Pathol. 2008;19(1):1–8.
138. Papotti M, Riella P, Montemurro F, Pietribiasi F, Bussolati G. Immunophenotypic heterogeneity of hyalinizing trabecular tumours of the thyroid. Histopathology. 1997;31(6):525–33.
139. Katoh R, Jasani B, Williams ED. Hyalinizing trabecular adenoma of the thyroid. A report of three cases with immunohistochemical and ultrastructural studies. Histopathology. 1989;15(3):211–24.
140. Leonardo E, Volante M, Barbareschi M, et al. Cell membrane reactivity of MIB-1 antibody to Ki67 in human tumors: fact or artifact? Appl Immunohistochem Mol Morphol. 2007;15(2):220–3.
141. LaGuette J, Matias-Guiu X, Rosai J. Thyroid paraganglioma: a clinicopathologic and immunohistochemical study of three cases. Am J Surg Pathol. 1997;21(7):748–53.
142. Yano Y, Nagahama M, Sugino K, Ito K, Kameyama K, Ito K. Paraganglioma of the thyroid: report of a male case with ultrasonographic imagings, cytologic, histologic, and immunohistochemical features. Thyroid. 2007;17(6):575–8.
143. Bockhorn M, Sheu SY, Frilling A, Molmenti E, Schmid KW, Broelsch CE. Paraganglioma-like medullary thyroid carcinoma: a rare entity. Thyroid. 2005;15(12):1363–7.
144. Magro G, Grasso S. Sustentacular cells in sporadic paraganglioma-like medullary thyroid carcinoma: report of a case with diagnostic and histogenetic considerations. Pathol Res Pract. 2000;196(1):55–9.
145. Ikeda T, Satoh M, Azuma K, Sawada N, Mori M. Medullary thyroid carcinoma with a paraganglioma-like pattern and melanin production: a case report with ultrastructural and immunohistochemical studies. Arch Pathol Lab Med. 1998;122(6):555–8.
146. Erem C, Kocak M, Nuhoglu I, Cobanoglu U, Ucuncu O, Okatan BK. Primary thyroid paraganglioma presenting with double thyroid nodule: a case report. Endocr. 2009;36(3):368–71.
147. Corrado S, Montanini V, De Gaetani C, Borghi F, Papi G. Primary paraganglioma of the thyroid gland. J Endocrinol Invest. 2004;27(8):788–92.
148. Gonzalez Poggioli N, Lopez Amado M, Pimentel MT. Paraganglioma of the thyroid gland: a rare entity. Endocr Pathol. 2009;20(1):62–5.
149. Johnson TL, Zarbo RJ, Lloyd RV, Crissman JD. Paragangliomas of the head and neck: immunohistochemical neuroendocrine and intermediate filament typing. Mod Pathol. 1988;1(3):216–23.
150. Montone KT, Baloch ZW, LiVolsi VA. The thyroid Hurthle (oncocytic) cell and its associated pathologic conditions: a surgical pathology and cytopathology review. Arch Pathol Lab Med. 2008;132(8):1241–50.
151. Abu-Alfa AK, Straus 2nd FH, Montag AG. An immunohistochemical study of thyroid Hurthle cells and their neoplasms: the roles of S-100 and HMB-45 proteins. Mod Pathol. 1994;7(5):529–32.

152. Erickson LA, Jin L, Goellner JR, et al. Pathologic features, proliferative activity, and cyclin D1 expression in Hurthle cell neoplasms of the thyroid. Mod Pathol. 2000;13(2):186–92.
153. Hoos A, Stojadinovic A, Singh B, et al. Clinical significance of molecular expression profiles of Hurthle cell tumors of the thyroid gland analyzed via tissue microarrays. Am J Pathol. 2002;160(1):175–83.
154. Bur M, Shiraki W, Masood S. Estrogen and progesterone receptor detection in neoplastic and non-neoplastic thyroid tissues. Mod Pathol. 1993;6(4):469–72.
155. Zaccheroni V, Vacirca A, Lucci E, et al. An immunohistochemical study of progesterone receptor in thyroidal Hurthle cells tumors. J Exp Clin Cancer Res. 1998;17(3):291–8.
156. Katoh R, Harach HR, Williams ED. Solitary, multiple, and familial oxyphil tumours of the thyroid gland. J Pathol. 1998;186(3):292–9.
157. Baloch ZW, Livolsi VA. Follicular-patterned lesions of the thyroid: the bane of the pathologist. Am J Clin Pathol. 2002;117(1):143–50.
158. Baloch ZW, LiVolsi VA. Unusual tumors of the thyroid gland. Endocrinol Metab Clin North Am. 2008;37(2):297–310. vii.
159. Baloch ZW, LiVolsi VA. Our approach to follicular-patterned lesions of the thyroid. J Clin Pathol. 2007;60(3):244–50.
160. Baloch ZW, LiVolsi VA. Microcarcinoma of the thyroid. Adv Anat Pathol. 2006;13(2):69–75.
161. Giorgadze TA, Baloch ZW, Pasha T, Zhang PJ, Livolsi VA. Lymphatic and blood vessel density in the follicular patterned lesions of thyroid. Mod Pathol. 2005;18(11):1424–31.
162. Thompson LD, Wieneke JA, Paal E, Frommelt RA, Adair CF, Heffess CS. A clinicopathologic study of minimally invasive follicular carcinoma of the thyroid gland with a review of the English literature. Cancer. 2001;91(3):505–24.
163. Lloyd RV, Erickson LA, Casey MB, et al. Observer variation in the diagnosis of follicular variant of papillary thyroid carcinoma. Am J Surg Pathol. 2004;28(10):1336–40.
164. Chan JK. Strict criteria should be applied in the diagnosis of encapsulated follicular variant of papillary thyroid carcinoma. Am J Clin Pathol. 2002;117(1):16–8.
165. Khan A, Baker SP, Patwardhan NA, Pullman JM. CD57 (Leu-7) expression is helpful in diagnosis of the follicular variant of papillary thyroid carcinoma. Virchows Arch. 1998;432(5):427–32.
166. Kawachi K, Matsushita Y, Yonezawa S, et al. Galectin-3 expression in various thyroid neoplasms and its possible role in metastasis formation. Hum Pathol. 2000;31(4):428–33.
167. Scognamiglio T, Hyjek E, Kao J, Chen YT. Diagnostic usefulness of HBME1, galectin-3, CK19, and CITED1 and evaluation of their expression in encapsulated lesions with questionable features of papillary thyroid carcinoma. Am J Clin Pathol. 2006;126(5):700–8.
168. Rezk S, Brynes RK, Nelson V, et al. Beta-Catenin expression in thyroid follicular lesions: potential role in nuclear envelope changes in papillary carcinomas. Endocr Pathol. 2004;15(4):329–37.
169. Kimura N, Nakazato Y, Nagura H, Sasano N. Expression of intermediate filaments in neuroendocrine tumors. Arch Pathol Lab Med. 1990;114(5):506–10.
170. Wang DG, Liu WH, Johnston CF, Sloan JM, Buchanan KD. Bcl-2 and c-Myc, but not bax and p53, are expressed during human medullary thyroid tumorigenesis. Am J Pathol. 1998;152(6):1407–13.
171. Colomer A, Martinez-Mas JV, Matias-Guiu X, et al. Sex-steroid hormone receptors in human medullary thyroid carcinoma. Mod Pathol. 1996;9(1):68–72.
172. Saad MF, Ordonez NG, Guido JJ, Samaan NA. The prognostic value of calcitonin immunostaining in medullary carcinoma of the thyroid. J Clin Endocrinol Metab. 1984;59(5):850–6.
173. Sikri KL, Varndell IM, Hamid QA, et al. Medullary carcinoma of the thyroid. An immunocytochemical and histochemical study of 25 cases using eight separate markers. Cancer. 1985;56(10):2481–91.
174. DeLellis RA, Rule AH, Spiler I, Nathanson L, Tashjian Jr AH, Wolfe HJ. Calcitonin and carcinoembryonic antigen as tumor markers in medullary thyroid carcinoma. Am J Clin Pathol. 1978;70(4):587–94.
175. Schmid KW, Fischer-Colbrie R, Hagn C, Jasani B, Williams ED, Winkler H. Chromogranin A and B and secretogranin II in medullary carcinomas of the thyroid. Am J Surg Pathol. 1987;11(7):551–6.
176. DeLellis RA, Moore FM, Wolfe HJ. Thyroglobulin immunoreactivity in human medullary thyroid carcinoma. Lab Invest. 1983;48:20A.
177. Ordonez NG. Thyroid transcription factor-1 is a marker of lung and thyroid carcinomas. Adv Anat Pathol. 2000;7(2):123–7.
178. Sanders Jr EM, LiVolsi VA, Brierley J, Shin J, Randolph GW. An evidence-based review of poorly differentiated thyroid cancer. World J Surg. 2007;31(5):934–45.
179. Agarwal S, Sharma MC, Aron M, Sarkar C, Agarwal N, Chumber S. Poorly differentiated thyroid carcinoma with rhabdoid phenotype: a diagnostic dilemma – report of a rare case. Endocr Pathol. 2006;17(4):399–405.
180. Akslen LA, LiVolsi VA. Poorly differentiated thyroid carcinoma – it is important. Am J Surg Pathol. 2000;24(2):310–3.
181. Tallini G, Garcia-Rostan G, Herrero A, et al. Downregulation of p27KIP1 and Ki67/Mib1 labeling index support the classification of thyroid carcinoma into prognostically relevant categories. Am J Surg Pathol. 1999;23(6):678–85.
182. DeLellis RA, Lloyd RV, Heitz PU, Eng C, editors. Pathology and Genetics, Tumours of Endocrine Organs, World Health Organization Classification Tumours. Lyon, France: IARC Press; 2004.
183. Decaussin M, Bernard MH, Adeleine P, et al. Thyroid carcinomas with distant metastases: a review of 111 cases with emphasis on the prognostic significance of an insular component. Am J Surg Pathol. 2002;26(8):1007–15.
184. Volante M, Landolfi S, Chiusa L, et al. Poorly differentiated carcinomas of the thyroid with trabecular, insular, and solid patterns: a clinicopathologic study of 183 patients. Cancer. 2004;100(5):950–7.
185. Hiltzik D, Carlson DL, Tuttle RM, et al. Poorly differentiated thyroid carcinomas defined on the basis of mitosis and necrosis: a clinicopathologic study of 58 patients. Cancer. 2006;106(6):1286–95.
186. Wang S, Wuu J, Savas L, Patwardhan N, Khan A. The role of cell cycle regulatory proteins, cyclin D1, cyclin E, and p27 in thyroid carcinogenesis. Hum Pathol. 1998;29(11):1304–9.
187. Fagin JA, Matsuo K, Karmakar A, Chen DL, Tang SH, Koeffler HP. High prevalence of mutations of the p53 gene in poorly differentiated human thyroid carcinomas. J Clin Invest. 1993;91(1):179–84.
188. Jossart GH, Epstein HD, Shaver JK, et al. Immunocytochemical detection of p53 in human thyroid carcinomas is associated with mutation and immortalization of cell lines. J Clin Endocrinol Metab. 1996;81(10):3498–504.
189. Ordonez NG, El-Naggar AK, Hickey RC, Samaan NA. Anaplastic thyroid carcinoma. Immunocytochemical study of 32 cases. Am J Clin Pathol. 1991;96(1):15–24.
190. Aratake Y, Nomura H, Kotani T, et al. Coexistent anaplastic and differentiated thyroid carcinoma: an immunohistochemical study. Am J Clin Pathol. 2006;125(3):399–406.
191. Fernandez PL, Merino MJ, Gomez M, et al. Galectin-3 and laminin expression in neoplastic and non-neoplastic thyroid tissue. J Pathol. 1997;181(1):80–6.
192. Quiros RM, Ding HG, Gattuso P, Prinz RA, Xu X. Evidence that one subset of anaplastic thyroid carcinomas are derived from papillary carcinomas due to BRAF and p53 mutations. Cancer. 2005;103(11):2261–8.

193. Venkatesh YS, Ordonez NG, Schultz PN, Hickey RC, Goepfert H, Samaan NA. Anaplastic carcinoma of the thyroid. A clinicopathologic study of 121 cases. Cancer. 1990;66(2):321–30.
194. Lacroix L, Mian C, Barrier T, et al. PAX8 and peroxisome proliferator-activated receptor gamma 1 gene expression status in benign and malignant thyroid tissues. Eur J Endocrinol. 2004;151(3):367–74.
195. LiVolsi VA, Brooks JJ, Arendash-Durand B. Anaplastic thyroid tumors. Immunohistology. Am J Clin Pathol. 1987;87(4):434–42.
196. Hurlimann J, Gardiol D, Scazziga B. Immunohistology of anaplastic thyroid carcinoma. A study of 43 cases. Histopathology. 1987;11(6):567–80.
197. Totsch M, Dobler G, Feichtinger H, Sandbichler P, Ladurner D, Schmid KW. Malignant hemangioendothelioma of the thyroid. Its immunohistochemical discrimination from undifferentiated thyroid carcinoma. Am J Surg Pathol. 1990;14(1):69–74.
198. Albores-Saavedra J, Nadji M, Civantos F, Morales AR. Thyroglobulin in carcinoma of the thyroid: an immunohistochemical study. Hum Pathol. 1983;14(1):62–6.
199. Ralfkiaer N, Gatter KC, Alcock C, Heryet A, Ralfkiaer E, Mason DY. The value of immunocytochemical methods in the differential diagnosis of anaplastic thyroid tumours. Br J Cancer. 1985;52(2):167–70.
200. Baloch ZW, Solomon AC, LiVolsi VA. Primary mucoepidermoid carcinoma and sclerosing mucoepidermoid carcinoma with eosinophilia of the thyroid gland: a report of nine cases. Mod Pathol. 2000;13(7):802–7.
201. Wenig BM, Adair CF, Heffess CS. Primary mucoepidermoid carcinoma of the thyroid gland: a report of six cases and a review of the literature of a follicular epithelial-derived tumor. Hum Pathol. 1995;26(10):1099–108.
202. Geisinger KR, Steffee CH, McGee RS, Woodruff RD, Buss DH. The cytomorphologic features of sclerosing mucoepidermoid carcinoma of the thyroid gland with eosinophilia. Am J Clin Pathol. 1998;109(3):294–301.
203. Sim SJ, Ro JY, Ordonez NG, Cleary KR, Ayala AG. Sclerosing mucoepidermoid carcinoma with eosinophilia of the thyroid: report of two patients, one with distant metastasis, and review of the literature. Hum Pathol. 1997;28(9):1091–6.
204. Shehadeh NJ, Vernick J, Lonardo F, et al. Sclerosing mucoepidermoid carcinoma with eosinophilia of the thyroid: a case report and review of the literature. Am J Otolaryngol. 2004;25(1):48–53.
205. Solomon AC, Baloch ZW, Salhany KE, Mandel S, Weber RS, LiVolsi VA. Thyroid sclerosing mucoepidermoid carcinoma with eosinophilia: mimic of Hodgkin disease in nodal metastases. Arch Pathol Lab Med. 2000;124(3):446–9.
206. Rhatigan RM, Roque JL, Bucher RL. Mucoepidermoid carcinoma of the thyroid gland. Cancer. 1977;39(1):210–4.
207. Monroe MM, Sauer DA, Samuels MH, Gross ND. Pathology quiz case 1. Coexistent conventional mucoepidermoid carcinoma of the thyroid (MECT) and papillary thyroid carcinoma. Arch Otolaryngol Head Neck Surg. 2009;135(7):720. 722.
208. Chan JK, Albores-Saavedra J, Battifora H, Carcangiu ML, Rosai J. Sclerosing mucoepidermoid thyroid carcinoma with eosinophilia. A distinctive low-grade malignancy arising from the metaplastic follicles of Hashimoto's thyroiditis. Am J Surg Pathol. 1991;15(5):438–48.
209. Miranda RN, Myint MA, Gnepp DR. Composite follicular variant of papillary carcinoma and mucoepidermoid carcinoma of the thyroid. Report of a case and review of the literature. Am J Surg Pathol. 1995;19(10):1209–15.
210. Cameselle-Teijeiro J, Febles-Perez C, Sobrinho-Simoes M. Papillary and mucoepidermoid carcinoma of the thyroid with anaplastic transformation: a case report with histologic and immunohistochemical findings that support a provocative histogenetic hypothesis. Pathol Res Pract. 1995;191(12):1214–21.
211. Viciana MJ, Galera-Davidson H, Martin-Lacave I, Segura DI, Loizaga JM. Papillary carcinoma of the thyroid with mucoepidermoid differentiation. Arch Pathol Lab Med. 1996;120(4):397–8.
212. Albores-Saavedra J, Gu X, Luna MA. Clear cells and thyroid transcription factor I reactivity in sclerosing mucoepidermoid carcinoma of the thyroid gland. Ann Diagn Pathol. 2003;7(6):348–53.
213. Franssila KO, Harach HR, Wasenius VM. Mucoepidermoid carcinoma of the thyroid. Histopathology. 1984;8(5):847–60.
214. Rocha AS, Soares P, Machado JC, et al. Mucoepidermoid carcinoma of the thyroid: a tumour histotype characterised by P-cadherin neoexpression and marked abnormalities of E-cadherin/catenins complex. Virchows Arch. 2002;440(5):498–504.
215. Guyetant S, Josselin N, Savagner F, Rohmer V, Michalak S, Saint-Andre JP. C-cell hyperplasia and medullary thyroid carcinoma: clinicopathological and genetic correlations in 66 consecutive patients. Mod Pathol. 2003;16(8):756–63.
216. Krueger JE, Maitra A, Albores-Saavedra J. Inherited medullary microcarcinoma of the thyroid: a study of 11 cases. Am J Surg Pathol. 2000;24(6):853–8.
217. Perry A, Molberg K, Albores-Saavedra J. Physiologic versus neoplastic C-cell hyperplasia of the thyroid: separation of distinct histologic and biologic entities. Cancer. 1996;77(4):750–6.
218. McDermott MB, Swanson PE, Wick MR. Immunostains for collagen type IV discriminate between C-cell hyperplasia and microscopic medullary carcinoma in multiple endocrine neoplasia, type 2a. Hum Pathol. 1995;26(12):1308–12.
219. Etit D, Faquin WC, Gaz R, Randolph G, DeLellis RA, Pilch BZ. Histopathologic and clinical features of medullary microcarcinoma and C-cell hyperplasia in prophylactic thyroidectomies for medullary carcinoma: a study of 42 cases. Arch Pathol Lab Med. 2008;132(11):1767–73.
220. Jakubiak-Wielganowicz M, Kubiak R, Sygut J, Pomorski L, Kordek R. Usefulness of galectin-3 immunohistochemistry in differential diagnosis between thyroid follicular carcinoma and follicular adenoma. Pol J Pathol. 2003;54(2):111–5.
221. Moyano L, Franco C, Carreno L, Robinson P, Sanchez G. HBME-1 and cyclin D1 as diagnostic markers for follicular thyroid carcinoma [in Spanish]. Rev Med Chil. 2004;132(3):279–84.
222. Xu XC, el-Naggar AK, Lotan R. Differential expression of galectin-1 and galectin-3 in thyroid tumors. Potential diagnostic implications. Am J Pathol. 1995;147(3):815–22.
223. Beesley MF, McLaren KM. Cytokeratin 19 and galectin-3 immunohistochemistry in the differential diagnosis of solitary thyroid nodules. Histopathology. 2002;41(3):236–43.
224. Martins L, Matsuo SE, Ebina KN, Kulcsar MA, Friguglietti CU, Kimura ET. Galectin-3 messenger ribonucleic acid and protein are expressed in benign thyroid tumors. J Clin Endocrinol Metab. 2002;87(10):4806–10.
225. Kovacs RB, Foldes J, Winkler G, Bodo M, Sapi Z. The investigation of galectin-3 in diseases of the thyroid gland. Eur J Endocrinol. 2003;149(5):449–53.
226. Bryson PC, Shores CG, Hart C, et al. Immunohistochemical distinction of follicular thyroid adenomas and follicular carcinomas. Arch Otolaryngol Head Neck Surg. 2008;134(6):581–6.
227. Savin S, Cvejic D, Isic T, Paunovic I, Tatic S, Havelka M. The efficacy of the thyroid peroxidase marker for distinguishing follicular thyroid carcinoma from follicular adenoma. Exp Oncol. 2006;28(1):70–4.
228. Nasr MR, Mukhopadhyay S, Zhang S, Katzenstein AL. Immunohistochemical markers in diagnosis of papillary thyroid carcinoma: utility of HBME1 combined with CK19 immunostaining. Mod Pathol. 2006;19(12):1631–7.
229. Rossi ED, Raffaelli M, Mule' A, et al. Simultaneous immunohistochemical expression of HBME-1 and galectin-3 differentiates papillary carcinomas from hyperfunctioning lesions of the thyroid. Histopathology. 2006;48(7):795–800.

230. Takano T, Yamada H. Trefoil factor 3 (TFF3): a promising indicator for diagnosing thyroid follicular carcinoma. Endocr J. 2009;56(1):9–16.
231. Takano T, Miyauchi A, Yoshida H, Kuma K, Amino N. Decreased relative expression level of trefoil factor 3 mRNA to galectin-3 mRNA distinguishes thyroid follicular carcinoma from adenoma. Cancer Lett. 2005;219(1):91–6.
232. Koo HL, Jang J, Hong SJ, Shong Y, Gong G. Renal cell carcinoma metastatic to follicular adenoma of the thyroid gland. A case report. Acta Cytol. 2004;48(1):64–8.
233. Ambrosiani L, Declich P, Bellone S, et al. Thyroid metastases from renal clear cell carcinoma: a cyto-histological study of two cases. Adv Clin Path. 2001;5(1–2):11–6.
234. Carcangiu ML, Sibley RK, Rosai J. Clear cell change in primary thyroid tumors. A study of 38 cases. Am J Surg Pathol. 1985;9(10):705–22.
235. Nakamura N, Erickson LA, Jin L, et al. Immunohistochemical separation of follicular variant of papillary thyroid carcinoma from follicular adenoma. Endocr Pathol. 2006;17(3):213–23.
236. Schelfhout LJ, Van Muijen GN, Fleuren GJ. Expression of keratin 19 distinguishes papillary thyroid carcinoma from follicular carcinomas and follicular thyroid adenoma. Am J Clin Pathol. 1989;92(5):654–8.
237. Guyetant S, Michalak S, Valo I, Saint-Andre JP. Diagnosis of the follicular variant of papillary thyroid carcinoma. Significance of immunohistochemistry [in French]. Ann Pathol. 2003;23(1):11–20.
238. Vasko VV, Gaudart J, Allasia C, et al. Thyroid follicular adenomas may display features of follicular carcinoma and follicular variant of papillary carcinoma. Eur J Endocrinol. 2004;151(6):779–86.
239. Laco J, Ryska A. The use of immunohistochemistry in the differential diagnosis of thyroid gland tumors with follicular growth pattern [in Czech]. Cesk Patol. 2006;42(3):120–4.
240. Matias-Guiu X, LaGuette J, Puras-Gil AM, Rosai J. Metastatic neuroendocrine tumors to the thyroid gland mimicking medullary carcinoma: a pathologic and immunohistochemical study of six cases. Am J Surg Pathol. 1997;21(7):754–62.
241. Lewis JS, Ritter JH, El-Mofty S. Alternative epithelial markers in sarcomatoid carcinomas of the head and neck, lung, and bladder-p63, MOC-31, and TTF-1. Mod Pathol. 2005;18(11):1471–81.
242. Al-Abbadi MA, Almasri NM, Al-Quran S, Wilkinson EJ. Cytokeratin and epithelial membrane antigen expression in angiosarcomas: an immunohistochemical study of 33 cases. Arch Pathol Lab Med. 2007;131(2):288–92.
243. Zhang PJ, Livolsi VA, Brooks JJ. Malignant epithelioid vascular tumors of the pleura: report of a series and literature review. Hum Pathol. 2000;31(1):29–34.
244. Folpe AL, Mentzel T, Lehr HA, Fisher C, Balzer BL, Weiss SW. Perivascular epithelioid cell neoplasms of soft tissue and gynecologic origin: a clinicopathologic study of 26 cases and review of the literature. Am J Surg Pathol. 2005;29(12):1558–75.
245. Wilson RW, Moran CA. Primary melanoma of the lung: a clinicopathologic and immunohistochemical study of eight cases. Am J Surg Pathol. 1997;21(10):1196–202.
246. Gupta D, Deavers MT, Silva EG, Malpica A. Malignant melanoma involving the ovary: a clinicopathologic and immunohistochemical study of 23 cases. Am J Surg Pathol. 2004;28(6):771–80.
247. Mills SE, Gaffey MJ, Watts JC, et al. Angiomatoid carcinoma and "angiosarcoma" of the thyroid gland. A spectrum of endothelial differentiation. Am J Clin Pathol. 1994;102(3):322–30.
248. Kim NR, Ko YH, Sung CO. A case of coexistent angiosarcoma and follicular carcinoma of the thyroid. J Korean Med Sci. 2003;18(6):908–13.
249. Prasad ML, Jungbluth AA, Iversen K, Huvos AG, Busam KJ. Expression of melanocytic differentiation markers in malignant melanomas of the oral and sinonasal mucosa. Am J Surg Pathol. 2001;25(6):782–7.
250. Bergman R, Azzam H, Sprecher E, et al. A comparative immunohistochemical study of MART-1 expression in Spitz nevi, ordinary melanocytic nevi, and malignant melanomas. J Am Acad Dermatol. 2000;42(3):496–500.
251. Deyrup AT, Miettinen M, North PE, et al. Angiosarcomas arising in the viscera and soft tissue of children and young adults: a clinicopathologic study of 15 cases. Am J Surg Pathol. 2009;33(2):264–9.
252. Heerema-McKenney A, Wijnaendts LC, Pulliam JF, et al. Diffuse myogenin expression by immunohistochemistry is an independent marker of poor survival in pediatric rhabdomyosarcoma: a tissue microarray study of 71 primary tumors including correlation with molecular phenotype. Am J Surg Pathol. 2008;32(10):1513–22.
253. Wang J, Tu X, Sheng W. Sclerosing rhabdomyosarcoma: a clinicopathologic and immunohistochemical study of five cases. Am J Clin Pathol. 2008;129(3):410–5.
254. Morotti RA, Nicol KK, Parham DM, et al. An immunohistochemical algorithm to facilitate diagnosis and subtyping of rhabdomyosarcoma: the Children's Oncology Group experience. Am J Surg Pathol. 2006;30(8):962–8.
255. Cessna MH, Zhou H, Perkins SL, et al. Are myogenin and myoD1 expression specific for rhabdomyosarcoma? A study of 150 cases, with emphasis on spindle cell mimics. Am J Surg Pathol. 2001;25(9):1150–7.
256. Sebire NJ, Malone M. Myogenin and MyoD1 expression in paediatric rhabdomyosarcomas. J Clin Pathol. 2003;56(6):412–6.
257. Nascimento AF, Fletcher CD. Spindle cell rhabdomyosarcoma in adults. Am J Surg Pathol. 2005;29(8):1106–13.
258. Furlong MA, Mentzel T, Fanburg-Smith JC. Pleomorphic rhabdomyosarcoma in adults: a clinicopathologic study of 38 cases with emphasis on morphologic variants and recent skeletal muscle-specific markers. Mod Pathol. 2001;14(6):595–603.
259. de Saint Aubain Somerhausen N, Fletcher CD. Leiomyosarcoma of soft tissue in children: clinicopathologic analysis of 20 cases. Am J Surg Pathol. 1999;23(7):755–63.
260. Oda Y, Miyajima K, Kawaguchi K, et al. Pleomorphic leiomyosarcoma: clinicopathologic and immunohistochemical study with special emphasis on its distinction from ordinary leiomyosarcoma and malignant fibrous histiocytoma. Am J Surg Pathol. 2001;25(8):1030–8.
261. Rubin BP, Fletcher CD. Myxoid leiomyosarcoma of soft tissue, an underrecognized variant. Am J Surg Pathol. 2000;24(7):927–36.
262. Matsumoto F, Fujii H, Abe M, et al. A novel tumor marker, Niban, is expressed in subsets of thyroid tumors and Hashimoto's thyroiditis. Hum Pathol. 2006;37(12):1592–600.
263. Liu J, Singh B, Tallini G, et al. Follicular variant of papillary thyroid carcinoma: a clinicopathologic study of a problematic entity. Cancer. 2006;107(6):1255–64.
264. Xing M, Westra WH, Tufano RP, et al. BRAF mutation predicts a poorer clinical prognosis for papillary thyroid cancer. J Clin Endocrinol Metab. 2005;90(12):6373–9.
265. Xing M, Vasko V, Tallini G, et al. BRAF T1796A transversion mutation in various thyroid neoplasms. J Clin Endocrinol Metab. 2004;89(3):1365–8.
266. Garcia-Rostan G, Zhao H, Camp RL, et al. ras mutations are associated with aggressive tumor phenotypes and poor prognosis in thyroid cancer. J Clin Oncol. 2003;21(17):3226–35.
267. Nikiforova MN, Lynch RA, Biddinger PW, et al. RAS point mutations and PAX8-PPAR gamma rearrangement in thyroid tumors: evidence for distinct molecular pathways in thyroid follicular carcinoma. J Clin Endocrinol Metab. 2003;88(5):2318–26.
268. Santoro M, Papotti M, Chiappetta G, et al. RET activation and clinicopathologic features in poorly differentiated thyroid tumors. J Clin Endocrinol Metab. 2002;87(1):370–9.
269. Nonaka D. A study of parathyroid transcription factor Gcm2 expression in parathyroid lesions [USCAP abstract 579]. Mod Pathol. 2010;23(Suppl 1s):131A.

270. Pesce C, Tobia F, Carli F, Antoniotti GV. The sites of hormone storage in normal and diseased parathyroid glands: a silver impregnation and immunohistochemical study. Histopathology. 1989;15(2):157–66.
271. Schmid KW, Hittmair A, Ladurner D, Sandbichler P, Gasser R, Totsch M. Chromogranin A and B in parathyroid tissue of cases of primary hyperparathyroidism: an immunohistochemical study. Virchows Arch A Pathol Anat Histopathol. 1991;418(4):295–9.
272. Miettinen M, Clark R, Lehto VP, Virtanen I, Damjanov I. Intermediate-filament proteins in parathyroid glands and parathyroid adenomas. Arch Pathol Lab Med. 1985;109(11):986–9.
273. Hadar T, Shvero J, Yaniv E, Ram E, Shvili I, Koren R. Expression of p53, Ki-67 and Bcl-2 in parathyroid adenoma and residual normal tissue. Pathol Oncol Res. 2005;11(1):45–9.
274. Naccarato AG, Marcocci C, Miccoli P, et al. Bcl-2, p53 and MIB-1 expression in normal and neoplastic parathyroid tissues. J Endocrinol Invest. 1998;21(3):136–41.
275. Parfitt AM, Wang Q, Palnitkar S. Rates of cell proliferation in adenomatous, suppressed, and normal parathyroid tissue: implications for pathogenesis. J Clin Endocrinol Metab. 1998;83(3):863–9.
276. Farnebo F, Auer G, Farnebo LO, et al. Evaluation of retinoblastoma and Ki-67 immunostaining as diagnostic markers of benign and malignant parathyroid disease. World J Surg. 1999;23(1):68–74.
277. Vargas MP, Vargas HI, Kleiner DE, Merino MJ. The role of prognostic markers (MiB-1, RB, and bcl-2) in the diagnosis of parathyroid tumors. Mod Pathol. 1997;10(1):12–7.
278. Delellis RA. Challenging lesions in the differential diagnosis of endocrine tumors: parathyroid carcinoma. Endocr Pathol. 2008;19(4):221–5.
279. Howell VM, Gill A, Clarkson A, et al. Accuracy of combined protein gene product 9.5 and parafibromin markers for immunohistochemical diagnosis of parathyroid carcinoma. J Clin Endocrinol Metab. 2009;94(2):434–41.
280. Gill AJ, Clarkson A, Gimm O, et al. Loss of nuclear expression of parafibromin distinguishes parathyroid carcinomas and hyperparathyroidism-jaw tumor (HPT-JT) syndrome-related adenomas from sporadic parathyroid adenomas and hyperplasias. Am J Surg Pathol. 2006;30(9):1140–9.
281. Tan MH, Morrison C, Wang P, et al. Loss of parafibromin immunoreactivity is a distinguishing feature of parathyroid carcinoma. Clin Cancer Res. 2004;10(19):6629–37.
282. Cetani F, Ambrogini E, Viacava P, et al. Should parafibromin staining replace HRTP2 gene analysis as an additional tool for histologic diagnosis of parathyroid carcinoma? Eur J Endocrinol. 2007;156(5):547–54.
283. DeLellis RA. Parathyroid carcinoma: an overview. Adv Anat Pathol. 2005;12(2):53–61.
284. DeLellis RA, Mazzaglia P, Mangray S. Primary hyperparathyroidism: a current perspective. Arch Pathol Lab Med. 2008;132(8): 1251–62.
285. Lloyd RV, Carney JA, Ferreiro JA, et al. Immunohistochemical analysis of the Cell cycle-associated antigens Ki-67 and retinoblastoma protein in parathyroid carcinomas and adenomas. Endocr Pathol. 1995;6(4):279–87.
286. Erickson LA, Jin L, Papotti M, Lloyd RV. Oxyphil parathyroid carcinomas: a clinicopathologic and immunohistochemical study of 10 cases. Am J Surg Pathol. 2002;26(3):344–9.
287. Erickson LA, Jin L, Wollan P, Thompson GB, van Heerden JA, Lloyd RV. Parathyroid hyperplasia, adenomas, and carcinomas: differential expression of p27Kip1 protein. Am J Surg Pathol. 1999;23(3):288–95.
288. Stojadinovic A, Hoos A, Nissan A, et al. Parathyroid neoplasms: clinical, histopathological, and tissue microarray-based molecular analysis. Hum Pathol. 2003;34(1):54–64.
289. Futrell JM, Roth SI, Su SP, Habener JF, Segre GV, Potts Jr JT. Immunocytochemical localization of parathyroid hormone in bovine parathyroid glands and human parathyroid adenomas. Am J Pathol. 1979;94(3):615–22.
290. Woodard GE, Lin L, Zhang JH, Agarwal SK, Marx SJ, Simonds WF. Parafibromin, product of the hyperparathyroidism-jaw tumor syndrome gene HRPT2, regulates cyclin D1/PRAD1 expression. Oncogene. 2005;24(7):1272–6.
291. Danks JA, Ebeling PR, Hayman J, et al. Parathyroid hormone-related protein: immunohistochemical localization in cancers and in normal skin. J Bone Miner Res. 1989;4(2):273–8.
292. Rosol TJ, Capen CC. Tumors of the parathyroid gland and circulating parathyroid hormone-related protein associated with persistent hypercalcemia. Toxicol Pathol. 1989;17(2):346–56.
293. Hellman P, Karlsson-Parra A, Klareskog L, et al. Expression and function of a CD4-like molecule in parathyroid tissue. Surgery. 1996;120(6):985–92.
294. Ordonez NG, Ibanez ML, Samaan NA, Hickey RC. Immunoperoxidase study of uncommon parathyroid tumors. Report of two cases of nonfunctioning parathyroid carcinoma and one intrathyroid parathyroid tumor-producing amyloid. Am J Surg Pathol. 1983;7(6):535–42.
295. Saggiorato E, Bergero N, Volante M, et al. Galectin-3 and Ki-67 expression in multiglandular parathyroid lesions. Am J Clin Pathol. 2006;126(1):59–66.
296. Fernandez-Ranvier GG, Khanafshar E, Tacha D, et al. Defining a molecular phenotype for benign and malignant parathyroid tumors. Cancer. 2009;115(2):334–44.

Chapter 12
Adrenal Gland

Hanna G. Kaspar

Abstract This chapter is an overview of frequently used markers in the differential diagnosis of both common and rare tumors of the adrenal gland, with a focus on the effective markers employed for differentiating primary adrenal tumors and their mimics including metastatic renal cell carcinoma, hepatocellular carcinoma, and malignant melanoma. Other useful panels in the differential diagnosis of pheochromocytoma, adrenal cortical neoplasms, and small blue cell tumors are also addressed. There are 19 tables in this chapter with immunohistochemical markers answering questions that may arise when examining hematoxylin and eosin-stained tumor sections. A summary of useful and frequently used markers is also provided, in addition to some representative photomicrographs, and the author's experience with a few tested antibodies. The effective diagnostic panels of antibodies for several entities are outlined.

Keywords Adrenal cortical neoplasms • Adrenal cortical adenoma • Adrenal cortical carcinoma • Pheochromocytoma • Neuroblastoma • Angiomyolipoma

H.G. Kaspar (✉)
Clinical Professor, Department of Pathology and Laboratory Medicine, Temple University School of Medicine, Philadelphia, PA, Staff Pathologist, Geisinger Wyoming Valley Medical Center, 1000 East Mountain Blvd., Wilkes-Barre, PA 18711, USA
e-mail: hgkaspar@geisinger.edu

FREQUENTLY ASKED QUESTIONS

F. Lin and J. Prichard (eds.), *Handbook of Practical Immunohistochemistry: Frequently Asked Questions*, DOI 10.1007/978-1-4419-8062-5_12, © Springer Science+Business Media, LLC 2011

Table 12.1 Summary of markers frequently used in adrenal glands

Antibodies	Staining pattern	Function	Key applications and pitfalls
MART-1	C	Melanoma marker cross reacts with an epitope present in steroid producing cells	Used in identifying adrenal cortical neoplasms and distinguishing them from adrenal medullary and metastatic neoplasms
Inhibin A	C	Dimeric glycoprotein produced by the gonads; inhibits FSH secretion by the pituitary	More sensitive but less specific than MART-1 in identifying adrenal cortical tumors
Bcl-2	C	B cell lymphoma 6 protein can interact with a variety of POZ-containing proteins that function as transcription corepressors	Suggested to be of help in the differential between adrenal cortical (reactive) and medullary tumors (unreactive), but antigen retrieval methodologies may produce conflicting results
Calretinin	N + C	Calcium binding protein detected in over two-thirds of adrenal cortical neoplasms	Used in identifying adrenal cortical neoplasms and distinguishing them from adrenal medullary neoplasms
NFP		Intermediate filaments found specifically in neurons	Expression is correlated with the differentiation into committed neurons or neoplasia
Vimentin	C	Intermediate filament	Frequently positive in both adrenal cortical neoplasms and pheochromocytomas
NSE	C	No specific neuroendocrine marker	Found in all pheochromocytomas, paragangliomas and most neuroblastomas, and may be present in other small, round, blue cell tumors
Synaptophysin	C	Present in neurotransmitter dense-core secretory vesicles	Found in all pheochromocytomas and paragangliomas
Chromogranin A	C	Present in neurotransmitter dense-coresecretory vesicles	Found in most pheochromocytomas, neuroblastomas paragangliomas; usually negative in cortical neoplasms
S100	N + C	Belongs to the family of S100 calcium-binding proteins	Identifies sustentacular cells in the adrenal medulla
CD56	M + C	Neuron adhesion molecules	Pheochromocytomas are typically strongly positive Focal positivity noted in adrenal cortical carcinomas Positive in neuroendocrine tumor including small cell carcinoma and a subset of non-small cell carcinoma with neuroendocrine differentiation
EMA	M	Epithelial marker	Typically negative in pheochromocytomas/paragangliomas and adrenal cortical neoplasms
CD99	M	Differentiation of primitive neuroectodermal cells	Reactive in most ES-PNET but not in neuroblastomas

References: [1–27]

Table 12.2 Summary of useful markers in common tumors

Antibodies	ACN	PCC	NB	GN
MART-1	+	–	–	–
Calretinin	+	–	–	– or +
Inhibin-alpha	+	– or +	–	–
Chromogranin	–	+	+	+
Synaptophysin	+	+	+ or –	+
Vimentin	+	– or +	+ or –	+
S100	–	+ or –	– or +	+
GFAP	–	+ or –	–	+ or –
NSE	+	+	+	+
Ad-4BP	+	–	–	–
CD99	–	–	–	–
HMB-45	–	–	–	–
Actin-HHF35	–	–	–	–
Pan-CK	– or +	– or +	–	–
AE1/AE3	– or +	– or focal +	–	–
CK7	–	–	–	–
EMA	–	–	– or +	–
CD56		+	+	
NFP	–	+	+	
NB84	–	–	+	–

ACN adrenal cortical neoplasms, *PCC* pheochromocytoma, *NB* neuroblastoma, *GN* ganglioneuroma

References: [3–6, 8, 9, 11, 13–16, 23–25, 28–46]

Table 12.3 Markers for adrenal cortical neoplasms

Antibodies	Literature	GML data
AD4BP	+	ND
Calretinin	+	24/24
Inhibin-A	+	10/24
Synaptophysin	+	10/24
Chromogranin	–	0/24
CD56	+	24/24
MART-1	+	24/24
NSE	+	22/24
Vimentin	+	10/24
Pan-CK	– or +	0/24
Bcl-2	– or +	0/24
CAM 5.2	– or +	0/24
35bH11	– or +	0/24
CD31	– or +	0/24
Ki-67	– or +	V
CD5	– or +	0/24
p53	–	ND
EMA	–	0/24
CK7	–	0/24
CK20	–	0/24

Note: *v* variable, *MITF* microphthalmia-associated transcription factor

Our study based on 24 cases of adrenal cortical adenoma on TMA sections shows that MART-1 and calretinin tend to demonstrate diffuse and strong immunoreactivity; in contrast, inhibin-alpha is usually weak and focal. Epithelial markers (AE1/AE3, CAM 5.2, CA7, CK20, CK5/6, CK903, and EMA) are negative in our experience. Other markers including TTF1, S100, Hep Par1, and CD10 are negative as well. The immunostaining results from a small number of adrenal cortical carcinomas ($N = 5$) are similar to that of cortical adenomas, with the exception of two cases being positive for CD10 and all cases positive for vimentin. An example of adrenal cortical carcinoma expressing vimentin, MART-1, inhibin-alpha, CD10, and a high MIB1 (Ki-67) proliferation index is shown in Fig. 12.1a–e

References: [3–6, 10–12, 14, 15, 19–21, 23, 24, 35, 38, 40, 43, 46–53]

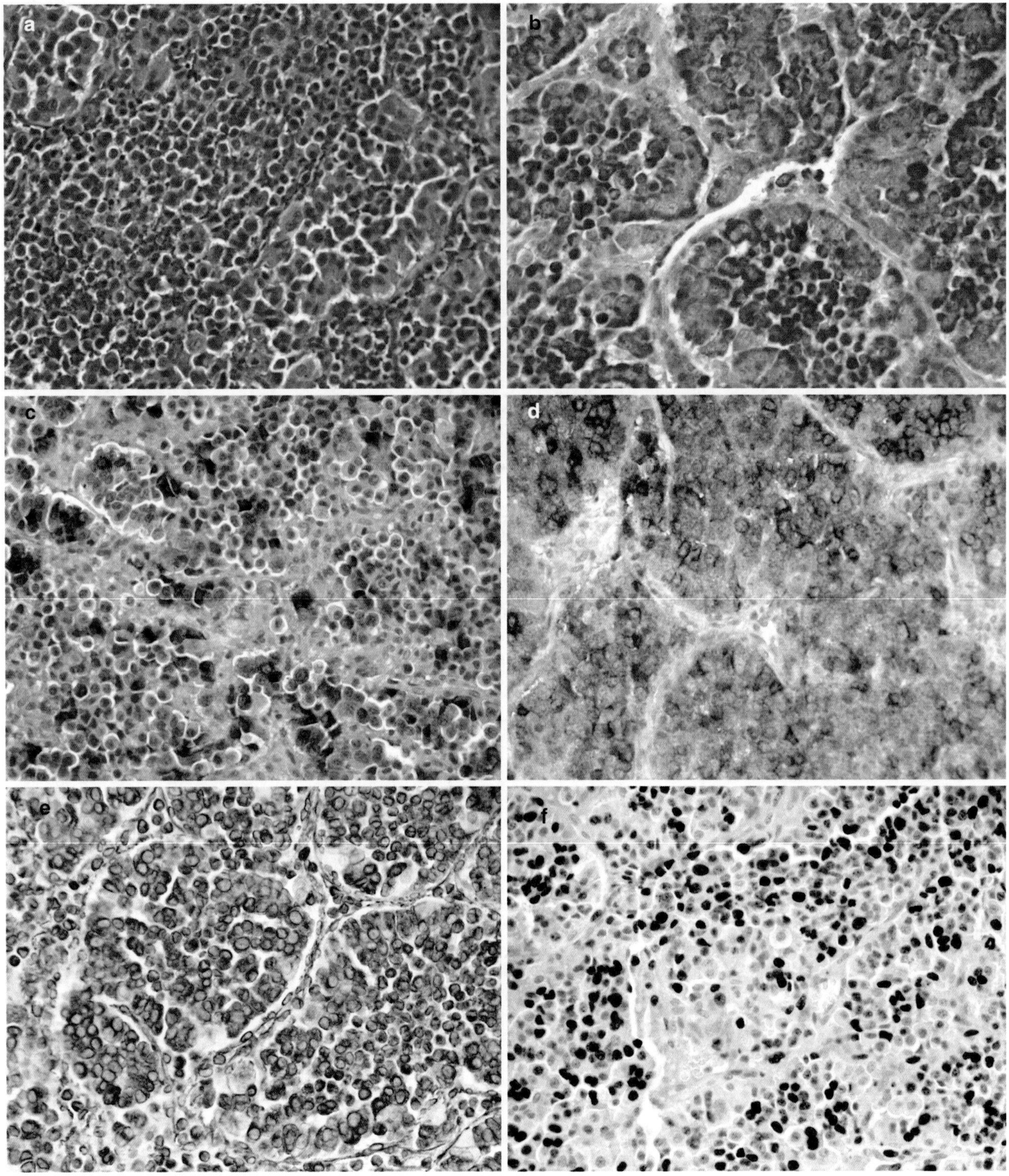

Fig. 12.1 Adrenal cortical carcinoma on H&E-stained section (**a**) with positive immunostaining for MART-1 (**b**), inhibin-alpha (**c**), CD10 (**d**), vimentin (**e**), and a high Ki-67 proliferative index (**f**)

Table 12.4 Markers for pheochromocytoma

Antibodies	Literature	GML data
Synaptophysin	+	13/13
Chromogranin	+	13/13
Inhibin-A	+	1/13 (Focal only)
MART-1	–	0/13
CD56	+	13/13
NFP	+	ND
Bcl-2	+	3/13
S100*	+ or –	9/13
GFAP	+ or –	0/13
Vimentin	– or +	11/13
p53	– or +	0/13
Pan-CK	– or +	1/13 (<1+)
Somatostatin	– or +	ND
Calcitonin	– or +	2/13, Weak +
Calretinin	–	0/13
CD99	–	ND
BNH9	–	ND

Note: A typical pheochromocytoma is positive for neuroendocrine markers (chromogranin, synaptophysin, CD56, and NSE), vimentin, and negative for cytokeratins, inhibin-alpha, and MART-1. Positive immunoreactivity for cytokeratins, inhibin-alpha, CD10, and calcitonin can be seen. An example is shown in Fig. 12.2a–f (H&E, chromogranin, calcitonin, S100 with three different staining patterns)

*Staining of sustentacular cells surrounding Zellballen is decreased in malignant neoplasms. *ND* no data

References: [54–56, 57–60]

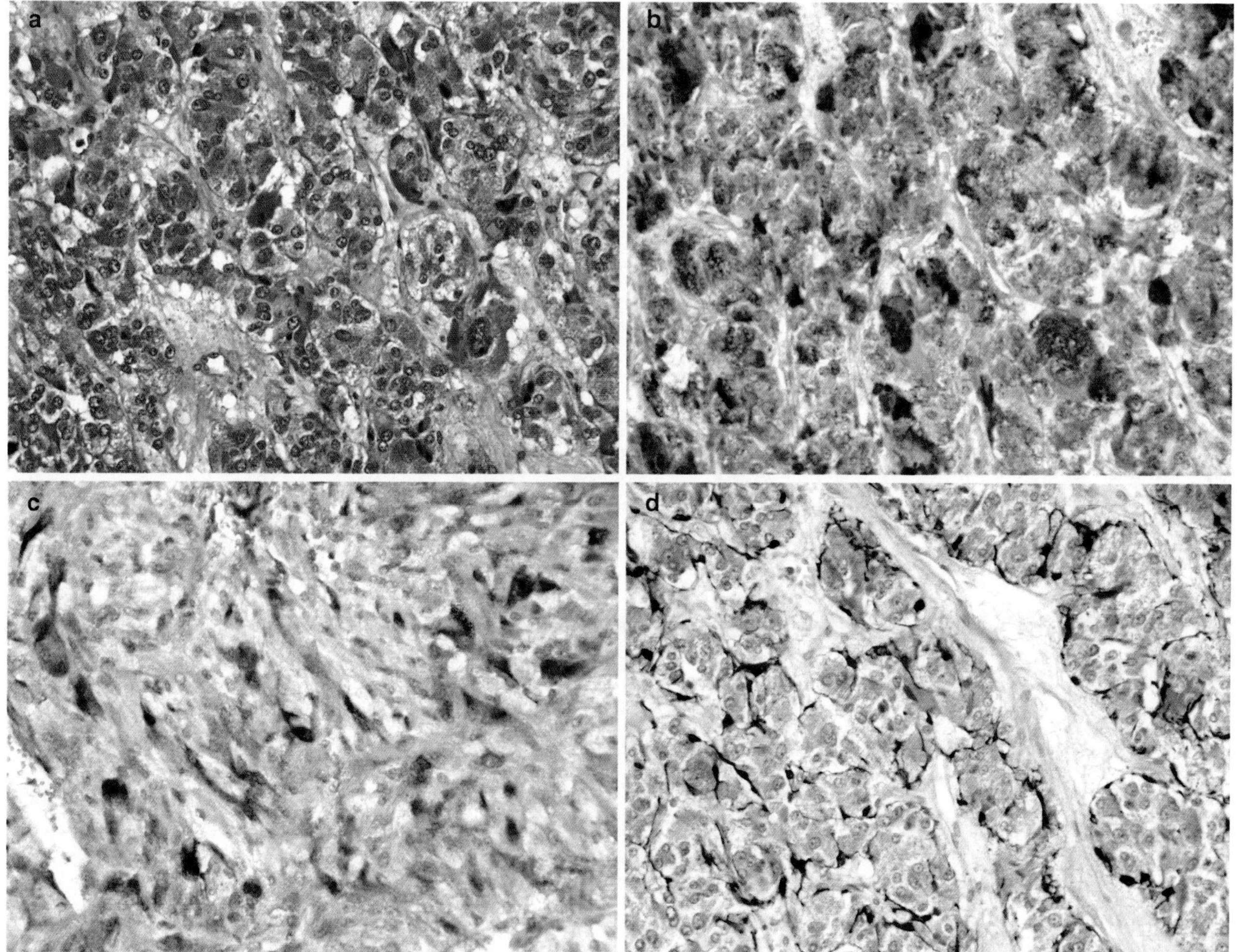

Fig. 12.2 Pheochromocytoma on H&E-stained section (**a**) with positive immunostaining for chromogranin (**b**), calcitonin (**c**), and three different staining patterns for sustentacular cells in diffuse pattern (**d**), patchy (**e**), and also staining tumor cells (**f**)

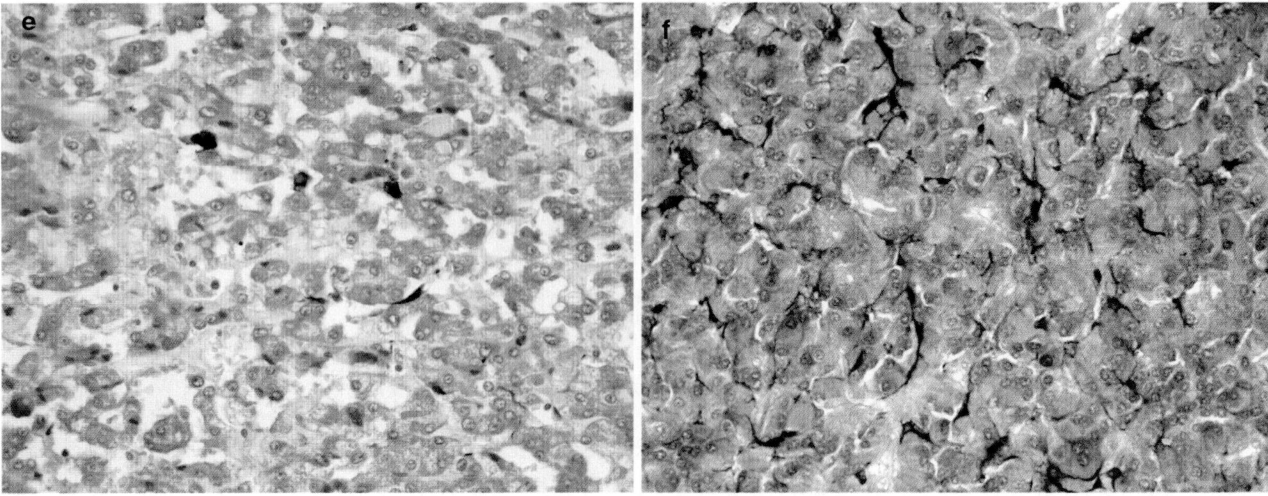

Fig. 12.2 (continued)

Table 12.5 Markers for neuroblastoma

Antibodies	Literature
NSE	+
CD56	+
Chromogranin	+
NB84	+
NFP	+
ALK-1	+
CD57	+
Synaptophysin	+ or –
Vimentin	+ or –
EMA	– or +
S100	– or +
WT1	– or +
CD57	– or +

Note: The following markers are usually negative: LCA, MyoD1, SMA, myogenin, actin-HHF35, desmin, GFAP, CK, Hep Par1, CD99, CD34, and PAX5

CD44 expressed in favorable histology NB and non-expression is associated with unfavorable histology

References: [26, 45, 59, 61–67]

Table 12.6 Markers for ganglioneuroma

Antibodies	Literature
Vimentin	+
NFP	+
S100	+
NSE	+
Chromogranin	+
Synaptophysin	+
GFAP	+ or –
Actin-HHF35	–
Desmin	–
CD99	–
AE1/AE3	–

References: [25, 26, 41, 44, 45]

Table 12.7 Markers for ganglioneuroblastoma

Antibodies	Literature
NFP	+
NSE	+
S100	+
Chromogranin	+
GFAP	+ or –
Synaptophysin	+ or –
CD68	–

References: [34, 67–69]

Table 12.8 Markers for angiomyolipoma

Antibodies	Literature
Calponin	+
CD63	+
F8RAG	+
HMB50	+
Actin-HHF35	+
MART-1	+
SMA	+
Vimentin	+
Desmin	+ or –
MITF	+ or –
ER	– or +
PR	– or +
CD34	– or +
S100	– or +
Tyrosinase	– or +
CD117	– or +
NSE	– or +

Note: The following markers are usually negative: Hep Par1, chromogranin, CAM 5.2, EMA, Pan-CK, and AE1/AE3

References: [70–85]

Table 12.9 Adrenal cortical neoplasm vs. pheochromocytoma

Antibodies	Cortical neoplasm	Pheochromocytoma
Calretinin	+	–
MART-1	+	–
Inhibin	+	
Chromogranin	–	+
S100	–	+
Synaptophysin	+	+
Vimentin	+	– or +
p53	–	– or +
Bcl-2	– or +	+
Somatostatin	–	– or +
BNH9	+	–
CD5	– or +	–
CD31	– or +	–
CD34	–	–
CD56	+	+
CD138	– or +	–
Pan-CK	– or +	– or +

Note: The following markers are usually negative: Hep Par1, TTF1, EMA, CK7, and CK20

References: [4, 11, 16, 24, 29, 33, 37, 38, 46–49, 86]

Table 12.10 Adrenal cortical neoplasm vs. metastatic renal cell carcinoma

Antibodies	Cortical neoplasm	Renal cell carcinoma
CD10	–	+
CD56	+	– or +
MART-1	+	–
Calretinin	+	–
Inhibin	+	– or +
Synaptophysin	+	–
EMA	–	+
Pan-CK	– or +	+
RCCMa	–	+
MUC1	–	+
AE1/AE3	– or +	+
CK19	–	– or +
CAM 5.2	– or +	+
PKK1	–	+ or –
Cyclin D1	–	– or +
35bH11	– or +	– or +
S100	–	– or +
BNH9	+	–
CD31	– or +	–
CD34	–	– or +
NSE	+	+ or –
pCEA	– or +	–
Ber-EP4	–	– or +
CK7	–	– or +
mCEA	–	– or +
MITF	–	– or +
CK5/6	–	– or +
CD5	– or +	–
CD63	– or +	– or +
Vimentin	+	+

Note: The following markers are usually negative: Hep Par1, p53, CD163, CD117, TTF1, mesothelin, CK14, and CK20

References: [3, 4, 7, 8, 11, 15, 16, 18, 22, 24, 29, 33, 35–38, 40, 43, 46, 47, 49, 51, 87–99]

Table 12.11 Adrenal cortical neoplasm vs. metastatic hepatocellular carcinoma

Antibodies	Adrenal cortical neoplasm	Hepatocellular carcinoma
Calretinin	+	–
MART-1	+	–
Inhibin	+	–
PKK1	–	+
Synaptophysin	+	– or +
Hep Par1	–	+
AE3	+	– or +
CAM 5.2	– or +	+
CD56	+	– or +
TTF1 C	–	+ or –
CD10	–	+ or –
CD117	–	+ or –
Pan-CK	– or +	+
35bH11	– or +	+
Vimentin	+	– or +
Glypican 3	–	+ or –
Bcl-2	– or +	–
EMA	–	– or +
AE1	–	– or +
p27	+	+ or –
CD138	– or +	+ or –
p53	–	– or +
MFG	–	– or +
AFP	–	– or +
pCEA	– or +	+
CD34	–	– or +
CK20	–	– or +
CK7	–	– or +
p21	+ or –	+ or –
AE1/AE3	– or +	– or +
CD31	– or +	–
CK19	–	– or +
CD5	– or +	–

Note: The following markers are usually negative in both: chromogranin, MUC1, S100, mesothelin, CEA, CK5/6, and TTF1

References: [3, 4, 8, 15, 16, 24, 26, 29, 35, 37, 38, 41, 46, 47, 49, 51, 89, 92, 93, 99–116]

Table 12.12 Ganglioneuroma vs. neurofibroma

Antibodies	Ganglioneuroma	Neurofibroma
Synaptophysin	+	–
NSE	+	–
Chromogranin	+	–
GFAP	+ or –	–
NFP	+	+ or –
CD57	+	+
S100	+	+
PGP 9.5	+	+
Vimentin	+	+
P75NTR	+	+
CD68	–	+ or –
Calretinin	– or +	– or +

Note: The following markers are usually negative in both: SMA, CD99, desmin, pan-CK, AE1/AE3, HMB-45, and actin-HHF35

References: [41, 42, 44]

Table 12.13 Neuroblastoma vs. ganglioneuroblastoma

Antibodies	Neuroblastoma	Ganglioneuroblastoma
S100	– or +	+
NSE	+	+
Chromogranin	+	+
NFP	+	+
Synaptophysin	+ or –	+ or –
Vimentin	+ or –	–
GFAP	–	+ or –
BNH9	+ or –	–
EMA	– or +	–
CD57	– or +	–

Note: The following markers are usually negative in both: SMA, AE1/AE3, CD99, CD34, and HMB-45

References: [21, 25, 26, 30, 33, 34, 44, 69, 117, 118]

Table 12.14 Ganglioneuroblastoma vs. ganglioneuroma[a]

Antibodies	Ganglioneuroblastoma	Ganglioneuroma
Synaptophysin	+ or –	+
SMA	–	–
Vimentin	–	+
NSE	+	+
GFAP	+ or –	+ or –
Chromogranin	+	+
NFP	+	+
S100	+	+
AE1/AE3	–	–
CD99	–	–
CD68	–	–

[a]**Note**: A satisfactory differentiating panel does not exist

References: [21, 25, 26, 30, 33, 34, 44, 69]

Table 12.15 Neuroblastoma vs. rhabdomyosarcoma

Antibodies	Neuroblastoma	Rhabdomyosarcoma
Synaptophysin	+ or –	–
Chromogranin	+	–
PLAP	–	+
Actin-HHF35	–	+
Myogenin	–	+
Desmin	–	+
NB84	+	–
CD99	–	– or +
S100	– or +	–
NSE	+	– or +
WT1	– or +	+ or –
NFP	+	– or +
CD117	+ or –	– or +
Vimentin	+ or –	+
BNH9	+ or –	–
SMA	–	– or +
PGP 9.5	+	+
CD57	– or +	–
EMA	– or +	– or +
CD34	–	– or +
CD56	+	+
Pan-CK	–	– or +
AE1/AE3	–	– or +
CAM 5.2	–	– or +
pCEA	+ or –	–

Note: The following markers are usually negative in both: Hep Par1, HMB-45, CD163, FLI-1, GFAP, and CD45

References: [25, 64, 69, 117–123]

Table 12.16 Neuroblastoma vs. lymphoma

Antibodies	Neuroblastoma	Lymphoma
CD45	–	+
CD56	+	–
Synaptophysin	+ or –	–
NSE	+	–
CD99	–	– or +
CD20	–	+
PAX5	–	+
CD117	+ or –	– or +
Chromogranin	+	–
NFP	+	–
CD57	– or +	– or +
S100	– or +	– or +
Vimentin	+ or –	+
Desmin	–	–
AE1/AE3	–	– or +
EMA	– or +	– or +
PLAP	–	– or +
Actin-HHF35	–	– or +
CD163	–	– or +
pCEA	+ or –	–
BNH9	+ or –	–

Note: CD5, Hep Par1, CD34, SMA, Pan-CK, CAM 5.2, and HMB-45 are usually negative in both

References: [25, 30, 33, 42, 44, 117, 124–128]

Table 12.17 Neuroblastoma vs. Ewing sarcoma

Antibodies	Ewing sarcoma	Neuroblastoma
Chromogranin	–	+
Synaptophysin	–	+ or –
CD56	– or +	+
CD99	+	–
NB84	– or +	+
NFP	– or +	+
S100	– or +	– or +
Vimentin	+	– or +
NSE	– or +	+
Beta-2 microglobulin	– or +	–
Pan-CK	– or +	–
AE1/AE3	– or +	–
EMA	– or +	– or +
CD57	– or +	– or +
CD117	–	+ or –
BNH9	–	+ or –
PGP 9.5	+	+
WT1	–	– or +

Note: CAM 5.2, LCA, CD20, GFAP, Actin-HHF35, CD163, desmin, myogenin, SMA, and HMB-45 are usually negative in both

References: [9, 13, 17, 28, 42, 129–134]

Table 12.18 Pigmented cortical adenoma vs. malignant melanoma

Antibodies	Cortical adenoma	Malignant melanoma
S100	–	+
HMB-45	–	+
Tyrosinase	–	+
MITF	–	+
Synaptophysin	+	– or +
CD56	+	– or +
Calretinin	+	– or +
CD63	– or +	+
Bcl-2	– or +	+
MART-1	+	+
CAM 5.2	– or +	–
Chromogranin	–	–
p53	–	– or +
Vimentin	+	+
mCEA	–	–
pCEA	– or +	– or +
Ki-67	– or +	+ or –
p27	– or +	+ or –
Her-2/neu	–	–
Cyclin D1	–	– or +
Desmin	–	–
NSE	+	+ or –
CD5	– or +	– or +
CD10	–	– or +
CD31	– or +	–
CD117	–	– or +
CD138	– or +	– or +
Pan-CK	– or +	–
AE1/AE3	– or +	–
Hep Par1	–	– or +

Note: CD34, CK7, CK20, CD163, AFP, TTF1 are usually negative in both

References: [1, 2, 4, 15, 27, 29, 35, 64, 135–137]

Table 12.19 Pigmented pheochromocytoma vs. malignant melanoma

Antibodies	Pheochromocytoma	Malignant melanoma
Chromogranin	+	–
MART-1	– or +	+
NFP	+	–
CD56	+	– or +
Synaptophysin	+	– or +
Vimentin	– or +	+
Pan-CK	– or +	–
p53	– or +	– or +
GFAP	+ or –	–
S100	+ or –	+
Bcl-2	+	+
CD5	–	– or +
CD63	+	+
CD68	+	+ or –
CD99	–	– or +
CD117	– or +	– or +
CD138	–	– or +
Cathepsin B	+	+
Calretinin	–	– or +
Inhibin	–	– or +
Hep Par1	–	– or +

Note: CD31, CD34, CD163, CK7, CK20, EMA, BNH9, F8RAG are usually negative in both

References: [39, 138–140]

Note for All Tables

Note: "+" – usually greater than 70% of cases are positive; "–" – less than 5% of cases are positive; "+ or –" – usually more than 50% of cases are positive; "– or +" – less than 50% of cases are positive.

References

1. Boyle JL, Haupt HM, Stern JB, Multhaupt HA. Tyrosinase expression in malignant melanoma, desmoplastic melanoma, and peripheral nerve tumors. Arch Pathol Lab Med. 2002;126(7):816–22.
2. Brat DJ, Giannini C, Scheithauer BW, Burger PC. Primary melanocytic neoplasms of the central nervous systems. Am J Surg Pathol. 1999;23(7):745–54.
3. Brown FM, Gaffey TA, Wold LE, Lloyd RV. Myxoid neoplasms of the adrenal cortex: a rare histologic variant. Am J Surg Pathol. 2000;24(3):396–401.
4. Busam KJ, Iversen K, Coplan KA, et al. Immunoreactivity for A103, an antibody to melan-A (Mart-1), in adrenocortical and other steroid tumors. Am J Surg Pathol. 1998;22(1):57–63.
5. Chetty R, Pillay P, Jaichand V. Cytokeratin expression in adrenal phaeochromocytomas and extra-adrenal paragangliomas. J Clin Pathol. 1998;51(6):477–8.
6. Cho EY, Ahn GH. Immunoexpression of inhibin alpha-subunit in adrenal neoplasms. Appl Immunohistochem Mol Morphol. 2001;9(3):222–8.
7. Chu P, Wu E, Weiss LM. Cytokeratin 7 and cytokeratin 20 expression in epithelial neoplasms: a survey of 435 cases. Mod Pathol. 2000;13(9):962–72.
8. Chu PG, Arber DA, Weiss LM. Expression of T/NK-cell and plasma cell antigens in nonhematopoietic epithelioid neoplasms. An immunohistochemical study of 447 cases. Am J Clin Pathol. 2003;120(1):64–70.
9. Collini P, Mezzelani A, Modena P, et al. Evidence of neural differentiation in a case of post-therapy primitive neuroectodermal tumor/Ewing sarcoma of bone. Am J Surg Pathol. 2003;27(8):1161–6.
10. Fetsch PA, Powers CN, Zakowski MF, Abati A. Anti-alpha-inhibin: marker of choice for the consistent distinction between adrenocortical carcinoma and renal cell carcinoma in fine-needle aspiration. Cancer. 1999;87(3):168–72.

11. Fogt F, Vortmeyer AO, Poremba C, Minda M, Harris CA, Tomaszewski JE. bcl-2 Expression in normal adrenal glands and in adrenal neoplasms. Mod Pathol. 1998;11(8):716–20.
12. Ghorab Z, Jorda M, Ganjei P, Nadji M. Melan A (A103) is expressed in adrenocortical neoplasms but not in renal cell and hepatocellular carcinomas. Appl Immunohistochem Mol Morphol. 2003;11(4):330–3.
13. Gluer S, Zense M, von Schweinitz D. Cell adhesion molecules and intermediate filaments on embryonal childhood tumors. Pathol Res Pract. 1998;194(11):773–80.
14. Jorda M, De MB, Nadji M. Calretinin and inhibin are useful in separating adrenocortical neoplasms from pheochromocytomas. Appl Immunohistochem Mol Morphol. 2002;10(1):67–70.
15. Lin BT, Bonsib SM, Mierau GW, Weiss LM, Medeiros LJ. Oncocytic adrenocortical neoplasms: a report of seven cases and review of the literature. Am J Surg Pathol. 1998;22(5):603–14.
16. Lugli A, Forster Y, Haas P, et al. Calretinin expression in human normal and neoplastic tissues: a tissue microarray analysis on 5233 tissue samples. Hum Pathol. 2003;34(10):994–1000.
17. Mahfouz S, Aziz AA, Gabal SM, el-Sheikh S. Immunohistochemical study of CD99 and EMA expression in ependymomas. Medscape J Med. 2008;10(2):41.
18. Matsuki Y, Tanimoto A, Hamada T, Sasaguri Y. Histidine decarboxylase expression as a new sensitive and specific marker for small cell lung carcinoma. Mod Pathol. 2003;16(1):72–8.
19. McCluggage WG, Maxwell P. Adenocarcinomas of various sites may exhibit immunoreactivity with anti-inhibin antibodies. Histopathology. 1999;35(3):216–20.
20. McCluggage WG, Maxwell P, Patterson A, Sloan JM. Immunohistochemical staining of hepatocellular carcinoma with monoclonal antibody against inhibin. Histopathology. 1997;30(6): 518–22.
21. Miettinen M, Lehto VP, Virtanen I. Immunofluorescence microscopic evaluation of the intermediate filament expression of the adrenal cortex and medulla and their tumors. Am J Pathol. 1985;118(3):360–6.
22. Miettinen M, Lindenmayer AE, Chaubal A. Endothelial cell markers CD31, CD34, and BNH9 antibody to H- and Y-antigens–evaluation of their specificity and sensitivity in the diagnosis of vascular tumors and comparison with von Willebrand factor. Mod Pathol. 1994;7(1):82–90.
23. Munro LM, Kennedy A, McNicol AM. The expression of inhibin/activin subunits in the human adrenal cortex and its tumours. J Endocrinol. 1999;161(2):341–7.
24. Pelkey TJ, Frierson Jr HF, Mills SE, Stoler MH. The alpha subunit of inhibin in adrenal cortical neoplasia. Mod Pathol. 1998;11(6):516–24.
25. Viswanathan S, George S, Ramadwar M, Medhi S, Arora B, Kurkure P. Evaluation of pediatric abdominal masses by fine-needle aspiration cytology: a clinicoradiologic approach. Diagn Cytopathol. 2010;38(1):15–27.
26. Wirnsberger GH, Becker H, Ziervogel K, Hofler H. Diagnostic immunohistochemistry of neuroblastic tumors. Am J Surg Pathol. 1992;16(1):49–57.
27. Zubovits J, Buzney E, Yu L, Duncan LM. HMB-45, S-100, NK1/C3, and MART-1 in metastatic melanoma. Hum Pathol. 2004;35(2):217–23.
28. Abramowsky CR, Katzenstein HM, Alvarado CS, Shehata BM. Anaplastic large cell neuroblastoma. Pediatr Dev Pathol. 2009;12(1):1–5.
29. Alsabeh R, Mazoujian G, Goates J, Medeiros LJ, Weiss LM. Adrenal cortical tumors clinically mimicking pheochromocytoma. Am J Clin Pathol. 1995;104(4):382–90.
30. Argani P, Erlandson RA, Rosai J. Thymic neuroblastoma in adults: report of three cases with special emphasis on its association with the syndrome of inappropriate secretion of antidiuretic hormone. Am J Clin Pathol. 1997;108(5):537–43.
31. Arola J, Liu J, Heikkila P, et al. Expression of inhibin alpha in adrenocortical tumours reflects the hormonal status of the neoplasm. J Endocrinol. 2000;165(2):223–9.
32. Clarke MR, Weyant RJ, Watson CG, Carty SE. Prognostic markers in pheochromocytoma. Hum Pathol. 1998;29(5):522–6.
33. Franquemont DW, Mills SE, Lack EE. Immunohistochemical detection of neuroblastomatous foci in composite adrenal pheochromocytoma–neuroblastoma. Am J Clin Pathol. 1994;102(2):163–70.
34. Hachitanda Y, Tsuneyoshi M, Enjoji M. An ultrastructural and immunohistochemical evaluation of cytodifferentiation in neuroblastic tumors. Mod Pathol. 1989;2(1):13–9.
35. Hoang MP, Ayala AG, Albores-Saavedra J. Oncocytic adrenocortical carcinoma: a morphologic, immunohistochemical and ultrastructural study of four cases. Mod Pathol. 2002;15(9):973–8.
36. Kimura N, Nakazato Y, Nagura H, Sasano N. Expression of intermediate filaments in neuroendocrine tumors. Arch Pathol Lab Med. 1990;114(5):506–10.
37. Komminoth P, Roth J, Schroder S, Saremaslani P, Heitz PU. Overlapping expression of immunohistochemical markers and synaptophysin mRNA in pheochromocytomas and adrenocortical carcinomas. Implications for the differential diagnosis of adrenal gland tumors. Lab Invest. 1995;72(4):424–31.
38. Loy TS, Phillips RW, Linder CL. A103 immunostaining in the diagnosis of adrenal cortical tumors: an immunohistochemical study of 316 cases. Arch Pathol Lab Med. 2002;126(2):170–2.
39. Mackenzie IS, Ashby MJ, Donovan T, Voutnis DD, Brown MJ. Bilateral adrenal masses: phaeochromocytoma or melanoma? J R Soc Med. 2006;99(3):153–5.
40. Sbragia L, Oliveira-Filho AG, Vassallo J, Pinto GA, Guerra-Junior G, Bustorff-Silva J. Adrenocortical tumors in Brazilian children: immunohistochemical markers and prognostic factors. Arch Pathol Lab Med. 2005;129(9):1127–31.
41. Shekitka KM, Sobin LH. Ganglioneuromas of the gastrointestinal tract. Relation to Von Recklinghausen disease and other multiple tumor syndromes. Am J Surg Pathol. 1994;18(3):250–7.
42. Smithey BE, Pappo AS, Hill DA. C-kit expression in pediatric solid tumors: a comparative immunohistochemical study. Am J Surg Pathol. 2002;26(4):486–92.
43. Stojadinovic A, Brennan MF, Hoos A, et al. Adrenocortical adenoma and carcinoma: histopathological and molecular comparative analysis. Mod Pathol. 2003;16(8):742–51.
44. Thomas JO, Olu-Eddo AA. Immunocytochemistry in the diagnosis of small blue cell tumours of childhood. West Afr J Med. 2006;25(3):199–204.
45. Wang LL, Perlman EJ, Vujanic GM, et al. Desmoplastic small round cell tumor of the kidney in childhood. Am J Surg Pathol. 2007;31(4):576–84.
46. Zhang PJ, Genega EM, Tomaszewski JE, Pasha TL, LiVolsi VA. The role of calretinin, inhibin, melan-A, BCL-2, and C-kit in differentiating adrenal cortical and medullary tumors: an immunohistochemical study. Mod Pathol. 2003;16(6):591–7.
47. Gaffey MJ, Traweek ST, Mills SE, et al. Cytokeratin expression in adrenocortical neoplasia: an immunohistochemical and biochemical study with implications for the differential diagnosis of adrenocortical, hepatocellular, and renal cell carcinoma. Hum Pathol. 1992;23(2):144–53.
48. Miettinen M. Neuroendocrine differentiation in adrenocortical carcinoma. New immunohistochemical findings supported by electron microscopy. Lab Invest. 1992;66(2):169–74.
49. Renshaw AA, Granter SR. A comparison of A103 and inhibin reactivity in adrenal cortical tumors: distinction from hepatocellular carcinoma and renal tumors. Mod Pathol. 1998;11(12):1160–4.
50. Schmitt A, Saremaslani P, Schmid S, et al. IGFII and MIB1 immunohistochemistry is helpful for the differentiation of benign from malignant adrenocortical tumours. Histopathology. 2006;49(3): 298–307.

51. Shin SJ, Hoda RS, Ying L, DeLellis RA. Diagnostic utility of the monoclonal antibody A103 in fine-needle aspiration biopsies of the adrenal. Am J Clin Pathol. 2000;113(2):295–302.
52. Vargas MP, Vargas HI, Kleiner DE, Merino MJ. Adrenocortical neoplasms: role of prognostic markers MIB-1, P53, and RB. Am J Surg Pathol. 1997;21(5):556–62.
53. Wick MR, Cherwitz DL, McGlennen RC, Dehner LP. Adrenocortical carcinoma. An immunohistochemical comparison with renal cell carcinoma. Am J Pathol. 1986;122(2):343–52.
54. Grignon DJ, Ro JY, Mackay B, et al. Paraganglioma of the urinary bladder: immunohistochemical, ultrastructural, and DNA flow cytometric studies. Hum Pathol. 1991;22(11):1162–9.
55. Lloyd RV, Blaivas M, Wilson BS. Distribution of chromogranin and S100 protein in normal and abnormal adrenal medullary tissues. Arch Pathol Lab Med. 1985;109(7):633–5.
56. Lloyd RV, Shapiro B, Sisson JC, Kalff V, Thompson NW, Beierwaltes WA. An immunohistochemical study of pheochromocytomas. Arch Pathol Lab Med. 1984;108(7):541–4.
57. Shipley WR, Hammer RD, Lennington WJ, Macon WR, et al. Paraffin immunohistochemical detection of CD56, a useful marker for neural cell adhesion molecule (NCAM) in normal and neoplastic fixed tissues. Appl Immunohistochem. 1997;5(2):87–93.
58. Sikri KL, Varndell IM, Hamid QA, et al. Medullary carcinoma of the thyroid. An immunocytochemical and histochemical study of 25 cases using eight separate markers. Cancer. 1985;56(10):2481–91.
59. Stevenson AJ, Chatten J, Bertoni F. CD99 (p30/32MIC2) neuroectodermal/Ewing's sarcoma antigen as an immunohistochemical marker: review of more than 600 tumors and the literature experience. Appl Immunohistochem. 1994;2:231–40.
60. Verhofstad AAJ, Steinbusch HWM, Joosten JWJ, Penke B, Varga J, Goldstein M. Immunocytochemical localization of noradrenaline, adrenaline and serotonin. In: Polak JM, Van Noorden S, editors. Immunocytochemistry: practical applications in pathology and biology. Bristol, England: Wright-PSG; 1983. p. 143.
61. DeLellis RA. Proliferation markers in neuroendocrine tumors: useful or useless? A critical reappraisal. Verh Dtsch Ges Pathol. 1997;81:53–61.
62. Fellinger EJ, Garin-Chesa P, Triche TJ, Huvos AG, Rettig WJ. Immunohistochemical analysis of Ewing's sarcoma cell surface antigen p30/32MIC2. Am J Pathol. 1991;139(2):317–25.
63. Hess E, Cohen C, DeRose PB, Yost B, Costa MD. Nonspecificity of p30/p32MIC2 immunolocalization with the 013 monoclonal antibody in the diagnosis of Ewing's sarcoma: application of an algorithmic immunohistochemical analysis. Appl Immunohistochem. 1997;5:94–103.
64. Miettinen M, Chatten J, Paetau A, Stevenson A. Monoclonal antibody NB84 in the differential diagnosis of neuroblastoma and other small round cell tumors. Am J Surg Pathol. 1998;22(3): 327–32.
65. Ordonez NG. Desmoplastic small round cell tumor: II: an ultrastructural and immunohistochemical study with emphasis on new immunohistochemical markers. Am J Surg Pathol. 1998;22(11): 1314–27.
66. Scotlandi K, Serra M, Manara MC, et al. Immunostaining of the p30/32MIC2 antigen and molecular detection of EWS rearrangements for the diagnosis of Ewing's sarcoma and peripheral neuroectodermal tumor. Hum Pathol. 1996;27(4):408–16.
67. Weidner N, Tjoe J. Immunohistochemical profile of monoclonal antibody O13: antibody that recognizes glycoprotein p30/32MIC2 and is useful in diagnosing Ewing's sarcoma and peripheral neuroepithelioma. Am J Surg Pathol. 1994;18(5):486–94.
68. Kurtin PJ, Bonin DM. Immunohistochemical demonstration of the lysosome-associated glycoprotein CD68 (KP-1) in granular cell tumors and schwannomas. Hum Pathol. 1994;25(11):1172–8.
69. Trojanowski JQ, Lee VM, Schlaepfer WW. An immunohistochemical study of human central and peripheral nervous system tumors, using monoclonal antibodies against neurofilaments and glial filaments. Hum Pathol. 1984;15(3):248–57.
70. Aydin H, Magi-Galluzzi C, Lane BR, et al. Renal angiomyolipoma: clinicopathologic study of 194 cases with emphasis on the epithelioid histology and tuberous sclerosis association. Am J Surg Pathol. 2009;33(2):289–97.
71. Davis CJ, Barton JH, Sesterhenn IA. Cystic angiomyolipoma of the kidney: a clinicopathologic description of 11 cases. Mod Pathol. 2006;19(5):669–74.
72. Eble JN, Amin MB, Young RH. Epithelioid angiomyolipoma of the kidney: a report of five cases with a prominent and diagnostically confusing epithelioid smooth muscle component. Am J Surg Pathol. 1997;21(10):1123–30.
73. Fetsch PA, Fetsch JF, Marincola FM, Travis W, Batts KP, Abati A. Comparison of melanoma antigen recognized by T cells (MART-1) to HMB-45: additional evidence to support a common lineage for angiomyolipoma, lymphangiomyomatosis, and clear cell sugar tumor. Mod Pathol. 1998;11(8):699–703.
74. Fujii T, Zen Y, Sato Y, et al. Podoplanin is a useful diagnostic marker for epithelioid hemangioendothelioma of the liver. Mod Pathol. 2008;21(2):125–30.
75. Hoon V, Thung SN, Kaneko M, Unger PD. HMB-45 reactivity in renal angiomyolipoma and lymphangioleiomyomatosis. Arch Pathol Lab Med. 1994;118(7):732–4.
76. Jimenez RE, Eble JN, Reuter VE, et al. Concurrent angiomyolipoma and renal cell neoplasia: a study of 36 cases. Mod Pathol. 2001;14(3):157–63.
77. L'Hostis H, Deminiere C, Ferriere JM, Coindre JM. Renal angiomyolipoma: a clinicopathologic, immunohistochemical, and follow-up study of 46 cases. Am J Surg Pathol. 1999;23(9):1011–20.
78. Makhlouf HR, Ishak KG, Shekar R, Sesterhenn IA, Young DY, Fanburg-Smith JC. Melanoma markers in angiomyolipoma of the liver and kidney: a comparative study. Arch Pathol Lab Med. 2002;126(1):49–55.
79. Makhlouf HR, Remotti HE, Ishak KG. Expression of KIT (CD117) in angiomyolipoma. Am J Surg Pathol. 2002;26(4):493–7.
80. Martignoni G, Pea M, Bonetti F, et al. Carcinomalike monotypic epithelioid angiomyolipoma in patients without evidence of tuberous sclerosis: a clinicopathologic and genetic study. Am J Surg Pathol. 1998;22(6):663–72.
81. Miettinen M, Fernandez M, Franssila K, Gatalica Z, Lasota J, Sarlomo-Rikala M. Microphthalmia transcription factor in the immunohistochemical diagnosis of metastatic melanoma: comparison with four other melanoma markers. Am J Surg Pathol. 2001;25(2):205–11.
82. Roma AA, Magi-Galluzzi C, Zhou M. Differential expression of melanocytic markers in myoid, lipomatous, and vascular components of renal angiomyolipomas. Arch Pathol Lab Med. 2007;131(1):122–5.
83. Sturtz CL, Dabbs DJ. Angiomyolipomas: the nature and expression of the HMB45 antigen. Mod Pathol. 1994;7(8):842–5.
84. Tsui WM, Colombari R, Portmann BC, et al. Hepatic angiomyolipoma: a clinicopathologic study of 30 cases and delineation of unusual morphologic variants. Am J Surg Pathol. 1999;23(1): 34–48.
85. Zavala-Pompa A, Folpe AL, Jimenez RE, et al. Immunohistochemical study of microphthalmia transcription factor and tyrosinase in angiomyolipoma of the kidney, renal cell carcinoma, and renal and retroperitoneal sarcomas: comparative evaluation with traditional diagnostic markers. Am J Surg Pathol. 2001;25(1):65–70.
86. Srivastava A, Padilla O, Fischer-Colbrie R, Tischler AS, Dayal Y. Neuroendocrine secretory protein-55 (NESP-55) expression discriminates pancreatic endocrine tumors and pheochromocytomas from gastrointestinal and pulmonary carcinoids. Am J Surg Pathol. 2004;28(10):1371–8.
87. Chu PG, Ishizawa S, Wu E, Weiss LM. Hepatocyte antigen as a marker of hepatocellular carcinoma: an immunohistochemical

comparison to carcinoembryonic antigen, CD10, and alpha-fetoprotein. Am J Surg Pathol. 2002;26(8):978–88.

88. De Young BR, Frierson Jr HF, Ly MN, Smith D, Swanson PE. CD31 immunoreactivity in carcinomas and mesotheliomas. Am J Clin Pathol. 1998;110(3):374–7.
89. Fan Z, van de Rijn M, Montgomery K, Rouse RV. Hep par 1 antibody stain for the differential diagnosis of hepatocellular carcinoma: 676 tumors tested using tissue microarrays and conventional tissue sections. Mod Pathol. 2003;16(2):137–44.
90. Higgins JP, Montgomery K, Wang L, et al. Expression of FKBP12 in benign and malignant vascular endothelium: an immunohistochemical study on conventional sections and tissue microarrays. Am J Surg Pathol. 2003;27(1):58–64.
91. Kaufmann O, Koch S, Burghardt J, Audring H, Dietel M. Tyrosinase, melan-A, and KBA62 as markers for the immunohistochemical identification of metastatic amelanotic melanomas on paraffin sections. Mod Pathol. 1998;11(8):740–6.
92. Kornstein MJ, Rosai J. CD5 labeling of thymic carcinomas and other nonlymphoid neoplasms. Am J Clin Pathol. 1998;109(6):722–6.
93. Lugli A, Tornillo L, Mirlacher M, Bundi M, Sauter G, Terracciano LM. Hepatocyte paraffin 1 expression in human normal and neoplastic tissues: tissue microarray analysis on 3,940 tissue samples. Am J Clin Pathol. 2004;122(5):721–7.
94. O'Connell FP, Pinkus JL, Pinkus GS. CD138 (syndecan-1), a plasma cell marker immunohistochemical profile in hematopoietic and nonhematopoietic neoplasms. Am J Clin Pathol. 2004;121(2):254–63.
95. Oliveira AM, Tazelaar HD, Myers JL, Erickson LA, Lloyd RV. Thyroid transcription factor-1 distinguishes metastatic pulmonary from well-differentiated neuroendocrine tumors of other sites. Am J Surg Pathol. 2001;25(6):815–9.
96. Petri BJ, Speel EJ, Korpershoek E, et al. Frequent loss of 17p, but no p53 mutations or protein overexpression in benign and malignant pheochromocytomas. Mod Pathol. 2008;21(4):407–13.
97. Srodon M, Westra WH. Immunohistochemical staining for thyroid transcription factor-1: a helpful aid in discerning primary site of tumor origin in patients with brain metastases. Hum Pathol. 2002;33(6):642–5.
98. Thompson LD. Pheochromocytoma of the adrenal gland scaled score (PASS) to separate benign from malignant neoplasms: a clinicopathologic and immunophenotypic study of 100 cases. Am J Surg Pathol. 2002;26(5):551–66.
99. Wieczorek TJ, Pinkus JL, Glickman JN, Pinkus GS. Comparison of thyroid transcription factor-1 and hepatocyte antigen immunohistochemical analysis in the differential diagnosis of hepatocellular carcinoma, metastatic adenocarcinoma, renal cell carcinoma, and adrenal cortical carcinoma. Am J Clin Pathol. 2002;118(6):911–21.
100. Frierson Jr HF, Moskaluk CA, Powell SM, et al. Large-scale molecular and tissue microarray analysis of mesothelin expression in common human carcinomas. Hum Pathol. 2003;34(6):605–9.
101. Iezzoni JC, Mills SE, Pelkey TJ, Stoler MH. Inhibin is not an immunohistochemical marker for hepatocellular carcinoma. An example of the potential pitfall in diagnostic immunohistochemistry caused by endogenous biotin. Am J Clin Pathol. 1999;111(2):229–34.
102. Kaiserling E, Xiao JC, Ruck P, Horny HP. Aberrant expression of macrophage-associated antigens (CD68 and Ki-M1P) by Schwann cells in reactive and neoplastic neural tissue. Light- and electron-microscopic findings. Mod Pathol. 1993;6(4):463–8.
103. Kakar S, Muir T, Murphy LM, Lloyd RV, Burgart LJ. Immunoreactivity of Hep Par 1 in hepatic and extrahepatic tumors and its correlation with albumin in situ hybridization in hepatocellular carcinoma. Am J Clin Pathol. 2003;119(3):361–6.
104. Lau SK, Prakash S, Geller SA, Alsabeh R. Comparative immunohistochemical profile of hepatocellular carcinoma, cholangiocarcinoma, and metastatic adenocarcinoma. Hum Pathol. 2002;33(12):1175–81.
105. Lau SK, Weiss LM, Chu PG. Differential expression of MUC1, MUC2, and MUC5AC in carcinomas of various sites: an immunohistochemical study. Am J Clin Pathol. 2004;122(1):61–9.
106. Lee ES, Han EM, Kim YS, et al. Occurrence of c-kit+ tumor cells in hepatitis B virus-associated hepatocellular carcinoma. Am J Clin Pathol. 2005;124(1):31–6.
107. Lee MJ, Lee HS, Kim WH, Choi Y, Yang M. Expression of mucins and cytokeratins in primary carcinomas of the digestive system. Mod Pathol. 2003;16(5):403–10.
108. Micchelli ST, Vivekanandan P, Boitnott JK, Pawlik TM, Choti MA, Torbenson M. Malignant transformation of hepatic adenomas. Mod Pathol. 2008;21(4):491–7.
109. Minervini MI, Demetris AJ, Lee RG, Carr BI, Madariaga J, Nalesnik MA. Utilization of hepatocyte-specific antibody in the immunocytochemical evaluation of liver tumors. Mod Pathol. 1997;10(7):686–92.
110. Murakata LA, Ishak KG, Nzeako UC. Clear cell carcinoma of the liver: a comparative immunohistochemical study with renal clear cell carcinoma. Mod Pathol. 2000;13(8):874–81.
111. Ordonez NG. Application of mesothelin immunostaining in tumor diagnosis. Am J Surg Pathol. 2003;27(11):1418–28.
112. Pan CC, Chen PC, Tsay SH, Chiang H. Cytoplasmic immunoreactivity for thyroid transcription factor-1 in hepatocellular carcinoma: a comparative immunohistochemical analysis of four commercial antibodies using a tissue array technique. Am J Clin Pathol. 2004;121(3):343–9.
113. Sasaki M, Tsuneyama K, Ishikawa A, Nakanuma Y. Intrahepatic cholangiocarcinoma in cirrhosis presents granulocyte and granulocyte-macrophage colony-stimulating factor. Hum Pathol. 2003;34(12):1337–44.
114. Terracciano LM, Glatz K, Mhawech P, et al. Hepatoid adenocarcinoma with liver metastasis mimicking hepatocellular carcinoma: an immunohistochemical and molecular study of eight cases. Am J Surg Pathol. 2003;27(10):1302–12.
115. Tickoo SK, Zee SY, Obiekwe S, et al. Combined hepatocellular-cholangiocarcinoma: a histopathologic, immunohistochemical, and in situ hybridization study. Am J Surg Pathol. 2002;26(8):989–97.
116. Yamauchi N, Watanabe A, Hishinuma M, et al. The glypican 3 oncofetal protein is a promising diagnostic marker for hepatocellular carcinoma. Mod Pathol. 2005;18(12):1591–8.
117. Hasegawa T, Hirose T, Ayala AG, et al. Adult neuroblastoma of the retroperitoneum and abdomen: clinicopathologic distinction from primitive neuroectodermal tumor. Am J Surg Pathol. 2001;25(7):918–24.
118. Pituch-Noworolska A, Zaremba M, Wieczorek A. Expression of proteins associated with therapy resistance in rhabdomyosarcoma and neuroblastoma tumour cells. Pol J Pathol. 2009;60(4):168–73.
119. Goldsmith JD, Pawel B, Goldblum JR, et al. Detection and diagnostic utilization of placental alkaline phosphatase in muscular tissue and tumors with myogenic differentiation. Am J Surg Pathol. 2002;26(12):1627–33.
120. Hasegawa T, Matsuno Y, Niki T, et al. Second primary rhabdomyosarcomas in patients with bilateral retinoblastoma: a clinicopathologic and immunohistochemical study. Am J Surg Pathol. 1998;22(11):1351–60.
121. Heerema-McKenney A, Wijnaendts LC, Pulliam JF, et al. Diffuse myogenin expression by immunohistochemistry is an independent marker of poor survival in pediatric rhabdomyosarcoma: a tissue microarray study of 71 primary tumors including correla-

tion with molecular phenotype. Am J Surg Pathol. 2008;32(10): 1513–22.
122. Nascimento AF, Fletcher CD. Spindle cell rhabdomyosarcoma in adults. Am J Surg Pathol. 2005;29(8):1106–13.
123. Wang J, Tu X, Sheng W. Sclerosing rhabdomyosarcoma: a clinicopathologic and immunohistochemical study of five cases. Am J Clin Pathol. 2008;129(3):410–5.
124. Gustafson S, Medeiros LJ, Kalhor N, Bueso-Ramos CE. Anaplastic large cell lymphoma: another entity in the differential diagnosis of small round blue cell tumors. Ann Diagn Pathol. 2009;13(6): 413–27.
125. Kagami Y, Suzuki R, Taji H, et al. Nodal cytotoxic lymphoma spectrum: a clinicopathologic study of 66 patients. Am J Surg Pathol. 1999;23(10):1184–200.
126. Osajima-Hakomori Y, Miyake I, Ohira M, Nakagawara A, Nakagawa A, Sakai R. Biological role of anaplastic lymphoma kinase in neuroblastoma. Am J Pathol. 2005;167(1):213–22.
127. Passoni L, Longo L, Collini P, et al. Mutation-independent anaplastic lymphoma kinase overexpression in poor prognosis neuroblastoma patients. Cancer Res. 2009;69(18):7338–46.
128. Rassidakis GZ, Georgakis GV, Oyarzo M, Younes A, Medeiros LJ. Lack of c-kit (CD117) expression in CD30+ lymphomas and lymphomatoid papulosis. Mod Pathol. 2004;17(8):946–53.
129. Folpe AL, Goldblum JR, Rubin BP, et al. Morphologic and immunophenotypic diversity in Ewing family tumors: a study of 66 genetically confirmed cases. Am J Surg Pathol. 2005;29(8): 1025–33.
130. Frostad B, Tani E, Brosjo O, Skoog L, Kogner P. Fine needle aspiration cytology in the diagnosis and management of children and adolescents with Ewing sarcoma and peripheral primitive neuroectodermal tumor. Med Pediatr Oncol. 2002;38(1):33–40.
131. Macak J, Mukensnabl P, Kawano N, Bobot L, Duskova M, Vacha P. Intra-abdominal desmoplastic small-cell tumor of the peritoneum [in Czech]. Cesk Patol. 2003;39(2):69–75.
132. Olsen SH, Thomas DG, Lucas DR. Cluster analysis of immunohistochemical profiles in synovial sarcoma, malignant peripheral nerve sheath tumor, and Ewing sarcoma. Mod Pathol. 2006;19(5):659–68.
133. Terrier-Lacombe MJ, Guillou L, Chibon F, et al. Superficial primitive Ewing's sarcoma: a clinicopathologic and molecular cytogenetic analysis of 14 cases. Mod Pathol. 2009;22(1):87–94.
134. Wong NA, Melegh Z. Antigen retrieval and primary antibody type affect sensitivity but not specificity of CD117 immunohistochemistry. Histopathology. 2009;54(5):529–38.
135. Beaty MW, Fetsch P, Wilder AM, Marincola F, Abati A. Effusion cytology of malignant melanoma. A morphologic and immunocytochemical analysis including application of the MART-1 antibody. Cancer. 1997;81(1):57–63.
136. Hitchcock MG, McCalmont TH, White WL. Cutaneous melanoma with myxoid features: twelve cases with differential diagnosis. Am J Surg Pathol. 1999;23(12):1506–13.
137. King R, Busam K, Rosai J. Metastatic malignant melanoma resembling malignant peripheral nerve sheath tumor: report of 16 cases. Am J Surg Pathol. 1999;23(12):1499–505.
138. Bastide C, Arroua F, Carcenac A, Anfossi E, Ragni E, Rossi D. Primary malignant melanoma of the adrenal gland. Int J Urol. 2006;13(5):608–10.
139. Nonaka D, Laser J, Tucker R, Melamed J. Immunohistochemical evaluation of necrotic malignant melanomas. Am J Clin Pathol. 2007;127(5):787–91.
140. Wilson RW, Moran CA. Primary melanoma of the lung: a clinicopathologic and immunohistochemical study of eight cases. Am J Surg Pathol. 1997;21(10):1196–202.

Chapter 13
Salivary Gland and Other Head and Neck Structures

Conrad Schuerch

Abstract This chapter is designed as an easy reference for the practicing pathologist aiming to solve diagnostic problems in head and neck pathology by immunohistochemistry (IHC). It is a collection of 38 practical tables including tables for commonly used antibodies, IHC reactions in normal salivary gland, IHC reactions in common salivary gland and head and neck tumors, and IHC reactions to resolve differential diagnostic challenges. Also included are practical footnotes and photographic illustrations.

Keywords Head and neck pathology • Immunohistochemistry • Salivary gland tumors • Antibodies

Summary of frequently used antibodies (Table 13.1) (pp. 174–177)

FREQUENTLY ASKED QUESTIONS

Salivary Gland

1. Markers in normal salivary gland (Fig. 13.1, Table 13.2) (p. 178)
2. Markers for selected benign salivary gland tumors (Fig. 13.2, Table 13.3) (p. 179)
3. Markers for Warthin's tumor (Fig. 13.3a, b, Table 13.4) (p. 180)
4. Markers for oncocytoma (Table 13.5) (p. 180)
5. Markers for mucoepidermoid carcinoma (Table 13.6) (p. 180)
6. Markers for polymorphous low-grade adenocarcinoma (Fig. 13.4, Table 13.7) (p. 181)
7. Markers for adenoid cystic carcinoma (Table 13.8) (p. 181)
8. Markers for acinic cell carcinoma (Table 13.9) (p. 181)
9. Markers for salivary duct adenocarcinoma (Fig. 13.5a, b, Table 13.10) (p. 182)
10. Markers for basal cell adenocarcinoma (Table 13.11) (p. 182)
11. Markers for myoepithelioma, epithelial–myoepithelial carcinoma (Table 13.12) (p. 182)
12. Markers for hyalinizing clear cell carcinoma (Fig. 13.6a, b, Table 13.13) (p. 183)
13. Markers for small cell neuroendocrine carcinoma (Table 13.14) (p. 183)
14. Adenoid cystic carcinoma (ACC) vs. polymorphic low-grade adenocarcinoma (PLGA) vs. basal cell adenoma (BCA) or pleomorphic adenoma (PA) (benign mixed tumor) (Table 13.15) (p. 183)
15. Clear cell epithelial tumors, differential diagnosis: hyalinizing clear cell carcinoma (HCCC) vs. metastatic renal cell carcinoma (MRCC) vs. oncocytoma with clear cell features (Ons) vs. mucoepidermoid carcinoma (OMEC) (Fig. 13.7a, b, Table 13.16) (p. 184)
16. Hyalinizing clear cell carcinoma (HCCC) vs. clear cells in epithelial–myoepithelial carcinoma (CMEC) vs. clear cell myoepithelioma (CCM) (Table 13.17) (p. 184)
17. Oncocytic epithelial tumors, differential diagnosis: oncocytoma and oncocytic carcinoma (O) vs. oncocytic mucoepidermoid carcinoma (OMEC) vs. acinic cell carcinoma (AC) vs. metastatic renal cell carcinoma (RCC) vs. salivary duct carcinoma (SDC) (Table 13.18) (p. 185)
18. Mucoepidermoid carcinoma, high grade (MECHG) vs. squamous carcinoma (SC) (Table 13.19) (p. 185)

Tumors of Larynx, Nasopharynx, and Oropharynx

1. Markers for normal nonkeratinized squamous mucosal epithelium (NLSq), keratosis with dysplasia (KD), invasive squamous carcinoma (Table 13.20) (p. 185)
2. Markers for spindle cell squamous carcinoma (SSC) or carcinosarcoma (Fig. 13.8, Table 13.21) (p. 186)
3. Markers for basaloid squamous carcinoma (BSC) vs. adenoid cystic carcinoma (ACC) vs. small cell carcinoma, neuroendocrine type (SCN) (Fig. 13.9, Table 13.22) (p. 186)
4. Markers for squamous carcinoma (SC), basaloid squamous carcinoma (BSC), and lymphoepithelial (nasopharyngeal) carcinoma (LEC) (Fig. 13.10, Table 13.23) (p. 186)
5. *NUT* midline carcinoma (NMC) vs. sinonasal undifferentiated carcinoma (SNUC) vs. nasopharyngeal carcinoma

C. Schuerch (✉)
Department of Pathology and Laboratory Medicine, Geisinger Medical Center, 100 N. Academy Avenue, Danville, PA 17822, USA
e-mail: cschuerch@geisinger.edu

F. Lin and J. Prichard (eds.), *Handbook of Practical Immunohistochemistry: Frequently Asked Questions*,
DOI 10.1007/978-1-4419-8062-5_13, © Springer Science+Business Media, LLC 2011

(NPC) vs. small cell neuroendocrine carcinoma (SCN) (Table 13.24) (p. 187)
6. Markers for Kaposi's sarcoma and angiosarcoma (Table 13.25) (p. 187)
7. Markers for small cell carcinoma of other sites vs. Merkel cell carcinoma (Table 13.26) (p. 187)
8. Markers for neuroendocrine tumors of the larynx: carcinoid, atypical carcinoid, small cell carcinoma (Fig. 13.11a, b, Table 13.27) (p. 187)

Nose and Nasal Sinus

1. Markers for olfactory neuroblastoma (Table 13.28) (p. 188)
2. Markers for sinonasal hemangiopericytoma (Table 13.29) (p. 188)
3. Markers for intestinal-type sinonasal adenocarcinoma (Table 13.30) (p. 188)
4. Markers for sinonasal teratocarcinosarcoma (Table 13.31) (p. 188)
5. Markers for lymphomas of upper aerodigestive tract (Table 13.32) (p. 188)
6. Poorly differentiated sinonasal tumors: olfactory neuroblastoma (ONB), sinonasal undifferentiated carcinoma (SNUC), lymphoepithelial (or poorly differentiated nasopharyngeal) carcinoma (LEC), melanoma (M), lymphoma (L) (Table 13.33) (p. 189)
7. Differential of small blue cell tumors of the head and neck: olfactory neuroblastoma (ONB), alveolar rhabdomyosarcoma (ARS), embryonal rhabdomyosarcoma (ERS), small cell neuroendocrine carcinoma (SCN), lymphoma (LYM), Ewings sarcoma/PNET (ES/PNET), synovial sarcoma (SS), mesenchymal chondrosarcoma (MC) (Table 13.34) (p. 190)

Middle Ear

1. Middle ear adenoma (MEA) vs. paraganglioma (PG) vs. endolymphatic sac tumor (EST) (Fig. 13.12, Table 13.35) (p. 190)
2. Markers for endolymphatic sac tumor (EST) vs. choroid plexus papilloma (CPP) (Table 13.36) (p. 190)

Jaws

1. Markers for clear cell odontogenic carcinoma (Table 13.37) (p. 190)
2. Odontogenic keratocyst (keratocystic odontogenic tumor [KCOT]) vs. dentigerous cyst vs. cystic ameloblastoma (Table 13.38) (p. 190)

Table 13.1 Summary of frequently used antibodies

Antibodies	Staining pattern	Function	Key applications and pitfalls
34BetaE12 (CK903)	M + C	High molecular wt. cytokeratin cocktail including CK1, 5, 10, and 14	Basal cell marker
Alpha amylase	C	Enzyme which hydrolyses polysaccharides to simple sugars	Pancreatic and salivary gland acinar cells
Alpha-SMA	C	Contractile protein	Smooth muscle, myofibroblasts, myoepithelial cells. Variable staining in myoepithelial cells
AR	N	Androgen receptor	Positive in salivary duct adenocarcinoma, carcinoma ex pleomorphic adenoma, and occasionally in other salivary tumors. Has been reported in acinic cells
B72.3	M + C	Tumor-associated glycoprotein	Widely distributed in adenocarcinomas but present in few normal epithelia
Bcl2	M + C + N	Membrane protein, oncogene product, apoptosis inhibitor	Expressed in follicular-derived B-cell lymphomas and many other tumors. Present in normal T-cells and B-cell subsets and other tissues
BerEP4, MOC 31	M + C	Epithelial cell adhesion molecule	Expressed in most epithelia but not in normal adult squamous epithelium and hepatocytes
c-kit, KIT, CD117	M	Transmembrane receptor-type tyrosine kinase	Positive in adenoid cystic carcinoma, mucosal melanoma; often positive in basaloid squamous cell carcinoma, basal cell adenocarcinoma
Calcitonin	C	Calcium regulatory hormone produced by the C-cells of the thyroid	Present in medullary thyroid cancer, often in atypical carcinoid of the larynx, and occasional, in neuroendocrine tumors
Calponin	C	Calcium-binding protein; inhibits smooth muscle ATPase	Marker for smooth muscle, myofibroblasts, myoepithelial cells
Calretinin	C or N + C	Calcium-binding protein	Present in mesothelial cells, adipocytes, neural cells, and sex cord tumors
CD2	M	Cell adhesion molecule	T cells and natural killer cells
CD3	M	Part of T-cell antigen receptor complex	T cells

(continued)

Table 13.1 (continued)

Antibodies	Staining pattern	Function	Key applications and pitfalls
CD10	M	Neprilisyn. Zinc-dependent membrane metalol-endo-peptidase, also known as common acute lympho-blastic leukemia antigen	Stains follicular center cells, acute lymphocytic leukemia, and some renal cell carcinomas
CD20	M	Nonglycosylated phosphopro-tein on cell membrane	B cells
CD31	M + C	Platelet endothelial cell adhesion marker, PECAM-1	Endothelial marker. Also expressed on hematopoietic cells
CD34	C + M	Surface glycoprotein, adhesion molecule	Marker for myeloblasts, lymphoblasts, endothelial cells. Positive in several types of soft tissue tumors
CD38	M	Activation antigen on lymphocytes	Positive on plasma cells, natural killer cells
CD45 (LCA)	M + C	Leukocyte common antigen. Transmembrane protein phosphatase receptor C	Reacts with all leukocytes except plasma cells. Isoforms, e.g., CD45RA, have more restricted leukocyte distributions
CD56	M + C	Neural cell adhesion molecule	Positive in neuroendocrine tumors, natural killer cells
CD57	M	Adhesion molecule	Marker for NK cells, T-cell subset, neuroendocrine cells
CD68	C + M	Glycoprotein that binds to low density lipoprotein	Marker for monocytes, macrophages, histiocytes, granulocytes
CD79a	C	Ig-alpha protein of B-cell surface receptor complex	B cells and plasma cells
CD99	M	MIC2 gene glycoprotein product	Marker for immature T-cells. Positive in several primitive small blue cell tumors
CD138	C + M	Syndecan 1	Marker for plasma cells, some epithelial cells
CD141, Thrombomodulin	M	Membrane protein on endothelial cells which binds thrombin	Endothelial marker; also binds a subset of dendritic cells
CDX2	N	A caudal related homeobox transcription factor	Expressed in intestinal epithelium
CEA	M, C	Glycoprotein adhesion molecule normally encountered in fetal tissues	Luminal/acinar differentiation
Chromogranin	C	Neuroendocrine secretory protein	Present in neurosecretory granules
CKAE1/AE3	M + C	Pankeratin cocktail containing high and low molecular weight keratins	Identifies epithelial cells
CK1	C	Basic, high molecular weight keratin	Spinous and intermediate cells of the epidermis
CK5/6	M + C	Basic keratins	Squamous and basal cells
CK7	M + C	Basic, low molecular weight keratin	+ Simple epithelia. + In many salivary tumors, adenocarci-nomas, and a subgroup of squamous carcinomas
CK8 (CAM5.2)	C	Low molecular weight keratin	Luminal ductal, acinar cells
CK10	C	Acidic, high molecular weight keratin	Positive in keratinizing epithelia
CK13	C	Acidic, high molecular weight keratin	Positive on esophageal and other internal stratified epithelia
CK14	C	Acidic, high molecular weight keratin	Basal cells, myoepithelium and some epithelium in tumors
CK17	C	Acidic, low molecular weight keratin	Positive in nail beds, hair follicles, sebaceous glands, and epidermal appendages
CK18	C	Acidic, low molecular weight keratin	Luminal/acinar epithelium
CK19	C	Acidic, low molecular weight keratin	Simple epithelia, some basal cells. Ductal elements in salivary tumors
CK20	M + C	Acidic, low molecular weight keratin	+ In Merkel cell carcinoma, small cell carcinoma of salivary gland, intestinal type sinonasal adenocarci-noma. Negative in most other head and neck tumors

(continued)

Table 13.1 (continued)

Antibodies	Staining pattern	Function	Key applications and pitfalls
D2-40, Podoplanin	M, C	Podoplanin, a mucin-type transmembrane glycoprotein	Positive normally in lymphatic endothelial cells, mesothelial cells, and basal cells of some benign squamous epithelia. Positive in premalignant and maligant squamous lesions of the head and neck and other tumors
Desmin	C	Intermediate filament related to the sarcomere	Positive in smooth, skeletal, and cardiac muscle
EBER ISH, EBV		Demonstration by in situ hybridization of the presence of Epstein–Barr Virus (EBV)-encoded early RNA	Positive in nasopharyngeal carcinoma, Burkitt, T/NK, plasmablastic and posttransplant lymphomas
Estrogen receptor	N	Estrogen receptors	Present in metastatic breast cancer, occasionally in salivary duct carcinoma
Factor XIIIa	C	Subunit of plasma clotting factor XII	Dermal dendrocyte marker
Fascin	C	Actin cross-link binding protein	Marker of dysplasia in inverted papillomas. Upregulated in carcinomas from several other sites
FLI1	N	Nuclear transcription factor	Endothelial marker and positive in Ewing sarcoma/PNET
GCDFP-15	C	Gross cystic disease fluid protein 15	Glycoprotein associated with apocrine differentiation
GFAP	C	Intermediate filament of cytoskeleton	Marker of astrocytes. Also positive in pleomorphic adenoma, some myoepitheliomas, and myoepithelial carcinomas
h-Caldesmon	C	Protein thought to regulate cellular contraction	Found in smooth muscle cells
HER2/neu	M	Human epidermal growth factor receptor 2. Receptor tyrosine kinase involved in signal transduction leading to cell growth and differentiation	Prognostic marker in breast cancer. Positive in some salivary duct adenocarcinomas
HHV8	N	Latent nuclear antigen of human herpesvirus type 8	Positive in Kaposi's sarcoma, primary effusion lymphoma
HMB45	C	Recognizes the antigen gp100 on melanosomes	Positive in melanoma and PEComas
HPV ISH	N	Demonstration of HPV by in situ hybridization	The identification of squamous carcinomas induced by high-risk HPV types is becoming clinically important
Ki67 (Mib1)	N	Proliferation marker	Expressed in cells in G1, M, G2, and S phases of the cell cycle (i.e., all phases except the resting phase)
Lactoferrin	C	Globular protein	Antimicrobial protein found in milk, tears, and saliva
Laminin	Extracellular	Protein in the basal lamina (basement membrane)	Endothelial, smooth muscle, and Schwann cells are surrounded by basement membrane
Maspin	C	Serine protease inhibitor	Stains basal cells in normal salivary gland. Related to prognosis in oral squamous cell carcinoma and salivary carcinomas
MelanA (MART1)	C	Protein, micropthalmia-associated transcription factor	Expressed in melanoma
Metallothionein		Heavy metal binding protein family	Found in myoepithelial cells, and basal cells of squamous epithelium. Inducible in normal elements adjacent to tumors. Present in a wide variety of tumors
Antimitochondrial	C	Mitochondria	In salivary gland, staining is limited to striated ducts. Positive in oncocytic cells, mucoepidermoid carcinoma
MSA	C	Contractile protein	Muscle marker
MUC1, EMA	M	Membrane-bound mucin (transmembrane glycoprotein)	Wide anatomic distribution. Highlights luminal, acinar differentiation in salivary tumors
MUC2	C	Secreted mucin	Found in goblet cells
MUC3		Membrane-bound mucin	Intestinal-associated mucin
MUC4	M	Membrane-bound mucin	Positive in endodermal-derived epithelia

(continued)

Table 13.1 (continued)

Antibodies	Staining pattern	Function	Key applications and pitfalls
MUC5AC	C	Secreted mucin	Respiratory tract
MUC6	C	Secreted mucin	Upper GI, salivary glands
MyoD1	N	Protein which regulates muscle differentiation	Present in immature skeletal muscle cells. Marker for rhabdomyosarcoma. Cytoplasmic staining is not specific for skeletal muscle differentiation
Myogenin	N	Transcription factor, member of the MyoD family involved in skeletal muscle development and repair	Marker for rhabdomyosarcoma. Cytoplasmic staining is not specific for skeletal muscle
NFP	C	Neurofilament protein intermediate filament	Found in neurons and neuronal-derived tumors
NSE	C	Neuron-specific enolase	Marker for neuronal cells and cells with neuroendocrine differentiation. Not specific as the antibody reacts with many other tissues. Additional markers are always needed to support a diagnosis of neuroendocrine or neural tumor
NUT		Recombinant *NUT* gene protein product	Marker for NUT midline carcinoma
P16	N	Cell cycle checkpoint regulator	Overexpressed in squamous carcinoma/dysplasia related to HPV infection
P53	N	Tumor suppressor protein. With P53 gene mutation abnormal forms may accumulate	Positive in many squamous cell carcinomas and some squamous dysplasia. In salivary tumors, P53 expression may indicate dedifferentiation, e.g., in dedifferentiated acinic cell carcinoma, basal cell adenocarcinoma, hybrid carcinomas, and epithelial–myoepithelial carcinomas
P63	N	Member of P53 family of transcription factors	Basal cells of squamous epithelium, and of salivary striated and excretory ducts. Some myoepithelial cells
Pankeratin	C	Several keratins	Epithelial cells
Progesterone receptor	N	Progesterone receptors	Present in meningioma, rarely in other head and neck tumors
PPAR γ	C	Peroxisome proliferator–activator receptor gamma, a nuclear hormone receptor	Expressed in salivary duct carcinoma, adipose tissue, and several carcinomas from other sites
pVHL	M	Von Hippel–Lindau gene product, a tumor suppressor protein	Positive in renal cell carcinoma, oncocytoma
RCC	C + M	Glycoprotein	Present in most renal cell carcinomas
S100 protein	N, C	Calcium binding proteins	Dendritic, antigen presenting cells, myoepithelial cells, melanocytes, chondrocytes, neural elements, lipocytes, some epithelial cells. Not specific or universally expressed in myoepithelium. Various isoforms have different patterns of reactivity
SMM heavy chain (SSMHC)	C	Contractile protein subunit	Smooth muscle, myofibroblasts, myoepithelial cells
Synaptophysin	C	Synaptic vesicle membrane protein	Present in secretory granules of neuroendocrine and neural cells
Transthyretin	C	Protein carrier of thyroxine	Positive in choroid plexus and liver
TTF1	N	Thyroid transcription factor-1, protein that regulates transcription of genes specific to thyroid, lung, and diencephalon	Thyroid cells, pulmonary alveolar lining cells, and their neoplastic counterparts. Small cell carcinoma especially of the lung and salivary gland
Vimentin	C	Intermediate filament of cytoskeleton	Mesenchymal cells, myoepithelial cells, spindled carcinoma cells, melanocytes, endocrine cells, endothelial cells, and many others
WT1	N, C	Tumor suppressor gene product	Positive in Wilms' tumor and a variety of other tumors

Note: *N* nuclear staining, *M* membranous staining, *C* cytoplasmic staining

References: [1–27]

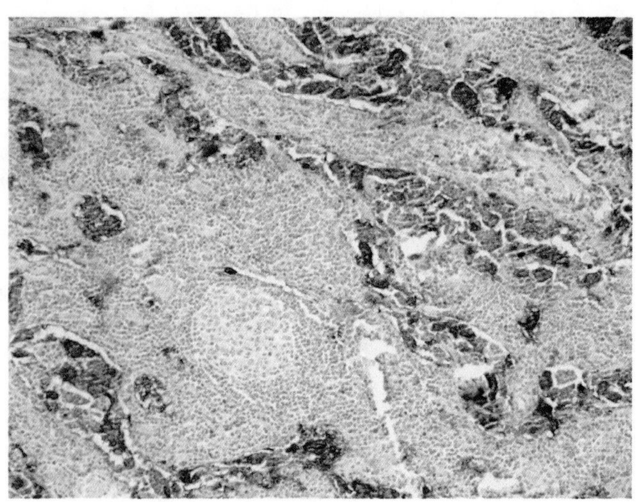

Fig. 13.1 S100 staining of sinus histiocytes in Rosai-Dorfman disease in cervical lymph node of a 7-year-old girl

Table 13.2 Markers in normal salivary gland

	Interlobular/ excretory duct luminal cell	Interlobular/ excretory duct basal cell	Striated duct cell	Intercalated (intralobular) duct luminal cell	Intercalated duct myoepithelial cell	Acinar epithelial cell	Periacinar myoepithelial cell
Alpha-SMA	–	–	–	–	+	–	+
Calponin	–	–	–	–	+	–	+
CEA	+ Luminal	–	–	+	–	+	–
CK5	nd	+	nd	nd	+	nd	+
CK7	+	+ Weak	+	+	+ Weak	+	+ Weak/–
CK8	–	–/Weak	+	+	–	+	–
CK13	+	–	nd	–	–	–	–
CK14	nd	+	nd	+/–	+	–	+
CK18	+	–/Weak	+	+	–	+	–
CK19	+	+ Weak	+	+	–/Weak	–/Weak	–/Weak
CK20	–	–	–	–	–	–	–
EMA	+ Luminal	–	–	+	–	+	nd
GFAP	–	–	–/+	–	–	–	–
h-Caldesmon	–	–	–	–	+	–	+
Lactoferrin	–	–	–	–	–	+	–
Mitochondrial Ag	–	–	+	–	–	–	–
MUC1	+ Apical	–	nd	+ Apical	–	–/+ Rare, focal	nd
MUC2	+ Focal	–	nd	nd	–	–	nd
MUC4	+ Apical	–	+/– Apical	nd	–	–/+ Weak, focal	nd
MUC5AC	+ Focal	–	nd	–/+	–	–	nd
P63	–	+	–	–	+	–	+/–
pVHL[a]	+	–	+	+	+	–	–
S100	–	–	–	+	+	–	+
SMMHC	–	–	–	–	+	–	+
Vimentin	–	–	–	–	+	–	+
WT1	–	–	–	–	–	–	–

Note: Striated ducts are present only in the major salivary glands

Note: Antibodies to various isoforms of S100 protein have very different staining patterns, some strongly positive in ductal luminal cells

[a] Geisinger experience with pVHL

References: [28–52]

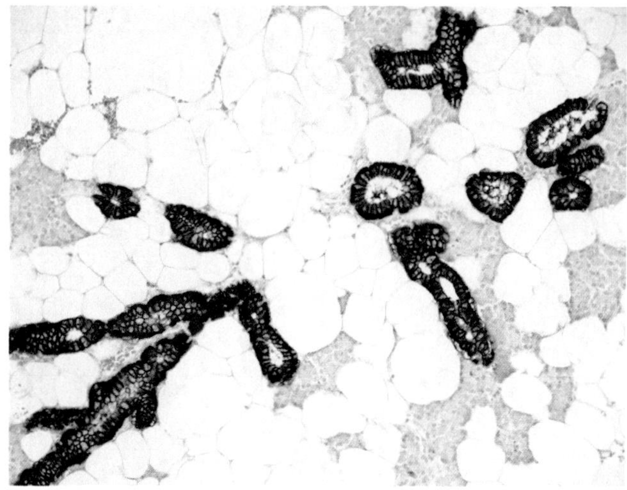

Fig. 13.2 Benign parotid tissue stained for pVHL shows strong positivity of intralobular and striated ducts, no staining of acini

Table 13.3 Markers for selected benign salivary gland tumors

Antibodies	Canalicular adenoma	Basal cell adenoma	Pleomorphic adenoma (benign mixed tumor)[a]	Myoepithelioma
Alpha-SMA	–	+ In peripheral and abluminal layers[b]	+	+
Calponin	–	+ In peripheral and abluminal cells[b]	+	+
CEA	–	+	+ Luminal	–
CKAE1/AE3	+	+	+	+
CK7	+	+ Luminal and solid areas	+ Luminal	+/–
CK14	–/+	+	+ Luminal, + abluminal	+
CK19	+	+ Luminal and solid	+ Luminal	+ Ductal
CK20	–	–	–	–
Desmin	–	–	–	–
EMA	–/+ Focal	+	nd	–
GFAP	–/Rare	–	Focal +/–	Focal +/–
MSA	–	–/+ Nonluminal	Focal –/+	
P63	–/+	+[c]	+	+
S100	+	Focal +	+	+
SMMHC	–	Focal +	Focal +	Focal +
Vimentin	–	+ Outer layers of epithelial nests	+	+
WT1[d]	nd	nd	+	nd

[a] In pleomorphic adenomas, there is a spectrum of myoepithelial differentiation. Outer tubular cells stain consistently with myoepithelial markers but modified myoepithelium (myxoid, cartilaginous, or hyaline) or transformed myoepithelium (epithelioid sheets and basaloid) stain less consistently

[b] This pattern is present in trabecular, tubular, solid, and membranous types of basal cell adenomas. In the membranous type, cells surrounding the hyaline cylinders are also positive

[c] Basal cell adenomas and canalicular adenomas of the upper lip were negative for P63 in the study by Edwards et al.

[d] Recently, WT-1 has been reported to stain more consistently across the spectrum of neoplastic myoepithelial differentiation in pleomorphic adenomas. WT-1 is not expressed in normal salivary tissue

References: [21, 29, 40, 43, 44, 51, 53–63]

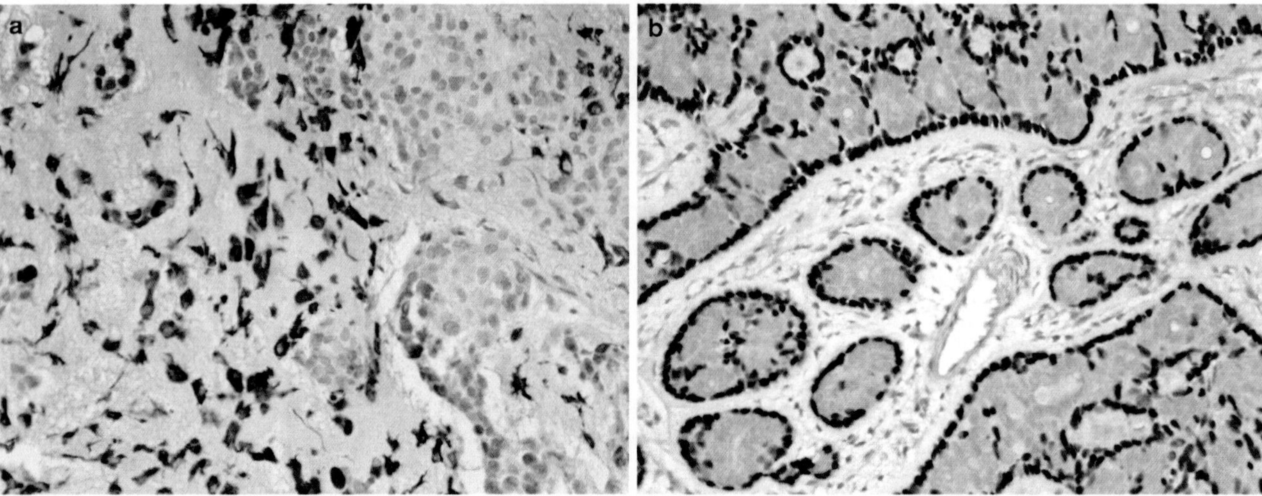

Fig. 13.3 (**a**) GFAP staining of some myoepithelial elements of a mixed tumor. (**b**) P63 staining of basal cell adenoma

Table 13.4 Markers for Warthin's tumor

Antibodies	Literature
Antimitochondrial antibody	+
CEA	+ Luminal
CK7	+
CK8	+
CK10	–
CK13	–
CK14	+ Basal cells
CK17	+ Basal cells
CK18	+
CK19	+
CK20	–
Keratins	+
Lymphoid markers	+ Lymphocytes
P63	+ Basal cells
S100	– In epithelium, + dendritic cells
Secretory component	+ Luminal

References: [43, 64–66]

Table 13.5 Markers for oncocytoma

Antibody	Literature
pVHL	+
CK5/6	+ Basal
CK7	+
CK8/18	+
CK10/13	+
CK19	+
EMA	+
MIB1	+ Cytoplasmic[a]
Antimitochondrial	+
Myoepithelial markers	–
P63	+ Basal

[a]This reaction is possibly a cross-reactive phenomenon

References: [43, 67–70]

Table 13.6 Markers for mucoepidermoid carcinoma

Antibodies	Literature
Apocrine marker	Negative
CK7	+ Luminal cells, intermediate cells, mucous cells, +/– squamous cells, clear cells
CK8	+ Intermediate cells. Focally basal cells
CK10	–
CK14	+ In squamous cells, outer rim of basaloid cells, + focally in intermediate cells
CK18	+/– In squamous cells, –/+intermediate cells
CK19	+/– In intermediate cells
CK20	– Or rare intermediate cells + only
Mitochondrial Ag	+ In epidermoid, intermediate, and basaloid cells
MUC1	+ Glandular cell cytoplasm and membranous staining of intermediate, clear, and squamous cells [a]
MUC2	–/+ Intermediate cell cytoplasm
MUC3	–
MUC4	+ Glandular cell cytoplasm and membranous staining of clear, intermediate, and squamous cells
MUC5AC	+ Intermediate cells
MUC6	–/+
Myoepithelial markers	Occasional intermediate cells may be +. Otherwise –
P63	+ In epidermoid, intermediate, and clear cells

Among the keratins, CK7 is strongly and reliably expressed in most elements of MEC. CK14 highlights principally the squamous elements. Staining for other keratins shows expression among the different cell types in MEC but the consistency appears inadequate for diagnostic purposes

[a]Higher expression of MUC1 has been related to worse prognosis

References: [1, 2, 43, 46, 47, 71, 72]

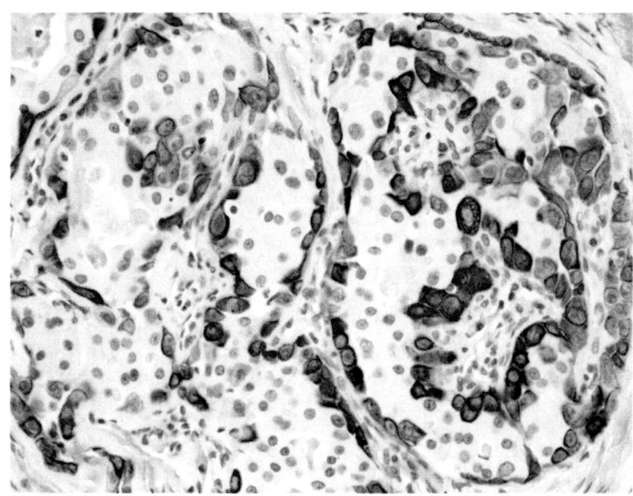

Fig. 13.4 Cytokeratin 14 staining of oncocytic mucoepidermoid carcinoma. The oncocytic cells are negative while the squamous elements are positive

Table 13.7 Markers for polymorphous low-grade adenocarcinoma

Antibodies	Literature
CKAE1/AE3	+
CEA	+ Mainly luminal
CK7	+
CK8	+
CK10	–
CK13	–
CK14	+/–
CK18	+
CK19	–/+
Myoepithelial markers	– Or rare focal positivity
P63	+ (Around 25% of cells, no definite pattern of positivity)
S100	+
Vimentin	+

References: [42, 43, 56, 73]

Table 13.8 Markers for adenoid cystic carcinoma

Antibodies	Tubular, trabecular	Cribriform	Solid
c-kit, KIT, CD117	+	+	+
CK7	+	+	+
CEA	+ Luminal cells	Occasional cells +	Occasional cells +
CK14	+ Inner cell layer	+ Luminal, –/+ pseudocyst	+/–
CK19	+ Inner cell layer	+ Luminal, – pseudocyst	+/–
MUC3	–	–	–
MUC5AC	–	–	–
Myoepithelial markers	+ Outer cell layer	+ Pseudocyst cylinder cells	–/+ Heterogeneous
P63	+ Outer cell layer	+	+/–
S100	+	+	+/–
Vimentin	+ Outer cell layer	+ Pseudocyst cylinder cells	+/– Heterogeneous
P16	+ Inner cell layer	+ Inner cells	+ Intermixed cells

Dedifferentiation of adenoid cystic carcinoma may be accompanied by p53 positivity, cyclin D1 positivity, overexpression of Her2/neu, increased Ki67 labeling index, and/or loss of myoepithelial markers

References: [9, 23, 40, 42, 50, 53, 56, 71, 74–77]

Table 13.9 Markers for acinic cell carcinoma

Antibodies	Literature
Alpha amylase	Weak/–
CK7	+/–
CK8	+/–
CK14	–/+ Rare peripheral cell clusters
CK19	–
CK18	+ Membranous pattern
CK20	–
c-kit, KIT, CD117	+
Lactoferrin	Focal +/–
MUC3	+
MUC5AC	–
Myoepithelial markers	–
P63	Compartmentalized: + peripheral cells Or interspersed + and – cells
Secretory piece	Focal +/–
Vimentin	–

A recently described tumor of salivary gland should be distinguished from acinic cell carcinoma. The mammary analog secretory carcinoma contains the ETV6-NTRK3 fusion gene characteristic of mammary secretory carcinoma: it is morphologically like the mammary tumor and is positive for MUC1, MUC4, vimentin, and S100 protein

References: [1, 23, 71, 78–82]

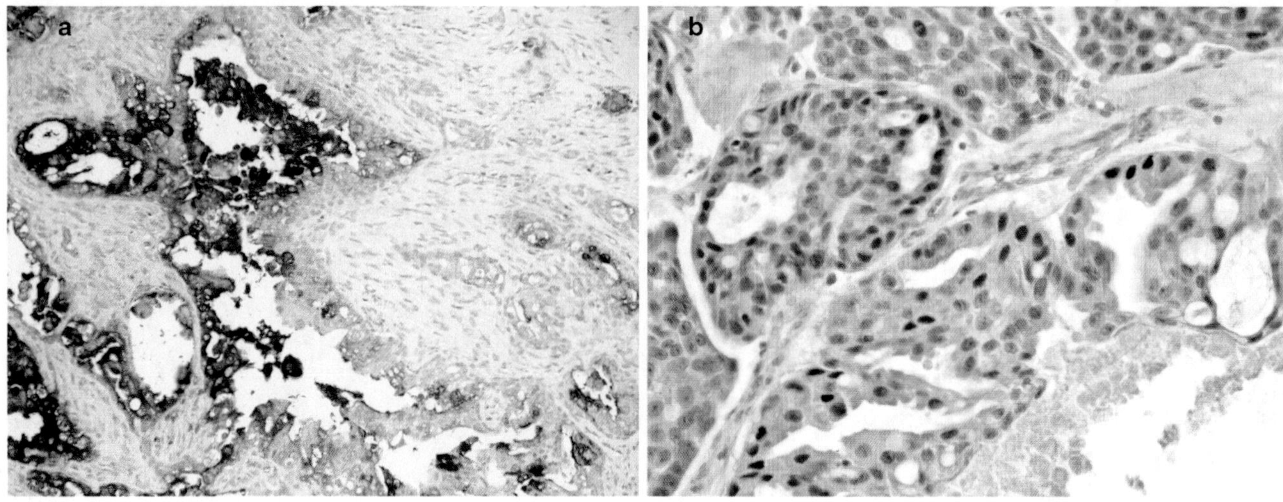

Fig. 13.5 (**a**) gross cystic disease fluid protein in salivary duct adenocarcinoma. (**b**) Androgen receptor in salivary duct adenocarcinoma

Table 13.10 Markers for salivary duct adenocarcinoma

Antibodies	Literature
Androgen receptor	+
CK7	+
CK20	–/+
GCDFP-15	+
HER2/neu	+[a]
P63	–
Estrogen receptor	–
Progesterone receptor	–/+
Prostatic acid phosphatase	+/–
Prostatic specific antigen	–/+
PPARγ	+
S100	+

Low-grade salivary duct carcinoma, an intraductal carcinoma, is Her2 negative

[a] Her2 expression does not correspond with gene amplification. One study reported all cases expressing HER2/neu did poorly

References: [25, 26, 31, 38, 83–90]

Table 13.11 Markers for basal cell adenocarcinoma

Antibodies	Literature
c-kit, KIT, CD117	+/–
CKAE1/AE3	+
CEA	+/–
CK7	+
CK20	–
EMA	+/– Focal
S100	+/– Focal
SMA	–/+ Focal
Vimentin	+/– Focal

References: [9, 91–94]

Table 13.12 Markers for myoepithelioma, epithelial–myoepithelial carcinoma

Antibodies	Myoepithelioma and myoepithelial carcinoma	Epithelial–myoepithelial carcinoma
Calponin	+	+ Myoepithelial cell component
CAM5.2	+/–	+ Strong in epithelial, weak in myoepithelial cells
CKAE1/AE3	+	+ Strong in epithelial, weaker in myoepithelial cells
CK14	+/–	nd
CK7	–/+	+
GFAP	–/+	+/– In myoepithelial cells
P63	+	+ In myoepithelial cells, – in epithelial cells
S100	+	+ In myoepithelial, –/+ in epithelial cells
SMA	+/–	+ In myoepithelial cells, – in epithelial cells
Vimentin	+	+ In myoepithelial cells, – in epithelial cells

References: [23, 43, 57, 95–102]

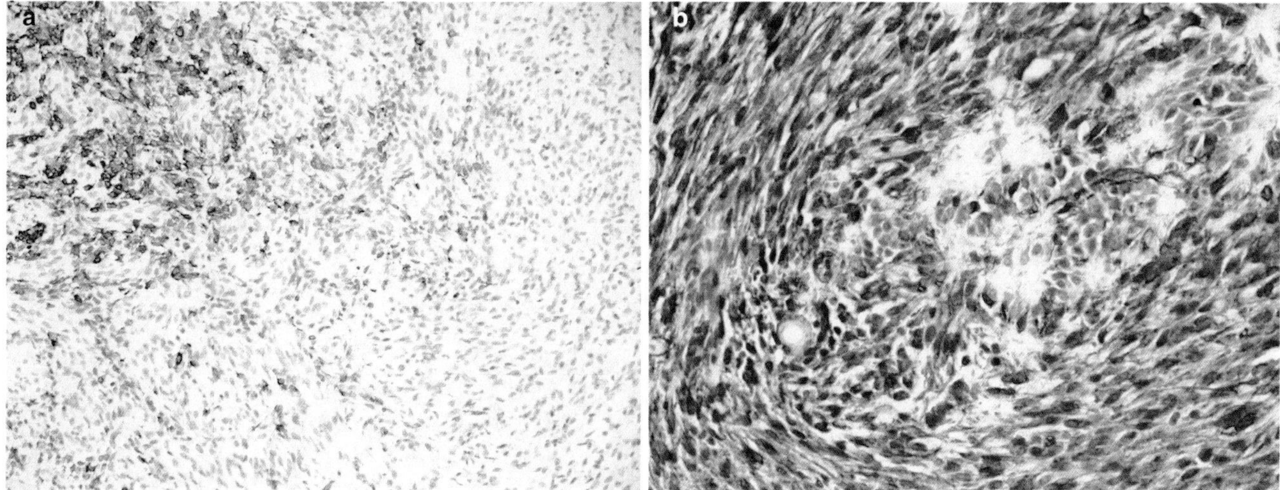

Fig. 13.6 (**a**) Keratin AE1/AE3 cocktail staining unevenly on myoepithelioma. (**b**) S-100 strong staining of myoepithelioma

Table 13.13 Markers for hyalinizing clear cell carcinoma

Antibodies	Literature
CAM5.2	+
CEA	–/+
CKAE1/AE3	+
CK20	–
EMA	+/–
MSA	–
P63	+
S100	–/+
SMA	–
Vimentin	–

HMB45 has been reported positive in two cases

References: [103–106]

Table 13.14 Markers for small cell neuroendocrine carcinoma

Antibodies	Literature
CD56	+
CD57	+/–
CKAE1/AE3	+
CK20	Usually + in SCC of salivary gland and skin, elsewhere usually –
Synaptophysin	+/–

Table 13.15 Adenoid cystic carcinoma (ACC) vs. polymorphic low-grade adenocarcinoma (PLGA) vs. basal cell adenoma (BCA) or pleomorphic adenoma (PA) (benign mixed tumor)

Antibodies	ACC	PLGA	BCA/PA[a]
c-kit, KIT, CD117	+	–/+	–/+
Calponin	+	–/+ Focal	+
CEA	+	+ Focal, variable	+ Focal, weak
CK7	+ Luminal cells	+ All cells	+ Luminal
CK14	+ Luminal cells	+ All cells	+
MIB1[b]	>10%[c]	<5%[d]	<5%
Metallothionein	+	–/+	nd
P63	+	+/–	+
S100	+	+	–/Focal/+
SMA	+	–	+
SMMHC	+	–	+

[a] See Table 13.3 for the patterns of expression of myoepithelial markers in BCA and PA. There is often incomplete or absent expression of myoepithelial markers in transformed myoepithelium

[b] As many as 20% of ACC have MIB1 indices less than 10%

[c] MIB1 index has been related to grade of ACC

[d] Rare cases PLGA have been reported with higher MIB1 index

References: [14, 62, 107–112]

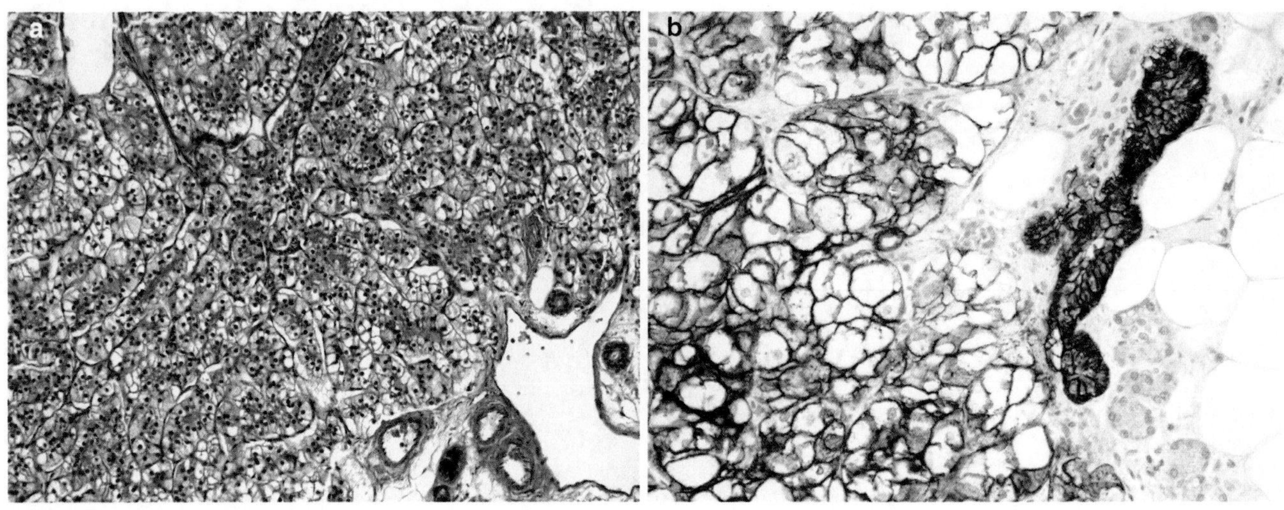

Fig. 13.7 (**a**) Clear cell oncocytoma of parotid in a patient with multiple bilateral nodules. (**b**) Same case of clear cell oncocytoma stained with pVHL. Normal duct and acini at right

Table 13.16 Clear cell epithelial tumors, differential diagnosis[a]: hyalinizing clear cell carcinoma (HCCC) vs. metastatic renal cell carcinoma (MRCC) vs. oncocytoma with clear cell features (Onc) vs. mucoepidermoid carcinoma (OMEC)

Antibodies	HCCC	MRCC	Onc	MEC
Calponin	–	–	–	–
CK5/6	+	+/–	+ Basal	+
CK7	+	–/+	+	+
CD10[b]	–	+/–	–/+ Focal	–
CK20	–	–	–/+	–
P63	+	–	+ Basal	+
RCC	–	–/+	–	–
S100	–/+	+/–	–	–
SMA	–	–	–	–
Vimentin	–	+	–/+	–/+ Focal

[a] The differential diagnosis of clear cell tumors in the head and neck includes myoepithelioma, myoepithelial carcinoma, and epithelial–myoepithelial carcinoma (see Table 13.17). More than one of the following markers P63, S100, calponin, MSA, or other myoepithelial markers should be present in these tumors. For tumors located in the jaw, clear cell odontogenic carcinoma should be included in the differential (see Table 13.37)

[b] CD10 may be expressed in myoepithelial tumors, a fact to consider in the differential with metastatic renal cell carcinoma

References: [68, 72, 97, 104–106, 113–119]

Table 13.17 Hyalinizing clear cell carcinoma (HCCC) vs. clear cells in epithelial–myoepithelial carcinoma (CMEC) vs. clear cell myoepithelioma (CCM)

Antibodies	HCCC	CMEC epithelial	CMEC myoepithelial	CCM
Calponin	–	–	+/–	+/–
CD10	–		+	–/+
CKAE1/AE3	+	+	–/+	+
GFAP	–	–	–/+	–/+
P63	+	–	+	+
S100	–/+	–/+	+	+/–
SMA	–	–	+	–/+
Vimentin	–	–	+	+

To enlarge the differential diagnosis of clear cell tumors see Table 13.16

References: [43, 103–106, 120, 121]

Table 13.18 Oncocytic epithelial tumors, differential diagnosis[a]: oncocytoma and oncocytic carcinoma (O) vs. oncocytic mucoepidermoid carcinoma (OMEC) vs. acinic cell carcinoma (AC) vs. metastatic renal cell carcinoma (RCC) vs. salivary duct carcinoma (SDC)

Antibodies	O	OMEC	AC	RCC	SDC
Androgen receptor	–	–	–	–	+
EMA	+	nd	–	+	nd
CD10	–/+ Focal	nd	–	+ Diffuse/–	nd
CK7	+	+	+	–/+	+
CK20	+/–	–	–	–	–/+
P63	+ Peripheral cells only	+ Diffuse	–/+	–	–
pVHL	+	nd	–	+/–	nd
RCC	–	–	–	+	–
S100	–	–	+ Focal	+/–	+
Antimitochondrial	+	+	–	+	nd
Vimentin	–/+	–/Rare +	–/+	+/–	nd

[a]This differential diagnostic challenge is mainly found in fine needle aspirates. Oncocytic myoepithelioma and oncocytic differentiation within pleomorphic adenoma are in the differential diagnosis of oncocytic tumors. Both may be S100+, however, in contrast to the tumors in this table, they should be positive for some myoepithelial markers

References: [1, 48, 68, 69, 72, 103, 122–129]

Table 13.19 Mucoepidermoid carcinoma, high grade (MECHG) vs. squamous carcinoma (SC)

Antibodies	MECHG	SC
c-kit, KIT, CD117	–	+/–
CK7	+	–/+
CK8	+ Scattered cells	–
CK10	–	+ Focal
CK13	+ Luminal and squamous	–
CK14	+ Scattered cells	+ Strong, diffuse
CK19	+ Scattered cells	–
MUC5AC	+/–	–

References: [31, 36, 47, 71]

Table 13.20 Markers for normal nonkeratinized squamous mucosal epithelium (NLSq), keratosis with dysplasia (KD), invasive squamous carcinoma (SCC)

Antibodies	NLSq	KD	SCC
BerEP4	–	+ Basal, suprabasal	+ Basal, nonkeratinized cells
CAM5.2	–	nd	+/–
CK1	+/– Intermediary cell layers[a]	+/–	–/+
CK5/6	+ Basal	nd	+/–
CK7	–	–	–/+
CK8/18	–	–/+	+/–
CK10	+/– Intermediary cell layers[a]	+/–	+/–
CK14	+ Basal	nd	–/+
CK19	+/– Basal, – suprabasal	–/+ Suprabasal	–/+
CK20	–	–	–
HPV ISH[b]	–	–/+	+/– Oropharynx, –/+ other H&N sites
P16[c]	–	–/+	+/– Oropharynx, +/– other H&N sites
P63	Basal cells	+ Basal	+ In peripheral layers. Diffusely positive in basaloid squamous cell carcinoma
Vimentin	–	–/Rare	–/+ Occasionally, especially spindle cell carcinoma

Fillies et al. suggest that the expression of CK8/18 or CK19 in benign mucosa or leukoplakia may be a marker for increased potential of tumor development

[a]According to Dale et al., CK1 and ten stain intermediate cells of the palate mucosa but not the buccal mucosa. There is variation in the expression of specific keratins in different squamous epithelial sites in the upper aerodigestive tract. CK19 stains the basal cells of buccal mucosa but not those of the palate. Similar findings of variation in keratin expression by anatomic location were demonstrated by Morgan et al.

[b]HPV is demonstrable by PCR in about 15–25% of squamous carcinomas of the head and neck and is thought to be causative in many of these cancers. The highest percentages of HPV-associated cancers are in Waldeyer's ring (70%) and most are associated with the HPV16 subtype. HPV-associated SCC is often poorly differentiated and nonkeratinizing, but has a better overall prognosis than SCC not associated with HPV

[c]P16 is strongly expressed in most cases of SCC in which HPV is demonstrable. Weaker expression of P16 is not specific for HPV and there is no consensus on a practical cutoff for use of P16 as a surrogate for HPV infections. P16 is mainly associated with high risk HPV subtypes and is not expressed strongly in most squamous papillomas

References: [6, 11, 58, 82, 130–144]

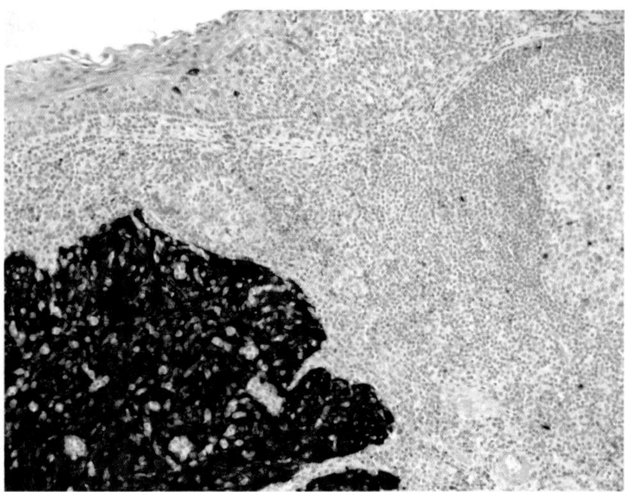

Fig. 13.8 P16 positive squamous cell carcinoma of tonsil

Table 13.21 Markers for spindle cell squamous carcinoma (SSC)[a] or carcinosarcoma

Antibodies	Differentiated squamous elements	SSC spindled areas
CKAE1/AE3	+	+/–
Desmin	–	–/+
EMA	+	+/–
MSA	–	–/+
Pankeratin	+	+/–
SMA	–	–/+
Vimentin	–	+

The WHO classifies all tumors of epithelial origin with squamous and spindle elements as "spindle cell squamous carcinoma" regardless of the presence of heterologous elements. When chondrosarcomatous, osteosarcomatous, or rhabdomyoblastic elements are present, the term "carcinosarcoma" is commonly used

References: [91, 145–148]

Table 13.22 Markers for basaloid squamous carcinoma (BSC) vs. adenoid cystic carcinoma (ACC) vs. small cell carcinoma, neuroendocrine type (SCN)

Antibodies	BSC	ACC	SCN
34BetaE12	+	+	–/+ Focal
CAM 5.2	+/–	+	+
CD56	–	+	+
CK5/6	+	+	–/+ Focal
Myoepithelial markers	–	+a	–
P63	+ Diffusely	+ In peripheral cells or segregated cells	+ Focal and weak
S100	–/+	+ Peripheral cells, myoepithelial	–
Synaptophysin	–	–	+/–
Vimentin	–	+	–

[a] May be negative in solid areas

References: [4, 74, 146–155]

Table 13.23 Markers for squamous carcinoma (SC), basaloid squamous carcinoma (BSC), and lymphoepithelial (nasopharyngeal) carcinoma (LEC)

Antibodies	SC	BSC	LEC
BerEP 4	+/– Basal, nonkeratinized cells	+ Diffuse	nd
c-kit, KIT, CD117	–	–/+	–/+
CK14	+	+/–	–
CK5/6	+	+	+
CK7	–/+	+/–	–
EBER, EBV ISH	–	–	+
Ki67	+ Basal layers	+ Diffuse	+ Diffuse
P16	–/+ Weak, focal	+ Diffuse	
P63	+ Basal layers	+	+

References: [6, 11, 43, 140, 156–160]

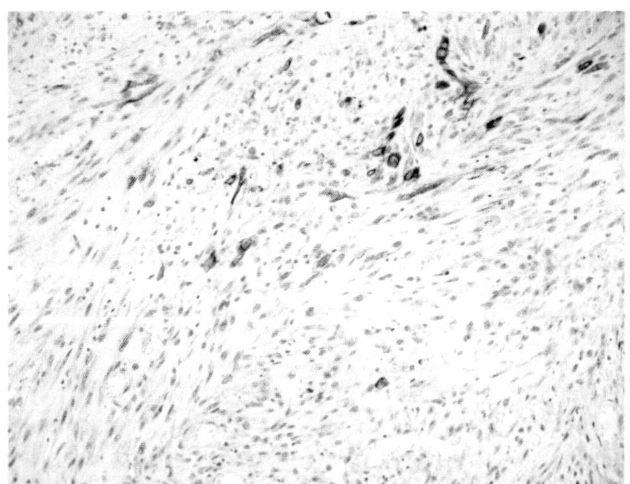

Fig. 13.9 Pankeratin stain in spindle cell squamous carcinoma. Keratin expression may be focal or absent

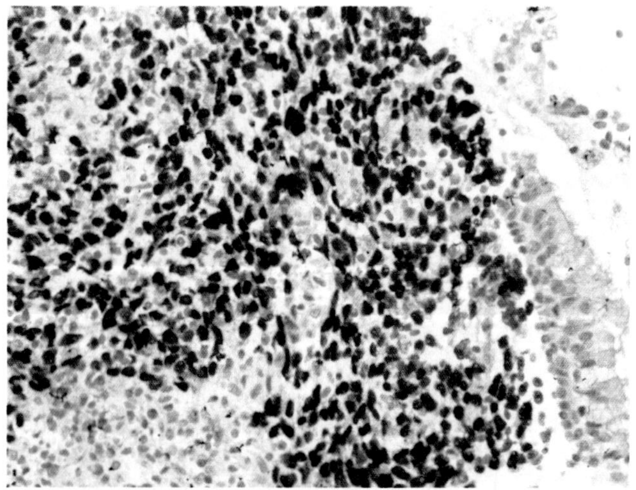

Fig. 13.10 Lymphoepithelial carcinoma of nasopharynx: in situ hybridization for EBV is positive (*black* nuclear chromogen)

Table 13.24 *NUT* midline carcinoma (NMC) vs. sinonasal undifferentiated carcinoma (SNUC) vs. nasopharyngeal carcinoma (NPC) vs. small cell neuroendocrine carcinoma (SCN)

	NMC	SNUC	NPC	SCN
CD34	+/–	nd	–	nd
Cytokeratin	+	+	+	+
EBV	–	–	+	–
NUT	+	–	–	–
P63	+	–/+	+	–/+

NUT (Nuclear Protein in Testis) midline carcinoma is a rare, clinically aggressive, high-grade carcinoma defined by a translocation involving the *NUT* gene of chromosome 15. The tumors often involve young patients (median age in the upper teens), occur most frequently in the head and neck or thorax, and are associated with survivals measured in months. Histologically, they are undifferentiated or poorly differentiated with focal squamous differentiation

In this table, "NUT" signifies a demonstrated translocation of the *NUT* gene by FISH or by immunohistochemical demonstration of a recombinant NUT polypeptide as was reported by Haak et al.

References: [161–165]

Table 13.25 Markers for Kaposi's sarcoma and angiosarcoma

Antibodies	Kaposi's sarcoma	Angiosarcoma
CD31	+/–	+
CD34	+	+
FLI1	+	+
HHV-8	+	–
Keratins	–	–/+
CD141, thrombomodulin	+	+

References: [10, 166–168]

Table 13.26 Markers for small cell carcinoma of other sites vs. Merkel cell carcinoma

Antibodies	Small cell carcinoma[a]	Merkel cell carcinoma[b]
CKAE1/AE3	+	+
CD56	+	+
Chromogranin	+/–	+/–
CK20	+/– For salivary gland primary;otherwise–	+
Synaptophysin	+	+
TTF1	–/+	–

[a]See Chap. 19

[b]See Chap. 32 for more extensive information on Merkel cell carcinoma

References: [169, 170]

Table 13.27 Markers for neuroendocrine tumors of the larynx: carcinoid, atypical carcinoid, and small cell carcinoma

Antibodies	Carcinoid	Atypical carcinoid	Small cell carcinoma
CKAE1/AE3	+	+	+
Calcitonin	–/+	+	–
Chromogranin	+	+	–/+
EMA	+	+	+
K homology domain containing protein	–	–	+
Other peptide hormones	–/+	–/+	–/+
Synaptophysin	+	+	+/–
TTF1		–/+ Weak, focal[a]	–/+

[a]TTF1 is strongly and diffusely positive in thyroid medullary carcinoma, which can be useful in distinguishing it from atypical carcinoid of the larynx

References: [91, 171–173]

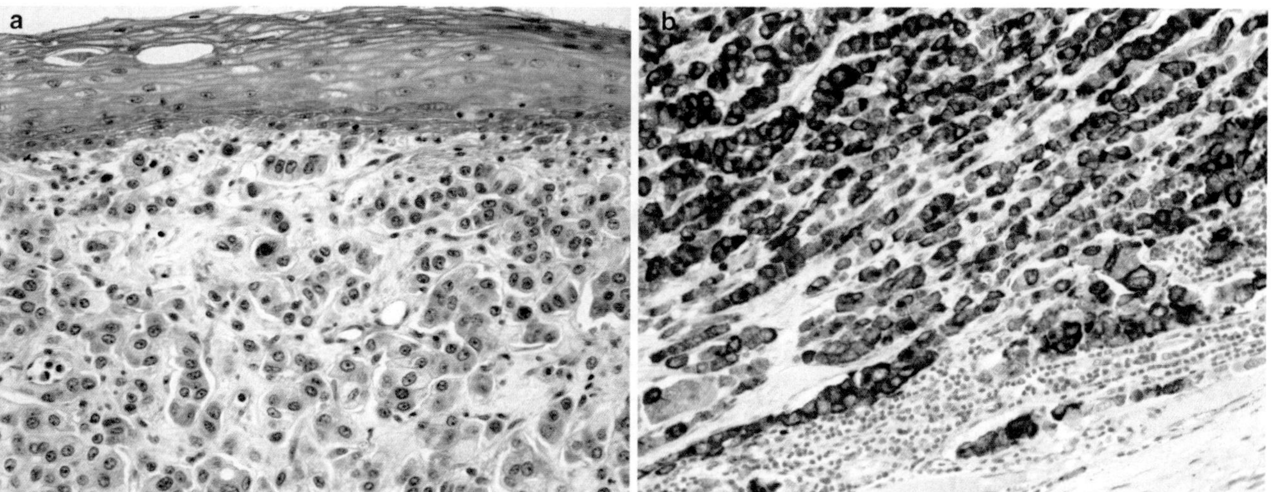

Fig. 13.11 (**a**) Atypical carcinoid of larynx, H&E. (**b**) Calcitonin positivity in lymph node metastasis of atypical carcinoid from larynx (same case). No tumor was present in the fully resected thyroid gland

Table 13.28 Markers for olfactory neuroblastoma

Antibodies	Literature
CAM5.2	–/+
CKAE1/AE3	–
Ber-Ep4	–/+
CD56	+
CD57	+
NFP	–/+
CD99	–
Desmin	–
EMA	–
HMB45	–
NSE	+
S100	+ In sustentacular cells, occasionally in tumor cells

[a]Rare cases of olfactory neuroblastoma are focally positive for epithelial markers

References: [146–148, 174]

Table 13.29 Markers for sinonasal hemangiopericytoma

Antibodies	Literature
Bcl2	–
c-kit, KIT, CD117	–
CD31	–
CD34	–/+ Focal
CD68	–
CKAE1/AE3	–
Desmin	–
Factor XIIIa	+
Laminin	+/–
MSA	+
S100	–
SMA	+
Vimentin	+

Reference: [175]

Table 13.30 Markers for intestinal-type sinonasal adenocarcinoma

Antibodies	Literature
B72.3	+
BerEP4	+
CDX2	+
Chromogranin	+/– Focal
CK7	+/–
CK20	+
MUC2	+

References: [91, 176, 177]

Table 13.31 Markers for sinonasal teratocarcinosarcoma

Antibodies	Literature
CD99	+ Undifferentiated areas
Synaptophysin	–/+ Undifferentiated areas
Vimentin	+ Spindle cell areas
Desmin	–/+ Spindle cell areas
NSE	+ Neuroepithelial areas
Cytokeratins	+ Epithelial areas
EMA	+ Epithelial areas
S100 protein	–/+
GFAP	–/+

Reference: [91]

Table 13.32 Markers for lymphomas of upper aerodigestive tract

Antibodies	Extranodal NK/T cell	Most B-cell lymphomas	Extramedullary plasmacytoma	Plasmablastic lymphoma
CD2	+	–	–	–
CD3	+ C	–	–	–
CD20	–	+	–	–/+
CD38	nd	–/+	+	+
CD56	+/–	–	+	–/+
CD79a	–	+	–/+	–/+
CD138	–	–	+	+
Clonal light chain	–	+/– SIg	+ CIg	+/– CIg
EBV ISH	+	–	–	+
EMA	–	–	+/–	+/–
LCA	+	+	–/+	–/+

C cytoplasmic, *SIg* surface immunoglobulin, *CIg* cytoplasmic immunoglobulin

References: [91, 146–148, 178–180]

Table 13.33 Poorly differentiated sinonasal tumors: olfactory neuroblastoma (ONB), sinonasal undifferentiated carcinoma (SNUC), lymphoepithelial (or poorly differentiated nasopharyngeal) carcinoma (LEC), melanoma (M), lymphoma (L)[a]

Antibodies	ONB	SNUC	LEC	M	L
CD45 and lymphocyte markers	–	–	–	–	+
CD56	–	–/+	–	–	–/+
EMA	–	+/–	+	–	–
CKAE1/AE3	–/Rare +	+	+	–	–
CK5/6	–	–	+	–	–
CK7	nd	+/–	–	–	–
EBV	–	–	+/–	–	–/+
HMB45	–	–	–	+	–
MelanA	–	–	–	+/–	–
NFP	+/–	–	–	–	–
CD99	–	–/+	–	–	–/+
NSE	+	–/+	–	–	–
S100	+ In peripheral sustentacular cells only	–	–	+	–
Synaptophysin	+/–	–/+	–	–	–

[a]To expand the differential diagnoses see Table 13.34. Differential of small blue cell tumors of the head and neck

References: [4, 91, 156, 160, 174, 181–188]

Table 13.34 Differential of small blue cell tumors of the head and neck: olfactory neuroblastoma (ONB), alveolar rhabdomyosarcoma (ARS), embryonal rhabdomyosarcoma (ERS), small cell neuroendocrine carcinoma (SCN), lymphoma (LYM), Ewings sarcoma/PNET (ES/PNET), synovial sarcoma (SS), mesenchymal chondrosarcoma (MC)

Antibodies	ONB	ARS	ERS	SCN[a]	LYM	ES/PNET	SS	MC
Bcl2	+/–	–	–	nd	+/–	–/+	+	
CD45 and lymphoid markers	–	–	–	–	+	–	–	–
CD56	+	+/–	+/–	+	–/+	–/+	–/+	–
CD99	–	–	–	–	–/+	+ M	+/–	+
CKAEI/AE3	–	–/+	–	+	–	–/+	+/–	–
Desmin	–	+	+	–	–	–/+	–	–/+ Rare
EBV ISH	–	nd	–	–	–/+	–	–	–
EMA	–	–	–	+	–/+ Rare	–	+	–
FLI1	–	–	–	–/+	nd	+	nd	–/+
MyoD1	–	+	+	–	–	–	–	–/+ Rare
Myogenin	–	+	+	–	–	–	–	–/+ Rare
S100	+ Sustentacular cells	–	–	–	–	–/+	–/+	+
Synaptophysin	+	–/+	–	+/–	–	–/+		–
Vimentin	–	+	+	–	–/+	+	+	+
WT1	nd	+ C	+ C	nd	nd	–/+	nd	+ C

Metastatic neuroblastoma and retinoblastoma have histochemical profiles similar to olfactory neuroblastoma.

Sinonasal desmoplastic small round cell tumor has been reported, which would also be within the differential of small blue cell tumors

A benign diagnosis to keep in the differential is extrasellar pituitary adenoma, which is positive for CAM5.2, neuroendocrine markers, and pituitary hormones

Weak, granular cytoplasmic staining for CD99 is occasionally seen in rhabdomyosarcoma

To expand the differential diagnosis see Table 13.33, poorly differentiated sinonasal tumors

[a] Small cell neuroendocrine carcinoma is extremely rare in the sinonasal region and its immunohistochemical profile has been documented mainly for the lung and other sites

References: [4, 10, 22, 183, 187–201]

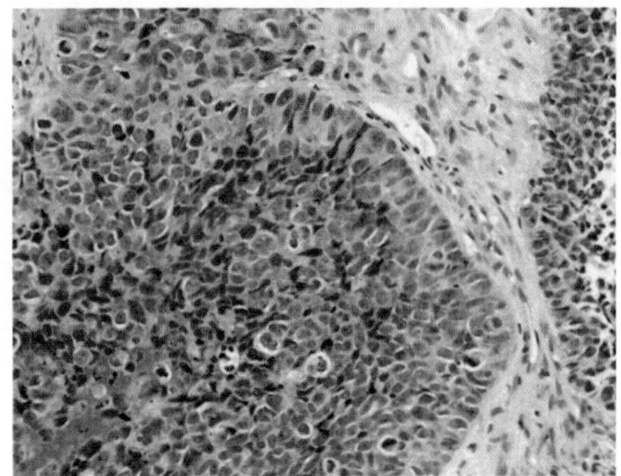

Fig. 13.12 Small cell neuroendocrine carcinoma of the nose in a 67-year-old male. The tumor was positive for cytokeratin, synaptophysin, and vimentin

Table 13.35 Middle ear adenoma (MEA) vs. paraganglioma (PG) vs. endolymphatic sac tumor (EST)

Antibodies	MEA	PG	EST
Chromogranin	+	+	–
CKAE1/AE3	+	–/+	+
EMA	+	–	+
GFAP	nd	–	–/+
S100	–	–/+ In chief cells. + in sustentacular cells	+/–
Synaptophysin	+	+	–
Vimentin	+	–/+	+

References: [91, 202–204]

Table 13.36 Markers for endolymphatic sac tumor (EST) vs. choroid plexus papilloma (CPP)

	EST	CPP
Transthyretin	–	+
GFAP	–/+	+/–
Cytokeratin	+	+
S100	+/–	+
EMA	+	+/–

References: [202, 203]

Table 13.37 Markers for clear cell odontogenic carcinoma

Antibodies	Literature
CK8	+
CK13	+
CK14	+
CK18	+
CK19	+
Desmin	–
EMA	+
HMB45	–
S100	–
SMA	–
Vimentin	–

References: [91, 205]

Table 13.38 Odontogenic keratocyst (keratocystic odontogenic tumor [KCOT])[a] vs. dentigerous cyst vs. cystic ameloblastoma

Antibodies	KCOT	Dentigerous cyst	Cystic ameloblastoma
Calretinin	–[b]	–	+ Groups of cells in superficial and stellate reticulum like areas
D2-40d	+Basal and suprabasal	– Except when inflamed	+ Peripheral cell layers
Ki67	Increased suprabasal positivity	Little (<1.5%) suprabasal positivity	Increased suprabasal positivity
P53	–/+	–	+
P63	More diffuse staining of epithelium	Basal, parabasal[c]	+

[a] Orthokeratinized odontogenic cysts (OOC) have recently been separated from KCOT. They have lower recurrence rate, lower proliferative activity, and are negative for podoplanin (D2-40)

[b] A study by Piatelli et al. found positivity to calretinin in the parabasal-intermediate cell layers in 8 of 12 parakeratinized odontogenic keratocysts and negativity in 10 orthokeratinized keratocysts

[c] Inflammation may increase the expression of P63 and Ki67

[d] According to Okamoto et al., stromal inflammation induces podoplanin (D2-40) expression in basal cells of dentigerous cysts, OOC, and gingiva

References: [206–219]

Notes for All Tables

Note: "+" = usually greater than 70% of cases are positive; "–" = less than 5% of cases are positive; "+/–" = usually more than 50% of cases are positive; "–/+" = less than 50% of cases are positive; "nd" = indicates no data currently available.

References

1. Foschini MP, Marucci G, Eusebi V. Low-grade mucoepidermoid carcinoma of salivary glands: characteristic immunohistochemical profile and evidence of striated duct differentiation. Virchows Arch. 2002;440(5):536–42.
2. Azevedo RS, de Almeida OP, Kowalski LP, Pires FR. Comparative cytokeratin expression in the different cell types of salivary gland mucoepidermoid carcinoma. Head Neck Pathol. 2008;2:257.
3. Lazard D, Sastre X, Frid MG, Glukhova MA, Thiery JP, Koteliansky VE. Expression of smooth muscle-specific proteins in myoepithelium and stromal myofibroblasts of normal and malignant human breast tissue. Proc Natl Acad Sci U S A. 1993; 90(3):999–1003.
4. Dabbs DJ. Diagnostic immunohistochemistry. 3rd ed. Philadelphia, PA: Churchill Livingstone Elsevier; 2010. Accessed 14 Mar 2010.
5. Kennedy M, Jordan R, Berean K, et al. Expression pattern of CK7, CK20, CDX-2, and villin in intestinal-type sinonasal adenocarcinoma. J Clin Pathol. 2004;57:932.
6. Regauer S, Beham A, Mannweiler S. CK7 expression in carcinomas of the Waldeyer's ring area. Hum Pathol. 2000;31:1096.
7. Xia W, Yiu-Kueng L, Hu M, et al. High tumoral maspin expression is associated with improved survival of patients with oral squamous cell carcinoma. Oncogene. 2000;19(20):2398.
8. Iwafuchi H, Mori N, Takahashi T, Yatabe Y. Phenotypic composition of salivary gland tumors: an application of principal [corrected] component analysis to tissue microarray data. Mod Pathol. 2004;17(7):803–10.
9. Mino M, Pilch BZ, Faquin WC. Expression of KIT (CD117) in neoplasms of the head and neck: an ancillary marker for adenoid cystic carcinoma. Mod Pathol. 2003;16(12):1224.
10. Rossi S, Orvieto E, Furlanetto A, Laurino L, Ninfo V, Dei Tos AP. Utility of the immunohistochemical detection of FLI-1 expression in round cell and vascular neoplasm using a monoclonal antibody. Mod Pathol. 2004;17(5):547–52.
11. Winter MJ, Nagtegaal ID, van Krieken JH, Litvinov SV. The epithelial cell adhesion molecule (Ep-CAM) as a morphoregulatory molecule is a tool in surgical pathology. Am J Pathol. 2003;163(6):2139–48.
12. Viacava P, Naccarato AG, Bevilacqua G. Spectrum of GCDFP-15 expression in human fetal and adult normal tissues. Virchows Arch. 1998;432(3):255–60.
13. Watanabe K, Tajino T, Sekiguchi M, Suzuki T. h-Caldesmon as a specific marker for smooth muscle tumors. Comparison with other smooth muscle markers in bone tumors. Am J Clin Pathol. 2000;113(5):663–8.
14. Alves SM, Cardoso SV, de Fatima Bernardes V, et al. Metallothionein immunostaining in adenoid cystic carcinomas of the salivary glands. Oral Oncol. 2007;43(3):252.
15. Dutsch-Wicherek M, Popiela TJ, Klimek M, et al. Metallothionein stroma reaction in tumour adjacent healthy tissue in head and neck squamous cell carcinoma and breat adenocarcinoma. Neuro Endocrinol Lett. 2005;26(5):567.
16. Cherian MG, Jayasurya A, Bay BH. Metallothioneins in human tumors and potential roles in carcinogenesis. Mutat Res. 2003;533(1–2):201–9.
17. Sundelin K, Jadner M, Norberg-Spaak L, Davidsson A, Hellquist HB. Metallothionein and Fas (CD95) are expressed in squamous cell carcinoma of the tongue. Eur J Cancer. 1997;33(11): 1860–4.
18. Gao Y, Han Z, Liu X. Megallothionein expression and its significance in salivary gland tumors. Zhonghua Kou Qiang Yi Xue Za Zhi. 1997;32(5):282.
19. Marioni G, Staffieri A, Bertolin A, et al. Laryngeal carcinoma lymph node metastasis and disease-free survival correlate with MASPIN nuclear expression but not with EGFR expression: a series of 108 cases. Eur Arch Otorhinolaryngol. 2010;267(7):1103–10.
20. Schwarz S, Ettl T, Kleinsasser N, Hartmann A, Reichert TE, Driemel O. Loss of Maspin expression is a negative prognostic factor in common salivary gland tumors. Oral Oncol. 2008;44(6): 563–70.
21. Meer S, Altini M. CK7+/CK20– immunoexpression profile is typical of salivary gland neoplasia. Histopathology. 2007; 51(1):26.
22. Nakatsuka S, Oji Y, Horiuchi T, et al. Immunohistochemical detection of WT1 protein in a variety of cancer cells. Mod Pathol. 2006;19(6):804–14.
23. Chu PG, Weiss LM. Keratin expression in human tissues and neoplasms. Histopathology. 2002;40(5):403–39.
24. Wu HH, Zafar S, Huan Y, Yee H, Chiriboga L, Wang BY. Fascin over expression is associated with dysplastic changes in sinonasal inverted papillomas: a study of 47 cases. Head Neck Pathol. 2009;3:212–6.
25. Mukunyadzi P, Ai L, Portilla D, Barnes EL, Fan CY. Expression of peroxisome proliferator-activated receptor gamma in salivary duct carcinoma: immunohistochemical analysis of 15 cases. Mod Pathol. 2003;16(12):1218–23.
26. Barnes L, Rao U, Contis L, Krause J, Schwartz A, Scalamogna P. Salivary duct carcinoma. Part II. Immunohistochemical evaluation of 13 cases for estrogen and progesterone receptors, cathepsin D, and c-erbB-2 protein. Oral Surg Oral Med Oral Pathol. 1994;78(1): 74–80.
27. Pires FR, da Cruz Perez DE, de Almeida OP, Kowalski LP. Estrogen receptor expression in salivary gland mucoepidermoid carcinoma and adenoid cystic carcinoma. Pathol Oncol Res. 2004;10(3):166–8.
28. Huang JW, Ming Z, Shrestha P, et al. Immunohistochemical evaluation of the Ca(2+)-binding S-100 proteins S-100A1, S-100A2, S-100A4, S-100A6 and S-100B in salivary gland tumors. J Oral Pathol Med. 1996;25(10):547–55.
29. Savera AT, Gown AM, Zarbo RJ. Immunolocalization of three novel smooth muscle-specific proteins in salivary gland pleomorphic adenoma: assessment of the morphogenetic role of myoepithelium. Mod Pathol. 1997;10(11):1093–100.
30. Seethala RR, LiVolsi VA, Zhang PJ, Pasha TL, Baloch ZW. Comparison of P63 and P73 expression in benign and malignant salivary gland lesions. Head Neck. 2005;27:696.
31. Nikitakis NG, Tosios KI, Papanikolaou VS, Rivera H, Papanicolaou SI, Ioffe OB. Immunohistochemical expression of cytokeratins 7 and 20 in malignant salivary gland tumors. Mod Pathol. 2004;17(4):407–15.
32. Azumi N, Battifora H. The cellular composition of adenoid cystic carcinoma. An immunohistochemical study. Cancer. 1987;60(7): 1589–98.
33. Weber A, Langhanki L, Schutz A, et al. Expression profiles of p53, p63, and p73 in benign salivary gland tumors. Virchows Arch. 2002;441(5):428–36.
34. Darling MR, Schneider JW, Phillips VM. Polymorphous low-grade adenocarcinoma and adenoid cystic carcinoma: a review and

comparison of immunohistochemical markers. Oral Oncol. 2002;38(7):641–5.
35. de Araujo VC, de Sousa SO. Expression of different keratins in salivary gland tumours. Eur J Cancer B Oral Oncol. 1996;32B(1): 14–8.
36. Sobral AP, Loducca SV, Kowalski LP, et al. Immunohistochemical distinction of high-grade mucoepidermoid carcinoma and epidermoid carcinoma of the parotid region. Oral Oncol. 2002;38(5): 437–40.
37. Su L, Morgan PR, Harrison DL, Waseem A, Lane EB. Expression of keratin mRNAs and proteins in normal salivary epithelia and pleomorphic adenomas. J Pathol. 1993;171(3):173–81.
38. Zarbo RJ. Salivary gland neoplasia: a review for the practicing pathologist. Mod Pathol. 2002;15(3):298–323.
39. Foschini MP, Scarpellini F, Gown AM, Eusebi V. Differential expression of myoepithelial markers in salivary, sweat and mammary glands. Int J Surg Pathol. 2000;8(1):29.
40. Ogawa Y, Toyosawa S, Ishida T, Ijuhin N. Keratin 14 immunoreactive cells in pleomorphic adenomas and adenoid cystic carcinomas of salivary glands. Virchows Arch. 2000;437(1):58–68.
41. Tsukitani K, Nakai M, Tatemoto Y, Hikosaka N, Mori M. Histochemical studies of obstructive adenitis in human submandibular salivary glands. I. Immunohistochemical demonstration of lactoferrin, lysozyme and carcinoembryonic antigen. J Oral Pathol. 1985;14:631.
42. Epivatianos A, Iordanides S, Zaraboukas T, Antoniades D. Adenoid cystic carcinoma and polymorphous low-grade adenocarcinoma of minor salivary glands: a comparative immunohistochemical study using the epithelial membrane and carcinoembryonic antibodies. Oral Dis. 2005;11(3):175–80.
43. Bilal H, Handra-Luca A, Bertrand JC, Fouret PJ. P63 is expressed in basal and myoepithelial cells of human normal and tumor salivary gland tissues. J Histochem Cytochem. 2003;51(2): 133–9.
44. Langman G, Andrews CL, Weissferdt A. WT-1 Expression in salivary gland pleomorphic adenomas: a reliable marker of neoplastic myoepithelium. 2010. Modern pathol. 2011 Feb, 24(2):168–74.
45. Gonzalez-Alva P, Tanaka A, Oku Y, et al. Enhanced expression of podoplanin in ameloblastomas. J Oral Pathol Med. 2010; 39(1):103.
46. Alos L, Lujan B, Castillo M, et al. Expression of membrane-bound mucins (MUC1 and MUC4) and secreted mucins (MUC2, MUC5AC, MUC5B, MUC6 and MUC7) in mucoepidermoid carcinomas of salivary glands. Am J Surg Pathol. 2005;29(6): 806–13.
47. Handra-Luca A, Lamas G, Bertrand JC, Fouret P. MUC1, MUC2, MUC4, and MUC5AC expression in salivary gland mucoepidermoid carcinoma: diagnostic and prognostic implications. Am J Surg Pathol. 2005;29(7):881–9.
48. Shi J, Huang Y, Liu H, Lin F. The von Hipple–Lindau gene product (Pvhl) is a useful marker in differentiating salivary acinar cell carcinoma from oncocytoma. Mod. Pathol. 2009;Suppl 22:96A.
49. Ogawa Y. Immunocytochemistry of myoepithelial cells in the salivary glands. Prog Histochem Cytochem. 2003;38(4):343–426.
50. Itoiz ME, Lanfranchi HE, Cabrini RL, Dominguez FV. Immunocytochemical detection of carcinoembryonic antigen in salivary gland tumors. Int J Oral Surg. 1983;12(5):340–3.
51. Nakazato Y, Ishida Y, Takahashi K, Suzuki K. Immunohistochemical distribution of S-100 protein and glial fibrillary acidic protein in normal and neoplastic salivary glands. Virchows Arch A Pathol Anat Histopathol. 1985;405(3):299–310.
52. DeRoche TC, Hoschar AP, Hunt JL. Immunohistochemical evaluation of androgen receptor, HER-2/neu, and p53 in benign pleomorphic adenomas. Arch Pathol Lab Med. 2008;132(12):1907–11.
53. Edwards PC, Bhuiya T, Kelsch RD. Assessment of p63 expression in the salivary gland neoplasms adenoid cystic carcinoma, polymorphous low-grade adenocarcinoma, and basal cell and canalicular adenomas. Oral Surg Oral Med Oral Pathol Oral Radiol Endod. 2004;97(5):613–9.
54. Zarbo RJ, Prasad AR, Regezi JA, Gown AM, Savera AT. Salivary gland basal cell and canalicular adenomas: immunohistochemical demonstration of myoepithelial cell participation and morphogenetic considerations. Arch Pathol Lab Med. 2000;124(3):401–5.
55. de Araujo VC, de Sousa SO, Carvalho YR, de Araujo NS. Application of immunohistochemistry to the diagnosis of salivary gland tumors. Appl Immunohistochem Mol Morphol. 2000;8(3): 195–202.
56. Prasad AR, Savera AT, Gown AM, Zarbo RJ. The myoepithelial immunophenotype in 135 benign and malignant salivary gland tumors other than pleomorphic adenoma. Arch Pathol Lab Med. 1999;123(9):801–6.
57. Alos L, Cardesa A, Bombi JA, Mallofre C, Cuchi A, Traserra J. Myoepithelial tumors of salivary glands: a clinicopathologic, immunohistochemical, ultrastructural, and flow-cytometric study. Semin Diagn Pathol. 1996;13(2):138–47.
58. Takahashi H, Tsuda N, Tezuka F, Okabe H. Immunohistochemical localization of carcinoembryonic antigen in carcinoma in pleomorphic adenoma of salivary gland: use in the diagnosis of benign and malignant lesions. Tohoku J Exp Med. 1986;149(3):329–40.
59. Ferreiro JA. Immunohistochemistry of basal cell adenoma of the major salivary glands. Histopathology. 1994;24(6):539–42.
60. Pereira MC, Pereira AA, Hanemann JA. Immunohistochemical profile of canalicular adenoma of the upper lip: a case report. Med Oral Patol Oral Cir Bucal. 2007;12(1):E1–3.
61. Yuri T, Mitsuyoshi H, Yoshiaki N, Hiromi K, Takeshi O, Chotatsu T. Morphology of myoepithelial cells seen in pleomorphic adenoma of the salivary gland. J Japan Soc Clin Cytol. 1999; 38(5):403.
62. Cavalcante RB, Lopes FF, Ferreira AS, Freitas Rde A, de Souza LB. Immunohistochemical expression of vimentin, calponin and HHF-35 in salivary gland tumors. Braz Dent J. 2007;18(3):192–7.
63. Korsrud FR, Brandtzaeg P. Immunofluorescence study of secretory epithelial markers in pleomorphic adenomas. Virchows Arch A Pathol Anat Histopathol. 1984;403(3):291–300.
64. Dardick I, Claude A, Parks WR, et al. Warthin's tumor: an ultrastructural and immunohistochemical study of basilar epithelium. Ultrastruct Pathol. 1988;12(4):419–32.
65. Segami N, Fukuda M, Manabe T. Immunohistological study of the epithelial components of Warthin's tumor. Int J Oral Maxillofac Surg. 1989;18(3):133–7.
66. Schwerer MJ, Kraft K, Baczako K, Maier H. Cytokeratin expression and epithelial differentiation in Warthin's tumour and its metaplastic (infarcted) variant. Histopathology. 2001;39(4): 347–52.
67. Zhou CX, Gao Y. Oncocytoma of the salivary glands: a clinicopathologic and immunohistochemical study. Oral Oncol. 2009;45(12):e232.
68. McHugh JB, Hoschar AP, Dvorakova M, Parwani AV, Barnes EL, Seethala RR. p63 Immunohistochemistry differentiates salivary gland oncocytoma and oncocytic carcinoma from metastatic renal cell carcinoma. Head Neck Pathol. 2007;1(2):123.
69. Weiler C, Reu S, Zengel P, Kirchner T, Ihrler S. Obligate basal cell component in salivary oncocytoma facilitates distinction from acinic cell carcinoma. Pathol Res Pract. 2009;205(12):838–42.
70. Thompson LD, Wenig BM, Ellis GL. Oncocytomas of the submandibular gland. A series of 22 cases and a review of the literature. Cancer. 1996;78(11):2281–7.
71. Lee JH, Lee JH, Kim A, Kim I, Chae YS. Unique expression of MUC3, MUC5AC and cytokeratins in salivary gland carcinomas. Pathol Int. 2005;55(7):386–90.
72. Loyola A, de Sousa SO, Araujo NS, Araujo VC. Study of minor salivary gland mucoepidermoid carcinoma differentiation based

on immunohistochemical expression of cytokeratins, vimentin and muscle-specific actin. Oral Oncol. 1998;34(2):112.
73. Araujo V, Sousa S, Jaeger M, et al. Characterization of the cellular component of polymorphous low-grade adenocarcinoma by immunohistochemistry and electron microscopy. Oral Oncol. 1999;35(2):164–72.
74. Klijanienko J, el-Naggar A, Ponzio-Prion A, Marandas P, Micheau C, Caillaud JM. Basaloid squamous carcinoma of the head and neck. Immunohistochemical comparison with adenoid cystic carcinoma and squamous cell carcinoma. Arch Otolaryngol Head Neck Surg. 1993;119(8):887–90.
75. Furuse C, Cury PR, de Araujo NS, de Araujo VC. Application of two different clones of vimentin to the diagnosis of salivary gland tumors. Appl Immunohistochem Mol Morphol. 2006;14(2): 217–9.
76. Nagao T, Gaffey TA, Serizawa H, et al. Dedifferentiated adenoid cystic carcinoma: a clinicopathologic study of 6 cases. Mod Pathol. 2003;16(12):1265–72.
77. Watanabe Y, Wato M. Expression of p16 and p73 in adenoid cystic carcinoma of the salivary gland. J Osaka Dental Univ. 2007;41(1):1.
78. Skalova A, Vanecek T, Sima R, et al. Mammary analogue secretory carcinoma of salivary glands, containing the ETV6-NTRK3 fusion gene: a hitherto undescribed salivary gland tumor entity. Am J Surg Pathol. 2010;34(5):599–608.
79. Ihrler S, Blasenbreu-Vogt S, Sendelhofert A, Lang S, Zietz C, Lohrs U. Differential diagnosis of salivary acinic cell carcinoma and adenocarcinoma (NOS). A comparison of (immuno-) histochemical markers. Pathol Res Pract. 2002;198(12): 777–83.
80. Crivelini MM, de Sousa SO, de Araujo VC. Immunohistochemical study of acinic cell carcinoma of minor salivary gland. Oral Oncol. 1997;33(3):204–8.
81. Warner TF, Seo IS, Azen EA, Hafez GR, Zarling TA. Immunocytochemistry of acinic cell carcinomas and mixed tumors of salivary glands. Cancer. 1985;56(9):2221–7.
82. Emanuel P, Wang B, Wu M, Burstein DE. p63 Immunohistochemistry in the distinction of adenoid cystic carcinoma from basaloid squamous cell carcinoma. Mod Pathol. 2005;18:645.
83. Skalova A, Starek I, Vanecek T, et al. Expression of HER-2/neu gene and protein in salivary duct carcinomas of parotid gland as revealed by fluorescence in-situ hybridization and immunohistochemistry. Histopathology. 2003;42(4):348–56.
84. Moriki T, Ueta S, Takahashi T, Mitani M, Ichien M. Salivary duct carcinoma: cytologic characteristics and application of androgen receptor immunostaining for diagnosis. Cancer. 2001;93(5): 344–50.
85. Johnson CJ, Barry MB, Vasef MA, Deyoung BR. Her-2/neu expression in salivary duct carcinoma: an immunohistochemical and chromogenic in situ hybridization study. Appl Immunohistochem Mol Morphol. 2008;16(1):54–8.
86. Etges A, Pinto Jr DS, Kowalski LP, Soares FA, Araujo VC. Salivary duct carcinoma: immunohistochemical profile of an aggressive salivary gland tumour. J Clin Pathol. 2003;56(12):914–8.
87. Kawahara A, Harada H, Akiba J, Kage M. Salivary duct carcinoma cytologically diagnosed distinctly from salivary gland carcinomas with squamous differentiation. Diagn Cytopathol. 2008; 36(7):485–93.
88. Brandwein-Gensler M, Hille J, Wang BY, et al. Low-grade salivary duct carcinoma: description of 16 cases. Am J Surg Pathol. 2004;28(8):1040–4.
89. Sygut D, Bien S, Ziolkowska M, Sporny S. Immunohistochemical expression of androgen receptor in salivary gland cancers. Polish J Pathol. 2008;59(4):205–10.
90. Nasser SM, Faquin WC, Dayal Y. Expression of androgen, estrogen, and progesterone receptors in salivary gland tumors. Frequent expression of androgen receptor in a subset of malignant salivary gland tumors. Am J Clin Pathol. 2003;119(6):801–6.
91. Barnes L, Eveson JW, Reichart P, Sidransky D. WHO classification of tumours pathology & genetics head and neck tumours. Lyon: International Agency for Research on Cancer; 2005. p. 430. Accessed 19 Apr 2010.
92. Farrell T, Chang YL. Basal cell adenocarcinoma of minor salivary gland. Arch Pathol Lab Med. 2007;131(10):1602.
93. Quddus MR, Henley JD, Affify AM, et al. Basal cell adenocarcinoma of the salivary gland. An ultrastructural and immunohistochemical study. Oral Surg Oral Med Oral Pathol Oral Radiol Endod. 1999;87:485.
94. Parashar P, Baron E, Papadimitriou JC, Ord RA, Nikitakis NG, University of Maryland. Basal cell adenocarcinoma of the oral minor salivary glands: review of the literature and presentation of two cases. Oral Surg Oral Med Oral Pathol Oral Radiol Endod. 2007;103:77.
95. Seethala RR, Barnes EL, Hunt JL. Epithelial-myoepithelial carcinoma: a review of the clinicopathologic spectrum and immunophenotypic characteristics in 61 tumors of the salivary glands and upper aerodigestive tract. Am J Surg Pathol. 2007;31(1):44–57.
96. Dardick I, Thomas MJ, van Nostrand AW. Myoepithelioma – new concepts of histology and classification: a light and electron microscopic study. Ultrastruct Pathol. 1989;13(2–3):187–224.
97. Ramraje S, Bharambe B, Zode R. Epithelial myoepithelial carcinoma of the submandibular salivary gland. Bombay Hosp J. 2010;52(1):141.
98. Nagao T, Sugano I, Ishida Y, et al. Salivary gland malignant myoepithelioma: a clinicopathologic and immunohistochemical study of ten cases. Cancer. 1998;83(7):1292–9.
99. Di Palma S, Guzzo M. Malignant myoepithelioma of salivary glands: clinicopathological features of ten cases. Virchows Arch A Pathol Anat Histopathol. 1993;423(5):389–96.
100. Hornick JL, Fletcher CD. Myoepithelial tumors of soft tissue: a clinicopathologic and immunohistochemical study of 101 cases with evaluation of prognostic parameters. Am J Surg Pathol. 2003; 27(9):1183.
101. Savera AT, Sloman A, Huvos AG, Klimstra DS. Myoepithelial carcinoma of the salivary glands: a clinicopathologic study of 25 patients. Am J Surg Pathol. 2000;24(6):761–74.
102. Jones H, Moshtael F, Simpson RH. Immunoreactivity of alpha smooth muscle actin in salivary gland tumours: a comparison with S100 protein. J Clin Pathol. 1992;45(10):938–40.
103. Takahashi H, Tsuda N, Tezuka F, Okabe H. An immunoperoxidase investigation of S-100 protein in the epithelial component of Warthin's tumor. Oral Surg Oral Med Oral Pathol Oral Radiol Endod. 1986;62(1):57.
104. Solar AA, Schmidt BL, Jordan RC. Hyalinizing clear cell carcinoma: case series and comprehensive review of the literature. Cancer. 2009;115(1):75–83.
105. O'Sullivan-Meja ED, Massey HD, Faquin WC, Powes CN. Hylanizing clear cell carcinoma: report of eight cases and a review of literature. Head Neck Pathol. 2009;3:179.
106. Wang B, Brandwein M, Gordon R, Robinson R, Urken M, Zarbo RJ. Primary salivary clear cell tumors – a diagnostic approach: a clinicopathologic and immunohistochemical study of 20 patients with clear cell carcinoma, clear cell myoepithelial carcinoma, and epithelial–myoepithelial carcinoma. Arch Pathol Lab Med. 2002;126:676.
107. Vargas H, Sudilovsky D, Kaplan M, Regezi J, Weidner N. Mixed tumor, polymorphous low-grade adenocarcinoma and adenoid cystic carcinoma of the salivary gland: pathogenic implications and differential diagnosis by Ki-67 (MIB1), BCL2, and S-100 immunohistochemistry. Appl Immunohistochem. 1997;5(1):8.
108. Beltran D, Faquin WC, Gallagher G, August M. Selective immunohistochemical comparison of polymorphous low-grade adeno-

carcinoma and adenoid cystic carcinoma. J Oral Maxillofac Surg. 2006;64(3):415–23.
109. Prasad ML, Barbacioru CC, Rawal YB, Husein O, Wen P. Hierarchical cluster analysis of myoepithelial/basal cell markers in adenoid cystic carcinoma and polymorphous low-grade adenocarcinoma. Mod Pathol. 2008;21(2):105–14.
110. Shibata R, Martiniuk F, Qian Y, et al. Immunohistochemical expression of *c-kit* (CD117) in mucosal melanomas of the head and neck. Lab Investig. 2010;90(11):280A.
111. Araujo VC, Loducca SV, Sousa SO, Williams DM, Araujo NS. The cribriform features of adenoid cystic carcinoma and polymorphous low-grade adenocarcinoma: cytokeratin and integrin expression. Ann Diagn Pathol. 2001;5(6):330–4.
112. Gnepp DR, Chen JC, Warren C. Polymorphous low-grade adenocarcinoma of minor salivary gland. An immunohistochemical and clinicopathologic study. Am J Surg Pathol. 1988;12(6): 461–8.
113. Kawahara A, Harada H, Yokoyama T, Kage M. p63 Expression of clear myoepithelial cells in epithelial–myoepithelial carcinoma of the salivary gland: a useful marker for naked myoepithelial cells in cytology. Cancer. 2005;105(4):240–5.
114. Ellis GL. "Clear cell" oncocytoma of salivary gland. Hum Pathol. 1988;19(7):862–7.
115. Lai G, Nemolato S, Lecca S, Parodo G, Medda C, Faa G. The role of immunohistochemistry in the diagnosis of hyalinizing clear cell carcinoma of the minor salivary gland: a case report. Eur J Histochem. 2008;52(4):251–4.
116. Pires FR, Azevedo RS, Guiseppe F, et al. Metastatic renal cell carcinoma to the oral cavity and clear cell mucoepidermoid carcinoma: comparative clinicopathologic and immunohistochemical study. Oral Surg Oral Med Oral Pathol Oral Radiol Endod. 2009;109(4):e22–7.
117. Lueck N, Robinson RA. High levels of expression of cytokeratin 5 are strongly correlated with poor survival in higher grades of mucoepidermoid carcinoma. J Clin Pathol. 2008;61(7):837.
118. Zarbo RJ, Regezi JA, Batsakis JG. S-100 protein in salivary gland tumors: an immunohistochemical study of 129 cases. Head Neck Surg. 1986;8(4):268–75.
119. Saqi A, Giorgadze TA, Eleazar J, Remotti F, Vazquez MF. Clear cell and eosinophilic oncocytomas of salivary gland: cytological variants or parallels? Diagn Cytopathol. 2007;35(3):158–63.
120. Neves C, Soares A, Costa A, et al. CD10 (neutral endopeptidase) expression in myoepithelial cells of salivary neoplasms. Appl Immunohistochem Mol Morphol. 2010;18(2):172.
121. Angiero F, Sozzi D, Seramondi R, Valente MG. Epithelial–myoepithelial carcinoma of the minor salivary glands: immunohistochemical and morphological · features. Anticancer Res. 2009;29(11):4703–9.
122. Lin F, Wannian Y, Betten M, Bin T, Yang XJ. Expression of S-100 protein in renal cell neoplasms. Hum Pathol. 2006;37(4):462.
123. Ozolek J, Bastacky S, Myers E, Hunt J. Immunophenotypic comparison of salivary gland oncocytoma and metastatic renal cell carcinoma. Laryngoscope. 2005;115:1097.
124. Skalova A, Michal M, Ryska A, et al. Oncocytic myoepithelioma and pleomorphic adenoma of the salivary glands. Virchows Arch. 1999;434(6):537–46.
125. Liu H, Shi J, Liang K, Meschter S, Lin F. Loss of or reduced expression of the Von Hipple–Lindau gene product (pVHL) in malignant salivary epithelial neoplasms – with an implication of its role in tumorigenesis. Mod Pathol. 2008;21(Suppl):1089.
126. Gustafsson H, Virtanen I, Thornell LE. Expression of cytokeratins and vimentin in salivary gland carcinomas as revealed with monoclonal antibodies. Virchows Arch. 1988;412(6):515.
127. Faquin WC, Powers CN. Salivary gland cytopathology, Essentials in cytopathology, vol. 5. US: Springer; 2008. p. 156. Accessed 19 May 2010.
128. Tickoo SK, Amin MB, Linden MD, Lee MW, Zarbo RJ. Antimitochondrial antibody (113-1) in the differential diagnosis of granular renal cell tumors. Am J Surg Pathol. 1997;21(8):922–30.
129. Weinreb I, Seethala RR, Perez-Ordonez B, Chetty R, Hoschar AP, Hunt JL. Oncocytic mucoepidermoid carcinoma: clinicopathologic description in a series of 12 cases. Am J Surg Pathol. 2009;33(3):409–16.
130. Dale BA, Salonen J, Jones AH. New approaches and concepts in the study of differentiation of oral epithelia. Crit Rev Oral Biol Med. 1990;1(3):167–90.
131. Morgan P, Leigh I, Purkis P, et al. Site variations in keratin expression in human oral epithelia: an immunohistochemical study of individual keratins. Epithelia. 1987;1:31.
132. Ogden GR, Lane EB, Hopwood DV, Chisholm DM. Evidence for field change in oral cancer based on cytokeratin expression. Br J Cancer. 1993;67:1324.
133. Fillies T, Jogschies M, Kleinheinz J, Brandt B, Joos U, Buerger H. Cytokeratin alteration in oral leukoplakia and oral squamous cell carcinoma. Oncol Rep. 2007;18:639.
134. Fillies T, Werkmeister R, Packeisen J, et al. Cytokeratin 8/18 expression indicates a poor prognosis in squamous cell carcinomas of the oral cavity. BMC Cancer. 2006;6(10):1471.
135. Ram Prassad VV, Nirmala NR, Kotian MS. Immunohistochemical evaluation of expression of cytokeratin 19 in different histological grades of leukoplakia and oral squamous cell carcinoma. Indian J Dent Res. 2005;16(1):6.
136. Gillison M, Koch W, Capone R, et al. Evidence for a causal association between human papillomavirus and a subset of head and neck cancers. J Natl Cancer Inst. 2000;92(9):709.
137. Syrjanen S. Human papillomavirus (HPV) in head and neck cancer. J Clin Virol. 2005;32 Suppl 1:S59.
138. McKaig RG, Baric RS, Olshan AF. Human papillomavirus and head and neck cancer: epidemiology and molecular biology. Head Neck. 1998;20(3):250.
139. Chernock R, El-Mofty SK, Thorstad WL, Parvin CA, Lewis JS. HPV-related nonkeratinizing squamous cell carcinoma of the oropharynx: utility of microscopic features in predicting patient outcome. Head Neck Pathol. 2009;3(3):186–94.
140. Winters R, Naud S, Evans M, Trotman W, Kasznica P, Elhosseiny A. Ber-EP4, CK1, CK7 and CK14 are useful markers for basaloid squamous carcinoma: a study of 45 cases. Head Neck Pathol. 2008;2(4):265.
141. van der Velden LA, Schaafsman HE, Manni JJ, Ramaekers FC, Kuijpers W. Expression of cytokeratin subtypes and vimentin in squamous cell carcinoma of the floor of the mouth and the mobile tongue. Otorhinolaryngol Nova. 2001;11:186.
142. van der Velden LA, Schaafsma HE, Manni JJ, Ruiter DJ, Ramaekers FC, Kuijpers W. Cytokeratin and vimentin expression in normal epithelium and squamous cell carcinomas of the larynx. Eur Arch Otorhinolaryngol. 1997;254(8):376–83.
143. Fregonesi PA, Teresa DB, Duarte RA, Neto CB, de Oliveira MR, Soares CP. p16(INK4A) immunohistochemical overexpression in premalignant and malignant oral lesions infected with human papillomavirus. J Histochem Cytochem. 2003;51(10):1291–7.
144. Singhi A, Westra W. Comparison of human papillomavirus in situ hybridization and p16 immunohistochemistry in the detection of human papillomavirus-associated head and neck cancer based on a prospective clinical experience. Cancer. 2010;116(9):2166–73.
145. Leonardi E, Dalri P, Pusiol T, Valdagni R, Piscioli F. Spindle-cell squamous carcinoma of head and neck region: a clinicopathologic and immunohistochemical study of eight cases. ORL J Otorhinolaryngol Relat Spec. 1986;48(5):275–81.
146. Barnes L. Surgical pathology of the head and neck, vol. 1. 2nd ed. New York, NY: Marcel Kekker Ag; 2001. p. 786.
147. Barnes L. Surgical pathology of the head and neck, vol. 2. 2nd ed. New York, NY: Marcel Dekker AG; 2001. p. 649.

148. Barnes L. Surgical pathology of the head and neck, vol. 3. 2nd ed. New York, NY: Marcel Dekker AG; 2001. p. 772.
149. Serrano MF, El-Mofty SK, Gnepp DR, Lewis Jr JS. Utility of high molecular weight cytokeratins, but not p63, in the differential diagnosis of neuroendocrine and basaloid carcinomas of the head and neck. Hum Pathol. 2008;39(4):591–8.
150. Chapman-Fredricks J, Jorda M, Gomez-Fernandez C. A limited immunohistochemical panel helps differentiate small cell epithelial malignancies of the sinonasal cavity and nasopharynx. Applied Immunohistochem Mol Morphol. 2009;17(3):207.
151. Banks ER, Frierson Jr HF, Mills SE, George E, Zarbo RJ, Swanson PE. Basaloid squamous cell carcinoma of the head and neck. A clinicopathologic and immunohistochemical study of 40 cases. Am J Surg Pathol. 1992;16(10):939–46.
152. Hutcheson JA, Vural E, Korourian S, Hanna E. Neural cell adhesion molecule expression in adenoid cystic carcinoma of the head and neck. Laryngoscope. 2009;110(6):946.
153. Gandour-Edwards R, Kapadia SB, Barnes L, Donald PJ, Janecka IP. Neural cell adhesion molecule in adenoid cystic carcinoma invading the skull base. Otolaryngol Head Neck Surg. 1997;117(5):453–8.
154. Morice WG, Ferreiro JA. Distinction of basaloid squamous cell carcinoma from adenoid cystic and small cell undifferentiated carcinoma by immunohistochemistry. Hum Pathol. 1998;29(6):609–12.
155. Lee JS, Ko IJ, Jun SY, Kim JY. Basaloid squamous cell carcinoma in nasal cavity. Clin Exp Otorhinolaryngol. 2009;2(4):207.
156. Franchi A, Moroni M, Massi D, Paglierani M, Santucci M. Sinonasal undifferentiated carcinoma, nasopharyngeal-type undifferentiated carcinoma, and keratinizing and nonkeratinizing squamous cell carcinoma express different cytokeratin patterns. Am J Surg Pathol. 2002;26(12):1597–604.
157. El-Mofty SK, Patil S. Human papillomavirus (HPV)-related oropharyngeal nonkeratinizing squamous cell carcinoma: characterization of a distinct phenotype. Oral Surg Oral Med Oral Pathol Oral Radiol Endod. 2006;101:339.
158. Friedrich RE, Bartel-Friedrich S, Lobeck H, Niedobitek G, Arps H. Epstein–Barr virus DNA and epithelial markers in nasopharyngeal carcinoma. Med Microbiol Immunol (Berl). 2003;192(3):141–4.
159. Bar-Sela G, Kuten A, Ben-Eliezer S, Gov-Ari E, Ben-Izhak O. Expression of HER2 and C-KIT in nasopharyngeal carcinoma: implications for a new therapeutic approach. Mod Pathol. 2003; 16(10):1035–40.
160. Jeng YM, Sung MT, Fang CL, et al. Sinonasal undifferentiated carcinoma and nasopharyngeal-type undifferentiated carcinoma: two clinically, biologically, and histopathologically distinct entities. Am J Surg Pathol. 2002;26(3):371–6.
161. Bellizzi AM, Bruzzi C, French CA, Stelow EB. The cytologic features of NUT midline carcinoma. Cancer Cytopathol. 2009;117(6):508–15.
162. French CA, Kutok JL, Faquin WC, et al. Midline carcinoma of children and young adults with NUT rearrangement. J Clin Oncol. 2004;22(20):4135–9.
163. Haack H, Johnson LA, Fry CJ, et al. Diagnosis of NUT midline carcinoma using a NUT-specific monoclonal antibody. Am J Surg Pathol. 2009;33(7):984–91.
164. Stelow EB, Bellizzi AM, Taneja K, et al. NUT rearrangement in undifferentiated carcinomas of the upper aerodigestive tract. Am J Surg Pathol. 2008;32(6):828–34.
165. French CA. Molecular pathology of NUT midline carcinomas. J Clin Pathol. 2010;63(6):492–6.
166. Russell-Jones R, Orchard G, Zelger B, Wilson-Jones E. Immunostaining for CD31 and CD34 in Kaposi sarcoma. J Clin Pathol. 1995;48:1011.
167. Zhang YM, Bachmann S, Hemmer C, et al. Vascular origin of Kaposi's sarcoma. Expression of leukocyte adhesion molecule-1, thrombomodulin, and tissue factor. Am J Pathol. 1994;144(1):51–9.
168. Manning T, Smoller BR, Horn TD, et al. Evaluation of anti-thrombomodulin antibody as a tumor marker for vascular neoplasms. J Cutan Pathol. 2004;31(10):652–6.
169. Chan JK, Suster S, Wenig BM, Tsang WY, Chan JB, Lau AL. Cytokeratin 20 immunoreactivity distinguishes Merkel cell (primary cutaneous neuroendocrine) carcinomas and salivary gland small cell carcinomas from small cell carcinomas of various sites. Am J Surg Pathol. 1997;21(2):226–34.
170. Nagao T, Gaffey TA, Olsen KD, Serizawa H, Lewis JE. Small cell carcinoma of the major salivary glands: clinicopathologic study with emphasis on cytokeratin 20 immunoreactivity and clinical outcome. Am J Surg Pathol. 2004;28(6):762.
171. Woodruff JM, Senie RT. Atypical carcinoid tumor of the larynx. A critical review of the literature. ORL J Otorhinolaryngol Relat Spec. 1991;53(4):194–209.
172. Ferlito A, Rinaldo A. Primary and secondary small cell neuroendocrine carcinoma of the larynx: a review. Head Neck. 2008;30(4): 518–24.
173. Hirsch MS, Faquin WC, Krane JF. Thyroid transcription factor-1, but not p53, is helpful in distinguishing moderately differentiated neuroendocrine carcinoma of the larynx from medullary carcinoma of the thyroid. Mod Pathol. 2004;17(6):631–6.
174. Faragalla H, Weinreb I. Olfactory neuroblastoma: a review and update. Adv Anat Pathol. 2009;16(5):322–31.
175. Thompson LD, Miettinen M, Wenig BM. Sinonasal-type hemangiopericytoma: a clinicopathologic and immunophenotypic analysis of 104 cases showing perivascular myoid differentiation. Am J Surg Pathol. 2003;27(6):737–49.
176. McKinney CD, Mills SE, Franquemont DW. Sinonasal intestinal-type adenocarcinoma: immunohistochemical profile and comparison with colonic adenocarcinoma. Mod Pathol. 1995;8(4):421–6.
177. Jo VY, Mills SE, Cathro HP, Carlson DL, Stelow EB. Low-grade sinonasal adenocarcinomas: the association with and distinction from respiratory epithelial adenomatoid hamartomas and other glandular lesions. Am J Surg Pathol. 2009;33(3):401–8.
178. Vega F, Chang CC, Medeiros LJ, et al. Plasmablastic lymphomas and plasmablastic plasma cell myelomas have nearly identical immunophenotypic profiles. Mod Pathol. 2005;18(6):806–15.
179. Colomo L, Loong F, Rives S, et al. Diffuse large B-cell lymphomas with plasmablastic differentiation represent a heterogeneous group of disease entities. Am J Surg Pathol. 2004;28(6):736–47.
180. Taddesse-Heath L, Meloni-Ehrig A, Scheerle J, Kelly JC, Jaffe ES. Plasmablastic lymphoma with *MYC* translocation: evidence for a common pathway in the generation of plasmablastic features. Mod Pathol. 2010;23(7):991–9.
181. Cerilli LA, Holst VA, Brandwein MS, Stoler MH, Mills SE. Sinonasal undifferentiated carcinoma: immunohistochemical profile and lack of EBV association. Am J Surg Pathol. 2001;25(2):156–63.
182. Thompson S. Sinonasal carcinomas. 2006;12(1):40. [2 Apr 2010].
183. Iezzoni JC, Mills SE. "Undifferentiated" small round cell tumors of the sinonasal tract: differential diagnosis update. Am J Clin Pathol. 2005;124(Suppl):S110–21.
184. Hirano T. Immunohistochemical study of malignant melanoma. Acta Pathol Jpn. 1986;36(5):733–43.
185. Carbone A, Gloghini A, Rinaldo A, Devaney KO, Tubbs R, Ferlito A. True identity by immunohistochemistry and molecular morphology of undifferentiated malignancies of the head and neck. Head Neck. 2009;31(7):949–61.
186. Ejaz A, Wenig BM. Sinonasal undifferentiated carcinoma: clinical and pathologic features and a discussion on classification, cellular differentiation, and differential diagnosis. Adv Anat Pathol. 2005;12(3):134–43.
187. Cordes B, Williams MD, Tirado Y, et al. Molecular and phenotypic analysis of poorly differentiated sinonasal neoplasms: an integrated approach for early diagnosis and classification. Hum Pathol. 2009;40(3):283–92.

188. Sung CO, Ko YH, Park S, Kim K, Kim W. Immunoreactivity of CD99 in non-Hodgkin's lymphoma: unexpected frequent expression in ALK-positive anaplastic large cell lyphoma. J Korean Med Sci. 2005;20(6):952.
189. Finke NM, Lae ME, Lloyd RV, Gehani SK, Nascimento AG. Sinonasal desmoplastic small round cell tumor: a case report. Am J Surg Pathol. 2002;26(6):799–803.
190. Hirakawa N, Naka T, Yamamoto I, Fukuda T, Tsuneyoshi M. Overexpression of bcl-2 protein in synovial sarcoma: a comparative study of other soft tissue spindle cell sarcomas and an additional analysis by fluorescence in situ hybridization. Hum Pathol. 1996;27(10):1060–5.
191. Kim JW, Kong IG, Lee CH, et al. Expression of Bcl-2 in olfactory neuroblastoma and its association with chemotherapy and survival. Otolaryngol Head Neck Surg. 2008;139(5):708–12.
192. Olsen SH, Thomas DG, Lucas DR. Cluster analysis of immunohistochemical profiles in synovial sarcoma, malignant peripheral nerve sheath tumor, and Ewing sarcoma. Mod Pathol. 2006; 19:659.
193. Sebire NJ, Gibson S, Rampling D, Williams S, Malone M, Ramsay AD. Immunohistochemical findings in embryonal small round cell tumors with molecular diagnostic confirmation. Appl Immunohistochem Mol Morphol. 2005;13(1):1–5.
194. Liu Q, Ohshima K, Sumie A, Suzushima H, Iwasaki H, Kikuchi M. Nasal CD56 positive small round cell tumors. Differential diagnosis of hematological, neurogenic, and myogenic neoplasms. Virchows Arch. 2001;438(3):271–9.
195. Folpe AL, Schmidt RA, Chapman D, Gown AM. Poorly differentiated synovial sarcoma: immunohistochemical distinction from primitive neuroectodermal tumors and high-grade malignant peripheral nerve sheath tumors. Am J Surg Pathol. 1998;22(6): 673–82.
196. Gu M, Antonescu CR, Guiter G, Huvos AG, Ladanyi M, Zakowski MF. Cytokeratin immunoreactivity in Ewing's sarcoma: prevalence in 50 cases confirmed by molecular diagnostic studies. Am J Surg Pathol. 2000;24(3):410–6.
197. Creager A. Immunohisothemical, molecular, and cytogenetic analysis of bone and soft tissue tumors. In: Diagnostic musculoskeletal surgical pathology. 1st ed. New York: Elsevier; 2004. Accessed 19 May 2010.
198. Yasuda T, Perry KD, Nelson M, et al. Alveolar rhabdomyosarcoma of the head and neck region in older adults: genetic characterization and a review of the literature. Hum Pathol. 2009;40(3): 341–8.
199. Bahrami A, Gown AM, Baird GS, Hicks MJ, Folpe AL. Aberrant expression of epithelial and neuroendocrine markers in alveolar rhabdomyosarcoma: a potentially serious diagnostic pitfall. Mod Pathol. 2008;21(7):795–806.
200. Weiss SW, Goldblum JR. Enzinger and Weiss's soft tissue tumors. 5th ed. Philadelphia, PA, USA: Mosby Elsevier; 2008. p. 1257. Accessed 21 May 2010.
201. Carpentieri DF, Nichols K, Chou PM, Matthews M, Pawel B, Huff D. The expression of WT1 in the differentiation of rhabdomyosarcoma from other pediatric small round blue cell tumors. Mod Pathol. 2002;15(10):1080–6.
202. Megerian CA, Pilch BZ, Bhan AK, McKenna MJ. Differential expression of transthyretin in papillary tumors of the endolymphatic sac and choroid plexus. Laryngoscope. 1997;107(2): 216–21.
203. Devaney KO, Ferlito A, Rinaldo A. Endolymphatic sac tumor (low-grade papillary adenocarcinoma) of the temporal bone. Acta Otolaryngol. 2003;123(9):1022.
204. Johnson TL, Zarbo RJ, Lloyd RV, Crissman JD. Paragangliomas of the head and neck: immunohistochemical neuroendocrine and intermediate filament typing. Mod Pathol. 1988;1(3):216–23.
205. Li TJ, Yu SF, Gao Y, Wang EB. Clear cell odontogenic carcinoma: a clinicopathologic and immunocytochemical study of 5 cases. Arch Pathol Lab Med. 2001;125(12):1566–71.
206. Dong Q, Pan S, Sun LS, Li TJ. Orthokeratinized odontogenic cyst: a clinicopathologic study of 61 cases. Arch Pathol Lab Med. 2010;134(2):271–5.
207. Piattelli A, Fioroni M, Iezzi G, Rubini C, Dental School, University of Chieti, Italy. Calretinin expression in odontogenic cysts. J Endod. 2003;29(6):394.
208. Ogden GR, Chisholm DM, Kiddie RA, et al. p53 Protein in odontogenic cysts: increased expression in some odontogenic keratocysts. J Clin Pathol. 1992;45:1007.
209. Malcic A, Jukic S, Anic I, et al. Alterations of FHIT and P53 genes in keratocystic odontogenic tumor, dentigerous and radicular cyst. J Oral Pathol Med. 2008;37(5):294.
210. Altini M, Coleman H, Doglioni C, Favia G, Maiorano E. Calretinin expression in ameloblastomas. Histopathology. 2000;37(1):27–32.
211. DeVilliers P, Liu H, Suggs C, et al. Calretinin expression in the differential diagnosis of human ameloblastoma and keratocystic odontogenic tumor. Am J Surg Pathol. 2008;32(2):256–60.
212. Devilliers P, Liu H, Suggs C, et al. Calretinin in ameloblastoma of KCOT. Mod. Pathol. 2006 June Seg. 81.
213. Okamoto E, Kikuchi K, Miyazaki Y, et al. Significance of podoplanin expression in keratocystic odontogenic tumor. J Oral Pathol Med. 2010;39(1):110.
214. Piattelli A, Lezzi G, Fioroni M, Santinelli A, Rubini C. Ki-67 expression in dentigerous cysts, unicystic ameloblastomas, and ameloblastomas arising from dental cysts. J Endod. 2002; 28(2):55–8.
215. Osman M, Ferriera P. Ki 47 immunoreactivity in odontogenic keratocysts and orthokertinized jaw cysts. 2007. abstract:http// iadr.confex.com/iadr/2007orleans/techprogram/abstract_88699. html.
216. Gurgel C, Ramos E, Azevedo R, Sarmento V, Carvalho A, Santos J. Expression of Ki-67, p53 and p63 proteins in keratocyst odontogenic tumours: an immunohistochemical study. Journal of molecular Histology 2008;39(3):311–316.
217. Eslami M, Eshghyar N, Tirgari F, Rezvani G. Ki-67 expression. Journal of Dentistry 2004;17(1).
218. Lo Muzio L, Santarelli A, Caltabiano R, et al. p63 Expression in odontogenic cysts. Int J Oral Maxillofac Surg. 2005;34(6): 668–73.
219. Coleman H, Altini M, Ali H, Doglioni C, Favia G, Maiorano E. Use of calretinin in the differential diagnosis of unicystic ameloblastomas. Histopathology. 2001;38(4):312–7.

Chapter 14
Lung, Pleura, and Mediastinum

Kai Zhang and Phillip Cagle

Abstract The chapter contains 51 frequently asked immunohistochemical questions with answers addressed with tables and concise note and representative pictures in the diagnosis of common and uncommon pleuropulmonary and mediastinal tumors. The questions and selected frequently used antibodies or antibody panels come from a review of numerous published literatures, books, and book chapters incorporated with authors' own practicing experience, which reflects up to date information in practicing immunohistochemistry in the field. Many of the antibodies have been tested, evaluated, and verified in author's institution on tissue microarray and tissue sections. In lights of recent progress in diagnosing and treating nonsmall cell lung carcinomas (NSCLC), the most useful diagnostic antibody panels have been highlighted in the chapter. For example, to differentiate pulmonary adenocarcinoma from squamous cell carcinoma, a panel of antibodies including (CK7, CK20, CK5/6, p63, TTF-1) has been recommended. Napsin A has been increasingly used together with TTF-1 to confirm NSCLC since a small subset of NSCLC may be only positive for Napsin A while being negative for TTF-1. Furthermore, immunophenotypes of various cell types of normal lung tissue have been described.

Keywords Nonsmall cell lung carcinoma • Adenocarcinoma • Squamous cell carcinoma • Small cell lung carcinoma • TTF-1 (thyroid transcription factor-1) • Napsin A • CK5/6 and p63

FREQUENTLY ASKED QUESTIONS

Pulmonary Tumors

K. Zhang (✉)
Department of Pathology and Laboratory Medicine,
Geisinger Medical Center, 100 North Academy Avenue,
Danville, PA 17822, USA

F. Lin and J. Prichard (eds.), *Handbook of Practical Immunohistochemistry: Frequently Asked Questions*,
DOI 10.1007/978-1-4419-8062-5_14,

Differential Diagnosis

Pleural Tumors

Mediastinal Tumors

Table 14.1 Markers commonly used in diagnosing pleuropulmonary neoplasms

Antibodies	Staining pattern	Function	Key applications and pitfalls
AE1/AE3	M + C	Epithelial marker	Positive in lung carcinoma and EM
Pan-CK	M + C	Epithelial marker	Positive in lung carcinoma and EM
CK7	M + C	Epithelial marker	Positive in lung AC including non-m-BAC and m-BAC and EM; usually negative in SQCC
CK20	M + C	Epithelial marker	Positive in m-BAC and goblet cell type of primary lung MC; negative in other AC, including non-m-BAC
CK5/6	M + C	Epithelial marker	Positive in SQCC and adenosquamous cell carcinoma and EM and negative in AC; also positive in a subset of breast and gynecologic malignancies
p63	N	A p53-homologous protein in the regulation of stem cell commitment in squamous and other epithelia	Positive in normal basal cell and SQCC; and variably positive in subset of BAC, AC, and large cell carcinoma; negative for carcinoid tumor and small cell carcinoma
CK903 (34betaE12)	M + C	Epithelial marker (high molecular weight cytokeratins, including CK1, 5, 10, and 14)	Positive in normal squamous epithelium and SQCC and basaloid carcinoma; negative in neuroendocrine tumors
TTF-1 (thyroid transcription factor-1)	N	A homeodomain-containing nuclear transcription protein of Nkx2 gene family	Positive in AC including non-m-BAC and signet ring cell type and goblet cell type of primary lung MC and small cell carcinoma and typically negative for m-BAC and SQCC and basaloid carcinoma; also positive in thyroid carcinomas
Napsin A	C + M	An aspartic protease with a molecular weight of approximately 38 kDa expressed in type-II pneumocytes and is involved in the N- and C-terminal processing of proSP-B in type-II pneumocytes	Positive in AC, including non-m-BAC and clear cell renal cell carcinoma; typically negative for SQCC
SP-A and SP-B (surfactant proteins A and B)	C	Surfactant proteins A and B for function and hemostasis of pulmonary surfactant, reducing the surface tension of the alveolar interface	Positive in 50% of ACs; but not as sensitive as TTF-1; however, also found to be positive in metastatic breast carcinoma to the lung
MOC-31	M	Expressed in various adenocarcinomas and normal glandular epithelium; usually negative in mesothelioma	Positive in AC and a subset of SQCC
Ber-EP4	M + C	Expressed in various adenocarcinomas and normal glandular epithelium; usually negative in diffuse malignant mesothelioma	Positive in lung AC; usually negative but occasionally positive in SQCC; negative in EM
TAG 72 (B72.3)	M + C	Expressed in various adenocarcinomas and normal glandular epithelium	Positive in lung adenocarcinoma, rarely positive in squamous cell carcinoma; negative in epithelial mesothelioma
CEA (carcino-embryonic antigen)	C	Expressed in various adenocarcinomas and normal glandular epithelium	Positive in lung adenocarcinoma, positive in squamous cell carcinoma; negative in epithelial mesothelioma
ES1	M or C	A variant of CEA-related cell adhesion molecule 6 (CEACAM6)	Positive in AC
CD15 (LeuM1)	M + C	Expressed in various adenocarcinomas	Positive in lung adenocarcinoma
Calretinin	C or N + C	Calcium-binding protein expressed in a variety of tissues, including mesothelial cells, adipocytes, neural tissue, and sex cord tumors	International Meso Panel and USCMRP recognize nuclear staining for calretinin as relatively specific for EM vs. pulmonary AC; nuclear staining for calretinin may be seen in other neoplasms, for example, synovial sarcoma; cytoplasmic staining for calretinin is nonspecific and may be seen in many tumors including some pulmonary AC
Mesothelin	M + C	A 40-kDa protein expressed in normal mesothelium and overexpressed in some cancers, such as EM, ovarian carcinoma, and DAC	Positive in EM; negative in AC

(continued)

Table 14.1 (continued)

Antibodies	Staining pattern	Function	Key applications and pitfalls
D2-40/Podoplanin	M + C	Lymphatic endothelial cells	Positive in mesothelial cells and EM and variably positive in SM; negative in AC
HBME-1	M	Surface microvilli of mesothelial cells	HBME-1 stains membrane of both EM and AC – the difference is qualitative. EM tend to have thick, continuous membranous staining, whereas AC have thin, discontinuous staining
WT1	N	Transcription factor	Positive in EM; negative in AC; also positive in ovarian and peritoneal serous carcinoma
Thrombomodulin	C + M	Surface glycoprotein	Positive in 80% of EM; positive in SQCC and urothelial carcinomas
CD56	M + C	Neuron adhesion molecules	Positive in neuroendocrine tumor including small cell carcinoma and a subset of nonsmall cell carcinoma with neuroendocrine differentiation
Synaptophysin	C	Present in the cores of amine and peptide hormone and neurotransmitter dense-core secretory vesicles	Positive in neuroendocrine tumor including small cell carcinoma and a subset of nonsmall cell carcinoma with neuroendocrine differentiation
Chromogranin	C	Present in the cores of amine and peptide hormone and neurotransmitter dense-core secretory vesicles	Positive in neuroendocrine tumor including small cell carcinoma and a subset of nonsmall cell carcinoma with neuroendocrine differentiation. Because this stains the secretory dense-core granules, it may not be positive in small cell carcinomas with scant granules
NSE (neuron-specific enolase)	C		Very nonspecific and, hence, not often used for this purpose; positive in neuroendocrine tumor including small cell carcinoma and nonsmall cell carcinoma with or without neuroendocrine differentiation
DC-LAMP		Dendritic cell marker	Positive in pulmonary carcinoma with Clara cell differentiation
Villin	Brush border pattern		Marker of adenocarcinoma of intestinal origin
CDX-2	N	A caudal-related homeobox transcription factor expressed in intestinal epithelium	Negative in AC including non-m-BAC and signet ring cell type and primary lung MC; positive for m-BAC and goblet cell type of primary lung MC and metastatic colorectal adenocarcinoma. Also reported in a few other nonpulmonary cell types
MUC2	C + M	A membrane-associated glycoprotein expressed in various tumor types	
MUC5AC	C + M	A membrane-associated glycoprotein expressed in various tumor types	

Note: *N* nuclear staining, *M* membranous staining, *C* cytoplasmic staining, *EM* epithelial diffuse malignant mesothelioma, *AC* adenocarcinoma of the lung (mixed subtype), *non-m-BAC* non-mucinous bronchioloalveolar adenocarcinoma, *m-BAC* mucinous bronchioloalveolar adenocarcinoma, *BAC* bronchioloalveolar adenocarcinoma, *MC* mucinous carcinoma, *SQCC* squamous cell carcinoma of the lung, *SM* sarcomatoid diffuse malignant mesothelioma

References: [1–123]

Table 14.2 Markers for normal lung

Markers	Bronchial and bronchiolar basal (reserve) cells	Bronchial epithelium in conducting airway	Bronchiolar epithelium	Alveolar epithelium (pneumocytes, type I and II)	Clara cells (nonciliated)
CK7	–	+	+	+	+?
CK20	–	–	–	–	–
CK5/6	+	–	–	–	–
p63	+	–	–	–	–
CK903 (34betaE12)	+	–	–	–	–
CK17	+	–	–	–	–
CK19	–	+ (Variable)	–	–	–
TTF-1	–	+/–	+ (Small-sized bronchioles and TRU)	+	+
SP-A	–	–	–	+	+
Villin	–	–	–	–	–
ER/PR	–	–	–	–	–
GCDFP-15	–	–	–	–	–
DC-LAMP (PE10)	–	–	+	+ (Diffuse staining pattern)	+ (Apical granular pattern)
CDX-2	–	–	–	–	–
MUC1	–	–	–	–	–
MUC2	–	–	–	–	–
MUC5AC	–	–/+	–	–	–
Inhibin-alpha	–	–	–	–	–

Note: *CK* cytokeratin, *TTF-1* thyroid transcription factor-1, *SP-A* surfactant protein A, *TRU* terminal respiratory unit (alveoli, alveolar sacs, ducts, and respiratory bronchioles), *GCDFP-15* gross cystic disease fluid protein-15, *ER* estrogen receptor, *DC-LAMP* a molecule expressed in mature dendritic cells

We have tested 19 cases of normal lung for these markers at GML (Geisinger Medical Laboratories), and the findings are similar to the published results

CK7 also stained submucosal seromucinous glands. CK20 stained <5% of bronchial epithelium. CK903 stained bronchial scattered, vertically oriented, non-mucinous cells, and bronchiolar basal cells as well as cuboidal and columnar cells of bronchial ducts. CK5/6 stained bronchiolar basal (reserve) cells; the positive staining is attenuated when bronchioles become smaller in size, whereas p63+ basal cells of bronchioles largely remain. Squamous metaplasia and myoepithelial cells from submucosal bronchial glands stained positively with p63. CK17 staining pattern is similar to CK5/6. CK19 stained submucosal seromucinous glands. MUC1 stained submucosal seromucinous glands showing an apical brush pattern. Occasional stromal cells of interstitial areas and large peribronchial areas show weak positivity for ER and PR. TTF-1 staining is quite uniform, but TTF-1 does not stain bronchial epithelium, bronchial glandular epithelium, vessels, fibrocytes/fibroblasts, or infiltrating inflammatory cells. SP-A stained alveolar epithelium, nonciliated Clara cells, and some cells of tracheobronchial epithelium and glands. MUC5AC stained the cytoplasm of scattered mucinous cells of the main bronchi and the mucin-rich cells of the associated bronchial glands. Villin shows positive staining in the brush border. DC-LAMP stained a subset of adenocarcinoma

Basal cells can give rise to the differentiated ciliated cells and mucous goblet cells in bronchi and bronchioles. Basal cells are capable of proliferating and differentiating into basal cell hyperplasia, followed by squamous cell metaplasia, squamous cell dysplasia, and squamous cell carcinoma. The tumors derived from these basal cell precursors (squamous cell carcinoma) are epidemiologically related to tobacco smoke, following multistep carcinogenesis. Basal cells are also capable of proliferating and differentiating into goblet cell hyperplasia, followed by adenocarcinoma with goblet cell features (mucinous bronchioloalveolar carcinoma or other MUC5AC-expressing adenocarcinoma)

References: [12, 62, 86, 90, 96, 97, 102, 108, 115, 120–124]

Table 14.3 Markers for mixed adenocarcinoma and adenocarcinoma with papillary or micropapillary features

Antibodies	Literature	AC, mixed subtype (N = 54)	AC, papillary, and/or micropapillary features (N = 10)
CK7	+	96% (52/54)	90% (9/10)
CK20	– or +	4% (2/54)	0% (0/10)
TTF-1	+	89% (48/54)	90% (9/10)
Napsin A	+	93% (50/54)	90% (9/10)
CK5/6	–	4% (2/54)	10% (1/10)
p63	–	2% (53/54)	20% (2/10)
SP-A (PE-10)	– or + (46% +)	ND	ND
SP-B (polyclonal)	+ or – (52% +)	ND	ND
GCDFP-15	– or + (5.2%)	2% (1/54) (Very focal)	0% (0/54)
ER	Variable (<10 or >80%)	0% (0/54)	ND
PR	Variable (<10 or >80%)	0% (0/54)	ND
Villin	6–68% (Variable)	6% (3/54)	0% (0/10)
DC-LAMP	+ (Clara cell differentiation)	ND	ND
Inhibin-alpha	–/+	6% (3/54)	0% (0/10)

Note: *ND* not done, *UK* unknown, *SP-A* surfactant protein A, *SP-B* surfactant protein B, *GCDFP-15* gross cystic disease fluid protein-15, *ER* estrogen receptor, *PR* progesterone receptor

GML data are based on TMA sections containing 54 cases of mixed or acinar lung adenocarcinoma and 10 cases of adenocarcinoma with papillary and/or micropapillary features

Detection of ER is dependent upon the antibody clone that is used

GML data show approximately 6% of mixed adenocarcinomas that are focally and weakly positive for villin

In cases where a diagnosis of adenocarcinoma vs. squamous cell carcinoma cannot be made on routine H&E, immunohistochemistry may be useful to distinguish the cell type. Although there is currently no consensus on the best immunohistochemistry panel for this purpose, TTF-1 and Napsin A for adenocarcinoma and CK5/6 and p63 for squamous cell carcinoma have been advocated as a panel by some investigators

Lung acinar adenocarcinoma shows membranous and cytoplasmic staining for CK7 (Fig. 14.1) and CK19 (Fig. 14.2); nuclear staining for TTF-1 (Fig. 14.3); membranous and cytoplasmic staining for Napsin A (Fig. 14.4); membranous and cytoplasmic staining for MOC-31 (Fig. 14.5); membranous and cytoplasmic s taining for KOC (Fig. 14.6); cytoplasmic staining for inhibin-alpha (Fig. 14.7); and positive staining for villin with apical pattern (Fig. 14.8). Lung adenocarcinoma shows cytoplasmic staining for ALK-1 (Fig. 14.9a) and H&E (Fig. 14.9b)

References: [5, 11, 26, 56, 57, 71, 90, 100, 101, 106, 115, 118, 121–123]

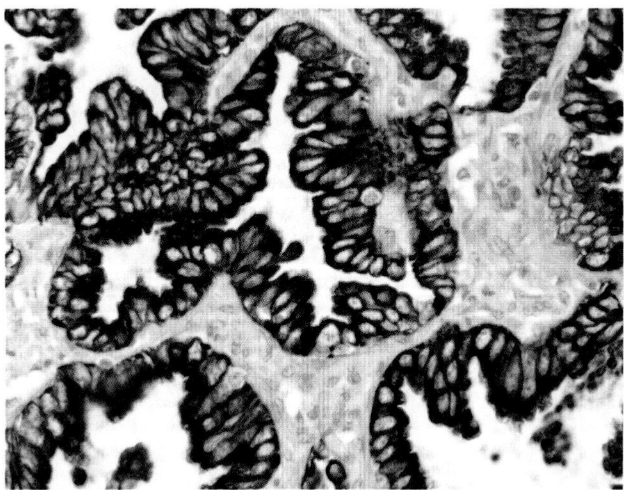

Fig. 14.1 Lung acinar adenocarcinoma shows membranous and cytoplasmic staining for CK7

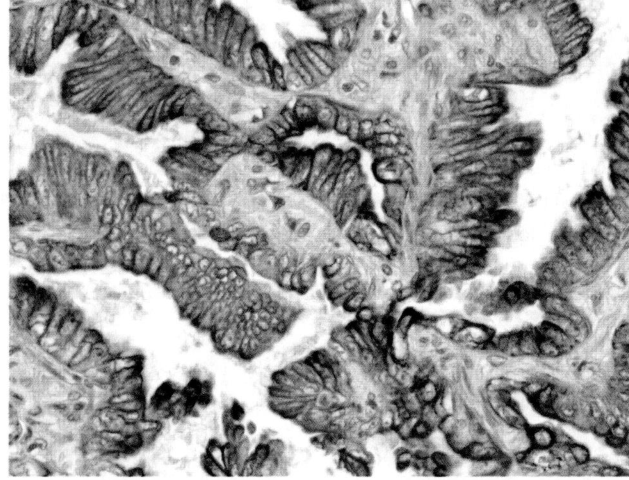

Fig. 14.2 Lung acinar adenocarcinoma shows membranous and cytoplasmic staining for CK19

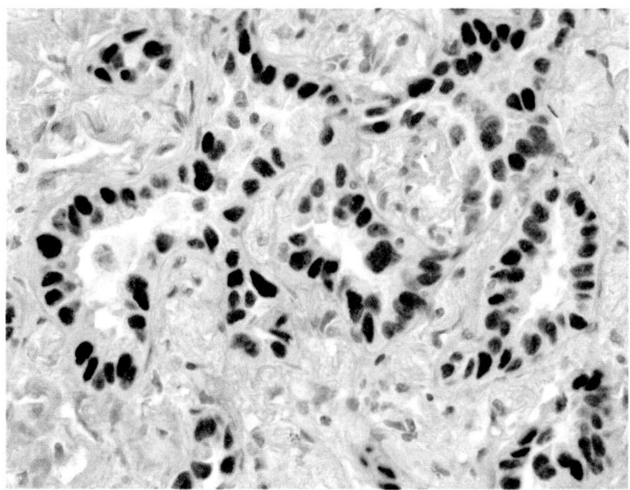

Fig. 14.3 Lung acinar adenocarcinoma show nuclear staining for TTF-1

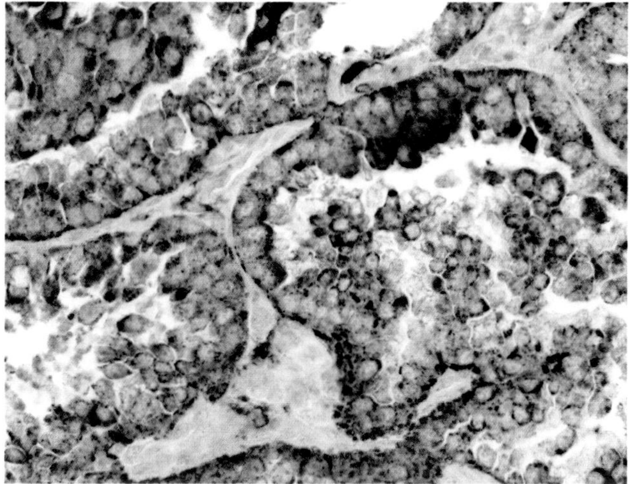

Fig. 14.4 Lung acinar adenocarcinoma shows membranous and cytoplasmic staining for Napsin A

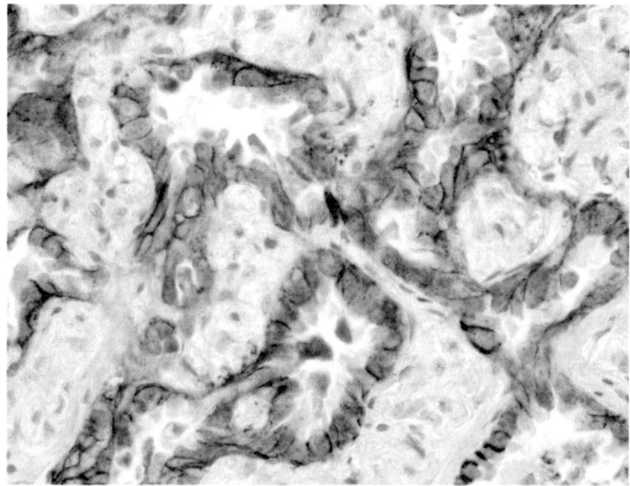

Fig. 14.5 Lung acinar adenocarcinoma shows membranous and cytoplasmic staining for MOC-31

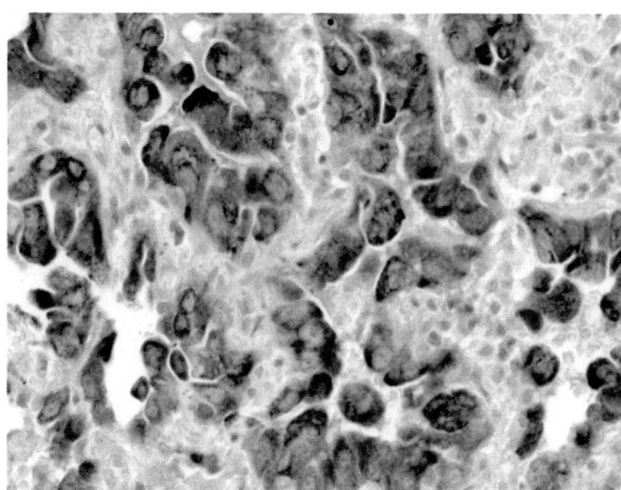

Fig. 14.6 Lung acinar adenocarcinoma shows membranous and cytoplasmic staining for KOC

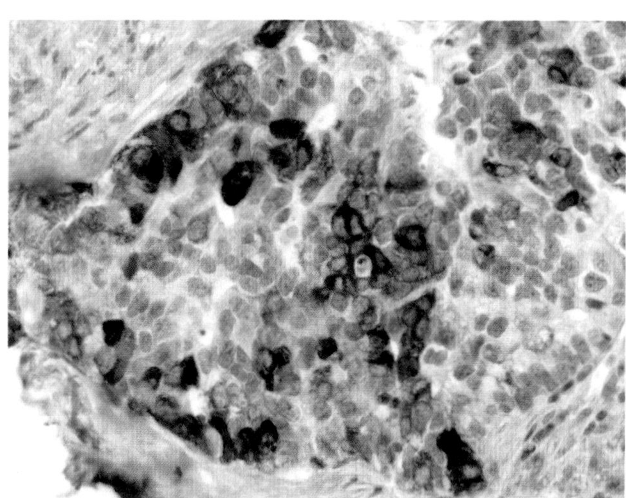

Fig. 14.7 Lung acinar adenocarcinoma shows cytoplasmic staining for inhibin-alpha

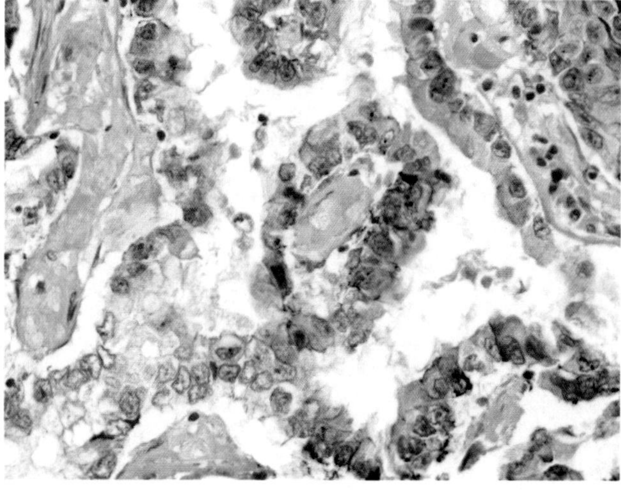

Fig. 14.8 Lung acinar adenocarcinoma shows positive staining for villin with apical pattern

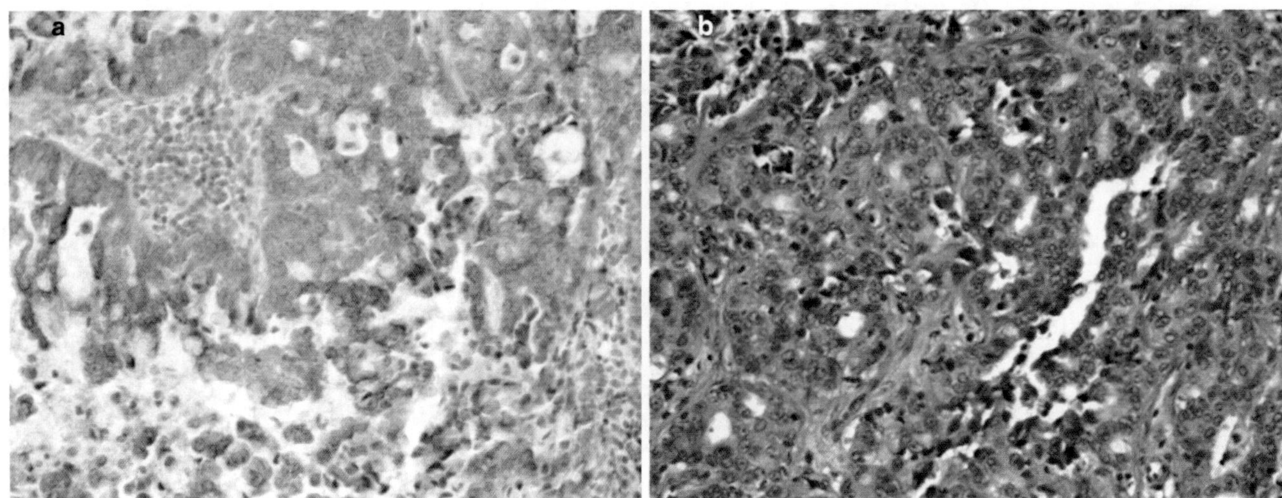

Fig. 14.9 Lung adenocarcinoma shows cytoplasmic staining for ALK-1 (**a**) and H&E (**b**)

Table 14.4 Markers for pure non-mucinous bronchioloalveolar carcinoma (non-m-BAC)

Antibodies	Literature	GML data (N = 3)
CK7	+	100% (3/3)
CK20	– or +	0% (0/3)
TTF-1	+	100% (3/3)
Napsin A	+	100% (3/3)
CEA	UK	100% (3/3)
p63	–	0% (0/3)
SP-A	+ or – (57% +)	ND
SP-B	+ or – (64% +)	ND
MOC-31	UK	100% (3/3)
CEA	UK	100% (3/3)

Note: *ND* not done, *UK* unknown, *SP-A* surfactant protein A, *SP-B* surfactant protein B

The limited GML data (N = 3) show similar findings compared to the published literature

References: [11, 31, 52, 86, 90, 101, 106, 110, 111, 113, 121–123]

Table 14.5 Markers for mucinous bronchioloalveolar carcinoma (m-BAC)

Antibodies	Literature	GML data (N = 10)
CK7	+ (Diffuse or patchy)	100% (10/10) (Usually diffusely and strongly)
CK20	+/– (Patchy)	30% (3/10) (When positive usually patchy)
TTF-1	–	20% (2/10) (When positive, usually focal)
CDX-2	–	30% (3/10) (When positive, very focal)
CK5/6	– or +	0% (0/10)
p63	–	0% (0/10)

Note: GML data are based on ten cases of TMA sections and routine sections

Lung mucinous bronchioloalveolar carcinoma shows membranous and cytoplasmic staining for CK7 (Fig. 14.10a), CK20 (Fig. 14.10b), nuclear staining for CDX-2 (Fig. 14.10c), and membranous and cytoplasmic staining for MUC5AC (Fig. 14.10d)

Note: CK20 and CDX-2 staining are usually patchy

References: [11, 20, 49, 86, 101, 106, 111, 121–123]

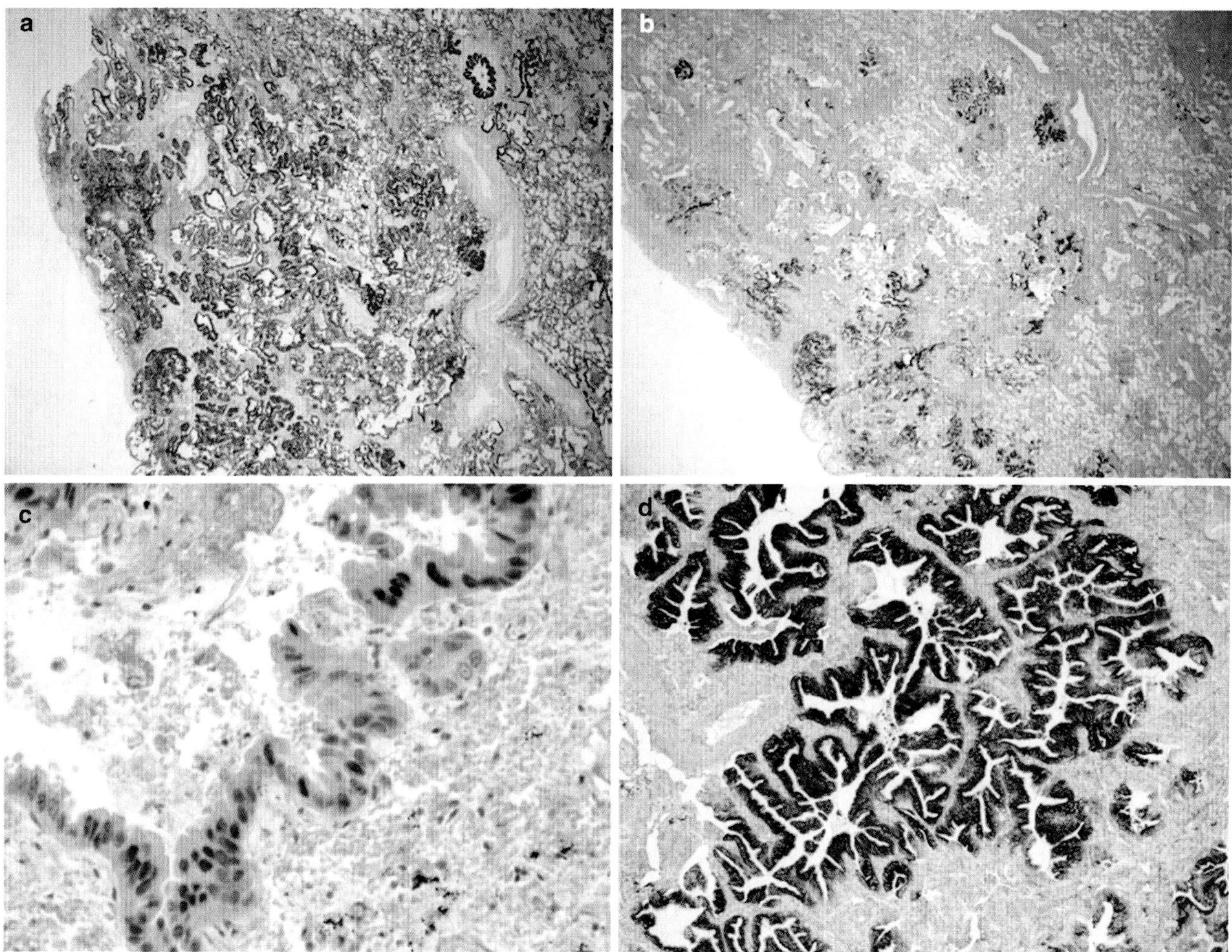

Fig. 14.10 Lung mucinous bronchioloalveolar carcinoma show membranous and cytoplasmic staining for CK7 (**a**), CK20 (**b**), CDX-2 (**c**), and MUC5AC (**d**). *Note*: CK20 and CDX-2 staining are usually patchy

Table 14.6 Markers for primary lung mucinous (colloid) carcinoma (goblet cell and signet ring cell type)

	Literature	
Antibodies	Goblet cell type	Signet ring cell type
Pan-CK	UK	+
CK7	+	+
CK20	+	–
TTF-1	+ or –	+
CDX-2	+	–
MUC1	UK	+
MUC2	+	–
MUC5AC	– or +	+
CEA	UK	+
ER/PR	UK	–
GCDFP-15	UK	–

Note: *UK* unknown

References: [11, 20, 49, 86, 101, 106, 111, 121–123]

Table 14.7 Markers for squamous cell carcinoma

Antibodies	Literature	GML data (N = 41)
CK7	–	34% (11/41)
CK20	–	<1% (1/41)
TTF-1	–	<1% (1/41)
p63	+	100% (41/41)
Napsin A	–	2% (1/41)
CK5/6	+	82% (35/41)
CD56	– or +	0% (0/41)

Note: *UK* unknown

GML data are based on TMA sections containing 41 cases

Immunohistochemistry has not proven useful in determining the origin of SQCC (i.e., primary lung SQCC or metastatic SQCC of extrapulmonary sites to lung)

In cases where a diagnosis of adenocarcinoma vs. squamous cell carcinoma cannot be made on routine H&E, immunohistochemistry may be useful to distinguish the cell type. Although there is currently no consensus on the best immunohistochemistry panel for this purpose, TTF-1 and Napsin A for adenocarcinoma and CK5/6 and p63 for squamous cell carcinoma have been advocated as a panel by some investigators

Today, oncologists need diagnosis of a specific cell type (adenocarcinoma vs. squamous cell carcinoma) in order to initiate targeted molecular lung cancer therapies. Diagnosing only "nonsmall cell carcinoma" is no longer as sufficient as it was in years past. The diagnosis "nonsmall cell carcinoma" should not be made whenever possible. Patients with adenocarcinomas may respond to bevacizumab therapy. Patients with squamous cell carcinoma who receive bevacizumab therapy are at risk of developing severe, even life-threatening, hemorrhage. Advanced stage adenocarcinomas, but not squamous cell carcinomas, may respond to pemetrexed therapy. Other potential targets of molecular targeted therapy tend to have histologic associations, for example, K-ras mutations in mucinous adenocarcinomas and epidermal growth factor receptor mutations in nonmucinous bronchioloalveolar carcinomas in specific populations

Lung squamous cell carcinoma shows membranous and cytoplasmic staining for CK5/6 (Fig. 14.11); nuclear staining for p63 (Fig. 14.12); membranous and cytoplasmic staining for CK903 (Fig. 14.13) and for Maspin (Fig. 14.14)

References: [11, 54, 97, 101, 106, 109, 112, 119, 121–123]

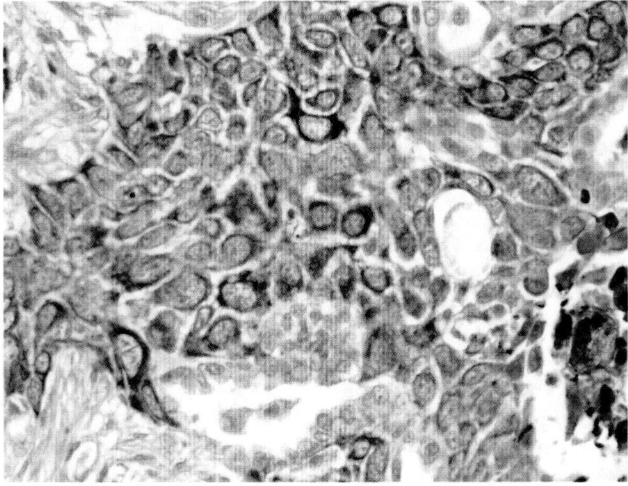

Fig. 14.11 Lung squamous cell carcinoma show membranous and cytoplasmic staining for CK5/6

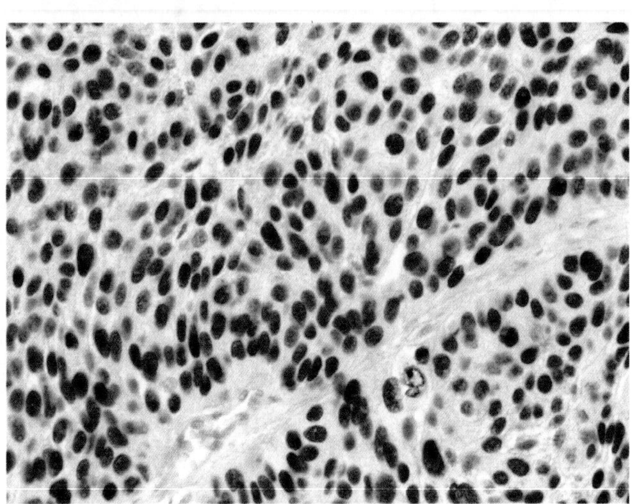

Fig. 14.12 Lung squamous cell carcinoma show nuclear staining for p63

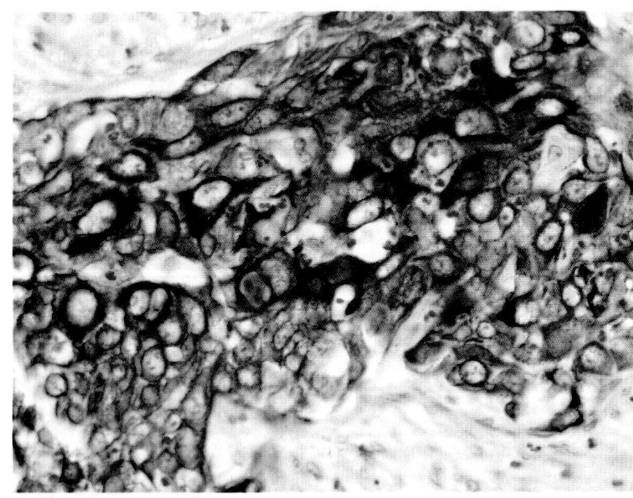

Fig. 14.13 Lung squamous cell carcinoma show membranous and cytoplasmic staining for CK903

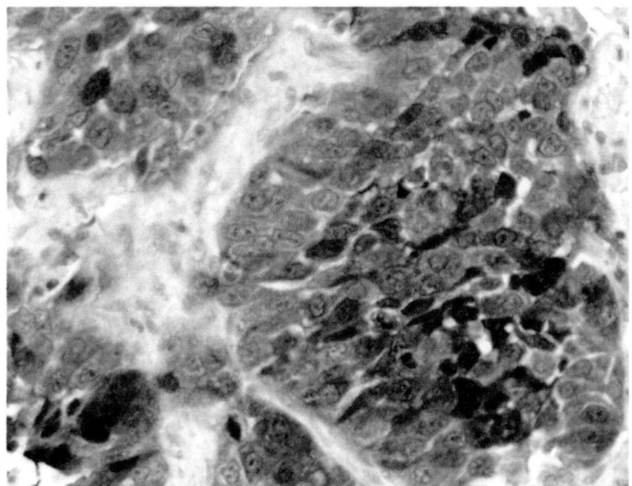

Fig. 14.14 Lung squamous cell carcinoma show membranous and cytoplasmic staining for Maspin

Table 14.8 Markers for adenosquamous carcinoma of the lung

Antibodies	Literature
CK7	+
CK20	–
TTF-1	+
CK5/6	+
p63	+
CK903	+
CK19	+
CEA	+
CA19.9	+

Note: Adenocarcinoma component is positive for CK7, TTF-1, and CEA, while squamous carcinoma component is positive for CK5/6, p63, and CK903

References: [5, 11, 26, 56, 57, 71, 78, 100, 101, 106, 108, 112, 115, 119, 121–123]

Table 14.9 Markers for large cell carcinoma (LCC), not otherwise specified (NOS)

Antibodies	Literature	GML data (N = 19)
CK7	+	47% (9/19)
CK20	–	0% (0/19)
CK5/6	–	5% (1/19)
p63	– or +	10% (2/19)
TTF-1	– or +	63% (12/19)
CK17	UK	5% (1/19)
CK19	UK	10% (4/19)
CK903	UK	10% (2/19)
Napsin A	+	5% (1/19)

Note: *UK* unknown

GML data are based on 19 cases of LCC NOS

Diagnosis of LCC is by far a morphologic diagnosis since no single marker is specific for LCC

References: [54, 78, 106, 108, 109, 112, 121–123]

Table 14.10 Markers for large cell carcinoma NOS vs. poorly differentiated adenocarcinoma vs. poorly differentiated squamous cell carcinoma

Antibodies	Adenocarcinoma	Squamous cell carcinoma	Large cell carcinoma
CK7	+	– or +	+
TTF-1	+	–	+ or –
CK5/6	–	+	– or focal +
p63	–	+	– or +
Mucicarmine stain	+ or –	–	–

References: [5, 11, 26, 56, 57, 71, 78, 100, 101, 106, 108, 112, 115, 119, 121–123]

Table 14.11 Markers for basaloid carcinoma (a subtype of large cell carcinoma)

Antibodies	Literature
CK7	+
CK20	–
CK903	+
TTF-1	–
CD56	V
Synaptophysin	V

Note: *V* variably positive

A subset of basaloid carcinoma can have variable positivity for CD56 or synaptophysin (less than 20% of tumor cells), suggesting focal neuroendocrine differentiation

References: [97, 106, 121–123]

Table 14.12 Markers for lymphoepithelioma-like carcinoma

Antibodies	Literature
AE1/AE3	+
EBER-1 by ISH	+

Note: *EBER-1* Epstein–Barr virus early RNA-1, *ISH* in situ hybridization

References: [48, 106, 121–123]

Table 14.13 Markers for typical and atypical carcinoid tumors

	Literature	
Antibodies	Typical carcinoid	Atypical carcinoid
AE1/AE3	+	+
CK7	– or +	+ or –
CK20	–	–
TTF-1	– or +	+ or –
CD56	+	+
CD57	+	+
Synaptophysin	+	+
Chromogranin	+	+
Ki-67	Low	Moderate to high
CDX-2	–	–
CD99	+	UK
PTEN	+	UK
ER	+ or –	+
PR	– or +	– or +
PDX1	–	UK
NESP-55	– or +	UK

Note: *UK* unknown, *PDX1* pancreatic and duodenal homeobox factor-1, *NESP-55* neuroendocrine secretory protein-55

CK7 and CD20 subsets are of limited value in diagnosing pulmonary neuroendocrine carcinoma since typical cases are negative for both CK7 and CK20, with a subset of cases CK7+ and rarely CK20+. TTF-1+ stain in typical and atypical carcinoid tumors appears to be correlative with pulmonary origin, although it is not specific for a primary pulmonary origin as it is in adenocarcinoma

References: [2, 9, 11, 40, 43, 55, 65, 73, 88, 93, 95, 101, 106, 121–123]

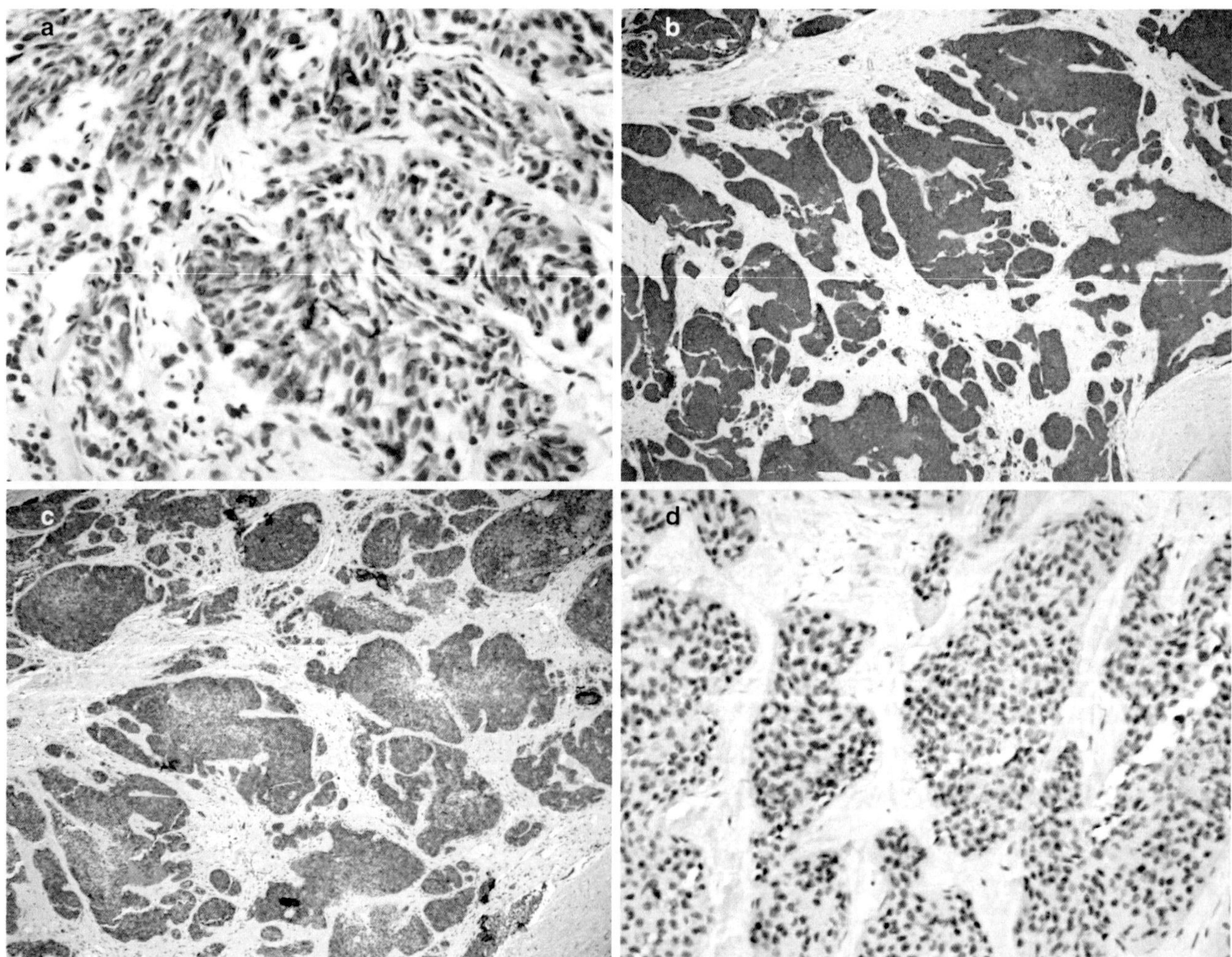

Fig. 14.15 Carcinoid tumor shows positive staining for CKAE1/3. Weak staining (**a**), synaptophysin (**b**), chromogranin (**c**), and TTF-1 (**d**)

Table 14.14 Markers for large cell neuroendocrine carcinoma (LCNEC)

Antibodies	Literature
CK7	+
CK20	–
TTF-1	– or +
CD56	+ or –
Synaptophysin	+
Chromogranin	+ or –
Ki-67	High
MASH1	+ or –
NeuroD	+ or –
p16	+ or –
PTEN	– or +
p63	– or +

Note: LCNEC is defined by a combination of histologic (i.e., neuroendocrine morphology, necrosis) and cytologic (i.e., large cell size, cytoplasm, nucleoli, coarse chromatin, and high mitotic rate) criteria as well as the presence of neuroendocrine differentiation demonstrated by immunohistochemistry

References: [11, 43, 65, 73, 101, 106, 121–123]

Table 14.15 Nonsmall cell lung carcinoma with neuroendocrine differentiation (NSCLC-ND) of various types vs. large cell neuroendocrine carcinoma (LCNEC)

	Literature			
Antibodies	NSCLC-ND-adenocarcinoma	NSCLC-ND-squamous cell carcinoma	NSCLC-ND-large cell carcinoma	LCNEC
CK7	+	– or +	+	+
CK20	–	–	–	– or +
TTF-1	+	–	– or +	– or +
CD56	– or +	– or +	– or +	+ or –
Synaptophysin	– or +	–	– or +	+
Chromogranin	–	–	–	+ or –

Note: NSCLC-ND only detected by immunohistochemistry or electron microscopy is a distinct entity in which no histologic features of neuroendocrine differentiation (growth pattern, nuclear chromatin change, etc.) are appreciated on routine H&E stain

References: [11, 43, 51, 54, 101, 106, 121–123]

Table 14.16 Markers for small cell lung carcinoma (SCLC)

Antibodies	Literature
CK1/3	+ (Weak to moderate)
TTF-1	+ (>90% of cases)
CD56	+
p63	–
Synaptophysin	+ or –
Chromogranin	– or +
Ki-67	High (>90%)
CAM 5.2	+
CK7	– or + (Focal)
CK20	–
CK903	–
MASH1	+
NeuroD	– or +
p16	+
PTEN	– or +

Note: Diagnosis of SCLC is largely a morphologic exercise, and SCLC is defined on the basis of cytologic criteria, with typically weak to moderate intensity staining in perinuclear rim and dot-like patterns for cytokeratins AE1/AE3 and CAM 5.2. Positive stain for neuroendocrine markers (CD56, synaptophysin, and chromogranin) is supportive of a morphologic diagnosis of SCLC; however, use extreme caution when discriminating between SCLC and nonsmall cell lung carcinoma, particularly on small crushed biopsy samples, since none of these markers is specific for SCLC. Extremely low Ki-67 index in tumor cells strongly militates against the diagnosis of SCLC

References: [11, 51, 54, 78, 101, 106, 108, 119, 121–123]

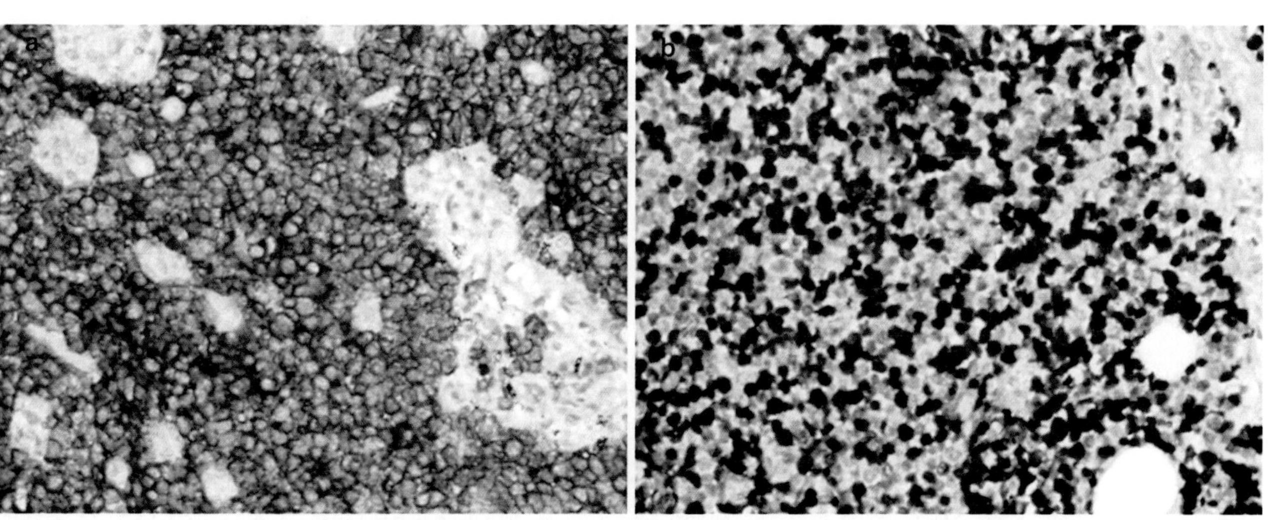

Fig. 14.16 Lung small cell carcinoma shows positive staining for CD56 (**a**) and Ki-67 (approaching 100% MIB-1 proliferation index) (**b**)

Table 14.17 Markers for carcinosarcoma

Antibodies	Literature
Pan-CK	+ In epithelial component
AE1/AE3	+ In epithelial component
EMA	+ In epithelial component
TTF-1	– or +
SP-A	–
S100	+ In chondrosarcoma
Muscle markers	+ In rhabdomyosarcoma

References: [11, 86, 101, 106, 121–123]

Table 14.18 Markers for pulmonary blastoma

Antibodies	Literature
AE1/AE3	+ In the component of fetal adenocarcinoma
EMA	+ In the component of fetal adenocarcinoma
CEA	+ In the component of fetal adenocarcinoma
Chromogranin	+ or –
Hormones (calcitonin, gastric releasing peptide, bombesin, leucine, methionine, enkephalin, somatostatin, and serotonin)	+ In the component of fetal adenocarcinoma
Vimentin	+ In stromal cells of blastomas
SMA	+ In stromal cells of blastomas
Desmin, myoglobulin	+ In striated muscle
S100	+ Cartilage

References: [58, 72, 106, 117, 121–123]

Table 14.19 Markers for pulmonary Langerhans cell histiocytosis

Antibodies	Literature
CD1a	+
S100	+
Langerin	+

References: [11, 91, 101, 106, 121–123]

Table 14.20 Markers for pulmonary Lymphangioleiomyomatosis

Antibodies	Literature
Vimentin	+
Desmin	+
Alpha-SMA	+
HMB-45	+
Estrogen or progesterone receptors	+

References: [11, 14, 16, 101, 106, 121–123]

Table 14.21 Markers for inflammatory myofibroblastic tumor

Antibodies	Literature
AE1/AE3	Focal +
Vimentin	+ In spindle cells
SMA	+ In spindle cells
ALK-1	+ In 40% cases
S100	–
Desmin	– or rare +
Myogenin	–
Myoglobulin	–

References: [9, 11, 21–23, 27, 30, 53, 82, 101, 106, 116, 121–123]

Table 14.22 Markers for sclerosing hemangioma

Antibodies	Round cells (% of cases)	Surface cells (% of cases)
Pan-cytokeratin	–	+
EMA	+	+
CAM 5.2	+ Focal (17%)	+
CK7	+ Focal (31%)	+
CK20	–	–
CK5/6 and CK903	–	–
TTF-1	+ (92%)	+ (97%)
Pro-SP-A and SP-B	–	+
Clara cell antigen	–	+
Vimentin	+	+
S100	–	–
SMA	–	–
Factor VIII	–	–
Calretinin	–	–
ER	+ (7%)	–
PR	+ (61%)	–
Chromogranin	–	–
Synaptophysin	–	–
Leu7	–	–

References: [11, 36, 101, 106, 121–123]

Table 14.23 Lung adenocarcinoma vs. metastatic pancreatic ductal carcinoma

Antibodies	Adenocarcinoma	Pancreatic ductal carcinoma
CK7	+	+
CK20	–	+ or –
CK17	– or + (13%)	+ or – (60%)
CK19	+ (80%)	+ (75%)
TTF-1	+ (78%)	– (0%)
Maspin	+ or – (51%)	+ (100%)
CA19.9	– or + (28%)	+ (84%)
MUC1	+ (100%)	+ (95%)
MUC2	– (0%)	– (4%)
MUC4	– or + (28%)	+ or – (50%)
DPC4/SMAD4	+ (95%)	– or + (41%)

Note: Percentage of positivity for each marker is based on TMA block containing 55 cases of mixed adenocarcinoma and 70 cases of pancreatic ductal carcinoma. CD20+ can be seen in certain subtypes of mucinous carcinoma, including mucinous BAC of the lung. CK7+ and CD20+ carcinoma include carcinomas originating from pancreas, ampulla, urinary bladder, and ovary

References: [11, 36, 101, 106, 121–123]

Table 14.24 Pulmonary carcinoid vs. gastrointestinal carcinoid tumors and pancreatic neuroendocrine tumor (PNET)

	Literature			
	TTF-1	CDX-2	PDX1	NESP-55
Pulmonary	– or +	–	–	– or +
Stomach	–	–	+ or –	–
Duodenum	–	–	+	–
Small intestine	–	+	–	–
Appendix	–	+	+ or –	–
Colon	–	+	?	?
Rectum	–	– or +	– or +	– or +
Pancreatic NET	–	–	– or +	– or +

Note: *PDX1* pancreatic and duodenal homeobox factor, *NESP-55* neuroendocrine secretory protein-55

TTF-1-positive stain in typical and atypical carcinoid tumors appears to be correlative with pulmonary origin, although it is not specific for a primary pulmonary origin as it is in adenocarcinoma. CDX-2-positive stain in neuroendocrine tumors suggests gastrointestinal origin

References: [11, 42, 65, 73, 101, 106, 121–123]

Table 14.25 Small cell lung carcinoma vs. small cell variant of squamous cell carcinoma (SQCC) of the lung

Antibodies	Small cell carcinoma	Small cell variant of SQCC
TTF-1	+	–
p63	–	+
CK903	–	+
CAM 5.2	+	–
Synaptophysin	+	–
Chromogranin A	– or +	–

Note: These markers are very helpful if the differential diagnosis is between SCLC and poorly differentiated SQCC, including small cell variant. On small crushed biopsy samples, caution should be taken since none of these markers is entirely specific. For example, SCLC can be negative for TTF-1 and neuroendocrine markers, and p63-positive stain has been found in a small subset of SCLC

References: [11, 78, 101, 106, 108, 112, 119, 121–123]

Table 14.26 Small cell lung carcinoma (SCLC) vs. nonsmall cell lung carcinoma

Antibodies	Small cell carcinoma	Nonsmall cell carcinoma
AE1/AE3	+ (Focal and weak)	+
CK7	– or +	+ or –
TTF-1	+	+ or –
p63	–	+ or –
CD56	+	– or +
Synaptophysin	+ or –	– or +
Chromogranin	– or +	–
Ki-67	High (>90%)	<90%

Note: Diagnosis of SCLC is first and foremost a morphologic diagnosis. Immunohistochemical interpretation should be cautioned since no single marker is positive for SCLC and absent in NSCLC; p63 is positive in most squamous cell carcinoma, subsets of adenocarcinoma, large cell carcinoma, and poorly differentiated neuroendocrine tumors

References: [5, 78, 101, 106, 108, 112, 119, 121–123]

Table 14.27 Small cell carcinoma vs. large cell neuroendocrine carcinoma (LCNEC)

Antibodies	Small cell carcinoma	LCNEC
Chromogranin A	– or +	+or–
Synaptophysin	+ or –	+
CD56	+	+ or –
CK903	–	–
MASH1	+	+ or –
TTF-1	+	+ or –
p16	+	+ or –
p63	–	– or +
PTEN	– or +	– or +
NeuroD	– or +	+ or –

Note: SCLC and LCNEC overlap in their immunophenotypic, clinical, histopathologic, and genetic characteristics making separation difficult. CK903 (34betaE12) shows focal positivity in a small subset of small cell carcinoma and LCNEC

References: [5, 43, 101, 106, 121–123]

Table 14.28 Small cell lung carcinoma (SCLC) vs. extrapulmonary small cell carcinoma of various organs

	Literature				
Antibodies	SCLC	Prostate	Bladder	Liver	Others
TTF-1	+	+	– or +	– or +	– But can be + in GI tract (2/12) and cervix: 1/3
CK20	–	– or +	– or +	–	–
CD56	+	+		+	
Synaptophysin	+ or –	+	+ or –	+	
Chromogranin	– or +	+ or –	– or +	+ or –	
AE1/AE3	V (Focal and weak)	+	UK	+	UK
CAM 5.2	?	+ (Cytoplasmic dot-like)	UK	UK	UK
CK7	– or + (Focal)	– or +	–	–	
CK903 (34betaE12)	–	– or +	UK	UK	UK
p63	–	– or +	UK	UK	UK
Ki-67	High (>90%)	High (>90%)	UK	UK	UK
PSA	–	– or +	UK	UK	UK
PSAP	UK	– or +	UK	UK	UK
P504S	UK	– or +	UK	UK	UK

Note: *UK* unknown

Others – gastrointestinal tract, sinonasal, thyroid gland, salivary gland, uterine cervix, and pancreas

TTF-1-positive stain on extrapulmonary SCC is not specific for pulmonary origin since SCC of primary arising in other organs can also be TTF-1-positive

References: [2, 3, 11, 25, 76, 101, 106, 121–123]

Table 14.29 Small cell carcinoma vs. Merkel cell carcinoma

Antibodies	Small cell carcinoma	Merkel callcarcinoma
CK20	–	+
TTF-1	+	–
Neurofilaments	–	+
MASH1	+	–
CD56	+	+
Chromogranin	+ or –	+
Synaptophysin	+	+

Note: *MASH1* mammalian or human achaete–scute complex homolog-1 (MASH1, HASH1)

CK20+ in a dot-like pattern

References: [11, 15, 18, 81, 101, 106, 121–123]

Table 14.30 Markers for sarcomatoid carcinoma (pleomorphic, spindle, and giant cell)

Antibodies	Literature
Pan-CK	+ or –
AE1/AE3	+ or –
CK7	+ or –
EMA	+ or –
CEA	+ or –
TTF-1	– (But can be + in giant cell carcinoma)
SP-A	– or + (Epithelial component)
Vimentin	+
SMA	– or +

Note: Expression of epithelial markers in the spindle and/or giant cell component of a pleomorphic carcinoma is not required for the diagnosis so long as there is a component of squamous cell carcinoma, adenocarcinoma, or large cell carcinoma. A wide immunohistochemical overlap exists among sarcomatoid carcinoma, sarcomatoid mesothelioma, and sarcoma. Generally, carcinomatous or epithelial elements retain expression of cytokeratin; whereas sarcomatoid/spindle components tend to lose cytokeratin with more variable expression. Sometimes cytokeratin stain may be weak or focal and need multiple antibodies. Positive keratin stain supports the diagnosis of carcinoma in the setting of a lung mass otherwise typical of a lung primary

References: [1, 7, 11, 24, 41, 86, 101, 106, 121–123]

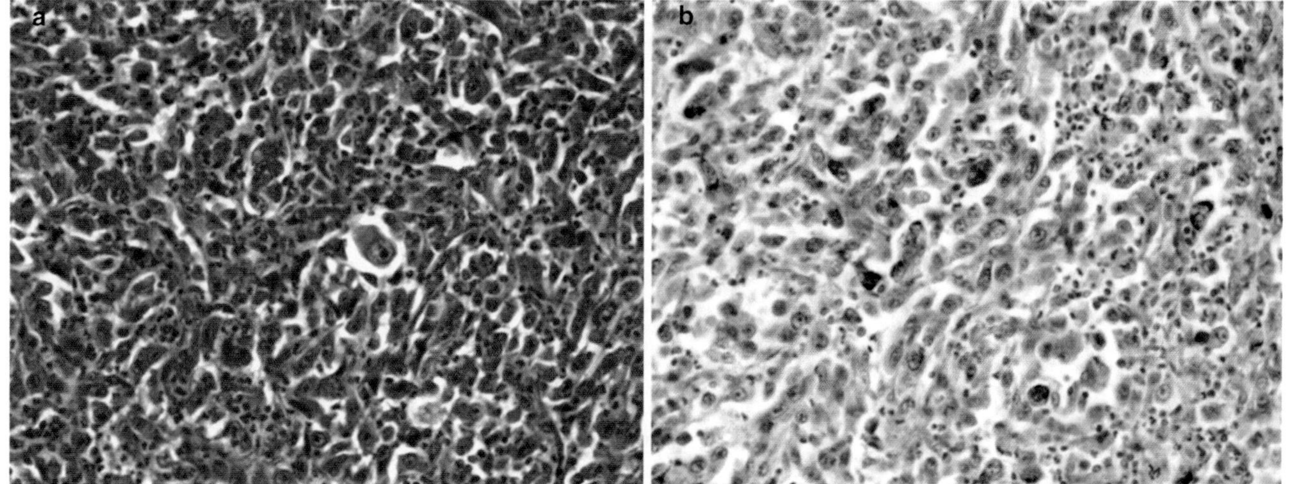

Fig. 14.17 Lung sarcomatoid carcinoma with giant and spindle cell feature [(**a**), H&E] and shows focally positive staining for CKAE1/3 (**b**)

Table 14.31 Markers for certain types of lung sarcoma

Antibodies	Angiosarcoma including Kaposi's	Leiomyosarcoma	MFH
Cytokeratin	– or +(Focal)	–	–
Vimentin	+	+	+
Desmin	–	+	–
Actin	–	+	+
CD31	+	–	–
CD34	+	–	–
Factor VIII	– or +	UK	UK
Fli and FKBP12	+	UK	UK
CD68	–	–	+
CD99	–	–	–

Note: *UK* unknown, *MFH* malignant fibrohistiocytoma

References: [4, 11, 38, 67, 75, 83, 84, 101, 106, 121–123]

Table 14.32 Benign clear cell tumor, granular cell tumor vs. clear cell carcinoma (primary and metastatic) vs. metastatic clear cell sarcoma or melanoma

Antibodies	Benign clear cell tumor/ "sugar tumor"/PEComa	Lung clear cell carcinoma	Granular cell tumor	Metastatic clear cell sarcoma or melanoma
S100	+	– or +	+	– or +
HMB-45	+	–	–	–
AE1/AE3	–	+	–	+
Diastase-sensitive PAS positivity	+	–	–	–
History of tumor	–	– or +	–	+ or –

References: [4, 11, 38, 67, 70, 75, 77, 83, 84, 101, 104, 106, 121–123]

Table 14.33 Lung nonsmall cell carcinoma with clear cell features vs. metastatic clear cell renal cell carcinoma vs. epithelial diffuse malignant mesothelioma with clear cell features

Antibodies	Nonsmall cell carcinoma with clear cell features	Renal cell carcinoma (clear cell type)	Epithelial diffuse malignant mesothelioma with clear cell features
CK7	+	– or +	+
CK20	–	–	–
Calretinin	–	–	+
CK5/6	– or +	–	+
WT1	–	–	+
Mesothelin	–	–	+
TTF-1	+ or –	–	
CD10	–	+	– or +
RCC	–	+	–

Note: CK5/6+ in squamous cell carcinoma with clear cell features

References: [6, 7, 11, 19, 24, 38, 41, 67, 70, 75, 77, 83, 84, 86, 101, 104, 106, 121–123]

Table 14.34 Mucosa-associated lymphoid tissue (MALT) lymphoma vs. small lymphocytic lymphoma (SLL) vs. mantle cell lymphoma (MCL) vs. follicular lymphoma (FL)

Antibodies	MALT lymphoma	SLL	MCL	FL
CD20	+	+ (Weak)	+	+
CD79a	+	+	+	–
PAX5	+	+	+	+
CD5	–	+	+	–
CD23	–	+	–	–
CD10	–	–	– or rare +	+
Bcl-6	–	–	–	+
CD43	– or +	+ or –	+ or –	–
Bcl-2	+	+	+	+
Ki-67	<10%	<10%	>10%	<10% In grade 1 FL or >20% in higher grade FL

Note: A subset of grade 1 FL can have a high MIB-1 proliferation index

References: [99, 106, 121–123]

Table 14.35 Diffuse large B cell lymphoma (DLBCL) vs. anaplastic large cell lymphoma (ALCL) vs. classical Hodgkin's lymphoma (CHL) vs. carcinoma vs. germ cell tumor (GCT)

Antibodies	DLBCL	ALCL	CHL	Carcinoma	GCT
AE1/AE3	–	–	–	+	–
CD45	+	+	–	–	–
CD20	+	–	– or +	–	–
CD79a	+	–	–	–	–
PAX5	+	–	+ or –	–	–
CD15	–	–	+	– or +	–
CD30	– or +	+	+	– or focal +	– or + in embryonal carcinoma
ALK-1	–	+ In ALK-1+ ALCL	–	–	–
CD117	–	–	–	–	+ In seminoma
EBER-1	+ In LYG	–	–	–	–

Note: *ERER-1* Epstein–Barr virus early RNA-1, *LYG* lymphomatoid granulomatosis

References: [99, 106, 121–123]

Table 14.36 Pulmonary adenocarcinoma vs. common metastatic carcinomas to lung

Antibodies	Lung adenocarcinoma	Breast carcinoma	Upper GI carcinoma	Lower GI carcinoma	Prostate carcinoma	Thyroid carcinoma	Hepato-cellular carcinoma	Adreno-cortical carcinoma
CK7	+	+	+	–	–	+	–	–
CK20	–	–	+ or –	+	–	–	–	–
TTF-1	+	–	–	–	–	+	–	–
GCDFP-15	+	+ or –						
ER	+ or –	– or +						
PR	+ or –	– or +						
Mammaglobin	–	+						
CDX-2	–		+ or –	+				
Villin	– or +		+	+				
PSA					+			
PAP					+			
Thyroglobulin						+		
Hepatocyte-1							+	
Inhibin-alpha								+

Note: *V* variably positive, *PSA* prostate-specific antigen, *PAP* placental acid phosphatase

E-cadherin is used in separating ductal carcinoma from lobular carcinoma but not used for supporting breast primary; 80% of lung carcinomas express E-cadherin. Similarly, Her-2/neu is a nonspecific marker and is expressed in a variety of malignancies, including 30% of lung carcinomas. CDX-2 may be positive in certain subtypes of lung adenocarcinoma

References: [11, 26, 33, 56, 66, 89, 101, 102, 106, 111, 121–123]

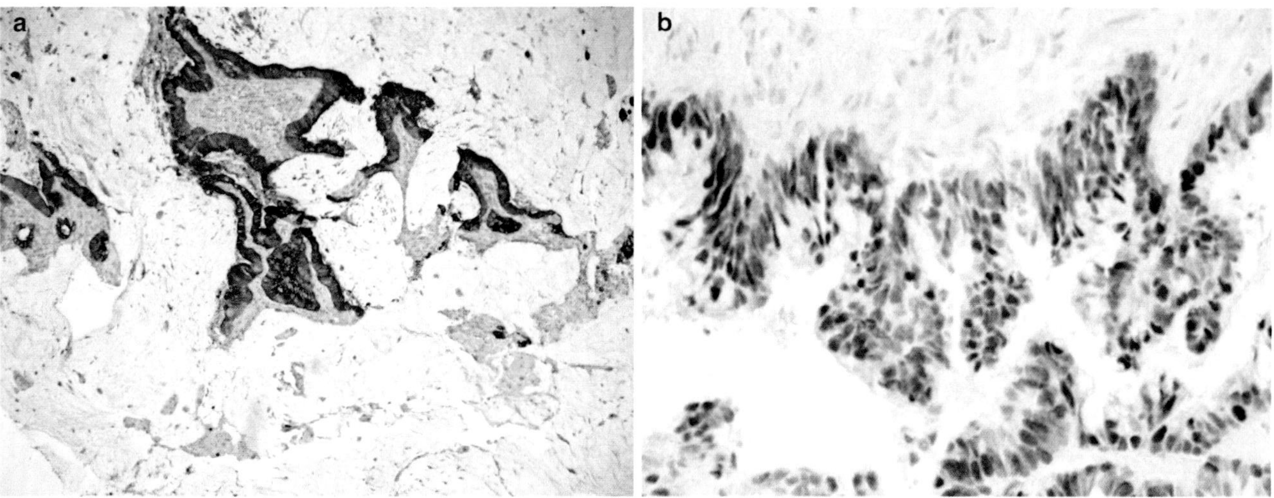

Fig. 14.18 Metastatic colonic carcinoma shows positive staining for CK20 (**a**) and CDX-2 (**b**)

Table 14.37 Lung adenocarcinoma vs. metastatic ovarian carcinoma

Antibodies	Adenocarcinoma	Ovarian non-mucinous carcinoma	Ovarian mucinous carcinoma
CK7	+	+	+
CK20	–	+ or –	+
TTF-1	+	–	–
CDX-2	–	–	+
WT1	–	+	–
ER	– or +	+	+
Inhibin-alpha	– or +	+ or –	+ or –

Note: *V* variably positive

CD20+ can be seen in certain subtypes of mucinous carcinoma, including mucinous BAC of the lung. CK7+ and CD20+ carcinoma include carcinomas originating from the pancreas, ampulla, urinary bladder, and ovary

References: [11, 26, 33, 101, 106]

Table 14.38 Markers for pleural epithelial diffuse malignant mesothelioma

Antibodies	Pleural epithelial diffuse malignant mesothelioma
Pan-CK	+
Calretinin	+ (Nuclear)
CK5/6	+
TTF-1	–
WT1	+
CEA	–
CD15	–
Ber-EP4	–
TAG 72 (B72.3)	–
MOC-31	–
D2-40	+

References: [7, 8, 11, 19, 24, 38, 41, 42, 64, 67, 70, 72, 80, 83, 86, 101, 106, 121–123]

Table 14.39 Markers for epithelial diffuse malignant mesothelioma vs. pulmonary adenocarcinoma

Antibodies	Pleural epithelial diffuse malignant mesothelioma	Pulmonary adenocarcinoma
Pan-CK	+	+
Calretinin	+	–
CK5/6	+	–
TTF-1	–	+
WT1	+	–
CEA	–	+
CD15	–	+
Ber-EP4	–	+
TAG 72 (B72.3)	–	+
MOC-31	–	– or +
D2-40	+	–

Note: *V* variably positive

References: [7, 11, 19, 24, 38, 41, 42, 64, 67, 70, 72, 80, 83, 84, 86, 101, 106, 121–123]

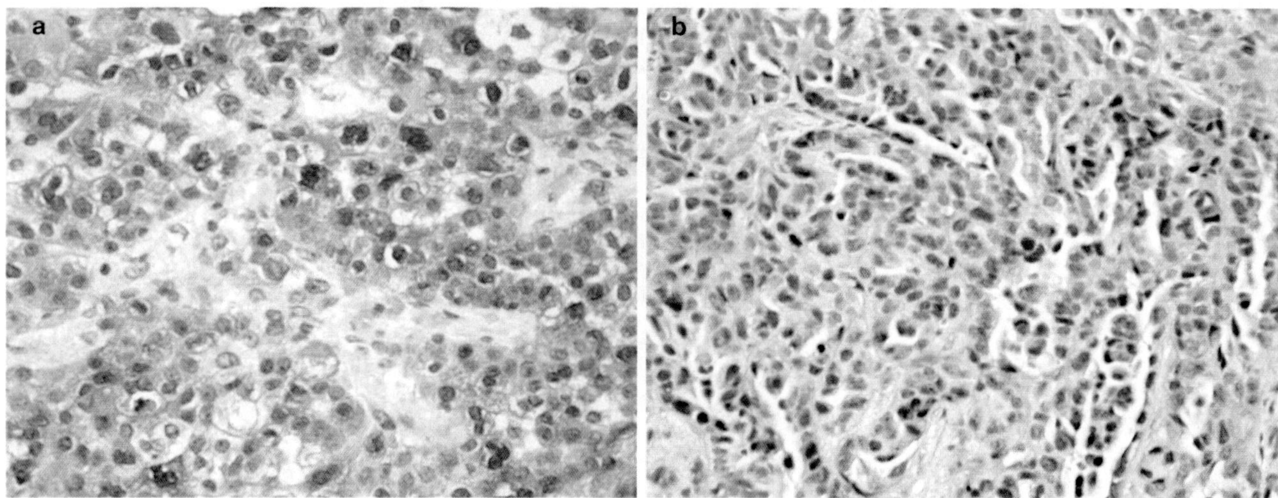

Fig. 14.19 Pleural epithelial mesothelioma shows nuclear and cytoplasmic staining for calretinin (**a**). Pleural epithelial mesothelioma shows nuclear staining for WT1 (**b**)

Table 14.40 Markers for sarcomatoid diffuse malignant mesothelioma vs. biphasic diffuse malignant mesothelioma vs. sarcomatoid carcinoma

Antibodies	Sarcomatoid mesothelioma	Biphasic mesothelioma	Sarcomatoid carcinoma
Pan-CK	+	+	+
Calretinin	– or +	+ or –	– or rare +
CK5/6	– or rare +	+ In epithelial component	–
WT1	– or rare +	+ In epithelial component	–
D2-40	+ or –	+	–
CEA	–	–	–
CD15	–	–	–
Ber-EP4	–	–	–
TAG 72 (B72.3)	–	–	–
MOC-31	–	–	–

References: [7, 11, 19, 24, 38, 41, 42, 64, 67, 70, 75, 80, 83, 84, 86, 101, 106, 121–123]

Table 14.41 Markers for pleuropulmonary synovial sarcomas (SS)

Antibodies	Literature
EMA	+ or –
AE1/AE3	+ or –
CK7	+ or –
CK19	+ or –
CK5/6	+ or –
CAM 5.2	+ or –
Ber-EP4	+ or –
CD99	+ or –
Bcl-2	+
CD56	+
Calretinin	– or +
WT1	–
CD15 (LeuM1)	– or +
HBME-1	+ or –
Thrombomodulin (CD141)	– or +
S100	– or +
CD34	–

Note: Markers for synovial sarcoma vary with whether they are biphasic or monophasic. Primary pleural SS are usually biphasic and primary pulmonary SS are usually sarcomatous monophasic

Biphasic SS shows a higher percentage of positivity for cytokeratins and mesothelial-related markers (calretinin, CK5/6) and Ber-EP4 than monophasic or spindle cell SS

References: [11, 70, 94, 98, 101, 106, 121–123]

Table 14.42 Markers for sarcomatoid carcinoma vs. sarcomatoid diffuse malignant mesothelioma vs. synovial sarcoma (SS) vs. sarcoma of the lung

Antibodies	Sarcomatoid carcinoma	Sarcomatoid diffuse malignant mesothelioma	Synovial sarcoma	Sarcoma
Pan-CK	+	+	+ or –	–
CK1/3	+	+	V (often weak)	–
CK5/6	Rare +	–	–	–
WT1	Rare +	–	–	–
D2-40	– or +	–	?	?
Bcl-2	–	?	+	?
Vimentin	+	+		+
Actin	–	+		V
CD31	–	–		V
CD34	–	–		V
Desmin	–	–		V
S100	–	–		V
Calretinin	– or +	+ or –	– or +	– or +
t(X;18)	–	–	+	–

Note: *V* variably positive depending on type of sarcoma

Markers for synovial sarcoma vary with whether they are biphasic or monophasic. Primary pleural SSs are usually biphasic and primary pulmonary SSs are usually sarcomatous monophasic

References: [7, 11, 19, 24, 38, 41, 43, 64, 67, 70, 75, 80, 83, 84, 86, 94, 98, 101, 106, 121–123]

Table 14.43 Markers for solitary fibrous tumor (SFT)

Antibodies	Literatures
AE1/AE3	–
CD34	+
Bcl-2	+

References: [11, 19, 42, 64, 67, 70, 76, 80, 83, 86, 101, 106, 121–123]

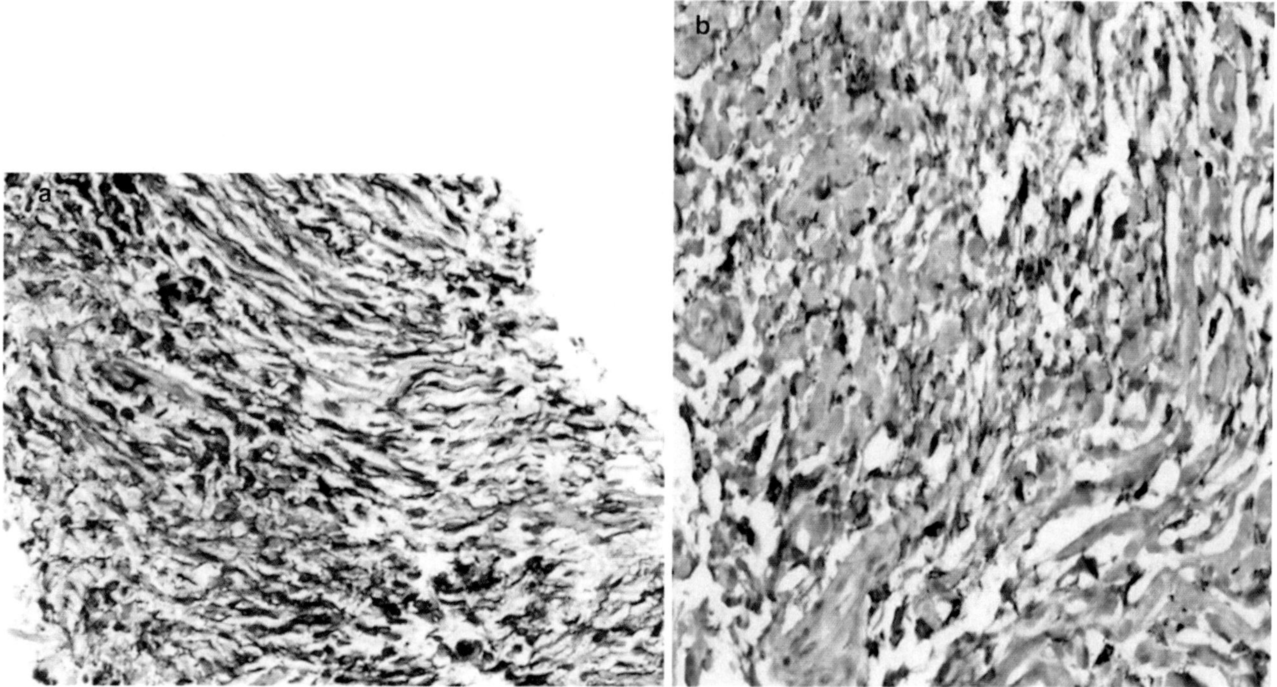

Fig. 14.20 Pleural solitary fibrous tumor shows positive staining for CD34 (**a**) and Bcl-2 (**b**)

Table 14.44 Markers for desmoplastic small round cell tumor (DRCT) of the pleura

Antibodies	DRCT
Cytokeratins	+
EMA	+
Desmin	+ (Dot-like pattern)
Vimentin	+
WT1	+
NSE	+
CD15	+
t(11; 22)/WT1-EWS	+

References: [11, 106, 121–123, 125]

Table 14.45 Markers for primary effusion lymphoma

Antibodies	Literature
CD45	+
CD20	–
CD79a	–
CD19	–
PAX5	–
CD3, CD7, or CD56	– or +
CD138	+
CD38	+
Surface or cytoplasmic light chain	–
CD30	+
Bcl-6/CD10	–
MUM1	
HHV8	+
EBER	+
LMP1 and 2	–
EBNA1	+
EBNA2	–

References: [99, 106, 121–123]

Table 14.46 Markers for pyothorax-associated lymphoma

Antibodies	Literature
CD45	+
CD20	+ or – in plasmacytoid differentiation
CD79a	+ or – in plasmacytoid differentiation
CD2, CD3, CD4, and CD7	– or aberrantly +
CD138	– or + in plasmacytoid differentiation
CD38	– or + in plasmacytoid differentiation
Cytoplasmic Ig light chain	+
CD30	+
Bcl-6/CD10	–
MUM1	+
EBER	+
LMP1 and 2	Rare +
EBNA1	– or +
EBNA2	+
HHV8	–

References: [99, 106, 121–123]

Table 14.47 Markers for thymoma

Antibodies	Literature
AE1/AE3	+ In all subtypes of thymoma
CK19, CK5/6, CAM 5.2, CK7, CK14, and CD18	+ (In the type B1, B2, and B3 thymoma)
CD57 and EMA	– or + (variable and focal in type A thymoma); but CD57+ in type B1, B2, and B3 thymoma. EMA+ in type B3 thymoma
Metallothionein	+ (Type A thymoma)
PE35	+ (Type A thymoma)
Ki-67 index	Low (in type A tumor cells)
CK20, CD5, CD70, TTF-1, and Bcl-2	– (In all subtypes of thymoma except some cases of type B3 with CD5+)
CD20	– or + (variable and focal)
Admixed cortical immature T cells	+ For CD1a, CD99, CD3, CD4, CD5, and CD8 and TdT
Admixed medullary mature T lymphocytes	+ For CD3 and CD5, but – for CD1a, CD99, and TdT

References: [106, 121–123]

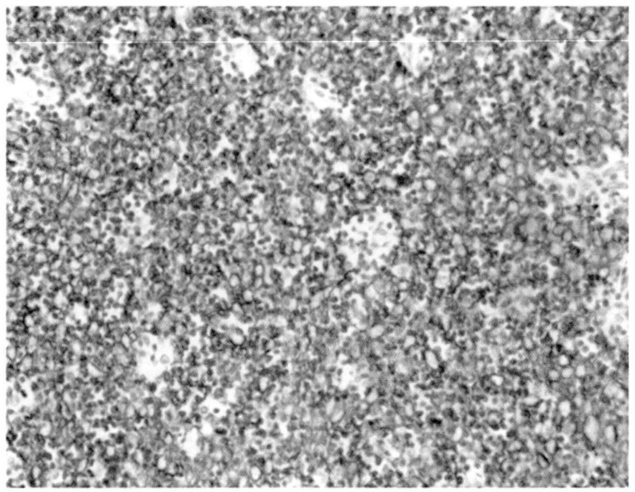

Fig. 14.21 Mediastinal thymoma (type A) shows positive staining for CKAE1/3

Table 14.48 Markers for thymic carcinoma

	Literature		
Antibodies	Squamous cell carcinoma	Basaloid carcinoma	Lymphoepithelioma-like carcinoma
AE1/AE3	+	+	+
CD5, CD70, and CD117	+	Can be CD5+	CD5+ (focal)/−
Chromogranin, synaptophysin, and CD56	+/−	−	UK
S100	UK	−	UK
Bcl-2	UK	UK	+
Admixed T lymphocytes	−	−	+ For CD3 and CD5, but − for CD1a, CD99, and TdT
EBV by CISH	−	−	+

Note: *UK* unknown

Squamous cell carcinomas (SQCC) of other organs are negative for CD5 and CD70, useful for confirming a diagnosis of anterior mediastinal SQCC. Nasopharyngeal carcinoma and Hodgkin's lymphoma may be CD70+. Thymic mucoepidermoid carcinoma is rare, closely resembling mucoepidermoid carcinomas of other organs (see related chapters). Diagnosis of thymic sarcomatoid carcinoma relies on demonstration of some CK+ and/or EMA+ tumor cells by immunohistochemistry and exclusion of sarcoma. Histochemical and immunohistochemical features of thymic clear cell carcinoma include d-PAS+, keratin+, EMA−/+, CD5−/+; negative for vimentin, PLAP, CEA, S100; and containing no immature T cells. Thymic papillary carcinoma shows variable positivity for CD15, Ber-EP4, and CEA. It may be CD5+, while negative for CD20, thyroglobulin, pulmonary surfactant, and calretinin, and contain no CD99+ immature T cells. Thymic nonpapillary adenocarcinomas, carcinomas with t(15;19) and undifferentiated carcinomas are rare tumors, and the former (nonpapillary adenocarcinomas) include adenocarcinoma with glandular differentiation arising in thymic cyst, adenoid cystic carcinoma, and mucinous (colloid) carcinoma. Immunohistochemical features of these tumors are not well characterized in the literature. Preferential expression of CD5, CD70, and CD117 in thymic carcinoma (approximately 60%) is used to differentiate thymic carcinoma from thymomas that are negative for these markers

References: [106, 121–123]

Table 14.49 Markers for thymic neuroendocrine tumor (NET) vs. metastatic NET from lung and other sites

	Literature		
Antibodies	Thymic carcinoid tumor and LCNEC	Pulmonary carcinoid tumor and LCNEC	Other sites (gastrointestinal and pancreatic NET)
TTF-1	−	+/−	−

Classification of thymic NET is similar to pulmonary NET, including carcinoid, atypical carcinoid, large cell neuroendocrine carcinoma (LCNEC), and small cell carcinoma. Hormones (ACTH, HCG, somatostatin, beta-endorphin, cholecystokinin, neurotensin, and calcitonin) can be detected in a variable number of tumor cells. The utility of TTF-1 in differentiating thymic small cell carcinoma from pulmonary small cell carcinoma is unclear. Thymic carcinomas with neuroendocrine cells usually exhibit focal positivity or scattered positive cells, whereas thymic neuroendocrine carcinoma exhibits a diffuse positive staining pattern. Thymic carcinoid tumors with spindle cell morphology should be differentiated from type A thymomas and synovial sarcomas that are negative for neuroendocrine markers. Nerve sheath tumors are positive for CD56 but negative for synaptophysin and chromogranin. Paraganglioma positive for neuroendocrine markers can be difficult to distinguish from pulmonary carcinoid tumors that can be focally positive for S100 protein

References: [106, 121–123]

Table 14.50 Markers for germ cell tumors

Antibodies	Seminoma	Embryonal carcinoma	Choriocarcinoma	Yolk sac tumor
Pan-CK	+ (Focal; weak, paranuclear)		+	
LMWCK		+		+
CAM 5.2			+	
CEA	–	–	–	
EMA	–	–		
PLAP	+	+ In scattered tumor cells or small foci	-	
CD117	+ (Membranous or paranuclear pattern)			+ (Focal)
CD30	–	+ (Membranous/cytoplasmic; uniform and strong)	–	
Beta-hCG	Only scattered syncytiotrophoblastic cells+; 5%+	Scattered syncytiotrophoblastic cells+	Scattered syncytiotrophoblastic cells+	
AFP	–	+ In scattered tumor cells or small foci	–	+
Vimentin	+ (70%)	–	–	

References: [106, 121–123]

Table 14.51 Markers for mediastinal lymphoma

Antibodies	Primary mediastinal large B cell lymphoma (PMLBCL)	Classical Hodgkin lymphoma (CHL)	B cell lymphoma, unclassifiable, with features between diffuse large B cell lymphoma and classical Hodgkin lymphoma/mediastinal gray zone lymphoma
CD45	+	–	+
CD20	+	– or +	+
CD79a	+	–	+
PAX5	+	+ (Usually weak)	+
OCT2	+	–/+	+
BOB.1	+	–/+	+
PU.1	+	–	
CD30	+ (Usually weak and heterogenous)	+	+
CD15	– Occasionally present	+	+/–
IRF4/MUM1	+	+	+
Bcl-6	+	+/–	+/–
CD10	–/+	–/+	–
Bcl-2	+/–	+/–	+ V
MAL	+	–/+	–/+

Note: *V* variably positive

There is no consensus for the interpretation of immunostaining for Bcl-6, and there is some variability in the criteria used by various authors. However, most have used a threshold of 10 or 20% positive nuclei. Expression of transcription factors, such as BOB.1, OCT2, and PU.1, is more commonly seen in PMLBCL than in CHL. PAX5 is expressed weakly by Hodgkin or Reed–Sternberg (RS) cells but strongly by the tumor cells in PMLBCL. There are significant overlapping immunophenotypic features among PMLBCL, CHL, and mediastinal gray zone lymphoma (MGZL). Expression of TRAF-1 (tumor necrosis factor receptor-associated factor-1) and nuclear c-Rel has been reported to be useful in distinguishing PMLBCL from other types of diffuse large B cell lymphoma

References: [99, 106, 121–123]

References

1. Abutaily AS, Addis BJ, Roche WR. Immunohistochemistry in the distinction between malignant mesothelioma and pulmonary adenocarcinoma: a critical evaluation of new antibodies. J Clin Pathol. 2002;55(9):662–8.
2. Agoff SN, Lamps LW, Philip AT, et al. Thyroid transcription factor-1 is expressed in extrapulmonary small cell carcinomas but not in other extrapulmonary neuroendocrine tumors. Mod Pathol. 2000;13(3):238–42.
3. Alijo Serrano F, Sanchez-Mora N, Angel Arranz J, Hernandez C, Alvarez-Fernandez E. Large cell and small cell neuroendocrine bladder carcinoma: immunohistochemical and outcome study in a single institution. Am J Clin Pathol. 2007;128(5):733–9.
4. Allen TC, Cagle PT, Churg AM, et al. Localized malignant mesothelioma. Am J Surg Pathol. 2005;29(7):866–73.
5. Amin MB, Tamboli P, Merchant SH, et al. Micropapillary component in lung adenocarcinoma: a distinctive histologic feature with possible prognostic significance. Am J Surg Pathol. 2002;26(3):358–64.

6. Andrion A, Mazzucco G, Gugliotta P, Monga G. Benign clear cell (sugar) tumor of the lung. A light microscopic, histochemical, and ultrastructural study with a review of the literature. Cancer. 1985;56(11):2657–63.
7. Attanoos RL, Papagiannis A, Suttinont P, Goddard H, Papotti M, Gibbs AR. Pulmonary giant cell carcinoma: pathological entity or morphological phenotype? Histopathology. 1998;32(3):225–31.
8. Bakir K, Kocer NE, Deniz H, Guldur ME. TTF-1 and surfactant-B as co-adjuvants in the diagnosis of lung adenocarcinoma and pleural mesothelioma. Ann Diagn Pathol. 2004;8(6):337–41.
9. Barbareschi M, Ferrero S, Aldovini D, et al. Inflammatory pseudotumour of the lung. Immunohistochemical analysis on four new cases. Histol Histopathol. 1990;5(2):205–11.
10. Barbareschi M, Roldo C, Zamboni G, et al. CDX-2 homeobox gene product expression in neuroendocrine tumors: its role as a marker of intestinal neuroendocrine tumors. Am J Surg Pathol. 2004;28(9):1169–76.
11. Beasley MB. Immunohistochemistry of pulmonary and pleural neoplasia. Arch Pathol Lab Med. 2008;132(7):1062–72 [erratum appears in Arch Pathol Lab Med 2008;132(9):1384].
12. Bejarano PA, Baughman RP, Biddinger PW, et al. Surfactant proteins and thyroid transcription factor-1 in pulmonary and breast carcinomas. Mod Pathol. 1996;9(4):445–52.
13. Bejarano PA, Nikiforov YE, Swenson ES, Biddinger PW. Thyroid transcription factor-1, thyroglobulin, cytokeratin 7, and cytokeratin 20 in thyroid neoplasms. Appl Immunohistochem Mol Morphol. 2000;8(3):189–94.
14. Berger U, Khaghani A, Pomerance A, Yacoub MH, Coombes RC. Pulmonary lymphangioleiomyomatosis and steroid receptors. An immunocytochemical study. Am J Clin Pathol. 1990;93(5):609–14.
15. Bobos M, Hytiroglou P, Kostopoulos I, Karkavelas G, Papadimitriou CS. Immunohistochemical distinction between Merkel cell carcinoma and small cell carcinoma of the lung. Am J Dermatopathol. 2006;28(2):99–104.
16. Bonetti F, Chiodera PL, Pea M, et al. Transbronchial biopsy in lymphangiomyomatosis of the lung. HMB45 for diagnosis. Am J Surg Pathol. 1993;17(11):1092–102.
17. Butnor KJ, Nicholson AG, Allred DC, et al. Expression of renal cell carcinoma-associated markers erythropoietin, CD10, and renal cell carcinoma marker in diffuse malignant mesothelioma and metastatic renal cell carcinoma. Arch Pathol Lab Med. 2006;130(6):823–7.
18. Byrd-Gloster AL, Khoor A, Glass LF, et al. Differential expression of thyroid transcription factor 1 in small cell lung carcinoma and Merkel cell tumor. Hum Pathol. 2000;31(1):58–62.
19. Cagle PT, Truong LD, Roggli VL, Greenberg SD. Immunohistochemical differentiation of sarcomatoid mesotheliomas from other spindle cell neoplasms. Am J Clin Pathol. 1989;92(5):566–71.
20. Castro CY, Moran CA, Flieder DG, Suster S. Primary signet ring cell adenocarcinomas of the lung: a clinicopathological study of 15 cases. Histopathology. 2001;39(4):397–401.
21. Cerfolio RJ, Allen MS, Nascimento AG, et al. Inflammatory pseudotumors of the lung. Ann Thorac Surg. 1999;67(4):933–6.
22. Cessna MH, Zhou H, Sanger WG, et al. Expression of ALK1 and p80 in inflammatory myofibroblastic tumor and its mesenchymal mimics: a study of 135 cases. Mod Pathol. 2002;15(9):931–8.
23. Chan JK, Cheuk W, Shimizu M. Anaplastic lymphoma kinase expression in inflammatory pseudotumors. Am J Surg Pathol. 2001;25(6):761–8.
24. Chejfec G, Candel A, Jansson DS, et al. Immunohistochemical features of giant cell carcinoma of the lung: patterns of expression of cytokeratins, vimentin, and the mucinous glycoprotein recognized by monoclonal antibody A-80. Ultrastruct Pathol. 1991;15(2):131–8.
25. Choi SJ, Kim JM, Han JY, et al. Extrapulmonary small cell carcinoma of the liver: clinicopathological and immunohistochemical findings. Yonsei Med J. 2007;48(6):1066–71.
26. Chu P, Wu E, Weiss LM. Cytokeratin 7 and cytokeratin 20 expression in epithelial neoplasms: a survey of 435 cases. Mod Pathol. 2000;13(9):962–72.
27. Coffin CM, Patel A, Perkins S, Elenitoba-Johnson KS, Perlman E, Griffin CA. ALK1 and p80 expression and chromosomal rearrangements involving 2p23 in inflammatory myofibroblastic tumor. Mod Pathol. 2001;14(6):569–76.
28. Coffin CM, Watterson J, Priest JR, Dehner LP. Extrapulmonary inflammatory myofibroblastic tumor (inflammatory pseudotumor). A clinicopathologic and immunohistochemical study of 84 cases. Am J Surg Pathol. 1995;19(8):859–72.
29. Colley MH, Geppert E, Franklin WA. Immunohistochemical detection of steroid receptors in a case of pulmonary lymphangioleiomyomatosis. Am J Surg Pathol. 1989;13(9):803–7.
30. Cook JR, Dehner LP, Collins MH, et al. Anaplastic lymphoma kinase (ALK) expression in the inflammatory myofibroblastic tumor: a comparative immunohistochemical study. Am J Surg Pathol. 2001;25(11):1364–71.
31. Copin MC, Buisine MP, Leteurtre E, et al. Mucinous bronchioloalveolar carcinomas display a specific pattern of mucin gene expression among primary lung adenocarcinomas. Hum Pathol. 2001;32(3):274–81.
32. Corson JM, Weiss LM, Banks-Schlegel SP, Pinkus GS. Keratin proteins and carcinoembryonic antigen in synovial sarcomas: an immunohistochemical study of 24 cases. Hum Pathol. 1984;15(7):615–21.
33. Dabbs DJ, Bhargava R, Chivukula M. Lobular versus ductal breast neoplasms: the diagnostic utility of p120 catenin. Am J Surg Pathol. 2007;31(3):427–37.
34. Dabbs DJ, Landreneau RJ, Liu Y, et al. Detection of estrogen receptor by immunohistochemistry in pulmonary adenocarcinoma. Ann Thorac Surg. 2002;73(2):403–5.
35. de Leval L, Ferry JA, Falini B, Shipp M, Harris NL. Expression of bcl-6 and CD10 in primary mediastinal large B-cell lymphoma: evidence for derivation from germinal center B cells? Am J Surg Pathol. 2001;25(10):1277–82.
36. Devouassoux-Shisheboran M, Hayashi T, Linnoila RI, Koss MN, Travis WD. A clinicopathologic study of 100 cases of pulmonary sclerosing hemangioma with immunohistochemical studies: TTF-1 is expressed in both round and surface cells, suggesting an origin from primitive respiratory epithelium. Am J Surg Pathol. 2000;24(7):906–16.
37. Dixon AY, Moran JF, Wesselius LJ, McGregor DH. Pulmonary mucinous cystic tumor. Case report with review of the literature. Am J Surg Pathol. 1993;17(7):722–8.
38. Doglioni C, Dei Tos AP, Laurino L, et al. Calretinin: a novel immunocytochemical marker for mesothelioma. Am J Surg Pathol. 1996;20(9):1037–46.
39. Du EZ, Goldstraw P, Zacharias J, et al. TTF-1 expression is specific for lung primary in typical and atypical carcinoids: TTF-1-positive carcinoids are predominantly in peripheral location. Hum Pathol. 2004;35(7):825–31.
40. Erickson LA, Papouchado B, Dimashkieh H, Zhang S, Nakamura N, Lloyd RV. Cdx2 as a marker for neuroendocrine tumors of unknown primary sites. Endocr Pathol. 2004;15(3):247–52.
41. Fishback NF, Travis WD, Moran CA, Guinee Jr DG, McCarthy WF, Koss MN. Pleomorphic (spindle/giant cell) carcinoma of the lung. A clinicopathologic correlation of 78 cases. Cancer. 1994;73(12):2936–45.
42. Folpe AL, Chand EM, Goldblum JR, Weiss SW. Expression of Fli-1, a nuclear transcription factor, distinguishes vascular neoplasms from potential mimics. Am J Surg Pathol. 2001;25(8):1061–6.
43. Folpe AL, Gown AM, Lamps LW, et al. Thyroid transcription factor-1: immunohistochemical evaluation in pulmonary neuroendocrine tumors. Mod Pathol. 1999;12(1):5–8.

44. Gaffey MJ, Mills SE, Askin FB, et al. Clear cell tumor of the lung. A clinicopathologic, immunohistochemical, and ultrastructural study of eight cases. Am J Surg Pathol. 1990;14(3):248–59.
45. Gaffey MJ, Mills SE, Zarbo RJ, Weiss LM, Gown AM. Clear cell tumor of the lung. Immunohistochemical and ultrastructural evidence of melanogenesis. Am J Surg Pathol. 1991;15(7):644–53.
46. Gal AA, Koss MN, Hochholzer L, Chejfec G. An immunohistochemical study of benign clear cell ('sugar') tumor of the lung. Arch Pathol Lab Med. 1991;115(10):1034–8.
47. Griffin CA, Hawkins AL, Dvorak C, Henkle C, Ellingham T, Perlman EJ. Recurrent involvement of 2p23 in inflammatory myofibroblastic tumors. Cancer Res. 1999;59(12):2776–80.
48. Han AJ, Xiong M, Gu YY, Lin SX, Xiong M. Lymphoepithelioma-like carcinoma of the lung with a better prognosis. A clinicopathologic study of 32 cases. Am J Clin Pathol. 2001;115(6):841–50.
49. Hayashi H, Kitamura H, Nakatani Y, Inayama Y, Ito T, Kitamura H. Primary signet-ring cell carcinoma of the lung: histochemical and immunohistochemical characterization. Hum Pathol. 1999;30(4):378–83.
50. Higashiyama M, Doi O, Kodama K, Yokouchi H, Tateishi R. Cystic mucinous adenocarcinoma of the lung. Two cases of cystic variant of mucus-producing lung adenocarcinoma. Chest. 1992;101(3):763–6.
51. Hiroshima K, Iyoda A, Shida T, et al. Distinction of pulmonary large cell neuroendocrine carcinoma from small cell lung carcinoma: a morphological, immunohistochemical, and molecular analysis. Mod Pathol. 2006;19(10):1358–68.
52. Honda T, Ota H, Ishii K, Nakamura N, Kubo K, Katsuyama T. Mucinous bronchioloalveolar carcinoma with organoid differentiation simulating the pyloric mucosa of the stomach: clinicopathologic, histochemical, and immunohistochemical analysis. Am J Clin Pathol. 1998;109(4):423–30.
53. Hussong JW, Brown M, Perkins SL, Dehner LP, Coffin CM. Comparison of DNA ploidy, histologic, and immunohistochemical findings with clinical outcome in inflammatory myofibroblastic tumors. Mod Pathol. 1999;12(3):279–86.
54. Ionescu DN, Treaba D, Gilks CB, et al. Nonsmall cell lung carcinoma with neuroendocrine differentiation – an entity of no clinical or prognostic significance. Am J Surg Pathol. 2007;31(1):26–32.
55. Jaffee IM, Rahmani M, Singhal MG, Younes M. Expression of the intestinal transcription factor CDX2 in carcinoid tumors is a marker of midgut origin. Arch Pathol Lab Med. 2006;130(10):1522–6.
56. Jerome Marson V, Mazieres J, Groussard O, et al. Expression of TTF-1 and cytokeratins in primary and secondary epithelial lung tumours: correlation with histological type and grade. Histopathology. 2004;45(2):125–34.
57. Kaufmann O, Dietel M. Thyroid transcription factor-1 is the superior immunohistochemical marker for pulmonary adenocarcinomas and large cell carcinomas compared to surfactant proteins A and B. Histopathology. 2000;36(1):8–16.
58. Koss MN, Hochholzer L, O'Leary T. Pulmonary blastomas. Cancer. 1991;67(9):2368–81.
59. Kuhnen C, Harms D, Niessen KH, Diehm T, Müller KM. Congenital pulmonary fibrosarcoma. Differential diagnosis of infantile pulmonary spindle cell tumors. Pathologe. 2001;22(2):151–6 [in German].
60. Lantuejoul S, Isaac S, Pinel N, Negoescu A, Guibert B, Brambilla E. Clear cell tumor of the lung: an immunohistochemical and ultrastructural study supporting a pericytic differentiation. Mod Pathol. 1997;10(10):1001–8.
61. Lantuejoul S, Moro D, Michalides RJ, Brambilla C, Brambilla E. Neural cell adhesion molecules (NCAM) and NCAM-PSA expression in neuroendocrine lung tumors. Am J Surg Pathol. 1998;22(10):1267–76.
62. Lau SK, Chu PG, Weiss LM. Immunohistochemical expression of estrogen receptor in pulmonary adenocarcinoma. Appl Immunohistochem Mol Morphol. 2006;14(1):83–7.
63. Lee WJ, Kim CH, Chang SE, et al. Cutaneous metastasis from large-cell neuroendocrine carcinoma of the urinary bladder expressing CK20 and TTF-1. Am J Dermatopathol. 2009;31(2):166–9.
64. Lin BT, Colby T, Gown AM, et al. Malignant vascular tumors of the serous membranes mimicking mesothelioma. A report of 14 cases. Am J Surg Pathol. 1996;20(12):1431–9.
65. Lin X, Saad RS, Luckasevic TM, Silverman JF, Liu Y. Diagnostic value of CDX-2 and TTF-1 expressions in separating metastatic neuroendocrine neoplasms of unknown origin. Appl Immunohistochem Mol Morphol. 2007;15(4):407–14.
66. Loy TS, Calaluce RD. Utility of cytokeratin immunostaining in separating pulmonary adenocarcinomas from colonic adenocarcinomas. Am J Clin Pathol. 1994;102(6):764–7.
67. Lucas DR, Pass HI, Madan SK, et al. Sarcomatoid mesothelioma and its histological mimics: a comparative immunohistochemical study. Histopathology. 2003;42(3):270–9.
68. Mai KT, Perkins DG, Zhang J, Mackenzie CR. ES1, a new lung carcinoma antibody – an immunohistochemical study. Histopathology. 2006;49(5):515–22.
69. Miettinen M. Keratin subsets in spindle cell sarcomas. Keratins are widespread but synovial sarcoma contains a distinctive keratin polypeptide pattern and desmoplakins. Am J Pathol. 1991;138(2):505–13.
70. Miettinen M, Fetsch JF. Distribution of keratins in normal endothelial cells and a spectrum of vascular tumors: implications in tumor diagnosis. Hum Pathol. 2000;31(9):1062–7.
71. Nakamura N, Miyagi E, Murata S, Kawaoi A, Katoh R. Expression of thyroid transcription factor-1 in normal and neoplastic lung tissues. Mod Pathol. 2002;15(10):1058–67.
72. Nakatani Y, Dickersin GR, Mark EJ. Pulmonary endodermal tumor resembling fetal lung: a clinicopathologic study of five cases with immunohistochemical and ultrastructural characterization. Hum Pathol. 1990;21(11):1097–107.
73. Oliveira AM, Tazelaar HD, Myers JL, Erickson LA, Lloyd RV. Thyroid transcription factor-1 distinguishes metastatic pulmonary from well-differentiated neuroendocrine tumors of other sites. Am J Surg Pathol. 2001;25(6):815–9.
74. Ordonez NG. The diagnostic utility of immunohistochemistry in distinguishing between mesothelioma and renal cell carcinoma: a comparative study. Hum Pathol. 2004;35(6):697–710.
75. Ordonez NG. Application of mesothelin immunostaining in tumor diagnosis. Am J Surg Pathol. 2003;27(11):1418–28.
76. Ordonez NG. Value of thyroid transcription factor-1 immunostaining in distinguishing small cell lung carcinomas from other small cell carcinomas. Am J Surg Pathol. 2000;24(9):1217–23.
77. Ordonez NG. Value of calretinin immunostaining in differentiating epithelial mesothelioma from lung adenocarcinoma. Mod Pathol. 1998;11(10):929–33.
78. Pelosi G, Pasini F, Olsen Stenholm C, et al. p63 Immunoreactivity in lung cancer: yet another player in the development of squamous cell carcinomas? J Pathol. 2002;198(1):100–9.
79. Pettinato G, Manivel JC, Wick MR, Dehner LP. Classical and cellular (atypical) congenital mesoblastic nephroma: a clinicopathologic, ultrastructural, immunohistochemical, and flow cytometric study. Hum Pathol. 1989;20(7):682–90.
80. Purdy LJ, Colby TV, Yousem SA, Battifora H. Pulmonary Kaposi's sarcoma. Premortem histologic diagnosis. Am J Surg Pathol. 1986;10(5):301–11.
81. Ralston J, Chiriboga L, Nonaka D. MASH1: a useful marker in differentiating pulmonary small cell carcinoma from Merkel cell carcinoma. Mod Pathol. 2008;21(11):1357–62.
82. Ramachandra S, Hollowood K, Bisceglia M, Fletcher CD. Inflammatory pseudotumour of soft tissues: a clinicopathological

and immunohistochemical analysis of 18 cases. Histopathology. 1995;27(4):313–23.

83. Rdzanek M, Fresco R, Pass HI, Carbone M. Spindle cell tumors of the pleura: differential diagnosis. Semin Diagn Pathol. 2006;23(1):44–55.
84. Roberts F, McCall AE, Burnett RA. Malignant mesothelioma: a comparison of biopsy and postmortem material by light microscopy and immunohistochemistry. J Clin Pathol. 2001;54(10):766–70.
85. Rodig SJ, Savage KJ, LaCasce AS, et al. Expression of TRAF1 and nuclear c-Rel distinguishes primary mediastinal large cell lymphoma from other types of diffuse large B-cell lymphoma. Am J Surg Pathol. 2007;31(1):106–12.
86. Rossi G, Cavazza A, Sturm N, et al. Pulmonary carcinomas with pleomorphic, sarcomatoid, or sarcomatous elements: a clinicopathologic and immunohistochemical study of 75 cases. Am J Surg Pathol. 2003;27(3):311–24.
87. Rossi G, Murer B, Cavazza A, et al. Primary mucinous (so-called colloid) carcinomas of the lung: a clinicopathologic and immunohistochemical study with special reference to CDX-2 homeobox gene and MUC2 expression. Am J Surg Pathol. 2004;28(4):442–52.
88. Saqi A, Alexis D, Remotti F, Bhagat G. Usefulness of CDX2 and TTF-1 in differentiating gastrointestinal from pulmonary carcinoids. Am J Clin Pathol. 2005;123(3):394–404.
89. Sasaki E, Tsunoda N, Hatanaka Y, Mori N, Iwata H, Yatabe Y. Breast-specific expression of MGB1/mammaglobin: an examination of 480 tumors from various organs and clinicopathological analysis of MGB1-positive breast cancers. Mod Pathol. 2007;20(2):208–14.
90. Shah RN, Badve S, Papreddy K, Schindler S, Laskin WB, Yeldandi AV. Expression of cytokeratin 20 in mucinous bronchioloalveolar carcinoma. Hum Pathol. 2002;33(9):915–20.
91. Sholl LM, Hornick JL, Pinkus JL, Pinkus GS, Padera RF. Immunohistochemical analysis of langerin in langerhans cell histiocytosis and pulmonary inflammatory and infectious diseases. Am J Surg Pathol. 2007;31(6):947–52.
92. Siami K, McCluggage WG, Ordonez NG, et al. Thyroid transcription factor-1 expression in endometrial and endocervical adenocarcinomas. Am J Surg Pathol. 2007;31(11):1759–63.
93. Sica G, Wagner PL, Altorki N, et al. Immunohistochemical expression of estrogen and progesterone receptors in primary pulmonary neuroendocrine tumors. Arch Pathol Lab Med. 2008;132(12):1889–95.
94. Smith TA, Machen SK, Fisher C, Goldblum JR. Usefulness of cytokeratin subsets for distinguishing monophasic synovial sarcoma from malignant peripheral nerve sheath tumor. Am J Clin Pathol. 1999;112(5):641–8.
95. Srivastava A, Hornick JL. Immunohistochemical staining for CDX-2, PDX-1, NESP-55, and TTF-1 can help distinguish gastrointestinal carcinoid tumors from pancreatic endocrine and pulmonary carcinoid tumors. Am J Surg Pathol. 2009;33(4):626–32.
96. Striebel JM, Dacic S, Yousem SA. Gross cystic disease fluid protein-(GCDFP-15): expression in primary lung adenocarcinoma. Am J Surg Pathol. 2008;32(3):426–32.
97. Sturm N, Rossi G, Lantuejoul S, et al. 34BetaE12 expression along the whole spectrum of neuroendocrine proliferations of the lung, from neuroendocrine cell hyperplasia to small cell carcinoma. Histopathology. 2003;42(2):156–66.
98. Suster S, Fisher C, Moran CA. Expression of bcl-2 oncoprotein in benign and malignant spindle cell tumors of soft tissue, skin, serosal surfaces, and gastrointestinal tract. Am J Surg Pathol. 1998;22(7):863–72.
99. Swerdlow SH, Campo E, Harris N, et al. WHO classification of tumours of haematopoietic and lymphoid tissues. 4th ed. Lyon, France: International Agency for Research on Cancer (IARC); 2008. p. 439.
100. Tan D, Li Q, Deeb G, et al. Thyroid transcription factor-1 expression prevalence and its clinical implications in non-small cell lung cancer: a high-throughput tissue microarray and immunohistochemistry study. Hum Pathol. 2003;34(6):597–604.
101. Tan D, Zander DS. Immunohistochemistry for assessment of pulmonary and pleural neoplasms: a review and update. Int J Clin Exp Pathol. 2008;1(1):19–31.
102. Tan J, Sidhu G, Greco MA, Ballard H, Wieczorek R. Villin, cytokeratin 7, and cytokeratin 20 expression in pulmonary adenocarcinoma with ultrastructural evidence of microvilli with rootlets. Hum Pathol. 1998;29(4):390–6.
103. Tot T. Cytokeratins 20 and 7 as biomarkers: usefulness in discriminating primary from metastatic adenocarcinoma. Eur J Cancer. 2002;38(6):758–63.
104. Tot T. The value of cytokeratins 20 and 7 in discriminating metastatic adenocarcinomas from pleural mesotheliomas. Cancer. 2001;92(10):2727–32.
105. Traverse-Glehen A, Pittaluga S, Gaulard P, et al. Mediastinal gray zone lymphoma: the missing link between classic Hodgkin's lymphoma and mediastinal large B-cell lymphoma. Am J Surg Pathol. 2005;29(11):1411–21.
106. Travis WD, Brambilla E, Muller-Hermelink HK, Harris CC. Tumours of the lung, pleura, thymus and heart. Lyon, France: IARC Press; 2004. p. 341.
107. Uzaslan E, Stuempel T, Ebsen M, et al. Surfactant protein A detection in primary pulmonary adenocarcinoma without bronchioloalveolar pattern. Respiration. 2005;72(3):249–53.
108. Wang BY, Gil J, Kaufman D, Gan L, Kohtz DS, Burstein DE. P63 in pulmonary epithelium, pulmonary squamous neoplasms, and other pulmonary tumors. Hum Pathol. 2002;33(9):921–6.
109. Wang J, Weiss LM, Hu B, et al. Usefulness of immunohistochemistry in delineating renal spindle cell tumours. A retrospective study of 31 cases. Histopathology. 2004;44(5):462–71.
110. Warson C, Van De Bovenkamp JH, Korteland-Van Male AM, et al. Barrett's esophagus is characterized by expression of gastric-type mucins (MUC5AC, MUC6) and TFF peptides (TFF1 and TFF2), but the risk of carcinoma development may be indicated by the intestinal-type mucin, MUC2. Hum Pathol. 2002;33(6):660–8.
111. Werling RW, Yaziji H, Bacchi CE, Gown AM. CDX2, a highly sensitive and specific marker of adenocarcinomas of intestinal origin: an immunohistochemical survey of 476 primary and metastatic carcinomas. Am J Surg Pathol. 2003;27(3):303–10.
112. Wu M, Wang B, Gil J, et al. p63 and TTF-1 immunostaining. A useful marker panel for distinguishing small cell carcinoma of lung from poorly differentiated squamous cell carcinoma of lung. Am J Clin Pathol. 2003;119(5):696–702.
113. Yamamoto H, Bai YQ, Yuasa Y. Homeodomain protein CDX2 regulates goblet-specific MUC2 gene expression. Biochem Biophys Res Commun. 2003;300(4):813–8.
114. Yao JL, Madeb R, Bourne P, et al. Small cell carcinoma of the prostate: an immunohistochemical study. Am J Surg Pathol. 2006;30(6):705–12.
115. Yatabe Y, Mitsudomi T, Takahashi T. TTF-1 expression in pulmonary adenocarcinomas. Am J Surg Pathol. 2002;26(6):767–73.
116. Yousem SA, Shaw H, Cieply K. Involvement of 2p23 in pulmonary inflammatory pseudotumors. Hum Pathol. 2001;32(4):428–33.
117. Yousem SA, Wick MR, Randhawa P, Manivel JC. Pulmonary blastoma. An immunohistochemical analysis with comparison with fetal lung in its pseudoglandular stage. Am J Clin Pathol. 1990;93(2):167–75.
118. Zamecnik J, Kodet R. Value of thyroid transcription factor-1 and surfactant apoprotein A in the differential diagnosis of pulmonary carcinomas: a study of 109 cases. Virchows Arch. 2002;440(4):353–61.
119. Zhang H, Liu J, Cagle PT, Allen TC, Laga AC, Zander DS. Distinction of pulmonary small cell carcinoma from poorly

differentiated squamous cell carcinoma: an immunohistochemical approach. Mod Pathol. 2005;18(1):111–8.

120. Zhu LC, Yim J, Chiriboga L, Cassai ND, Sidhu GS, Moreira AL. DC-LAMP stains pulmonary adenocarcinoma with bronchiolar Clara cell differentiation. Hum Pathol. 2007;38(2): 260–8.

121. Chu PG, Weiss LM. Modern immunohistochemistry. New York, NY: Cambridge University Press; 2009.

122. Dabbs DJ. Diagnostic immunohistochemistry. 3rd ed. Philadelphia, PA: Churchill Livingstone Elsevier; 2010.

123. Taylor C, Cote R. Immunomicroscopy a diagnostic tool for the surgical pathologist, Major problems in pathology, vol. 19. 3rd ed. Philadelphia, PA: Saunders Elsevier; 2006.

124. Chilosi M, Murer B. Mixed adenocarcinomas of the lung: place in new proposals in classification, mandatory for target therapy. Arch Pathol Lab Med. 2010;134(1):55–65.

125. Gerald WL, Ladanyi M, de Alava E, et al. Clinical, pathologic, and molecular spectrum of tumors associated with t(11;22)(p13;q12): desmoplastic small round-cell tumor and its variants. J Clin Oncol. 1998;16(9):3028–36.

Chapter 15
Breast

Haiyan Liu

Abstract Immunohistochemistry plays a crucial role in the routine practice of breast pathology. This chapter answers questions about immunohistochemistry many applications to topics including stromal invasion, columnar cell lesions, intraductal proliferations, papillary lesions, sclerosing lesions, spindle cell lesions, nipple neoplasia and Paget's disease, fibroepithelial lesions, prognostic and predictive factors, and genomic phenotypes (luminal A, B, basal, and Her-2). Photomicrographs demonstrate the characteristic staining patterns of common stains such as nuclear and cytoplasmic myoepithelial markers, membranous E-cadherin and p^{120} catenin proteins in lobular neoplasia and D2-40 in lymphatic invasion. Images also show novel dual color staining techniques such as p63 and c-kit staining of adenoid cystic carcinoma.

Keywords Breast • Ductal • Lobular • Columnar cell • Flat epithelial atypia • Stromal invasion • Lymphatic invasion • Medullary • Metaplastic • Tubulolobular • Micropapillary • Mucinous • Adenoid cystic • Luminal • Basal-like • Fibroepithelial • Myoepithelial • Prognostic • Predictive • Paget's disease • Nipple • p63 • E-cadherin • p^{120} Catenin • D2-40 • Calponin • Smooth muscle myosin heavy chain • Estrogen • Progesterone • Her-2 • Androgen

FREQUENTLY ASKED QUESTIONS

General Questions of Breast Lesion/Neoplasm

H. Liu (✉)
Department of Pathology and Laboratory Medicine,
Geisinger Medical Center, 100 North Academy Avenue, Danville, PA 17822, USA
e-mail: hliu1@geisinger.edu

F. Lin and J. Prichard (eds.), *Handbook of Practical Immunohistochemistry: Frequently Asked Questions*,
DOI 10.1007/978-1-4419-8062-5_15, © Springer Science+Business Media, LLC 2011

25. Prognostic and predictive markers of breast carcinoma (Table 15.25) (p. 239).

Differential Diagnosis

26. The differentiation of columnar cell lesions (including flat epithelial atypia) vs. normal/usual ductal hyperplasia (Table 15.26) (p. 239).
27. The differentiation of usual duct hyperplasia vs. atypical duct hyperplasia/ductal carcinoma in situ (Table 15.27) (p. 239).
28. The differentiation of lobular carcinoma vs. ductal carcinoma (Table 15.28) (p. 240).
29. The differentiation of tubular carcinoma vs. sclerosing adenosis and microglandular adenosis (Table 15.29) (p. 240).
30. The differentiation of adenoid cystic carcinoma, tubular carcinoma, and cribriform carcinoma (Table 15.30) (p. 240).
31. The differentiation of spindle cell neoplasm of breast (Fig. 15.9, Table 15.31) (pp. 240–241).
32. Differentiation of micropapillary patterned carcinoma: ovarian vs. breast (Table 15.32) (p. 241).
33. The differentiation of primary breast vs. metastatic adenocarcinoma (Table 15.33) (p. 241).

Neoplasm of Nipple

34. The evaluation of mammary Paget's disease (Table 15.34) (p. 242).
35. The evaluation of nipple adenoma (syringomatous adenoma of nipple), large duct papilloma, and low-grade ductal/tubular carcinoma (Table 15.35) (p. 242).
36. The differentiation of Paget's disease, Bowen's disease, and malignant melanoma (Table 15.36) (p. 242).

Table 15.1 Summary of frequently used antibodies

Markers	Localization (N, M, C)	Function	Application and pitfalls
AE1/AE3	M	Pankeratin peptides	Both epithelia and myoepithelia are reactive; Useful used in combination with p63 to confirm small foci of carcinomas
Pan-CK	M	Pankeratin peptides	Both epithelia and myoepithelia are reactive; Similar utility as AE1/AE3
CK7	M	A 54 kDa type II simple keratin	Both epithelia and myoepithelia are reactive; May be used in the work-up of metastatic disease. Majority of breast carcinomas (over 95%) are positive
CAM 5.2	M, C	LMWCK, simple keratin peptide, recognize CK8 and CK18	Positive in epithelia; Used in the work-up of spindle cell lesions (positive for sarcomatoid carcinoma – carcinosarcoma, spindle cell carcinoma, and metaplastic carcinoma)
CK8/18	M, C	LMWCK, same as CAM 5.2	Positive in epithelia; Luminal-type carcinomas are reactive
CK19	M, C	A 43 kDa simple keratin	Positive in epithelia; Luminal-type carcinomas are reactive
CK903	M, C	HMWCK	Both epithelia and myoepithelia are reactive; Used as a basal marker to identified basal-like carcinoma; Useful in the differentiation of UDH (diffuse membrane staining) vs. ADH/DCIS (negative); Limited utility in the evaluation of stromal invasion due to low sensitivity to myoepithelial cells and the reactivity in epithelium
CK5/6	M	HMWCK	Both epithelia and myoepithelia are reactive; Similar utility as CK903; Used as a basal marker
CK14	M	HMWCK	Both epithelia and myoepithelia are reactive; Used as a basal marker
CK17	M	HMWCK	Both epithelia and myoepithelia are reactive; Used as a basal marker
EMA	M	T transmembrane glycoprotein	A general epithelial marker (membrane stain); Normal breast demonstrates an apical membranous staining pattern while breast carcinoma a circumferential membranous staining pattern
CEA	C	A 180 kDa glycoprotein	Breast carcinomas are often CEA positive
p63	N	A homologue of the tumor suppressor protein p53	Positive in myoepithelium; The most specific marker for myoepithelial cells, useful in the evaluation of stromal invasion; Reported 5–12% of invasive carcinomas (esp. high grade) and UDH show scattered staining
SMM-HC	C	A 200 kDa, unique structural component of myosin	Positive in myoepithelium; An excellent marker for myoepithelial cells, no or few cross-reaction with myofibroblasts, useful in the evaluation of stromal invasion
Calponin	C	A 34 kDa, smooth muscle-restricted regulatory protein	Positive in myoepithelium; A good marker for myoepithelial cells, with lesser degree of cross-reaction with myofibroblasts in the stroma

(continued)

Table 15.1 (continued)

Markers	Localization (N, M, C)	Function	Application and pitfalls
SMA	C	Micro-filamentous contractile polypeptide	Positive in myoepithelium; With cross-reaction to myofibroblasts in the stroma, making it difficult to identify the myoepithelium in cases of DCIS with periductal desmoplasia
HHF-35	C	Anti-muscle-specific actin	Positive in myoepithelium
S100	N, C	A calcium flux regulator	One of the earliest myoepithelial markers, also labeling normal and neoplastic luminal epithelial cells; No longer used for the purpose of detecting breast myoepithelial cells
CD10	M, C	A type II integral membrane glycoprotein	Myoepithelial cell marker, less sensitive than others; also labeling luminal cells of the terminal duct lobular unit and tumor cells
Maspin	N + C	A member of the serpin family of serine proteases	Positive in myoepithelium; Myoepithelial cell marker, also label luminal cells of the terminal duct lobular unit and tumor cells
P-cadherin	M, C	A calcium-dependent cellular adhesion molecule	Reported positive in myoepithelium. Normal breast luminal cells are nonreactive; Frequently expressed in high-grade breast carcinoma
WT1	N	Antibody to the carboxy-terminal (C-terminal) region of WT gene	Positive in myoepithelium; An earlier basal marker, labeling myoepithelial cells
MNF116	C	Pan-CK	Positive in myoepithelium and epithelium
EGFR	M	Receptor tyrosine kinases	Frequently overexpressed in variety of carcinomas; as a marker to identified basal-like carcinoma
Vimentin	C	A 57-kDa protein, member of the intermediate filament family	Not a cell type-specific marker, useful to serve as a "control marker" to ensure tissue proper handling; Often coexpressed in metaplastic carcinoma
CA-125	C	A high molecular weight glycoprotein	Gynecologic carcinomas and mesotheliomas are positive; Breast carcinomas are nonreactive
TTF1	N	A transcription factor	Expressed in thyroid, diencephalon and lung; Breast carcinomas are nonreactive
NSE	C	Enolase enzymes	Expressed in a variety of normal and neoplastic neuroendocrine cells, with poor specificity
CD56	C + M	Neural cell adhesion molecule	The prototypic natural killer cell marker, also found in subsets of CD4- and CD8-positive T cells; A broad-spectrum neuroendocrine marker
Synap	C	A glycoprotein in NE secretory granule	A broad-spectrum neuroendocrine marker
Chrom	C	Main protein extract of NE granules of NE cells	A neuroendocrine marker, more specific than Synap
E-cadherin	M	A calcium-dependent transmembrane adhesion protein	A negative membranous marker for lobular neoplasia
p^{120}ctn	C or M	A member of the transmembrane E-cadherin proteins	A positive marker for lobular neoplasia; Membranous pattern for ductal neoplasia and cytoplasmic pattern for lobular neoplasia
GCDFP-15	C	Androgen and prolactin responsive protein	Expressed in benign and malignant human breast tumors, salivary gland, and skin adnexal tumors; Lower sensitivity but higher specificity for breast primary compared with MGB
MGB	C	A glycoprotein of the secreto-globin family	Positive in breast and gynecologic tumors; Higher sensitivity but lower specificity for breast primary compared with GDCFP-15
D2-40	C	A 40-kDa sialoglycoprotein against an oncofetal antigen – M2A	A marker labeling lymphatic endothelia and mesothelium; Used to identify lymphatic invasion. Pitfall: Weakly reactive to myoepithelium, may mistake small duct for lymphatic space
CD31	M	A 130 kDa integral membrane protein mediating cell-to-cell adhesion	Expressed on the surface of endothelial cells, weakly on peripheral leukocytes and platelets; Used to identify vascular invasion or vascular neoplasm
CD34	M	A single-chain transmembrane glycoprotein	Expressed on immature hematopoietic precursor cells, also capillary endothelial cells
c-kit	M	Transmembrane type 3 receptor tyrosine kinase	Expressed in 90–100% GISTs; A marker for adenoid cystic carcinoma, decorating the luminal cells; High level of c-kit expression is also seen in malignant phyllodes tumor
MUC1	C	A high molecular weight glycoprotein	Normal ductal/lobular epithelium and majority of breast carcinomas (over 95%) are positive
MUC2	C	A high molecular weight glycoprotein	Normal ductal/lobular epithelium and breast carcinomas are negative

(continued)

Table 15.1 (continued)

Markers	Localization (N, M, C)	Function	Application and pitfalls
MUC4	C	A high molecular weight glycoprotein	Normal ductal/lobular epithelium and majority of breast carcinomas (over 95%) are negative
MUC5AC	C	A high molecular weight glycoprotein	Normal ductal/lobular epithelium and majority of breast carcinomas (over 95%) are negative
MUC6	C	A high molecular weight glycoprotein	Normal ductal/lobular epithelium and majority of breast carcinomas (over 90%) are negative
p53	N	A tumor-suppressor and transcription factor	p53 is frequently mutated or inactivated in carcinomas; Used as a prognostic marker, associated with high-grade tumor and worse prognosis. High immunoreactivity was reported in apocrine carcinomas, especially in situ carcinoma
MIB-1	N	A nuclear antigen associated with cell proliferation	Expressed in all proliferating cells which are in the active phases of the cell cycle (late G1, S, G2, and mitosis); Used as a prognostic marker, associated with worse prognosis
ARP	N	A nuclear protein belonging to the steroid receptor family	Positive for apocrine lesions, both benign and malignant
ER	N	A nuclear protein belonging to the steroid receptor family	A favorable prognostic marker for breast carcinoma; Also used in metastatic disease, as a marker for breast and gynecologic primary
PR	N	A nuclear protein belonging to the steroid receptor family	A favorable prognostic marker for breast carcinoma
Her-2/neu	M	Transmembrane tyrosine kinase belongs to the ErbB receptor family	An unfavorable prognostic marker for breast carcinoma, usually overexpressed in high-grade tumor

Note: *HMWCK* high molecular weight cytokeratin, *LMWCK* low molecular weight cytokeratin CK903 or 34βE12, *EMA* epithelial membrane antigen, *CEA* carcinoembryonic antigen, *S100* S100 protein, *CD10 (CALLA)* acute lymphocyte leukemia antigen, *EGFR* epidermal growth factor receptor, *Vim* vimentin, *Synap* synaptophysin, *Chrom* chromogranin, *NSE* neuron-specific enolase, *NE* neuroendocrine, *MGB* mammaglobin, *GCDFP-15* gross cystic disease fluid protein-15, *CD31* also known as PECAM-1 (platelet endothelial cell adhesion molecule-1), *$p^{120}ctn$* p^{120} catenin, *ARP* androgen receptor protein, *ER* estrogen receptor, *PR* progesterone receptor

References: [1–215]

Table 15.2 Epithelial markers of breast tissue/neoplasm

Marker	Pattern	Target	Comment
AE1/AE3	M, C	Luminal epithelium; myoepithelium	Breast carcinomas are positive
Pan-CK	M, C	Luminal epithelium; myoepithelium	Breast carcinomas are positive
CK7	M	Luminal epithelium; myoepithelium	Majority of breast carcinomas (over 95%) are positive
CAM 5.2	M	Luminal epithelium	Positive for luminal-type and sarcomatoid carcinoma (carcinosarcoma, spindle cell carcinoma, and metaplastic carcinoma)
CK8/18	M	Luminal epithelium	Positive for luminal-type carcinoma
CK19	M	Luminal epithelium	Positive for luminal-type carcinoma
CK5/6	M	Myoepithelium; benign hyperplastic luminal epithelium	Basal-type cytokeratin, positive for basal-like carcinoma
CK14	M, C	Myoepithelium; benign hyperplastic luminal epithelium	Basal-type cytokeratin, positive for basal-like carcinoma
CK17	M, C	Myoepithelium	Basal-type cytokeratin, positive for basal-like carcinoma
CK903	M, C	Myoepithelium; basal-like carcinoma	Positive for basal-like carcinoma and lobular carcinomas

References: [1, 5–8, 11–14]

Table 15.3 Myoepithelial markers of breast tissue/neoplasm

Marker	Pattern	Component	Comment
p63	N	Myoepithelium; rare tumor cells	A very sensitive and specific myoepithelial marker, demonstrating continuous "dot-like" pattern in normal ducts; focally discontinuous "dotted" line in in situ carcinomas; nonreactive or attenuated in invasive or papillary carcinomas
SMM-HC	C	Myoepithelium; blood vessel; occasional myofibroblasts	Very sensitive myoepithelial marker, but slightly less specific than p63; Nonreactive in invasive carcinomas; Positive with gap in in-situ carcinomas; positive and intact in normal ducts
Calponin	C	Myoepithelium; myofibroblast; blood vessel; rare tumor cells	A good marker of myoepithelial cells, demonstrating continuous cytoplasmic linear pattern
SMA	C	Myoepithelium; myofibroblast; blood vessels; rare epithelium	A myoepithelial marker, not very specific
CK14	C, M	Myoepithelium; hyperplastic luminal epithelium; rare myofibroblasts	A HMWCK used as a myoepithelial or basal marker; mosaic pattern in hyperplastic luminal epithelium. Nonreactive in majority of invasive carcinomas and DCIS, except basaloid phenotype or high-grade DCIS (frequent coexpression of luminal and basal markers)
CK5/6	C, M	Myoepithelium; hyperplastic luminal epithelium	Similar to CK14
CD10	C, M	Myoepithelium; fibroblasts; epithelium	Negative or attenuated in invasive carcinoma or papillary carcinoma. Positive in normal ducts and in situ carcinomas
S100 protein	C, N	Epithelium, myoepithelium	Invasive breast carcinomas: reported 48% positive
Maspin	N	Myoepithelium, tumor cells	Sensitive myoepithelial marker, but limited utility due to the staining of tumor cells
P-cadherin	C	Myoepithelium; epithelial proliferation	Myoepithelial marker, also stain some tumor cells

Note: Although being considered as one of the best myoepithelial markers, p63 also labels the following breast carcinomas in a diffuse fashion: adenoid cystic carcinomas and metaplastic carcinomas of the squamous component. A small subset of ductal carcinomas of the NOS type demonstrates p63 reactivity in a minor fraction of tumor cells

The combination of p63 and SMM-HC or p63 and calponin had been recommended in the literature for the evaluation of invasion. Examples of p63 and calponin immunostains in normal tissue are illustrated in Fig. 15.1a, b

References: [1–6, 11, 14–25]

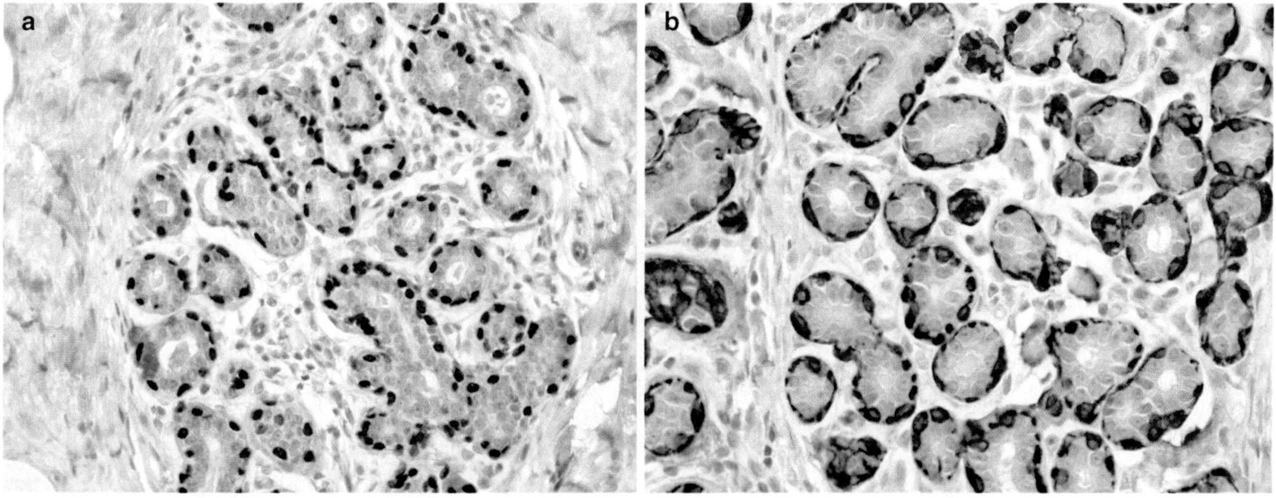

Fig. 15.1 (**a**) p63 nuclear staining for myoepithelial cells in normal breast tissue, continuous "dot-like" pattern. (**b**) Calponin cytoplasmic staining for myoepithelial cells in normal breast tissue, continuous linear pattern

Table 15.4 Phenotype of normal breast ductal/lobular epithelium

Marker	Pattern
AE1/AE3	+, M, C
CK7, CK8/18, CK19	+, M
CK5/6, CK14, CK903	–
E-cadherin	+, M
p^{120} Catenin	+, M
ER, PR	+, N, Scattered
Her-2/neu	–

Note: Normal breast epithelium (ductal and lobular) demonstrates intense linear membranous staining pattern for E-cadherin and p^{120} catenin. In lobular neoplasia, mutation of the E-cadherin gene leads to a complete absence of E-cadherin protein or abnormal localization (apical or perinuclear). Immunohistochemically, lobular neoplasia is negative for E-cadherin and cytoplasmic staining pattern with the loss of membranous staining for p^{120} catenin

Examples of E-cadherin (Fig. 15.2a–c) and p^{120} catenin (Fig. 15.3a–c) in normal breast tissue, invasive ductal, and lobular carcinoma are illustrated

References: [1, 5–8, 14, 15, 26–29]

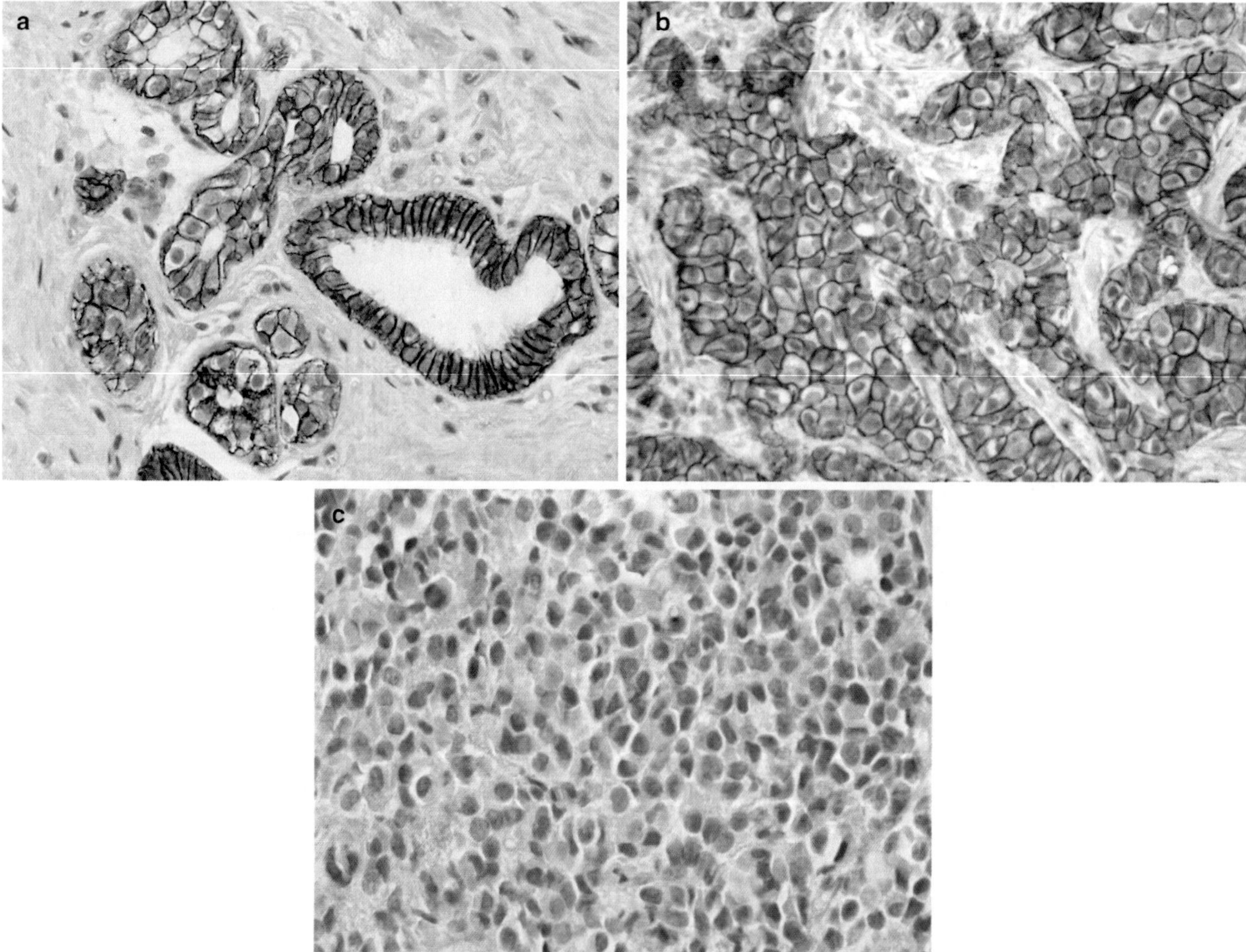

Fig. 15.2 (**a**) E-cadherin membranous staining pattern in normal ductal and lobular epithelium. (**b**) E-cadherin membranous staining pattern in ductal carcinoma. (**c**) E-cadherin, the loss of expression in lobular carcinoma

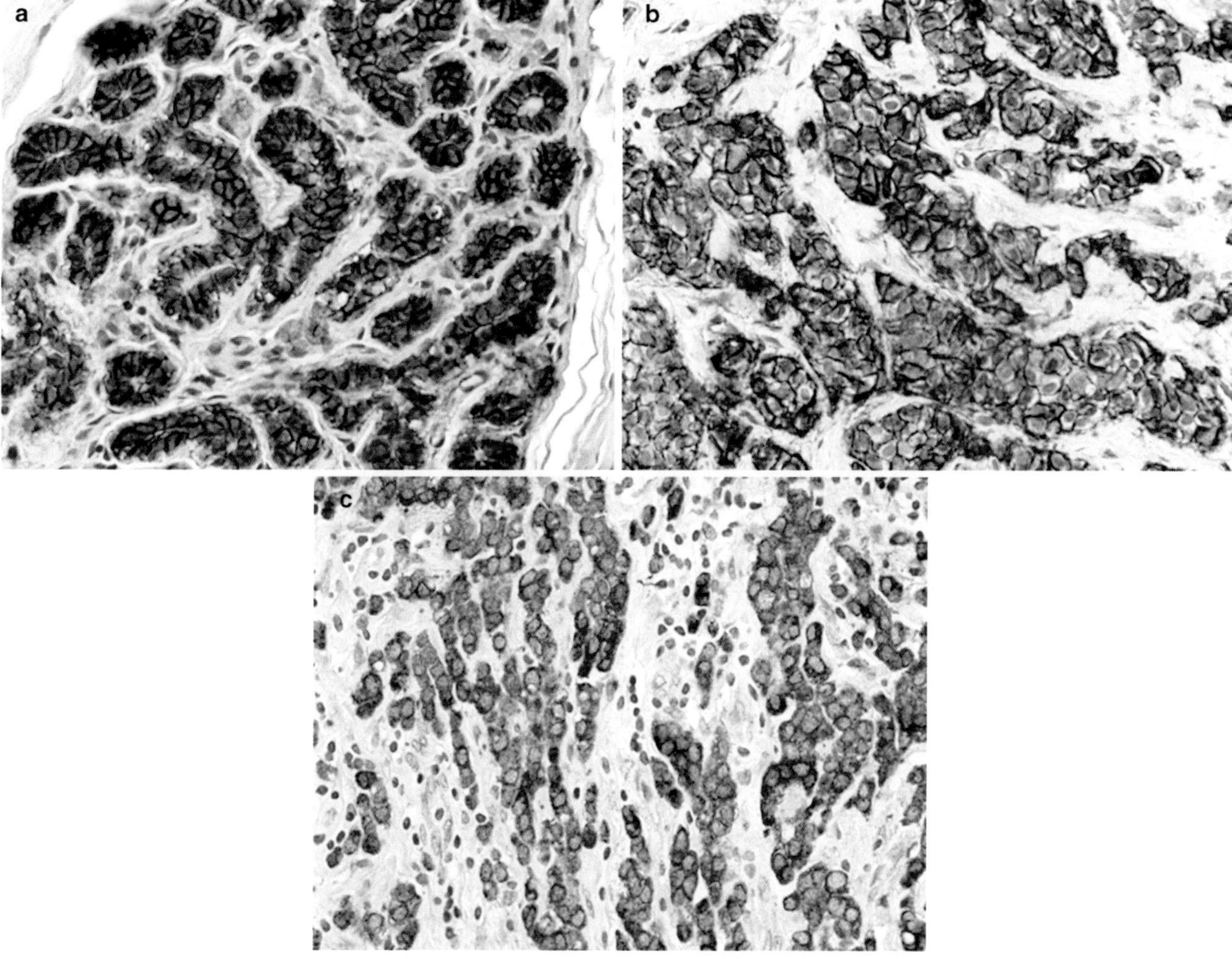

Fig. 15.3 (**a**) p120 Catenin membranous staining pattern in normal ductal and lobular epithelium. (**b**) p120 Catenin membranous staining pattern in ductal carcinoma. (**c**) p120 Catenin perinuclear, cytoplasmic staining pattern in lobular carcinoma

Table 15.5 Phenotype of columnar cell lesions (columnar cell changes/hyperplasia)

Marker	Pattern
LMWCK (CK8/18, CK19)	+
HMWCK (CK5/6, CK903, CK14)	–
ER, PR	+, N, strong and diffuse
E-cadherin	+, M
Her-2/neu	–
p53	–
MIB-1	Low

Note: HMWCKs are nonreactive in columnar cell lesions, except in lesions with hyperplasia, which usually show a central luminal position – the residual luminal cells

HMWCK and ER/PR immunostains are not helpful in the differentiation of atypical vs. non-atypical columnar cell lesions

References: [1–7, 14, 28, 30–34]

Table 15.6 Phenotype of flat epithelial atypia (FEA)

Marker	Pattern
LMWCK (CK8/18, CK19)	+, M
HMWCK (CK903, CK5/6)	–
ER, PR	+, N, strong and diffuse
Bcl-2	+, C, strong and diffuse
Cyclin D1	+, Variable
MIB-1	Very low

Note: HMWCK may show intense staining in the residual luminal epithelial cells adherent along the luminal surface

References: [3, 4, 30, 35–39]

Table 15.7 The evaluation of stromal invasion

Marker	Pattern	Comment
p63	N	Negative in invasive carcinoma. "Dotted" line surrounding normal ducts and in situ carcinomas
SMM-HC	C	Negative in invasive carcinoma. Present in normal ducts and in situ carcinomas
Calponin	C	Negative in invasive carcinoma. Present in normal ducts and in situ carcinomas
SMA	C	Negative in invasive carcinoma. Present in normal ducts and in situ carcinomas

Note: The presence of an intact peripheral myoepithelial cell layer characterizes normal, benign, and in situ lesions. The loss of myoepithelial cell layer is the hallmark of invasive carcinoma. Several myoepithelial markers have been used to assess invasion. p63, SMM-HC, calponin, and SMA are most commonly used for this purpose. Studies report using a combination of p63 and SMM-HC or p63 and calponin is helpful

Other myoepithelial markers, such as CD10, P-cadherin, S100 protein, maspin, and HMWCK can also be used

References: [1–6, 11, 14–17, 22–25, 40]

Table 15.8 The evaluation of angiolymphatic invasion

Marker	Pattern	Comment
CD31	Cytoplasmic	Positive for endothelial cells of vascular channels
CD34	Cytoplasmic	Positive for endothelial cells of vascular channels
D2-40	Cytoplasmic	Positive for endothelial cells of lymphatics

Note: D2-40 is a selective lymphatic endothelial marker, usually stains very intensely. A pitfall is weak to occasionally moderate staining for ducts, which may be mistaken for lymphatic invasion. An example of D2-40 immunostain is illustrated in Fig. 15.4a, b

References: [1–6, 14, 41–43]

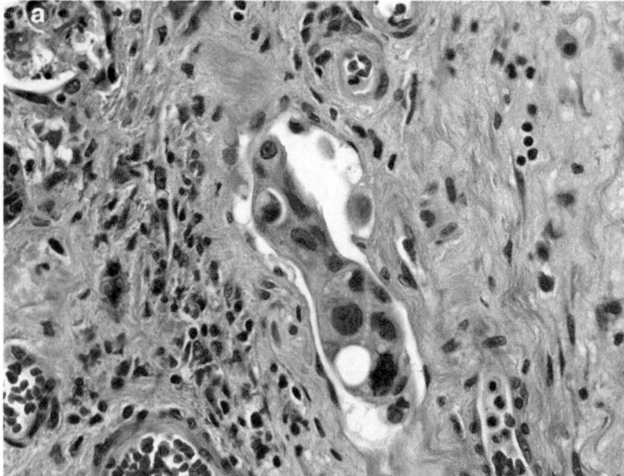

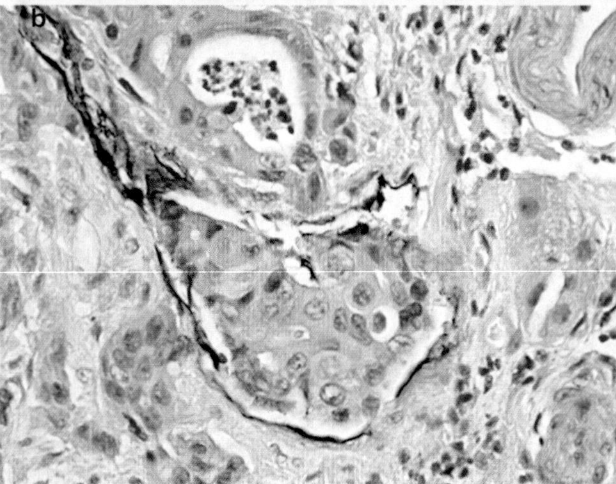

Fig. 15.4 (**a**) H&E, lymphatic invasion. (**b**) Immunostain for D2-40, highlighting the endothelial cells of the lymphatic channel, with very strong stain

Table 15.9 The phenotype of ductal carcinoma of breast

Marker	Literature	GHL data (%), *n* = 176
CK903	–	ND
E-cadherin	+, M	ND
p120 Catenin	+, M	94.6, M
CK7	+	91.7
ER	+/–	59.1
CK8	+, Peripheral-predominant membranous pattern	98.8
GCDFP-15	–/+	31.4
Mammaglobin	–/+	42.2

Note: *ND* no data

The majority of breast ductal carcinomas are nonreactive to CK903, except basal-like phenotype. CK8/18 demonstrates a peripheral-predominant membranous staining pattern in ductal carcinoma, as illustrated in Fig. 15.5a

E-cadherin, a negative marker for lobular neoplasia of breast, decorates ductal carcinomas in a membranous pattern, as illustrated in Fig. 15.2b. p120 Catenin, a positive marker for lobular neoplasia of the breast, decorates ductal carcinomas in a membranous pattern, as illustrated in Fig. 15.3b

References: [1–6, 14, 26, 27, 45]

Table 15.10 The phenotype of lobular carcinoma of breast

Marker	Literature	GHL data (%), *n* = 76
CK903	+	96.3
E-cadherin	–	0
p120 Catenin	+, C	100
CK7	+	90
ER	+	83.7
CK8	+, Perinuclear, ring-like, cytoplasmic pattern	100
GCDFP-15	–/+	28.3
Mammaglobin	+/–	69.5

Note: *ND* no data

E-cadherin is a negative membranous marker for lobular neoplasia of breast. The majority of lobular carcinomas demonstrate the loss of E-cadherin expression (negative staining for E-cadherin), as illustrated in Fig. 15.2c

p120 Catenin is a useful positive marker for lobular neoplasia of breast, with a cytoplasmic staining pattern, as illustrated in Fig. 15.3c

CK8/18 demonstrates perinuclear, ring-like, cytoplasmic staining pattern in lobular carcinoma, as illustrated in Fig. 15.5b

References: [1–6, 14, 26, 27, 45]

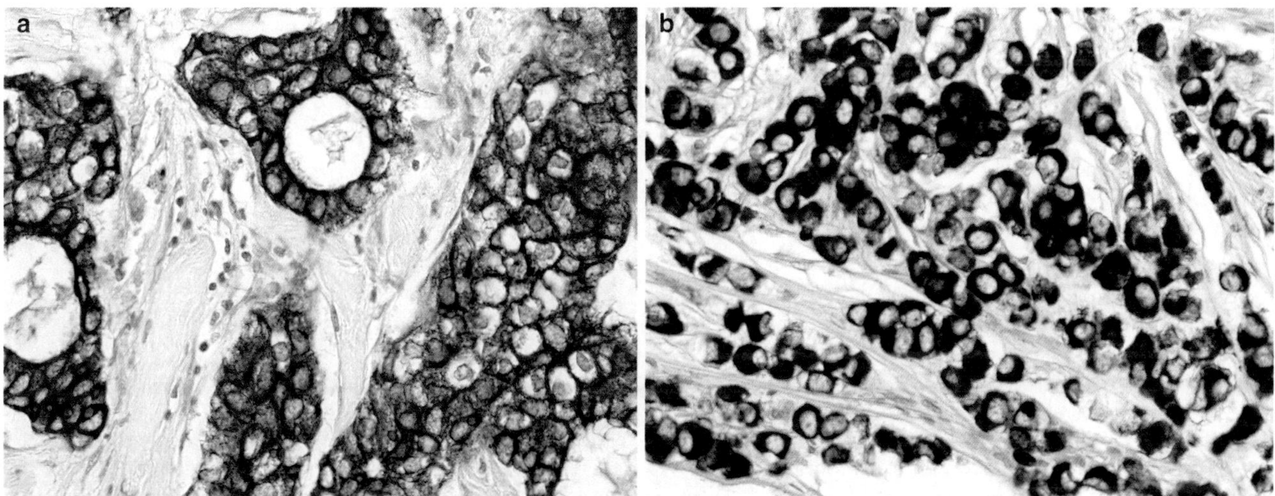

Fig. 15.5 (**a**) Immunostain for CK8/18 in ductal carcinoma, demonstrating peripheral-predominant membranous staining pattern. (**b**) Immunostain for CK8/18 in lobular carcinoma, demonstrating perinuclear, ring-like, cytoplasmic staining pattern

Table 15.11 Phenotype of medullary carcinoma of breast

Marker	Pattern
ER, PR, Her-2/neu	–
p53	+/–
MIB-1	High
CK5/6, CK14, CK903	+/–
EMA	+
AE1/AE3	+
CAM 5.2	+
S100 protein	+
Vimentin	–/+

Note: Medullary carcinomas are usually ER–, PR–, Her-2– tumors exhibiting basal-like phenotype, high-proliferative activity, p53 overexpression and frequent BRCA1 mutation, or protein deficiency

References: [1–6, 14, 44, 46–57]

Table 15.12 Markers used in the evaluation of metaplastic carcinoma

Marker	Literature
Pan-CK (MNF-116)	+
HMWCK (CK5/6, CK14, CK17, CK903)	+
Myoepithelial markers (p63, CD10, SMA)	+
AE1/AE3	+/–
CAM 5.2	+/–
CK7	+
Vimentin	+
EGFR	+
ER, PR, Her-2/neu	–

Note: Reported cytokeratin immunoreactivity ranges widely in metaplastic carcinoma, both epithelial or spindle cell elements, usually in an unpredictable fashion. CK7 was reported in epithelial element only. A panel of cytokeratins, including pan-CK (MNF116), HMWCK (CK5/6, CK14, CK903), and LMWCK (CAM 5.2) should be performed when encountering a spindle cell lesion of the breast. Myoepithelial markers (p63, calponin, and CD10) are often expressed in metaplastic carcinoma in the spindle cell element and should be included in the panel. An example of metaplastic carcinoma of the breast is illustrated in Fig. 15.6a–c

Immunohistochemical and molecular studies of metaplastic carcinoma reveal that the majority of metaplastic carcinomas exhibit EGFR overexpression (reported 57–87%), associated with EGFR gene amplification (about one-third of those cases)

References: [1–6, 14, 58–68]

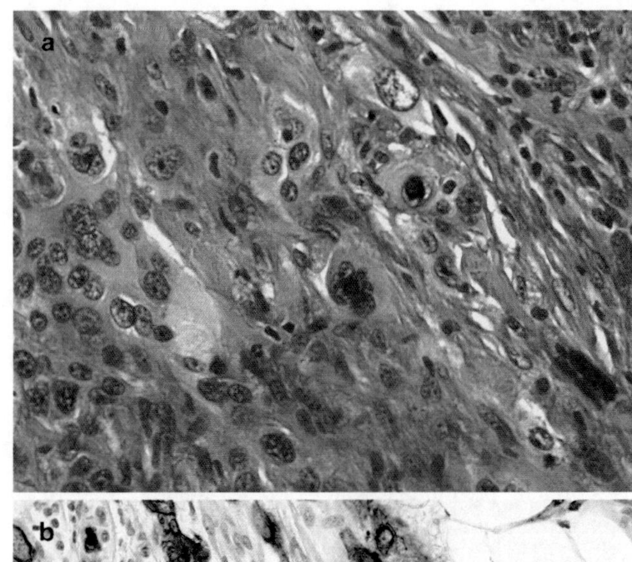

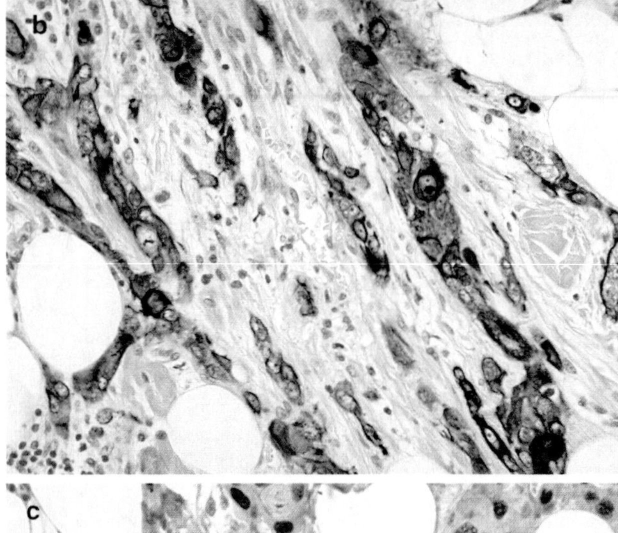

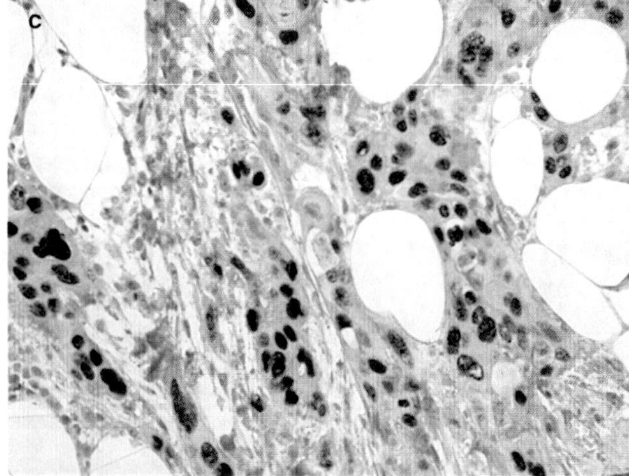

Fig. 15.6 (**a**) Metaplastic carcinoma of breast, H&E stain. (**b**) Metaplastic carcinoma of breast demonstrates cytoplasmic staining for CK903. (**c**) Metaplastic carcinoma of breast demonstrates nuclear st aining for p63

Table 15.13 Phenotype of tubulolobular carcinoma of breast

Marker	Pattern
ER, PR	+
Her-2/neu	–
E-cadherin	+
CK903	+
Beta-catenin	+/–
Alpha-catenin	–/+

Note: Tubulolobular carcinoma of breast is a tumor with a hybrid morphology and immunoprofile, exhibiting features of both ductal and lobular differentiation. This tumor is usually ER+, PR+, Her-2–, but rare cases may be Her-2+

References: [1, 2, 4–6, 14, 69–74]

Table 15.14 Phenotype of micropapillary carcinoma of breast

Marker	Pattern
EMA	+, M, "inside-out" pattern
MUC1	+, External surface adjacent to stroma
E-cadherin	+, M, mainly between tumor cells
N-cadherin	+/–
CK7	+
CK5/6	–
ER, PR, Her-2/neu	–/+
p53	–/+
EGFR, c-kit	–

Note: Micropapillary carcinoma is considered to behave aggressively; it is frequently associated with vascular invasion and axillary lymph node metastases, but not associated with poorer survival rates

Studies reported that micropapillary carcinomas have a higher level of p53 expression, higher Her-2/neu overexpression rate (reported 36–100%), and lower frequency of ER expression (reported 19–75%) compared with invasive ductal carcinoma, NOS type. The cytokeratin expression profile is not different from ductal carcinoma of the NOS type. The differentiation of invasive ductal carcinoma (IDC) with retraction artifact vs. micropapillary carcinoma (MC) may be achieved by immunohistochemical study of epithelial membrane antigen (EMA) or MUC1. IDC demonstrates an apical or cytoplasmic staining for EMA or MUC1, while MC showing an "inside-out" staining pattern: accentuation of the basal surface (stromal facing or periphery) of the tumor cells. The E-cadherin stain shows accentuation between carcinoma cells but not the contiguous surfaces

References: [1–3, 75–82]

Table 15.15 Phenotype of mucinous (colloid) carcinoma of breast

Marker	Pattern
CK7	+
ER, PR	+
Her-2/neu	–
MUC2	+
MUC6	+/–
CK20	–
WT1	+/–, N
CEA	+/–
EGFR	–

Note: Mucinous carcinoma of breast is usually ER+, PR+, and Her-2–. By gene profiling, mucinous carcinoma is of luminal subtype. Cytokeratin expression profile is similar to ductal carcinoma, NOS type. Studies revealed an increased expression of MUC1, MUC6, and WT1 in mucinous carcinoma of breast

Our data (invasive ductal carcinoma, NOS, $n = 175$; mucinous carcinoma, $n = 2$) showed that MUC2 is positive in 2.3% (4/175) of invasive ductal carcinomas, NOS, and both cases of mucinous carcinoma (Fig. 15.7)

References: [1–6, 14, 83–89]

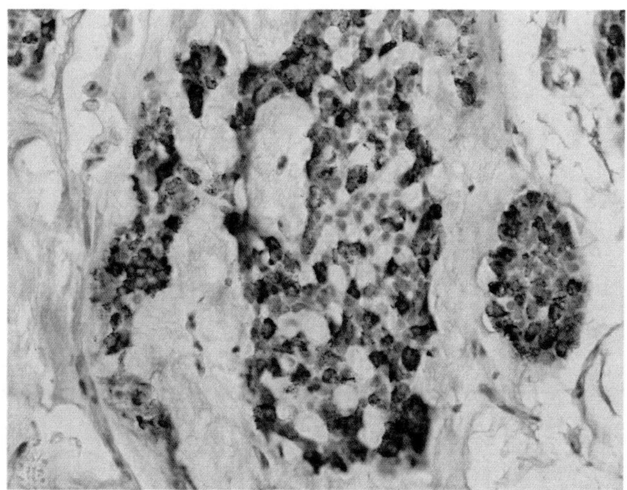

Fig. 15.7 Mucinous carcinoma of breast demonstrates positive stain for MUC2

Table 15.16 Phenotype of apocrine carcinoma of breast

Marker	Pattern
GCDFP-15	+, C
ARP	+, N
ER, PR	–
Her-2/neu	–/+
p53	+/–, N
MIB-1	High
EGFR	+/–, M
E-cadherin	+, M
AE1/AE3, CK7	+, M, C
CEA	+, M, C
S100 protein	–

Note: Apocrine carcinomas are usually androgen receptor (AR) positive and triple negative (ER–, PR–, and Her-2–), or Her-2/neu overexpression (ER–, PR–, and Her-2+) tumors. Nearly all of the apocrine lesions are positive for GCDFP-15, however, which also decorates nonapocrine breast epithelial cells

Apocrine carcinoma is frequently positive for p53, especially in situ carcinoma. Benign apocrine lesions are nonreactive to p53. It has been reported that EGFR expression is much higher in apocrine carcinoma (88%) than in conventional ductal carcinoma

Positive, membranous staining for E-cadherin has been reported a marker to distinguish apocrine carcinoma from pleomorphic lobular carcinoma

Special stains for PAD-D, Toluidine blue, and Trichrome reveal cytoplasmic, granular staining in apocrine neoplasms. The cytoplasmic secretion is occasionally positive for mucicarmine

References: [1–6, 14, 90–98]

Table 15.17 Phenotype of secretory carcinoma of breast

Marker	Pattern
ER, PR, Her-2/neu	–
S100 protein	+
CK5/6	+, Diffuse or focal
E-cadherin	+
CK8/18	+
Vim	+
GCDFP-15	–
p63	–

Note: A typical finding of secretory carcinoma is the presence of intracellular or extracellular secretory material, which is positive for PAS-D and Alcian blue, and negative for mucicarmine

Secretory carcinomas are typically low-grade morphology and triple negative (ER–, PR–, and Her-2–) with the expression of basal markers (CK5/6 or CK14)

References: [1–7, 14, 99–102]

Table 15.18 Phenotype of adenoid cystic carcinoma of breast

Marker	Pattern
ER, PR, Her-2/neu	–
c-kit	+
P63	+
E-cadherin	+
S100	+
CK8/18	+, Luminal cells
Beta-catenin	+
CK903, CK5/6	+

Note: Adenoid cystic carcinoma is typically a triple negative (ER–, PR–, and Her-2–), basal-like carcinoma

Adenoid cystic carcinoma is composed of both luminal and myoepithelial cells. p63 is a specific myoepithelial marker, labeling the peripheral or area of solid myoepithelial cells

p63 and c-kit are useful adjunct in differentiation adenoid cystic carcinoma from other types of ductal carcinomas. c-kit labels ductal luminal cells, not the myoepithelial cells; therefore, the solid area (which is composed of myoepithelial cells) is nonreactive

Figure 15.8a, b demonstrate immunostaining pattern of adenoid cystic carcinoma with double stain for p63 and c-kit

References: [1–6, 14, 103–108]

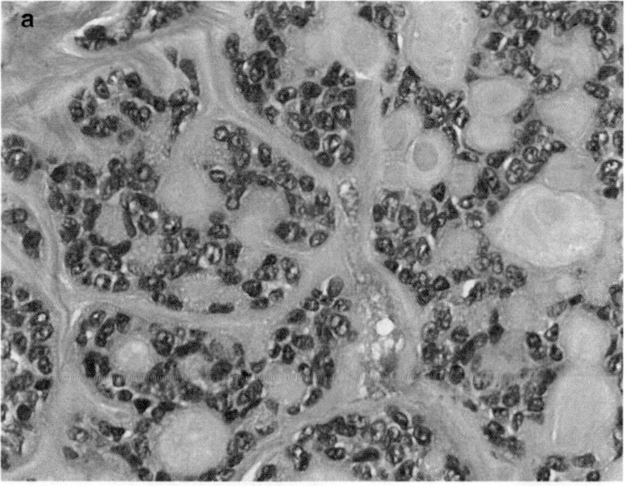

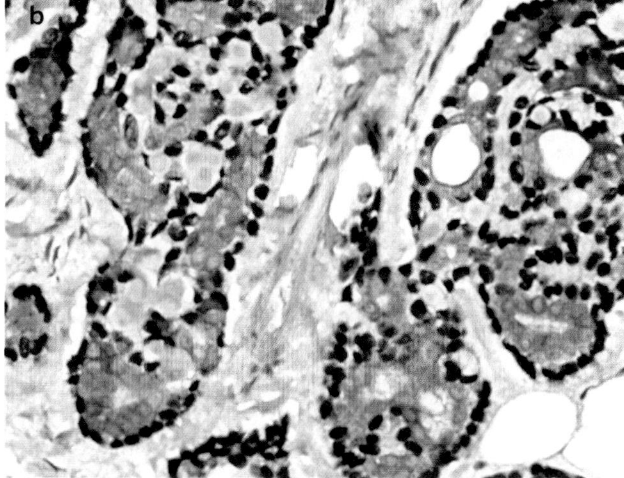

Fig. 15.8 (**a**) Adenoid cystic carcinoma of breast, H&E stain. (**b**) Adenoid cystic carcinoma of breast demonstrates double stain for p63 (*brown* nuclear stain, peripheral myoepithelial cells) and c-kit (*pink* cytoplasmic stain, luminal ductal cells)

Table 15.19 Phenotype of small cell carcinoma of breast

Marker	Pattern
CK7	+
CK20	–
NSE	+
Bcl-2	+
E-cadherin	+
AE1/AE3, CAM 5.2	+
CD56, Synap, Chrom	+/–
TTF1	– or few +
ER, PR	+/–
Her-2/neu	–

Note: The diagnosis of primary small cell carcinoma of breast can only be made with confidence, if a non-mammary primary is excluded or if an in situ component can be demonstrated

More than half of the reported mammary small cell carcinomas are ER and PR positive; all cases reported are Her-2/neu negative

CK7 and CK20 immunostaining pattern aids in the differentiation of pulmonary vs. breast primary. Neuroendocrine markers showed variable staining pattern in mammary small cell carcinoma, except NSE, which is positive in all reported cases

The majority of primary small cell carcinomas of breast are positive for E-cadherin, suggesting a form of ductal carcinoma. However, rare E-Cadherin-negative mammary small cell carcinoma had been reported

References: [1–4, 14, 109–113]

Table 15.20 Phenotype of basal-like carcinoma

Marker	Pattern
Basal keratins (CK5/6, CK14, CK17, CK903)	+
ER, PR, Her-2/neu	–
EGFR	+
p53	+/–
MIB-1	High
p63	+/–
P-cadherin, Nestin	+

Note: Basal-like cancers are identified by gene expression profiling (GEP). Immunohistochemical surrogates are developed, including basal cytokeratins and epidermal growth factor receptor (EGFR). Currently, there is no international consensus on biomarkers to identified tumors as basal-like subtype. The most widely used immunohistochemical surrogate to define a tumor as basal-like is that proposed by Nielsen and colleagues, where basal-like carcinomas were defined as those with ER–, Her-2–, and cytokeratin 5/6 and/or Her1(EGFR)+ phenotype

Basal-like cancers are usually ER–, PR–, and Her-2– (triple-negative), expressing basal cytokeratins (CK5, 5/6; CK14, CK17, CK903), EGFR, vimentin, p53, and myoid differentiation (such as p63, P-cadherin, Nestin, and CD10)

References: [1–6, 14, 114–124]

Table 15.21 The evaluation of papillary neoplasm

Marker	Benign papillary neoplasm	Malignant papillary neoplasm
p63	+	– or scattered +
CK5/6, CK14, CK903	+, Diffuse or mosaic pattern	–
SMM-HC	+	– or scattered +
Calponin	+	– or scattered +
CD10	+	– or scattered +

Note: Benign papillary neoplasms include papilloma and papilloma with florid epithelial hyperplasia. Malignant papillary neoplasms include invasive papillary carcinoma, papillary carcinoma in situ (intracystic papillary carcinoma), and DCIS involving papilloma

High molecular weight cytokeratins (CK5/6, CK14, and CK903) decorate luminal cells (especially hyperplastic) and myoepithelial cells in diffuse or mosaic pattern in benign papillary neoplasms, nonreactive in malignant papillary neoplasms. Myoepithelial markers (p63, SMM-HC, calponin, CD10, myosin, S100, and SMA) highlight myoepithelial cells at the basement membrane in benign papillary neoplasm, which is absent in malignant papillary neoplasm. Scattered tumor cells may stain for p63

References: [1–6, 11, 14, 40, 125–130]

Table 15.22 The evaluation of fibroepithelial neoplasms

Marker	Fibroadenoma	Benign PT	Borderline PT	Malignant PT
Mitosis	Unusual	<2/10 hpf	2–5/10 hpf	>5/10 hpf
p53	Few	Few	Increased	High
MIB-1	Very low	Few	Increased	High
CD117	+, Scattered	+, Scattered	Increased	High
PR	+, Stromal cells	+, Stromal cells	+, Stromal cells	+, Stromal cells
CK5/6, CK903	–	–	–	–

Note: *PT* phyllodes tumor

No definitive consensus exists on the number of mitoses required for the classification of PTs into three subgroups. The numeric figures listed in the table above are recommendations by some authors. The World Health Organization classification of PT requires more than ten mitoses per 10 hpf for malignant PT but provides no numeric figure for benign and borderline PTs

Studies using a variety of immunohistochemical markers demonstrated a good correlation between MIB-1 index and histologic category or grade of phyllodes tumors, as did p53 expression. However, those markers are not independent predictors of outcome, such as local recurrence or metastases

CD117 and VEGF have been reported with higher expression in malignant than in benign PT

References: [1–4, 14, 131–144]

Table 15.23 The evaluation of myoepithelial neoplasms

Marker	Adenomyoepithelioma, benign	Myoepithelioma	Myoepithelial carcinoma
Myoepithelial markers	–, Glandular cells +, Myoepithelial cells	+	+
AE1/AE3, CAM 5.2	+, Glandular cells –, Myoepithelial cells	–	–
EMA	+, Luminal surface of glandular cells	–	–
MIB-1	Low (≤2/hpf)	Low (≤2/hpf)	High
ER	+, Glandular cells –, Myoepithelial cells	–	–

Note: Myoepithelial markers: include p63, SMA, calponin, caldesmon, SMM-HC, CD10, maspin, and HMWCKs (CK5/6 and CK14)

Adenomyoepithelioma is composed of both glandular and myoepithelial elements. There are PAS or mucicarmine-positive secretions within the glands, which are also positive for CEA

Myoepithelial neoplasms are nonreactive to PR, desmin, and CD34

References: [1–6, 14, 145–153]

Table 15.24 Genomic phenotype of breast carcinoma (luminal A, B, basal, and Her-2)

Marker	Luminal A	Luminal B	Basal-like	Her-2
ER	+	+	–	–
PR	+	+	–	–
Her-2/neu	–	+	–/+	+
CK5/6	–	–	+	–
EGFR	–	–	+	–
Ki-67	≤14%	≥14% (if Her-2–)	High	High

Note: DNA microarray profiling studies categorize breast carcinomas into ER+/luminal, normal breast-like, Her-2 overexpressing, and basal-like subtypes. Basal-like and Her-2 overexpressing subtypes are frequently having *Tp53* mutation and worse prognoses. It had been described an association with BRCA-1-associated carcinomas in basal-like subtype of breast carcinoma

References: [1–6, 14, 114, 116–122, 154–158]

Table 15.25 Prognostic and predictive markers

Marker	Pattern	Comment
ER, PR	+, N	Good prognostic factor
Her-2/neu	+, M	Worse prognostic factor
p53	+, N	High expression associated with high-grade tumor and worse prognosis
MIB-1	+, N	High Ki67 relates to poor outcome. Post-therapy Ki67 is a strong predictor of outcome for patients not achieving a pathological complete response
AR	+, N	Studies suggest ER and AR are coexpressed in the majority of breast tumor cells. Low level of AR in ER-positive breast carcinoma is a worse prognostic factor

References: [1–6, 14, 159–167]

Table 15.26 The differentiation of columnar cell lesions (including flat epithelial atypia-FEA) vs. normal/UDH

Marker	CCL (include FEA)	NL or UDH
CK5/6, CK14, CK903	–	+, Mosaic or diffuse
ER, PR	+, N, diffuse	–/+, N, scattered
AR	+	–/+, Rare
CK19	+	+
E-cadherin	+	+
Her-2/neu	–	–
MIB-1, Cyclin D1	Higher	Lower
Bcl-2	Decreased	High

Note: Normal/UDH demonstrates mixed staining pattern for high molecular weight cytokeratins (CK903, CK14, and CK5/6), and usually scattered nuclear staining for ER/PR

References: [1–6, 14, 28, 130–139, 171]

Table 15.27 The differentiation of usual duct hyperplasia (UDH) vs. atypical duct hyperplasia (ADH) or ductal carcinoma in situ (DCIS)

Marker	UDH	ADH or DCIS
CK5/6, CK903	+, Diffuse	– or focal w+
ER, PR	+, Scattered	+, Diffuse
CK8/18/19	+	+

Note: High molecular weight cytokeratins, CK5/6 and CK903, are reported useful in the differentiation of UDH (usual ductal hyperplasia) vs. AHD (atypical ductal hyperplasia) or DCIS (ductal carcinoma in situ), demonstrating diffuse reactivity in UDH vs. nonreactive in ADH or DCIS (except rare residual luminal epithelial cells in ADH and basal layer in DCIS or basaloid DCIS). Basaloid DCIS (positive for HMWCK, a reported incidence of 3.7%) is often a high-grade, triple-negative tumor with necrosis, easily recognized by morphology

ER and PR often show diffuse nuclear staining in ADH and DCIS, especially in low-grade lesions; only scattered nuclear staining in UDH

References: [1–6, 10, 13, 30, 35–38, 168–174]

Table 15.28 The differentiation of lobular vs. ductal carcinomas

Marker	Ductal carcinoma	Lobular carcinoma
E-cadherin	+	–
p120 Catenin	+, M	+, C
CK903	–*	+
CK8	+, Peripheral-predominant membranous pattern	+, Perinuclear, ring-like, cytoplasmic pattern

Note: p120 Catenin stains both lobular and ductal carcinomas with different staining patterns: membrane stain for ductal carcinoma and cytoplasmic stain for lobular carcinoma

*Ductal carcinoma is negative for CK903 except basaloid type

CK8 decorates ductal and lobular carcinomas in different patterns, which have been described as tumor cells "molding" to each other in ductal carcinoma and a "bag of marbles" appearance in lobular carcinoma

References: [1–6, 13, 27, 45, 175–182]

Table 15.29 The differentiation of tubular carcinoma (TC) vs. sclerosing adenosis (SA) and microglandular adenosis (MA)

Marker	TC	SA	MA
Myoepithelial markers	–	+	–
Markers of basement membrane	–	+	+

Note: Myoepithelial markers: p63, SMM-HC, CD10, myosin, and calponin

Markers of basement membrane: laminin, Type IV collagen, reticulin, and periodic acid-Schiff (PAS)

Both tubular carcinoma and microglandular adenosis lack myoepithelium. Laminin, type IV collagen, reticulin, and PAS decorate basement membrane, which is present in microglandular adenosis and absent in tubular carcinoma

Myoepithelial cells are usually proliferating in sclerosing adenosis, demonstrating more intense staining for myoepithelial markers

References: [1–6, 14, 22–24, 29, 183–185]

Table 15.30 The differentiation of adenoid cystic carcinoma (ACC) vs. tubular carcinoma (TC) vs. cribriform carcinoma (CC)

Markers	ACC	TC	CC
c-kit	+	–	–
p63	+	–	–
ER, PR	–/+	+	+
Her-2/neu	–	–	–
E-cadherin	+	+	+

Note: In general, adenoid cystic carcinomas are triple negative (ER–, PR–, and Her-2–) tumors, but tubular and cribriform carcinomas are low-grade ductal carcinomas, often positive for ER, PR and negative for Her-2/neu (ER+, PR+, and Her-2–). A reported 15% of ACCs are ER/PR positive, and 15% of TCs and CCs show weak, incomplete membranous staining for Her-2/neu

References: [1–6, 14, 22–24, 103–108]

Table 15.31 The differentiation of spindle cell tumors of breast

Marker	ME	MFB	SpCC	MPT	MM
Pan-CK (MNF-116)	+	–	+	–	–
CK5/6, CK14, CK903	+	–	+	–	–
AE1/AE3	–	–	–/+	–	–
CAM 5.2	–	–	–/+	–	–
p63	+	–	+/–	–	–
Calponin	+	+/–	–/+	–	–
SMA	–	+	+/–	+/–	–
CD34	–	+	–	–/+	–
Desmin	–	+	–	+/–	–
S100	+	–/+	–	–	+
HMB-45	–	–	–	–	+

Note: *ME* myoepithelioma, *MFB* myofibroblastoma, *SpCC* spindle cell carcinoma, *MPT* malignant phyllodes tumor, *PS* primary sarcoma, *MM* malignant melanoma

Primary breast sarcomas with spindle cell morphology (other than high-grade angiosarcoma) are exceedingly rare and therefore not included in this table

When encountering a spindle cell neoplasm of the breast, a battery of cytokeratins, including pan-CK, HMWCK (CK5/6, CK14, CK903), and LMWCK (CAM 5.2) should be applied to detect spindle cell carcinoma, which is far more common than primary spindle cell sarcoma. Many studies showed myoepithelial differentiation in spindle cell carcinoma of breast. p63, a specific and sensitive myoepithelial marker, was proposed to including in the work-up panel for spindle cell neoplasm. Phyllodes tumors (benign or malignant) are negative for p63 except the normal myoepithelial cells surrounding ductal structure

Myofibroblastoma is reported positive for CD34, desmin, SMA, bcl2, vimentin, and steroid receptors. An example of myofibroblastoma is illustrated in Fig. 15.9a–d

References: [1–6, 14, 58–63, 65–68, 186–193]

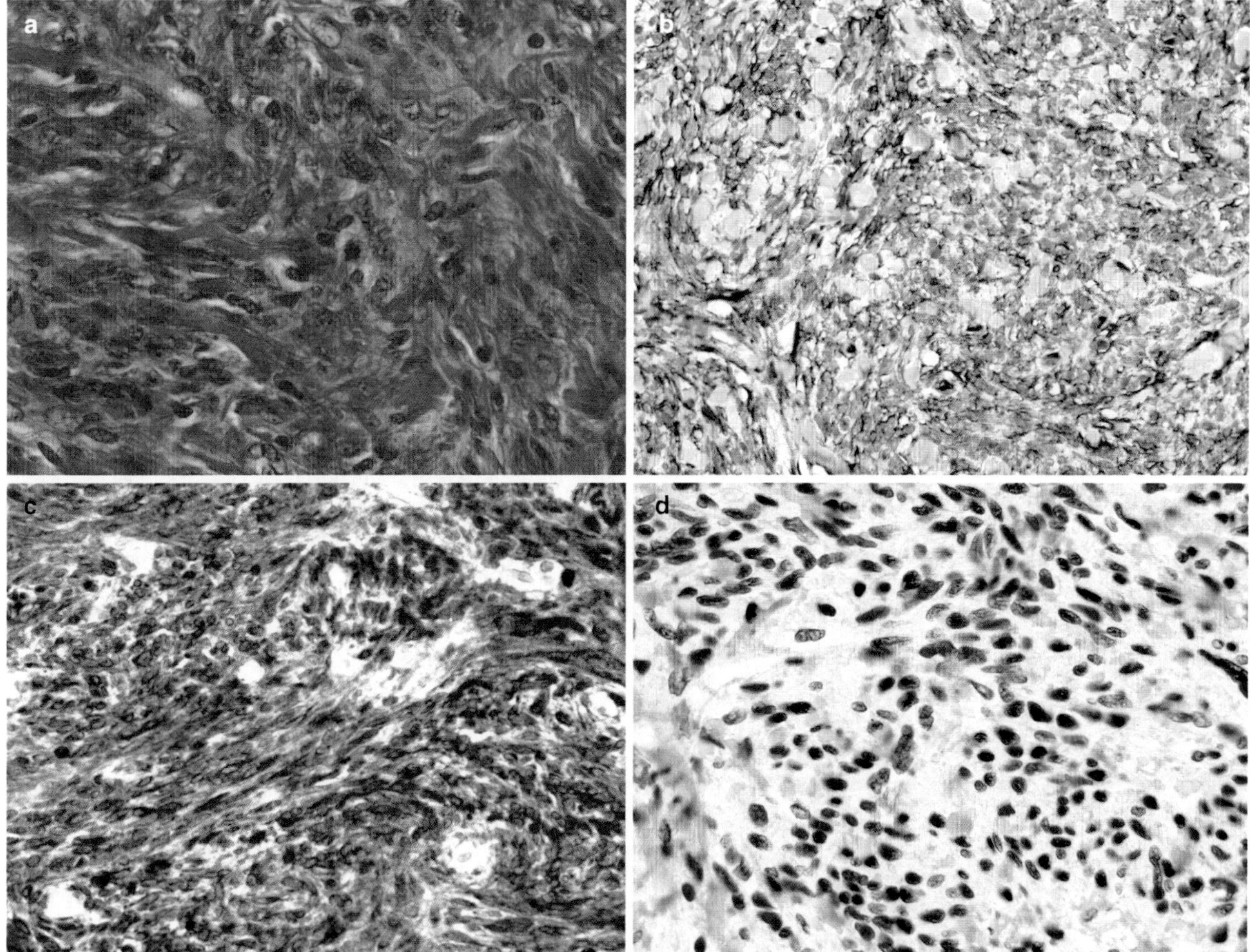

Fig. 15.9 (**a**) Myofibroblastoma, H&E stain. (**b**) Myofibroblastoma, demonstrating positive staining for CD34. (**c**) Myofibroblastoma, demonstrating positive staining for Bcl2. (**d**) Myofibroblastoma, demonstrating positive nuclear staining for AR

Table 15.32 The differentiation of micropapillary patterned carcinoma (ovarian vs. breast)

Marker	Ovarian serous carcinoma	Micropapillary carcinoma of breast
WT1	+	–
CA-125	+	–
GCDFP-15	–	+/–
PAX8	+	–

Note: Diffuse nuclear stain for WT1 and cytoplasmic stain for CA-125 (>90%) favor a metastatic papillary ovarian carcinoma. A small percentage of micropapillary carcinomas of breast is reactive to WT1 (3–26%) and CA-125 (21%)

References: [1–4, 14, 79, 82, 194–198]

Table 15.33 Markers used in the evaluation of metastatic breast carcinoma

Marker	Pattern
MGB	+
GCDFP-15	+/–
CK7	+
CK20	–
ER, PR	+/–
Her-2/neu	–/+
P^{120}-catenin	+

Note: Breast carcinomas are CK7+ and CK20–. GCDFP-15 and mammaglobin (MGB) are used as markers of breast differentiation. The sensitivities for breast carcinoma were reported 35–74% for GCDFP-15 and 50–84% for MGB. Our data (invasive ductal and lobular carcinoma, $n = 252$) reveals a sensitivity of 30.6% for GCDFP-15 and 50.6% for MGB. But, GCDFP-15 is reported to be more specific than mammaglobin (MGB)

p^{120} Catenin, as a positive marker of lobular neoplasia, may be helpful including in the work-up panel for metastatic lobular carcinoma

References: [1–6, 14, 194–198]

Table 15.34 The evaluation of mammary Paget's disease

Marker	Pattern
CK7	+
LMWCK (CAM 5.2)	+
AR	+
ER, PR	–
Her-2/neu	+
EMA	+
HMFG	+
CK20	–
HMWCK	–
Mucicarmine	+
Alcian blue-PAS stains	+

Note: *HMFG* human milk-fat globule

The majority of mammary Paget's diseases are AR+, ER–, and Her-2+. CK7 and CK20 profile is different from extramammary Paget's disease, which is positive for both

References: [1–6, 14, 199–215]

Table 15.35 The evaluation of nipple adenoma (syringomatous adenoma of nipple), large duct papilloma, and low-grade ductal/tubular carcinoma

Marker	Nipple (syringomatous) adenoma	Large duct papilloma	Low-grade ductal/ tubular carcinoma
p63	+	+	–
Calponin	+	+	–
SMM-HC	+	+	–
SMA	+	+	–
ER	–	+/–	+
PR	–	+/–	+

Note: Both nipple adenoma and papilloma are benign lesions, with an intact myoepithelial cell layer. p63 is an excellent marker of myoepithelial cells, and also reactive to cells of squamous differentiation

References: [1–6, 11, 14, 22–24, 29]

Table 15.36 The differentiation of Paget's disease vs. Bowen's disease vs. malignant melanoma

Marker	Paget's disease	Bowen's disease	Malignant melanoma
CK7	+	–	–
CAM 5.2	+	–	–
HMB-45	–	–	+
S100 protein	–	–	+
HMFG	+	–	–
EMA	+	–	–
AR	+/–	–	–
ER	–/+	–	–
Her-2/neu	+	–/+	–
GCDFP-15	+	–	–
CEA	–/+	–	–
Mucicarmine	+	–	–

Note: *HMFG* human milk-fat globule membrane antigen

References: [1–5, 14, 199–214]

Note for All Tables

Note: "+" – usually greater than 70% of cases are positive; "–" – less than 5% of cases are positive; "+ or –" – usually more than 50% of cases are positive; "– or +" – less than 50% of cases are positive.

References

1. Dabbs DJ. Diagnostic immunohistochemistry. 3rd ed. Philadelphia, PA: Churchill Livingstone Elsevier; 2010.
2. Rosen PP. Rosen's breast pathology. 3rd ed. Philadelphia, PA: Lippincott, Williams & Wilkins; 2008.
3. Tavassoli FA, Devilee P. WHO classification of tumours: pathology & genetics tumors of the breast and female genital organs. Lyon, France: IARC; 2003.
4. Collins LC. Surgical pathology clinics: current concepts in breast pathology, vol. 2. Philadelphia, PA: WB Saunders; 2009.
5. Yeh IT, Mies C. Application of immunohistochemistry to breast lesions. Arch Pathol Lab Med. 2008;132(3):349–58.
6. Lerwill MF. Current practical applications of diagnostic immunohistochemistry in breast pathology. Am J Surg Pathol. 2004;28(8):1076–91.
7. Bocker W, Bier B, Freytag G, et al. An immunohistochemical study of the breast using antibodies to basal and luminal keratins, alpha-smooth muscle actin, vimentin, collagen IV and laminin. Part II: epitheliosis and ductal carcinoma in situ. Virchows Arch A Pathol Anat Histopathol. 1992;421(4):323–30.
8. Bocker W, Bier B, Freytag G, et al. An immunohistochemical study of the breast using antibodies to basal and luminal keratins, alpha-smooth muscle actin, vimentin, collagen IV and laminin. Part I: normal breast and benign proliferative lesions. Virchows Arch A Pathol Anat Histopathol. 1992;421(4):315–22.
9. Ichihara S, Koshikawa T, Nakamura S, Yatabe Y, Kato K. Epithelial hyperplasia of usual type expresses both S100-alpha and S100-beta in a heterogeneous pattern but ductal carcinoma in situ can express only S100-alpha in a monotonous pattern. Histopathology. 1997;30(6):533–41.
10. Lacroix-Triki M, Mery E, Voigt JJ, Istier L, Rochaix P. Value of cytokeratin 5/6 immunostaining using D5/16 B4 antibody in the spectrum of proliferative intraepithelial lesions of the breast. A comparative study with 34betaE12 antibody. Virchows Arch. 2003;442(6):548–54.
11. Tse GM, Tan PH, Moriya T. The role of immunohistochemistry in the differential diagnosis of papillary lesions of the breast. J Clin Pathol. 2009;62(5):407–13.
12. Moriya T, Kasajima A, Ishida K, et al. New trends of immunohistochemistry for making differential diagnosis of breast lesions. Med Mol Morphol. 2006;39(1):8–13.
13. Tang P, Wang X, Schiffhauer L, et al. Relationship between nuclear grade of ductal carcinoma in situ and cell origin markers. Ann Clin Lab Sci. 2006;36(1):16–22.
14. Bhargava R, Dabbs DJ. Use of immunohistochemistry in diagnosis of breast epithelial lesions. Adv Anat Pathol. 2007;14(2):93–107.
15. Heatley M, Maxwell P, Whiteside C, Toner P. Cytokeratin intermediate filament expression in benign and malignant breast disease. J Clin Pathol. 1995;48(1):26–32.
16. Werling RW, Hwang H, Yaziji H, Gown AM. Immunohistochemical distinction of invasive from noninvasive breast lesions: a comparative study of p63 versus calponin and smooth muscle myosin heavy chain. Am J Surg Pathol. 2003;27(1):82–90.

17. Barbareschi M, Pecciarini L, Cangi MG, et al. p63, a p53 homologue, is a selective nuclear marker of myoepithelial cells of the human breast. Am J Surg Pathol. 2001;25(8):1054–60.
18. Moritani S, Kushima R, Sugihara H, Bamba M, Kobayashi TK, Hattori T. Availability of CD10 immunohistochemistry as a marker of breast myoepithelial cells on paraffin sections. Mod Pathol. 2002;15(4):397–405.
19. Kovacs A, Walker RA. P-cadherin as a marker in the differential diagnosis of breast lesions. J Clin Pathol. 2003;56(2):139–41.
20. Jones C, Nonni AV, Fulford L, et al. CGH analysis of ductal carcinoma of the breast with basaloid/myoepithelial cell differentiation. Br J Cancer. 2001;85(3):422–7.
21. Dwarakanath S, Lee AK, Delellis RA, Silverman ML, Frasca L, Wolfe HJ. S-100 protein positivity in breast carcinomas: a potential pitfall in diagnostic immunohistochemistry. Hum Pathol. 1987;18(11):1144–8.
22. Ribeiro-Silva A, Zambelli Ramalho LN, Britto Garcia S, Zucoloto S. The relationship between p63 and p53 expression in normal and neoplastic breast tissue. Arch Pathol Lab Med. 2003;127(3): 336–40.
23. Reis-Filho JS, Milanezi F, Amendoeira I, Albergaria A, Schmitt FC. Distribution of p63, a novel myoepithelial marker, in fine-needle aspiration biopsies of the breast: an analysis of 82 samples. Cancer. 2003;99(3):172–9.
24. Stefanou D, Batistatou A, Nonni A, Arkoumani E, Agnantis NJ. p63 expression in benign and malignant breast lesions. Histol Histopathol. 2004;19(2):465–71.
25. Kalof AN, Tam D, Beatty B, Cooper K. Immunostaining patterns of myoepithelial cells in breast lesions: a comparison of CD10 and smooth muscle myosin heavy chain. J Clin Pathol. 2004;57(6):625–9.
26. Dabbs DJ, Bhargava R, Chivukula M. Lobular versus ductal breast neoplasms: the diagnostic utility of p120 catenin. Am J Surg Pathol. 2007;31(3):427–37.
27. Dabbs DJ, Kaplai M, Chivukula M, Kanbour A, Kanbour-Shakir A, Carter GJ. The spectrum of morphomolecular abnormalities of the E-cadherin/catenin complex in pleomorphic lobular carcinoma of the breast. Appl Immunohistochem Mol Morphol. 2007;15(3):260–6.
28. Dabbs DJ, Carter G, Fudge M, Peng Y, Swalsky P, Finkelstein S. Molecular alterations in columnar cell lesions of the breast. Mod Pathol. 2006;19(3):344–9.
29. Gusterson BA, Warburton MJ, Mitchell D, Ellison M, Neville AM, Rudland PS. Distribution of myoepithelial cells and basement membrane proteins in the normal breast and in benign and malignant breast diseases. Cancer Res. 1982;42(11):4763–70.
30. Simpson PT, Gale T, Reis-Filho JS, et al. Columnar cell lesions of the breast: the missing link in breast cancer progression? A morphological and molecular analysis. Am J Surg Pathol. 2005;29(6):734–46.
31. Abdel-Fatah TM, Powe DG, Hodi Z, Reis-Filho JS, Lee AH, Ellis IO. Morphologic and molecular evolutionary pathways of low nuclear grade invasive breast cancers and their putative precursor lesions: further evidence to support the concept of low nuclear grade breast neoplasia family. Am J Surg Pathol. 2008;32(4):513–23.
32. Dessauvagie BF, Zhao W, Heel-Miller KA, Harvey J, Bentel JM. Characterization of columnar cell lesions of the breast: immunophenotypic analysis of columnar alteration of lobules with prominent apical snouts and secretions. Hum Pathol. 2007;38(2): 284–92.
33. Rosen PP. Columnar cell hyperplasia is associated with lobular carcinoma in situ and tubular carcinoma. Am J Surg Pathol. 1999;23(12):1561.
34. Fraser JL, Raza S, Chorny K, Connolly JL, Schnitt SJ. Columnar alteration with prominent apical snouts and secretions: a spectrum of changes frequently present in breast biopsies performed for microcalcifications. Am J Surg Pathol. 1998;22(12):1521–7.
35. Collins LC, Achacoso NA, Nekhlyudov L, et al. Clinical and pathologic features of ductal carcinoma in situ associated with the presence of flat epithelial atypia: an analysis of 543 patients. Mod Pathol. 2007;20(11):1149–55.
36. O'Malley FP, Mohsin SK, Badve S, et al. Interobserver reproducibility in the diagnosis of flat epithelial atypia of the breast. Mod Pathol. 2006;19(2):172–9.
37. Schnitt SJ. The diagnosis and management of pre-invasive breast disease: flat epithelial atypia – classification, pathologic features and clinical significance. Breast Cancer Res. 2003;5(5):263–8.
38. Otterbach F, Bankfalvi A, Bergner S, Decker T, Krech R, Boecker W. Cytokeratin 5/6 immunohistochemistry assists the differential diagnosis of atypical proliferations of the breast. Histopathology. 2000;37(3):232–40.
39. Allred DC, Mohsin SK, Fuqua SA. Histological and biological evolution of human premalignant breast disease. Endocr Relat Cancer. 2001;8(1):47–61.
40. Collins LC, Carlo VP, Hwang H, Barry TS, Gown AM, Schnitt SJ. Intracystic papillary carcinomas of the breast: a reevaluation using a panel of myoepithelial cell markers. Am J Surg Pathol. 2006;30(8):1002–7.
41. Kahn HJ, Bailey D, Marks A. Monoclonal antibody D2-40, a new marker of lymphatic endothelium, reacts with Kaposi's sarcoma and a subset of angiosarcomas. Mod Pathol. 2002;15(4): 434–40.
42. Chu AY, Litzky LA, Pasha TL, Acs G, Zhang PJ. Utility of D2-40, a novel mesothelial marker, in the diagnosis of malignant mesothelioma. Mod Pathol. 2005;18(1):105–10.
43. Rabban JT, Chen YY. D2-40 expression by breast myoepithelium: potential pitfalls in distinguishing intralymphatic carcinoma from in situ carcinoma. Hum Pathol. 2008;39(2):175–83.
44. Rodriguez-Pinilla SM, Rodriguez-Gil Y, Moreno-Bueno G, et al. Sporadic invasive breast carcinomas with medullary features display a basal-like phenotype: an immunohistochemical and gene amplification study. Am J Surg Pathol. 2007;31(4):501–8.
45. Liu H, Shi J, Xu Y, Zhang K, Kaspar H, Lin F. Reevaluation of diagnostic value of p120 catenin in differentiating lobular carcinoma from low-grade ductal carcinoma of the breast [CAP Poster #28]. Arch Pathol Lab Med. 2009;10(October 2009):1635.
46. Holck S, Pedersen L, Schiodt T, Zedeler K, Mouridsen H. Vimentin expression in 98 breast cancers with medullary features and its prognostic significance. Virchows Arch A Pathol Anat Histopathol. 1993;422(6):475–9.
47. Kajiwara M, Toyoshima S, Yao T, Tanaka M, Tsuneyoshi M. Apoptosis and cell proliferation in medullary carcinoma of the breast: a comparative study between medullary and non-medullary carcinoma using the TUNEL method and immunohistochemistry. J Surg Oncol. 1999;70(4):209–16.
48. Rosen PP, Lesser ML, Arroyo CD, Cranor M, Borgen P, Norton L. p53 in node-negative breast carcinoma: an immunohistochemical study of epidemiologic risk factors, histologic features, and prognosis. J Clin Oncol. 1995;13(4):821–30.
49. Marchetti A, Buttitta F, Pellegrini S, et al. p53 mutations and histological type of invasive breast carcinoma. Cancer Res. 1993;53(19):4665–9.
50. Davidoff AM, Herndon 2nd JE, Glover NS, et al. Relation between p53 overexpression and established prognostic factors in breast cancer. Surgery. 1991;110(2):259–64.
51. Xu R, Feiner H, Li P, et al. Differential amplification and overexpression of HER-2/neu, p53, MIB1, and estrogen receptor/progesterone receptor among medullary carcinoma, atypical medullary carcinoma, and high-grade invasive ductal carcinoma of breast. Arch Pathol Lab Med. 2003;127(11):1458–64.
52. Jacquemier J, Padovani L, Rabayrol L, et al. Typical medullary breast carcinomas have a basal/myoepithelial phenotype. J Pathol. 2005;207(3):260–8.
53. Flucke U, Flucke MT. Distinguishing medullary carcinoma of the breast from high-grade hormone receptor-negative invasive ductal

carcinoma: an immunohistochemical approach. Histopathology. 2010;56(7):852–9.
54. Marginean F, Rakha EA, Ho BC, Ellis IO, Lee AH. Histological features of medullary carcinoma and prognosis in triple-negative basal-like carcinomas of the breast. Mod Pathol. 2010. doi: 10.1038/modpathol.2010.123.
55. Kleer CG. Carcinoma of the breast with medullary-like features: diagnostic challenges and relationship with BRCA1 and EZH2 functions. Arch Pathol Lab Med. 2009;133(11):1822–5.
56. Vincent-Salomon A, Gruel N, Lucchesi C, et al. Identification of typical medullary breast carcinoma as a genomic sub-group of basal-like carcinomas, a heterogeneous new molecular entity. Breast Cancer Res. 2007;9(2):R24.
57. Bertucci F, Finetti P, Cervera N, et al. Gene expression profiling shows medullary breast cancer is a subgroup of basal breast cancers. Cancer Res. 2006;66(9):4636–44.
58. Wargotz ES, Deos PH, Norris HJ. Metaplastic carcinomas of the breast. II. Spindle cell carcinoma. Hum Pathol. 1989;20(8): 732–40.
59. Pitts WC, Rojas VA, Gaffey MJ, et al. Carcinomas with metaplasia and sarcomas of the breast. Am J Clin Pathol. 1991;95(5):623–32.
60. Ellis IO, Bell J, Ronan JE, Elston CW, Blamey RW. Immunocytochemical investigation of intermediate filament proteins and epithelial membrane antigen in spindle cell tumours of the breast. J Pathol. 1988;154(2):157–65.
61. Santeusanio G, Pascal RR, Bisceglia M, Costantino AM, Bosman C. Metaplastic breast carcinoma with epithelial phenotype of pseudosarcomatous components. Arch Pathol Lab Med. 1988;112(1):82–5.
62. Meis JM, Ordonez NG, Gallager HS. Sarcomatoid carcinoma of the breast: an immunohistochemical study of six cases. Virchows Arch A Pathol Anat Histopathol. 1987;410(5):415–21.
63. Oberman HA. Metaplastic carcinoma of the breast. A clinicopathologic study of 29 patients. Am J Surg Pathol. 1987;11(12):918–29.
64. Leibl S, Moinfar F. Mammary NOS-type sarcoma with CD10 expression: a rare entity with features of myoepithelial differentiation. Am J Surg Pathol. 2006;30(4):450–6.
65. Leibl S, Moinfar F. Metaplastic breast carcinomas are negative for Her-2 but frequently express EGFR (Her-1): potential relevance to adjuvant treatment with EGFR tyrosine kinase inhibitors? J Clin Pathol. 2005;58(7):700–4.
66. Reis-Filho JS, Milanezi F, Carvalho S, et al. Metaplastic breast carcinomas exhibit EGFR, but not HER2, gene amplification and overexpression: immunohistochemical and chromogenic in situ hybridization analysis. Breast Cancer Res. 2005;7(6):R1028–35.
67. Reis-Filho JS, Pinheiro C, Lambros MB, et al. EGFR amplification and lack of activating mutations in metaplastic breast carcinomas. J Pathol. 2006;209(4):445–53.
68. Reis-Filho JS, Milanezi F, Steele D, et al. Metaplastic breast carcinomas are basal-like tumours. Histopathology. 2006;49(1):10–21.
69. Wheeler DT, Tai LH, Bratthauer GL, Waldner DL, Tavassoli FA. Tubulolobular carcinoma of the breast: an analysis of 27 cases of a tumor with a hybrid morphology and immunoprofile. Am J Surg Pathol. 2004;28(12):1587–93.
70. Esposito NN, Chivukula M, Dabbs DJ. The ductal phenotypic expression of the E-cadherin/catenin complex in tubulolobular carcinoma of the breast: an immunohistochemical and clinicopathologic study. Mod Pathol. 2007;20(1):130–8.
71. Kuroda H, Tamaru J, Takeuchi I, et al. Expression of E-cadherin, alpha-catenin, and beta-catenin in tubulolobular carcinoma of the breast. Virchows Arch. 2006;448(4):500–5.
72. Bratthauer GL, Moinfar F, Stamatakos MD, et al. Combined E-cadherin and high molecular weight cytokeratin immunoprofile differentiates lobular, ductal, and hybrid mammary intraepithelial neoplasias. Hum Pathol. 2002;33(6):620–7.
73. Green I, McCormick B, Cranor M, Rosen PP. A comparative study of pure tubular and tubulolobular carcinoma of the breast. Am J Surg Pathol. 1997;21(6):653–7.
74. Kanter MH. Tubulolobular carcinoma of the breast. Am J Surg Pathol. 1998;22(6):776.
75. Kim MJ, Gong G, Joo HJ, Ahn SH, Ro JY. Immunohistochemical and clinicopathologic characteristics of invasive ductal carcinoma of breast with micropapillary carcinoma component. Arch Pathol Lab Med. 2005;129(10):1277–82.
76. Nassar H, Pansare V, Zhang H, et al. Pathogenesis of invasive micropapillary carcinoma: role of MUC1 glycoprotein. Mod Pathol. 2004;17(9):1045–50.
77. Paterakos M, Watkin WG, Edgerton SM, Moore 2nd DH, Thor AD. Invasive micropapillary carcinoma of the breast: a prognostic study. Hum Pathol. 1999;30(12):1459–63.
78. Nagi C, Guttman M, Jaffer S, et al. N-cadherin expression in breast cancer: correlation with an aggressive histologic variant – invasive micropapillary carcinoma. Breast Cancer Res Treat. 2005;94(3): 225–35.
79. Marchio C, Iravani M, Natrajan R, et al. Genomic and immunophenotypical characterization of pure micropapillary carcinomas of the breast. J Pathol. 2008;215(4):398–410.
80. Pettinato G, Manivel CJ, Panico L, Sparano L, Petrella G. Invasive micropapillary carcinoma of the breast: clinicopathologic study of 62 cases of a poorly recognized variant with highly aggressive behavior. Am J Clin Pathol. 2004;121(6):857–66.
81. Luna-More S, Gonzalez B, Acedo C, Rodrigo I, Luna C. Invasive micropapillary carcinoma of the breast. A new special type of invasive mammary carcinoma. Pathol Res Pract. 1994;190(7):668–74.
82. Li YS, Kaneko M, Sakamoto DG, Takeshima Y, Inai K. The reversed apical pattern of MUC1 expression is characteristics of invasive micropapillary carcinoma of the breast. Breast Cancer. 2006;13(1):58–63.
83. Domfeh AB, Carley AL, Striebel JM, et al. WT1 immunoreactivity in breast carcinoma: selective expression in pure and mixed mucinous subtypes. Mod Pathol. 2008;21(10):1217–23.
84. O'Connell JT, Shao ZM, Drori E, Basbaum CB, Barsky SH. Altered mucin expression is a field change that accompanies mucinous (colloid) breast carcinoma histogenesis. Hum Pathol. 1998;29(12):1517–23.
85. Coady AT, Shousha S, Dawson PM, Moss M, James KR, Bull TB. Mucinous carcinoma of the breast: further characterization of its three subtypes. Histopathology. 1989;15(6):617–26.
86. Diab SG, Clark GM, Osborne CK, Libby A, Allred DC, Elledge RM. Tumor characteristics and clinical outcome of tubular and mucinous breast carcinomas. J Clin Oncol. 1999;17(5):1442–8.
87. Schmitt FC, Pereira MB, Reis CA. MUC 5 expression in breast carcinomas. Hum Pathol. 1999;30(10):1270–1.
88. Matsukita S, Nomoto M, Kitajima S, et al. Expression of mucins (MUC1, MUC2, MUC5AC and MUC6) in mucinous carcinoma of the breast: comparison with invasive ductal carcinoma. Histopathology. 2003;42(1):26–36.
89. Rakha EA, Boyce RW, Abd El-Rehim D. Expression of mucins (MUC1, MUC2, MUC3, MUC4, MUC5AC and MUC6) and their prognostic significance in human breast cancer. Mod Pathol. 2005;18(10):1295–304.
90. Eusebi V, Betts C, Haagensen Jr DE, Gugliotta P, Bussolati G, Azzopardi JG. Apocrine differentiation in lobular carcinoma of the breast: a morphologic, immunologic, and ultrastructural study. Hum Pathol. 1984;15(2):134–40.
91. Pagani A, Sapino A, Eusebi V, Bergnolo P, Bussolati G. PIP/GCDFP-15 gene expression and apocrine differentiation in carcinomas of the breast. Virchows Arch. 1994;425(5):459–65.
92. Leal C, Henrique R, Monteiro P, et al. Apocrine ductal carcinoma in situ of the breast: histologic classification and expression of biologic markers. Hum Pathol. 2001;32(5):487–93.
93. Moriya T, Sakamoto K, Sasano H, et al. Immunohistochemical analysis of Ki-67, p53, p21, and p27 in benign and malignant apocrine lesions of the breast: its correlation to histologic findings in 43 cases. Mod Pathol. 2000;13(1):13–8.

94. Mossler JA, Barton TK, Brinkhous AD, McCarty KS, Moylan JA, McCarty Jr KS. Apocrine differentiation in human mammary carcinoma. Cancer. 1980;46(11):2463–71.
95. Miller WR, Telford J, Dixon JM, Hawkins RA. Androgen receptor activity in human breast cancer and its relationship with oestrogen and progestogen receptor activity. Eur J Cancer Clin Oncol. 1985;21(4):539–42.
96. Vranic S, Tawfik O, Palazzo J, et al. EGFR and HER-2/neu expression in invasive apocrine carcinoma of the breast. Mod Pathol. 2010;23(5):644–53.
97. Gatalica Z. Immunohistochemical analysis of apocrine breast lesions. Consistent over-expression of androgen receptor accompanied by the loss of estrogen and progesterone receptors in apocrine metaplasia and apocrine carcinoma in situ. Pathol Res Pract. 1997;193(11–12):753–8.
98. Bundred NJ, Stewart HJ, Shaw DA, Forrest AP, Miller WR. Relation between apocrine differentiation and receptor status, prognosis and hormonal response in breast cancer. Eur J Cancer. 1990;26(11–12):1145–7.
99. Hartman AW, Magrish P. Carcinoma of breast in children; case report: six-year-old boy with adenocarcinoma. Ann Surg. 1955;141(6):792–8.
100. Lamovec J, Bracko M. Secretory carcinoma of the breast: light microscopical, immunohistochemical and flow cytometric study. Mod Pathol. 1994;7(4):475–9.
101. Akhtar M, Robinson C, Ali MA, Godwin JT. Secretory carcinoma of the breast in adults. Light and electron microscopic study of three cases with review of the literature. Cancer. 1983;51(12): 2245–54.
102. Lae M, Freneaux P, Sastre-Garau X, Chouchane O, Sigal-Zafrani B, Vincent-Salomon A. Secretory breast carcinomas with ETV6-NTRK3 fusion gene belong to the basal-like carcinoma spectrum. Mod Pathol. 2009;22(2):291–8.
103. Mastropasqua MG, Maiorano E, Pruneri G, et al. Immunoreactivity for c-kit and p63 as an adjunct in the diagnosis of adenoid cystic carcinoma of the breast. Mod Pathol. 2005;18(10):1277–82.
104. Azoulay S, Lae M, Freneaux P, et al. KIT is highly expressed in adenoid cystic carcinoma of the breast, a basal-like carcinoma associated with a favorable outcome. Mod Pathol. 2005;18(12): 1623–31.
105. Rabban JT, Swain RS, Zaloudek CJ, Chase DR, Chen YY. Immunophenotypic overlap between adenoid cystic carcinoma and collagenous spherulosis of the breast: potential diagnostic pitfalls using myoepithelial markers. Mod Pathol. 2006;19(10): 1351–7.
106. Kasami M, Olson SJ, Simpson JF, Page DL. Maintenance of polarity and a dual cell population in adenoid cystic carcinoma of the breast: an immunohistochemical study. Histopathology. 1998;32(3):232–8.
107. Due W, Herbst WD, Loy V, Stein H. Characterisation of adenoid cystic carcinoma of the breast by immunohistology. J Clin Pathol. 1989;42(5):470–6.
108. Morice WG, Ferreiro JA. Distinction of basaloid squamous cell carcinoma from adenoid cystic and small cell undifferentiated carcinoma by immunohistochemistry. Hum Pathol. 1998;29(6):609–12.
109. Adegbola T, Connolly CE, Mortimer G. Small cell neuroendocrine carcinoma of the breast: a report of three cases and review of the literature. J Clin Pathol. 2005;58(7):775–8.
110. Papotti M, Gherardi G, Eusebi V, Pagani A, Bussolati G. Primary oat cell (neuroendocrine) carcinoma of the breast. Report of four cases. Virchows Arch A Pathol Anat Histopathol. 1992;420(1): 103–8.
111. Shin SJ, DeLellis RA, Rosen PP. Small cell carcinoma of the breast – additional immunohistochemical studies. Am J Surg Pathol. 2001;25(6):831–2.
112. Bergman S, Hoda SA, Geisinger KR, Creager AJ, Trupiano JK. E-cadherin-negative primary small cell carcinoma of the breast. Report of a case and review of the literature. Am J Clin Pathol. 2004;121(1):117–21.
113. Shin SJ, DeLellis RA, Ying L, Rosen PP. Small cell carcinoma of the breast: a clinicopathologic and immunohistochemical study of nine patients. Am J Surg Pathol. 2000;24(9):1231–8.
114. Rakha EA, Reis-Filho JS, Ellis IO. Basal-like breast cancer: a critical review. J Clin Oncol. 2008;26(15):2568–81.
115. Dabbs DJ, Chivukula M, Carter G, Bhargava R. Basal phenotype of ductal carcinoma in situ: recognition and immunohistologic profile. Mod Pathol. 2006;19(11):1506–11.
116. Bhargava R, Dabbs DJ. Luminal B breast tumors are not HER2 positive. Breast Cancer Res. 2008;10(5):404.
117. Laakso M, Loman N, Borg A, Isola J. Cytokeratin 5/14-positive breast cancer: true basal phenotype confined to BRCA1 tumors. Mod Pathol. 2005;18(10):1321–8.
118. Lerma E, Peiro G, Ramon T, et al. Immunohistochemical heterogeneity of breast carcinomas negative for estrogen receptors, progesterone receptors and Her2/neu (basal-like breast carcinomas). Mod Pathol. 2007;20:1200–7.
119. Livasy CA, Karaca G, Nanda R, et al. Phenotypic evaluation of the basal-like subtype of invasive breast carcinoma. Mod Pathol. 2006;19:264–71.
120. Nielsen TO, Hsu FD, Jensen K, et al. Immunohistochemical and clinical characterization of the basal-like subtype of invasive breast carcinoma. Clin Cancer Res. 2004;10(16):5367–74.
121. Li H, Cherukuri P, Li N, et al. Nestin is expressed in the basal/myoepithelial layer of the mammary gland and is a selective marker of basal epithelial breast tumors. Cancer Res. 2007;67(2): 501–10.
122. Cheang MC, Voduc D, Bajdik C, et al. Basal-like breast cancer defined by five biomarkers has superior prognostic value than triple-negative phenotype. Clin Cancer Res. 2008;14(5):1368–76.
123. Lakhani SR, Reis-Filho JS, Fulford L, et al. Prediction of BRCA1 status in patients with breast cancer using estrogen receptor and basal phenotype. Clin Cancer Res. 2005;11(14):5175–80.
124. Kuroda H, Ishida F, Nakai M, Ohnisi K, Itoyama S. Basal cytokeratin expression in relation to biological factors in breast cancer. Hum Pathol. 2008;39(12):1744–50.
125. Esposito NN, Dabbs DJ, Bhargava R. Are encapsulated papillary carcinomas of the breast in situ or invasive? A basement membrane study of 27 cases. Am J Clin Pathol. 2009;131(2):228–42.
126. Zhang C, Zhang P, Hao J, Quddus MR, Steinhoff MM, Sung CJ. High nuclear grade, frequent mitotic activity, cyclin D1 and p53 overexpression are associated with stromal invasion in mammary intracystic papillary carcinoma. Breast J. 2005;11(1):2–8.
127. Tan PH, Aw MY, Yip G, et al. Cytokeratins in papillary lesions of the breast: is there a role in distinguishing intraductal papilloma from papillary ductal carcinoma in situ? Am J Surg Pathol. 2005;29(5):625–32.
128. Saddik M, Lai R. CD44s as a surrogate marker for distinguishing intraductal papilloma from papillary carcinoma of the breast. J Clin Pathol. 1999;52(11):862–4.
129. Tse GM, Tan PH, Ma TK, Gilks CB, Poon CS, Law BK. CD44s is useful in the differentiation of benign and malignant papillary lesions of the breast. J Clin Pathol. 2005;58(11):1185–8.
130. Hill CB, Yeh IT. Myoepithelial cell staining patterns of papillary breast lesions: from intraductal papillomas to invasive papillary carcinomas. Am J Clin Pathol. 2005;123(1):36–44.
131. Kleer CG, Giordano TJ, Braun T, Oberman HA. Pathologic, immunohistochemical, and molecular features of benign and malignant phyllodes tumors of the breast. Mod Pathol. 2001;14(3): 185–90.
132. Kocova L, Skalova A, Fakan F, Rousarova M. Phyllodes tumour of the breast: immunohistochemical study of 37 tumours using MIB1 antibody. Pathol Res Pract. 1998;194(2):97–104.
133. Kuenen-Boumeester V, Henzen-Logmans SC, Timmermans MM, et al. Altered expression of p53 and its regulated proteins in phyllodes tumours of the breast. J Pathol. 1999;189(2):169–75.

134. Umekita Y, Yoshida H. Immunohistochemical study of MIB1 expression in phyllodes tumor and fibroadenoma. Pathol Int. 1999;49(9):807–10.
135. Shpitz B, Bomstein Y, Sternberg A, et al. Immunoreactivity of p53, Ki-67, and c-erbB-2 in phyllodes tumors of the breast in correlation with clinical and morphologic features. J Surg Oncol. 2002;79(2):86–92.
136. Millar EK, Beretov J, Marr P, et al. Malignant phyllodes tumours of the breast display increased stromal p53 protein expression. Histopathology. 1999;34(6):491–6.
137. Feakins RM, Mulcahy HE, Nickols CD, Wells CA. p53 expression in phyllodes tumours is associated with histological features of malignancy but does not predict outcome. Histopathology. 1999;35(2):162–9.
138. Tse GM, Putti TC, Kung FY, et al. Increased p53 protein expression in malignant mammary phyllodes tumors. Mod Pathol. 2002;15(7):734–40.
139. Tse GM, Lui PC, Scolyer RA, et al. Tumour angiogenesis and p53 protein expression in mammary phyllodes tumors. Mod Pathol. 2003;16(10):1007–13.
140. Tan PH, Jayabaskar T, Yip G, et al. p53 and c-kit (CD117) protein expression as prognostic indicators in breast phyllodes tumors: a tissue microarray study. Mod Pathol. 2005;18(12):1527–34.
141. Tse GM, Putti TC, Lui PC, et al. Increased c-kit (CD117) expression in malignant mammary phyllodes tumors. Mod Pathol. 2004;17(7):827–31.
142. Esposito NN, Mohan D, Brufsky A, Lin Y, Kapali M, Dabbs DJ. Phyllodes tumor: a clinicopathologic and immunohistochemical study of 30 cases. Arch Pathol Lab Med. 2006;130(10):1516–21.
143. Tan PH. 2005 Galloway memorial lecture: breast phyllodes tumours – morphology and beyond. Ann Acad Med Singapore. 2005;34(11):671–7.
144. Giri D. Recurrent challenges in the evaluation of fibroepithelial lesions. Arch Pathol Lab Med. 2009;133(5):713–21.
145. Rosen PP. Adenomyoepithelioma of the breast. Hum Pathol. 1987;18(12):1232–7.
146. Weidner N, Levine JD. Spindle-cell adenomyoepithelioma of the breast. A microscopic, ultrastructural, and immunocytochemical study. Cancer. 1988;62(8):1561–7.
147. Vielh P, Thiery JP, Validire P, de Maublanc Annick M, Woto G. Adenomyoepithelioma of the breast: fine-needle sampling with histologic, immunohistologic, and electron microscopic analysis. Diagn Cytopathol. 1993;9(2):188–93.
148. Tamura G, Monma N, Suzuki Y, Satodate R, Abe H. Adenomyoepithelioma (myoepithelioma) of the breast in a male. Hum Pathol. 1993;24(6):678–81.
149. Erlandson RA, Rosen PP. Infiltrating myoepithelioma of the breast. Am J Surg Pathol. 1982;6(8):785–93.
150. Bigotti G, Di Giorgio CG. Myoepithelioma of the breast: histologic, immunologic, and electromicroscopic appearance. J Surg Oncol. 1986;32(1):58–64.
151. Schurch W, Potvin C, Seemayer TA. Malignant myoepithelioma (myoepithelial carcinoma) of the breast: an ultrastructural and immunocytochemical study. Ultrastruct Pathol. 1985;8(1):1–11.
152. Thorner PS, Kahn HJ, Baumal R, Lee K, Moffatt W. Malignant myoepithelioma of the breast. An immunohistochemical study by light and electron microscopy. Cancer. 1986;57(4):745–50.
153. Cartagena Jr N, Cabello-Inchausti B, Willis I, Poppiti Jr R. Clear cell myoepithelial neoplasm of the breast. Hum Pathol. 1988;19(10):1239–43.
154. Cheang MC, Chia SK, Voduc D, et al. Ki67 index, HER2 status, and prognosis of patients with luminal B breast cancer. J Natl Cancer Inst. 2009;101(10):736–50.
155. Perou CM, Sorlie T, Eisen MB, et al. Molecular portraits of human breast tumours. Nature. 2000;406(6797):747–52.
156. Sorlie T, Perou CM, Tibshirani R, et al. Gene expression patterns of breast carcinomas distinguish tumor subclasses with clinical implications. Proc Natl Acad Sci USA. 2001;98(19): 10869–74.
157. Carey LA, Perou CM, Livasy CA, et al. Race, breast cancer subtypes, and survival in the Carolina Breast Cancer Study. JAMA. 2006;295(21):2492–502.
158. Rakha E, Reis-Filho JS. Basal-like breast carcinoma: from expression profiling to routine practice. Arch Pathol Lab Med. 2009;133(6):860–8.
159. Flanagan MB, Dabbs DJ, Brufsky AM, Beriwal S, Bhargava R. Histopathologic variables predict oncotype DX recurrence score. Mod Pathol. 2008;21(10):1255–61.
160. Fitzgibbons PL, Page DL, Weaver D, et al. Prognostic factors in breast cancer. College of American Pathologists Consensus Statement 1999. Arch Pathol Lab Med. 2000;124(7):966–78.
161. Schmitz KJ, Grabellus F, Callies R, et al. Relationship and prognostic significance of phospho-(serine 166)-murine double minute 2 and Akt activation in node-negative breast cancer with regard to p53 expression. Virchows Arch. 2006;448(1):16–23.
162. Schmitz KJ, Otterbach F, Callies R, et al. Prognostic relevance of activated Akt kinase in node-negative breast cancer: a clinicopathological study of 99 cases. Mod Pathol. 2004;17(1):15–21.
163. Lark AL, Livasy CA, Dressler L, et al. High focal adhesion kinase expression in invasive breast carcinomas is associated with an aggressive phenotype. Mod Pathol. 2005;18(10):1289–94.
164. Schmitz KJ, Callies R, Wohlschlaeger J, et al. Overexpression of cyclo-oxygenase-2 is an independent predictor of unfavourable outcome in node-negative breast cancer, but is not associated with protein kinase B (Akt) and mitogen-activated protein kinase (ERK1/2, p38) activation or with Her-2/neu signalling pathways. J Clin Pathol. 2006;59(7):685–91.
165. Shim JY, An HJ, Lee YH, Kim SK, Lee KP, Lee KS. Overexpression of cyclooxygenase-2 is associated with breast carcinoma and its poor prognostic factors. Mod Pathol. 2003;16(12):1199–204.
166. Peters AA, Buchanan G, Ricciardelli C, et al. Androgen receptor inhibits estrogen receptor-alpha activity and is prognostic in breast cancer. Cancer Res. 2009;69(15):6131–40.
167. Jones RL, Salter J, A'Hern R, et al. The prognostic significance of Ki67 before and after neoadjuvant chemotherapy in breast cancer. Breast Cancer Res Treat. 2009;116(1):53–68.
168. Moinfar F, Man YG, Bratthauer GL, Ratschek M, Tavassoli FA. Genetic abnormalities in mammary ductal intraepithelial neoplasia-flat type ("clinging ductal carcinoma in situ"): a simulator of normal mammary epithelium. Cancer. 2000;88(9):2072–81.
169. Lee S, Mohsin SK, Mao S, Hilsenbeck SG, Medina D, Allred DC. Hormones, receptors, and growth in hyperplastic enlarged lobular units: early potential precursors of breast cancer. Breast Cancer Res. 2006;8(1):R6.
170. Moinfar F, Man YG, Lininger RA, Bodian C, Tavassoli FA. Use of keratin 35betaE12 as an adjunct in the diagnosis of mammary intraepithelial neoplasia-ductal type – benign and malignant intraductal proliferations. Am J Surg Pathol. 1999;23(9):1048–58.
171. Boecker W, Moll R, Dervan P, et al. Usual ductal hyperplasia of the breast is a committed stem (progenitor) cell lesion distinct from atypical ductal hyperplasia and ductal carcinoma in situ. J Pathol. 2002;198(4):458–67.
172. Bankfalvi A, Ludwig A, De-Hesselle B, Buerger H, Buchwalow IB, Boecker W. Different proliferative activity of the glandular and myoepithelial lineages in benign proliferative and early malignant breast diseases. Mod Pathol. 2004;17(9):1051–61.
173. Rabban JT, Koerner FC, Lerwill MF. Solid papillary ductal carcinoma in situ versus usual ductal hyperplasia in the breast: a potentially difficult distinction resolved by cytokeratin 5/6. Hum Pathol. 2006;37(7):787–93.
174. Pinder SE, Ellis IO. The diagnosis and management of pre-invasive breast disease: ductal carcinoma in situ (DCIS) and atypical ductal hyperplasia (ADH) – current definitions and classification. Breast Cancer Res. 2003;5(5):254–7.

175. Da Silva L, Parry S, Reid L, et al. Aberrant expression of E-cadherin in lobular carcinomas of the breast. Am J Surg Pathol. 2008;32(5):773–83.
176. Reis-Filho JS, Simpson PT, Turner NC, et al. FGFR1 emerges as a potential therapeutic target for lobular breast carcinomas. Clin Cancer Res. 2006;12(22):6652–62.
177. Acs G, Lawton TJ, Rebbeck TR, LiVolsi VA, Zhang PJ. Differential expression of E-cadherin in lobular and ductal neoplasms of the breast and its biologic and diagnostic implications. Am J Clin Pathol. 2001;115(1):85–98.
178. Goldstein NS, Bassi D, Watts JC, Layfield LJ, Yaziji H, Gown AM. E-cadherin reactivity of 95 noninvasive ductal and lobular lesions of the breast. Implications for the interpretation of problematic lesions. Am J Clin Pathol. 2001;115(4):534–42.
179. Choi YJ, Pinto MM, Hao L, Riba AK. Interobserver variability and aberrant E-cadherin immunostaining of lobular neoplasia and infiltrating lobular carcinoma. Mod Pathol. 2008;21(10):1224–37.
180. Jacobs TW, Pliss N, Kouria G, Schnitt SJ. Carcinomas in situ of the breast with indeterminate features: role of E-cadherin staining in categorization. Am J Surg Pathol. 2001;25(2):229–36.
181. Kovacs A, Dhillon J, Walker RA. Expression of P-cadherin, but not E-cadherin or N-cadherin, relates to pathological and functional differentiation of breast carcinomas. Mol Pathol. 2003;56(6):318–22.
182. Lehr HA, Folpe A, Yaziji H, Kommoss F, Gown AM. Cytokeratin 8 immunostaining pattern and E-cadherin expression distinguish lobular from ductal breast carcinoma. Am J Clin Pathol. 2000;114(2):190–6.
183. Joshi MG, Lee AK, Pedersen CA, Schnitt S, Camus MG, Hughes KS. The role of immunocytochemical markers in the differential diagnosis of proliferative and neoplastic lesions of the breast. Mod Pathol. 1996;9(1):57–62.
184. Dabbs DJ, Gown AM. Distribution of calponin and smooth muscle myosin heavy chain in fine-needle aspiration biopsies of the breast. Diagn Cytopathol. 1999;20(4):203–7.
185. Flotte TJ, Bell DA, Greco MA. Tubular carcinoma and sclerosing adenosis: the use of basal lamina as a differential feature. Am J Surg Pathol. 1980;4(1):75–7.
186. Carter MR, Hornick JL, Lester S, Fletcher CD. Spindle cell (sarcomatoid) carcinoma of the breast: a clinicopathologic and immunohistochemical analysis of 29 cases. Am J Surg Pathol. 2006;30(3):300–9.
187. Sneige N, Yaziji H, Mandavilli SR, et al. Low-grade (fibromatosis-like) spindle cell carcinoma of the breast. Am J Surg Pathol. 2001;25(8):1009–16.
188. Koker MM, Kleer CG. p63 expression in breast cancer: a highly sensitive and specific marker of metaplastic carcinoma. Am J Surg Pathol. 2004;28(11):1506–12.
189. Wargotz ES, Weiss SW, Norris HJ. Myofibroblastoma of the breast. Sixteen cases of a distinctive benign mesenchymal tumor. Am J Surg Pathol. 1987;11(7):493–502.
190. Magro G, Bisceglia M, Michal M, Eusebi V. Spindle cell lipoma-like tumor, solitary fibrous tumor and myofibroblastoma of the breast: a clinico-pathological analysis of 13 cases in favor of a unifying histogenetic concept. Virchows Arch. 2002;440(3):249–60.
191. Magro G. Epithelioid-cell myofibroblastoma of the breast: expanding the morphologic spectrum. Am J Surg Pathol. 2009;33(7):1085–92.
192. Magro G. Mammary myofibroblastoma: a tumor with a wide morphologic spectrum. Arch Pathol Lab Med. 2008;132(11):1813–20.
193. Meguerditchian AN, Malik DA, Hicks DG, Kulkarni S. Solitary fibrous tumor of the breast and mammary myofibroblastoma: the same lesion? Breast J. 2008;14(3):287–92.
194. Lee AH, Paish EC, Marchio C, et al. The expression of Wilms' tumour-1 and Ca125 in invasive micropapillary carcinoma of the breast. Histopathology. 2007;51(6):824–8.
195. Bhargava R, Beriwal S, Dabbs DJ. Mammaglobin vs GCDFP-15: an immunohistologic validation survey for sensitivity and specificity. Am J Clin Pathol. 2007;127(1):103–13.
196. Mazoujian G, Bodian C, Haagensen Jr DE, Haagensen CD. Expression of GCDFP-15 in breast carcinomas. Relationship to pathologic and clinical factors. Cancer. 1989;63(11):2156–61.
197. Tornos C, Soslow R, Chen S, et al. Expression of WT1, CA 125, and GCDFP-15 as useful markers in the differential diagnosis of primary ovarian carcinomas versus metastatic breast cancer to the ovary. Am J Surg Pathol. 2005;29(11):1482–9.
198. Nonaka D, Chiriboga L, Soslow RA. Expression of pax8 as a useful marker in distinguishing ovarian carcinomas from mammary carcinomas. Am J Surg Pathol. 2008;32(10):1566–71.
199. Vanstapel MJ, Gatter KC, De Wolf-Peeters C, Millard PR, Desmet VJ, Mason DY. Immunohistochemical study of mammary and extra-mammary Paget's disease. Histopathology. 1984;8(6): 1013–23.
200. Liegl B, Horn LC, Moinfar F. Androgen receptors are frequently expressed in mammary and extramammary Paget's disease. Mod Pathol. 2005;18(10):1283–8.
201. Ordonez NG, Awalt H, Mackay B. Mammary and extramammary Paget's disease. An immunocytochemical and ultrastructural study. Cancer. 1987;59(6):1173–83.
202. Jones RR, Spaull J, Gusterson B. The histogenesis of mammary and extramammary Paget's disease. Histopathology. 1989;14(4): 409–16.
203. Chaudary MA, Millis RR, Lane EB, Miller NA. Paget's disease of the nipple: a ten year review including clinical, pathological, and immunohistochemical findings. Breast Cancer Res Treat. 1986;8(2): 139–46.
204. Shah KD, Tabibzadeh SS, Gerber MA. Immunohistochemical distinction of Paget's disease from Bowen's disease and superficial spreading melanoma with the use of monoclonal cytokeratin antibodies. Am J Clin Pathol. 1987;88(6):689–95.
205. Smith KJ, Tuur S, Corvette D, Lupton GP, Skelton HG. Cytokeratin 7 staining in mammary and extramammary Paget's disease. Mod Pathol. 1997;10(11):1069–74.
206. Lundquist K, Kohler S, Rouse RV. Intraepidermal cytokeratin 7 expression is not restricted to Paget cells but is also seen in Toker cells and Merkel cells. Am J Surg Pathol. 1999;23(2):212–9.
207. Gusterson BA, Machin LG, Gullick WJ, et al. Immunohistochemical distribution of c-erbB-2 in infiltrating and in situ breast cancer. Int J Cancer. 1988;42(6):842–5.
208. Wolber RA, Dupuis BA, Wick MR. Expression of c-erbB-2 oncoprotein in mammary and extramammary Paget's disease. Am J Clin Pathol. 1991;96(2):243–7.
209. Meissner K, Riviere A, Haupt G, Loning T. Study of neu-protein expression in mammary Paget's disease with and without underlying breast carcinoma and in extramammary Paget's disease. Am J Pathol. 1990;137(6):1305–9.
210. Keatings L, Sinclair J, Wright C, et al. c-erbB-2 oncoprotein expression in mammary and extramammary Paget's disease: an immunohistochemical study. Histopathology. 1990;17(3): 243–7.
211. Lloyd J, Flanagan AM. Mammary and extramammary Paget's disease. J Clin Pathol. 2000;53(10):742–9.
212. Reed W, Oppedal BR, Eeg Larsen T. Immunohistology is valuable in distinguishing between Paget's disease, Bowen's disease and superficial spreading malignant melanoma. Histopathology. 1990;16(6):583–8.
213. Wood WS, Hegedus C. Mammary Paget's disease and intraductal carcinoma. Histologic, histochemical, and immunocytochemical comparison. Am J Dermatopathol. 1988;10(3):183–8.
214. Anderson JM, Ariga R, Govil H, et al. Assessment of Her-2/Neu status by immunohistochemistry and fluorescence in situ hybridization in mammary Paget disease and underlying carcinoma. Appl Immunohistochem Mol Morphol. 2003;11(2):120–4.
215. Bianco MK, Vasef MA. HER-2 gene amplification in Paget disease of the nipple and extramammary site: a chromogenic in situ hybridization study. Diagn Mol Pathol. 2006;15(3):131–5.

Chapter 16
Uterus

Hanna G. Kaspar

Abstract This chapter is an overview of frequently used markers in the differential diagnosis of both common and less common tumors of the uterine cervix and corpus, with a focus on the effective markers employed to differentiate adenocarcinoma of the endocervix vs. endometrium, low-grade vs. high-grade endometrial neoplasms, and benign vs. malignant mimics of cervical and endometrial lesions. Other useful panels in the differential diagnosis of gestational trophoblastic lesions in addition to the less common carcinomas of the cervix are also addressed. There are 41 tables in this chapter with immunohistochemical markers answering questions that may arise when examining hematoxylin and eosin-stained sections. A summary of useful and frequently used markers with potential pitfalls is also provided, in addition to some representative photomicrographs. The effective diagnostic panels of antibodies for several entities are highlighted in several tables.

Keywords Endocervical adenocarcinoma • Small cell undifferentiated cervical tumors • Endometrial serous carcinoma • Endometrial clear cell carcinoma • Gestational trophoblastic tumors • Placental site trophoblastic tumor • Endometrial stromal tumors

FREQUENTLY ASKED QUESTIONS

H.G. Kaspar (✉)
Clinical Professor, Department of Pathology and Laboratory Medicine, Temple University School of Medicine, Philadelphia PA, Staff Pathologist, Geisinger Wyoming Valley Medical Center, 1000 East Mountain Blvd., Wilkes-Barre, PA 18711, USA
e-mail: hgkaspar@geisinger.edu

F. Lin and J. Prichard (eds.), *Handbook of Practical Immunohistochemistry: Frequently Asked Questions*, DOI 10.1007/978-1-4419-8062-5_16, © Springer Science+Business Media, LLC 2011

Table 16.1 Summary of applications and limitations of useful markers

Antibodies	Stain pattern	Function	Key applications and pitfalls
Epithelial markers			
CK (AE1, AE3)	C	• Helps to confirm the epithelial lineage of a neoplasm	• Uterine smooth muscle tumors and endometrial stromal neoplasms may also be weakly reactive • Also expressed in the sarcomatous portion of carcinosarcomas • Simple confirmation of the presence of an implantation site (trophoblast positive; decidual cells negative) • Not useful in the evaluation of trophoblastic disease
CK5/6	C	• Usually reacts with normal, reactive and neoplastic mesothelial cells	• To distinguish benign and malignant mesothelial from benign, borderline, and malignant epithelial (especially serous) proliferations
CK7	C	• Type 2 filament protein	• Simultaneous CK7 and K20 reactivity in most metastatic neoplasms from the stomach, pancreas, biliary tree or urinary bladder • CK7 positive and CK20 negative in endometrial, and endocervical adenocarcinomas and also in breast and pulmonary adenocarcinoma • Otherwise, differential CK staining is limited in the evaluation of primary vs. metastatic adenocarcinoma
CK20	C	• Type 1 filament protein	
CAM5.2	C	• Reactive against CK8 and CK18 • Usually positive in glandular epithelium • Does not react against normal squamous epithelium	• To exclude mimics of Paget's cells in the vulva • Paget's cells usually are positive, while squamous cells, melanocytic tumors, Mycosis Fungoidis, and pagetoid Bowen's are negative
EMA	M	• Glycoprotein in human milk fat globule membranes • Helps confirm the epithelial lineage of a neoplasm • Non-neoplastic and neoplastic trophoblast is also reactive	• Usually negative in stromal and smooth muscle neoplasms that may express CAM5.2 and CK (AE1, AE3) • Unreactive in the female adnexal tumor of probable wolffian origin (FATWO) in the differential diagnosis of an epithelial neoplasm (EMA positive)
BerEP4	M	• Epithelial-specific antigen to a membrane-bound glycoprotein	• Useful in distinguishing a serous adenocarcinoma of the ovary or peritoneum and implants in the peritoneum (positive) from mesothelial-derived lesions (negative)

(continued)

Table 16.1 (continued)

Antibodies	Stain pattern	Function	Key applications and pitfalls
Mesenchymal cell markers			
Vimentin	C	• Intermediate filament expressed in most endometrial carcinomas, normal proliferative endometrial glands, stroma and mesenchymal tissue, and neoplasms	• Used in the differential diagnosis of endometrial (positive) and endocervical (negative) adenocarcinomas • To distinguish between tuboendometrioid metaplasia and endometriosis (usually positive) and adenocarcinoma in-situ (AIS) (usually negative)
Alpha-SMA	C	• Identifies smooth muscle cells	Also may be positive in endometrial stromal cells
SMSA	C	• Identifies smooth muscle cells • Also in endometrial stromal cells	Also may be positive in endometrial stromal cells
h-Caldesmon	C	• Mediator of the inhibition of Ca^{2+}-dependent smooth muscle contraction More specific marker that identifies smooth muscle cells	• Specific marker for differentiation between endometrial stromal neoplasms (negative) and smooth muscle neoplasms (positive) • May be expressed in endometrial stromal neoplasms with smooth muscle differentiation
Desmin	C	• Identifies smooth muscle cells	• To demonstrate the rhabdomyoblastic differentiation in carcinosarcomas • In confirming the diagnosis of rhabdomyosarcoma
myoD1	N	• Skeletal muscle marker	• To demonstrate the rhabdomyoblastic differentiation in carcinosarcomas • In confirming the diagnosis of rhabdomyosarcoma
Myogenin	N	• Skeletal muscle marker	• To demonstrate the rhabdomyoblastic differentiation in carcinosarcomas • In confirming the diagnosis of rhabdomyosarcoma
CD10	C/M	• Benign and neoplastic endometrial stromal cells	• May be expressed in myometrium surrounding invasive endometrial cancer cells • May be expressed in smooth muscle neoplasms • May not be expressed in less differentiated endometrial stromal neoplasms • In the distinction between a metastatic renal clear cell carcinoma (positive) and metastatic clear cell carcinoma of the ovary (negative)
Calretinin	C/N	• Calcium-binding protein • More sensitive but less specific marker of ovarian sex-cord-stromal tumors • Positive in FATWO • Positive in uterine tumor resembling ovarian sex-cord tumors • Positive in both benign and malignant mesonephric lesions within the cervix and female genital tract • Positive in adenomatoid tumors	• As a part of a panel including BerEp4 in distinguishing mesothelioma (calretinin positive, BerEp4 negative) and serous epithelial neoplasms (calretinin negative, BerEp4 positive)
CD34	M	• A single chain transmembrane glycoprotein leukocyte differentiation antigen • Expressed by hematopoietic progenitor cells, endothelial cells, and fixed connective tissue cells • Potential indicator of vascular differentiation	• Solitary fibrous tumors (rare) • In differentiating endometrial stromal neoplasms (negative) from metastatic reactive mimics (such as metastatic GIST, and primary GIST arising in the vulvovaginal region and rectovaginal septum
Trophoblastic markers			
HCG	C	• Reacts against syncytiotrophoblast but not cytotrophoblast	• Strong and diffuse reactivity in choriocarcinoma • (PSTT and ETT are less reactive) • Highlights trophoblastic elements in mixed germ cell tumors • May be reactive in cervical squamous cell carcinoma
PLAP	C	• A heterogeneous group of glycoproteins that are usually confined to the cell surface	• Stronger reactivity in lesions of chorion-type intermediate trophoblast (placental site nodule) • Only focally positivity in lesions of implantation site intermediate trophoblast • Metastatic ovarian dysgerminoma is also reactive

(continued)

Table 16.1 (continued)

Antibodies	Stain pattern	Function	Key applications and pitfalls
HPL	C	• A member of the gene family that includes human growth hormone and human prolactin • Expressed in intermediate trophoblast	• To diagnose trophoblastic neoplasms • Stronger and more diffuse expression in placental site trophoblastic tumor than in choriocarcinoma • Identification of implantation site
HLA-G	C/M	• Present in all implantation-types and chorion-types of intermediate trophoblast • Expressed in all benign and malignant trophoblastic lesions • Negative in non-trophoblastic uterine neoplasms	• In the differentiation of trophoblastic (positive) vs. non-trophoblastic (negative) lesions of the uterus • Positivity is reported in ovarian carcinomas
CD146 (MEL-CAM)	C/N/M	• Expressed in implantation site intermediate trophoblastic cells • Chorion-type intermediate trophoblastic cells are usually unreactive or focally reactive	• PSTT and exaggerated placental site (positive) • Placental site nodules and epithelioid trophoblastic tumor (negative) • MIB-1 distinguishes PSTT and exaggerated placental site reaction
Melanocytic markers			
HMB45	C	• Melanosome-associated marker	• Specific marker to identify malignant melanoma • PEComa of the uterus is characteristically reactive • May also be reactive with clear cell uterine epithelioid leiomyosarcoma
MELANA (MART1)	C	• Melanocytic marker	• Used in identifying malignant melanoma • Sex-cord stromal tumors of the ovary are also reactive
S100	N/C	• Dimeric protein • Ca^{2+} flux regulator • Wide distribution in human tissues	• Used for the diagnosis of malignant melanoma at all sites of the female genital tract • Also expressed in the cartilaginous areas of carcinosarcoma and sex-cord stromal tumors of the ovary
Tumor markers			
CA125 (OC125)	C+M	• A glycoprotein (mucin-like) antibody to an ovarian carcinoma antigen	• Used to distinguish between a primary and a metastatic ovarian adenocarcinoma • Expressed in ovarian, breast, lung, cervix, and uterine corpus adenocarcinoma • Mesotheliomas and benign mesothelial cells are commonly reactive • Primary ovarian mucinous carcinomas and colorectal adenocarcinomas are unreactive
CA19.9	C	• An antigen of sialyl Lewis(a) containing glycoprotein	• Used to identify pancreatic, biliary, or colorectal adenocarcinoma metastatic to the genital tract • Mucinous neoplasms of the ovary may be focally reactive, whereas most primary ovarian adenocarcinomas are negative
CEA	C+L	• A heterogeneous family of related oncofetal glycoproteins secreted in the glycocalyceal surface of gastrointestinal cells • The monoclonal antibody to CEA is derived from antibodies to tumor cells of hepatic metastasis of colorectal carcinoma	• As a component of a panel that differentiates endometrioid endometrial adenocarcinoma (negative) from endocervical adenocarcinoma (positive) • Usually differentiates cervical AIS (positive) and benign endocervical glandular lesions (negative) • When used as part of a panel, monoclonal CEA helps distinguish non-mucinous ovarian adenocarcinomas (usually negative) from colorectal adenocarcinoma (usually positive) • A proportion of primary endometrial mucinous adenocarcinomas are positive
Inhibin	C	• Peptide hormone expressed by granulosa and theca cells	• Variably expressed by FATWO, cervical mesonephric adenocarcinoma, uterine tumor resembling ovarian sex-cord tumor, and sex-cord-like areas within endometrial stromal neoplasms • Also reactive in some trophoblastic cell populations, syncytiotrophoblast and some intermediate trophoblastic cells • Cytotrophoblast is unreactive • Choriocarcinoma, PSTT and ETT, may be positive

(continued)

Table 16.1 (continued)

Antibodies	Stain pattern	Function	Key applications and pitfalls
OCT4	N	• Octamer transcription factor	• Predominantly in dysgerminoma, embryonal carcinoma of the ovary and in the germ cell component of gonadoblastoma
HIK1083	C	• Monoclonal antibody against gastric gland cell mucin	• Reactive in minimal deviation adenocarcinoma of the cervix • Normal endocervical glands are not reactive • Focal reactivity is encountered in some of the usual adenocarcinoma, and benign endocervical glandular lesion
CDX2	N	• A homeobox domain-containing transcription factor involved in the differentiation of the intestines	• Marker for colorectal adenocarcinoma • AIS and adenocarcinoma of the cervix may also be reactive • Occasionally expressed in ovarian mucinous neoplasms
HepPar1	C	• Specific marker of hepatocytic differentiation in paraffin-embedded tissue	• Expressed in hepatocellular carcinoma • Occasional adenocarcinoma and squamous cell carcinoma of the cervix may be positive • Also expressed in several primary hepatoid ovarian carcinomas, ovarian hepatoid yolk sac tumors, and metastatic carcinomas from other organs with hepatoid features
AFP	C	• Glycoprotein present in yolk sac tumors and cases of hepatocellular carcinoma	• In differentiating metastatic hepatocellular carcinoma and hepatoid carcinomas from other primary carcinomas of the genital tract
CD99	M	• MIC2 gene product • Cell surface glycoprotein involved in cell adhesion	• Part of a panel for the diagnosis of small round blue cell tumor • In the diagnosis of PNET (rare in the female genital system) • Reactivity in sex-cord-like areas in endometrial stromal neoplasms and uterine tumors resembling ovarian sex-cord tumors
MUC5AC	C+M	• High molecular weight glycoprotein	• Distinguishes primary ovarian carcinoma (positive) from metastatic colonic adenocarcinoma (negative) • Pancreatic and appendiceal tumors are positive • Reactive in endocervical glands
MUC2	C+M	• High molecular weight glycoprotein	• Reactivity in vulvar Paget's disease favors an underlying colorectal adenocarcinoma
Tumor suppressor genes markers			
WT1	N	• In smooth muscle tumors and • Benign and neoplastic endometrial stromal cells • In serous carcinomas primarily arising in the ovary, peritoneum, and fallopian tube and • Uterine serous carcinomas are primarily unreactive or focally positive	• Differentiates most endometrioid, clear cell, and mucinous carcinomas (negative) from metastatic or extending ovarian (positive) • Does not differentiate endometrial stromal sarcomas from smooth muscle tumor
DPC4	N+C	• Deleted in pancreatic cancer, locus 4	• Helpful in differentiating metastatic pancreatic adenocarcinoma to the genital tract (negative) from primary mucinous benign or malignant lesions of the genital tract primarily ovary (reactive)
PTEN		• Mutation associated with loss of reactivity	• Loss of reactivity in most endometrioid adenocarcinomas of the endometrium and their precursors • Loss of reactivity is also encountered in normal cyclical and secretory endometrium
p53	N	• Mutations cause conformational changes and stabilization of this nuclear protein involved in regulating cell growth, which allows for immunohistochemical detection	• Predominantly in distinguishing serous adenocarcinoma, EIC, and clear cell carcinoma from benign papillary endometrial proliferations and metaplasias • In distinguishing uterine serous carcinoma (diffuse intense positive) from endometrioid adenocarcinoma (absent, weak, or focal positive) • Significant p53 positivity is reported in some endometrioid adenocarcinomas and an occasional serous carcinoma may be negative • Much more commonly reactive in leiomyosarcomas than benign smooth muscle neoplasms

(continued)

Table 16.1 (continued)

Antibodies	Stain pattern	Function	Key applications and pitfalls
p63	N	• Transcription factor that belongs to the p53 family	• Reactive in immature basal and reserve squamous cells of the cervix • Distinguishes small cell non-keratinizing squamous cell carcinoma of the cervix (diffusely reactive) from small cell neuroendocrine carcinoma (negative or focally positive)
Cell cycle and nuclear proliferation			
MIB1 (Ki67)	N	• Identifies cells in non-G0 phases of the cell cycle	• In benign cervical and vulvar squamous epithelium, reactivity confined to basal and parabasal layers • In CIN and VIN reactivity increases in upper layers • To distinguish cauterized cervical margins with CIN3 from non-dysplastic epithelium • Part of a panel to distinguish AIS from benign mimics • Part of a panel to distinguish endometrioid adenocarcinoma (lower index) and serous and clear cell carcinoma (higher index) • May distinguish exaggerated placental site (nearly absent) from PSTT (elevated)
p16	N+C	• Binds to cyclin D-CDK4/6 complex to control the cell cycle at G_1-S interphase	• Diffuse nuclear and cytoplasmic staining in high-grade squamous dysplasia and AIS • Used to distinguish dysplastic squamous and glandular lesions of the cervix from benign mimics • Used to distinguish cervical (diffuse strong reactivity) from endometrial (absent or focally positive) adenocarcinoma • Some endometrioid and serous carcinomas of the endometrium may express diffuse reactivity
P57	N	• Cell cycle inhibitor of proliferation • Expressed only when maternal DNA is present	• Absent in the villous cytotrophoblast of the complete hydatidiform mole • Reactivity present in decidua and extravillous trophoblast
Proto-oncogenes markers			
Bcl2	C	• A proto-oncogene, encoding a 25 kDa protein localized to the inner mitochondrial membrane, blocks apoptosis, and extends cell survival	• Used to differentiates tuboendometrial metaplasia and endometriosis of the cervix (diffusely positive) from AIS (usually negative) • Diffusely expressed in the gland cell cytoplasm in proliferative endometrium • Reduced expression in the glands of both atypical hyperplasia and endometrioid-adenocarcinomas • Positive in the basal cell layer of the normal squamous epithelium of the cervix
CD117 (cKIT)	C	• Transmembrane tyrosine kinase receptor	• Metastatic GIST • Primary rectovaginal septum • Uterine leiomyosarcoma • Occasionally expressed in uterine carcinosarcoma and ovarian serous carcinomas and germ cell tumors
Hormone receptors			
ER and PR	N	• DNA-binding transcription factor that regulates gene expression • Other functions independent of DNA binding	• In distinguishing endometrial endometrioid adenocarcinoma (reactive) from endocervical adenocarcinoma (negative) • In distinguishing type 2 endometrial adenocarcinoma (focal or unreactive) from the less aggressive variant type 1 (diffusely reactive) • In distinguishing some benign papillary proliferations of the endometrium (reactive) from small serous carcinomas or precursors (EIN) (unreactive) • Positive in ESS, uterine smooth muscle proliferations, and vulvovaginal mesenchymal lesions

(continued)

Table 16.1 (continued)

Antibodies	Stain pattern	Function	Key applications and pitfalls
AR	N	• DNA-binding transcription factor that regulates gene expression • Other functions include maintenance of the male sexual phenotype	• Reactive in mesonephric remnants and ectopic prostate present in both cervix and vagina • Fibroblasts in cervix and vagina are reactive • Also reactive in endometrial adenocarcinoma, FATWO, mesonephric carcinoma of cervix, and endometrial stromal sarcoma
Oxytocin receptor	M	• Receptor for the hormone and neurotransmitter oxytocin	• In distinguishing uterine smooth muscle tumors (reactive) from endometrial stromal neoplasms (unreactive)
Neuroendocrine markers			
CD56 Chromogranin Synaptophysin PGP9.5			• To establish neuroendocrine differentiation in a tumor • Establish the diagnosis of large cell neuroendocrine carcinoma of cervix • Small cell neuroendocrine carcinoma is not reactive
Lymphoid antibodies			
B and T lymphoid markers			• Used in the diagnosis of the rare lymphoma or leukemia in the genital tact • CD20 and CD79a may help in the diagnosis of low-grade endometritis • ISH for kappa and lambda light chain may assist in the diagnosis of endometritis

References: [6–65]

Table 16.2 Summary of useful markers in common tumors

Antibodies	SCCx	AdenoCx	AdenoEM	SerEM	CCEM	ESS	LMS
CK (AE1, AE3)	+	+	+	+	+	– or +	– or +
EMA	+	+	+	+	+	–	– or +
CK7	+	+	+	+	+	– or +	– or +
CK20	–	– or +	– or +	–	–	–	–
CEA	+ or –	+	– or +	– or +	– or +	–	–
CD10	–	–	–	–	–	+	– or +
ER	–	– or +	+	– or +	– or +	+	– or +
PR	–	– or +	+	– or +	– or +	+	+ or –
Vimentin	–	–	+	+	+	+	+
Calponin	–	–	–	–	–	+ or –	+
Desmin	–	–	–	–	–	– or +	+
h-Caldesmon	–	–	–	–	–	– or+	+
SMA	–	–	–	–	–	+ or –	+
S100	–	–	–	–	–	–	– or +
HMB45	–	–	–	–	–	–	– or +
Inhibin	–	–	– or +	–		–	–
MART-1	–	–	–	–	–	– or +	–
p16	+	+	– or +	+ or –	+ or –	–	+ or –
p53	+ or –	– or +	– or +	+	+ or –	– or +	– or +
p63	+	– or +	– or +	– or +	– or +	–	–
WT1		+ or –	– or +	– or +	–		– or +

Note: *SCCx* cervical squamous cell carcinoma, *AdenoCx* cervical adenocarcinoma, *AdenoEM* endometrial endometrioid adenocarcinoma, *SerEM* endometrial serous carcinoma, *CCEM* endometrial clear cell carcinoma, *ESS* endometrial stromal cell sarcoma, *LMS* leiomyosarcoma, and *CC* choriocarcinoma

References: [1–3, 6–9, 11–14, 17, 20–22, 27, 28, 30, 31, 33, 34, 39, 42–44, 48, 52, 53, 64, 66–97]

Table 16.3 Markers for normal and non-neoplastic lesions of the cervix

Marker	CG	CS	MH	MRH	FDG
ER	– or +	+ or –	– or +	–	– or +
PR	– or +	+ or –	+ or –	–	– or +
CEA	+	–	–	–	–
Vimentin	–	+ or –	– or +	+ or –	– or +
CD10		– or + (W)	– or + (W)	+ (A + L)	–
AE1,AE3	+	– or +	+	+	+
EMA	+	–	+	+	+
CK7	+	–	+	+	+
CK20	–	–	– or +	–	–
p16	–	–	– (F)	– (F)	–

CG endocervical glands, *CS* endocervical stroma, *MH* microglandular hyperplasia, *MRH* mesonephric remnant hyperplasia, *FDG* florid deep glands, *W* weakly positive, *A + L* apical and luminal, and *F* may be focally positive

References: [34, 42, 70, 85, 86, 98–102]

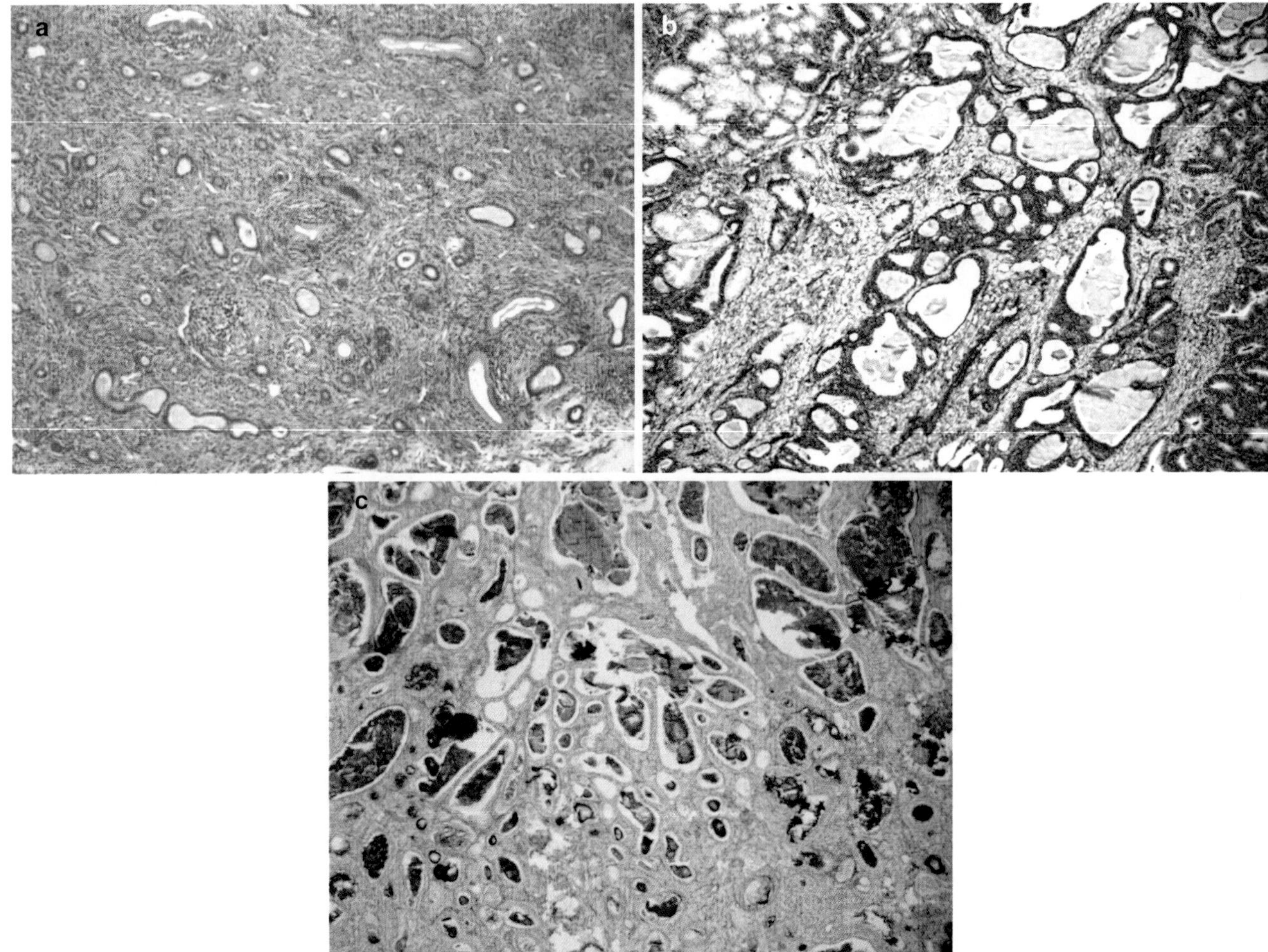

Fig. 16.1 Mesonephric remnant hyperplasia (**a**), with diffuse positive vimentin (**b**), and luminal CD10 positivity (**c**)

Table 16.4 Markers for normal and non-neoplastic lesions of the endometrium

Marker	EG	ES	SME	ASR	E
ER	+ or −	− or +	+ or −	− or +	+ or −
PR	+ or −	− or +	+ or −	+ or −	+ or −
CEA	− or +	−	−	−	−
Vimentin	+	+	− or +	+	+
CD10	−	+	−	−	+ (S)
AE1, AE3	+	− or +	+	+	+
EMA	+	−	+	+	+
CK7	+	−	+	+	+
CK20	−	−	−	−	−
p16	−	−	− or +	− or +	− or +

EG endometrial glands, *ES* endometrial stroma, *SME* squamous metaplasia of endometrium, *ASR* Arias-Stella reaction, *E* Endometriosis, and *S* Stromal

References: [34, 65, 85]

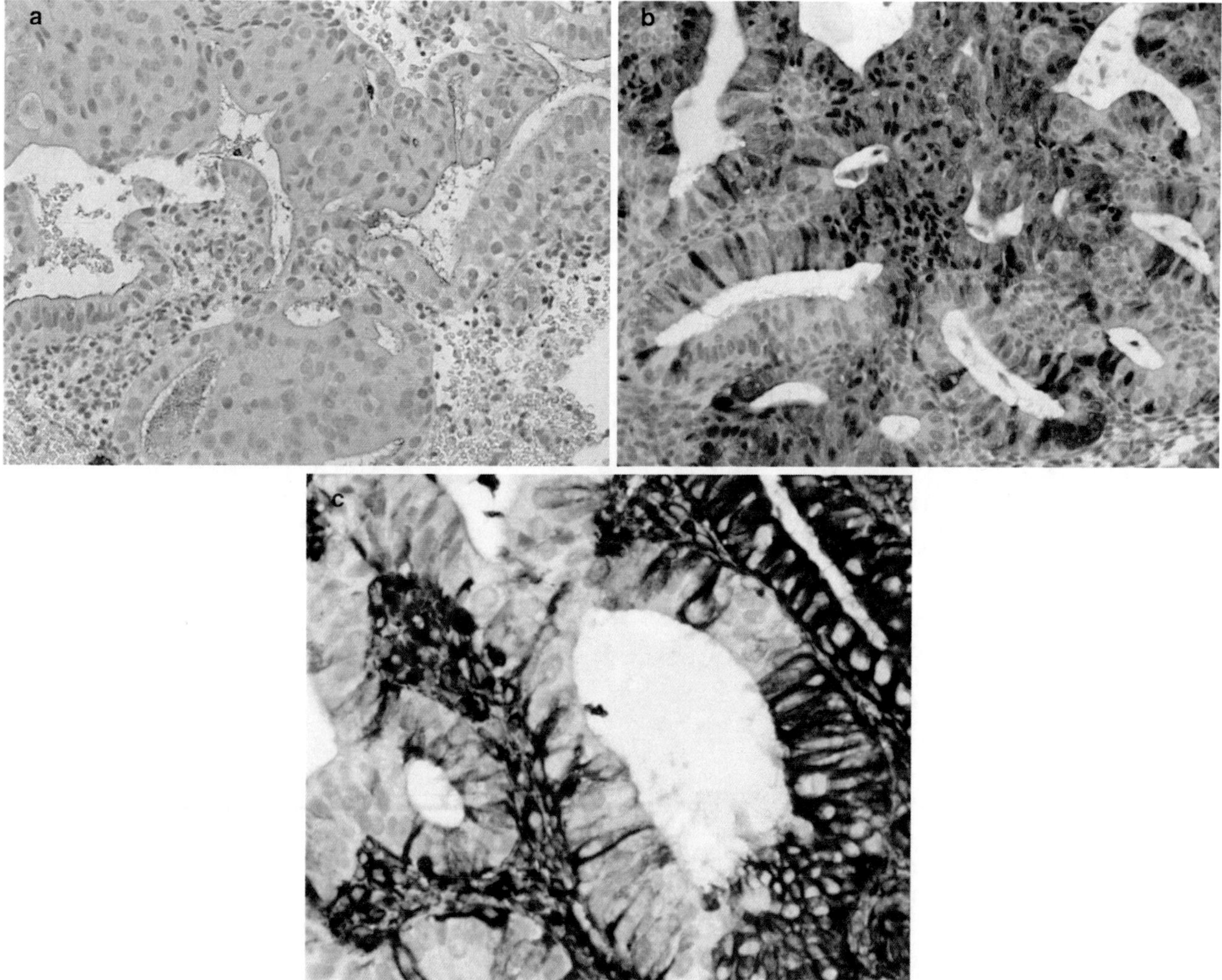

Fig. 16.2 Endometrial squamous metaplasia with lack of CEA staining (**a**), patchy staining pattern with p16 (**b**), and lack of staining with vimentin in the metaplastic foci (**c**)

Table 16.5 Markers for cervical high-grade squamous intraepithelial lesion

Antibodies	Literature
p16	+[a]
Ki67	+[b]
HPV	+[c]

Notes:

[a]p16 usually shows strong nuclear and cytoplasmic staining of at least two-third thickness of the involved mucosa

[b]Ki67 usually shows strong nuclear staining of at least two-third thickness of the involved mucosa

[c]HPV by in situ hybridization

References: [8, 34, 43, 45, 51, 60, 63, 77, 78, 80, 81, 86, 103–108]

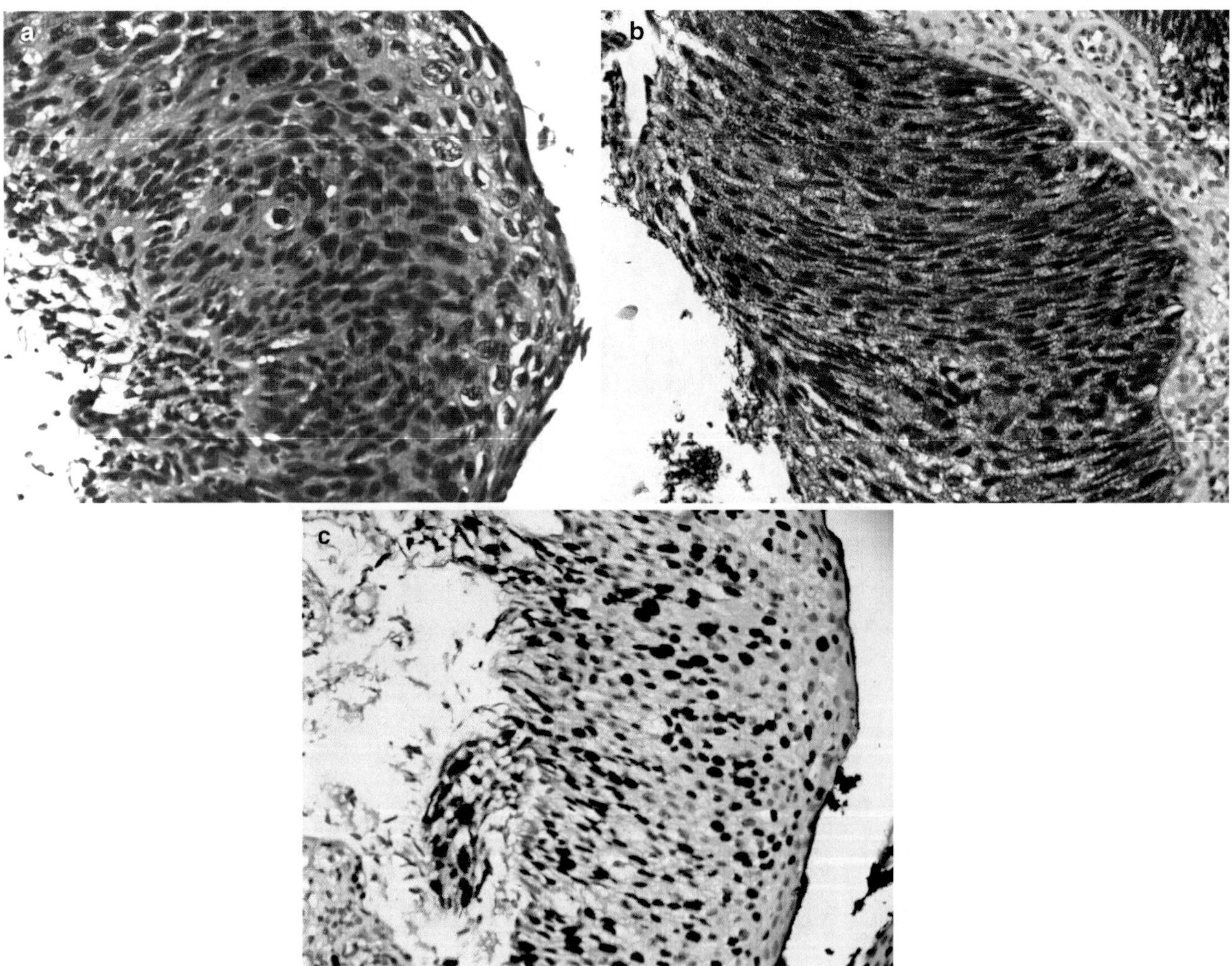

Fig. 16.3 High-grade SIL on H&E (**a**), with full thickness and intense nuclear staining with p16 (**b**), and increased Ki-67 proliferative index involving upper layers (**c**)

Table 16.6 Markers for endocervical in situ adenocarcinoma

Antibodies	Literature
p16	+[a]
Ki67	+[b]
p53	+ or −
Bcl2	− or +
CEA	+ or −
CA125	−[c]
ER (glands)	− or +
PR (glands)	− or +
ER (stromal cells)	+[d]
Alpha-SMA (stromal cells)	+
Vimentin (crypts)	−
CD10 (stroma)	−
ESA	−[e]
HPV	+
PAX-2	−

Notes:

[a]p16 positivity is usually strong and diffuse in in-situ adenocarcinoma. Focal reactivity is encountered in normal cervix, lower-grade glandular intra-epithelial lesions, tubo-endometrioid metaplasia, and other reactive and malignant conditions

[b]High Ki67 proliferative index is also encountered in inflammation, proliferative endometrium, and other conditions

[c]In in-situ adenocarcinoma, CA125 is absent or localized to the perinuclear region of the cytoplasm as an accumulation of atypical coarse granules. CA125 is encountered in the secretory products of the uninvolved endocervical glands on the luminal surfaces

[d]The stromal cells surrounding crypts/glands are estrogen receptor (ER) positive and alpha-smooth muscle actin negative in in-situ adenocarcinoma. The stomal cells associated with invasive adenocarcinoma show an opposite pattern

[e]Epithelial-specific antigen (ESA) shows diffuse cytoplasmic and membranous staining in lower grades glandular lesions and in in-situ adenocarcinoma. It is confined to the basolateral membrane of uninvolved endocervical cells

References: [28, 34, 43, 52, 63, 70, 71, 77, 78, 80, 82, 84, 86, 100, 103–106, 108–111]

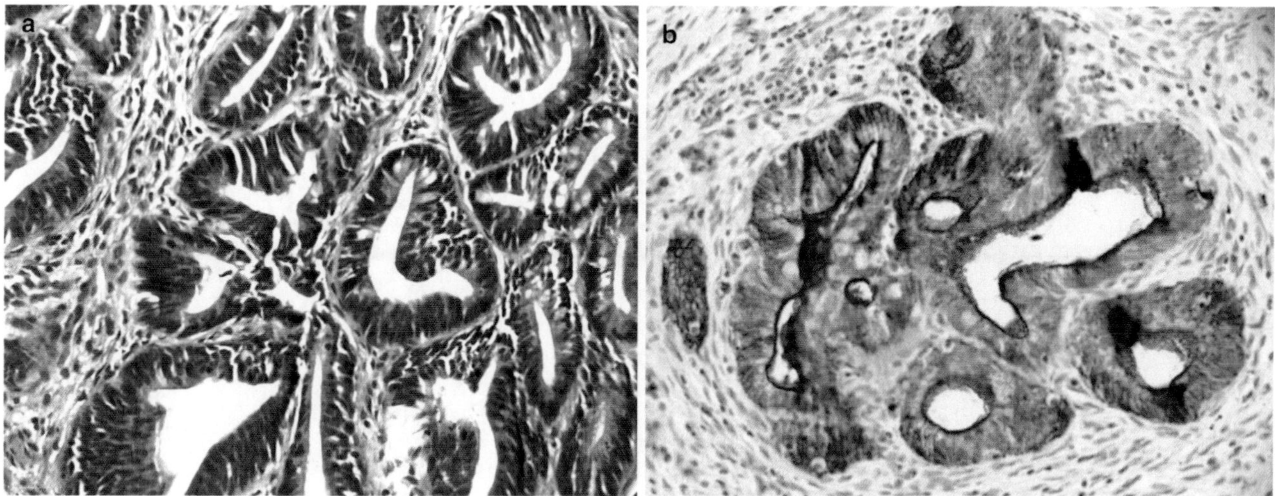

Fig. 16.4 Adenocarcinoma in situ of the endocervix on H&E (**a**), with CEA positive staining (**b**), diffuse and intense p16 nuclear and cytoplasmic staining (**c**), and increased Ki-67 proliferative index (**d**)

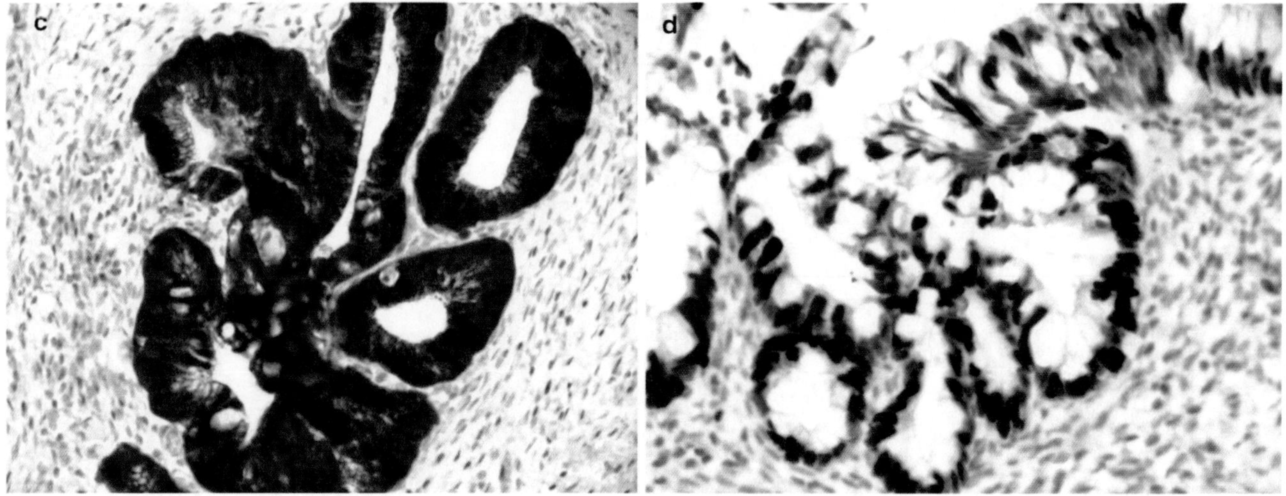

Fig. 16.4 (continued)

Table 16.7 Markers for invasive squamous cell carcinoma of the cervix

Antibodies	Literature
CK (AE1, AE3)	+
p63	+
p16	+
P14ARF	+
p53	+ or –
CEA-P	– or +
Bcl2	– or +
Synaptophysin	– or +
Chromogranin	–
HepPar1	–
CD-56	–

References: [34, 57, 60, 76, 78, 80, 86, 90, 106, 108, 110–112]

Table 16.8 Markers for invasive endocervical (mucinous) and endometrioid adenocarcinoma of the cervix

Antibodies	Literature
CK (AE1, AE3)	+
CK7	+
EMA	+
CEA-M	+
CEA-P	+
p16 INK4	+
pRB	+
MUC1	+
MUC5AC	+
HepPar1	+
WT1	+ or –
CA125	+ or –
CA 19-9	– or +
MUC 6	– or +
p53	– or +

References: [6, 8, 28, 34, 35, 42, 51, 52, 60, 63, 71, 80, 84, 86, 106, 108, 110, 113–115]

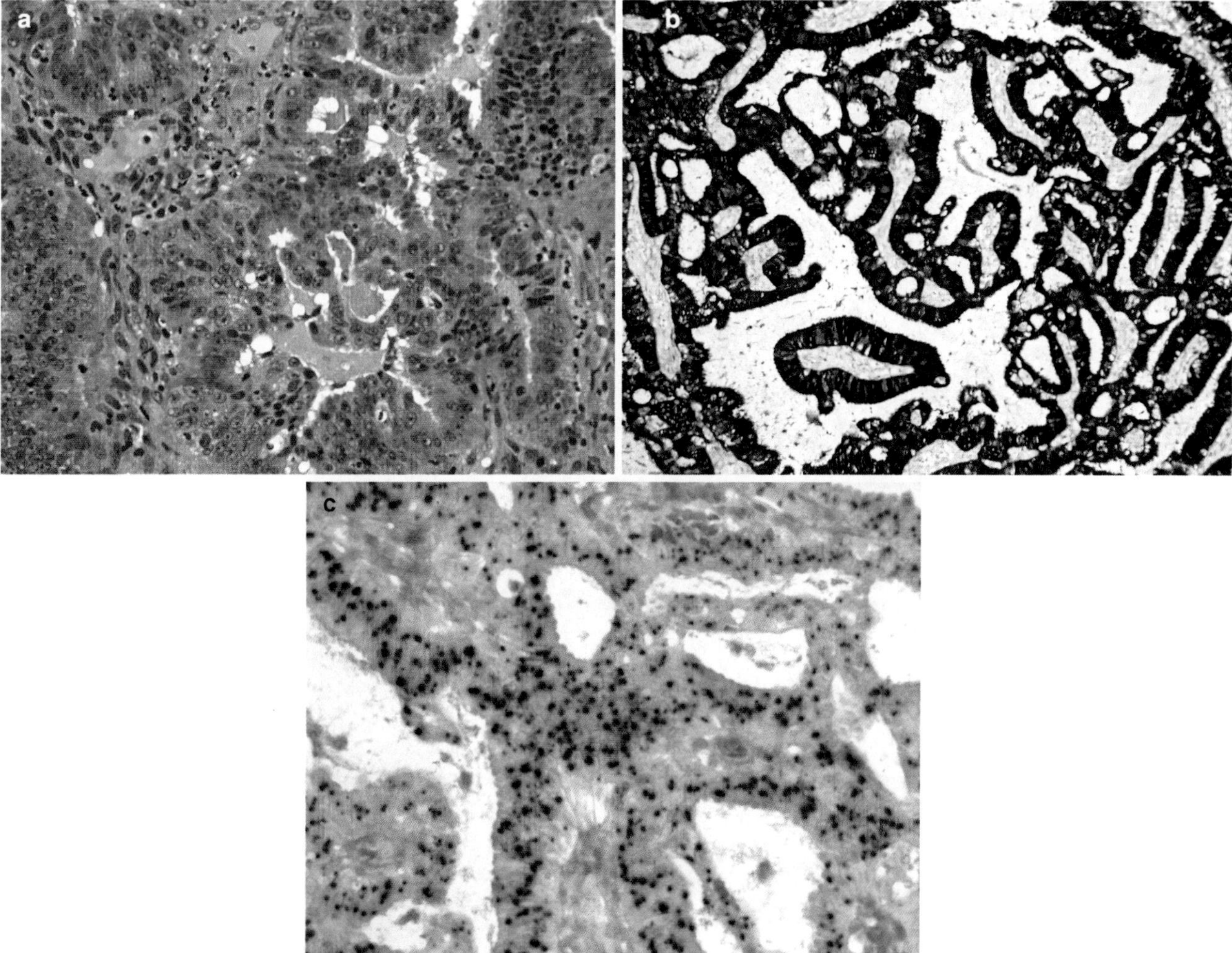

Fig. 16.5 Invasive endocervical adenocarcinoma on H&E (**a**), with p16 diffuse and intense positive staining (**b**) and positive inclusions by in-situ hybridization for HPV (c) [21–61]

Table 16.9 Markers for in-situ and invasive intestinal-type endocervical adenocarcinoma

Antibodies	Literature
CK (AE1, AE3)	+
CK7	+
CK20	–
CDX2	+
EMA	+
CEA-M	+
CEA-P	+
p16 INK4	+
pRB	+
MUC1	+
MUC5AC	+
WT1	+ or –
CA125	+ or –
CA 19-9	– or +
MUC6	– or +
p53	– or +

References: [8, 28, 34, 42, 51, 52, 60, 63, 71, 78, 80, 84, 86, 106, 108, 110, 113, 114]

Table 16.10 Markers for minimal deviation adenocarcinoma of the cervix

Antibodies	Literature
HIK1083	+
PAX-2	–
p16	–
CEA	– or +
p53	– or +
Ki-67	– or +
ER	–
PR	–
HPV	–
CD10	–
HPV	–

References: [86, 98, 100, 110, 116–118]

Table 16.11 Markers for small cell undifferentiated carcinomas of the uterine cervix

Marker	NEC	SCNKSCC	BC	PNET	Melanoma	ERMS
Chromogranin-A	+ or –	–	–	–	–	–
Synaptophysin	+ or –	–	–	– or +	– or +	–
NSE	+	– or +	– or +	+ or –	+ or –	– or +
p63	– or +	+	+	– or +	–	
Desmin	–	–	–	–	–	+
Actin-HHF-35	–	–	–	–	–	+
SMA	–	–	–	–	– or +	– or +
BerEp4/EpCAM	+	+ or –	+		–	–
EMA/MUC1	+	+	+ or –	– or +	–	– or +
p16	+ or –	+ or –	+	– or +	+ or –	– or +
CK7	+	–	+	– or +	–	–
CK20	– or +	–	–		–	–
PAX5	+	–	+ or –	–	–	–
PLAP	– or +	–	–	–	–	+
Vimentin	– or +	+ or –	– or +	+	+	+
S100	– or +	–	+ or –	– or +	+	–
HMB45	–	–	–	– or +	+	–
MART-1		–	–	– or +	+	–
CD99	– or +	– or +	+ or –	+	+ or –	– or +
TTF1	– or +	–	–	–	–	–

Note: *NEC* neuroendocrine carcinoma, *SCNKSCC* small cell non-keratinizing squamous cell carcinoma, *BC* basaloid carcinoma, *PNET* peripheral neuroendocrine tumor, and *ERMS* embryonal rhabdomyosarcoma

References: [9, 23, 34, 60, 63, 72, 80, 86, 89, 108]

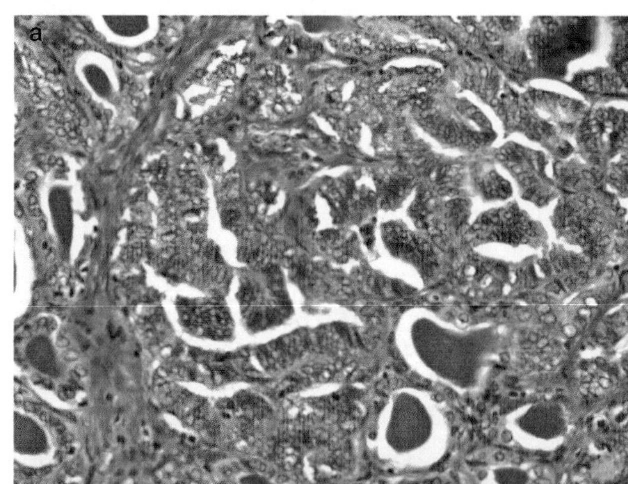

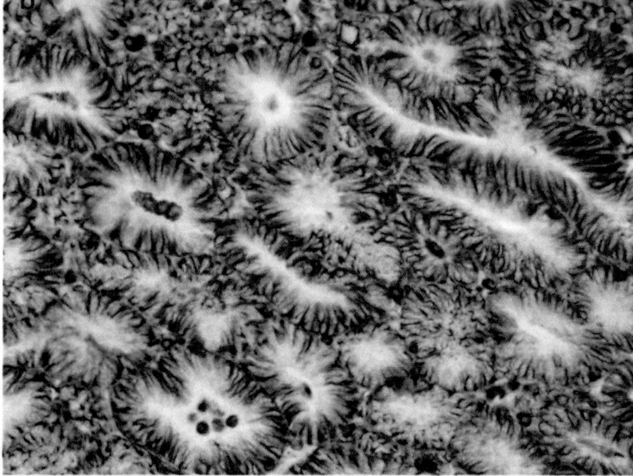

Fig. 16.6 Mesonephric carcinoma on H&E (**a**) and positive vimentin (**b**)

Table 16.12 Markers for mesonephric (adeno)carcinoma of cervix

Antibodies	Literature
CAM5.2	One case +
CK7	+
CK20	–
EMA	+
Calretinin	+ or –
Vimentin	+ or –
mCEA	–
ER	–
PR	–
CD10	+ or –
PAX2	–

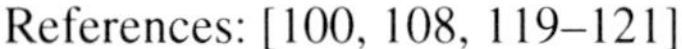

References: [100, 108, 119–121]

Table 16.13 Markers for endometrioid adenocarcinoma of the endometrium (type 1 or tumors without serous, clear cell or undifferentiated features)

Antibodies	Literature
CAM5.2	+
BerEP4	+
CK (AE1, AE3)	+
HMSH2	+
CD64	+
EMA	+
CK7	+
CA125	+
HMLH-1	+
ER	+
PR	+
BAX	+
Vimentin	+
Cyclin D1	+
CK5/6	+ or –
CA19-9	+ or –
Beta-catenin	– or +[a]
Mesothelin	+ or –
p53	– or +[b]
WT1	– or +
PTEN	– or +
CD56	– or +
Bcl2	– or +
Antibodies	Literature
CDX2	– or +
Calretinin	– or +
TTF1	– or +
CEA-P	– or +
CEA-M	– or +
MUC5AC	– or +
p63	– or +
CD57	– or +
CD5	– or +
TAG72	– or +
P27_KIP1	– or +
GFI-1	– or +
IMP3	– or +
CDX2	– or +[c]

Note: Additional negative markers include: CK20, CD10, HepPar-1, GCDFP-15, MUC-2, PAP, and thrombomodulin

References: [6, 14, 15, 20, 21, 26, 31, 37, 53, 67, 74, 82, 93, 106, 112, 122–133]

[a]Nuclear staining is encountered in approximately one-third of FIGO 1 and 2 cases of adenocarcinomas, in particular cases with squamous an morular metaplasias

[b]Weak reactivity with p53 in less than 50% of tumor cells is common in type 1 endometrioid adenocarcinoma

[c]Found in squamous morular metaplasia

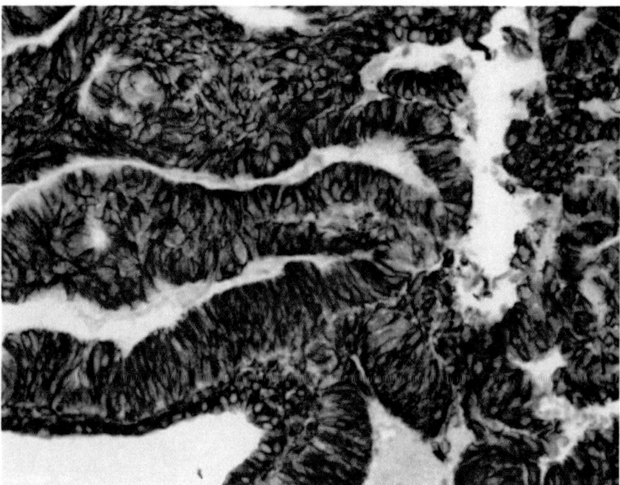

Fig. 16.7 Intense vimentin staining in endometrioid adenocarcinoma

Table 16.14 Markers for serous carcinoma of the endometrium and putative precursors EIC

Antibodies	Literature
PanCK	+
EMA	+
BerEP4	+
CK7	+
CA125	+
B72.3	+
Vimentin	+
Ki67	+[a]
IMP3	+
p53	+[b]
p16	+ or –[c]
WT1	– or +
CEA-M	– or +
ER	– or +
PR	– or +
Bcl2	– or +
Her2neu	– or +
P21-WAF1	– or +
B-catenin	–
CK20	–
Loss of PTEN	Almost never
Loss of MLH1	Almost never
Loss of MSH2	Almost never
Loss of MSH6	Almost never
Loss of PMS2	Almost never

Notes:

[a]Very high-proliferative index exceeding 70%

[b]Intense nuclear staining in over 90% of tumor cells (L2) [98, 119, 120, 124, 125]

[c]Diffuse and intense staining including nuclear staining is encountered in almost every cell

References: [6, 10, 14, 21, 31, 42, 53, 67, 74, 93, 106, 122, 123, 125, 127, 129, 134–141]

Table 16.15 Markers for clear cell carcinoma of the endometrium

Antibodies	Literature
PanCK	+
EMA	+
BerEP4	+
CK7	+
CA125	+
B72.3	+
Vimentin	+
HNF-1beta	+
p53	+ or −
p16	+ or −
Ki67	+ or −
ER	− or +
PR	− or +
CK20	−
WT1	−
CEA	− or +
Loss of MSH6	Rare
Loss of PMS2	Rare

References: [6, 15, 86, 92, 120, 142]

Table 16.16 Markers for carcinosarcoma of the endometrium[a]

Antibodies	Literature
CD10	+
CK (AE1, AE3)	+
p16	+
PLAP	− or +
Calretinin	− or +
Inhibin	−

[a]**Note**: Myogenin and Myo-D1 are also used to establish a rhabdomyoblastic differentiation

References: [73, 86]

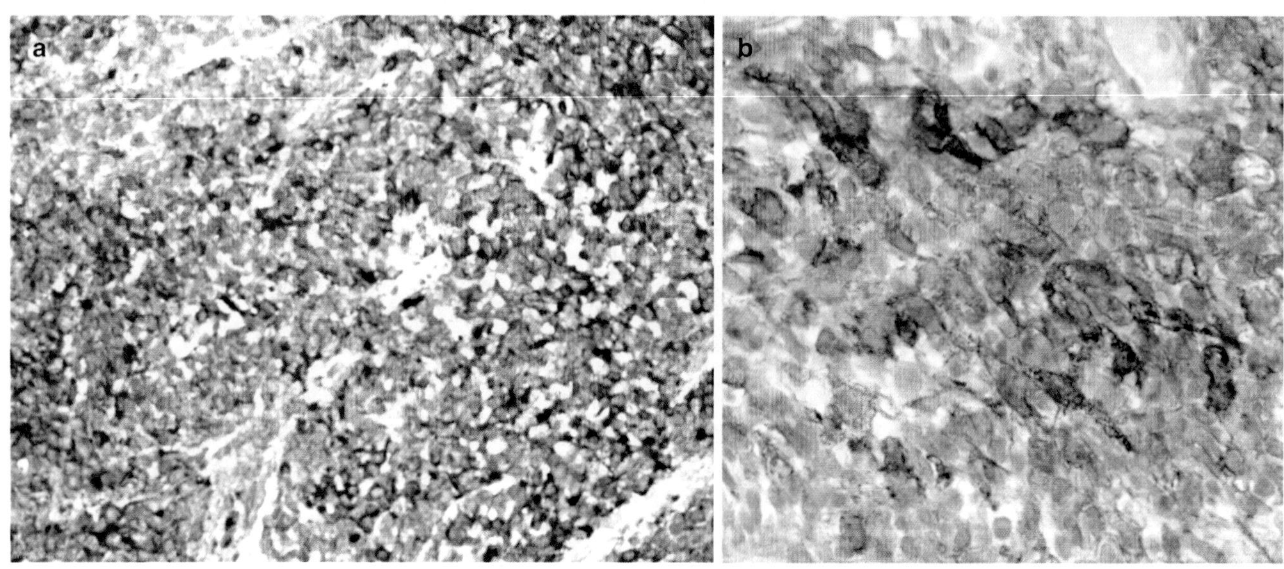

Fig. 16.8 CD10 in carcinosarcoma of the endometrium (**a**) and in low-grade endometrial stromal sarcoma (**b**)

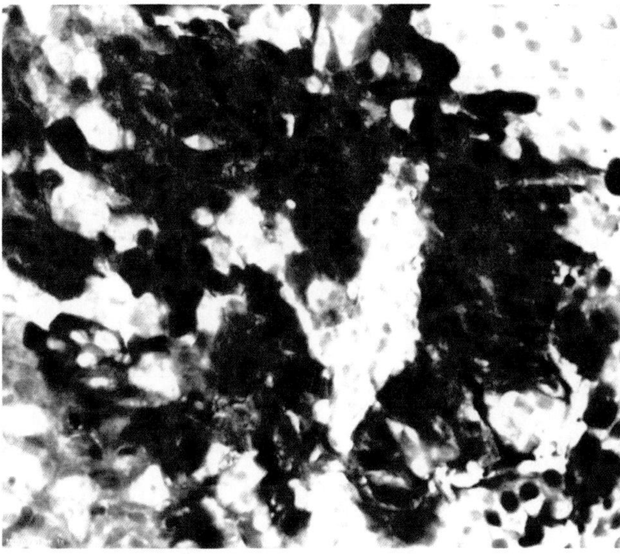

Fig. 16.9 Carcinosarcoma with intense and diffuse p16 staining

Table 16.18 Markers for endometrial stromal sarcoma[a,b]

Antibodies	Literature
CD10	+
(ER)	+
PR	+
Vimentin	+
WT1	+
Calponin	+ or −
SMA	+ or −
B-catenin	+ or −
CK (AE1, AE3)	− or +
Desmin	− or +
CAM5.2	− or +
Pan-CK	− or +
h-Caldesmon	− or +
ACTIN-HHF35	− or +
CD117	−
EMA	−
Inhibin	−
CD34	−
HMB45	−

Notes:

[a]The metaplastic elements lose the endometrial stromal immunophenotype and acquire the corresponding metaplastic tissue immunophenotype

[b]The above table reflects predominantly the low-grade variant of endometrial stromal component. The immunohistochemical profile of high-grade uterine sarcomas (undifferentiated sarcoma) is not defined. For the workup of an undifferentiated neoplasm, it is recommended to exclude melanoma, carcinoma, lymphoma, and leukemia before rendering the diagnosis of undifferentiated uterine sarcoma (Fig. 16.8b)

References: [7, 29, 30, 40, 64, 72, 75, 143–146]

Table 16.17 Markers for atypical polypoid adenomyoma

Antibodies	Literature
SMA[a]	+
Desmin[a]	+ or −
CD34[a]	+ or −
CK (AE1, AE3)[b]	+
CAM5.2[b]	+
ER[b]	+
PR[b]	+

Notes:

[a]In mesenchymal component

[b]In epithelial component

Table 16.19 Markers for low-grade Müllerian adenosarcoma (stromal component)

Antibodies	Literature
Vimentin	+
WT1	+
CD10	+[a]
ER	+[a]
PR	+[a]
CK (AE1, AE3)	+ or −
SMA	+ or −
AR	+ or −

[a]**Note**: Areas with sarcomatous overgrowth (müllerian adenosarcoma with sarcomatous overgrowth, MASO) are frequently negative for CD10, ER, and PR

References: [68, 110, 147, 148]

Table 16.20 Markers for uterine smooth muscle tumors

Antibodies	Leiomyoma	Leiomyosarcoma
Desmin	+	+ or −
SMA	+	+
ACTIN-HHF35	+	+
h-Caldesmon	+	+
Cyclin D1	+	+
Calponin	+	+
Vimentin	+	+
ER	+ or −	− or +
PR	+ or −	− or +
NSE	+ or −	
p16 INK4a	− or +	+ or −
Bcl2	− or +	− or +
HLA-DR	− or +	
p53	− or +	− or +
MITF	− or +	
CD10	− or +	− or +
CD30	− or +	− or +
CD34	− or +	− or +
CD57	− or +	
CD68	− or +	− or +
CD99	− or +	− or +
MDM-2	− or +	− or +
CAM5.2	− or +	− or +
E-cadherin	− or +	− or +
Calretinin	− or +	
CD34	− or +	
CLUSTERIN	− or +	− or +
AE1	− or +	− or +
CK (AE1, AE3)	− or +	− or +
Pan-CK	− or +	− or +
HMB45	− or +	− or +
EMA	− or +	− or +
CDK4	− or +	− or +

Note: Additional negative markers include: S100, Alk1, p63, beta-catenin (nuclear), CD31, CD117, CD163, tyrosinase, myogenin, inhibin, myoglobulin, MelanA 103, GFAP, NFP, factor VIIIR AG, actin-SARC, CK19, actin-SARC, and HepPar-1

References: [3, 11, 13, 27, 29, 32, 38, 41, 50, 69, 73, 80, 94–96, 110, 114, 149–153]

Table 16.21 Markers for adenomatoid tumor

Antibodies	Literature
Calretinin	+
Pan-CK	+
WT1	+
Vimentin	+ or −
BerEP4	− or +
CEA-P	−
CEA-M	−
TAG72	−
CD34	−
CD15	−
POU5F1	−

References: [87, 154]

Table 16.22 Markers for PECOMAs

Antibodies	Literature
HMB45	+
MelanA	+
MiTF	+ or −
S100	−
Inhibin	−
Pan-CK	−
HMB50	+
Actin	+
Calponin	+
Vimentin	+
FVIIIRAG	+
h-Caldesmon	+ or −
Desmin	+ or −
S100	− or +
NSE	− or +
CD117	− or +
CD34	− or +
PR	− or +
ER	− or +
CD68	− or +
Tyrosinase	− or +
Synaptophysin	−
Chromogranin	−
GFAP	−
NFP	−
CEA-P	−
EMA	−
CAM5.2	−
CK (AE1, AE3)	−
HepPar1	−
CD57	−

References: [11, 38, 49, 73, 155]

Table 16.23 Markers for gestational trophoblastic lesions

Marker	PSN	PSTT	ETT	CC
CK (AE1, AE3)	+	+	+	+
CK18	+	+	+	+
EMA	+	+	+	+ or −
Beta-HCG	+ or −	− or +	− or +	+
HPL	+ or −	+	− or +	+
Inhibin	+	+	+	+
HLA-G	+	+	−	+
p16	−	−	−	− or +
CD146	+ or −	+	− or +	+
PLAP	+	− or +	+	− or +
E-cadherin	+		+	
CD68	−	−	−	−
CEA-P	+	+	+	− or +
p63	+	− or +	+	+ or −
Vimentin	+	+ or −	−	−
CD10	+	+	+	+
Ki-67 index	≤10%	15–25%	10–25%	>50–70%

PSN placental site nodule, *PSTT* placental site trophoblastic tumor, *ETT* epithelioid trophoblastic tumor, *CC* choriocarcinoma

References: [1, 2, 46, 79, 120, 156–159]

Table 16.24 Differentiating high-grade SIL from benign mimics and low-grade SIL

Marker	HGSIL	AR	RC	AT	ISM	TM	LGSIL
p16	+[a]	–	–	–	–	–	+ or –[b]
Ki67	+[a]	– or +[b]	– or +[b]	– or +[b]	– or +[b]	– or +[b]	+[b]
HPV[c]	+	–	–	–	–	–	+

Notes:

[a]Diffuse, strong nuclear staining involving the superficial two-thirds of the involved mucosa

[b]Only the basal layer is involved

[c]By in situ hybridization

HGSIL high-grade squamous intraepithelial lesion, *AR* atypical repair, *RC* radiation change, *AT* atrophy, *ISM* immature squamous metaplasia, *TM* transitional metaplasia, and *LGSIL* low-grade squamous intraepithelial lesion

References: [8, 34, 45, 51, 80, 81, 84, 86, 106, 110, 114, 160]

Table 16.25 Differentiating endocervical in situ adenocarcinoma and endometriosis

Antibodies	In situ adenocarcinoma	Endometriosis
CEA-P	+	–
ER	– or +	+
PR	– or +	+
PAX-2	–	+
p16	+[a]	+ or –[b]
CD10	– or +	– or +
Vimentin	– or +	–
Chromogranin-A	– or +	–
EpCAM/BerEP4	+	+
CK7	+	+
CK20	– or +	–
p53	– or +	–
Ki67	+ or –	– or +

Notes:

[a]Strong, diffuse

[b]Patchy

References: [48, 70, 86, 99, 100, 106, 110, 111, 141, 161–163]

Table 16.26 Cervical microglandular hyperplasia vs. endometrial mucinous adenocarcinoma

Antibodies	Microglandular hyperplasia, cervix	Mucinous adenocarcinoma, endometrium
MIB1	Less than 1%	At least 10%
Vimentin	– or +	+
PAX-2	+	–
p16	–	+
CEA	–	+
CA19-9	–	
ER	– or +	+
PR	+ or –	+
CA125	+[a]	+
p53	–	–
CK7	+	+ (Focal or diffuse)
CK20	–	– or +[b]
CDX2	– or +	– or +[b]
CD10 (stromal cells)	– or + (Weak to moderate)	+ (Strong)
CD34 (stromal cells)	+ (Strong)	– or + (Weak)
p63	+ (Sub-columnar)	

Notes:

[a]In the luminal surface and secretory products

[b]Intensity correlates with intestinal differentiation

References: [42, 70, 85, 98–102]

Table 16.27 Cervical vs. endometrial adenocarcinoma

Antibodies	Cervix	Endometrium
CEA	+	–
Vimentin	–	+
ER	–	+
PR	–	+
p16	+	– or +
HPV DNA	+	–

References: [7, 20, 28, 52, 71, 80, 99, 110, 117, 164–167]

Table 16.28 Cervical minimal deviation adenocarcinoma of the mucinous type (adenoma malignum) vs. benign endocervical glandular lesions and cervical adenocarcinoma, NOS

Markers	MDA	BEGL	ACNOS
HIK 1083	+	– or +	–
PAX-2	–	+	–
p16	–	– or +	+
CEA-M	– or +	+	+
CEA-P	– or +	+	+
ER	–	–	–
PR	–	–	–
p53	– or +	–	– or +

Note: *MDA* minimal deviation adenocarcinoma of the mucinous type, *BEGL* benign endocervical glandular lesions, and *ACNOS* cervical adenocarcinoma, NOS

References: [42, 98, 100, 102, 116]

Table 16.29 Epithelioid trophoblastic tumor and cervical squamous cell carcinoma

Antibodies	Epithelioid trophoblastic tumor	Squamous cell carcinoma
Inhibin	+	–
HLA-G	+	–
CD146	+	–
p63	+	+
PLAP	+ or –	– or +
CK (AE1, AE3)	+	+
EMA/MUC1	+	+
AFP	–	–
Ki67	+	+
CEA-P	+	– or +

References: [1, 4, 86, 156]

Table 16.30 Cervical small cell carcinoma and neuroendocrine carcinoma

Antibodies	Cervical small cell carcinoma	Neuroendocrine carcinomas
CAM5.2	– or +	+
Pan-CK	– or +	+
Serotonin	– or +	+
Chromogranin A	+ or –	+
CEA-P	+	+ or –
NSE	+	+
CD99	–	– or +
CK (AE1, AE3)	+	+ or –
Rb	+	+ or –

References: [9, 89]

Table 16.31 Adenoid cystic carcinoma and basaloid squamous cell carcinoma of cervix

Antibodies	Adenoid cystic carcinoma	Basaloid squamous cell carcinoma
Vimentin	+	– or +
SMA	+	–
CEA-M	+	–
Actin-HHF-35	+ or –	–
CD117	+	+ or –
S100	+	– or +
p53	– or +	+ or –
CK8	+	–
CK14	+	+
CK19	+	+
CK (AE1, AE3)	+	+
EGFR	+	+
GFAP-15	–	–
CAM5.2	+	+
p63	+	+
Chromogranin A	–	–

References: [5, 23]

Table 16.32 Arias-Stella reaction and clear cell carcinoma of endometrium

Antibodies	Arias-Stella reaction	Clear cell carcinoma
MIB1	+ In less than 5% nuclei	+ In more than 5% nuclei
p53	+ In less than 25% nuclei	+ In more than 25% nuclei

References: [168, 169]

Table 16.33 Endometrial adenocarcinoma and carcinosarcoma (MMMT)

Antibodies	Adenocarcinoma	Carcinosarcoma
CD10	–	+ Usually M+C
CA125	+	–
Calretinin	–	– or +
CAM5.2	+ C	+ C
CEA-P	– or +	–
CK (AE1, AE3)	+	+
CK5/6	+ or –	–
CK7	+	+ or –
CK20	–	–
EMA	+	+
HepPar1	–	–
Inhibin	–	–
PLAP	– or +	– or +
S100	+	–
Thrombomodulin	–	–

References: [123, 147, 153]

Table 16.34 Clear cell carcinoma (CCC) vs. malignant neoplasms with clear cytoplasm (glycogen-rich squamous cell carcinoma (GRSCC), clear cell leiomyosarcoma (CCS), metastatic renal cell carcinoma (MCCRCC), and yolk sac tumor (YST))

Marker	CCC	GRSCC	CCS	MCCRCC	YST
Pan-CK	+	+	– or +		+
CK7	+	+	–	–	–
CK20	–	–	–	–	
BerEp4	+	+	–	–	
Vimentin	+	–	+	+	–
Desmin	–	–	–	–	–
MelanA	–	–	+	–	–
HMB45	–	–	+		–
S100		–	+	+	–
p16	+ or –	+	+ or –		
ER	– or +	–	– or +	–	–
PR	– or +	–	– or +	–	–
CEA	– or +	+	–	–	
p53	+ or –	–	– or +	–	
AFP	–	–	–	–	+
Glypican-3		–	–	–	+
CD10	–	–	– or +	+	–
RCC Ma	–	–	–	+	–

References: [6, 14, 47, 92, 120, 152, 168, 169]

Table 16.35 Endometrial serous vs. endometrioid adenocarcinoma

Antibodies	Serous	Endometrioid
p16	+	– or +
Beta-catenin	–	+ or –
IMP3	+	– or +
p53	+	– or +
ER	– or +	+
PR	– or +	+
Her2	– or +	– or +
BAX	– or +	+
CD44	– or +	+ or –
Vimentin	+	+
CK7	+	+
BerEP4	+	+
TTF1	– or +	– or +
Bcl2	+ or –	– or +
CEA-M	– or +	– or +
CK20	–	– or +

References: [6, 14, 21, 74, 122, 137]

Table 16.36 Leiomyosarcoma and endometrial stromal sarcoma (ESS)

Antibodies	Leiomyosarcoma	ESS
Actin-HHF-35	+	– or +
Bcl2	– or +	+
CD10	– or +	+
EGFR	– or +	+
Beta-catenin (N)[a]	–	+ or –
SMMHC[b]	+	+ or –
CK (AE1, AE3)	– or +	– or +
Vimentin	+	+
Desmin	+	– or +
SMA	+	+ or –
Calponin	+	+ or –
Cyclin-D1	+	– or +
ER	– or +	+
PR	– or +	+
CD99	– or +	–
WT1	– or +	+
p53	– or +	– or +
Pan-CK	– or +	– or +
EMA/MUC1	– or +	–
CAM5.2	– or +	– or +
Calretinin	–	– or +
S100	– or +	–
HMB45	– or +	–
ALK1	– or +	–
CD117	–	– or +
CD34	– or +	–
p63	– or +	–

Notes:

[a]*N* nuclear

[b]*SMMHC* smooth muscle myosin heavy chain

Additional negative markers for both tumors include: Myoglobin, HepPar-1, DOG-1, inhibin, and CD163

References: [3, 7, 13, 32, 33, 38, 40, 44, 50, 64, 69, 72, 75, 83, 94–96, 143, 145, 151, 153, 170]

Table 16.37 Leiomyosarcoma and PEComa

Antibodies	Leiomyosarcoma	PEComa
MelanA 103	–	+
FVIIIRAg	–	+
CD31	–	+
HMB45	– or +	+
S100	–	– or +
Vimentin	+	+
Desmin	+	+ or –
SMA	+	+
CD117	–	– or +
MITF	– or +	+
CD34	– or +	– or +
CD57	+	–
CD99	– or +	–
ER	– or +	– or +
PR	– or +	– or +
Tyrosinase	–	– or +
Pan-CK	– or +	–
EMA/MUC1	– or +	–
CK (AE1, AE3)	– or +	–
BerEP4	–	–
CAM5.2	– or +	–
ALK1	– or +	–
CD68	– or +	– or +
HepPar1	–	–
Calponin	+	+

References: [13, 38, 69, 149, 155]

Table 16.38 Complete hydatidiform and partial hydatidiform mole

Antibodies	Complete mole	Partial mole
p57 (N)	– or +	+

Note: *N* nuclear

References: [16, 19, 24, 94–96, 171–173]

Table 16.39 Epithelioid trophoblastic tumor and poorly differentiated endometrial adenocarcinoma

Antibodies	Epithelioid trophoblastic tumor	Poorly differentiated endometrial adenocarcinoma
Inhibin	+	–
HLA-G	+	–
E-cadherin	+	– or +
CEA-P	+	– or +
CD146	+	–
p63	+	– or +
Vimentin	–	+
EMA/MUC1	+	+
CK (AE1, AE3)	+	+
PLAP	+ or –	– or +
CD68	–	–
S100	–	+ or –
ER	+ or –	+ or –
EGFR	+	+ or –

References: [1, 2, 46, 156, 174]

Table 16.40 Differentiating placental site trophoblastic tumor and mimics

Marker	PSTT	EPS	ETT	CC	ESMT	MC	MM
HPL	+	+	– or +	+	–	–	–
CD146	+	+	– or +	+	–	–	–
HLA-G	+	+	+	+	–	–	–
CK (AE1, AE3)	+	+	+	+	+	+	–
CK18	+	+	+	+	– or +	+ or –	–
EMA	+	+	+	+	–	+	–
Inhibin	+	+	+	+	–	–	– or +
p63	–	+ or –	+	+ or –	–	+ or –	–
Beta-HCG	– or +	– or +	– or +	+	–	–	–
S100	–	–	–	–	+ or –	–	+
HMB45	–	–	–	–	+ or –	–	+
Ki67	+ >10%	<10%	+ or –	+ + +	+ or –	+	+ or –

EPS exaggerated placental site, *ETT* epithelioid trophoblastic tumor, *CC* Choriocarcinoma, *ESMT* epithelioid smooth muscle tumor, *MC* metastatic carcinoma, and *MM* malignant melanoma

References: [1, 2, 46, 66, 79, 86, 156, 158, 174–177]

Table 16.41 Summary of common markers of primary uterine carcinoma and the more common metastatic carcinomas

Marker	Cervix	Uterus	Ovary	Stomach	Breast	Colon	Kidney	Lung	Bladder
CK7	+	+	+	+	+	–	–	+	+
CK20	–	–	–	– or +	–	+	–	+	+ or –
CK5/6	+ or –	–	–	–	–	–	–	–	+
p63	+ or –	–	–	–	–	–	–	–	+
CK903	–	–	–	–	–	–	–	–	+
TTF1	–	–	–	–	–	–	–	+	–
CDX2	– or +	–	–	+ or –	–	+	–	–	–
ER	–	+	+	–	+	–	–	–	–
CD10	–	–	–	–	–	–	+	–	–
RCC Ma	–	–	–	–	–	–	+	–	–
Vimentin	–	+ or –	–	–	–	–	+	–	–

References: [22, 91, 124, 135, 178–180]

Note for All Tables

Note: "+" – usually greater than 70% of cases are positive; "–" – less than 5% of cases are positive; "+ or –" – usually more than 50% of cases are positive; "– or +" – less than 50% of cases are positive.

References

1. Kommoss F, Schmidt D, Coerdt W, Olert J, Muntefering H. Immunohistochemical expression analysis of inhibin-alpha and -beta subunits in partial and complete moles, trophoblastic tumors, and endometrial decidua. Int J Gynecol Pathol. 2001;20(4):380–5.
2. Daya D, Sabet L. The use of cytokeratin as a sensitive and reliable marker for trophoblastic tissue. Am J Clin Pathol. 1991;95(2): 137–41.
3. Rush DS, Tan J, Baergen RN, Soslow RA. h-Caldesmon, a novel smooth muscle-specific antibody, distinguishes between cellular leiomyoma and endometrial stromal sarcoma. Am J Surg Pathol. 2001;25(2):253–8.
4. Parwani AV, Smith Sehdev AE, Kurman RJ, Ronnett BM. Cervical adenoid basal tumors comprised of adenoid basal epithelioma associated with various types of invasive carcinoma: clinicopathologic features, human papillomavirus DNA detection, and P16 expression. Hum Pathol. 2005;36(1):82–90.
5. Grayson W, Taylor LF, Cooper K. Adenoid cystic and adenoid basal carcinoma of the uterine cervix: comparative morphologic, mucin, and immunohistochemical profile of two rare neoplasms of putative 'reserve cell' origin. Am J Surg Pathol. 1999;23(4):448–58.
6. Acs G, Pasha T, Zhang PJ. WT1 is differentially expressed in serous, endometrioid, clear cell, and mucinous carcinomas of the peritoneum, fallopian tube, ovary, and endometrium. Int J Gynecol Pathol. 2004;23(2):110–8.
7. Agoff SN, Grieco VS, Garcia R, Gown AM. Immunohistochemical distinction of endometrial stromal sarcoma and cellular leiomyoma. Appl Immunohistochem Mol Morphol. 2001;9(2):164–9.

8. Agoff SN, Lin P, Morihara J, Mao C, Kiviat NB, Koutsky LA. p16(INK4a) expression correlates with degree of cervical neoplasia: a comparison with Ki-67 expression and detection of high-risk HPV types. Mod Pathol. 2003;16(7):665–73.
9. Albores-Saavedra J, Latif S, Carrick KS, Alvarado-Cabrero I, Fowler MR. CD56 reactivity in small cell carcinoma of the uterine cervix. Int J Gynecol Pathol. 2005;24(2):113–7.
10. Ambros RA, Sherman ME, Zahn CM, Bitterman P, Kurman RJ. Endometrial intraepithelial carcinoma: a distinctive lesion specifically associated with tumors displaying serous differentiation. Hum Pathol. 1995;26(11):1260–7.
11. Atkins KA, Arronte N, Darus CJ, Rice LW. The use of p16 in enhancing the histologic classification of uterine smooth muscle tumors. Am J Surg Pathol. 2008;32(1):98–102.
12. Bayer-Garner IB, Korourian S. Plasma cells in chronic endometritis are easily identified when stained with syndecan-1. Mod Pathol. 2001;14(9):877–9.
13. Bodner-Adler B, Bodner K, Czerwenka K, Kimberger O, Leodolter S, Mayerhofer K. Expression of p16 protein in patients with uterine smooth muscle tumors: an immunohistochemical analysis. Gynecol Oncol. 2005;96(1):62–6.
14. Bussaglia E, del Rio E, Matias-Guiu X, Prat J. PTEN mutations in endometrial carcinomas: a molecular and clinicopathologic analysis of 38 cases. Hum Pathol. 2000;31(3):312–7.
15. Carcangiu ML, Dorji T, Radice P, et al. HNPCC-related endometrial carcinomas show a high frequency of non-endometroid types and of high FIGO grade endometrioid carcinomas. Mod Pathol. 2006;19:173A.
16. Castrillon DH, Sun D, Weremowicz S, Fisher RA, Crum CP, Genest DR. Discrimination of complete hydatidiform mole from its mimics by immunohistochemistry of the paternally imprinted gene product p57KIP2. Am J Surg Pathol. 2001;25(10):1225–30.
17. Cessna MH, Zhou H, Perkins SL, et al. Are myogenin and myoD1 expression specific for rhabdomyosarcoma? A study of 150 cases, with emphasis on spindle cell mimics. Am J Surg Pathol. 2001;25(9):1150–7.
18. Chu PG, Arber DA, Weiss LM, Chang KL. Utility of CD10 in distinguishing between endometrial stromal sarcoma and uterine smooth muscle tumors: an immunohistochemical comparison of 34 cases. Mod Pathol. 2001;14(5):465–71.
19. Crisp H, Burton JL, Stewart R, Wells M. Refining the diagnosis of hydatidiform mole: image ploidy analysis and p57KIP2 immunohistochemistry. Histopathology. 2003;43(4):363–73.
20. Dabbs DJ, Sturtz K, Zaino RJ. The immunohistochemical discrimination of endometrioid adenocarcinomas. Hum Pathol. 1996;27(2):172–7.
21. Darvishian F, Hummer AJ, Thaler HT, et al. Serous endometrial cancers that mimic endometrioid adenocarcinomas: a clinicopathologic and immunohistochemical study of a group of problematic cases. Am J Surg Pathol. 2004;28(12):1568–78.
22. Elishaev E, Gilks CB, Miller D, Srodon M, Kurman RJ, Ronnett BM. Synchronous and metachronous endocervical and ovarian neoplasms: evidence supporting interpretation of the ovarian neoplasms as metastatic endocervical adenocarcinomas simulating primary ovarian surface epithelial neoplasms. Am J Surg Pathol. 2005;29(3):281–94.
23. Emanuel P, Wang B, Wu M, Burstein DE. p63 Immunohistochemistry in the distinction of adenoid cystic carcinoma from basaloid squamous cell carcinoma. Mod Pathol. 2005;18(5):645–50.
24. Fukunaga M. Immunohistochemical characterization of p57(KIP2) expression in early hydatidiform moles. Hum Pathol. 2002;33(12):1188–92.
25. Goldblum JR, Hart WR. Perianal Paget's disease: a histologic and immunohistochemical study of 11 cases with and without associated rectal adenocarcinoma. Am J Surg Pathol. 1998;22(2):170–9.
26. Henderson GS, Brown KA, Perkins SL, Abbott TM, Clayton F. bcl-2 is down-regulated in atypical endometrial hyperplasia and adenocarcinoma. Mod Pathol. 1996;9(4):430–8.
27. Hurrell DP, McCluggage WG. Uterine leiomyosarcoma with HMB45+ clear cell areas: report of two cases. Histopathology. 2005;47(5):540–2.
28. Ishikawa M, Fujii T, Masumoto N, et al. Correlation of p16INK4A overexpression with human papillomavirus infection in cervical adenocarcinomas. Int J Gynecol Pathol. 2003;22(4):378–85.
29. Klein WM, Kurman RJ. Lack of expression of c-kit protein (CD117) in mesenchymal tumors of the uterus and ovary. Int J Gynecol Pathol. 2003;22(2):181–4.
30. Kurihara S, Oda Y, Ohishi Y, et al. Endometrial stromal sarcomas and related high-grade sarcomas: immunohistochemical and molecular genetic study of 31 cases. Am J Surg Pathol. 2008;32(8):1228–38.
31. Lax SF, Pizer ES, Ronnett BM, Kurman RJ. Comparison of estrogen and progesterone receptor, Ki-67, and p53 immunoreactivity in uterine endometrioid carcinoma and endometrioid carcinoma with squamous, mucinous, secretory, and ciliated cell differentiation. Hum Pathol. 1998;29(9):924–31.
32. Leitao MM, Soslow RA, Nonaka D, et al. Tissue microarray immunohistochemical expression of estrogen, progesterone, and androgen receptors in uterine leiomyomata and leiomyosarcoma. Cancer. 2004;101(6):1455–62.
33. Loddenkemper C, Mechsner S, Foss HD, et al. Use of oxytocin receptor expression in distinguishing between uterine smooth muscle tumors and endometrial stromal sarcoma. Am J Surg Pathol. 2003;27(11):1458–62.
34. McCluggage WG. Immunohistochemical and functional biomarkers of value in female genital tract lesions. In: Robboy SJ, Mutter GL, Prat J, Bentley R, Russell P, Anderson MC, editors. Robboy's pathology of the female reproductive tract. 2nd ed. Churchill Livingstone: London; 2009. p. 999–1010.
35. Mikami Y, Kiyokawa T, Hata S, et al. Gastrointestinal immunophenotype in adenocarcinomas of the uterine cervix and related glandular lesions: a possible link between lobular endocervical glandular hyperplasia/pyloric gland metaplasia and 'adenoma malignum'. Mod Pathol. 2004;17(8):962–72.
36. Mittal K. Utility of MIB-1 in evaluating cauterized cervical cone biopsy margins. Int J Gynecol Pathol. 1999;18(3):211–4.
37. Nascimento AF, Hirsch MS, Cviko A, Quade BJ, Nucci MR. The role of CD10 staining in distinguishing invasive endometrial adenocarcinoma from adenocarcinoma involving adenomyosis. Mod Pathol. 2003;16(1):22–7.
38. Norton AJ, Thomas JA, Isaacson PG. Cytokeratin-specific monoclonal antibodies are reactive with tumours of smooth muscle derivation. An immunocytochemical and biochemical study using antibodies to intermediate filament cytoskeletal proteins. Histopathology. 1987;11(5):487–99.
39. Oliva E. Pure mesenchymal and mixed mullerian tumors of the uterus. In: Nucci MR, Oliva E, editors. Gynecologic pathology. London: Churchill Livingstone Elsevier; 2009. p. 261–327.
40. Oliva E. CD10 expression in the female genital tract: does it have useful diagnostic applications? Adv Anat Pathol. 2004;11(6):310–5.
41. O'Neill CJ, McBride HA, Connolly LE, McCluggage WG. Uterine leiomyosarcomas are characterized by high p16, p53 and MIB1 expression in comparison with usual leiomyomas, leiomyoma variants and smooth muscle tumours of uncertain malignant potential. Histopathology. 2007;50(7):851–8.
42. Park KJ, Bramlage MP, Ellenson LH, Pirog EC. Immunoprofile of adenocarcinomas of the endometrium, endocervix, and ovary with mucinous differentiation. Appl Immunohistochem Mol Morphol. 2009;17(1):8–11.

43. Quade BJ, Yang A, Wang Y, et al. Expression of the p53 homologue p63 in early cervical neoplasia. Gynecol Oncol. 2001;80(1):24–9.
44. Raspollini MR, Paglierani M, Taddei GL, Villanucci A, Amunni G, Taddei A. The protooncogene c-KIT is expressed in leiomyosarcomas of the uterus. Gynecol Oncol. 2004;93(3):718.
45. Shi J, Liu H, Wilkerson M, et al. Evaluation of p16INK4a, minichromosome maintenance protein 2, DNA topoisomerase IIalpha, ProEX C, and p16INK4a/ProEX C in cervical squamous intraepithelial lesions. Hum Pathol. 2007;38(9):1335–44.
46. Shih IM, Kurman RJ. p63 expression is useful in the distinction of epithelioid trophoblastic and placental site trophoblastic tumors by profiling trophoblastic subpopulations. Am J Surg Pathol. 2004;28(9):1177–83.
47. Silva EG, Young RH. Endometrioid neoplasms with clear cells: a report of 21 cases in which the alteration is not of typical secretory type. Am J Surg Pathol. 2007;31(8):1203–8.
48. Sumathi VP, McCluggage WG. CD10 is useful in demonstrating endometrial stroma at ectopic sites and in confirming a diagnosis of endometriosis. J Clin Pathol. 2002;55(5):391–2.
49. Vang R, Kempson RL. Perivascular epithelioid cell tumor ('PEComa') of the uterus: a subset of HMB-45-positive epithelioid mesenchymal neoplasms with an uncertain relationship to pure smooth muscle tumors. Am J Surg Pathol. 2002;26(1):1–13.
50. Wang L, Felix JC, Lee JL, et al. The proto-oncogene c-kit is expressed in leiomyosarcomas of the uterus. Gynecol Oncol. 2003;90(2):402–6.
51. Yaziji H, Gown AM. Immunohistochemical analysis of gynecologic tumors. Int J Gynecol Pathol. 2001;20(1):64–78.
52. Zaino RJ. The fruits of our labors: distinguishing endometrial from endocervical adenocarcinoma. Int J Gynecol Pathol. 2002;21(1):1–3.
53. Zheng W, Cao P, Zheng M, Kramer EE, Godwin TA. p53 overexpression and bcl-2 persistence in endometrial carcinoma: comparison of papillary serous and endometrioid subtypes. Gynecol Oncol. 1996;61(2):167–74.
54. Disep B, Innes BA, Cochrane HR, Tijani S, Bulmer JN. Immunohistochemical characterization of endometrial leucocytes in endometritis. Histopathology. 2004;45(6):625–32.
55. Euscher E, Nuovo GJ. Detection of kappa- and lambda-expressing cells in the endometrium by in situ hybridization. Int J Gynecol Pathol. 2002;21(4):383–90.
56. Gendler SJ, Spicer AP. Epithelial mucin genes. Annu Rev Physiol. 1995;57:607–34.
57. Heatley MK. Cytokeratins and cytokeratin staining in diagnostic histopathology. Histopathology. 1996;28(5):479–83.
58. Kim MA, Lee HS, Yang HK, Kim WH. Cytokeratin expression profile in gastric carcinomas. Hum Pathol. 2004;35(5):576–81.
59. Leong AS, Vinyuvat S, Leong FJ, et al. Anti-CD38 and VS38 antibodies for detection of plasma cells in the diagnosis of chronic endometritis. Appl Immunohistochem. 1997;5:189.
60. McCluggage WG. Recent advances in immunohistochemistry in gynaecological pathology. Histopathology. 2002;40(4):309–26.
61. Moll R, Franke WW, Schiller DL, Geiger B, Krepler R. The catalog of human cytokeratins: patterns of expression in normal epithelia, tumors and cultured cells. Cell. 1982;31(1):11–24.
62. Quddus MR, Sung CJ, Zheng W, Lauchlan SC. p53 immunoreactivity in endometrial metaplasia with dysfunctional uterine bleeding. Histopathology. 1999;35(1):44–9.
63. Sano T, Oyama T, Kashiwabara K, Fukuda T, Nakajima T. Expression status of p16 protein is associated with human papillomavirus oncogenic potential in cervical and genital lesions. Am J Pathol. 1998;153(6):1741–8.
64. Adegboyega PA, Qiu S. Immunohistochemical profiling of cytokeratin expression by endometrial stroma sarcoma. Hum Pathol. 2008;39(10):1459–64.
65. Mylonas I, Makovitzky J, Friese K, Jeschke U. Immunohistochemical labelling of steroid receptors in normal and malignant human endometrium. Acta Histochem. 2009;111(4):349–59.
66. Al-Hussaini M, Stockman A, Foster H, McCluggage WG. WT-1 assists in distinguishing ovarian from uterine serous carcinoma and in distinguishing between serous and endometrioid ovarian carcinoma. Histopathology. 2004;44(2):109–15.
67. Alkushi A, Lim P, Coldman A, Huntsman D, Miller D, Gilks CB. Interpretation of p53 immunoreactivity in endometrial carcinoma: establishing a clinically relevant cut-off level. Int J Gynecol Pathol. 2004;23(2):129–37.
68. Amant F, Steenkiste E, Schurmans K, et al. Immunohistochemical expression of CD10 antigen in uterine adenosarcoma. Int J Gynecol Cancer. 2004;14(6):1118–21.
69. Brown DC, Theaker JM, Banks PM, Gatter KC, Mason DY. Cytokeratin expression in smooth muscle and smooth muscle tumours. Histopathology. 1987;11(5):477–86.
70. Cameron RI, Maxwell P, Jenkins D, McCluggage WG. Immunohistochemical staining with MIB1, bcl2 and p16 assists in the distinction of cervical glandular intraepithelial neoplasia from tubo-endometrial metaplasia, endometriosis and microglandular hyperplasia. Histopathology. 2002;41(4):313–21.
71. Castrillon DH, Lee KR, Nucci MR. Distinction between endometrial and endocervical adenocarcinoma: an immunohistochemical study. Int J Gynecol Pathol. 2002;21(1):4–10.
72. Chu P, Wu E, Weiss LM. Cytokeratin 7 and cytokeratin 20 expression in epithelial neoplasms: a survey of 435 cases. Mod Pathol. 2000;13(9):962–72.
73. Coosemans A, Nik SA, Caluwaerts S, et al. Upregulation of Wilms' tumour gene 1 (WT1) in uterine sarcomas. Eur J Cancer. 2007;43(10):1630–7.
74. Egan JA, Ionescu MC, Eapen E, Jones JG, Marshall DS. Differential expression of WT1 and p53 in serous and endometrioid carcinomas of the endometrium. Int J Gynecol Pathol. 2004;23(2): 119–22.
75. Farhood AI, Abrams J. Immunohistochemistry of endometrial stromal sarcoma. Hum Pathol. 1991;22(3):224–30.
76. Hameed A, Miller DS, Muller CY, Coleman RL, Albores-Saavedra J. Frequent expression of beta-human chorionic gonadotropin (beta-hCG) in squamous cell carcinoma of the cervix. Int J Gynecol Pathol. 1999;18(4):381–6.
77. Kalof AN, Evans MF, Simmons-Arnold L, Beatty BG, Cooper K. p16INK4A immunoexpression and HPV in situ hybridization signal patterns: potential markers of high-grade cervical intraepithelial neoplasia. Am J Surg Pathol. 2005;29(5):674–9.
78. Keating JT, Cviko A, Riethdorf S, et al. Ki-67, cyclin E, and p16INK4 are complimentary surrogate biomarkers for human papilloma virus-related cervical neoplasia. Am J Surg Pathol. 2001;25(7):884–91.
79. Mao TL, Kurman RJ, Huang CC, Lin MC, Shih I. Immunohistochemistry of choriocarcinoma: an aid in differential diagnosis and in elucidating pathogenesis. Am J Surg Pathol. 2007;31(11):1726–32.
80. Marjoniemi VM. Immunohistochemistry in gynaecological pathology: a review. Pathology. 2004;36(2):109–19.
81. Mittal K, Mesia A, Demopoulos RI. MIB-1 expression is useful in distinguishing dysplasia from atrophy in elderly women. Int J Gynecol Pathol. 1999;18(2):122–4.
82. McCluggage WG, Oliva E, Herrington CS, McBride H, Young RH. CD10 and calretinin staining of endocervical glandular lesions, endocervical stroma and endometrioid adenocarcinomas of the uterine corpus: CD10 positivity is characteristic of, but not specific for, mesonephric lesions and is not specific for endometrial stroma. Histopathology. 2003;43(2):144–50.
83. Nucci MR, O'Connell JT, Huettner PC, Cviko A, Sun D, Quade BJ. h-Caldesmon expression effectively distinguishes endometrial

stromal tumors from uterine smooth muscle tumors. Am J Surg Pathol. 2001;25(4):455–63.
84. Negri G, Egarter-Vigl E, Kasal A, Romano F, Haitel A, Mian C. p16INK4a is a useful marker for the diagnosis of adenocarcinoma of the cervix uteri and its precursors: an immunohistochemical study with immunocytochemical correlations. Am J Surg Pathol. 2003;27(2):187–93.
85. Qiu W, Mittal K. Comparison of morphologic and immunohistochemical features of cervical microglandular hyperplasia with low-grade mucinous adenocarcinoma of the endometrium. Int J Gynecol Pathol. 2003;22(3):261–5.
86. Rabban JT, Soslow R, Zaloudek C. Immunohistochemistry of the female genital tract. In: Dabbs DJ, editor. Diagnostic immunohistochemistry, theranostic and genomic applications. 3rd ed. Philadelphia: Elsevier Saunders; 2010. p. 690–720.
87. Schwartz EJ, Longacre TA. Adenomatoid tumors of the female and male genital tracts express WT1. Int J Gynecol Pathol. 2004;23(2):123–8.
88. Suresh UR, Hale RJ, Fox H, Buckley CH. Use of proliferation cell nuclear antigen immunoreactivity for distinguishing hydropic abortions from partial hydatidiform moles. J Clin Pathol. 1993;46(1):48–50.
89. Wang HL, Lu DW. Detection of human papillomavirus DNA and expression of p16, Rb, and p53 proteins in small cell carcinomas of the uterine cervix. Am J Surg Pathol. 2004;28(7):901–8.
90. Wang TY, Chen BF, Yang YC, et al. Histologic and immunophenotypic classification of cervical carcinomas by expression of the p53 homologue p63: a study of 250 cases. Hum Pathol. 2001;32(5):479–86.
91. Werling RW, Yaziji H, Bacchi CE, Gown AM. CDX2, a highly sensitive and specific marker of adenocarcinomas of intestinal origin: an immunohistochemical survey of 476 primary and metastatic carcinomas. Am J Surg Pathol. 2003;27(3):303–10.
92. Yamamoto S, Tsuda H, Aida S, Shimazaki H, Tamai S, Matsubara O. Immunohistochemical detection of hepatocyte nuclear factor 1beta in ovarian and endometrial clear-cell adenocarcinomas and nonneoplastic endometrium. Hum Pathol. 2007;38(7):1074–80.
93. Zheng W, Khurana R, Farahmand S, Wang Y, Zhang ZF, Felix JC. p53 immunostaining as a significant adjunct diagnostic method for uterine surface carcinoma: precursor of uterine papillary serous carcinoma. Am J Surg Pathol. 1998;22(12):1463–73.
94. Iwata J, Fletcher CD. Immunohistochemical detection of cytokeratin and epithelial membrane antigen in leiomyosarcoma: a systematic study of 100 cases. Pathol Int. 2000;50(1):7–14.
95. Fukunaga M, Nomura K, Endo Y, Ushigome S, Aizawa S. Carcinosarcoma of the uterus with extensive neuroectodermal differentiation. Histopathology. 1996;29(6):565–70.
96. Kanamori T, Takakura K, Mandai M, Kariya M, Fukuhara K, Sakaguchi M, et al. Increased expression of calcium-binding protein S100 in human uterine smooth muscle tumours. Mol Hum Reprod. 2004;10(10):735–42.
97. Liang SX, Patel K, Pearl M, Liu J, Zheng W, Tornos C. Sertoliform endometrioid carcinoma of the endometrium with dual immunophenotypes for epithelial membrane antigen and inhibin alpha: case report and literature review. Int J Gynecol Pathol. 2007;26(3): 291–7.
98. Xu JY, Hashi A, Kondo T, et al. Absence of human papillomavirus infection in minimal deviation adenocarcinoma and lobular endocervical glandular hyperplasia. Int J Gynecol Pathol. 2005;24(3):296–302.
99. Cina SJ, Richardson MS, Austin RM, Kurman RJ. Immunohistochemical staining for Ki-67 antigen, carcinoembryonic antigen, and p53 in the differential diagnosis of glandular lesions of the cervix. Mod Pathol. 1997;10(3):176–80.
100. Rabban JT, McAlhany S, Lerwill MF, Grenert JP, Zaloudek CJ. PAX2 distinguishes benign mesonephric and mullerian glandular lesions of the cervix from endocervical adenocarcinoma, including minimal deviation adenocarcinoma. Am J Surg Pathol. 2010;34(2):137–46.
101. Chekmareva M, Ellenson LH, Pirog EC. Immunohistochemical differences between mucinous and microglandular adenocarcinomas of the endometrium and benign endocervical epithelium. Int J Gynecol Pathol. 2008;27(4):547–54.
102. Mikami Y, Hata S, Fujiwara K, Imajo Y, Kohno I, Manabe T. Florid endocervical glandular hyperplasia with intestinal and pyloric gland metaplasia: worrisome benign mimic of "adenoma malignum". Gynecol Oncol. 1999;74(3):504–11.
103. Klaes R, Benner A, Friedrich T, et al. p16INK4a immunohistochemistry improves interobserver agreement in the diagnosis of cervical intraepithelial neoplasia. Am J Surg Pathol. 2002;26(11):1389–99.
104. Klaes R, Friedrich T, Spitkovsky D, et al. Overexpression of p16 (INK4A) as a specific marker for dysplastic and neoplastic epithelial cells of the cervix uteri. Int J Cancer. 2002;92:276.
105. Kruse AJ, Baak JP, Helliesen T, Kjellevold KH, Bol MG, Janssen EA. Evaluation of MIB-1-positive cell clusters as a diagnostic marker for cervical intraepithelial neoplasia. Am J Surg Pathol. 2002;26(11):1501–7.
106. Nucci MR, Castrillon DH, Bai H, et al. Biomarkers in diagnostic obstetric and gynecologic pathology: a review. Adv Anat Pathol. 2003;10(2):55–68.
107. McCluggage WG, Buhidma M, Tang L, Maxwell P, Bharucha H. Monoclonal antibody MIB1 in the assessment of cervical squamous intraepithelial lesions. Int J Gynecol Pathol. 1996;15(2):131–6.
108. Tringler B, Gup CJ, Singh M, et al. Evaluation of p16INK4a and pRb expression in cervical squamous and glandular neoplasia. Hum Pathol. 2004;35(6):689–96.
109. Lee KR, Sun D, Crum CP. Endocervical intraepithelial glandular atypia (dysplasia): a histopathologic, human papillomavirus, and MIB-1 analysis of 25 cases. Hum Pathol. 2000;31(6):656–64.
110. O'Neill CJ, McCluggage WG. p16 expression in the female genital tract and its value in diagnosis. Adv Anat Pathol. 2006;13(1): 8–15.
111. Pirog EC, Isacson C, Szabolcs MJ, Kleter B, Quint W, Richart RM. Proliferative activity of benign and neoplastic endocervical epithelium and correlation with HPV DNA detection. Int J Gynecol Pathol. 2002;21(1):22–6.
112. Horn LC, Richter CE, Einenkel J, Tannapfel A, Liebert UG, Leo C. p16, p14, p53, cyclin D1, and steroid hormone receptor expression and human papillomaviruses analysis in primary squamous cell carcinoma of the endometrium. Ann Diagn Pathol. 2006;10(4):193–6.
113. Wang NP, Zee S, Zarbo RJ, et al. Coordinate expression of cytokeratins 7 and 20 definte unique subsets of carcinomas. Appl Immunohistochem. 1995;3:99.
114. Riethdorf L, Riethdorf S, Lee KR, Cviko A, Loning T, Crum CP. Human papillomaviruses, expression of p16, and early endocervical glandular neoplasia. Hum Pathol. 2002;33(9):899–904.
115. Thamboo TP, Wee A. Hep Par 1 expression in carcinoma of the cervix: implications for diagnosis and prognosis. J Clin Pathol. 2004;57(1):48–53.
116. Gilks CB, Young RH, Aguirre P, DeLellis RA, Scully RE. Adenoma malignum (minimal deviation adenocarcinoma) of the uterine cervix. A clinicopathological and immunohistochemical analysis of 26 cases. Am J Surg Pathol. 1989;13(9):717–29.
117. Mikami Y, Kiyokawa T, Moriya T, Sasano H. Immunophenotypic alteration of the stromal component in minimal deviation adenocarcinoma ("adenoma malignum") and endocervical glandular hyperplasia: a study using oestrogen receptor and alpha-smooth muscle actin double immunostaining. Histopathology. 2005;46(2):130–6.
118. Utsugi K, Hirai Y, Takeshima N, Akiyama F, Sakurai S, Hasumi K. Utility of the monoclonal antibody HIK1083 in the diagnosis of

adenoma malignum of the uterine cervix. Gynecol Oncol. 1999;75(3):345–8.

119. Ordi J, Nogales FF, Palacin A, et al. Mesonephric adenocarcinoma of the uterine corpus: CD10 expression as evidence of mesonephric differentiation. Am J Surg Pathol. 2001;25(12):1540–5.

120. Ordi J, Romagosa C, Tavassoli FA, et al. CD10 expression in epithelial tissues and tumors of the gynecologic tract: a useful marker in the diagnosis of mesonephric, trophoblastic, and clear cell tumors. Am J Surg Pathol. 2003;27(2):178–86.

121. Silver SA, Devouassoux-Shisheboran M, Mezzetti TP, Tavassoli FA. Mesonephric adenocarcinomas of the uterine cervix: a study of 11 cases with immunohistochemical findings. Am J Surg Pathol. 2001;25(3):379–87.

122. Chiesa-Vottero AG, Malpica A, Deavers MT, Broaddus R, Nuovo GJ, Silva EG. Immunohistochemical overexpression of p16 and p53 in uterine serous carcinoma and ovarian high-grade serous carcinoma. Int J Gynecol Pathol. 2007;26(3):328–33.

123. Fukuchi T, Sakamoto M, Tsuda H, Maruyama K, Nozawa S, Hirohashi S. Beta-catenin mutation in carcinoma of the uterine endometrium. Cancer Res. 1998;58(16):3526–8.

124. Goldstein NS, Uzieblo A. WT1 immunoreactivity in uterine papillary serous carcinomas is different from ovarian serous carcinomas. Am J Clin Pathol. 2002;117(4):541–5.

125. Lax SF, Kendall B, Tashiro H, Slebos RJ, Hedrick L. The frequency of p53, K-ras mutations, and microsatellite instability differs in uterine endometrioid and serous carcinoma: evidence of distinct molecular genetic pathways. Cancer. 2000;88(4):814–24.

126. Mutter GL, Ince TA, Baak JP, Kust GA, Zhou XP, Eng C. Molecular identification of latent precancers in histologically normal endometrium. Cancer Res. 2001;61(11):4311–4.

127. Pallares J, Bussaglia E, Martinez-Guitarte JL, et al. Immunohistochemical analysis of PTEN in endometrial carcinoma: a tissue microarray study with a comparison of four commercial antibodies in correlation with molecular abnormalities. Mod Pathol. 2005;18(5):719–27.

128. Peiro G, Diebold J, Lohse P, et al. Microsatellite instability, loss of heterozygosity, and loss of hMLH1 and hMSH2 protein expression in endometrial carcinoma. Hum Pathol. 2002;33(3):347–54.

129. Schlosshauer PW, Ellenson LH, Soslow RA. Beta-catenin and E-cadherin expression patterns in high-grade endometrial carcinoma are associated with histological subtype. Mod Pathol. 2002;15(10):1032–7.

130. Siami K, McCluggage WG, Ordonez NG, et al. Thyroid transcription factor-1 expression in endometrial and endocervical adenocarcinomas. Am J Surg Pathol. 2007;31(11):1759–63.

131. Soslow RA, Shen PU, Chung MH, Isacson C, Baergen RN. Cyclin D1 expression in high-grade endometrial carcinomas–association with histologic subtype. Int J Gynecol Pathol. 2000;19(4):329–34.

132. Tashiro H, Blazes MS, Wu R, et al. Mutations in PTEN are frequent in endometrial carcinoma but rare in other common gynecological malignancies. Cancer Res. 1997;57(18):3935–40.

133. Wani Y, Notohara K, Saegusa M, Tsukayama C. Aberrant Cdx2 expression in endometrial lesions with squamous differentiation: important role of Cdx2 in squamous morula formation. Hum Pathol. 2008;39(7):1072–9.

134. Dupont J, Wang X, Marshall DS, et al. Wilms tumor gene (WT1) and p53 expression in endometrial carcinomas: a study of 130 cases using a tissue microarray. Gynecol Oncol. 2004;94(2):449–55.

135. Hashi A, Yuminamochi T, Murata S, Iwamoto H, Honda T, Hoshi K. Wilms tumor gene immunoreactivity in primary serous carcinomas of the fallopian tube, ovary, endometrium, and peritoneum. Int J Gynecol Pathol. 2003;22(4):374–7.

136. Liang SX, Chambers SK, Cheng L, Zhang S, Zhou Y, Zheng W. Endometrial glandular dysplasia: a putative precursor lesion of uterine papillary serous carcinoma. Part II: molecular features. Int J Surg Pathol. 2004;12(4):319–31.

137. McCluggage WG. WT1 is of value in ascertaining the site of origin of serous carcinomas within the female genital tract. Int J Gynecol Pathol. 2004;23(2):97–9.

138. Sherman ME, Bitterman P, Rosenshein NB, Delgado G, Kurman RJ. Uterine serous carcinoma. A morphologically diverse neoplasm with unifying clinicopathologic features. Am J Surg Pathol. 1992;16(6):600–10.

139. Slomovitz BM, Broaddus RR, Burke TW, et al. Her-2/neu overexpression and amplification in uterine papillary serous carcinoma. J Clin Oncol. 2004;22(15):3126–32.

140. Tashiro H, Isacson C, Levine R, Kurman RJ, Cho KR, Hedrick L. p53 gene mutations are common in uterine serous carcinoma and occur early in their pathogenesis. Am J Pathol. 1997;150(1):177–85.

141. Zheng W, Yi X, Fadare O, et al. The oncofetal protein IMP3: a novel biomarker for endometrial serous carcinoma. Am J Surg Pathol. 2008;32(2):304–15.

142. Lax SF, Pizer ES, Ronnett BM, Kurman RJ. Clear cell carcinoma of the endometrium is characterized by a distinctive profile of p53, Ki-67, estrogen, and progesterone receptor expression. Hum Pathol. 1998;29(6):551–8.

143. Jung CK, Jung JH, Lee A, et al. Diagnostic use of nuclear beta-catenin expression for the assessment of endometrial stromal tumors. Mod Pathol. 2008;21(6):756–63.

144. McCluggage WG, Sumathi VP, Maxwell P. CD10 is a sensitive and diagnostically useful immunohistochemical marker of normal endometrial stroma and of endometrial stromal neoplasms. Histopathology. 2001;39(3):273–8.

145. Oliva E, Young RH, Clement PB, Bhan AK, Scully RE. Cellular benign mesenchymal tumors of the uterus. A comparative morphologic and immunohistochemical analysis of 33 highly cellular leiomyomas and six endometrial stromal nodules, two frequently confused tumors. Am J Surg Pathol. 1995;19(7):757–68.

146. Sumathi VP, Al-Hussaini M, Connolly LE, Fullerton L, McCluggage WG. Endometrial stromal neoplasms are immunoreactive with WT-1 antibody. Int J Gynecol Pathol. 2004;23(3):241–7.

147. Mikami Y, Hata S, Kiyokawa T, Manabe T. Expression of CD10 in malignant mullerian mixed tumors and adenosarcomas: an immunohistochemical study. Mod Pathol. 2002;15(9):923–30.

148. Soslow RA, Ali A, Oliva E. Mullerian adenosarcomas: an immunophenotypic analysis of 35 cases. Am J Surg Pathol. 2008;32(7):1013–21.

149. Gannon BR, Manduch M, Childs TJ. Differential immunoreactivity of p16 in leiomyosarcomas and leiomyoma variants. Int J Gynecol Pathol. 2008;27(1):68–73.

150. Mittal K, Demopoulos RI. MIB-1 (Ki-67), p53, estrogen receptor, and progesterone receptor expression in uterine smooth muscle tumors. Hum Pathol. 2001;32(9):984–7.

151. Oliva E, Clement PB, Young RH. Epithelioid endometrial and endometrioid stromal tumors: a report of four cases emphasizing their distinction from epithelioid smooth muscle tumors and other oxyphilic uterine and extrauterine tumors. Int J Gynecol Pathol. 2002;21(1):48–55.

152. Silva EG, Deavers MT, Bodurka DC, Malpica A. Uterine epithelioid leiomyosarcomas with clear cells: reactivity with HMB-45 and the concept of PEComa. Am J Surg Pathol. 2004;28(2):244–9.

153. Winter 3rd WE, Seidman JD, Krivak TC, et al. Clinicopathological analysis of c-kit expression in carcinosarcomas and leiomyosarcomas of the uterine corpus. Gynecol Oncol. 2003;91(1):3–8.

154. Otis CN. Uterine adenomatoid tumors: immunohistochemical characteristics with emphasis on Ber-EP4 immunoreactivity and

distinction from adenocarcinoma. Int J Gynecol Pathol. 1996;15(2):146–51.

155. Fadare O. Perivascular epithelioid cell tumors (PEComas) and smooth muscle tumors of the uterus. Am J Surg Pathol. 2007;31(9): 1454–5.

156. Mao TL, Seidman JD, Kurman RJ, Shih I. Cyclin E and p16 immunoreactivity in epithelioid trophoblastic tumor – an aid in differential diagnosis. Am J Surg Pathol. 2006;30(9):1105–10.

157. McCluggage WG, Ashe P, McBride H, Maxwell P, Sloan JM. Localization of the cellular expression of inhibin in trophoblastic tissue. Histopathology. 1998;32(3):252–6.

158. Shih IM, Kurman RJ. The pathology of intermediate trophoblastic tumors and tumor-like lesions. Int J Gynecol Pathol. 2001;20(1):31–47.

159. Singer G, Kurman RJ, McMaster MT, Shih I. HLA-G immunoreactivity is specific for intermediate trophoblast in gestational trophoblastic disease and can serve as a useful marker in differential diagnosis. Am J Surg Pathol. 2002;26(7):914–20.

160. Pirog EC, Baergen RN, Soslow RA, et al. Diagnostic accuracy of cervical low-grade squamous intraepithelial lesions is improved with MIB-1 immunostaining. Am J Surg Pathol. 2002;26(1): 70–5.

161. McCluggage WG, Maxwell P. bcl-2 and p21 immunostaining of cervical tubo-endometrial metaplasia. Histopathology. 2002;40(1): 107–8.

162. McCluggage WG, Maxwell P, McBride HA, Hamilton PW, Bharucha H. Monoclonal antibodies Ki-67 and MIB1 in the distinction of tuboendometrial metaplasia from endocervical adenocarcinoma and adenocarcinoma in situ in formalin-fixed material. Int J Gynecol Pathol. 1995;14(3):209–16.

163. Marques T, Andrade LA, Vassallo J. Endocervical tubal metaplasia and adenocarcinoma in situ: role of immunohistochemistry for carcinoembryonic antigen and vimentin in differential diagnosis. Histopathology. 1996;28(6):549–50.

164. McCluggage WG, Sumathi VP, McBride HA, Patterson A. A panel of immunohistochemical stains, including carcinoembryonic antigen, vimentin, and estrogen receptor, aids the distinction between primary endometrial and endocervical adenocarcinomas. Int J Gynecol Pathol. 2002;21(1):11–5.

165. Kamoi S, AlJuboury MI, Akin MR, Silverberg SG. Immunohistochemical staining in the distinction between primary endometrial and endocervical adenocarcinomas: another viewpoint. Int J Gynecol Pathol. 2002;21(3):217–23.

166. McCluggage WG, Jenkins D. Immunohistochemical staining with p16 may assist in the distinction between endometrial and endocervical adenocarcinoma. Int J Gynecol Pathol. 2003;22:128.

167. Staebler A, Sherman ME, Zaino RJ, Ronnett BM. Hormone receptor immunohistochemistry and human papillomavirus in situ hybridization are useful for distinguishing endocervical and endometrial adenocarcinomas. Am J Surg Pathol. 2002;26(8):998–1006.

168. Vang R, Whitaker BP, Farhood AI, Silva EG, Ro JY, Deavers MT. Immunohistochemical analysis of clear cell carcinoma of the gynecologic tract. Int J Gynecol Pathol. 2001;20(3):252–9.

169. Vang R, Barner R, Wheeler DT, Strauss BL. Immunohistochemical staining for Ki-67 and p53 helps distinguish endometrial Arias-Stella reaction from high-grade carcinoma, including clear cell carcinoma. Int J Gynecol Pathol. 2004;23(3):223–33.

170. Oliva E, Young RH, Amin MB, Clement PB. An immunohistochemical analysis of endometrial stromal and smooth muscle tumors of the uterus: a study of 54 cases emphasizing the importance of using a panel because of overlap in immunoreactivity for individual antibodies. Am J Surg Pathol. 2002;26(4):403–12.

171. Fisher RA, Hodges MD, Rees HC, et al. The maternally transcribed gene p57(KIP2) (CDNK1C) is abnormally expressed in both androgenetic and biparental complete hydatidiform moles. Hum Mol Genet. 2002;11(26):3267–72.

172. Jun SY, Ro JY, Kim KR. p57kip2 is useful in the classification and differential diagnosis of complete and partial hydatidiform moles. Histopathology. 2003;43(1):17–25.

173. Sebire NJ, Rees HC, Peston D, Seckl MJ, Newlands ES, Fisher RA. p57(KIP2) immunohistochemical staining of gestational trophoblastic tumours does not identify the type of the causative pregnancy. Histopathology. 2004;45(2):135–41.

174. Ben-Izhak O, Stark P, Levy R, Bergman R, Lichtig C. Epithelial markers in malignant melanoma. A study of primary lesions and their metastases. Am J Dermatopathol. 1994;16(3):241–6.

175. Shih IM, Kurman RJ. Immunohistochemical localization of inhibin-alpha in the placenta and gestational trophoblastic lesions. Int J Gynecol Pathol. 1999;18(2):144–50.

176. Shih IM, Kurman RJ. Ki-67 labeling index in the differential diagnosis of exaggerated placental site, placental site trophoblastic tumor, and choriocarcinoma: a double immunohistochemical staining technique using Ki-67 and Mel-CAM antibodies. Hum Pathol. 1998;29(1):27–33.

177. Wong SC, Chan AT, Chan JK, Lo YM. Nuclear beta-catenin and Ki-67 expression in choriocarcinoma and its pre-malignant form. J Clin Pathol. 2006;59(4):387–92.

178. Irving JA, Catasus L, Gallardo A, et al. Synchronous endometrioid carcinomas of the uterine corpus and ovary: alterations in the beta-catenin (CTNNB1) pathway are associated with independent primary tumors and favorable prognosis. Hum Pathol. 2005;36(6):605–19.

179. Cappellari JO, Geisinger KR, Albertson DA, Wolfman NT, Kute TE. Malignant papillary cystic tumor of the pancreas. Cancer. 1990;66(1):193–8.

180. Lagendijk JH, Mullink H, Van Diest PJ, Meijer GA, Meijer CJ. Tracing the origin of adenocarcinomas with unknown primary using immunohistochemistry: differential diagnosis between colonic and ovarian carcinomas as primary sites. Hum Pathol. 1998;29(5):491–7.

Chapter 17
Ovary

Jeffrey Prichard, Haiyan Liu, and Myra Wilkerson

Abstract Although the majority of ovarian tumors are diagnosed purely on morphologic findings, this chapter identifies specific opportunities for the application of immunohistochemistry to the diagnosis of ovarian surface epithelial tumors, sex cord–stromal tumors, and germ cells tumors. This chapter addresses the use of newer markers such as SALL4 in yolk sac tumors and PAX8 in serous, clear cell and endometrioid carcinomas. Special attention is paid to ovarian versus appendiceal mucinous tumors in pseudomyxoma peritonei, metastatic Krukenberg tumors, and the differential diagnosis of primary and metastatic clear cell tumors. Illustrations demonstrate differential staining patterns such as is seen with p16 in müllerian tumors.

Keywords Ovary • Germ cell • Sex cord • Krukenberg • Pseudomyxoma • Granulosa • Serous • Clear cell • Endometrioid • Mucinous • Thecoma • Sertoli • Leydig • hCG • Inhibin • OCT4 • p16 • PAX8 • PLAP • SALL4 • WT1

FREQUENTLY ASKED QUESTIONS

Surface Epithelial Tumors

Sex Cord–Stromal Tumors

J. Prichard (✉)
Department of Pathology and Laboratory Medicine, Geisinger Medical Center, 100 N. Academy Ave, Danville, PA 17822, USA
e-mail: jwprichard@geisinger.edu

F. Lin and J. Prichard (eds.), *Handbook of Practical Immunohistochemistry: Frequently Asked Questions*,
DOI 10.1007/978-1-4419-8062-5_17, © Springer Science+Business Media, LLC 2011

26. The differentiation of diffuse adult granulose cell tumor (AGCT) versus endometrioid stromal sarcoma (ESS, primary or metastasis from uterus) (Fig. 17.29 and Table 17.26) (p. 293)
27. The differentiation of granulosa cell tumor (GCT) versus small cell carcinoma (SCC) versus undifferentiated carcinoma, nonsmall cell (neuroendocrine) type (UC) (Table 17.27) (p. 293)
28. The differentiation of Sertoli cell tumor (SCT) versus endometrioid tumor (EMT) versus carcinoid tumor (CT) (Table 17.28) (p. 294)

Germ Cell Tumors

29. Summary of markers in germ cell tumors of the ovary (Table 17.29) (p. 294)
30. Germ cell tumors versus ovarian adenocarcinoma (Table 17.30) (p. 294)
31. Yolk sac tumor versus clear cell carcinoma (Fig. 17.30 and Table 17.31) (p. 295)

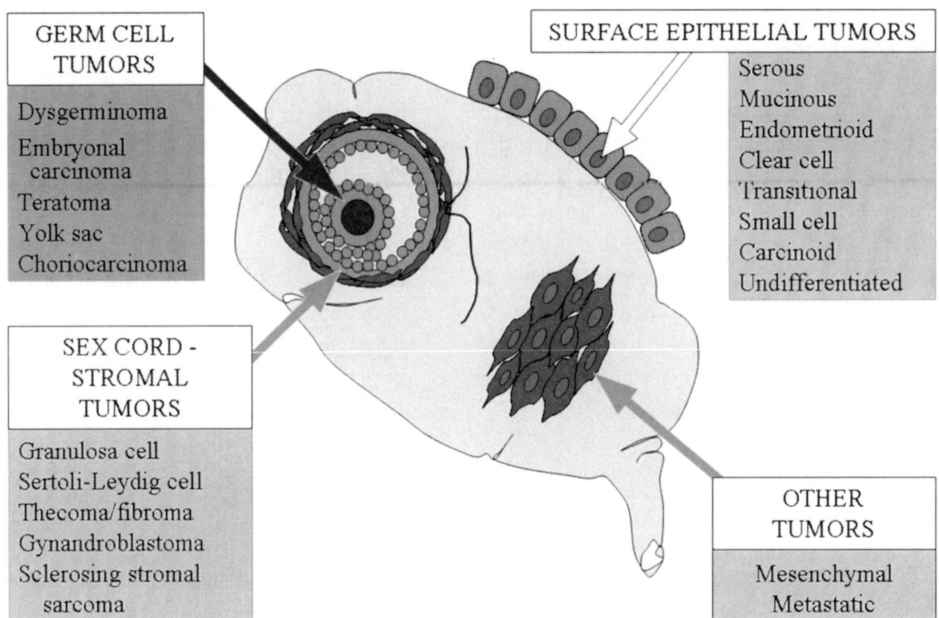

Fig. 17.1 The great diversity of tumor types that can arise from the ovary can be overwhelming to comprehend and diagnose. Being aware of the relationship between the different ovarian cell types and their corresponding tumors can help to put the challenge into perspective. The vast majority of ovarian tumor diagnoses are based on morphologic findings. But IHC has a role to play most frequently in the differential diagnoses between primary and metastatic carcinomas. The most elegant use of IHC may be in the differential diagnosis of germ cell tumors, most of which are shared with the testes and addressed more fully in Chap. 21

Table 17.1 Summary of uses and limitations of useful markers in ovarian pathology

Antibodies	Staining pattern	Function	Key applications and pitfalls
AE1/AE3	M, C	Intermediate filament in cytoskeleton	Pan-cytokeratin cocktail to identify epithelial tumors including most germ cell tumors except dysgerminoma. Typically does not stain sex cord–stromal tumor, but can stain 30–60% of granulosa cell tumors
AFP	C	Protein produced by fetal yolk sac, gastrointestinal epithelium, and liver	Useful marker in germ cell tumors, but also present in hepatocellular carcinoma and hepatoid ovarian carcinoma
CA-125	C	Transmembrane glycoprotein	Of limited value in ovarian IHC due to the lack of specificity. May stain both primary and metastatic epithelial tumors. Is negative in sex cord stromal tumors and germ cell tumors
Calretinin	C, N	Calcium binding protein	Used as a marker for mesothelioma in differential with carcinomas. May be positive in sex cord stromal tumors but is not specific and not as sensitive as inhibin
CAM5.2	M, C	LMWCK, simple keratin peptide, recognize CK8, and CK18	Low molecular weight cytokeratin used in combination with AE1/AE3 to screen for epithelial differentiation. Granulosa cell tumors may be positive as well

(continued)

Table 17.1 (continued)

Antibodies	Staining pattern	Function	Key applications and pitfalls
CD30	M, C	Transmembrane glycoprotein	Useful in diagnosis of embryonal carcinoma, but may be positive in anaplastic large cell lymphoma and Reed–Sternberg cells
CEA	C	Cell surface glycoprotein; produced by fetal gut epithelium; plays a role in cell adhesion	Adenocarcinoma-related marker more commonly expressed in metastatic tumors in the ovary. Rarely positive in serous carcinoma. May be positive in primary mucinous tumors
Chromogranin	C	Main protein extract of neuroendocrine granules of neuroendocrine cells	A neuroendocrine marker for carcinoid tumor, more specific than Synaptophysin
CK7	C	Intermediate filament protein in cytoskeleton	Expressed in all primary ovarian epithelial tumors and most metastatic adenocarcinomas except in gastrointestinal tract and prostate gland. Negativity in ovarian carcinoma suggests metastasis
CK8	C	Intermediate filament protein in cytoskeleton	Expressed in nonsquamous epithelium and in most adenocarcinomas
CK20	C	Intermediate filament protein in cytoskeleton	Expressed in gastrointestinal epithelium, urothelium, and Merkel cells. May be found in mucinous and transitional tumors of the ovary. Other primary epithelial tumors are negative
c-kit	M, C	Transmembrane glycoprotein receptor kinase	Commonly expressed in dysgerminoma, but may also be seen in renal carcinoma. Negative in embryonal carcinoma
D2-40	C, M	Oncofetal transmembrane mucoprotein	Expressed by fetal germ cells and germ cell tumors. Will also stain lymphatic endothelium and mesothelial cells
EMA	C, M	A transmembrane glycoprotein	A general epithelial marker, with increased expression in carcinomas. An important negative marker of sex cord–stromal tumors of ovary
ER	N	A nuclear protein belongs to steroid receptor family	Expressed in many serous and endometrioid tumors and some clear cell tumors of the ovary. Also often present in breast cancer metastatic to the ovary
hCG	C	Glycoprotein produced by syncytiotrophoblast	Seen diffusely in choriocarcinoma and focally in other germ cell tumors containing syncytiotrophoblasts
INHA	C	A glycoprotein (32 kDa) involving in regulation of the pituitary–gonadal feedback system. Inhibits release of follicle stimulating hormone	A sensitive and relatively specific marker of sex cord–stromal tumors of ovary. Luteinized stromal cells are reactive. Also produced by syncytiotrophoblast and adrenal neoplasms
MOC31	M	Membranous glycoprotein commonly found in carcinomas, lacking in mesotheliomas	MOC31 is expressed in most all adenocarcinoma. Not present in mesothelioma
MART-1	C	A melanocyte-specific transmembrane protein	Commonly used as a melanocytic marker. Steroid cell tumors are the only sex cord–stromal tumor reactive to MART-1
NSE	C	Neuronal form of a glycolytic enzyme	Expressed in germ cell tumors, and also in tumors of neural and neuroendocrine origin
OCT4	N	Stem cell transcriptional regulator	Useful in germ cell tumors
p16	C	Involved in cell cycle regulation	Expressed strongly and diffusely in endocervical carcinoma, but only patchy in endometrioid and serous carcinomas
p53	N	Tumor suppressor protein that plays a role in apoptosis, genetic stability, and inhibition of angiogenesis	In the ovary, p53 used strongly expressed in serous carcinomas and used to distinguish serous carcinoma from other primary epithelial tumors
PAX8	N	Member of the paired box (PAX) family of transcription factors involved in thyroid follicular cell development and expression of thyroid-specific genes	Marker associated with thyroid follicular tumors, but in the ovary strongly stains serous, clear cell, and endometrioid carcinomas
PLAP	C, M	Enzyme produced by syncytiotrophoblast	Useful in germ cell tumors; however, less specific than OCT4. PLAP is also in many carcinomas
PR	N	A nuclear protein belongs to steroid receptor family	Used similar to ER but less sensitive. Expressed in many serous and endometrioid tumors and some clear cell tumors of the ovary. Also often present in breast cancer metastatic to the ovary
SALL4	N	Sall4 modulates embryonic stem cell pluripotency and early embryonic development by the transcriptional regulation of Pou5f1	Useful for marking yolk sac tumor

(continued)

Table 17.1 (continued)

Antibodies	Staining pattern	Function	Key applications and pitfalls
SF1	N	A nuclear transcription factor regulates steroidogenesis and gonad/adrenal gland development	Claimed the most sensitive marker for sex cord–stromal tumor (SCST) lineage. Reported 100% of SCSTs are positive for SF1
Synaptophysin	C	A glycoprotein in neuroendocrine secretory granules	A sensitive broad-spectrum neuroendocrine marker
TM	M, C	Endothelial cell-associated cofactor for thrombin-mediated activator of protein C	Urothelial marker, and also positive in mesothelium, vascular tumors, and squamous cell carcinoma
UPIII	M, C	Urothelial transmembrane protein	Marker for Brenner tumor and transitional cell tumors. Only the luminal aspect of the umbrella cells should stain in normal urothelium, but entire membrane will stain in urothelial carcinoma
Vim	C	Intermediate filament in cytoskeleton	Coexpression of vimentin with epithelial markers occurs in both endometrioid and serous tumor of the ovary
WT1	C, N	Transcription factor involved in gonadal development	Positive in both serous and mesothelial tumors. Positive in all types of sex cord–stromal tumor except thecoma

Note: *N* nuclear staining, *M* membranous staining, *C* cytoplasmic staining, *SF1* steroidogenic factor 1 or adrenal 4-binding protein

References: [1–18]

Table 17.2 Markers for serous tumors

Antibody	Literature	GML data (*N* = 34)
AE1/AE3	+	100% (34/34)
BerEP4	+	97% (33/34)
CA125	+	79% (27/24)
Calretinin	−/+	24% (8/34)
CD56	−	9% (3/34)
CDX2	−	0% (0/34)
CEA	−	6% (2/34)
CK5/6	−	3% (1/34)
CK7	+	94% (32/34)
CK20	−	3% (1/34), focal
D2-40	−	0% (0/34)
ER	+/−	82% (28/34)
GCDFP-15	−	0% (0/34)
Glypican-3	−	0% (0/34)
HepPar1	−	0% (0/34)
IMP(KOC)	−	26% (9/34)
INHA	−	0% (0/34)
KIM-1	−	0% (0/34)
MOC31	+	100% (34/34)
MUC1	ND	82% (28/34)
MUC2	ND	0% (0/34)
MUC4	ND	11% (34)
MUC5AC	ND	0% (0/34)
NapsinA	ND	3% (1/34)
OCT4	−	0% (0/34)
p16	−	35% (12/34)
P504S	−	3% (1/34)
p53	−/+	29% (10/29)
PAX2	+	32% (11/34)
PAX8	+	85% (29/34)
PR	+/−	50%(17/34)
RCC	−	0% (0/34)
S100	−	0% (0/34)
TAG72	+	12% (4/34)
TTF1	−	0% (0/34)
VHL	ND	6% (2/34)
Vimentin	+	79% (27/34)
WT1	+	44% (15/34)

Note: *ND* no data

Serous tumors express PAX8 and epithelial markers including AE1/AE3, BerEP4, CK7, MOC31 in almost all cases. CA125 is slightly less sensitive as a screening marker. Mesothelial marker, calretinin, is present in some serous tumors but in a focal pattern. CEA is expressed in only few serous tumors. ER and PR are present in the majority of serous tumors. IMP3 (KOC), p16, and p53 are seen only in malignant serous tumors. PAX2 is expressed in serous adenomas and lacking in serous carcinomas. WT-1 is seen more frequently in malignant serous tumors

Examples of serous carcinoma staining are demonstrated in Figs. 17.2–17.10

References: [1–4, 19–27]

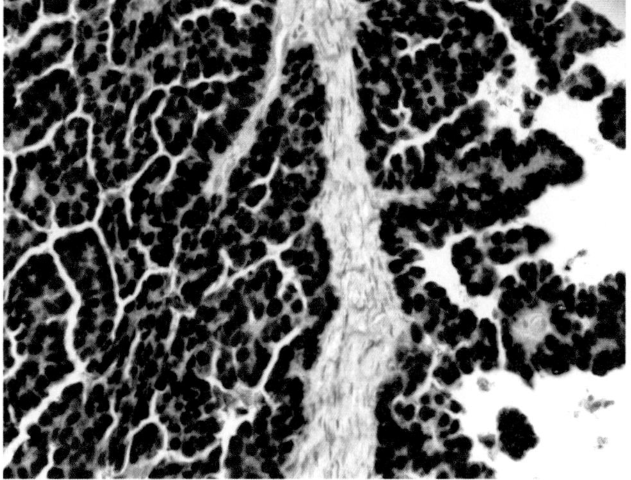

Fig. 17.2 Serous carcinoma – Strong diffuse nuclear staining with PAX 2

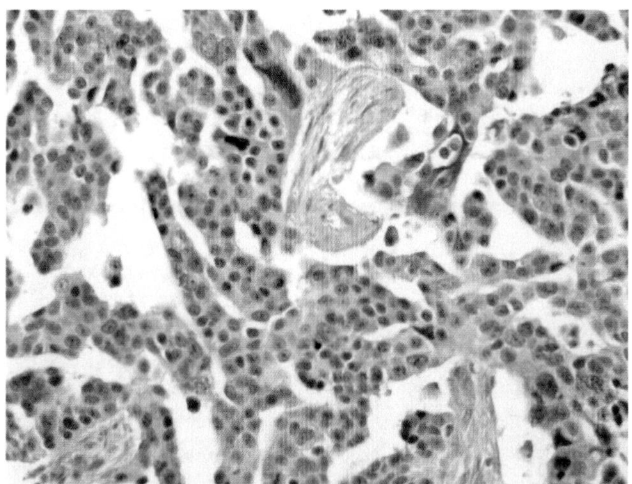

Fig. 17.3 Serous carcinoma – Diffuse nuclear staining with WT1

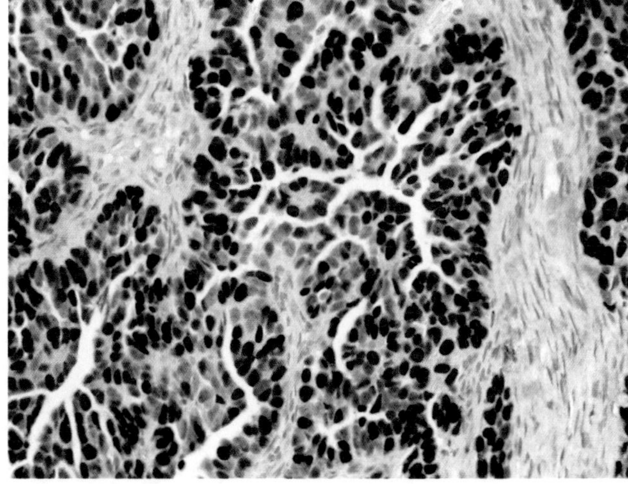

Fig. 17.4 Serous carcinoma – Strong diffuse nuclear staining with p53

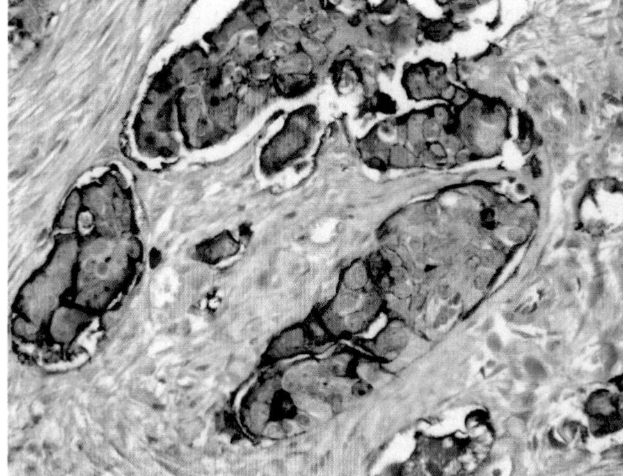

Fig. 17.5 Serous carcinoma – Strong cytoplasmic staining with PAX 2

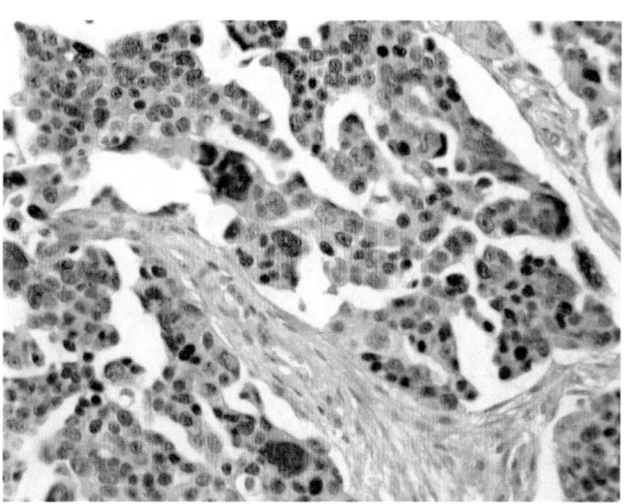

Fig. 17.6 Serous carcinoma – Diffuse nuclear staining with estrogen receptor

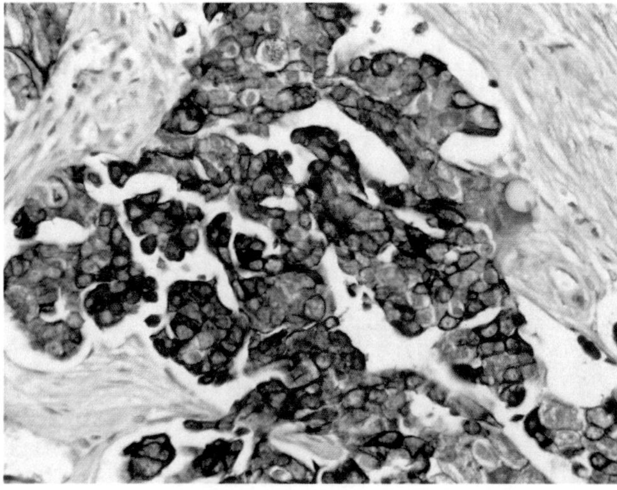

Fig. 17.7 Serous carcinoma – Strong cytoplasmic staining with CK7

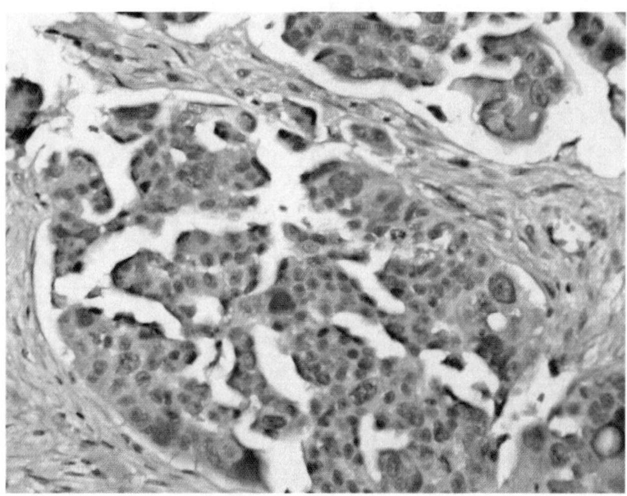

Fig. 17.8 Serous carcinoma – Negative staining with CK20

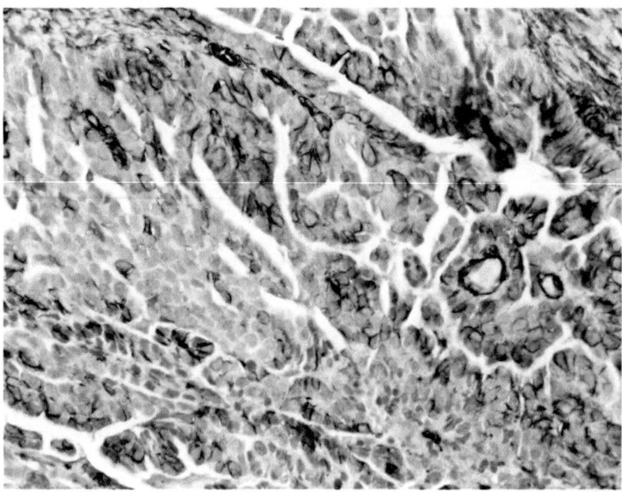

Fig. 17.9 Serous carcinoma – Variable cytoplasmic staining with vimentin

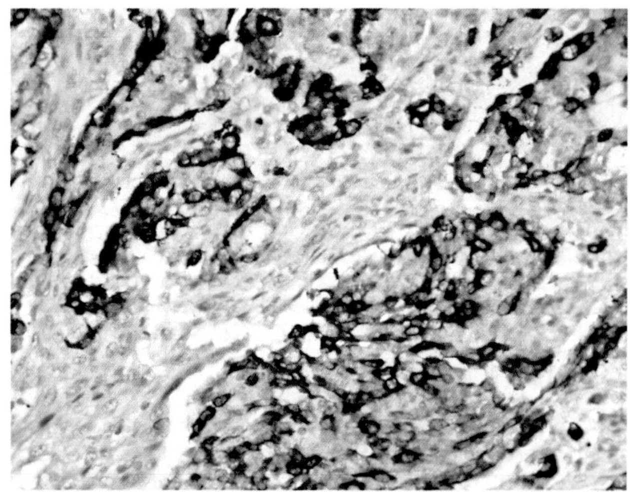

Fig. 17.10 Serous carcinoma – Variable cytoplasmic staining with MUC-4

Table 17.3 Markers for mucinous tumors

Antibody	Literature	GML data (*N* = 15)
AE1/AE3	+	100% (15/15)
BerEP4	+	87% (13/15)
CA125	–/+	33% (5/15)
Calretinin		20% (3/15)
CDX2	–/+	13% (2/15)
CEA	+/–	40% (6/15)
CK5/6	–	0% (0/15)
CK7	+	80% (12/15)
CK19	+	93% (14/15)
CK20	–/+	20% (3/15)
D2-40	–	0% (0/15)
ER	–/+	20% (3/15)
GCDFP-15	–	0% (0/15)
Glypican-3	–	7% (1/15)
HepPar1	–	7% (1/15)
IMP(KOC)	ND	20% (3/15)
INHA	–	0% (0/15)
KIM-1	ND	0% (0/15)
MOC31	+	100% (15/15)
MUC1	+	47% (7/15)
MUC2	+/–	7% (1/15)
MUC4	+/–	53% (8/15)
MUC5AC	+	47% (7/15)
NapsinA	ND	7% (1/15)
OCT4	–	0% (0/15)
p16	–/+	47% (7/15)
P504S	ND	20% (3/15)
p53	–/+	13% (2/15)
PAX2	ND	13% (2/15)
PAX8	–	40% (6/15)
RCC	–	0% (0/15)
S100	–	0% (0/15)
TTF1	–	0% (0/15)
VHL	ND	7% (1/15)
Vimentin	–	0% (0/15)
WT1	–	0% (0/15)

Note: *ND* no data

Mucinous ovarian tumors lack PAX8 but express epithelial markers including AE1/AE3, BerEP4, CK7, MOC31 in almost all cases. Ovarian mucinous tumors may express cytokeratin 20 but only in a focal pattern. CA125 and hormone receptors stain only a minority of mucinous ovarian tumors. Examples of mucinous tumor staining are demonstrated in Figs. 17.11–17.14

CK 20 is patchy when present

References: [1–4, 19, 28–34]

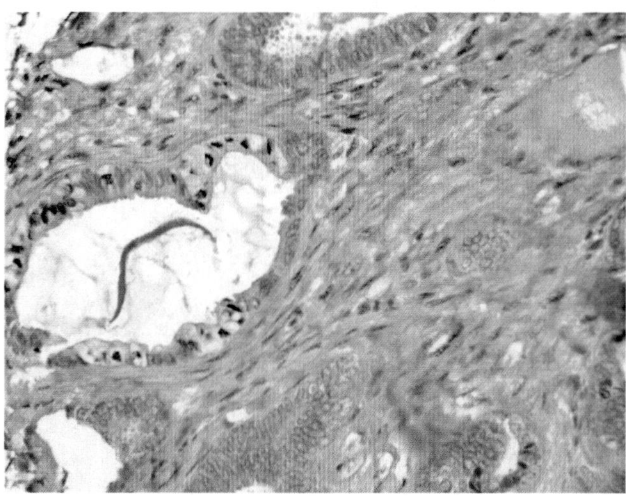

Fig. 17.11 Mucinous adenoma – Variable nuclear staining with estrogen receptor

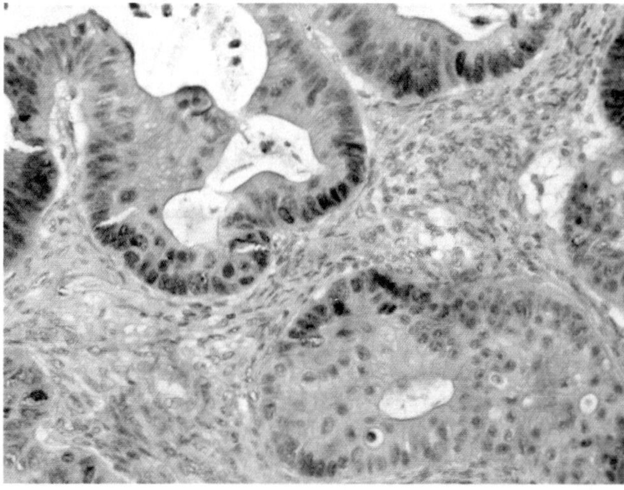

Fig. 17.12 Mucinous carcinoma – Strong nuclear staining with CDX-2

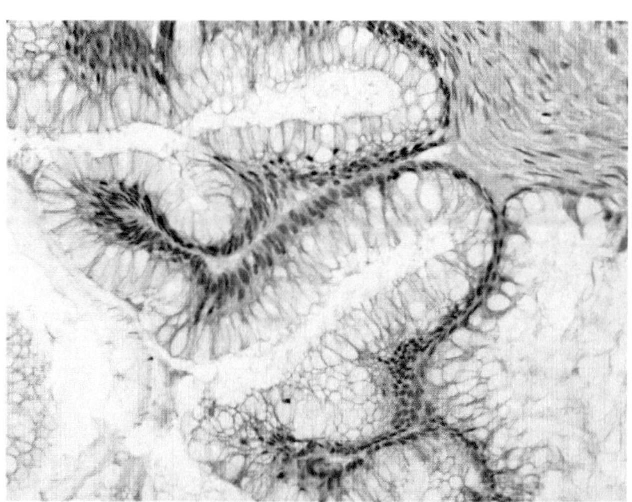

Fig. 17.13 Mucinous carcinoma – Nuclear CDX-2 staining in this well-differentiated mucinous carcinoma

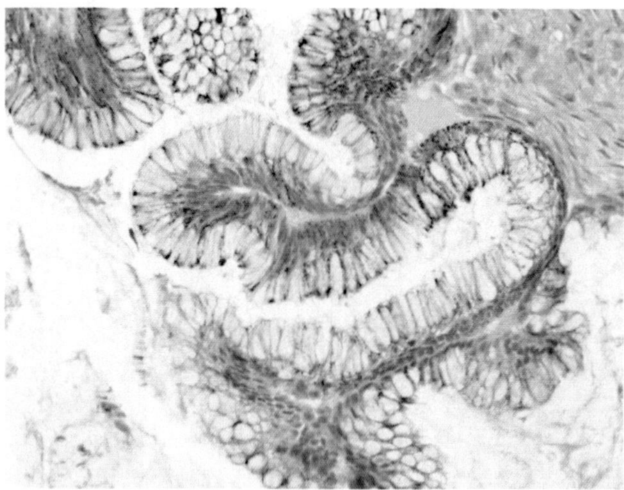

Fig. 17.14 Mucinous carcinoma – Uncharacteristic Heppar-1 staining occurred in this well-differentiated mucinous carcinoma

Table 17.4 Markers for clear cell carcinoma

Antibody	Literature
CK7	+
VHL	+
KIM-1	+
RCC	–/+
PAX8	+
CD15	+
p53	– or +
CK20	–
CD10	–
Inhibin-alpha	–
WT1	–
Glypican 3	+ or –
SALL4	–/+
ER	–/+

Note: *OCCC* ovarian clear cell carcinoma

Clear cell carcinomas of the ovary also express PAX 8 and epithelial marker common to ovarian epithelial tumors including AE1/AE3, CK7, and MOC31. Hormone receptors are expressed less commonly than in serous or endometrioid tumors. SALL4 is a useful marker in distinction between yolk sac tumor from ovarian clear cell carcinoma; it was reported that only 3 of 45. Examples of clear cell carcinoma staining are demonstrated in Figs. 17.15–17.18

References: [1–4, 19, 24, 25, 35–37]

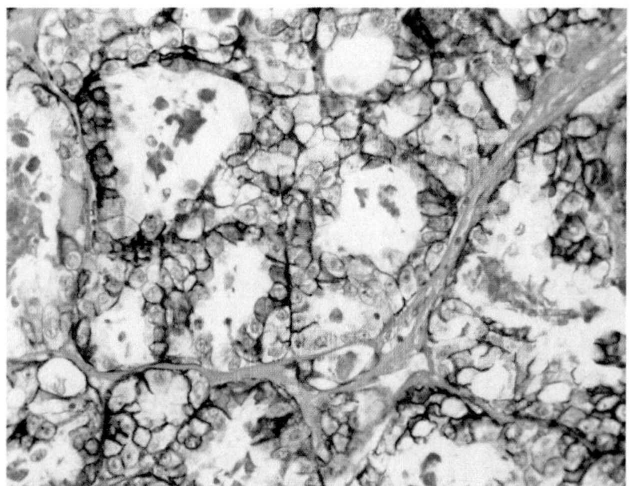

Fig. 17.15 Ovarian clear cell carcinoma – Strong cytoplasmic staining with pVHL. A marker shared with renal clear cell carcinoma

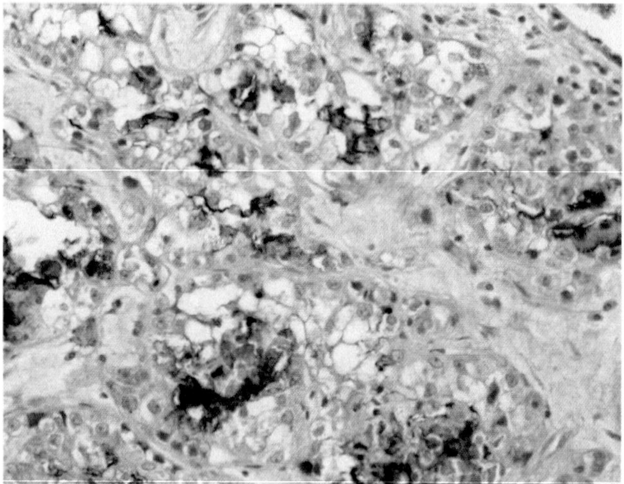

Fig. 17.16 Ovarian clear cell carcinoma – Variable cytoplasmic staining with CA125

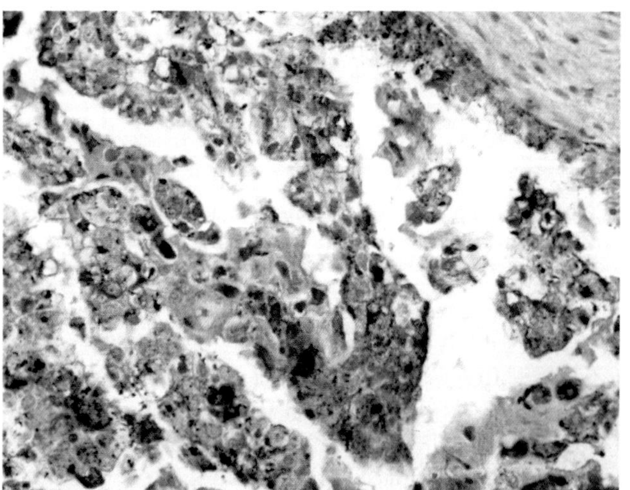

Fig. 17.17 Ovarian clear cell carcinoma – This positive staining for napsin A was unexpected in this ovarian clear cell carcinoma

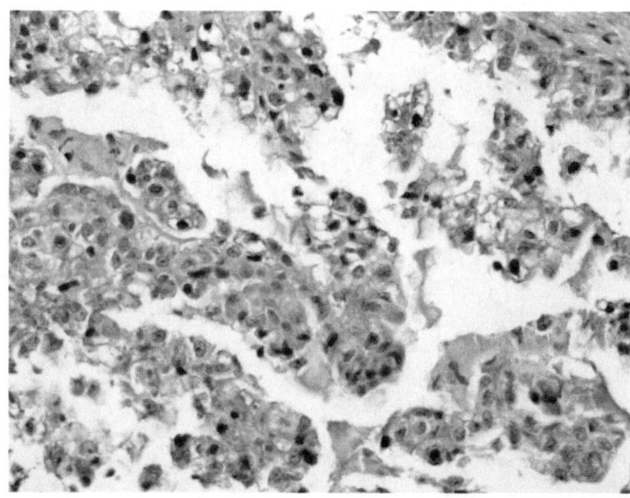

Fig. 17.18 Ovarian clear cell carcinoma – Negative TTF-1 staining in the same tumor seen in Fig. 17.17

Table 17.5 Markers for ovarian endometrioid carcinoma

Antibody	Literature
CK7	+
CK20	–
ER	+
P16	+ (patchy)
HPV-IS	–
WT1	–
P53	–/+

HPV-IS human papilloma virus in situ hybridization

Note: Ovarian endometrioid carcinomas have similar immunophenotype to the uterine endometrioid carcinoma. Endometrioid carcinomas share the frequent expression of PAX8 with serous and clear cell types. Low-grade endometrioid tumors usually strongly express hormone receptor proteins. Diffuse strong p53 staining is uncommon but may be seen in high-grade tumors. Negative HPV-IS and patchy rather than diffuse p16 staining distinguish endometrioid from endocervical carcinoma. Examples of endometrioid carcinoma staining are demonstrated in Figs. 17.19 and 17.20

References: [1–4, 38, 39]

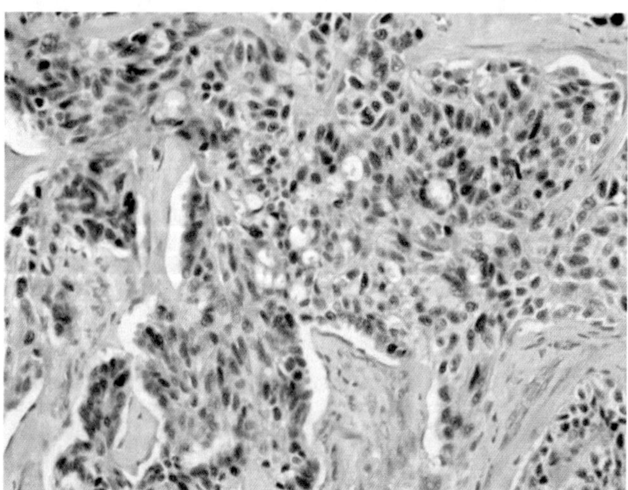

Fig. 17.19 Endometrioid carcinoma – Diffuse nuclear staining with estrogen receptor

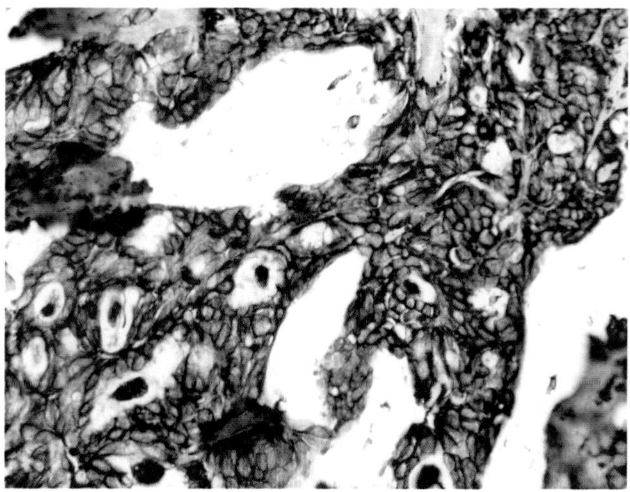

Fig. 17.20 Endometrioid carcinoma – Diffuse cytoplasmic staining with vimentin

Table 17.6 Differential panel for common ovarian epithelial tumors

Antibodies	WT1	p53	ER
Serous	+	+	+/–
Clear cell	–	+	–/+
Intestinal type mucinous	–	–/+	–
Endometrioid	–	–/+	+
Transitional	+	+	–

Note: A screening panel combining WT1, p53, and ER can distinguish among most types of primary surface epithelial carcinomas. WT1 staining identifies serous or transitional types. Endometrioid lacks WT-1 and the diffuse p53 staining of serous carcinoma and often strongly expresses ER. Additional specific markers for each type can be used to confirm any differentiation in question. Figure 17.21 shows the differential staining of WT1 I this group

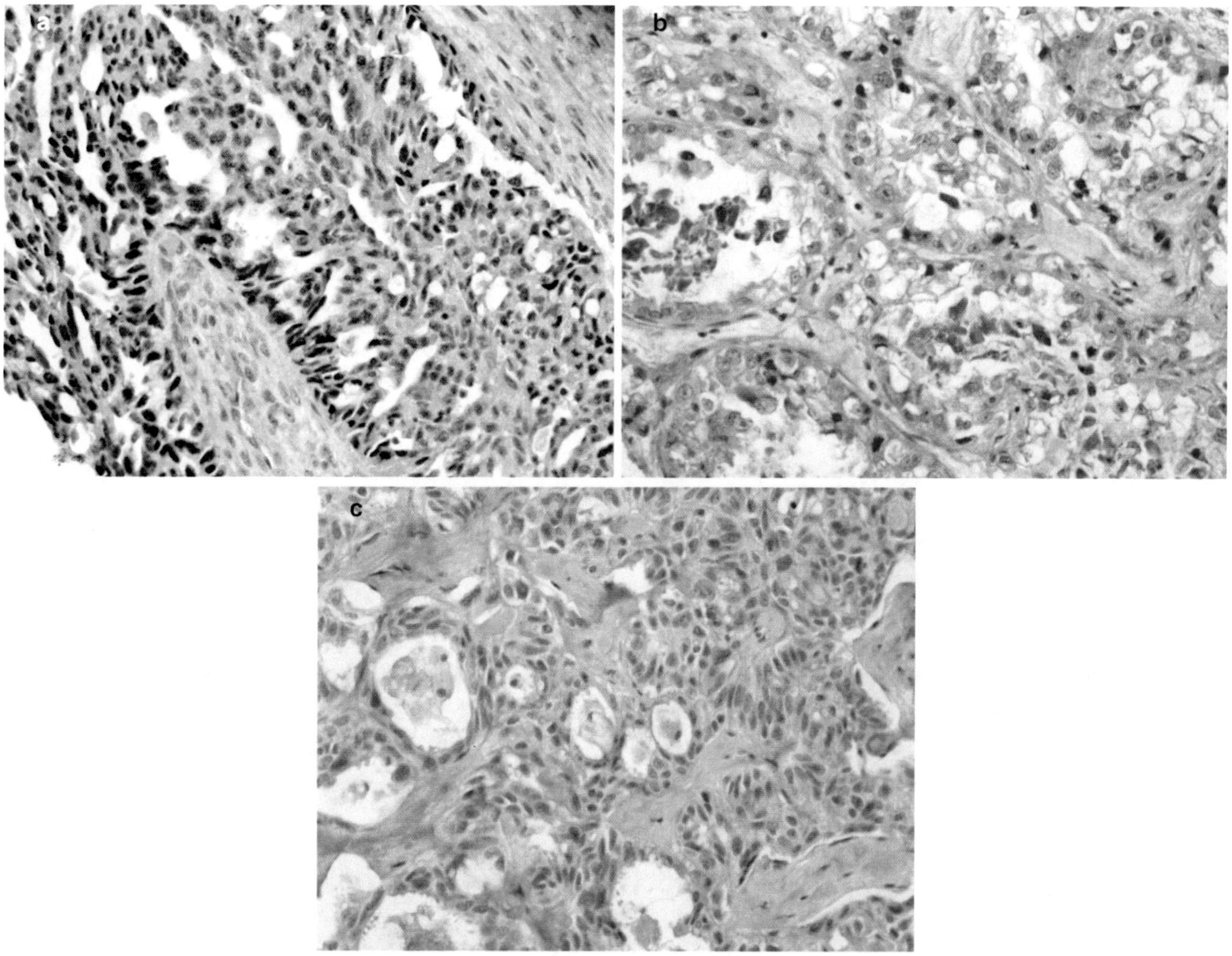

Fig. 17.21 Differential use of WT-1 staining in ovarian epithelial tumors. Diffuse nuclear staining of WT1 in serous carcinoma in (**a**). WT1 staining is lacking in clear cell carcinoma in (**b**) and endometrioid carcinoma in (**c**)

Table 17.7 Ovarian serous versus clear cell carcinoma

Antibody	Clear cell	Serous
WT1	–	+
p53	–/+	+
ER	–/+	+/–
KIM-1	+	–
pVHL	+	–

References: [1–4, 24]

Table 17.8 Endometrial versus ovarian serous carcinoma

Antibody	Ovarian serous	Endometrial serous
WT1	+	–

Note: Strong nuclear WT1 one expression characteristic of ovarian serous carcinoma is not seen in the uterine serous tumors

References: [1–4, 40–42]

Table 17.9 Primary versus metastatic intestinal type mucinous carcinoma

Antibody	Primary ovarian mucinous carcinoma	Colorectal carcinoma	Pancreatic carcinoma	Gastric carcinoma	Breast carcinoma
CK7	+	–[a]	+	+	+
CK20	+/–	+	+/–	–/+	–
MUC2	–/+	+	–	–	–
MUC5AC	+	–/+	+	+/–	–
CDX2	+/–	+	+/–	–/+	–
P504S	–	+/–	–	–/+	–
Beta-catenin	–/+	+/–	–	–/+	–
DPC4	+	+	–/+	+	ND
GCDFP-15	–	–	–	–	–/+
pVHL	–	–	–	–	ND
ER	–/+	–	–	–	+
WT1	–	–	–	–	–

Note: *ND* no data

Intestinal type carcinoma exhibits intracytoplasmic mucinous vacuoles in contrast to the homogeneous "picket fence" endocervical-type mucinous tumors. Primary ovarian mucinous carcinomas are rare and most often FIGO stage 1. The presence of a borderline ovarian mucinous tumor favors a primary ovarian carcinoma

Ovarian mucinous tumors are usually diffusely positive for CK7 and MUC5AC and negative for nuclear beta-catenin, which is opposite of colorectal carcinoma. Negative staining for DPC4 favors metastatic pancreas carcinoma. Positive GCDFP-15 and ER and negative CDX2 and CK20 indicate metastatic breast carcinoma

Examples of differential cytokeratin staining in primary and metastatic mucinous adenocarcinoma of the ovary are in Fig. 17.22

[a]Right sided colorectal carcinoma may express CK7 or lack CK20 and CDX2 when associated with microsatellite instability. Mucinous adenocarcinomas arising from teratomas may have an immunophenotype identical to colorectal adenocarcinoma

References: [1–4, 43]

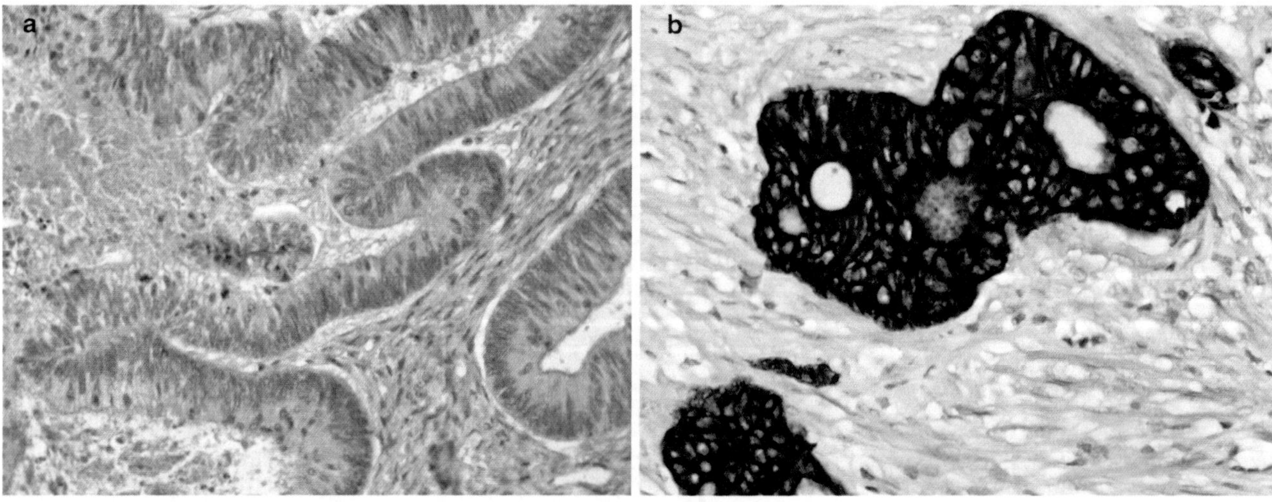

Fig. 17.22 (**a**) Colorectal carcinoma – negative CK7, (**b**) colorectal carcinoma – diffusely positive CK20, (**c**) ovarian mucinous adenocarcinoma – diffusely positive CK7, (**d**) ovarian mucinous adenocarcinoma – focally positive CK20

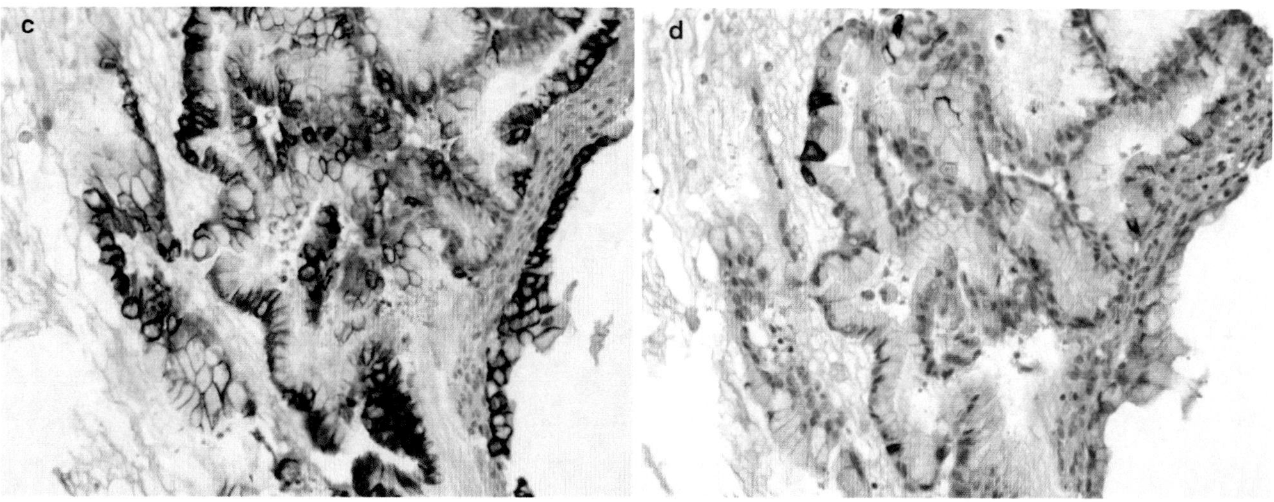

Fig. 17.22 (continued)

Table 17.10 Ovarian versus appendiceal mucinous tumors in pseudomyxoma peritonei

Antibody	Ovarian	Appendiceal
CK7	–	–
CK20	–	+
CEA	+/–	+
Beta-catenin, nuclear	–	+/–
P504S	–	+
MUC2	–/+	+/–
MUC5AC	–/+	+

Note: CK7 and CK20 are not helpful in distinguishing ovarian from appendiceal origin in the setting of pseudomyxoma peritonei. CEA may be useful because ovarian mucinous tumors may lack CEA, while it is almost always present in colorectal carcinoma. Recent studies show that the vast majority of tumors in this setting are appendiceal

References: [1–4, 44]

Table 17.11 Primary versus metastatic uterine mucinous carcinoma

Antibody	Ovarian mucinous carcinoma	Endometrioid carcinoma	Metastatic endocervical mucinous carcinoma
CK7	+	+	+
CK20	–/+	–	–
p16	–	+[a]	+[a]
HPV-IS	–	–	+
ER	–	+	–/+
Beta-catenin, nuclear	–	+	–

Note: Most all endocervical adenocarcinomas are positive for human papilloma virus (HPV) by in situ hybridization (IS)

References: [1–4, 45–47]

[a]p16 is diffusely positive in endocervical adenocarcinoma and patchy positive in endometrioid carcinoma. The presence of ovarian endometriosis favors an endometrioid tumor in this differential. Examples of p16 staining in primary and metastatic mucinous adenocarcinoma of the ovary are in Fig. 17.23

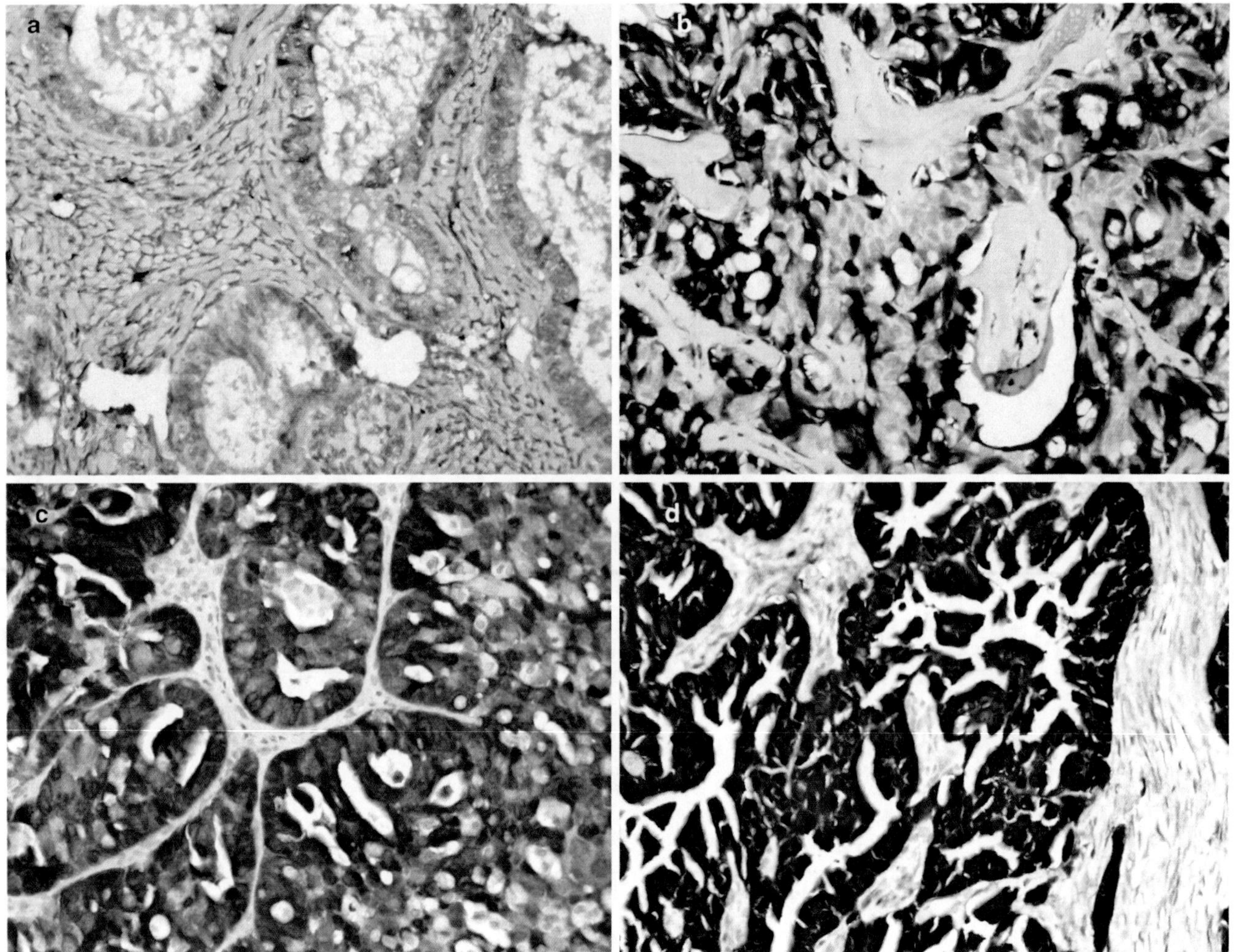

Fig. 17.23 (**a**) Ovarian mucinous adenocarcinoma – only rare cells stain weakly for p16, (**b**) endometrioid adenocarcinoma – strong but incomplete staining of all cells for p16, (**c**) metastatic endocervical adenocarcinoma – strong complete staining of all cells for p16, (**d**) ovarian serous adenocarcinoma – strong complete staining of all cells for p16

Table 17.12 Reactive mesothelium/mesothelioma versus serous implants/carcinoma

Antibody	Serous	Mesothelial
MOC31	+	–
BerEP4	+	–
CK5/6	–	+
Calretinin, nuclear	–	+
Thrombomodulin	–	+
ER	+/–	–
D240	+/–	+
CA-125	+	+/–
CK7	+	+

Note: A panel of markers is recommended for this differential diagnosis choosing two positive and two negative markers to establish the cell type. Examples of staining in serous adenocarcinoma of the ovary are in Figs. 17.24 and 17.25

References: [1–4, 48–50]

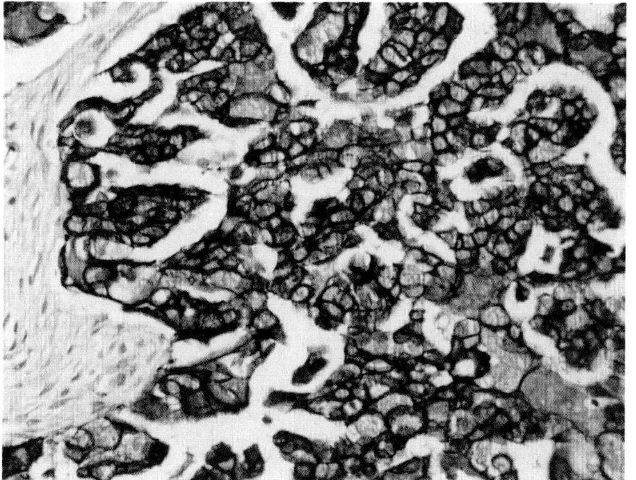

Fig. 17.24 Serous carcinoma – Diffuse membranous staining for MOC31

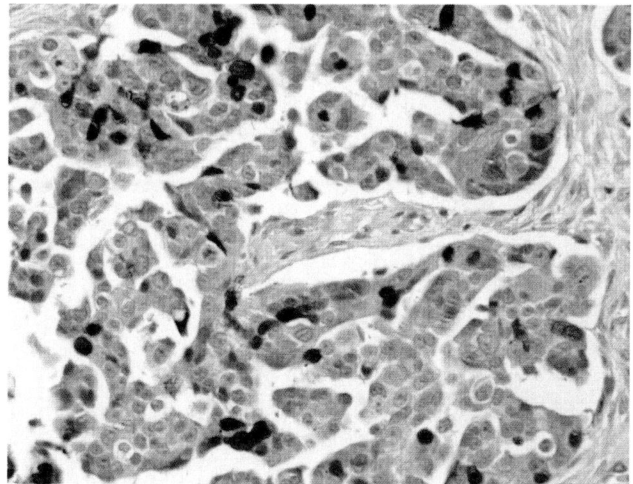

Fig. 17.25 Serous carcinoma – Focal cytoplasmic and nuclear staining for calretinin can occur in serous carcinoma use of a panel is recommended for differentiation from mesothelial proliferations

Table 17.13 Metastatic renal versus ovarian primary clear cell carcinoma

Antibody	Ovarian clear cell	Renal clear cell carcinoma
CK7	+	–/+
RCC	–	+
CD10	–	+
KIM-1	+	+
pVHL	+	+

Note: CD10 can be positive in clear cell and papillary renal cell carcinoma. Conventional clear cell renal carcinoma is negative for cytokeratin 7, though chromophobe renal cell carcinoma is positive for CK7. Clear cell carcinoma of the ovary share expression of VHL and KIM-1 with clear cell renal cell carcinoma (Figs. 17.26 and 17.27)

References: [1–4, 24, 25, 51]

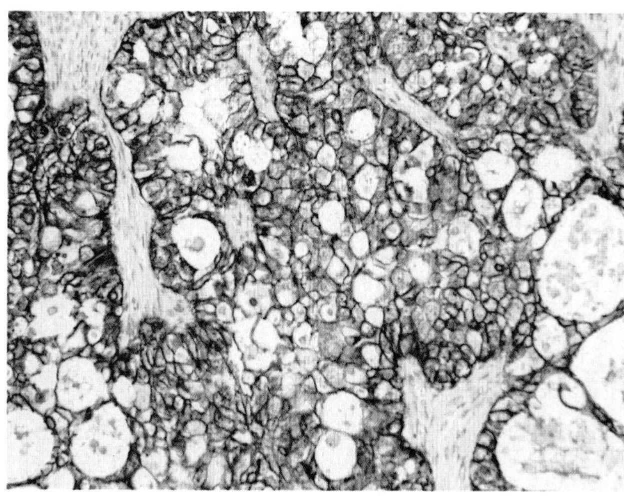

Fig. 17.26 Ovarian clear cell carcinoma – Strong diffuse cytoplasmic staining with VHL

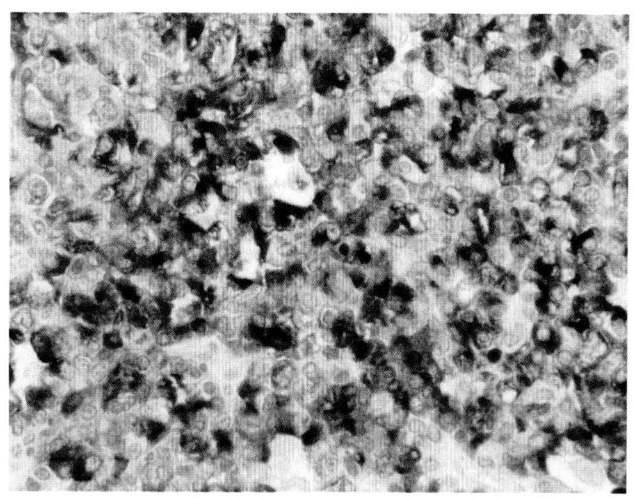

Fig. 17.27 Ovarian clear cell carcinoma – Strong diffuse cytoplasmic staining with KIM-1

Table 17.14 Ovarian adenocarcinoma versus sex cord–stromal tumor

Antibody	Ovarian adenocarcinoma	Sex cord–stromal tumor
CK7	+	–
Ber-EP4	+	–
EMA	+	–
Inhibin	–	+
Calretinin	–	+

References: [1–4, 52]

Table 17.15 Ovarian adenocarcinoma versus carcinoid tumor

Antibody	Ovarian adenocarcinoma	Sex cord–stromal tumor
Chromogranin	–	+
Synaptophysin	–	+
CD56	–	+

Note: Carcinoid in the ovary may be primary or a metastasis commonly from the appendix

References: [1–4, 53]

Table 17.16 Ovarian adenocarcinoma versus Sertoli cell tumor

Antibody	Ovarian adenocarcinoma	Sertoli cell tumor
CK7	+	–
EMA	+	–
Inhibin	–	+

References: [1–4, 52, 54]

Table 17.17 Ovarian small blue cell tumors

Antibody	Ovarian small cell carcinoma	Metastatic small cell carcinoma	Granulosa cell tumor	Lymphoma	Immature neural teratoma
AE1/AE3	+/–	+/–	–	–	–
TTF-1	–	+	–	–	–
Inhibin		–	+	–	–
LCA		–	–	+	–
Synaptophysin		+	–	–	+

Note: Small cell carcinoma of the ovary may be primary or metastatic

References: [1–4, 55, 56]

Table 17.18 Summary of markers in transitional cell tumors: primary ovarian tumors versus urinary bladder

	BT	BorBT	TCC-O	TCC-B	NU
CK7	+	+	+	+	+
CK20	– or +[a]	–	+	+	+[b]
TM	+	+ or –	+	+	+
UPIII	+	– or +	+ or –	+ or –	+
INHA	–	–	ND	ND	ND
CK8	+	ND	+	+	+
CK5/6	+	ND	+	+	+[c]
CK13	+	ND	–	+	+[d]
Vim	–	ND	+ or –	–	–
CA125	+ or –	ND	+	–	–
CEA	– or +	ND	– or +	+ or –	+ or –
WT1	– or +	ND	+	ND	ND

Abbreviations: *BT* benign Brenner tumor, *BorBT* borderline Brenner tumor, *TCC-O* primary ovarian transitional cell carcinoma, *TCC-B* primary urothelial (transitional cell) carcinoma of urinary bladder, *NU* normal urothelium

Notes:

[a]If staining is present, usually only focal

[b]Stains umbrella cells only

[c]Stains basal cell layers only

[d]Stains basal and intermediate cell layers

References: [1, 3, 10, 11, 18, 57–59]

Table 17.19 Summary of markers in the differential of Krukenberg tumors versus primary ovarian tumors

	Krukenberg tumors (metastatic; classic signet ring or tubule forming)					Primary ovarian tumors						
						Signet ring cell pattern					Tubule forming	
						Mucin (+)		Mucin (–)				
	CC	GC	AC	PC	BC	PM	MC	SR	SS	CO	SL	PE
AE1/AE3	+	+	+	+	+		+	–[a]	–	+	– or +[b]	+
CK7	– or +[c]	+	– or +	+	+	+		–	–	+	–	+
CK20	+	+ or –	+	+ or –	–	+[d]		–	–	–		–
EMA	+	+	+	+	+	+	–	–		–	–	+
Vim	–	–	–	–	–			+	+	– or +		– or +
INHA	–	–	–	–	–	–	–	+ or –	+	–	+	–
CDX2	+	+ or –[e]		– or +	–	– or +						– or +
MUC2	+	– or +[e]	+	–	–	+ or –						
MUC5AC	– or +[e]	+	+ or –	+	–	+ or –						+
P504s	+ or –	– or +		–	–	–						
BCAT	+[f]	– or +		–	–	– or +[g]						+[f]
DPC4	+	+	–	+ or –		+						
CEA	+[h]	+	+	+		+[d]	+[d]	–		+		–
CA125	–	–	–	– or +		– or +		–	–	+		+
Chrom							+				–	–
Synap							+					
CD10							–	–	+[d]	– or +	+ or –	– or +
CD99							–	–	+	– or +	+ or –	– or +
A103	–	–		–	–	–	–	–	+		+	–
Calret		–					–	+ or –	+	– or +	+	– or +
ER	–	–	–	–	+ or –	–		–	–	– or +	+ or –	+

Abbreviations: *CC* colorectal adenocarcinoma, *GC* gastric adenocarcinoma, *AC* appendiceal adenocarcinoma, *PC* pancreatic adenocarcinoma, *BC* breast adenocarcinoma, *PM* primary mucinous carcinoma of ovary, *MC* mucinous carcinoid, *SR* signet ring stromal tumor, *SS* sclerosing stromal cell tumor, *CO* clear cell carcinoma of ovary, *SL* Sertoli–Leydig cell tumor, *PE* primary endometrioid carcinoma of ovary

Notes:

[a]Rare case reported dot-like and membranous staining of tumor cells

[b]Sertoli–Leydig cell tumors are typically CK AE1/AE3 (–), but may be (+) in tubules, if they are present

[c]CK7 (+)/CK20 (–) phenotype may be seen in carcinomas from the right colon

[d]If positive, usually only focal

[e]May be strongly positive in pure signet ring cell pattern tumors

[f]Nuclear staining pattern

[g]If positive, demonstrates a membranous staining pattern

[h]Stains along glycocalyceal border and apical cytoplasm

References: [3, 12, 57, 60–82]

Table 17.20 Immunoprofile of granulosa cell tumor

Marker	Pattern
Alpha-inhibin	+
Calretinin	+
EMA	–
CK7	–
Vimentin	+
SF1	+
AE1/AE3, CAM5.2	+ or –
SMA	+
Desmin	–
CD99	+ or –, M
S100	+ or –
MIS	+ or –

Note: The typical immunostain profile of a granulose cell tumor is positive for alpha-inhibin and calretinin; negative for EMA and CK7. Studies suggested that calretinin is more sensitive, but less specific compared with alpha-inhibin in the immunostain of granulose cell tumors. In general, alpha-inhibin is a sensitive marker for sex cord–stromal tumors, but staining in a more patchy fashion. Calretinin is less sensitive, more specific marker compared with alpha-inhibin, but staining in a more diffuse fashion

A recent study suggested that SF1 is the most sensitive marker for sex cord–stromal tumor lineage. SF1 has not been studied extensively, there are only few studies in the literature regarding SF1 expression in ovarian epithelial tumors, with inconsistent results, from no expression in ovarian epithelial tumors (including benign, borderline, and malignant serous and mucinous tumors, clear cell carcinoma, transitional cell carcinoma and endometrioid carcinomas), to expression in 40–60% of benign, malignant, and borderline serous and mucinous tumors

References: [83–86]

Table 17.21 Immunoprofile of thecoma

Marker	Pattern
Alpha-inhibin	+
Calretinin	+
SF1	+
Vimentin	+
AE1/AE3	–
WT1	–
Reticulin	Investment of individual tumor cells by reticulin fibrils

Note: Inhibin staining is a characteristic of sex cord–stromal tumors including thecomas (Fig. 17.28)

References: [1, 3, 54, 87–89]

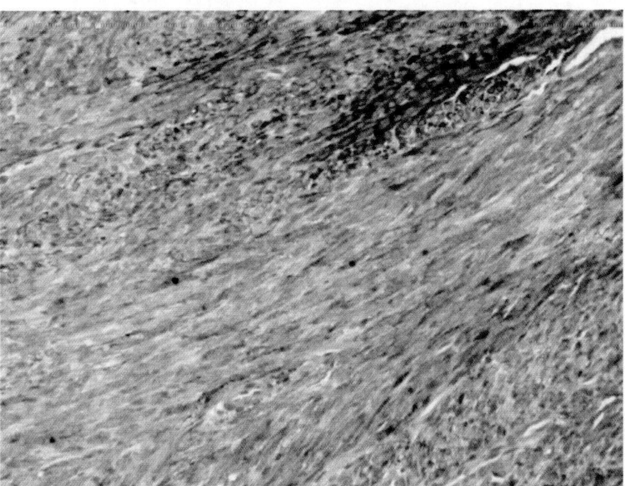

Fig. 17.28 Fibrothecoma – Diffuse cytoplasmic staining with inhibin-alpha

Table 17.22 Immunoprofile of fibroma

Marker	Pattern
Alpha-inhibin	– or +
Calretinin	+ or –
SF1	+
Vimentin	+
AE1/AE3	–

References: [57, 83, 90–92]

Table 17.23 Immunoprofile of Sertoli–Leydig cell tumor

Marker	Pattern
Alpha-inhibin	+
Calretinin	+
CD99	+, M, Sertoli cells
WT-1	+, Sertoli cells
SF1	+
Pan-CK	+, Sertoli cells –, Stromal cells and Leydig cells
CAM 5.2	+, Sertoli cells –, Stromal cells and Leydig cells
EMA	–
Vimentin	+

Note: Sertoli–Leydig cell tumors often contain heterologous elements, such as enteric epithelium (cytokeratin +, EMA +, alpha-inhibin –), hepatoid differentiation (CAM5.2 +, AFP +, alpha-inhibin –), carcinoid differentiation (chromogranin +, synaptophysin +), or rhabdomyoblastic differentiation (Desmin +, myogenin +)

Table 17.24 Immunoprofile of Sertoli cell tumor

Marker	Pattern
Alpha-inhibin	+
SF1	+
WT1	+
EMA	–
CK7	– or +
Pan-CK	+
Calretinin	+
ER, PR	– or +
Chrom, Synap	– or +
CD99	+ or –
CAM 5.2	– or +

Note: Majority cases of SCTs are negative for CK7, ER, and PR with few positive reports (in less than 15% of cases)

References: [1, 54, 87–89]

Table 17.25 Immunoprofile of steroid cell tumors

Marker	Pattern
Alpha-inhibin	+
Calretinin	+
MART-1	+
Vimentin	+
AE1/AE3, CAM5.2	– or +
SMA	– or +
Desmin	– or +
CD68	– or +
EMA	– or +
S100	– or +

Note: Steroid cell tumors include stromal luteoma, Leydig cell tumor, and adrenal cortical type. As a group, they are all positive for alpha-inhibin and calretinin. Leydig cell tumors show strong positivity for alpha-inhibin and vimentin

References: [87, 93]

Table 17.26 The differentiation of diffuse adult granulosa cell tumor (AGCT) versus endometrioid stromal sarcoma (ESS, primary or metastasis from uterus)

Marker	GCT	ESS
Alpha-inhibin	+	–
Calretinin	+ or –	–
CD10	–	+
Vimentin	+	+
Reticulin	None	Individual investment of tumor cells by reticulin fibrils
SMA	+	Focal +
CAM5.2	+ or –	Focal +

Note: Endometrioid stromal sarcoma is composed of cell resembling the stromal cells of normal proliferative endometrium (Fig. 17.29)

Reference: [64]

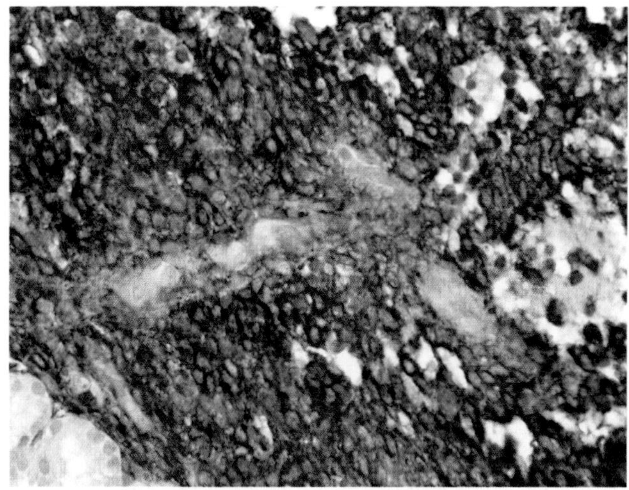

Fig. 17.29 Endometrioid stromal sarcoma – Diffuse cytoplasmic staining with CD10

Table 17.27 The differentiation of granulosa cell tumor (GCT) versus small cell carcinoma (SCC) versus undifferentiated carcinoma, nonsmall cell (neuroendocrine) type (UC)

Marker	GCT	SCC	UC
Alpha-inhibin	+	–	–
EMA	–	+	+
WT1	+	+	N/A
Vim	+	+ or –	–
P53	–	+	– or +
NSE	–	+ or –	+
Chrom	–	+ or –	+
SF1	+	N/A	N/A
CD99	+	–	N/A
CAM5.2	+ or –	+	+

Note: *GCT* granulosa cell tumor, *SCC* small cell carcinoma, *UC* undifferentiated carcinoma, nonsmall cell (neuroendocrine) type, *N/A* no data available in literature

References: [52, 53, 72, 94–101]

Table 17.28 The differentiation of Sertoli cell tumor (SCT) versus endometrioid tumor (EMT) versus carcinoid tumor (CT)

Marker	SCT	EMT	CT
Alpha-inhibin	+	–	–
SF1	+	–	–
WT1	+	–	–
CK7	– or +	+	– or +
ER, PR	– or +	+	–
Chromogranin	– or +	– or +	+
Synaptophysin	– or +	– or +	+
EMA	–	+	– or +
Calretinin	+ or –	– or +	–
CD99	+ or –	– or +	– or +
Pan-CK	+ or –	+	+
CAM 5.2	– or +	+	+

Note: Endometrioid tumors (EMT) includes endometrioid borderline tumor, sertoliform endometrioid carcinoma and well-differentiated endometrioid carcinoma

Majority of endometrioid tumors are positive for CK7, ER, PR, and EMA. Majority of carcinoid tumors are reactive to chromogranin and synaptophysin. Most of the Sertoli cell tumors are positive for alpha-inhibin, SF1, WT1, calretinin (about 60% of cases), while negative for EMA

References: [54, 88]

Table 17.29 Summary of markers in germ cell tumors of the ovary

	DYSG[a]	YST	EC	CC	GBL	Syn	ITr
PLAP	+	+ or –	+	+ or –	+[b]	+ or –	ND
OCT3/4	+	–	+	ND	+[b]	ND	ND
ckit	+	ND	ND	ND	+[b]	ND	ND
AFP	–	+ or –	– or +	–	ND	–	ND
D2-40	+	– or +	– or +	ND	ND	ND	ND
INHA	–	–	–	+	– or +[c]	+ or –	– or +
CD30	–	– or +	+	ND	ND	ND	ND
EMA	–	–	–	– or +	ND	ND	ND
NSE	+	+ or –	+	– or +	ND	ND	ND
AAT	–	– or +	–	–	ND	ND	ND
HCG	–	–	–	+	ND	+	+
CEA	–	–	–	–	ND	+ or –	– or +[d]
AE1/AE3[e]	– or +	+	+	+	ND	+ or –	+
Vim	– or +	–	–	–	ND	ND	ND
CK18	+ or –[f]	ND	ND	–	ND	+	+
CK7	+ or –	–	+	–	ND	ND	ND

Abbreviations: *DYSG* dysgerminoma, *YST* yolk sac tumor, *EC* embryonal carcinoma, *CC* choriocarinoma, *GBL* gonadoblastoma, *Syn* syncytiotrophoblast, *ITr* intermediate trophoblast

References: [1, 3, 13, 14, 102–106]

Notes:

[a] Dysgerminomas are negative for CK7, CK10, CK11, CK13, and CK19

[b] (+) Staining is in germ cell component; sex-cord stromal component is (–)

[c] (+) Staining is in sex-cord stromal component; germ cell component is (–)

[d] When present, usually only focal

[e] When present, cytokeratin staining often has a punctate pattern

[f] Staining is usually diffuse but can be fibrillary; may also stain a few spindle stromal cells

Table 17.30 Germ cell tumors versus ovarian adenocarcinoma

Antibody	Ovarian adenocarcinoma	Choriocarcinoma	Embryonal carcinoma	Yolk sac tumor	Dysgerminoma
CK7	+	+/–	+	–	–
hCG	–	+	–/+	–[a]	–[a]
AFP	–	–	+	+	–
OCT4, nuclear	–	–	+	+	+

Note: [a]May contain scattered HCG positive syncytiotrophoblasts

References: [2, 104, 107, 108]

Table 17.31 Yolk sac tumor versus ovarian clear cell carcinoma

Antibody	Clear cell carcinoma	Yolk sac tumor
Oct4	–	+
SALL4	–	+
EMA	+	–
ER	–/+	–
AFP	–	+/–
Glypican-3	–/+	+

Note: Glypican-3 staining is diffuse in yolk sac tumors and patchy in ovarian clear cell carcinomas when present (Fig. 17.30)

References: [26, 36, 107, 109–111]

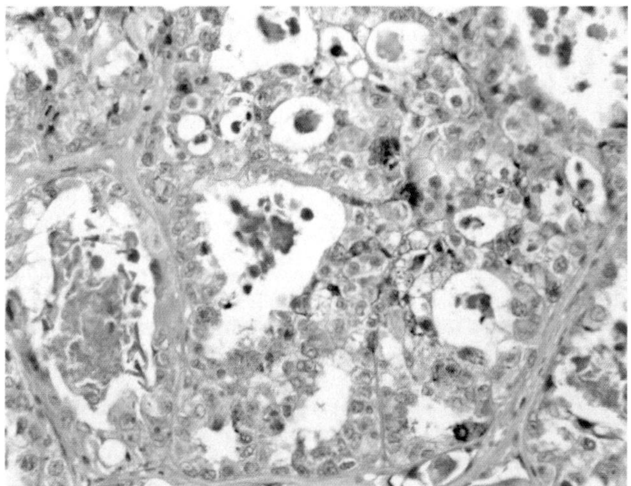

Fig. 17.30 Ovarian clear cell carcinoma – Weak focal cytoplasmic staining with glypican 3

Note for All Tables

Note: "+" – usually greater than 70% of cases are positive; "–" – less than 5% of cases are positive; "+ or –" – usually more than 50% of cases are positive; "– or +" – less than 50% of cases are positive.

References

1. McCluggage WG, Young RH. Immunohistochemistry as a diagnostic aid in the evaluation of ovarian tumors. Semin Diagn Pathol. 2005;22(1):3–32.
2. Soslow RA. Histologic subtypes of ovarian carcinoma: an overview. Int J Gynecol Pathol. 2008;27(2):161–74.
3. Baker PM, Oliva E. Immunohistochemistry as a tool in the differential diagnosis of ovarian tumors: an update. Int J Gynecol Pathol. 2005;24(1):39–55.
4. Mittal K, Soslow R, McCluggage WG. Application of immunohistochemistry to gynecologic pathology. Arch Pathol Lab Med. 2008;132(3):402–23.
5. Cathro HP, Stoler MH. Expression of cytokeratins 7 and 20 in ovarian neoplasia. Am J Clin Pathol. 2002;117(6):944–51.
6. Chu P, Wu E, Weiss LM. Cytokeratin 7 and cytokeratin 20 expression in epithelial neoplasms: a survey of 435 cases. Mod Pathol. 2000;13(9):962–72.
7. Moll R, Lowe A, Laufer J, Franke WW. Cytokeratin 20 in human carcinomas. A new histodiagnostic marker detected by monoclonal antibodies. Am J Pathol. 1992;140(2):427–47.
8. Lagendijk JH, Mullink H, van Diest PJ, Meijer GA, Meijer CJ. Immunohistochemical differentiation between primary adenocarcinomas of the ovary and ovarian metastases of colonic and breast origin. Comparison between a statistical and an intuitive approach. J Clin Pathol. 1999;52(4):283–90.
9. Wauters CC, Smedts F, Gerrits LG, Bosman FT, Ramaekers FC. Keratins 7 and 20 as diagnostic markers of carcinomas metastatic to the ovary. Hum Pathol. 1995;26(8):852–5.
10. Riedel I, Czernobilsky B, Lifschitz-Mercer B, et al. Brenner tumors but not transitional cell carcinomas of the ovary show urothelial differentiation: immunohistochemical staining of urothelial markers, including cytokeratins and uroplakins. Virchows Arch. 2001;438(2):181–91.
11. Ordonez NG. Transitional cell carcinomas of the ovary and bladder are immunophenotypically different. Histopathology. 2000;36(5):433–8.
12. McCluggage WG. My approach to and thoughts on the typing of ovarian carcinomas. J Clin Pathol. 2008;61(2):152–63.
13. Manivel JC, Niehans G, Wick MR, Dehner LP. Intermediate trophoblast in germ cell neoplasms. Am J Surg Pathol. 1987;11(9):693–701.
14. Kalhor N, Ramirez PT, Deavers MT, Malpica A, Silva EG. Immunohistochemical studies of trophoblastic tumors. Am J Surg Pathol. 2009;33(4):633–8. doi:10.1097/PAS.0b013e318191f2eb.
15. Southgate J, Harnden P, Trejdosiewicz LK. Cytokeratin expression patterns in normal and malignant urothelium: a review of the biological and diagnostic implications. Histol Histopathol. 1999;14(2):657–64.
16. McKenney JK, Desai S, Cohen C, Amin MB. Discriminatory immunohistochemical staining of urothelial carcinoma in situ and non-neoplastic urothelium: an analysis of cytokeratin 20, p53, and CD44 antigens. Am J Surg Pathol. 2001;25(8):1074–8.
17. Parker DC, Folpe AL, Bell J, et al. Potential utility of uroplakin III, thrombomodulin, high molecular weight cytokeratin, and cytokeratin 20 in noninvasive, invasive, and metastatic urothelial (transitional cell) carcinomas. Am J Surg Pathol. 2003;27(1):1–10.
18. Shevchuk MM, Fenoglio CM, Richart RM. Carcinoembryonic antigen localization in benign and malignant transitional epithelium. Cancer. 1981;47(5):899–905.
19. Nonaka D, Chiriboga L, Soslow RA. Expression of pax8 as a useful marker in distinguishing ovarian carcinomas from mammary carcinomas. Am J Surg Pathol. 2008;32(10):1566–71.
20. Roh MH, Kindelberger D, Crum CP. Serous tubal intraepithelial carcinoma and the dominant ovarian mass: clues to serous tumor origin? Am J Surg Pathol. 2009;33(3):376–83.
21. O'Neill CJ, Deavers MT, Malpica A, Foster H, McCluggage WG. An immunohistochemical comparison between low-grade and high-grade ovarian serous carcinomas: significantly higher expression of p53, MIB1, BCL2, HER-2/neu, and C-KIT in high-grade neoplasms. Am J Surg Pathol. 2005;29(8):1034–41.
22. Takeshima Y, Amatya VJ, Kushitani K, Inai K. A useful antibody panel for differential diagnosis between peritoneal mesothelioma and ovarian serous carcinoma in Japanese cases. Am J Clin Pathol. 2008;130(5):771–9.
23. Frierson Jr HF, Moskaluk CA, Powell SM, et al. Large-scale molecular and tissue microarray analysis of mesothelin expression in common human carcinomas. Hum Pathol. 2003;34(6):605–9.

24. Lin F, Shi J, Liu H, et al. Immunohistochemical detection of the von Hippel-Lindau gene product (pVHL) in human tissues and tumors: a useful marker for metastatic renal cell carcinoma and clear cell carcinoma of the ovary and uterus. Am J Clin Pathol. 2008;129(4):592–605.
25. Lin F, Zhang PL, Yang XJ, et al. Human kidney injury molecule-1 (hKIM-1): a useful immunohistochemical marker for diagnosing renal cell carcinoma and ovarian clear cell carcinoma. Am J Surg Pathol. 2007;31(3):371–81.
26. Tong GX, Chiriboga L, Hamele-Bena D, Borczuk AC. Expression of PAX2 in papillary serous carcinoma of the ovary: immunohistochemical evidence of fallopian tube or secondary Mullerian system origin? Mod Pathol. 2007;20(8):856–63.
27. Ordonez NG. Role of immunohistochemistry in distinguishing epithelial peritoneal mesotheliomas from peritoneal and ovarian serous carcinomas. Am J Surg Pathol. 1998;22(10):1203–14.
28. Maeda D, Ota S, Takazawa Y, et al. Glypican-3 expression in clear cell adenocarcinoma of the ovary. Mod Pathol. 2009;22(6): 824–32.
29. Boman F, Buisine MP, Wacrenier A, Querleu D, Aubert JP, Porchet N. Mucin gene transcripts in benign and borderline mucinous tumours of the ovary: an in situ hybridization study. J Pathol. 2001;193(3):339–44.
30. Tashiro Y, Yonezawa S, Kim YS, Sato E. Immunohistochemical study of mucin carbohydrates and core proteins in human ovarian tumors. Hum Pathol. 1994;25(4):364–72.
31. Ho SB, Niehans GA, Lyftogt C, et al. Heterogeneity of mucin gene expression in normal and neoplastic tissues. Cancer Res. 1993;53(3):641–51.
32. Vang R, Gown AM, Farinola M, et al. p16 expression in primary ovarian mucinous and endometrioid tumors and metastatic adenocarcinomas in the ovary: utility for identification of metastatic HPV-related endocervical adenocarcinomas. Am J Surg Pathol. 2007;31(5):653–63.
33. Tabrizi AD, Kalloger SE, Kobel M, et al. Primary ovarian mucinous carcinoma of intestinal type: significance of pattern of invasion and immunohistochemical expression profile in a series of 31 cases. Int J Gynecol Pathol. 2010;29(2):99–107.
34. Kappes S, Milde-Langosch K, Kressin P, et al. p53 mutations in ovarian tumors, detected by temperature-gradient gel electrophoresis, direct sequencing and immunohistochemistry. Int J Cancer. 1995;64(1):52–9.
35. Esheba GE, Pate LL, Longacre TA. Oncofetal protein glypican-3 distinguishes yolk sac tumor from clear cell carcinoma of the ovary. Am J Surg Pathol. 2008;32(4):600–7.
36. Cao D, Guo S, Allan RW, Molberg KH, Peng Y. SALL4 is a novel sensitive and specific marker of ovarian primitive germ cell tumors and is particularly useful in distinguishing yolk sac tumor from clear cell carcinoma. Am J Surg Pathol. 2009;33(6):894–904.
37. Cameron RI, Ashe P, O'Rourke DM, Foster H, McCluggage WG. A panel of immunohistochemical stains assists in the distinction between ovarian and renal clear cell carcinoma. Int J Gynecol Pathol. 2003;22(3):272–6.
38. Kong CS, Beck AH, Longacre TA. A panel of 3 markers including p16, ProExC, or HPV ISH is optimal for distinguishing between primary endometrial and endocervical adenocarcinomas. Am J Surg Pathol. 2010;34(7):915–26.
39. Madore J, Ren F, Filali-Mouhim A, et al. Characterization of the molecular differences between ovarian endometrioid carcinoma and ovarian serous carcinoma. J Pathol. 2010;220(3):392–400.
40. Euscher ED, Malpica A, Deavers MT, Silva EG. Differential expression of WT-1 in serous carcinomas in the peritoneum with or without associated serous carcinoma in endometrial polyps. Am J Surg Pathol. 2005;29(8):1074–8.
41. Hashi A, Yuminamochi T, Murata S, Iwamoto H, Honda T, Hoshi K. Wilms tumor gene immunoreactivity in primary serous carcinomas of the fallopian tube, ovary, endometrium, and peritoneum. Int J Gynecol Pathol. 2003;22(4):374–7.
42. Al-Hussaini M, Stockman A, Foster H, McCluggage WG. WT-1 assists in distinguishing ovarian from uterine serous carcinoma and in distinguishing between serous and endometrioid ovarian carcinoma. Histopathology. 2004;44(2):109–15.
43. Lin F, Shi J, Liu H, et al. Diagnostic utility of S100P and von Hippel-Lindau gene product (pVHL) in pancreatic adenocarcinoma-with implication of their roles in early tumorigenesis. Am J Surg Pathol. 2008;32(1):78–91.
44. O'Connell JT, Tomlinson JS, Roberts AA, McGonigle KF, Barsky SH. Pseudomyxoma peritonei is a disease of MUC2-expressing goblet cells. Am J Pathol. 2002;161(2):551–64.
45. Carico E, Fulciniti F, Giovagnoli MR, et al. Adhesion molecules and p16 expression in endocervical adenocarcinoma. Virchows Arch. 2009;455(3):245–51.
46. Vang R, Gown AM, Barry TS, Wheeler DT, Ronnett BM. Immunohistochemistry for estrogen and progesterone receptors in the distinction of primary and metastatic mucinous tumors in the ovary: an analysis of 124 cases. Mod Pathol. 2006;19(1):97–105.
47. Staebler A, Sherman ME, Zaino RJ, Ronnett BM. Hormone receptor immunohistochemistry and human papillomavirus in situ hybridization are useful for distinguishing endocervical and endometrial adenocarcinomas. Am J Surg Pathol. 2002;26(8):998–1006.
48. Lee ES, Leong AS, Kim YS, et al. Calretinin, CD34, and alpha-smooth muscle actin in the identification of peritoneal invasive implants of serous borderline tumors of the ovary. Mod Pathol. 2006;19(3):364–72.
49. Comin CE, Saieva C, Messerini L. h-caldesmon, calretinin, estrogen receptor, and Ber-EP4: a useful combination of immunohistochemical markers for differentiating epithelioid peritoneal mesothelioma from serous papillary carcinoma of the ovary. Am J Surg Pathol. 2007;31(8):1139–48.
50. Ordonez NG. Value of immunohistochemistry in distinguishing peritoneal mesothelioma from serous carcinoma of the ovary and peritoneum: a review and update. Adv Anat Pathol. 2006;13(1): 16–25.
51. Leroy X, Farine MO, Buob D, Wacrenier A, Copin MC. Diagnostic value of cytokeratin 7, CD10 and mesothelin in distinguishing ovarian clear cell carcinoma from metastasis of renal clear cell carcinoma. Histopathology. 2007;51(6):874–6.
52. Cathro HP, Stoler MH. The utility of calretinin, inhibin, and WT1 immunohistochemical staining in the differential diagnosis of ovarian tumors. Hum Pathol. 2005;36(2):195–201.
53. Veras E, Deavers MT, Silva EG, Malpica A. Ovarian nonsmall cell neuroendocrine carcinoma: a clinicopathologic and immunohistochemical study of 11 cases. Am J Surg Pathol. 2007;31(5): 774–82.
54. Zhao C, Bratthauer GL, Barner R, Vang R. Comparative analysis of alternative and traditional immunohistochemical markers for the distinction of ovarian sertoli cell tumor from endometrioid tumors and carcinoid tumor: a study of 160 cases. Am J Surg Pathol. 2007;31(2):255–66.
55. Engohan-Aloghe C, Aubain Sommerhausen Nde S, Noel JC. Ovarian involvement by desmoplastic small round cell tumor with leydig cell hyperplasia showing an unusual immunophenotype (cytokeratin negative, calretinin and inhibin positive) mimicking poorly differentiated sertoli leydig cell tumor. Int J Gynecol Pathol. 2009;28(6):579–83.
56. Carlson JW, Nucci MR, Brodsky J, Crum CP, Hirsch MS. Biomarker-assisted diagnosis of ovarian, cervical and pulmonary small cell carcinomas: the role of TTF-1, WT-1 and HPV analysis. Histopathology. 2007;51(3):305–12.
57. Kommoss F, Oliva E, Bhan AK, Young RH, Scully RE. Inhibin expression in ovarian tumors and tumor-like lesions: an immunohistochemical study. Mod Pathol. 1998;11(7):656–64.

58. Ordonez NG, Mackay B. Brenner tumor of the ovary: a comparative immunohistochemical and ultrastructural study with transitional cell carcinoma of the bladder. Ultrastruct Pathol. 2000;24(3):157–67.
59. Logani S, Oliva E, Amin MB, Folpe AL, Cohen C, Young RH. Immunoprofile of ovarian tumors with putative transitional cell (urothelial) differentiation using novel urothelial markers: histogenetic and diagnostic implications. Am J Surg Pathol. 2003; 27(11):1434–41.
60. Al-Agha OM, Nicastri AD. An in-depth look at Krukenberg tumor: an overview. Arch Pathol Lab Med. 2006;130(11):1725–30.
61. Hart WR. Diagnostic challenge of secondary (metastatic) ovarian tumors simulating primary endometrioid and mucinous neoplasms. Pathol Int. 2005;55(5):231–43.
62. Hart WR. Mucinous tumors of the ovary: a review. Int J Gynecol Pathol. 2005;24(1):4–25.
63. McCluggage WG, Wilkinson N. Metastatic neoplasms involving the ovary: a review with an emphasis on morphological and immunohistochemical features. Histopathology. 2005;47(3):231–47.
64. Prat J. Ovarian carcinomas, including secondary tumors: diagnostically challenging areas. Mod Pathol. 2005;18 Suppl 2:S99–111.
65. Hardisson D, Regojo RM, Marino-Enriquez A, Martinez-Garcia M. Signet-ring stromal tumor of the ovary: report of a case and review of the literature. Pathol Oncol Res. 2008;14(3):333–6.
66. Irving JA, Young RH. Microcystic stromal tumor of the ovary: report of 16 cases of a hitherto uncharacterized distinctive ovarian neoplasm. Am J Surg Pathol. 2009;33(3):367–75.
67. Ohishi Y, Kaku T, Oya M, Kobayashi H, Wake N, Tsuneyoshi M. CD56 expression in ovarian granulosa cell tumors, and its diagnostic utility and pitfalls. Gynecol Oncol. 2007;107(1):30–8.
68. Nolan LP, Heatley MK. The value of immunocytochemistry in distinguishing between clear cell carcinoma of the kidney and ovary. Int J Gynecol Pathol. 2001;20(2):155–9.
69. Gilks CB, Prat J. Ovarian carcinoma pathology and genetics: recent advances. Hum Pathol. 2009;40(9):1213–23.
70. Farinola MA, Gown AM, Judson K, et al. Estrogen receptor alpha and progesterone receptor expression in ovarian adult granulosa cell tumors and Sertoli-Leydig cell tumors. Int J Gynecol Pathol. 2007;26(4):375–82.
71. McCluggage WG, Young RH. Ovarian sertoli-leydig cell tumors with pseudoendometrioid tubules (pseudoendometrioid sertoli-leydig cell tumors). Am J Surg Pathol. 2007;31(4):592–7.
72. Riopel MA, Perlman EJ, Seidman JD, Kurman RJ, Sherman ME. Inhibin and epithelial membrane antigen immunohistochemistry assist in the diagnosis of sex cord-stromal tumors and provide clues to the histogenesis of hypercalcemic small cell carcinomas. Int J Gynecol Pathol. 1998;17(1):46–53.
73. Busam KJ, Iversen K, Coplan KA, et al. Immunoreactivity for A103, an antibody to melan-A (Mart-1), in adrenocortical and other steroid tumors. Am J Surg Pathol. 1998;22(1):57–63.
74. Baker PM, Oliva E, Young RH, Talerman A, Scully RE. Ovarian mucinous carcinoids including some with a carcinomatous component: a report of 17 cases. Am J Surg Pathol. 2001;25(5):557–68.
75. Alenghat E, Okagaki T, Talerman A. Primary mucinous carcinoid tumor of the ovary. Cancer. 1986;58(3):777–83.
76. Chu PG, Weiss LM. Immunohistochemical characterization of signet-ring cell carcinomas of the stomach, breast, and colon. Am J Clin Pathol. 2004;121(6):884–92.
77. Vang R, Bague S, Tavassoli FA, Prat J. Signet-ring stromal tumor of the ovary: clinicopathologic analysis and comparison with Krukenberg tumor. Int J Gynecol Pathol. 2004;23(1):45–51.
78. Shaco-Levy R, Kachko L, Mazor M, Piura B. Ovarian signet-ring stromal tumor: a potential diagnostic pitfall. Int J Surg Pathol. 2008;16(2):180–4.
79. Irving JA, McCluggage WG. Ovarian spindle cell lesions: a review with emphasis on recent developments and differential diagnosis. Adv Anat Pathol. 2007;14(5):305–19.
80. He Y, Yang KX, Jiang W, Wang DQ, Li L. Sclerosing stromal tumor of the ovary in a 4-year-old girl with characteristics of an ovarian signet-ring stromal tumor. Pathol Res Pract. 2010;206(5): 338–41.
81. Matsumoto M, Hayashi Y, Ohtsuki Y, et al. Signet-ring stromal tumor of the ovary: an immunohistochemical and ultrastructural study with a review of the literature. Med Mol Morphol. 2008;41(3):165–70.
82. McCluggage WG. Immunohistochemical and functional biomarkers of value in female genital tract lesions. Int J Gynecol Pathol. 2006;25(2):101–20.
83. Zhao C, Vinh TN, McManus K, Dabbs D, Barner R, Vang R. Identification of the most sensitive and robust immunohistochemical markers in different categories of ovarian sex cord-stromal tumors. Am J Surg Pathol. 2009;33(3):354–66.
84. Sasano H, Kaga K, Sato S, Yajima A, Nagura H. Adrenal 4-binding protein in common epithelial and metastatic tumors of the ovary. Hum Pathol. 1996;27(6):595–8.
85. Abd-Elaziz M, Moriya T, Akahira J, Nakamura Y, Suzuki T, Sasano H. Immunolocalization of nuclear transcription factors, DAX-1 and Ad4BP/SF-1, in human common epithelial ovarian tumors: correlations with StAR and steroidogenic enzymes in epithelial ovarian carcinoma. Int J Gynecol Pathol. 2005;24(2):153–63.
86. Matias-Guiu X, Pons C, Prat J. Mullerian inhibiting substance, alpha-inhibin, and CD99 expression in sex cord-stromal tumors and endometrioid ovarian carcinomas resembling sex cord-stromal tumors. Hum Pathol. 1998;29(8):840–5.
87. Oliva E, Alvarez T, Young RH. Sertoli cell tumors of the ovary: a clinicopathologic and immunohistochemical study of 54 cases. Am J Surg Pathol. 2005;29(2):143–56.
88. Zhao C, Barner R, Vinh TN, McManus K, Dabbs D, Vang R. SF-1 is a diagnostically useful immunohistochemical marker and comparable to other sex cord-stromal tumor markers for the differential diagnosis of ovarian sertoli cell tumor. Int J Gynecol Pathol. 2008;27(4):507–14.
89. Zhao C, Bratthauer GL, Barner R, Vang R. Diagnostic utility of WT1 immunostaining in ovarian sertoli cell tumor. Am J Surg Pathol. 2007;31(9):1378–86.
90. Irving JA, Alkushi A, Young RH, Clement PB. Cellular fibromas of the ovary: a study of 75 cases including 40 mitotically active tumors emphasizing their distinction from fibrosarcoma. Am J Surg Pathol. 2006;30(8):929–38.
91. Deavers MT, Malpica A, Liu J, Broaddus R, Silva EG. Ovarian sex cord-stromal tumors: an immunohistochemical study including a comparison of calretinin and inhibin. Mod Pathol. 2003;16(6): 584–90.
92. Movahedi-Lankarani S, Kurman RJ. Calretinin, a more sensitive but less specific marker than alpha-inhibin for ovarian sex cord-stromal neoplasms: an immunohistochemical study of 215 cases. Am J Surg Pathol. 2002;26(11):1477–83.
93. Seidman JD, Abbondanzo SL, Bratthauer GL. Lipid cell (steroid cell) tumor of the ovary: immunophenotype with analysis of potential pitfall due to endogenous biotin-like activity. Int J Gynecol Pathol. 1995;14(4):331–8.
94. Costa MJ, DeRose PB, Roth LM, Brescia RJ, Zaloudek CJ, Cohen C. Immunohistochemical phenotype of ovarian granulosa cell tumors: absence of epithelial membrane antigen has diagnostic value. Hum Pathol. 1994;25(1):60–6.
95. Young RH. Sex cord-stromal tumors of the ovary and testis: their similarities and differences with consideration of selected problems. Mod Pathol. 2005;18 Suppl 2:S81–98.
96. McCluggage WG, Oliva E, Connolly LE, McBride HA, Young RH. An immunohistochemical analysis of ovarian small cell carcinoma of hypercalcemic type. Int J Gynecol Pathol. 2004;23(4):330–6.
97. McCluggage WG. Ovarian neoplasms composed of small round cells: a review. Adv Anat Pathol. 2004;11(6):288–96.

98. Horny HP, Marx L, Krober S, Luttges J, Kaiserling E, Dietl J. Granulosa cell tumor of the ovary. Immunohistochemical evidence of low proliferative activity and virtual absence of mutation of the p53 tumor-suppressor gene. Gynecol Obstet Invest. 1999; 47(2):133–8.
99. Costa MJ, Walls J, Ames P, Roth LM. Transformation in recurrent ovarian granulosa cell tumors: Ki67 (MIB-1) and p53 immunohistochemistry demonstrates a possible molecular basis for the poor histopathologic prediction of clinical behavior. Hum Pathol. 1996;27(3):274–81.
100. Kuwashima Y, Uehara T, Kishi K, Shiromizu K, Matsuzawa M, Takayama S. Immunohistochemical characterization of undifferentiated carcinomas of the ovary. J Cancer Res Clin Oncol. 1994;120(11):672–7.
101. Eichhorn JH, Lawrence WD, Young RH, Scully RE. Ovarian neuroendocrine carcinomas of non-small-cell type associated with surface epithelial adenocarcinomas. A study of five cases and review of the literature. Int J Gynecol Pathol. 1996;15(4): 303–14.
102. Schacht V, Dadras SS, Johnson LA, Jackson DG, Hong YK, Detmar M. Up-regulation of the lymphatic marker podoplanin, a mucin-type transmembrane glycoprotein, in human squamous cell carcinomas and germ cell tumors. Am J Pathol. 2005;166(3): 913–21.
103. Cools M, Stoop H, Kersemaekers AM, et al. Gonadoblastoma arising in undifferentiated gonadal tissue within dysgenetic gonads. J Clin Endocrinol Metab. 2006;91(6):2404–13. doi:10.1210/ jc.2005-2554.
104. Niehans GA, Manivel JC, Copland GT, Scheithauer BW, Wick MR. Immunohistochemistry of germ cell and trophoblastic neoplasms. Cancer. 1988;62(6):1113–23.
105. Lifschitz-Mercer B, Walt H, Kushnir I, et al. Differentiation potential of ovarian dysgerminoma: an immunohistochemical study of 15 cases. Hum Pathol. 1995;26(1):62–6.
106. Ulbright TM. Germ cell tumors of the gonads: a selective review emphasizing problems in differential diagnosis, newly appreciated, and controversial issues. Mod Pathol. 2005;18 Suppl 2:S61–79.
107. Liu A, Cheng L, Du J, et al. Diagnostic utility of novel stem cell markers SALL4, OCT4, NANOG, SOX2, UTF1, and TCL1 in primary mediastinal germ cell tumors. Am J Surg Pathol. 2010;34(5):697–706.
108. Damjanov I, Osborn M, Miettinen M. Keratin 7 is a marker for a subset of trophoblastic cells in human germ cell tumors. Arch Pathol Lab Med. 1990;114(1):81–3.
109. Dabbs DJ. Diagnostic immunohistochemistry. 3rd ed. Philadelphia, PA: Churchill Livingstone; 2010.
110. Zynger DL, McCallum JC, Luan C, Chou PM, Yang XJ. Glypican 2 has a higher sensitivity than alpha-fetoprotein for testicular and ovarian yolk sac tumour: immunohistochemical investigation with analysis of histological growth patterns. Histopathology. 2010;56(6):750.
111. Cheng L, Zhang S, Talerman A, Roth LM. Morphologic, immunohistochemical, and fluorescence in situ hybridization study of ovarian embryonal carcinoma with comparison to solid variant of yolk sac tumor and immature teratoma. Hum Pathol. 2010;41(5):7 16–23.

Chapter 18
Prostate Gland

Haiyan Liu, Fan Lin, and Qihui (Jim) Zhai

Abstract This chapter provides a practical overview of frequently used markers in the diagnosis and differential diagnosis of both common and rare neoplasms of prostate gland with a specific focus on adenocarcinoma and its mimickers. The chapter contains 41 questions; each question is addressed with a table, concise note, and representative pictures if applicable. In addition to the literature review, the authors have included their own experience and tested numerous antibodies reported in the literature. The most effective diagnostic panels of antibodies have been recommended for many entities, such as CK7, PAX2, and MUC6 being suggested as the best diagnostic panel for distinguishing seminal vesicles from prostatic ductal adenocarcinoma and high-grade prostatic intraepithelial neoplasia. Furthermore, immunophenotypes of normal prostate and seminal vesicles have been described, which tend to be neglected in the literature.

Keywords Prostatic adenocarcinoma • P504S (AMACR) • PSA • PAX2 • PIN4 (triple stain)

FREQUENTLY ASKED QUESTIONS

Differential Diagnosis

H. Liu (✉)
Department of Pathology and Laboratory Medicine, Geisinger Medical Center, Danville, VA, USA
e-mail: hliu1@geisinger.edu

F. Lin and J. Prichard (eds.), *Handbook of Practical Immunohistochemistry: Frequently Asked Questions*,
DOI 10.1007/978-1-4419-8062-5_18, © Springer Science+Business Media, LLC 2011

Table 18.1 Summary of frequently used antibodies in prostate pathology

Markers	Localization (N, M, C)	Function	Application and pitfalls
PSA	C	34-kDa single-chain glycoprotein is a serine protease responsible for gel dissolution in freshly ejaculated semen	Prostate-specific marker, expressed in normal and malignant prostate tissue. Some poorly differentiated or metastatic carcinomas may lose expression (reported <15%). Reactivity in nonprostatic tissue (breast and salivary gland tumors) has been reported.
PSAP	C	100-kDa glycoprotein present in high concentration in prostate gland and its secretions	Prostate-specific marker, expressed in normal and neoplastic prostate tissue. Elevation of PSAP also reported in testicular tumors, lymphomas, and cirrhotic liver.
PSMA	C, M	Prostate-specific membrane antigen, 100-kDa type II membrane glycoprotein	Prostate-specific marker, expressed in benign and malignant prostate epithelial cells, most intense in prostatic adenocarcinoma of the highest grade. Negative for basal cells, stromal cells, vasculature, and urothelium.
P504S (AMACR)	C, granular	Overexpressed in prostate cancer, believed to be functionally important for prostate cancer cell growth	Relatively specific marker of prostate malignancy, but not prostate specific. Positive in majority of prostatic adenocarcinomas, high-grade PIN, and ductal carcinomas. Nonreactive or focally weakly reactive in normal and hyperplastic prostate tissue. Reported positive in carcinomas of colorectal (reported 92%), breast (reported 44%), and others (such as carcinomas of ovary, bladder, lung, and kidney, and dysplastic epithelium in Barrett's esophagus).
P501S	C, perinuclear	A 553-amino acid protein that is localized to the Golgi complex	Prostate-specific marker, positive in benign and malignant prostatic glandular (epithelial) cells. Decreased or lost expression in approximately 10% of metastatic prostatic carcinomas.
p63	N	Nuclear protein, homologous to the p53 tumor suppressor gene	Specific marker for basal cells. Studies suggested that p63 has better sensitivity and greater specificity compared with HMWCK.

(continued)

Table 18.1 (continued)

Markers	Localization (N, M, C)	Function	Application and pitfalls
CK903	C	HMWCK is a cytoplasmic marker for intermediate cytokeratin filaments in basal cells	Specific marker for basal cells used in combination with p63 and AMACR, known as PIN4, in the differentiation of atypical glands in prostate biopsy specimen
CK5/6	C	HMWCK	Specific for basal cells in prostate, with similar overall sensitivity, specificity, and diagnostic utility compared to 34β (beta)-E12
PAX2	N	A homeogene expressed in the development of the urogenital tract	Diffuse nuclear stain in SVED, none in PAs, HGPIN, and normal prostatic glands
S100A1	C + N	Belongs to a family of small acidic EF-hand calcium-binding proteins	A specific marker for nephrogenic adenoma
bcl2	N	A membrane-associated anti-apoptotic oncoprotein	Expressed in basal cell carcinoma and solitary fibrous tumor of the prostate
MUC1	C	A secretory mucin	Overexpressed in prostate carcinomas
MUC6	C	A secretory mucin originally isolated from a gastric cDNA library	Positive in seminal vesicles and negative in normal prostate and adenocarcinoma
CD44	M	A cell surface molecule proposed a prostate cancer stem cell marker	Expressed in basal cells of normal prostate tissue; reported strong and diffuse membranous staining in small cell carcinoma of the prostate
CK7	M, C	Epithelial marker	Negative in normal and neoplastic prostatic glandular epithelia
CK20	M, C	Epithelial marker	Negative in normal and neoplastic prostatic glandular epithelia

Note: *M* membranous; *C* cytoplasmic; *N* nuclear

PSA – prostate-specific antigen; PSAP – prostate-specific acid phosphatase; PSMA – prostate-specific membrane antigen; P504S – alpha-methylacyl-CoA racemase (AMACR) or 2-methylacyl-CoA racemase (RACE); P501S – prostein; HMWCK – high molecular weight cytokeratin. CK903 – 34β (beta)-E12

References: [1–95]

Table 18.2 Special markers of the prostate

Markers	Localization	Applications and pitfalls
PSA	Benign and malignant prostate epithelium	Prostate-specific marker. Most intense in benign prostate epithelium. Expressed in majority of prostatic adenocarcinoma (85–100%). Some poorly differentiated carcinoma or metastatic carcinoma may lose expression. Reactivity in some nonprostatic tissue (breast and salivary gland tumors) has been reported.
PSAP	Benign and malignant prostate epithelium	Similar to PSA
P501S	Benign and malignant prostate epithelium	Prostate-specific marker, expressed in the cytoplasm of benign and malignant prostatic glandular cells with granular, perinuclear staining pattern
PSMA	Benign and malignant prostate epithelium	Highly specific prostatic marker, especially for high-grade prostatic adenocarcinoma. Can be detected in colon, breast, bladder, pancreas, kidney, and melanoma.
P504S	Malignant prostate epithelium	Specific prostate carcinoma marker, not prostate specific. Overexpressed in over 90% of prostatic adenocarcinomas and 50% HGPIN.

Note: Using a panel of both PSA and P501S (prostein) increases the sensitivity in identifying a metastatic carcinoma of unknown primary, which is suspected to be of prostatic in origin

Both P501S and PSMA are prostate-specific markers, but positive stain in urothelial cell carcinoma has been reported (~10%) although usually lacking the typical prostatic carcinoma pattern (granular perinuclear stain – P501S, membrane stain – PSMA)

References: [4, 5, 7, 9–11, 14–22, 24, 25, 79–85]

Table 18.3 Markers for basal cells

Markers	Literature	GML data
p63	+	100% (25/25)
CK903	+	96% (24/25)
CK5/6	+	60% (15/25)
Maspin	+	100% (25/25)
S100A6	+	ND

Note: *ND* no data

p63 immunostaining is more consistent and less variable due to nuclear localization, demonstrating continuous "dotted" staining pattern. CK903 shows cytoplasmic "linear" staining pattern. Basal cell markers are subject to staining variability, including surgical procedure, tissue fixation, and antigen retrieval methods. Basal cell cocktail (CK903 + p63) improves the detection of prostate basal cells

p63 is usually used in combination with CK903 or CK5/6, and P504S, so-called triple stain, known as PIN4

References: [4, 5, 27–30, 73, 89–94, 96, 97]

Table 18.4 Markers for prostatic epithelial (secretory) cells

Markers	Literature	GML data
AE1/AE3	+	96% (24/25)
CAM 5.2	+	100% (25/25)
CK7	– or +	24% (6/25)
PSA	+	100% (25/25)
P504S	–	16% W+ (4/25)
EMA	–	– (0/25)
CK20	–	– (0/25)

Note: *W* weak

The immunoreactivity of CK7 and P504S in benign prostatic acinar cells tends to be weak and focal. MOC31 and BerEP4 are usually positive in normal acinar cells, whereas CEA and B72.3 are generally nonreactive

References: [4, 5, 7, 76, 83, 95]

Table 18.5 Markers for prostatic high-grade intraepithelial neoplasia

Antibody	Literature
p63	+ (basal layer)
CK903	+ (basal layer)
CK5/6	+ (basal layer)
P504S	+ or –
AE1/AE3	+
CAM 5.2	+
PSA	+
PSAP	+
KA4	+
UEA-1	+
Vimentin	– or +

Note: Immunostain for p63 frequently shows partial loss of basal cells in high-grade prostatic intraepithelial neoplasia (HGPIN), demonstrating a skipped nuclear staining pattern; in acini adjacent to prostatic adenocarcinoma, usually loss of basal cells. An example of HGPIN with triple stain (PIN4) is illustrated in Fig. 18.1

Over 60% of HGPIN are positive for P504S, with most intense staining in acini adjacent to prostatic adenocarcinoma

KA4 immunostain was reported positive in over 90% of cases of HGPIN and invasive carcinoma, but only in 4% of benign prostatic hypertrophy

References: [4–7, 21–23, 82–86, 92, 98–108]

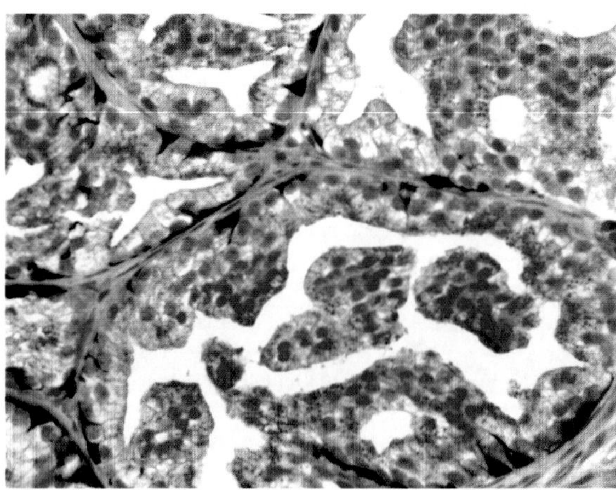

Fig. 18.1 High-grade prostatic intraepithelial neoplasia (HGPIN) demonstrates PIN4 (p63, CK903, and P504S) immunostaining. Note that the skipped brown nuclear (p63) and cytoplasmic (CK903) staining pattern for myoepithelial cells. The glandular epithelial cells show pink, granular, cytoplasmic staining (P504S)

Table 18.6 Markers for prostatic adenocarcinoma

Antibody	Literature	GML data (N = 136)
P504S	+	97.8% (133/136)
p63	–	– (0/136; basal layer)
CK5/6	–	– (0/136; basal layer)
CK903	–	– (0/136; basal layer)
PSA	+	100% (136/136)
CAM 5.2	+	100% (136/136)
AE1/AE3	+	88.4% (118/136)
CK7	– or +	3.7% (5/136)
CK20	–	2.9% (4/136)
MUC1	+	63% (86/136)

Note: Among the 136 cases of the GML tissue microarray data, 100 cases are prostatic adenocarcinomas Gleason score 3 + 3 and 36 cases are Gleason score 4 + 4. The staining results for these two groups (Gleason 3 + 3 and Gleason 4 + 4) are nearly identical, and the results have no statistical significance. In addition, a small number of cases of foamy gland carcinoma (11 cases of Gleason score 3 + 3 and 12 cases of Gleason score 4 + 4) also demonstrate similar findings

Expression of MUC1 is observed in 63% of cases and only seen in 36% of normal prostatic acini. Other mucin gene proteins (MUC2, MUC4, MUC5AC, and MUC6) are usually negative in both prostatic carcinoma and normal prostatic acini. In contrast, MUC6 is expressed in 100% of cases of seminal vesicles

CD10 is frequently positive in both benign and prostatic adenocarcinomas, with a strong intensity in carcinoma cases. MOC31 and BerEP4 are usually positive in both carcinoma and benign acini; in contrast, CEA and B72.3 are often negative in both

PAX2, PAX8, RCC, TTF-1, CDX2, S100P, VHL, ER, and PR are negative in both benign and carcinoma cases in our study. Androgen receptor (AR) is positive in 45% of carcinoma and 40% of normal acinar cells; however, the immunoreactivity is more diffuse and stronger in carcinomas. PSA is diffusely and strongly positive in both benign acinar cells and carcinomas. All carcinoma cases are diffusely and strongly positive for CAM 5.2; however, only 88% of cases for AE1/AE3. Therefore, caution should be taken when using AE1/AE3 as a screening marker for an epithelial lineage

An example of foamy gland carcinoma on H&E slide and the positive staining result for PIN4 (P504S, p63, and CK903) is shown in Fig. 18.2a, b. An example of immunoreactivity for P504S and PSA is shown in Figs. 18.3 and 18.4

References: [4, 5, 23, 24, 27–30, 76, 79–93, 109]

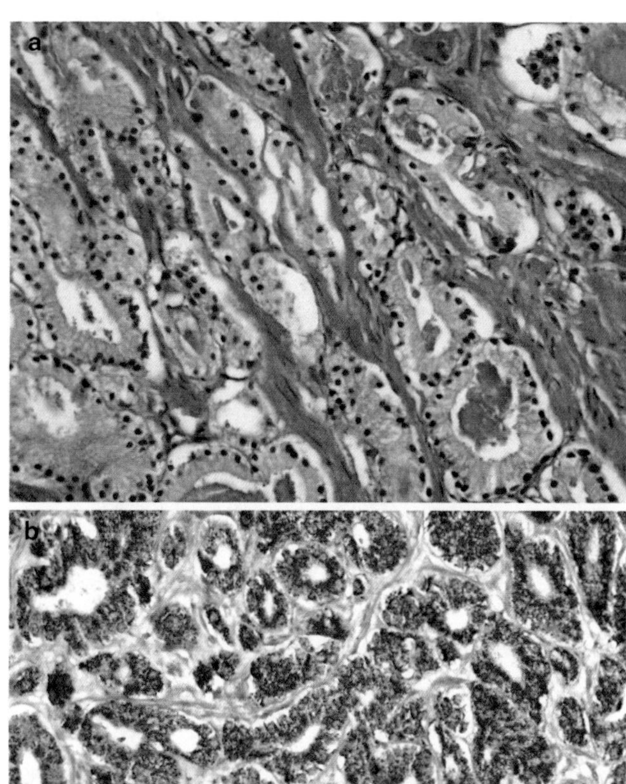

Fig. 18.2 (**a**) Prostate adenocarcinoma, foamy gland morphology, H&E. (**b**) Prostate adenocarcinoma, foamy gland morphology, immunostain for PIN4 (CK903, p63, P504S). Note that the tumor acini demonstrate lack of myoepithelial cells (negative for p63 and CK903) and strong, cytoplasmic, granular staining pattern for P504S

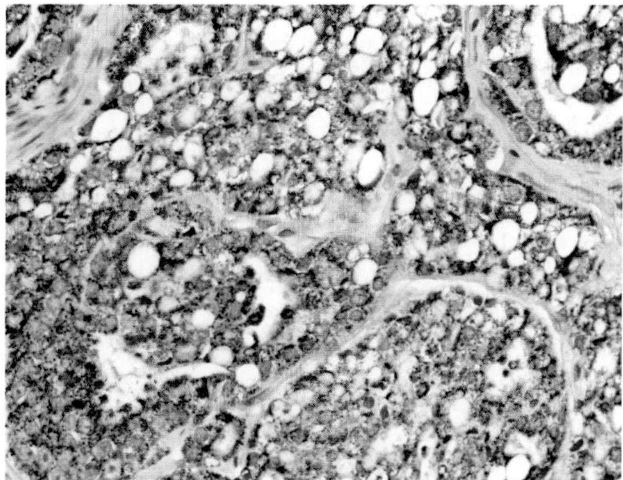

Fig. 18.3 Adenocarcinoma of the prostate demonstrates cytoplasmic granular staining for P504S

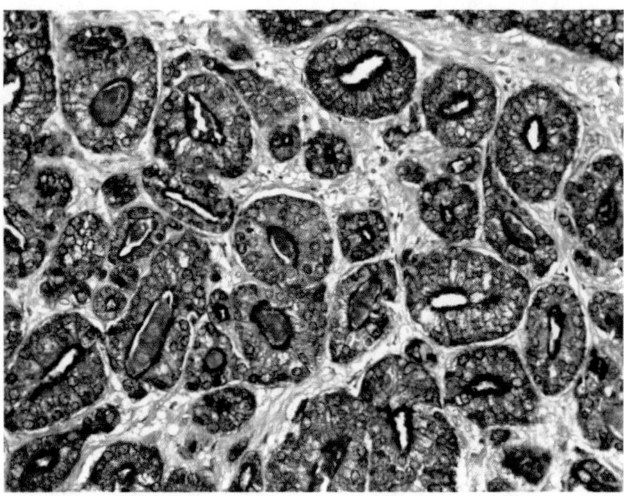

Fig. 18.4 Adenocarcinoma of the prostate, Gleason 3 + 3, demonstrates cytoplasmic staining for PSA

Table 18.7 Markers for prostatic ductal adenocarcinoma (PDA)

Antibody	Literature
P504S	+ or –
p63	– (absence of basal layer)
CK903	–
CK5/6	–
PSA	+ or –
PSAP	+ or –

Note: Basal cell markers are reported to be reactive in up to 30% of cases of PDA, which may represent intraductal carcinoma or intraductal involvement of the tumor. Staining patterns for P504S, PSA, and PSAP are similar to those of HGPIN

References: [4, 5, 19–21, 64, 68, 79–85, 110–118]

Table 18.8 Markers for basal cell carcinoma of the prostate

Antibody	Literature
p63	+
CK903	+
CK5/6	+
bcl2	+
P504S	–
PSA or PSAP	–
AE1/AE3	+
CK7	+
CK20	–

Note: A majority of the cases show multilayered basal staining; rare cases show some degree of P504S staining and focal staining for PSA or PSAP; CK7, AE1/AE3, and rarely PSA are positive in the cells of the center of the tumor nests

Basal cell carcinoma was reported demonstrating strong bcl2 positivity and high MIB-1 index

References: [4, 5, 7–9, 54–59]

Table 18.9 Markers for mucinous adenocarcinoma of the prostate

Antibody	Literature
PSA	+
PSAP	+
CEA	–
CDX2	–
CK7	–
CK20	–
CK903	–

References: [4, 5, 7–9, 35, 36, 119–122]

Table 18.10 Markers for signet ring cell carcinoma of the prostate

Antibody	Literature
PSA	+ or –
PSAP	+ or –
PAS-D	+
Mucicarmine	+ or –
Alcian blue	+ or –
AE1/AE3	+
CAM 5.2	+
CK903	–

Note: The phenotype of signet ring cell carcinoma is not different from high-grade prostatic carcinoma; about one-third of cases are negative for PSA and PSAP, and positive for intracytoplasmic neutral and acidic mucin stains, with most intense staining using PAS-D

References: [4, 5, 11, 12, 62, 123–132]

Table 18.11 Markers for small cell carcinoma of the prostate

Antibody	Literature
Chromogranin	+
CD56	+
TTF-1	+ or –
Synaptophysin	+
P501S, PSMA, PSA	– or +
CD44	+
AE1/AE3	+
CAM 5.2	+ or –
CK7	+ or –
CK20	–
p63	– or +
CK903	– or +
AR	– or +
c-kit (CD117)	+
bcl2	+
EGFR	+ or –

Note: A majority of small cell carcinomas of the prostate express at least one neuroendocrine marker; the two largest IHC studies of small cell carcinoma of the prostate report 52.3 and 83.3% of cases being positive for TTF-1; the majority of prostatic small cell carcinomas are negative for P504S, P501S, and PSA; diffuse, strong membranous staining for CD44 had been reported in small cell carcinoma of the prostate, but rare in small cell carcinomas of other sites and absent in majority of prostatic adenocarcinomas

References: [41–53, 133–139]

Table 18.12 Markers for squamous cell carcinoma of the prostate

Antibody	Literature
CK903	+
CK5/6	+
p63	+
PSA	–
PSAP	–
CK7	–
CK20	–

References: [4, 5, 7–9, 38, 95, 133, 140–142]

Table 18.13 Markers for sarcomatoid carcinoma of the prostate

Antibody	Literature
PSA	+
PSAP	+
AE1/AE3	+
Vimentin	+

Note: PSA, PSAP, and AE1/AE3 are usually only positive in the carcinomatous component, but negative in the sarcomatous component; vimentin is positive in the sarcomatous component

References: [4, 5, 7–9, 39, 95, 143–148]

Table 18.14 Benign prostatic lesions vs. malignant lesions

Markers	Benign	Malignant
p63	+ (basal layer)	–
CK903	+ (basal layer)	–
P504S	–	+

Note: When encounter a case of atypical glands of the prostate, using a cocktail of p63, P504S, and CK903 or CK5/6, known as PIN4, can significantly increase the specificity of the diagnosis of carcinoma

Rare prostate cancer cells (less than 0.3% of cases) show rare basal cell labeling, especially with CK903 and in high-grade carcinomas

Focal and weak P504S positivity can be seen in benign prostatic acini, up to 16% in our study

References: [27–30, 57, 60, 61, 79–85, 95, 109]

Table 18.15 Prostatic ductal (PDC) vs. acinar adenocarcinoma (PAC)

Antibody	PDC	PAC
Prolactin receptor	+, C	–/+
CK903, p63	–	–
P504S	+	+
PSA	+	+
PSAP	+	+

Note: Prolactin receptor demonstrates diffuse and strong cytoplasmic reactivity in a majority of ductal adenocarcinomas (75%); whereas only 20% of acinar adenocarcinomas show immunoreactivity, mainly in Gleason pattern 3

Patchy basal cell stains are identified in about 30% of prostatic ductal and cribriform acinar adenocarcinomas, as previously stated. It is rare in noncribriform prostatic acinar adenocarcinomas

P504S stain is positive in 80% of classic (noncribriform) acinar adenocarcinomas, similar to ductal adenocarcinomas (77%), and lower in foamy gland prostatic carcinomas (68%) and atrophic prostatic carcinomas (67%)

References: [26, 63–69, 79–85]

Table 18.16 Markers of basal cell hyperplasia (BCH) vs. basaloid carcinoma (BC)

Antibody	BCH	BC
bcl2	– or W+	S+
MIB-1 (Ki-67)	Low (~13.3/500)	High (~55/500)
CK903, CK14	+, multilayer	+/–
Calponin, SMA, SMMHC, S100 protein	–	–
PSA	–	–

Note: *SMA* smooth muscle actin; *SMMHC* smooth muscle myosin heavy chain; *W* weak; *S* strong

A high level of expression of bcl2 and MIB-1 helps establish the diagnosis of malignancy in basal cell lesions

References: [4, 5, 13–15, 54–59, 70–73, 77, 78]

Table 18.17 High-grade prostatic intraepithelial neoplasia (HGPIN) vs. seminal vesicles/ejaculatory duct epithelium (SV/EDE)

Antibody	HGPIN	SV/EDE	
		Literature	GML data
PAX2	–	+	100% (24/24)
P504S	+	–	W+, 41.7% (10/24)
PSA	+	–	– (0/24)
MUC6	–	+	95.8% (23/24)
CK7	– or +	+	100% (24/24)
p63, CK903, CK5/6	+ or discontinuous	+	100% (24/24)
AE1/AE3	+	+	100% (24/24)
CAM 5.2	+	+	100% (24/24)
CK20	–	–	– (0/24)

Note: PSA and PAP may be positive in distal SV/EDE. PAX2 is diffusely positive in SVED and nonreactive in PA, HGPIN, and normal prostatic tissue (except 10.5% of cases showed focal nuclear reactivity in central zone prostatic secretory epithelium)

In our study, 10 of the 24 cases of SV/EDE show weak staining for P504S. An example of the staining result in seminal vesicles for CK7, PAX2, MUC6, and P504S is shown in Figs. 18.5–18.9

References: [4, 5, 8–10, 87, 88, 149–153]

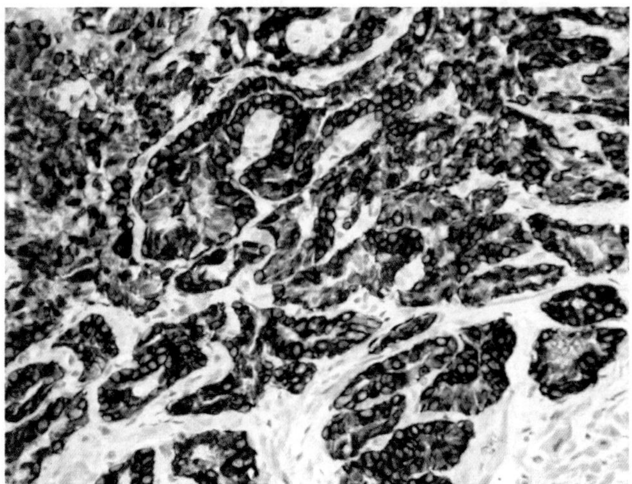

Fig. 18.6 Seminal vesicle demonstrates cytoplasmic and membranous staining for CK7

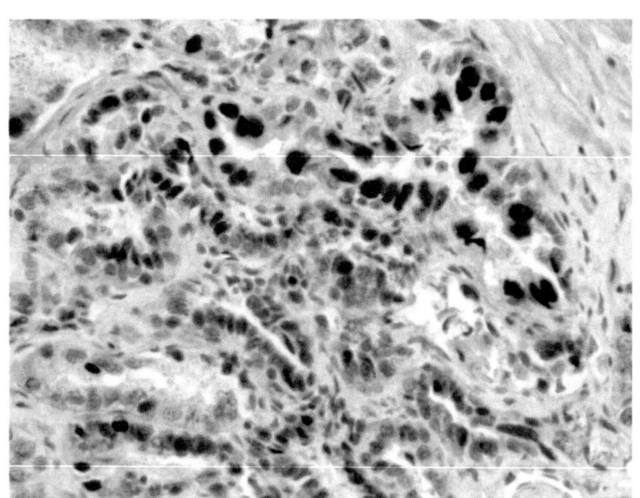

Fig. 18.7 Seminal vesicle demonstrates nuclear staining for Pax2

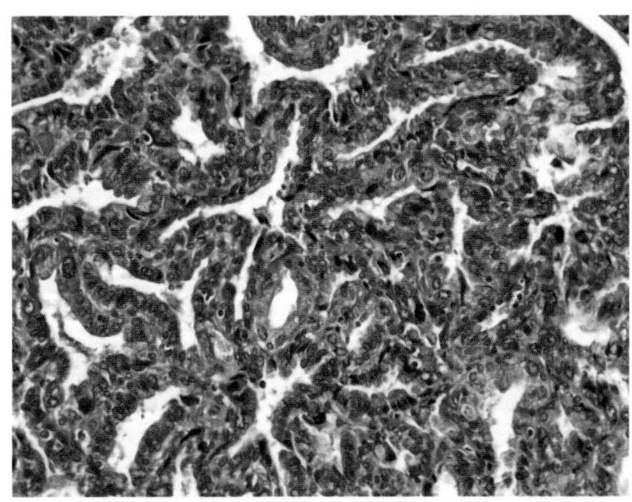

Fig. 18.5 Seminal vesicle, H&E

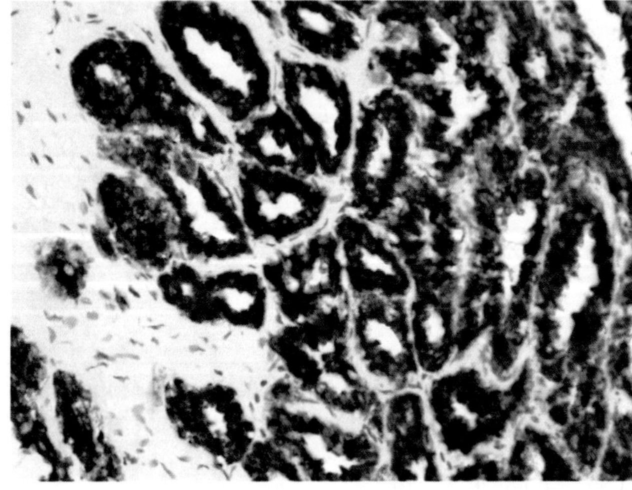

Fig. 18.8 Seminal vesicle demonstrates cytoplasmic staining for MUC6

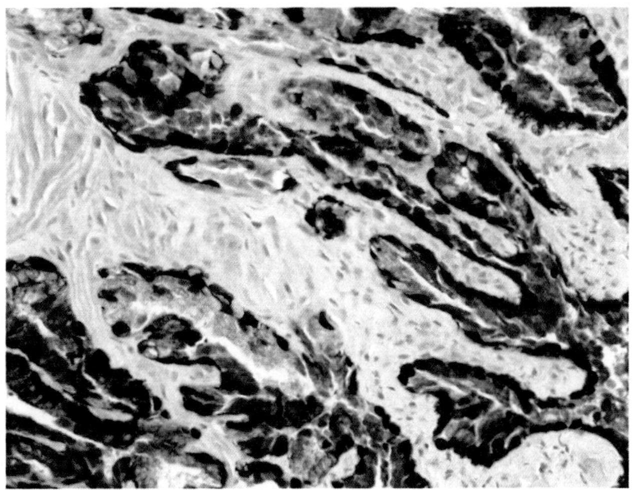

Fig. 18.9 Seminal vesicle demonstrates PIN4 staining. Note that the brown nuclear (p63) and brown cytoplasmic (CK903) staining of the myoepithelial cells, and the weak, pink cytoplasmic (P504S) staining of the luminal cells

Table 18.18 High-grade prostatic intraepithelial neoplasia (HGPIN) vs. basal cell hyperplasia (BCH)

Antibody	HGPIN	BCH
p63, CK903, CK5/6	+, −, discontinuous	+, multilayer, continuous
P504S	+ (50%)	−
CAM 5.2	+	−
Glutathione-*s*-transferase-pi (GST-π)	N/A	+

Note: Rare basal cell lesions may be negative for HMWCK, but positive for p63; therefore, both markers should be applied in the workup of basal cell lesions. GST-π shows decreased expression in prostate carcinoma and PIN, but immunostain is limited

References: [4–7, 21–24, 70–78, 82–86, 95]

Table 18.19 High-grade prostatic intraepithelial neoplasia (HGPIN) vs. prostatic adenocarcinoma (PA) with cribriform pattern

Markers	HGPIN	PA, cribriform pattern
p63	+	−
CK903	+	−
P504S	+ or −	+
PSA	+	+
PSAP	+	+

Note: HGPIN may show a discontinuous staining pattern for basal markers or loss of basal cells in acini adjacent to adenocarcinoma. Positive P504S staining is seen in 60% of HGPIN and over 90% of carcinomas

References: [4–7, 15–17, 21–23, 82–86, 95, 154, 155]

Table 18.20 High-grade prostatic intraepithelial neoplasia (HGPIN) vs. prostatic intraductal carcinoma (PIC)

Markers	HGPIN	PIC
p63	+	+
CK903	+	+
P504S	+	+

Note: Both show a similar immunostaining pattern. No reliable markers can differentiate these two entities. The diagnosis is based on histomorphology

References: [4, 5, 27, 30, 79–85, 89–95]

Table 18.21 High-grade prostatic intraepithelial neoplasia (HGPIN) vs. prostatic ductal adenocarcinoma (PDA)

Antibody	HGPIN	PDA
CK903	+	−
p63	+	−
P504S	+	+

References: [4, 5, 12–14, 79–85, 95, 110, 156–158]

Table 18.22 Low-grade prostatic adenocarcinoma (PA) vs. atypical adenomatous hyperplasia (AAH) or adenosis

Antibody	PA	AAH
CK903 or CK5/6	–	+, patchy
p63	–	+, patchy
P504S	+	– or +
PSA, PSAP	+	+

Note: Patchy basal stain is usually detected in AAH. Up to 18% of prostate cancers can be P504S-negative on core biopsy; for foamy gland and pseudohyperplastic type, the percentage is higher (up to 20–30%). A majority of AAHs are nonreactive to P504S. Focal staining for P504S had been reported in 10% of cases of AAH and diffuse staining in 7.5%

Our experience shows approximately 98% of prostatic adenocarcinomas are positive for P504S including Gleason 3 + 3, Gleason 4 + 4, and foamy gland carcinoma

References: [4, 5, 15–17, 26, 79–85, 95, 159–164]

Table 18.23 Low-grade prostatic adenocarcinoma (PA) vs. atrophy (simple atrophy and partial atrophy)

Markers	PA	Atrophy
CK903 or CK5/6	–	+
p63	–	+
P504S	+	–

Note: Partial atrophy, also referred to as postatrophic hyperplasia, is a benign mimicker of adenocarcinoma. In general, there is a continuous basal layer on immunostain and usually a lack of P504S staining. Some studies report an overlapping immunostain profile between PA and partial atrophy, but a majority of the cases of partial atrophy are positive for basal markers (reported 68.7%)

References: [4, 5, 12–14, 69, 79–85, 95, 165–167]

Table 18.24 Low-grade prostatic adenocarcinoma (PA) vs. basal cell hyperplasia (BCH) and high-grade prostatic intraepithelial neoplasia (HGPIN)

Antibody	PA	BCH	HGPIN
CK903 or CK5/6	–	+, C	+, C
p63	–	+, N	+, N
P504S	+, C	–	+, C

Note: BCH reveals multilayered staining for CK903 and p63 in some glands, while HGPIN shows single-cell layer staining

References: [4, 5, 54–59, 70–72, 78–85]

Table 18.25 Low-grade prostatic adenocarcinoma (PA) vs. nephrogenic adenoma (NA)

Antibody	PA	NA
PAX2	–	+
PAX8	–	+
S100A1	–	+
EMA	–	+
PSA	+	– or +
PSAP	+	– or +
CK7	– or +	+
CK903	–	– or +
p63	–	– or +
P504S	+	+ or –

Note: An example of nephrogenic adenoma is illustrated in Fig. 18.10a–e

References: [4, 5, 15–17, 79–85, 95, 168–174]

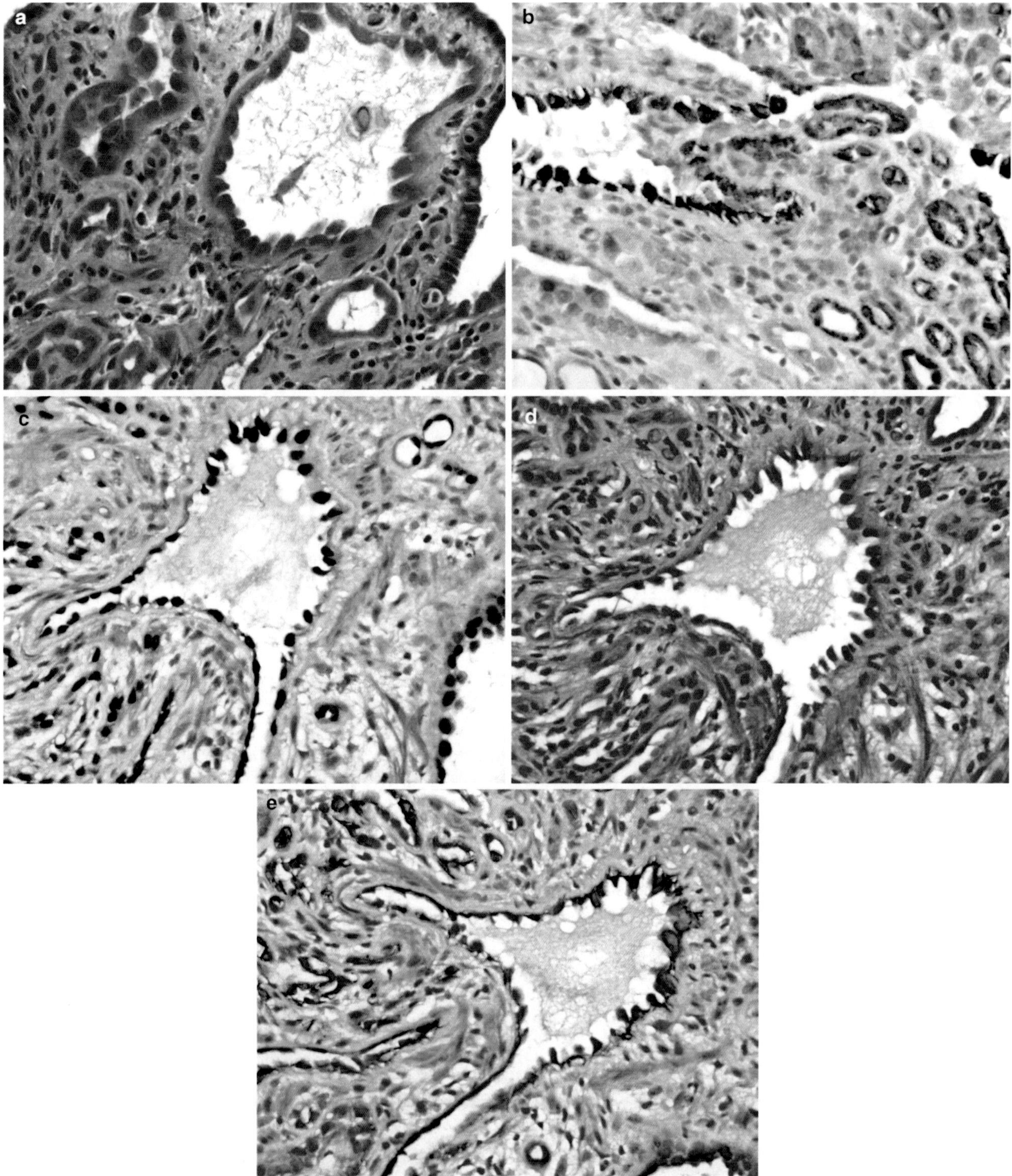

Fig. 18.10 (**a**) Nephrogenic adenoma, H&E. (**b**) Nephrogenic adenoma, demonstrating cytoplasmic staining for P504S. (**c**) Nephrogenic adenoma, demonstrating nuclear staining for PAX8. (**d**) Nephrogenic adenoma, demonstrating negative PSA staining. (**e**) Nephrogenic adenoma, demonstrating cytoplasmic staining for CK7

Table 18.26 Low-grade prostatic adenocarcinoma (PA) vs. radiation atypia (RA)

Antibody	PA	RA
CK903	–	+
CK5/6	–	+
p63	–	+
PSA	+	–
PSAP	+	–
P504S	+	–

Note: The profile of postradiation atypia of benign glands is similar to that of nonirradiated benign glands with a relative preponderance of high molecular weight cytokeratin (CK903)-positive basal cells and a paucity of PSA and PSAP-positive secretory acinar cells, which is of great diagnostic utility

References: [4, 5, 7–9, 95, 175–180]

Table 18.27 Low-grade prostatic adenocarcinoma (PA) vs. mesonephric hyperplasia (MH) and verumontanum mucosal gland hyperplasia (VMGH)

Antibody	PA	MH	VMGH
CK903	–	+	+
CK5/6	–	+	+
p63	–	+	+
PSA	+	–	–
PSAP	+	–	–
P504S	+	N/A	N/A

References: [4, 5, 8–10, 84, 85, 95, 181–186]

Table 18.28 Low-grade prostatic adenocarcinoma (PA) vs. normal structures (seminal vesicles, colonic mucosa, and Cowper's glands)

Antibody	PA	Seminal vesicle	Cowper's gland	Colonic mucosa
CK903	–	+	– or +	+
CK5/6	–	+	– or +	+
p63	–	+	– or +	+
SMA	–	–	+	–
P504S	+	–	N/A	N/A
PSA	+	–	– or +	–
PSAP	+	–	–	–
PAX2	–	+	N/A	N/A

Notes: Basal cell markers (CK903, CK5/6, and p63) identified the myoepithelial cells in benign structures. HMWCK stains the ductal epithelium of the Cowper's gland, but the acini are often negative, failing to reveal the attenuated myoepithelium; however, SMA is often positive

References: [4, 5, 10–13, 84, 87, 88, 95, 149–153, 187, 188]

Table 18.29 High-grade prostatic adenocarcinoma (PA) vs. clear cell cribriform hyperplasia (CCCH)

Antibody	PA	CCCH
CK903	–	+
CK5/6	–	+
p63	–	+
P504S	+	–

Note: The key feature for the diagnosis of CCCH is the preservation of a nodular configuration with a bland cytology and two cell populations lining the involved acini

References: [3–6, 84, 95, 189, 190]

Table 18.30 High-grade prostatic adenocarcinoma (PA) vs. nonspecific granulomatous prostatitis (NSGP) and xanthoma

Antibody	PA	NSGP and xanthoma
AE1/AE3	+	–
CAM 5.2	+	–
PSA	+	–
PSAP	+	–
P504S	+	–
CD68	–	+

Note: Rare cases of xanthoma may reactive to PSA and PAP (about 10%)

References: [4–7, 84, 95, 191–193]

Table 18.31 High-grade prostatic adenocarcinoma (PA) vs. sclerosing adenosis (SA)

Antibody	PA	SA
CK903	–	+
p63	–	+
MSA	–	+
S100	–	+

Note: Sclerosing adenosis demonstrates a dense spindle cell component and basally located cells with true myoepithelial differentiation (coexpression of cytokeratin, muscle-specific actin (MSA), and S100 protein). MSA and S100 protein are not expressed in normal basal cells

References: [4–7, 84, 95, 194–197]

Table 18.32 High-grade prostatic adenocarcinoma (PA) vs. paraganglia

Antibody	PA	Paraganglia
AE1/AE3	+	–
Synaptophysin	–	+
Chromogranin	–	+
NSE	–	+
S100	–	+*
PSA	+	–
PSAP	+	–

Note: * Sustentacular cells in paraganglia are positive for S100 protein

References: [4–7, 84, 95, 198–200]

Table 18.33 Prostatic adenocarcinoma (PA) vs. renal cell carcinoma (RCC)

Antibody	PA	RCC
PAX8	–	+
RCC	–	+
VHL	ND	+
Vimentin	–	+
PSA	+	–
PSAP	+	–
CD10	–[a]	+
P504S	+	+ or –

References: [4, 5, 21–23, 71, 79–85, 95, 174, 201–211]

[a]**Note**: A subset of high-grade prostatic adenocarcinoma (Gleason scores of 8, 9, and 10) with infiltrative patterns (angulated narrow nests, single files, or single cells) displays cytoplasmic and membranous expression of CD10. FLI-1 was reported positive in PA and negative in RCC

Table 18.34 Prostatic adenocarcinoma (PA) vs. urothelial carcinoma (UC)

	PA		UC	
Antibody	Literature	GMC	Literature	GMC
PSA	+	100% (136/136)	–	0 (0/40)
PSAP	+	ND	–	ND
p63	–	– (0/136)	+	98% (39/40)
S100P	–	– (0/136)	+	68% (27/40)
CK 903	–	– (0/136)	+ or –	93% (37/40)
CK5/6	–	– (0/136)	+ or –	45% (18/40)
Thrombomodulin	–	ND	+	38% (15/40)
P501S	+	ND	– or +	ND
P504S	+	97.8% (133/136)	– or+	8% (3/40)
CK7	– or +	3.7% (5/136)	+	98% (39/40)
CK20	–	2.9% (4/136)	+ or –	58% (23/40)
CK17	–	– (0/136)	+ or –	40% (16/40)
Uroplakin III	–	ND	+ or –	ND
p53	Rare	ND	– or +	50% (20/40)

Note: Metastatic prostatic adenocarcinoma may lose expression of PSA and P501S (less than 20%), but simultaneous loss of both is rare (3%)

References: [4, 5, 8, 9, 21–23, 34–36, 79–85, 95, 205, 212–218]

Table 18.35 Prostatic adenocarcinoma (PA) vs. small cell carcinoma (SCC)

Antibody	PA	SCC
Chromogranin	–	+
CD56	–	+
TTF-1	–	+ or –
CD44	–	+, M
PSA	+	– or +
PSMA	+	– or +
Synaptophysin	–	+
NSE	–	+
P501S	+	– or +
P504S	+	– or +
PSAP	+	– or +
AR	+	–
Leu 7	+	–

Note: TTF-1 was reported positive in 52.3 and 83.3% of small cell carcinoma of the prostate as previously stated (Table 18.11). CD44 immunostain shows strong membrane staining pattern in prostatic small cell carcinoma (see Table 18.11). A small proportion of prostatic small cell carcinomas (0–25%) shows reactivity to PSA, P501S, and PSMA

References: [41–53, 79–85, 133–139]

Table 18.36 Prostatic adenocarcinoma (PA) vs. basal cell carcinoma (BCC)

Antibody	PA	BCC
p63	–	+
CK903 or CK5/6	–	+
P504S	+	–
PSA or PSAP	+	–
CK7	– or +	+
bcl2	– or +	+

References: [4, 5, 14, 15, 17, 54–59, 79–85, 95]

Table 18.37 Prostatic adenocarcinoma (PA) vs. squamous cell carcinoma (SQCC)

Antibody	PA	SQCC
CK5/6	–	+
p63	–	+
P504S	+	–
PSA	+	–
PSAP	+	–
CK7	– or +	–

References: [41–43, 45–53, 79–85, 133–139]

Table 18.38 The evaluation of residual carcinoma status post hormonal and radiation therapy

Antibody	Residual carcinoma
AE1/AE3	+
PSA, PSMA	+
P504S	+
CK903	–
p63	–

References: [84, 95, 177, 187, 188, 194, 195, 219–221]

Table 18.39 Markers used in prostate mesenchymal lesions

Markers	Localization (N, M, C)	Function	Application and pitfalls
CD34	M	A 110-kDa heavily glycosylated transmembrane glycoprotein	Expressed in embryonic cells of the hematopoietic system and endothelia. Positive in vascular neoplasm, spindle cell lipoma, dermatofibrosarcoma protuberans, solitary fibrous tumor, and some leiomyosarcomas.
Vimentin	C	A 57-kDa cytoplasmic intermediate filament protein	Considered to be the "primordial" member of the intermediate filament protein family expressed in most fetal cells during early development. Not cell-type specific, with very limited diagnostic utility. Serves as a useful "control marker," ensuring properly preserved and processed tissue.
SMA	C	A cytoplasmic protein of the actin family	A marker of myogenetic differentiation. Positive for smooth muscle tissue or neoplasms, also for myofibroblasts, myoepithelial, and others.
HHF-35	C	A cytoplasmic protein of the actin family	A more specific, muscle-restricted marker
Desmin	C	A 53-kDa cytoplasmic intermediate filament protein	Characteristically found in muscle cells and in neoplasms associated with them
S100	N + C	Small dimeric member of the family of calcium-binding proteins	Widely distributed in human tissues, including glia, neurons, chondrocytes, Schwann cells, melanocytes, fixed phagocytic, or antigen-presenting mononuclear cells, Langerhans, histiocytes, myoepithelial cells, and various epithelia
Myogenin	N	A transcription factor	Positive for rhabdomyosarcoma
bcl2	C	A membrane-associated anti-apoptotic oncoprotein	Solitary fibrous tumors and GISTs are positive for bcl2
p53	N	Tumor suppressor gene	Not very specific. Inflammatory myofibroblastic tumors are positive.
Beta-catenin	M, N		About 33–50% of solitary fibrous tumors show nuclear stain for β-catenin
CD117	C	A member of the receptor tyrosine kinase family	Positive in GISTs. Rare positive in inflammatory myofibroblastic tumors.
ALK-1	C, N	The protein product of the anaplastic lymphoma kinase gene	May be expressed in inflammatory myofibroblastic tumors
PR	N	Progesterone receptor	Present in hormone-responsive tissue and their neoplasm, also reported in carcinomas of lung, stomach, and thyroid. STUMP and stromal sarcomas are positive for PR.
AR	N	A 11-kDa nuclear protein belonging to the family of activated class I steroid receptors	Frequently expressed in the stromal and epithelial components of stromal tumors of uncertain malignant potential, phyllodes type

Note: *SMA* smooth muscle actin; HHF-35 – or anti-muscle-specific actin; CD34 – or human hematopoietic progenitor cell antigen; *ALK-1* anaplastic lymphoma kinase-1; *GIST* gastrointestinal stromal tumor; *STUMP* stromal tumors of uncertain malignant potential

References: [39, 157, 222–249]

Table 18.40 Markers for the evaluation of benign or low-grade stromal tumors

Markers	SFT	Leiomyoma	STUMP	IMT	GIST
CD34	+	–	+	–	+
SMA	–	+	– or +	+	–
Desmin	–	+	– or +	+	–
PR	+ or –	– or +	+	N/A	–
ALK-1	–	–	–	+	–
CD117	–	–	–	– or +	+
Pan-CK	–	– or +	–	+	–
bcl2	+	–	–	N/A	+
p53	– or +	N/A	– or +	+	N/A
HHF-35	–	+	– or +	+	–
Beta-catenin	– or +	–	–	N/A	N/A
Vimentin	+	+	+	N/A	N/A

Note: *SFT* solitary fibrous tumor; *STUMP* stromal tumors of uncertain malignant potential; *IMT* inflammatory myofibroblastic tumor; *GIST* gastrointestinal stromal tumors

References: [39, 157, 222–249]

Table 18.41 Markers for the evaluation of malignant stromal tumors

Markers	SS	LMS	RMS
CD34	+	–	–
SMA	–	+	+
Desmin	–	+	+
Myogenin	–	–	+
PR	+	+ or –	–
MyoD1	–	–	+
Vimentin	+	+	+
Pan-CK, CAM 5.2	–	– or focal +	– or +
S100	–	–	–

Note: *SS* stromal sarcoma; *LMS* leiomyosarcoma; *RMS* rhabdomyosarcoma

Nuclear stain for p53 and β (beta)-catenin has been reported in a few high-grade stromal sarcomas. Focal cytokeratin expression is observed in about one-quarter of LMSs

References: [39, 157, 222–249]

Note for All Tables

Note: "+" – usually greater than 70% of cases are positive; "–" – less than 5% of cases are positive; "+ or –" – usually more than 50% of cases are positive; "– or +" – less than 50% of cases are positive.

References

1. Eble JN, Sauter G, Epstein JI, Sesterhenn IA, editors. Pathology and genetics of tumours of the urinary system and male genital organs. World Health Organization classifications of tumours. Lyon, France: IARC Press; 2004.
2. Fletcher CD, editor. Diagnostic histopathology of tumors. 3rd ed. Philadelphia, PA: Churchill Livingstone Elsevier; 2007.
3. Dabbs DJ. Diagnostic immunohistochemistry: theranostic and genomic applications. 3rd ed. Philadelphia, PA: Saunders Elsevier; 2010.
4. Paner GP, Luthringer DJ, Amin MB. Best practice in diagnostic immunohistochemistry: prostate carcinoma and its mimics in needle core biopsies. Arch Pathol Lab Med. 2008;132(9):1388–96.
5. Hammerich KH, Ayala GE, Wheeler TM. Application of immunohistochemistry to the genitourinary system (prostate, urinary bladder, testis, and kidney). Arch Pathol Lab Med. 2008;132(3):432–40.
6. Bostwick DG. Prostate-specific antigen. Current role in diagnostic pathology of prostate cancer. Am J Clin Pathol. 1994;102(4 Suppl 1):S31–7.
7. Bostwick DG, Pacelli A, Blute M, Roche P, Murphy GP. Prostate specific membrane antigen expression in prostatic intraepithelial neoplasia and adenocarcinoma: a study of 184 cases. Cancer. 1998;82(11):2256–61.
8. Sheridan T, Herawi M, Epstein JI, Illei PB. The role of P501S and PSA in the diagnosis of metastatic adenocarcinoma of the prostate. Am J Surg Pathol. 2007;31(9):1351–5.
9. Yin M, Dhir R, Parwani AV. Diagnostic utility of p501s (prostein) in comparison to prostate specific antigen (PSA) for the detection of metastatic prostatic adenocarcinoma. Diagn Pathol. 2007;2:41.
10. Chang SS, Reuter VE, Heston WD, Gaudin PB. Comparison of anti-prostate-specific membrane antigen antibodies and other immunomarkers in metastatic prostate carcinoma. Urology. 2001;57(6):1179–83.
11. Carder PJ, Speirs V, Ramsdale J, Lansdown MR. Expression of prostate specific antigen in male breast cancer. J Clin Pathol. 2005;58(1):69–71.
12. Cheng CW, Chan LW, Ng CF, Chan CK, Tse MK, Lai MM. Breast metastasis from prostate cancer and interpretation of immunoreactivity to prostate-specific antigen. Int J Urol. 2006;13(4): 463–5.
13. Gatalica Z, Norris BA, Kovatich AJ. Immunohistochemical localization of prostate-specific antigen in ductal epithelium of male breast. Potential diagnostic pitfall in patients with gynecomastia. Appl Immunohistochem Mol Morphol. 2000;8(2):158–61.
14. Sweat SD, Pacelli A, Murphy GP, Bostwick DG. Prostate-specific membrane antigen expression is greatest in prostate adenocarcinoma and lymph node metastases. Urology. 1998;52(4):637–40.
15. Silver DA, Pellicer I, Fair WR, Heston WD, Cordon-Cardo C. Prostate-specific membrane antigen expression in normal and malignant human tissues. Clin Cancer Res. 1997;3(1):81–5.
16. Kinoshita Y, Kuratsukuri K, Landas S, et al. Expression of prostate-specific membrane antigen in normal and malignant human tissues. World J Surg. 2006;30(4):628–36.
17. Murphy GP, Elgamal AA, Su SL, Bostwick DG, Holmes EH. Current evaluation of the tissue localization and diagnostic utility of prostate specific membrane antigen. Cancer. 1998;83(11): 2259–69.
18. Chang SS. Monoclonal antibodies and prostate-specific membrane antigen. Curr Opin Investig Drugs. 2004;5(6):611–5.
19. Mhawech-Fauceglia P, Zhang S, Terracciano L, et al. Prostate-specific membrane antigen (PSMA) protein expression in normal and neoplastic tissues and its sensitivity and specificity in prostate adenocarcinoma: an immunohistochemical study using multiple tumour tissue microarray technique. Histopathology. 2007;50(4):472–83.
20. Parwani AV, Marlow C, Demarzo AM, et al. Immunohistochemical staining of precursor forms of prostate-specific antigen (proPSA) in metastatic prostate cancer. Am J Surg Pathol. 2006;30(10): 1231–6.
21. Xu J, Kalos M, Stolk JA, et al. Identification and characterization of prostein, a novel prostate-specific protein. Cancer Res. 2001;61(4):1563–8.
22. Kalos M, Askaa J, Hylander BL, et al. Prostein expression is highly restricted to normal and malignant prostate tissues. Prostate. 2004;60(3):246–56.
23. Hameed O, Humphrey PA. Immunohistochemistry in diagnostic surgical pathology of the prostate. Semin Diagn Pathol. 2005; 22(1):88–104.
24. Goldstein NS. Immunophenotypic characterization of 225 prostate adenocarcinomas with intermediate or high Gleason scores. Am J Clin Pathol. 2002;117(3):471–7.
25. Friedman RS, Spies AG, Kalos M. Identification of naturally processed CD8 T cell epitopes from prostein, a prostate tissue-specific vaccine candidate. Eur J Immunol. 2004;34(4):1091–101.
26. Zhou M, Jiang Z, Epstein JI. Expression and diagnostic utility of alpha-methylacyl-CoA-racemase (P504S) in foamy gland and pseudohyperplastic prostate cancer. Am J Surg Pathol. 2003; 27(6):772–8.
27. Ali TZ, Epstein JI. False positive labeling of prostate cancer with high molecular weight cytokeratin: p63 a more specific immunomarker for basal cells. Am J Surg Pathol. 2008;32(12):1890–5.
28. Oliai BR, Kahane H, Epstein JI. Can basal cells be seen in adenocarcinoma of the prostate?: an immunohistochemical study using high molecular weight cytokeratin (clone 34betaE12) antibody. Am J Surg Pathol. 2002;26(9):1151–60.
29. Kahane H, Sharp JW, Shuman GB, Dasilva G, Epstein JI. Utilization of high molecular weight cytokeratin on prostate needle biopsies in an independent laboratory. Urology. 1995; 45(6):981–6.
30. Weinstein MH, Signoretti S, Loda M. Diagnostic utility of immunohistochemical staining for p63, a sensitive marker of prostatic basal cells. Mod Pathol. 2002;15(12):1302–8.
31. Gupta RK. Immunoreactivity of prostate-specific antigen in male breast carcinomas: two examples of a diagnostic pitfall in discriminating a primary breast cancer from metastatic prostate carcinoma. Diagn Cytopathol. 1999;21(3):167–9.
32. Holmes GF, Eisele DW, Rosenthal D, Westra WH. PSA immunoreactivity in a parotid oncocytoma: a diagnostic pitfall in discriminating primary parotid neoplasms from metastatic prostate cancer. Diagn Cytopathol. 1998;19(3):221–5.
33. van Krieken JH. Prostate marker immunoreactivity in salivary gland neoplasms. A rare pitfall in immunohistochemistry. Am J Surg Pathol. 1993;17(4):410–4.
34. Lane Z, Hansel DE, Epstein JI. Immunohistochemical expression of prostatic antigens in adenocarcinoma and villous adenoma of the urinary bladder. Am J Surg Pathol. 2008;32(9):1322–6.
35. Osunkoya AO, Epstein JI. Primary mucin-producing urothelial-type adenocarcinoma of prostate: report of 15 cases. Am J Surg Pathol. 2007;31(9):1323–9.

36. Curtis MW, Evans AJ, Srigley JR. Mucin-producing urothelial-type adenocarcinoma of prostate: report of two cases of a rare and diagnostically challenging entity. Mod Pathol. 2005;18(4):585–90.
37. Gopalan A, Sharp DS, Fine SW, et al. Urachal carcinoma: a clinicopathologic analysis of 24 cases with outcome correlation. Am J Surg Pathol. 2009;33(5):659–68.
38. Parwani AV, Kronz JD, Genega EM, Gaudin P, Chang S, Epstein JI. Prostate carcinoma with squamous differentiation: an analysis of 33 cases. Am J Surg Pathol. 2004;28(5):651–7.
39. Hansel DE, Epstein JI. Sarcomatoid carcinoma of the prostate: a study of 42 cases. Am J Surg Pathol. 2006;30(10):1316–21.
40. Parwani AV, Herawi M, Epstein JI. Pleomorphic giant cell adenocarcinoma of the prostate: report of 6 cases. Am J Surg Pathol. 2006;30(10):1254–9.
41. Wang W, Epstein JI. Small cell carcinoma of the prostate. A morphologic and immunohistochemical study of 95 cases. Am J Surg Pathol. 2008;32(1):65–71.
42. Simon RA, di Sant'Agnese PA, Huang LS, et al. CD44 expression is a feature of prostatic small cell carcinoma and distinguishes it from its mimickers. Hum Pathol. 2009;40(2):252–8.
43. Oesterling JE, Hauzeur CG, Farrow GM. Small cell anaplastic carcinoma of the prostate: a clinical, pathological and immunohistological study of 27 patients. J Urol. 1992;147(3 Pt 2):804–7.
44. Fan CY, Wang J, Barnes EL. Expression of androgen receptor and prostatic specific markers in salivary duct carcinoma: an immunohistochemical analysis of 13 cases and review of the literature. Am J Surg Pathol. 2000;24(4):579–86.
45. Agoff SN, Lamps LW, Philip AT, et al. Thyroid transcription factor-1 is expressed in extrapulmonary small cell carcinomas but not in other extrapulmonary neuroendocrine tumors. Mod Pathol. 2000;13(3):238–42.
46. Ordonez NG. Value of thyroid transcription factor-1 immunostaining in distinguishing small cell lung carcinomas from other small cell carcinomas. Am J Surg Pathol. 2000;24(9):1217–23.
47. Cheuk W, Kwan MY, Suster S, Chan JK. Immunostaining for thyroid transcription factor 1 and cytokeratin 20 aids the distinction of small cell carcinoma from Merkel cell carcinoma, but not pulmonary from extrapulmonary small cell carcinomas. Arch Pathol Lab Med. 2001;125(2):228–31.
48. Chan JK, Suster S, Wenig BM, Tsang WY, Chan JB, Lau AL. Cytokeratin 20 immunoreactivity distinguishes Merkel cell (primary cutaneous neuroendocrine) carcinomas and salivary gland small cell carcinomas from small cell carcinomas of various sites. Am J Surg Pathol. 1997;21(2):226–34.
49. di Sant'Agnese PA. Neuroendocrine differentiation in carcinoma of the prostate. Diagnostic, prognostic, and therapeutic implications. Cancer. 1992;70(1 Suppl):254–68.
50. di Sant'Agnese PA. Neuroendocrine differentiation in human prostatic carcinoma. Hum Pathol. 1992;23(3):287–96.
51. Ather MH, Abbas F, Faruqui N, Israr M, Pervez S. Correlation of three immunohistochemically detected markers of neuroendocrine differentiation with clinical predictors of disease progression in prostate cancer. BMC Urol. 2008;8:21.
52. Yao JL, Madeb R, Bourne P, et al. Small cell carcinoma of the prostate: an immunohistochemical study. Am J Surg Pathol. 2006;30(6):705–12.
53. Patrawala L, Calhoun T, Schneider-Broussard R, et al. Highly purified CD44+ prostate cancer cells from xenograft human tumors are enriched in tumorigenic and metastatic progenitor cells. Oncogene. 2006;25(12):1696–708.
54. McKenney JK, Amin MB, Srigley JR, et al. Basal cell proliferations of the prostate other than usual basal cell hyperplasia: a clinicopathologic study of 23 cases, including four carcinomas, with a proposed classification. Am J Surg Pathol. 2004;28(10):1289–98.
55. Yang XJ, McEntee M, Epstein JI. Distinction of basaloid carcinoma of the prostate from benign basal cell lesions by using immunohistochemistry for bcl-2 and Ki-67. Hum Pathol. 1998;29(12):1447–50.
56. Ali TZ, Epstein JI. Basal cell carcinoma of the prostate: a clinicopathologic study of 29 cases. Am J Surg Pathol. 2007;31(5): 697–705.
57. Begnami MD, Quezado M, Pinto P, Linehan WM, Merino M. Adenoid cystic/basal cell carcinoma of the prostate: review and update. Arch Pathol Lab Med. 2007;131(4):637–40.
58. Iczkowski KA, Ferguson KL, Grier DD, et al. Adenoid cystic/basal cell carcinoma of the prostate: clinicopathologic findings in 19 cases. Am J Surg Pathol. 2003;27(12):1523–9.
59. Montironi R, Mazzucchelli R, Stramazzotti D, Scarpelli M, Lopez Beltran A, Bostwick DG. Basal cell hyperplasia and basal cell carcinoma of the prostate: a comprehensive review and discussion of a case with c-erbB-2 expression. J Clin Pathol. 2005;58(3):290–6.
60. Parsons JK, Gage WR, Nelson WG, De Marzo AM. p63 Protein expression is rare in prostate adenocarcinoma: implications for cancer diagnosis and carcinogenesis. Urology. 2001; 58(4):619–24.
61. Osunkoya AO, Hansel DE, Sun X, Netto GJ, Epstein JI. Aberrant diffuse expression of p63 in adenocarcinoma of the prostate on needle biopsy and radical prostatectomy: report of 21 cases. Am J Surg Pathol. 2008;32(3):461–7.
62. Torbenson M, Dhir R, Nangia A, Becich MJ, Kapadia SB. Prostatic carcinoma with signet ring cells: a clinicopathologic and immunohistochemical analysis of 12 cases, with review of the literature. Mod Pathol. 1998;11(6):552–9.
63. Sanati S, Watson MA, Salavaggione AL, Humphrey PA. Gene expression profiles of ductal versus acinar adenocarcinoma of the prostate. Mod Pathol. 2009;22(10):1273–9.
64. Herawi M, Epstein JI. Immunohistochemical antibody cocktail staining (p63/HMWCK/AMACR) of ductal adenocarcinoma and Gleason pattern 4 cribriform and noncribriform acinar adenocarcinomas of the prostate. Am J Surg Pathol. 2007; 31(6):889–94.
65. Zaloudek C, Williams JW, Kempson RL. "Endometrial" adenocarcinoma of the prostate: a distinctive tumor of probable prostatic duct origin. Cancer. 1976;37(5):2255–62.
66. Christensen WN, Steinberg G, Walsh PC, Epstein JI. Prostatic duct adenocarcinoma. Findings at radical prostatectomy. Cancer. 1991;67(8):2118–24.
67. Bock BJ, Bostwick DG. Does prostatic ductal adenocarcinoma exist? Am J Surg Pathol. 1999;23(7):781–5.
68. Epstein JI, Woodruff JM. Adenocarcinoma of the prostate with endometrioid features. A light microscopic and immunohistochemical study of ten cases. Cancer. 1986;57(1):111–9.
69. Farinola MA, Epstein JI. Utility of immunohistochemistry for alpha-methylacyl-CoA racemase in distinguishing atrophic prostate cancer from benign atrophy. Hum Pathol. 2004; 35(10):1272–8.
70. Hosler GA, Epstein JI. Basal cell hyperplasia: an unusual diagnostic dilemma on prostate needle biopsies. Hum Pathol. 2005;36(5):480–5.
71. Yang XJ, Tretiakova MS, Sengupta E, Gong C, Jiang Z. Florid basal cell hyperplasia of the prostate: a histological, ultrastructural, and immunohistochemical analysis. Hum Pathol. 2003;34(5):462–70.
72. Rioux-Leclercq NC, Epstein JI. Unusual morphologic patterns of basal cell hyperplasia of the prostate. Am J Surg Pathol. 2002;26(2):237–43.
73. Zhou M, Magi-Galluzzi C, Epstein JI. Prostate basal cell lesions can be negative for basal cell keratins: a diagnostic pitfall. Anal Quant Cytol Histol. 2006;28(3):125–9.
74. Nakayama M, Bennett CJ, Hicks JL, et al. Hypermethylation of the human glutathione S-transferase-pi gene (GSTP1) CpG island

is present in a subset of proliferative inflammatory atrophy lesions but not in normal or hyperplastic epithelium of the prostate: a detailed study using laser-capture microdissection. Am J Pathol. 2003;163(3):923–33.

75. Lee WH, Morton RA, Epstein JI, et al. Cytidine methylation of regulatory sequences near the pi-class glutathione S-transferase gene accompanies human prostatic carcinogenesis. Proc Natl Acad Sci U S A. 1994;91(24):11733–7.
76. Nagle RB, Ahmann FR, McDaniel KM, Paquin ML, Clark VA, Celniker A. Cytokeratin characterization of human prostatic carcinoma and its derived cell lines. Cancer Res. 1987;47(1):281–6.
77. Thorson P, Swanson PE, Vollmer RT, Humphrey PA. Basal cell hyperplasia in the peripheral zone of the prostate. Mod Pathol. 2003;16(6):598–606.
78. Grignon DJ, Ro JY, Ordonez NG, Ayala AG, Cleary KR. Basal cell hyperplasia, adenoid basal cell tumor, and adenoid cystic carcinoma of the prostate gland: an immunohistochemical study. Hum Pathol. 1988;19(12):1425–33.
79. Jiang Z, Woda BA, Rock KL, et al. P504S: a new molecular marker for the detection of prostate carcinoma. Am J Surg Pathol. 2001;25(11):1397–404.
80. Luo J, Zha S, Gage WR, et al. Alpha-methylacyl-CoA racemase: a new molecular marker for prostate cancer. Cancer Res. 2002;62(8):2220–6.
81. Rubin MA, Zhou M, Dhanasekaran SM, et al. Alpha-methylacyl coenzyme A racemase as a tissue biomarker for prostate cancer. JAMA. 2002;287(13):1662–70.
82. Zhou M, Chinnaiyan AM, Kleer CG, Lucas PC, Rubin MA. Alpha-methylacyl-CoA racemase: a novel tumor marker over-expressed in several human cancers and their precursor lesions. Am J Surg Pathol. 2002;26(7):926–31.
83. Beach R, Gown AM, De Peralta-Venturina MN, et al. P504S immunohistochemical detection in 405 prostatic specimens including 376 18-gauge needle biopsies. Am J Surg Pathol. 2002;26(12):1588–96.
84. Evans AJ. Alpha-methylacyl CoA racemase (P504S): overview and potential uses in diagnostic pathology as applied to prostate needle biopsies. J Clin Pathol. 2003;56(12):892–7.
85. Srigley JR. Benign mimickers of prostatic adenocarcinoma. Mod Pathol. 2004;17(3):328–48.
86. Abrahams NA, Bostwick DG, Ormsby AH, Qian J, Brainard JA. Distinguishing atrophy and high-grade prostatic intraepithelial neoplasia from prostatic adenocarcinoma with and without previous adjuvant hormone therapy with the aid of cytokeratin 5/6. Am J Clin Pathol. 2003;120(3):368–76.
87. Quick CM, Gokden N, Sangoi AR, Brooks JD, McKenney JK. The distribution of PAX-2 immunoreactivity in the prostate gland, seminal vesicle, and ejaculatory duct: comparison with prostatic adenocarcinoma and discussion of prostatic zonal embryogenesis. Hum Pathol. 2010;41:1145–9. doi:10.1016/j.humpath.2010.01.010.
88. Leroy X, Ballereau C, Villers A, et al. MUC6 is a marker of seminal vesicle-ejaculatory duct epithelium and is useful for the differential diagnosis with prostate adenocarcinoma. Am J Surg Pathol. 2003;27(4):519–21.
89. Abrahams NA, Ormsby AH, Brainard J. Validation of cytokeratin 5/6 as an effective substitute for keratin 903 in the differentiation of benign from malignant glands in prostate needle biopsies. Histopathology. 2002;41(1):35–41.
90. Shah RB, Zhou M, LeBlanc M, Snyder M, Rubin MA. Comparison of the basal cell-specific markers, 34betaE12 and p63, in the diagnosis of prostate cancer. Am J Surg Pathol. 2002;26(9):1161–8.
91. Reis-Filho JS, Simpson PT, Martins A, Preto A, Gartner F, Schmitt FC. Distribution of p63, cytokeratins 5/6 and cytokeratin 14 in 51 normal and 400 neoplastic human tissue samples using TARP-4 multi-tumor tissue microarray. Virchows Arch. 2003;443(2): 122–32.
92. Wu HH, Lapkus O, Corbin M. Comparison of 34betaE12 and P63 in 100 consecutive prostate carcinoma diagnosed by needle biopsies. Appl Immunohistochem Mol Morphol. 2004;12(4): 285–9.
93. Shah RB, Kunju LP, Shen R, LeBlanc M, Zhou M, Rubin MA. Usefulness of basal cell cocktail (34betaE12 + p63) in the diagnosis of atypical prostate glandular proliferations. Am J Clin Pathol. 2004;122(4):517–23.
94. Hameed O, Sublett J, Humphrey PA. Immunohistochemical stains for p63 and alpha-methylacyl-CoA racemase, versus a cocktail comprising both, in the diagnosis of prostatic carcinoma: a comparison of the immunohistochemical staining of 430 foci in radical prostatectomy and needle biopsy tissues. Am J Surg Pathol. 2005;29(5):579–87.
95. Zhou M, Magi-Galluzi C. Prostatic adenocarcinoma, prostatic intraepithelial neoplasia, and intraductal carcinoma. Surgical Pathol Clin: Current Concepts in Genitourinary Pathology: Prostate and Bladder. 2008;1(1):43–75.
96. Novis DA, Zarbo RJ, Valenstein PA. Diagnostic uncertainty expressed in prostate needle biopsies. A College of American Pathologists Q-probes Study of 15,753 prostate needle biopsies in 332 institutions. Arch Pathol Lab Med. 1999;123(8):687–92.
97. Wojno KJ, Epstein JI. The utility of basal cell-specific anti-cytokeratin antibody (34 beta E12) in the diagnosis of prostate cancer. A review of 228 cases. Am J Surg Pathol. 1995;19(3):251–60.
98. Bostwick DG, Brawer MK. Prostatic intra-epithelial neoplasia and early invasion in prostate cancer. Cancer. 1987;59(4):788–94.
99. McNeal JE, Villers A, Redwine EA, Freiha FS, Stamey TA. Microcarcinoma in the prostate: its association with duct-acinar dysplasia. Hum Pathol. 1991;22(7):644–52.
100. Kronz JD, Allan CH, Shaikh AA, Epstein JI. Predicting cancer following a diagnosis of high-grade prostatic intraepithelial neoplasia on needle biopsy: data on men with more than one follow-up biopsy. Am J Surg Pathol. 2001;25(8):1079–85.
101. Nagle RB, Brawer MK, Kittelson J, Clark V. Phenotypic relationships of prostatic intraepithelial neoplasia to invasive prostatic carcinoma. Am J Pathol. 1991;138(1):119–28.
102. McNeal JE, Leav I, Alroy J, Skutelsky E. Differential lectin staining of central and peripheral zones of the prostate and alterations in dysplasia. Am J Clin Pathol. 1988;89(1):41–8.
103. Qian J, Jenkins RB, Bostwick DG. Detection of chromosomal anomalies and c-myc gene amplification in the cribriform pattern of prostatic intraepithelial neoplasia and carcinoma by fluorescence in situ hybridization. Mod Pathol. 1997;10(11): 1113–9.
104. McNeal JE, Alroy J, Leav I, Redwine EA, Freiha FS, Stamey TA. Immunohistochemical evidence for impaired cell differentiation in the premalignant phase of prostate carcinogenesis. Am J Clin Pathol. 1988;90(1):23–32.
105. Tamboli P, Amin MB, Xu HJ, Linden MD. Immunohistochemical expression of retinoblastoma and p53 tumor suppressor genes in prostatic intraepithelial neoplasia: comparison with prostatic adenocarcinoma and benign prostate. Mod Pathol. 1998;11(3): 247–52.
106. Tamboli P, Amin MB, Schultz DS, Linden MD, Kubus J. Comparative analysis of the nuclear proliferative index (Ki-67) in benign prostate, prostatic intraepithelial neoplasia, and prostatic carcinoma. Mod Pathol. 1996;9(10):1015–9.
107. Zeng L, Rowland RG, Lele SM, Kyprianou N. Apoptosis incidence and protein expression of p53, TGF-beta receptor II, p27Kip1, and Smad4 in benign, premalignant, and malignant human prostate. Hum Pathol. 2004;35(3):290–7.
108. Zhang PJ, Driscoll DL, Lee HK, Nolan C, Velagapudi SR. Decreased immunoexpression of prostate inhibin peptide in prostatic carcinoma: a study with monoclonal antibody. Hum Pathol. 1999;30(2):168–72.

109. Zhou M, Shah R, Shen R, Rubin MA. Basal cell cocktail (34betaE12 + p63) improves the detection of prostate basal cells. Am J Surg Pathol. 2003;27(3):365–71.
110. Tavora F, Epstein JI. High-grade prostatic intraepithelial neoplasialike ductal adenocarcinoma of the prostate: a clinicopathologic study of 28 cases. Am J Surg Pathol. 2008;32(7):1060–7.
111. Guo CC, Epstein JI. Intraductal carcinoma of the prostate on needle biopsy: histologic features and clinical significance. Mod Pathol. 2006;19(12):1528–35.
112. Shah RB, Magi-Galluzzi C, Han B, Zhou M. Atypical cribriform lesions of the prostate: relationship to prostatic carcinoma and implication for diagnosis in prostate biopsies. Am J Surg Pathol. 2010;34(4):470–7.
113. Han B, Suleman K, Wang L, et al. ETS gene aberrations in atypical cribriform lesions of the prostate: implications for the distinction between intraductal carcinoma of the prostate and cribriform high-grade prostatic intraepithelial neoplasia. Am J Surg Pathol. 2010;34(4):478–85.
114. Hameed O, Humphrey PA. Stratified epithelium in prostatic adenocarcinoma: a mimic of high-grade prostatic intraepithelial neoplasia. Mod Pathol. 2006;19(7):899–906.
115. Bostwick DG, Kindrachuk RW, Rouse RV. Prostatic adenocarcinoma with endometrioid features. Clinical, pathologic, and ultrastructural findings. Am J Surg Pathol. 1985;9(8):595–609.
116. Ro JY, Ayala AG, Wishnow KI, Ordonez NG. Prostatic duct adenocarcinoma with endometrioid features: immunohistochemical and electron microscopic study. Semin Diagn Pathol. 1988;5(3):301–11.
117. Millar EK, Sharma NK, Lessells AM. Ductal (endometrioid) adenocarcinoma of the prostate: a clinicopathological study of 16 cases. Histopathology. 1996;29(1):11–9.
118. Samaratunga H, Delahunt B. Ductal adenocarcinoma of the prostate: current opinion and controversies. Anal Quant Cytol Histol. 2008;30(4):237–46.
119. Epstein JI, Lieberman PH. Mucinous adenocarcinoma of the prostate gland. Am J Surg Pathol. 1985;9(4):299–308.
120. Tran KP, Epstein JI. Mucinous adenocarcinoma of urinary bladder type arising from the prostatic urethra. Distinction from mucinous adenocarcinoma of the prostate. Am J Surg Pathol. 1996;20(11):1346–50.
121. Ro JY, Grignon DJ, Ayala AG, Fernandez PL, Ordonez NG, Wishnow KI. Mucinous adenocarcinoma of the prostate: histochemical and immunohistochemical studies. Hum Pathol. 1990;21(6):593–600.
122. Osunkoya AO, Nielsen ME, Epstein JI. Prognosis of mucinous adenocarcinoma of the prostate treated by radical prostatectomy: a study of 47 cases. Am J Surg Pathol. 2008;32(3):468–72.
123. Matsuoka Y, Arai G, Ishimaru H, Takagi K, Ito Y. Primary signet-ring cell carcinoma of the prostate. Can J Urol. 2007;14(6):3764–6.
124. Ro JY, el-Naggar A, Ayala AG, Mody DR, Ordonez NG. Signet-ring-cell carcinoma of the prostate. Electron-microscopic and immunohistochemical studies of eight cases. Am J Surg Pathol. 1988;12(6):453–60.
125. Skodras G, Wang J, Kragel PJ. Primary prostatic signet-ring cell carcinoma. Urology. 1993;42(3):338–42.
126. Alline KM, Cohen MB. Signet-ring cell carcinoma of the prostate. Arch Pathol Lab Med. 1992;116(1):99–102.
127. Remmele W, Weber A, Harding P. Primary signet-ring cell carcinoma of the prostate. Hum Pathol. 1988;19(4):478–80.
128. Kuroda N, Yamasaki I, Nakayama H, et al. Prostatic signet-ring cell carcinoma: case report and literature review. Pathol Int. 1999;49(5):457–61.
129. Hayashi H, Kitamura H, Nakatani Y, Inayama Y, Ito T, Kitamura H. Primary signet-ring cell carcinoma of the lung: histochemical and immunohistochemical characterization. Hum Pathol. 1999;30(4):378–83.
130. Hejka AG, England DM. Signet ring cell carcinoma of prostate. Immunohistochemical and ultrastructural study of a case. Urology. 1989;34(3):155–8.
131. Saito S, Iwaki H. Mucin-producing carcinoma of the prostate: review of 88 cases. Urology. 1999;54(1):141–4.
132. Fujita K, Sugao H, Gotoh T, Yokomizo S, Itoh Y. Primary signet ring cell carcinoma of the prostate: report and review of 42 cases. Int J Urol. 2004;11(3):178–81.
133. Randolph TL, Amin MB, Ro JY, Ayala AG. Histologic variants of adenocarcinoma and other carcinomas of prostate: pathologic criteria and clinical significance. Mod Pathol. 1997;10(6):612–29.
134. Schron DS, Gipson T, Mendelsohn G. The histogenesis of small cell carcinoma of the prostate. An immunohistochemical study. Cancer. 1984;53(11):2478–80.
135. Ro JY, Tetu B, Ayala AG, Ordonez NG. Small cell carcinoma of the prostate. II. Immunohistochemical and electron microscopic studies of 18 cases. Cancer. 1987;59(5):977–82.
136. Tetu B, Ro JY, Ayala AG, Johnson DE, Logothetis CJ, Ordonez NG. Small cell carcinoma of the prostate. Part I. A clinicopathologic study of 20 cases. Cancer. 1987;59(10):1803–9.
137. Kallakury BV, Yang F, Figge J, et al. Decreased levels of CD44 protein and mRNA in prostate carcinoma. Correlation with tumor grade and ploidy. Cancer. 1996;78(7):1461–9.
138. Hagood PG, Johnson FE, Bedrossian CW, Silverberg AB. Small cell carcinoma of the prostate. Cancer. 1991;67(4):1046–50.
139. Grignon DJ. Unusual subtypes of prostate cancer. Mod Pathol. 2004;17(3):316–27.
140. Miller VA, Reuter V, Scher HI. Primary squamous cell carcinoma of the prostate after radiation seed implantation for adenocarcinoma. Urology. 1995;46(1):111–3.
141. Nabi G, Ansari MS, Singh I, Sharma MC, Dogra PN. Primary squamous cell carcinoma of the prostate: a rare clinicopathological entity. Report of 2 cases and review of literature. Urol Int. 2001;66(4):216–9.
142. Munoz F, Franco P, Ciammella P, et al. Squamous cell carcinoma of the prostate: long-term survival after combined chemo-radiation. Radiat Oncol. 2007;2:15.
143. Dundore PA, Cheville JC, Nascimento AG, Farrow GM, Bostwick DG. Carcinosarcoma of the prostate. Report of 21 cases. Cancer. 1995;76(6):1035–42.
144. Ordonez NG, Ayala AG, von Eschenbach AC, Mackay B, Hanssen G. Immunoperoxidase localization of prostatic acid phosphatase in prostatic carcinoma with sarcomatoid changes. Urology. 1982;19(2):210–4.
145. Nazeer T, Barada JH, Fisher HA, Ross JS. Prostatic carcinosarcoma: case report and review of literature. J Urol. 1991;146(5):1370–3.
146. Shannon RL, Ro JY, Grignon DJ, et al. Sarcomatoid carcinoma of the prostate. A clinicopathologic study of 12 patients. Cancer. 1992;69(11):2676–82.
147. Wick MR, Young RH, Malvesta R, Beebe DS, Hansen JJ, Dehner LP. Prostatic carcinosarcomas. Clinical, histologic, and immunohistochemical data on two cases, with a review of the literature. Am J Clin Pathol. 1989;92(2):131–9.
148. Ogawa K, Kim YC, Nakashima Y, Yamabe H, Takeda T, Hamashima Y. Expression of epithelial markers in sarcomatoid carcinoma: an immunohistochemical study. Histopathology. 1987;11(5):511–22.
149. Amin MB, Bostwick DG. Pigment in prostatic epithelium and adenocarcinoma: a potential source of diagnostic confusion with seminal vesicular epithelium. Mod Pathol. 1996;9(7):791–5.
150. Shidham VB, Lindholm PF, Kajdacsy-Balla A, Basir Z, George V, Garcia FU. Prostate-specific antigen expression and lipochrome pigment granules in the differential diagnosis of prostatic adenocarcinoma versus seminal vesicle-ejaculatory duct epithelium. Arch Pathol Lab Med. 1999;123(11):1093–7.

151. Ormsby AH, Haskell R, Jones D, Goldblum JR. Primary seminal vesicle carcinoma: an immunohistochemical analysis of four cases. Mod Pathol. 2000;13(1):46–51.
152. Varma M, Morgan M, O'Rourke D, Jasani B. Prostate specific antigen (PSA) and prostate specific acid phosphatase (PSAP) immunoreactivity in benign seminal vesicle\ejaculatory duct epithelium: a potential pitfall in the diagnosis of prostate cancer in needle biopsy specimens. Histopathology. 2004;44(4): 405–6.
153. Bartman AE, Buisine MP, Aubert JP, et al. The MUC6 secretory mucin gene is expressed in a wide variety of epithelial tissues. J Pathol. 1998;186(4):398–405.
154. Amin MB, Schultz DS, Zarbo RJ. Analysis of cribriform morphology in prostatic neoplasia using antibody to high-molecular-weight cytokeratins. Arch Pathol Lab Med. 1994;118(3):260–4.
155. McNeal JE, Reese JH, Redwine EA, Freiha FS, Stamey TA. Cribriform adenocarcinoma of the prostate. Cancer. 1986;58(8):1714–9.
156. Samaratunga H, Singh M. Distribution pattern of basal cells detected by cytokeratin 34 beta E12 in primary prostatic duct adenocarcinoma. Am J Surg Pathol. 1997;21(4):435–40.
157. Bostwick DG, Hossain D, Qian J, et al. Phyllodes tumor of the prostate: long-term followup study of 23 cases. J Urol. 2004;172(3):894–9.
158. Nelson RS, Epstein JI. Prostatic carcinoma with abundant xanthomatous cytoplasm. Foamy gland carcinoma. Am J Surg Pathol. 1996;20(4):419–26.
159. Yang XJ, Wu CL, Woda BA, et al. Expression of alpha-Methylacyl-CoA racemase (P504S) in atypical adenomatous hyperplasia of the prostate. Am J Surg Pathol. 2002;26(7):921–5.
160. Zhou M, Aydin H, Kanane H, Epstein JI. How often does alpha-methylacyl-CoA-racemase contribute to resolving an atypical diagnosis on prostate needle biopsy beyond that provided by basal cell markers? Am J Surg Pathol. 2004;28(2):239–43.
161. Armah HB, Parwani AV. Atypical adenomatous hyperplasia (adenosis) of the prostate: a case report with review of the literature. Diagn Pathol. 2008;3:34.
162. Qian J, Bostwick DG. The extent and zonal location of prostatic intraepithelial neoplasia and atypical adenomatous hyperplasia: relationship with carcinoma in radical prostatectomy specimens. Pathol Res Pract. 1995;191(9):860–7.
163. Cheng L, Bostwick DG. Atypical sclerosing adenosis of the prostate: a rare mimic of adenocarcinoma. Histopathology. 2010;56(5):627–31.
164. Bostwick DG, Qian J. Atypical adenomatous hyperplasia of the prostate. Relationship with carcinoma in 217 whole-mount radical prostatectomies. Am J Surg Pathol. 1995;19(5):506–18.
165. Wang W, Sun X, Epstein JI. Partial atrophy on prostate needle biopsy cores: a morphologic and immunohistochemical study. Am J Surg Pathol. 2008;32(6):851–7.
166. Hedrick L, Epstein JI. Use of keratin 903 as an adjunct in the diagnosis of prostate carcinoma. Am J Surg Pathol. 1989;13(5):389–96.
167. Cina SJ, Epstein JI. Adenocarcinoma of the prostate with atrophic features. Am J Surg Pathol. 1997;21(3):289–95.
168. Gupta A, Wang HL, Policarpio-Nicolas ML, et al. Expression of alpha-methylacyl-coenzyme A racemase in nephrogenic adenoma. Am J Surg Pathol. 2004;28(9):1224–9.
169. Skinnider BF, Oliva E, Young RH, Amin MB. Expression of alpha-methylacyl-CoA racemase (P504S) in nephrogenic adenoma: a significant immunohistochemical pitfall compounding the differential diagnosis with prostatic adenocarcinoma. Am J Surg Pathol. 2004;28(6):701–5.
170. Cossu-Rocca P, Contini M, Brunelli M, et al. S-100A1 is a reliable marker in distinguishing nephrogenic adenoma from prostatic adenocarcinoma. Am J Surg Pathol. 2009;33(7):1031–6.
171. Xiao GQ, Burstein DE, Miller LK, Unger PD. Nephrogenic adenoma: immunohistochemical evaluation for its etiology and differentiation from prostatic adenocarcinoma. Arch Pathol Lab Med. 2006;130(6):805–10.
172. Rahemtullah A, Oliva E. Nephrogenic adenoma: an update on an innocuous but troublesome entity. Adv Anat Pathol. 2006; 13(5):247–55.
173. Tong GX, Melamed J, Mansukhani M, et al. PAX2: a reliable marker for nephrogenic adenoma. Mod Pathol. 2006;19(3): 356–63.
174. Tong GX, Weeden EM, Hamele-Bena D, et al. Expression of PAX8 in nephrogenic adenoma and clear cell adenocarcinoma of the lower urinary tract: evidence of related histogenesis? Am J Surg Pathol. 2008;32(9):1380–7.
175. Magi-Galluzzi C, Sanderson H, Epstein JI. Atypia in nonneoplastic prostate glands after radiotherapy for prostate cancer: duration of atypia and relation to type of radiotherapy. Am J Surg Pathol. 2003;27(2):206–12.
176. Gaudin PB, Zelefsky MJ, Leibel SA, Fuks Z, Reuter VE. Histopathologic effects of three-dimensional conformal external beam radiation therapy on benign and malignant prostate tissues. Am J Surg Pathol. 1999;23(9):1021–31.
177. Brawer MK, Nagle RB, Pitts W, Freiha F, Gamble SL. Keratin immunoreactivity as an aid to the diagnosis of persistent adenocarcinoma in irradiated human prostates. Cancer. 1989;63(3): 454–60.
178. Ljung G, Norberg M, Holmberg L, Busch C, Nilsson S. Characterization of residual tumor cells following radical radiation therapy for prostatic adenocarcinoma; immunohistochemical expression of prostate-specific antigen, prostatic acid phosphatase, and cytokeratin 8. Prostate. 1997;31(2):91–7.
179. Grob BM, Schellhammer PF, Brassil DN, Wright Jr GL. Changes in immunohistochemical staining of PSA, PAP, and TURP-27 following irradiation therapy for clinically localized prostate cancer. Urology. 1994;44(4):525–9.
180. Mahan DE, Bruce AW, Manley PN, Franchi L. Immunohistochemical evaluation of prostatic carcinoma before and after radiotherapy. J Urol. 1980;124(4):488–91.
181. Gikas PW, Del Buono EA, Epstein JI. Florid hyperplasia of mesonephric remnants involving prostate and periprostatic tissue. Possible confusion with adenocarcinoma. Am J Surg Pathol. 1993;17(5):454–60.
182. Bostwick DG, Qian J, Ma J, Muir TE. Mesonephric remnants of the prostate: incidence and histologic spectrum. Mod Pathol. 2003;16(7):630–5.
183. Gagucas RJ, Brown RW, Wheeler TM. Verumontanum mucosal gland hyperplasia. Am J Surg Pathol. 1995;19(1):30–6.
184. Gaudin PB, Wheeler TM, Epstein JI. Verumontanum mucosal gland hyperplasia in prostatic needle biopsy specimens. A mimic of low grade prostatic adenocarcinoma. Am J Clin Pathol. 1995;104(6):620–6.
185. Gaudin PB, Reuter VE. Benign mimics of prostatic adenocarcinoma on needle biopsy. Anat Pathol. 1997;2:111–34.
186. Muezzinoglu B, Erdamar S, Chakraborty S, Wheeler TM. Verumontanum mucosal gland hyperplasia is associated with atypical adenomatous hyperplasia of the prostate. Arch Pathol Lab Med. 2001;125(3):358–60.
187. Cina SJ, Silberman MA, Kahane H, Epstein JI. Diagnosis of Cowper's glands on prostate needle biopsy. Am J Surg Pathol. 1997;21(5):550–5.
188. Saboorian MH, Huffman H, Ashfaq R, Ayala AG, Ro JY. Distinguishing Cowper's glands from neoplastic and pseudoneoplastic lesions of prostate: immunohistochemical and ultrastructural studies. Am J Surg Pathol. 1997;21(9):1069–74.
189. Frauenhoffer EE, Ro JY, el-Naggar AK, Ordonez NG, Ayala AG. Clear cell cribriform hyperplasia of the prostate. Immunohistochemical and DNA flow cytometric study. Am J Clin Pathol. 1991;95(4):446–53.

190. Ayala AG, Srigley JR, Ro JY, Abdul-Karim FW, Johnson DE. Clear cell cribriform hyperplasia of prostate. Report of 10 cases. Am J Surg Pathol. 1986;10(10):665–71.
191. Presti B, Weidner N. Granulomatous prostatitis and poorly differentiated prostate carcinoma. Their distinction with the use of immunohistochemical methods. Am J Clin Pathol. 1991;95(3): 330–4.
192. Sebo TJ, Bostwick DG, Farrow GM, Eble JN. prostatic xanthoma: a mimic of prostatic adenocarcinoma. Hum Pathol. 1994;25(4):386–9.
193. Chuang AY, Epstein JI. Xanthoma of the prostate: a mimicker of high-grade prostate adenocarcinoma. Am J Surg Pathol. 2007;31(8):1225–30.
194. Luque RJ, Lopez-Beltran A, Perez-Seoane C, Suzigan S. Sclerosing adenosis of the prostate. Histologic features in needle biopsy specimens. Arch Pathol Lab Med. 2003;127(1):e14–6.
195. Jones EC, Clement PB, Young RH. Sclerosing adenosis of the prostate gland. A clinicopathological and immunohistochemical study of 11 cases. Am J Surg Pathol. 1991;15(12):1171–80.
196. Meister P. Sclerosing adenosis of the prostate. Carcinoma simulation [in German]. Pathologe. 1996;17(2):157–62.
197. Ronnett BM, Epstein JI. A case showing sclerosing adenosis and an unusual form of basal cell hyperplasia of the prostate. Am J Surg Pathol. 1989;13(10):866–72.
198. Ostrowski ML, Wheeler TM. Paraganglia of the prostate. Location, frequency, and differentiation from prostatic adenocarcinoma. Am J Surg Pathol. 1994;18(4):412–20.
199. Howarth SM, Griffiths DF, Varma M. Paraganglion of the prostate gland: an uncommon mimic of prostate cancer in needle biopsies. Histopathology. 2005;47(1):114–5.
200. Kawabata K. Paraganglion of the prostate in a needle biopsy: a potential diagnostic pitfall. Arch Pathol Lab Med. 1997;121(5):515–6.
201. Skinnider BF, Folpe AL, Hennigar RA, et al. Distribution of cytokeratins and vimentin in adult renal neoplasms and normal renal tissue: potential utility of a cytokeratin antibody panel in the differential diagnosis of renal tumors. Am J Surg Pathol. 2005;29(6): 747–54.
202. Simic T, Mimic-Oka J, Ille K, Dragicevic D, Savic-Radojevic A. Glutathione S-transferase isoenzyme profile in non-tumor and tumor human kidney tissue. World J Urol. 2003;20(6):385–91.
203. Grignon DJ, Abdel-Malak M, Mertens WC, Sakr WA, Shepherd RR. Glutathione S-transferase expression in renal cell carcinoma: a new marker of differentiation. Mod Pathol. 1994;7(2):186–9.
204. May EE, Perentes E. Anti-Leu 7 immunoreactivity with human tumours: its value in the diagnosis of prostatic adenocarcinoma. Histopathology. 1987;11(3):295–304.
205. Genega EM, Hutchinson B, Reuter VE, Gaudin PB. Immunophenotype of high-grade prostatic adenocarcinoma and urothelial carcinoma. Mod Pathol. 2000;13(11):1186–91.
206. Tawfic S, Niehans GA, Manivel JC. The pattern of CD10 expression in selected pathologic entities of the prostate gland. Hum Pathol. 2003;34(5):450–6.
207. Tong GX, Yu WM, Beaubier NT, et al. Expression of PAX8 in normal and neoplastic renal tissues: an immunohistochemical study. Mod Pathol. 2009;22(9):1218–27.
208. Nonaka D, Tang Y, Chiriboga L, Rivera M, Ghossein R. Diagnostic utility of thyroid transcription factors Pax8 and TTF-2 (FoxE1) in thyroid epithelial neoplasms. Mod Pathol. 2008;21(2):192–200.
209. Gill R, O'Donnell RJ, Horvai A. Utility of immunohistochemistry for endothelial markers in distinguishing epithelioid hemangioendothelioma from carcinoma metastatic to bone. Arch Pathol Lab Med. 2009;133(6):967–72.
210. Folpe AL, Chand EM, Goldblum JR, Weiss SW. Expression of Fli-1, a nuclear transcription factor, distinguishes vascular neoplasms from potential mimics. Am J Surg Pathol. 2001;25(8):1061–6.
211. Kollermann J, Helpap B. Expression of vascular endothelial growth factor (VEGF) and VEGF receptor Flk-1 in benign, premalignant, and malignant prostate tissue. Am J Clin Pathol. 2001;116(1):115–21.
212. Bassily NH, Vallorosi CJ, Akdas G, Montie JE, Rubin MA. Coordinate expression of cytokeratins 7 and 20 in prostate adenocarcinoma and bladder urothelial carcinoma. Am J Clin Pathol. 2000;113(3):383–8.
213. Chuang AY, DeMarzo AM, Veltri RW, Sharma RB, Bieberich CJ, Epstein JI. Immunohistochemical differentiation of high-grade prostate carcinoma from urothelial carcinoma. Am J Surg Pathol. 2007;31(8):1246–55.
214. Mhawech P, Uchida T, Pelte MF. Immunohistochemical profile of high-grade urothelial bladder carcinoma and prostate adenocarcinoma. Hum Pathol. 2002;33(11):1136–40.
215. Mulders TM, Bruning PF, Bonfrer JM. Prostate-specific antigen (PSA). A tissue-specific and sensitive tumor marker. Eur J Surg Oncol. 1990;16(1):37–41.
216. Higgins JP, Kaygusuz G, Wang L, et al. Placental S100 (S100P) and GATA3: markers for transitional epithelium and urothelial carcinoma discovered by complementary DNA microarray. Am J Surg Pathol. 2007;31(5):673–80.
217. Esheba GE, Longacre TA, Atkins KA, Higgins JP. Expression of the urothelial differentiation markers GATA3 and placental S100 (S100P) in female genital tract transitional cell proliferations. Am J Surg Pathol. 2009;33(3):347–53.
218. Soslow RA, Rouse RV, Hendrickson MR, Silva EG, Longacre TA. Transitional cell neoplasms of the ovary and urinary bladder: a comparative immunohistochemical analysis. Int J Gynecol Pathol. 1996;15(3):257–65.
219. Kusumi T, Koie T, Tanaka M, et al. Immunohistochemical detection of carcinoma in radical prostatectomy specimens following hormone therapy. Pathol Int. 2008;58(11):687–94.
220. Chang SS, Reuter VE, Heston WD, Hutchinson B, Grauer LS, Gaudin PB. Short term neoadjuvant androgen deprivation therapy does not affect prostate specific membrane antigen expression in prostate tissues. Cancer. 2000;88(2):407–15.
221. Cheng L, Cheville JC, Bostwick DG. Diagnosis of prostate cancer in needle biopsies after radiation therapy. Am J Surg Pathol. 1999;23(10):1173–83.
222. Herawi M, Epstein JI. Specialized stromal tumors of the prostate: a clinicopathologic study of 50 cases. Am J Surg Pathol. 2006;30(6):694–704.
223. Herawi M, Montgomery EA, Epstein JI. Gastrointestinal stromal tumors (GISTs) on prostate needle biopsy: a clinicopathologic study of 8 cases. Am J Surg Pathol. 2006;30(11):1389–95.
224. Herawi M, Epstein JI. Solitary fibrous tumor on needle biopsy and transurethral resection of the prostate: a clinicopathologic study of 13 cases. Am J Surg Pathol. 2007;31(6):870–6.
225. Pins MR, Campbell SC, Laskin WB, Steinbronn K, Dalton DP. Solitary fibrous tumor of the prostate a report of 2 cases and review of the literature. Arch Pathol Lab Med. 2001;125(2): 274–7.
226. Mentzel T, Bainbridge TC, Katenkamp D. Solitary fibrous tumour: clinicopathological, immunohistochemical, and ultrastructural analysis of 12 cases arising in soft tissues, nasal cavity and nasopharynx, urinary bladder and prostate. Virchows Arch. 1997;430(6):445–53.
227. Wang X, Jones TD, Zhang S, et al. Amplifications of EGFR gene and protein expression of EGFR, Her-2/neu, c-kit, and androgen receptor in phyllodes tumor of the prostate. Mod Pathol. 2007;20(2):175–82.
228. Hansel DE, Herawi M, Montgomery E, Epstein JI. Spindle cell lesions of the adult prostate. Mod Pathol. 2007;20(1):148–58.
229. Cohen MB. Atypical prostatic stromal lesions. Adv Anat Pathol. 1998;5(6):359–66.

230. Hossain D, Meiers I, Qian J, MacLennan GT, Bostwick DG. Prostatic stromal hyperplasia with atypia: follow-up study of 18 cases. Arch Pathol Lab Med. 2008;132(11):1729–33.
231. Bierhoff E, Vogel J, Benz M, Giefer T, Wernert N, Pfeifer U. Stromal nodules in benign prostatic hyperplasia. Eur Urol. 1996;29(3):345–54.
232. Bierhoff E, Walljasper U, Hofmann D, Vogel J, Wernert N, Pfeifer U. Morphological analogies of fetal prostate stroma and stromal nodules in BPH. Prostate. 1997;31(4):234–40.
233. Gupta R, Singh S, Khurana N. Leiomyoma of the prostate – a rare mesenchymal tumor: a case report. Indian J Pathol Microbiol. 2007;50(2):403–5.
234. Srinivasan G, Campbell E, Bashirelahi N. Androgen, estrogen, and progesterone receptors in normal and aging prostates. Microsc Res Tech. 1995;30(4):293–304.
235. Montgomery EA, Shuster DD, Burkart AL, et al. Inflammatory myofibroblastic tumors of the urinary tract: a clinicopathologic study of 46 cases, including a malignant example inflammatory fibrosarcoma and a subset associated with high-grade urothelial carcinoma. Am J Surg Pathol. 2006;30(12):1502–12.
236. Gaudin PB, Rosai J, Epstein JI. Sarcomas and related proliferative lesions of specialized prostatic stroma: a clinicopathologic study of 22 cases. Am J Surg Pathol. 1998;22(2):148–62.
237. Young RH, Scully RE. Pseudosarcomatous lesions of the urinary bladder, prostate gland, and urethra. A report of three cases and review of the literature. Arch Pathol Lab Med. 1987;111(4):354–8.
238. Mobbs BG, Liu Y. Immunohistochemical localization of progesterone receptor in benign and malignant human prostate. Prostate. 1990;16(3):245–51.
239. Morikawa T, Goto A, Tomita K, et al. Recurrent prostatic stromal sarcoma with massive high-grade prostatic intraepithelial neoplasia. J Clin Pathol. 2007;60(3):330–2.
240. Dotan ZA, Tal R, Golijanin D, et al. Adult genitourinary sarcoma: the 25-year Memorial Sloan-Kettering experience. J Urol. 2006;176(5):2033–8.
241. Cheville JC, Dundore PA, Nascimento AG, et al. Leiomyosarcoma of the prostate. Report of 23 cases. Cancer. 1995;76(8):1422–7.
242. Janet NL, May AW, Akins RS. Sarcoma of the prostate: a single institutional review. Am J Clin Oncol. 2009;32(1):27–9.
243. Sexton WJ, Lance RE, Reyes AO, Pisters PW, Tu SM, Pisters LL. Adult prostate sarcoma: the M. D. Anderson Cancer Center Experience. J Urol. 2001;166(2):521–5.
244. Kelley TW, Borden EC, Goldblum JR. Estrogen and progesterone receptor expression in uterine and extrauterine leiomyosarcomas: an immunohistochemical study. Appl Immunohistochem Mol Morphol. 2004;12(4):338–41.
245. Fisher C, Goldblum JR, Epstein JI, Montgomery E. Leiomyosarcoma of the paratesticular region: a clinicopathologic study. Am J Surg Pathol. 2001;25(9):1143–9.
246. Parham DM. Pathologic classification of rhabdomyosarcomas and correlations with molecular studies. Mod Pathol. 2001;14(5):506–14.
247. Kuhnen C, Herter P, Muller O, et al. Beta-catenin in soft tissue sarcomas: expression is related to proliferative activity in high-grade sarcomas. Mod Pathol. 2000;13(9):1005–13.
248. Waring PM, Newland RC. Prostatic embryonal rhabdomyosarcoma in adults. A clinicopathologic review. Cancer. 1992;69(3):755–62.
249. Nabi G, Dinda AK, Dogra PN. Primary embryonal rhabdomyosarcoma of prostate in adults: diagnosis and management. Int Urol Nephrol. 2002;34(4):531–4.

Chapter 19
Urinary Bladder

Myra Wilkerson

Abstract Biopsies from the urinary bladder are challenging and it may be difficult to differentiate normal from benign or reactive processes, and even from low-grade neoplastic processes. This chapter addresses these common problems by profiling immunohistochemical stains that change their patterns of expression from that of normal urothelium, including both the cellular layers and cellular compartments in which markers are expressed. Morphologic patterns that cause diagnostic dilemmas are also included, including glandular lesions of both primary and metastatic origin, lesions with a nested growth pattern, and lesions with an inverted growth pattern. Although uncommon, the differential diagnosis of spindle cells lesions is also addressed.

Keywords Urinary bladder • Urachus • Nephrogenic-adenoma • Cytokeratins • Umbrella cells • Cystitis glandularis • Clear cell adenocarcinoma

FREQUENTLY ASKED QUESTIONS

M. Wilkerson (✉)
Department of Pathology and Laboratory Medicine, Geisinger Medical Center, 1000 East Mountain Blvd., Wilkes-Barre, PA 18711, USA
e-mail: mwilkerson@geisinger.edu

F. Lin and J. Prichard (eds.), *Handbook of Practical Immunohistochemistry: Frequently Asked Questions*,
DOI 10.1007/978-1-4419-8062-5_19,

Table 19.1 Antibodies frequently used in urothelium

Antibody	Localization in normal urothelium	Function	Applications and pitfalls
Bcl-2	NCM; B	Mitochondrial membrane protein that blocks apoptosis, particularly in lymphocytes	Stains nuclear membrane and mitochondrial membrane
Bcl-6	NC; U	Proto-oncogene expressed in normal germinal center B-cells; plays role in inflammatory response	
CD44	M; B	Transmembrane receptor for hyaluronate; involved in leukocyte adhesion	Focal staining only in normal urothelium
CEA	C	Cell surface glycoprotein; produced by fetal gut epithelium; plays a role in cell adhesion	Adenocarcinoma-related marker
CK13	C; BIU	Intermediate filament protein in cytoskeleton	
CK14	C; B	Intermediate filament protein in cytoskeleton	
CK17	C; B	Intermediate filament protein in cytoskeleton	
CK18	C; BIU	Intermediate filament protein in cytoskeleton	Expressed in non-squamous epithelia and in most adenocarcinomas
CK19	C; BIU	Intermediate filament protein in cytoskeleton	Often coexpressed with CK7
CK20	C; U	Intermediate filament protein in cytoskeleton	Expressed in gastrointestinal epithelium, urothelium, and Merkel cells
CK5	C; BIU	Intermediate filament protein in cytoskeleton	
CK7	C; BIU	Intermediate filament protein in cytoskeleton	Also expressed in glandular epithelia except in gastrointestinal tract and prostate gland
CK8	C; BIU	Intermediate filament protein in cytoskeleton	Expressed in non-squamous epithelia and in most adenocarcinomas
CK903	C; B	Intermediate filament protein in cytoskeleton	Antibody reacts with CK1, CK5, CK10, and CK14. Also positive in squamous, ductal, and other complex epithelia including basal cells of prostatic acini
EGFR	MC; BI	Tyrosine kinase receptor; expression in tumors correlates with poor prognosis	
ErbB-2	M; U	Tyrosine kinase receptor; expression in tumors correlates with poor prognosis	
Ki-67	N; B	Nuclear protein expressed in all phases of the active cell cycle (G1, S, G2, M)	
p53	N	Activation of p53 gene leads to cell cycle arrest and DNA repair or apoptosis	
p63	N	Activation of p63 gene can induce p53 and apoptosis	
TM	M(U, I) and C(U)	Endothelial cell-associated cofactor for thrombin-mediated activator of protein C	Urothelial marker, but also positive in mesothelium, vascular tumors, and squamous cell carcinoma
UPIII	M; U		Only the luminal aspect of the umbrella cells should stain

Abbreviations: *N* nuclear staining, *C* cytoplasmic staining, *M* membranous staining, *B* basal cell layers stain, *I* intermediate cell layers stain, *U* umbrella cell layer stains

References: [1–28]

Table 19.2 Markers for normal, reactive, and neoplastic urothelium

	NU	RA	UH	PLMP	LGD	H/CIS	LNIP	HNIP	LIUC	HIUC
ErbB-2	+ or –; U	ND	ND	ND	+	+	ND	ND	ND	ND
EGFR	– or +; BI	ND	ND	ND	– or +	+ or –	ND	ND	+ or –	+ or –
CK20	+[a]; U	+	ND	+ (U); + or –(I)	+; UIB	+; UIB	+ or –; UI	+; UI	+	+
Bcl-2	+[a]; B	+[a]	+[a]	ND	+; BI	+; BI	ND	ND	– or +	– or +
CK7	+; BIU	+	ND	ND	ND	ND	+	+	+	+
CK8	+; BIU	+	ND	ND	ND	ND	ND	ND	+	+
CK18	+; BIU	+	ND	ND	ND	ND	ND	ND	+	ND
CK19	+; BIU	+	ND	ND	ND	ND	ND	ND	ND	ND
CK17	+; B	+ or –	ND	ND	ND	ND	ND	ND	ND	ND
CK5	+; BIU	+	ND	ND	ND	ND	ND	ND	ND	ND
CK13	+; BIU	+	ND	ND	ND	ND	ND	ND	+	+
CK14	–	+ or –; BIU	ND	ND	ND	ND	ND	ND	+	
CD44	+; B[a]	+; BIU	+[b]	+[c]	ND	– or +	ND	ND	ND	ND
CK903	+; B	+ or –; BIU	ND	+; B	ND	ND	+ or –; BI	+ or –; BIU	+; BIU	+; BIU
Bcl-6	– or +; U	ND	ND	ND	ND	ND	ND	ND	+	– or +
p63	ND	ND	ND	ND	ND	ND	+	+ or –	– or +	– or +
UPIII	+; U[d]	ND	ND	+	ND	ND	+	+	– or +	+ or –[e]
TM	+; IU	ND	ND	+	ND	ND	+	+	+ or –	+ or –
CEA	+ or –	+ or –	ND	ND	ND	+ or –	+ or –	+ or –	+ or –	+ or –
Ki-67	– or +; B	Rare	– or +	– or +	– or +	+; BIU	– or +	+	+	+
p53	–	–	–	– or +	ND	+	– or +	+	ND	ND
Ki-67 index[f]	13.1	ND	1.1	<5	3–11	11–31	7.3	15.7	22.8	>40
p53 index[f]	ND	ND	ND	<5; B	3.2	6–50	2.9	25.7	ND	ND

Abbreviations: *B* basal cell layers stain, *I* intermediate cell layers stain, *U* umbrella cell layer stains, *NU* normal urothelium, *RA* reactive atypia, *UH* urothelial hyperplasia, *PLMP* papillary urothelial neoplasm of uncertain malignant potential, *LGD* low-grade urothelial dysplasia, *H/CIS* high-grade urothelial dysplasia/carcinoma in situ, *LNIP* low-grade noninvasive papillary urothelial carcinoma, *HNIP* high-grade noninvasive papillary urothelial carcinoma, *LIUC* low-grade invasive urothelial carcinoma, *HIUC* high-grade invasive urothelial carcinoma

See Figs. 19.1–19.10 for representative staining patterns of key markers

Notes:

[a]Focal or patchy staining only

[b]75% of cases show basal staining only; 25% show basal and intermediate

[c]12.5% of cases show basal staining only; 50% show basal and intermediate; 37.5% intermediate only

[d]Stains luminal aspect of umbrella cells

[e]Shows predominantly membranous staining, but can also be cytoplasmic; membranous staining pattern occurs more often in surface cells of a papillary tumor, but can be more widely distributed in an invasive lesion

[f]Mean percentage of cells that stain in literature

References: [1–28]

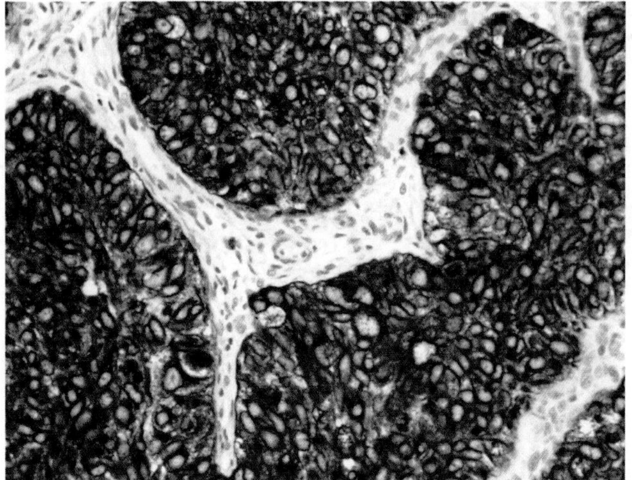

Fig. 19.1 Invasive urothelial carcinoma demonstrating diffuse and strong cytoplasmic staining for CK7

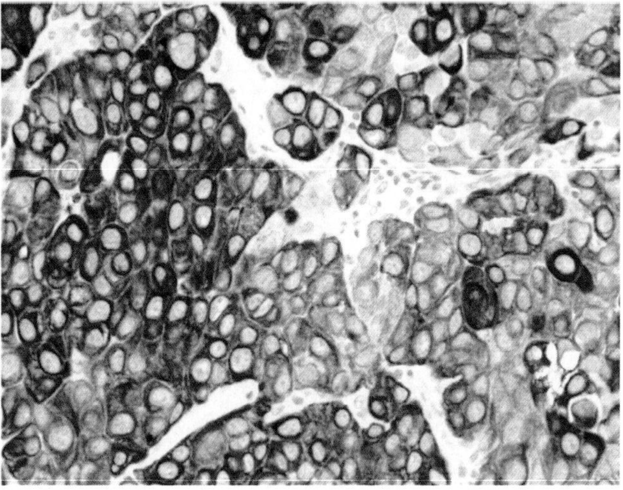

Fig. 19.2 Invasive urothelial carcinoma demonstrating diffuse and strong cytoplasmic staining for CK20

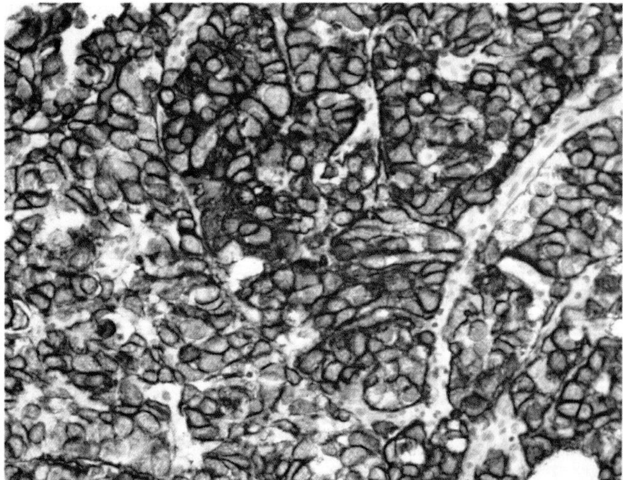

Fig. 19.3 Invasive urothelial carcinoma demonstrating diffuse and strong cytoplasmic and membranous staining for CK903

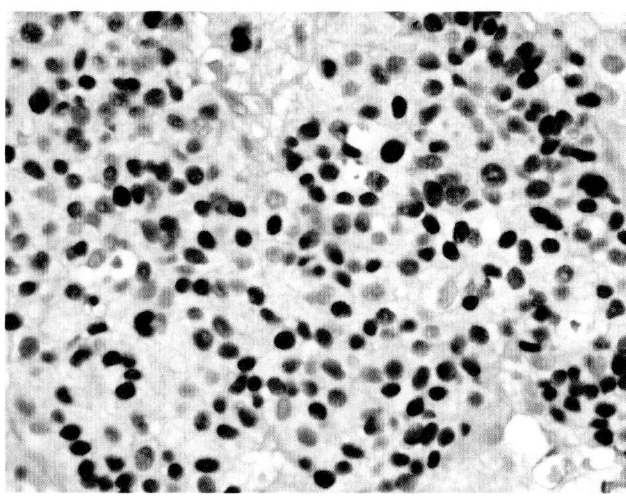

Fig. 19.4 Invasive urothelial carcinoma demonstrating strong nuclear staining for p63

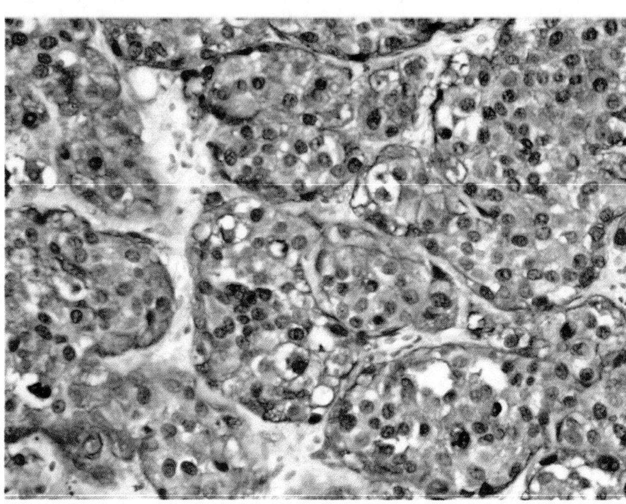

Fig. 19.5 Invasive urothelial carcinoma demonstrating diffuse and strong cytoplasmic and nuclear staining for S100P

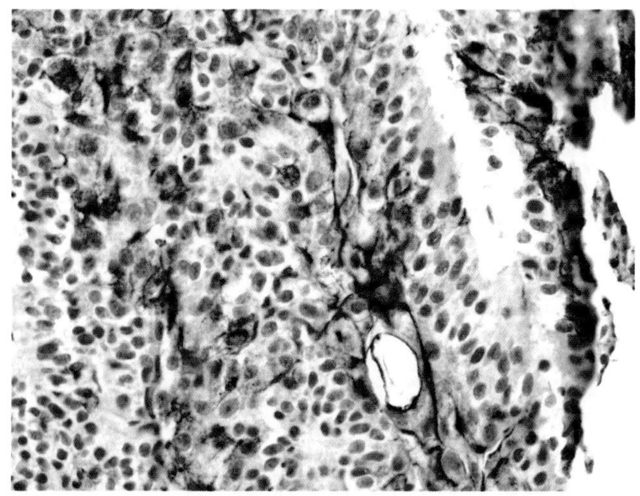

Fig. 19.6 Papillary urothelial carcinoma demonstrating typical membranous staining for Uroplakin III, as well as some fine granular cytoplasmic staining

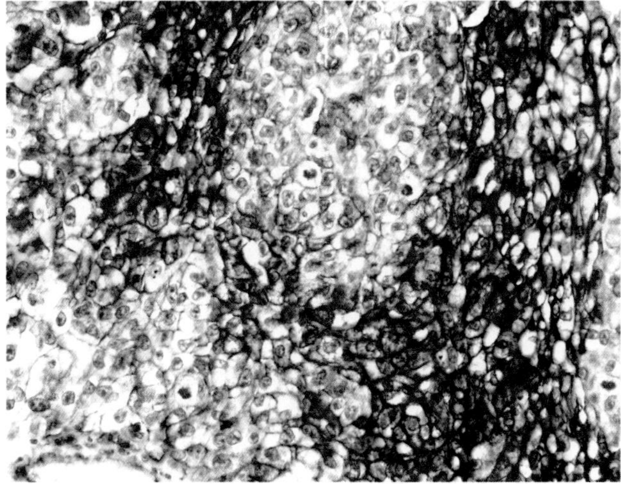

Fig. 19.7 Noninvasive, low-grade papillary urothelial carcinoma demonstrating predominantly membranous staining, as well as some cytoplasmic staining, for thrombomodulin

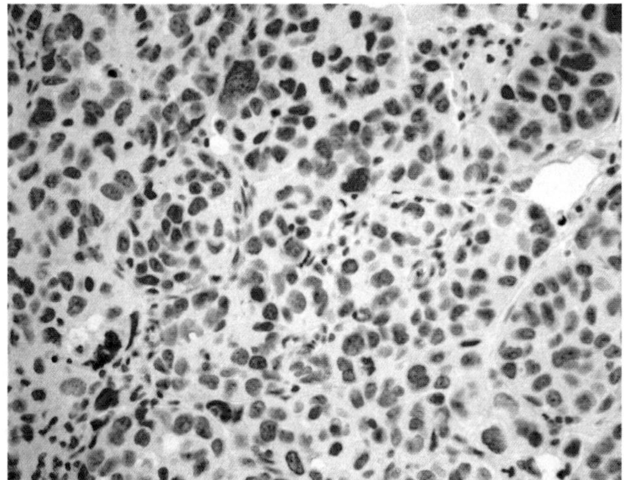

Fig. 19.8 Approximately 40% of urothelial carcinoma is negative for or only focally positive for CK20

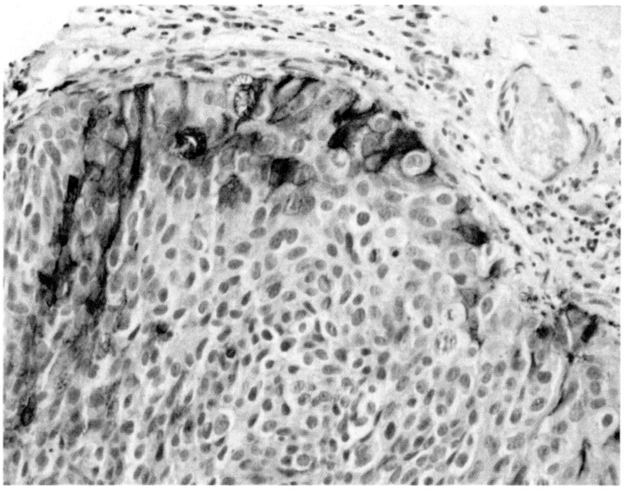

Fig. 19.9 Urothelial carcinoma may show staining for CEA

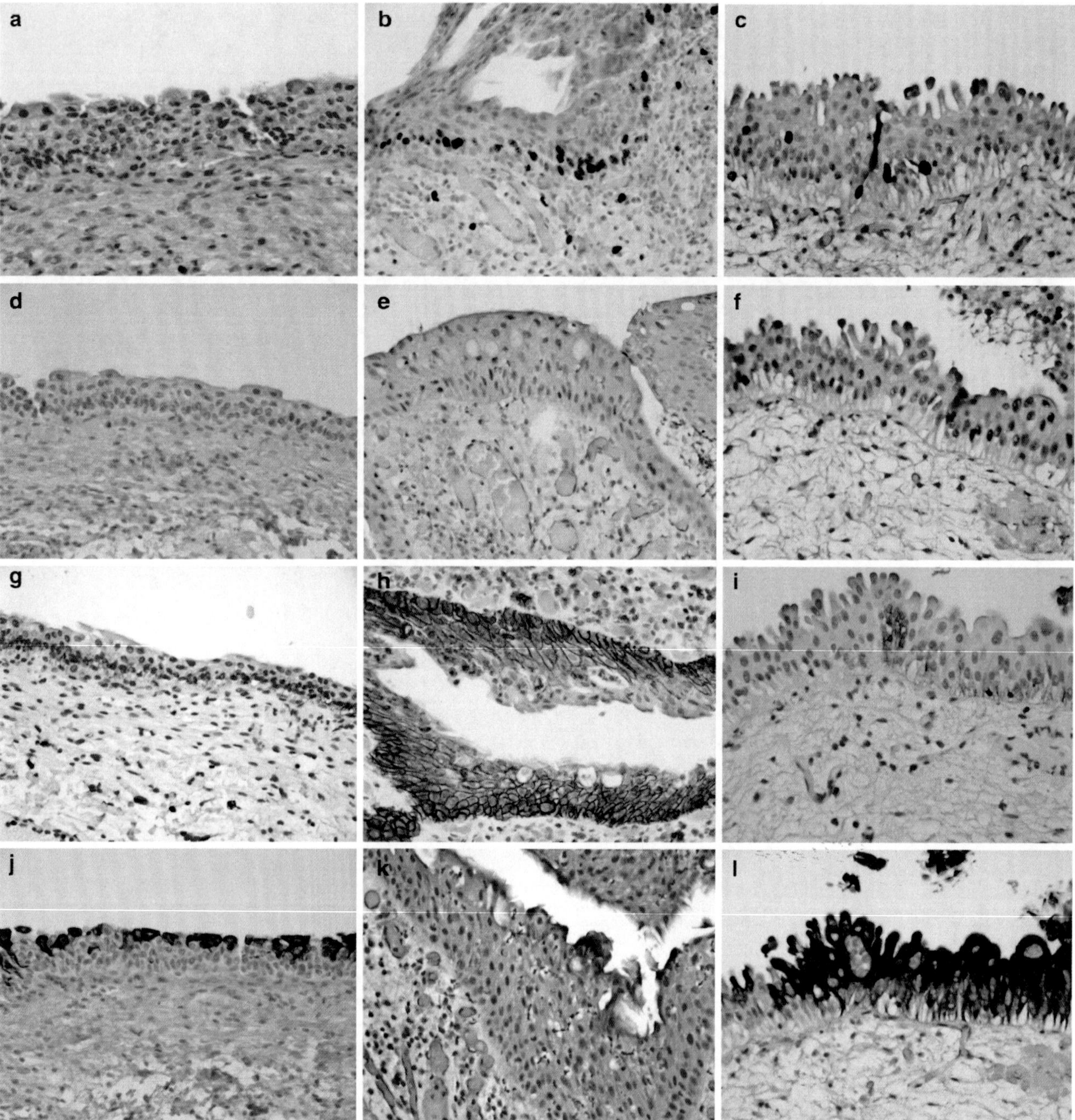

Fig. 19.10 A comparison of four antibodies in normal urothelium (NU), cystitis, and urothelial carcinoma in situ (CIS). Ki-67 is rare in NU (**a**), increased in the basal layers in cystitis (**b**; there is nonspecific staining of neutrophils in the urothelium here due to endogenous peroxidase), and increased in both basal and intermediate cell layers of CIS (**c**). Staining for p53 is similar to Ki-67 with only rare basal cells staining very weakly in NU (**d**), increased staining in cystitis (**e**), and increased staining of greater strength in CIS (**f**). CD44 is quite helpful as it normally demonstrates patchy staining of the basal cells in NU (**g**), diffuse and strong positivity of all cell layers in cystitis (**h**), but only focal and patchy staining of basal cells in CIS (**i**). CK20 demonstrates strong staining of umbrella cells in NU (**j**), but may only be patchy and react weakly in umbrella cells in cystitis (**k**), while often showing strong positivity in all cell layers of CIS (**l**)

Table 19.3 Markers for primary urinary bladder lesions with an inverted growth pattern

	von Brunn nests	Inverted urothelial papilloma	UC with inverted growth pattern
Ki-67	–	– or +[a]	+ or –
p53	–	– or +[b]	+ or –
CK20	ND	–	+ or –
UPIII	+	ND	+ or –
CEA	+	ND	ND

Abbreviation: *UC* urothelial carcinoma

Notes:

[a]In tumors that show any staining, approximately 10–12% of nuclei will stain

[b]In tumors that show any staining, approximately 12% of nuclei will stain

References: [25, 29–31]

Table 19.4 Markers used in primary glandular lesions of the urinary bladder

	Glmet	CyGl	UrcRem	UrcAC	PrBlAC	UCgl
Chrom	ND	+	+	– or +	+	ND
NSE	ND	–	–	– or +	–	ND
Synap	ND	–	–	ND	–	ND
UPIII	ND	ND	ND	–	ND	ND
CDX-2	+	–	ND	+	ND	ND
CK20	+	–	ND	+	+	+
CK7	– or +	+	ND	– or +	+ or –	+
PSA	ND	+	– or +	–	–	–
PSAP	ND	+	ND	–	–	ND
CA-125	ND	ND	ND	–	+ or –	+ or –
CEA	ND	+	ND	+	+ or –	ND

Abbreviations: *Glmet* glandular (intestinal) metaplasia, *CyGl* cystitis glandularis, *UrcRem* urachal remnants, *UrcAC* urachal adenocarcinoma, *PrBlAC* primary bladder adenocarcinoma, *UCgl* urothelial carcinoma with glandular differentiation

References: [1, 30, 32–43]

Table 19.5 Nephrogenic adenoma vs. prostate acini and adenocarcinoma vs. clear cell adenocarcinoma of bladder

	NAPU	NAB	NPA	PAC	CCU
P504S	+	– or +	– or +	+	ND
PSA	–	–	+	+	–
PAP	ND	ND	ND	ND	–
PSAP	ND	–	ND	+	–
CK903	– or +	– or +	ND	– or +	+ or –
p63	–	–	+	–	ND
CD10	ND	–	+ or –	– or +	ND
EMA	ND	+	– or +	–	ND
AE1	ND	+	ND	ND	+
AE3	ND	+	ND	ND	+
CAM 5.2	ND	+	ND	ND	+
S100	ND	+[a]	ND	ND	+ or –
CEA	ND	– or +	ND	– or +	+
Leu-M1	ND	+[a]	ND	ND	+
CA 19-9	ND	+[a]	ND	ND	+
Brst-3	ND	– or +	ND	ND	+ or –
PR	ND	–	ND	ND	–
ER	ND	– or +	ND	ND	–
Her-2/neu	ND	–	ND	– or +	–
Bcl-2	ND	+ or –	ND	ND	+ or –
p53	ND	– or +	ND	ND	+
CK20	ND	ND	ND	– or +	+
CK7	ND	ND	ND	–	+

Abbreviations: *NAPU* nephrogenic adenoma of prostatic urethra, *NAB* nephrogenic adenoma of bladder, *NPA* normal prostatic acini, *PAC* prostatic adenocarcinoma, *CCU* clear cell adenocarcinoma of bladder

Note:

[a]Sometimes only focal staining

References: [15, 35, 39, 44–53]

Table 19.6 Markers for primary urothelial carcinoma and adenocarcinoma vs. adenocarcinomas other than bladder origin

	UC	PrBlAC	CoAC	PAC	CxAC	OAC	EAC	UrAC	SVAC	RC
CK7	+	+ or –	– or +	–	+	+	+	– or +	+ or –	–
CK20	– or +	+ or –	+	– or +	+	+ or –	–	+	–	–
TM	+	+ or –	–	–	ND	– or +	ND	ND	ND	ND
UPIII	– or +	ND	–	–	–	–	–	–	–	–
Villin[a]	–	– or +	+	–	ND	+ or –	ND	+	ND	–
CDX-2	–	– or +	+	–	ND	– or +	– or +	+	ND	–
CK903	+	ND	–	– or +	ND	–	ND	+ or –	ND	–
PSA	–	–	–	+	–	–	–	–	–	–
PSAP	–	+ or –	–	+	–	–	–	–	ND	–
P504S	–	+ or –	+	+	ND	ND	ND	ND	ND	ND
PSMA	–	ND	ND	+	ND	ND	ND	–	ND	ND
PAP	ND	ND	ND	+	ND	ND	ND	ND	–	ND
CEA	+ or –	+	+	– or +	+ or –	– or +	– or +	+	– or +	–
CA-125	– or +	+ or –	– or +	–	+	+	+	–	+	–
Her-2/neu	– or +	ND	– or +	– or +	–	–	– or +	–	ND	ND
Vim	– or +	–	–	–	–	– or +	+ or –	–	ND	+
B-cat	[b]	[b]	[c]	ND	ND	ND	ND	[b]	ND	ND
p63	+	ND	ND	–	ND	ND	ND	ND	ND	ND
S100P	+ or –	ND	ND	– or +	ND	ND	ND	ND	ND	ND

Abbreviations: *UC* urothelial carcinoma, *PrBlAC* primary bladder adenocarcinoma, *CoAC* colonic adenocarcinoma, *PAC* prostatic adenocarcinoma, *CxAC* cervical adenocarcinoma, *OAC* ovarian adenocarcinoma, *EAC* endometrial adenocarcinoma, *UrcAC* urachal adenocarcinoma, *SVAC* seminal vesicle adenocarcinoma, *RC* renal carcinoma

Notes:

[a]Stains cytoplasm and brush border

[b]Demonstrates membranous or cytoplasmic staining only

[c]Demonstrates nuclear staining and sometimes membranous or cytoplasmic staining

References: [6, 15, 27, 30, 36, 37, 39–43, 48, 52–58]

Table 19.7 Markers for small cell carcinoma primary to bladder vs. poorly differentiated urothelial carcinoma

	SmCC	UC
p53	+ or −	ND
EMA	+	+
CAM 5.2	+[a]	+
NSE	+	−
Chrom	+ or −	−
Leu-7	− or +	ND
Synap	+ or −	− or +
AE1/AE3	+	ND
HMFG	+ or −	ND
Leu-M1	+ or −	− or +
VIP	− or +	ND
Serotonin	− or +	ND
S100	− or +	−
CK20	−	+
CK7	+ or −	+
CD44v6	− or +	+ or −
CD45	−	−
TTF-1	− or +	ND
UPIII	−	+ or −
c-kit	− or +	ND
EGFR	− or +	− or +
p63	+	+
CK903	− or +	+ or −

Abbreviations: *SmCC* small cell carcinoma, *UC* urothelial carcinoma

Note:

[a]Demonstrates a dot staining pattern in cytoplasm

References: [6, 13, 15, 20, 30, 32, 48, 59–70]

Table 19.8 Markers for von Brunn nests vs. nested variant of urothelial carcinoma

	von Brunn nests	Nested variant of UCa
Ki-67	Rare cells	− or +[a]
p53	Rare cells	− or +
p27	− or +	+[b]
Bcl-2	+	− or +
EGFR	ND	−
p21	ND	+[c]
Bcl-6	−	ND
CK8	+	ND
CK19, 18, 8	+[d]	ND
CK16, 13	+	ND
CK7	ND	+
CK20	ND	+
CK903	ND	+
p63	ND	+

Notes:

[a]If tumor stains, usually >15% of nuclei are positive

[b]Stains only superficial component of tumor

[c]May stain diffusely throughout tumor, but 50% stain base only

[d]Stains umbrella cells

References: [11, 31, 71, 72]

Table 19.9 Markers in tumors with a nested morphology

	Paraganglioma[a]	Carcinoid[b]	UC, nested variant[c]	Melanoma
AE1/AE3	–	+	+	–
CK7	–	– or +	+	–
CK20	–	–	+	–
Vim	+ or –	ND	ND	+
S100	+[d]	–	–	+
Chrom	+	+	–	–
Synap	+	+	–	–
NSE	+	ND	ND	ND
CAM 5.2	–	ND	ND	–
CEA	–	ND	ND	–
p53	[e]	ND	[e]	ND
Ki-67	Rare	ND	– or +	ND

Abbreviation: *UC* urothelial carcinoma

Notes:

[a]Paragangliomas: (+) for Leu7, adrenomedullin, VEGF; (+ or –) for met-enkephalin, leu-enkephalin, VIP; (– or +) for somatostatin, serotonin, calcitonin; (–) for p27, topoisomerase-2alpha, COX-2

[b]Carcinoids (– or +) for serotonin

[c]Nested variant of urothelial carcinoma will show some focal reactivity for p27

[d]Stains sustentacular cells only

[e]May show focal staining

References: [6, 31, 48, 62, 71, 73–77]

Table 19.10 Markers for spindle cell lesions of the urinary bladder

	IMFP	SFT	LMY	LMS	RMS	SarUC
AE1/AE3	– or +	–	–	+ or –	ND	+
EMA	– or +	–	–	– or +	–	+ or –
Vim	+	+	+	+ or –	+	+
Actin	+	+	+	+ or –	+	– or +
Desmin	+ or –	+ or –	+	+ or –	+	– or +
S100	–	–	–	–	–	–
CD34	–	+	+ or –	+ or –	ND	–
p53	+ or –	–	–	+	ND	+ or –
Caldesmon	+ or –	ND	ND	+	ND	–
ALK-1	+ or –	ND	ND	– or +	– or +	–
MyoD1	–	ND	ND	ND	+	ND
Myoglobin	–	ND	ND	ND	+	ND
PanCK	ND	ND	ND	–	–	+
CAM 5.2	ND	ND	ND	–	–	+
CK903	–	ND	ND	–	–	+ or –
CK19	ND	ND	ND	–	–	+
SMA	+ or –	ND	ND	+	–	– or +
E-cad	ND	ND	ND	–	–	+
CD44	ND	ND	ND	–	–	+ or –
CD44v6	ND	ND	ND	–	–	+
p63	–	ND	ND	– or +	ND	+ or –[a]

Abbreviations: *IMFP* inflammatory myofibroblastic proliferation, *SFT* solitary fibrous tumor, *LMY* leiomyoma, *LMS* leiomyosarcoma, *RMS* rhabdomyosarcoma, *SarUC* sarcomatoid urothelial carcinoma

Note:

[a]May be positive in spindle cell component

References: [6, 53, 78–81]

Note for All Tables

Note: "+" – usually greater than 70% of cases are positive; "–" – less than 5% of cases are positive; "+ or –" – usually more than 50% of cases are positive; "– or +" – less than 50% of cases are positive.

References

1. Wagner U, Sauter G, Moch H, et al. Patterns of p53, erbB-2, and EGF-r expression in premalignant lesions of the urinary bladder. Hum Pathol. 1995;26(9):970–8.
2. Mallofre C, Castillo M, Morente V, Sole M. Immunohistochemical expression of CK20, p53, and Ki-67 as objective markers of urothelial dysplasia. Mod Pathol. 2003;16(3):187–91.
3. Nakopoulou L, Vourlakou C, Zervas A, Tzonou A, Gakiopoulou H, Dimopoulos MA. The prevalence of bcl-2, p53, and Ki-67 immunoreactivity in transitional cell bladder carcinomas and their clinicopathologic correlates. Hum Pathol. 1998;29(2):146–54.
4. Southgate J, Harnden P, Trejdosiewicz LK. Cytokeratin expression patterns in normal and malignant urothelium: a review of the biological and diagnostic implications. Histol Histopathol. 1999;14(2):657–64.
5. McKenney JK, Desai S, Cohen C, Amin MB. Discriminatory immunohistochemical staining of urothelial carcinoma in situ and non-neoplastic urothelium: an analysis of cytokeratin 20, p53, and CD44 antigens. Am J Surg Pathol. 2001;25(8):1074–8.
6. McKenney JK, Amin MB. The role of immunohistochemistry in the diagnosis of urinary bladder neoplasms. Semin Diagn Pathol. 2005;22(1):69–87.
7. Cina SJ, Lancaster-Weiss KJ, Lecksell K, Epstein JI. Correlation of Ki-67 and p53 with the new World Health Organization/International Society of Urological Pathology Classification System for Urothelial Neoplasia. Arch Pathol Lab Med. 2001;125(5):646–51.
8. Desai S, Lim SD, Jimenez RE, et al. Relationship of cytokeratin 20 and CD44 protein expression with WHO/ISUP grade in pTa and pT1 papillary urothelial neoplasia. Mod Pathol. 2000;13(12):1315–23.
9. Laguna P, Smedts F, Nordling J, et al. Keratin expression profiling of transitional epithelium in the painful bladder syndrome/interstitial cystitis. Am J Clin Pathol. 2006;125(1):105–10.
10. Sarkis AS, Dalbagni G, Cordon-Cardo C, et al. Association of P53 nuclear overexpression and tumor progression in carcinoma in situ of the bladder. J Urol. 1994;152(2 Pt 1):388–92.
11. Lin Z, Kim H, Park H, Kim Y, Cheon J, Kim I. The expression of bcl-2 and bcl-6 protein in normal and malignant transitional epithelium. Urol Res. 2003;31(4):272–5.
12. Lu QL, Laniado M, Abel PD, Stamp GW, Lalani EN. Expression of bcl-2 in bladder neoplasms is a cell lineage associated and p53-independent event. Mol Pathol. 1997;50(1):28–33.
13. Yin H, Leong AS. Histologic grading of noninvasive papillary urothelial tumors: validation of the 1998 WHO/ISUP system by immunophenotyping and follow-up. Am J Clin Pathol. 2004;121(5):679–87.
14. Urist MJ, Di Como CJ, Lu ML, et al. Loss of p63 expression is associated with tumor progression in bladder cancer. Am J Pathol. 2002;161(4):1199–206.
15. Parker DC, Folpe AL, Bell J, et al. Potential utility of uroplakin III, thrombomodulin, high molecular weight cytokeratin, and cytokeratin 20 in noninvasive, invasive, and metastatic urothelial (transitional cell) carcinomas. Am J Surg Pathol. 2003;27(1):1–10.
16. Ordonez NG. Transitional cell carcinomas of the ovary and bladder are immunophenotypically different. Histopathology. 2000;36(5):433–8.
17. Ordonez NG, Mackay B. Brenner tumor of the ovary: a comparative immunohistochemical and ultrastructural study with transitional cell carcinoma of the bladder. Ultrastruct Pathol. 2000;24(3):157–67.
18. Alsheikh A, Mohamedali Z, Jones E, Masterson J, Gilks CB. Comparison of the WHO/ISUP classification and cytokeratin 20 expression in predicting the behavior of low-grade papillary urothelial tumors. World/Health Organization/International Society of Urologic Pathology. Mod Pathol. 2001;14(4):267–72.
19. Harnden P, Eardley I, Joyce AD, Southgate J. Cytokeratin 20 as an objective marker of urothelial dysplasia. Br J Urol. 1996;78(6):870–5.
20. Rotterud R, Nesland JM, Berner A, Fossa SD. Expression of the epidermal growth factor receptor family in normal and malignant urothelium. BJU Int. 2005;95(9):1344–50.
21. Petraki CD, Sfikas CP. Review. Non-papillary urothelial lesions of the urinary bladder: morphological classification and immunohistochemical markers. In Vivo. 2008;22(4):493–501.
22. Obama H, Obama K, Takemoto M, et al. Expression of Thrombomodulin in the epithelium of the urinary bladder: a possible source of urinary thrombomodulin. Anticancer Res. 1999;19(2A):1143–7.
23. Riedel I, Czernobilsky B, Lifschitz-Mercer B, et al. Brenner tumors but not transitional cell carcinomas of the ovary show urothelial differentiation: immunohistochemical staining of urothelial markers, including cytokeratins and uroplakins. Virchows Arch. 2001;438(2):181–91.
24. Soini Y, Turpeenniemi-Hujanen T, Kamel D, et al. p53 immunohistochemistry in transitional cell carcinoma and dysplasia of the urinary bladder correlates with disease progression. Br J Cancer. 1993;68(5):1029–35.
25. Shevchuk MM, Fenoglio CM, Richart RM. Carcinoembryonic antigen localization in benign and malignant transitional epithelium. Cancer. 1981;47(5):899–905.
26. Sun W, Zhang PL, Herrera GA. p53 protein and Ki-67 overexpression in urothelial dysplasia of bladder. Appl Immunohistochem Mol Morphol. 2002;10(4):327–31.
27. Olsburgh J, Harnden P, Weeks R, et al. Uroplakin gene expression in normal human tissues and locally advanced bladder cancer. J Pathol. 2003;199(1):41–9.
28. Lopez-Beltran A, Cheng L. Histologic variants of urothelial carcinoma: differential diagnosis and clinical implications. Hum Pathol. 2006;37(11):1371–88.
29. Jones TD, Zhang S, Lopez-Beltran A, et al. Urothelial carcinoma with an inverted growth pattern can be distinguished from inverted papilloma by fluorescence in situ hybridization, immunohistochemistry, and morphologic analysis. Am J Surg Pathol. 2007;31(12):1861–7.
30. Kaufmann O, Volmerig J, Dietel M. Uroplakin III is a highly specific and moderately sensitive immunohistochemical marker for primary and metastatic urothelial carcinomas. Am J Clin Pathol. 2000;113(5):683–7.
31. Volmar KE, Chan TY, De Marzo AM, Epstein JI. Florid von Brunn nests mimicking urothelial carcinoma: a morphologic and immunohistochemical comparison to the nested variant of urothelial carcinoma. Am J Surg Pathol. 2003;27(9):1243–52.
32. Bollito ER, Pacchioni D, Lopez-Beltran A, et al. Immunohistochemical study of neuroendocrine differentiation in primary glandular lesions and tumors of the urinary bladder. Anal Quant Cytol Histol. 2005;27(4):218–24.
33. Sung MT, Lopez-Beltran A, Eble JN, et al. Divergent pathway of intestinal metaplasia and cystitis glandularis of the urinary bladder. Mod Pathol. 2006;19(11):1395–401.

34. Nowels K, Kent E, Rinsho K, Oyasu R. Prostate specific antigen and acid phosphatase-reactive cells in cystitis cystica and glandularis. Arch Pathol Lab Med. 1988;112(7):734–7.
35. Oliva E, Amin MB, Jimenez R, Young RH. Clear cell carcinoma of the urinary bladder: a report and comparison of four tumors of mullerian origin and nine of probable urothelial origin with discussion of histogenesis and diagnostic problems. Am J Surg Pathol. 2002;26(2):190–7.
36. Wang HL, Lu DW, Yerian LM, et al. Immunohistochemical distinction between primary adenocarcinoma of the bladder and secondary colorectal adenocarcinoma. Am J Surg Pathol. 2001;25(11):1380–7.
37. Werling RW, Yaziji H, Bacchi CE, Gown AM. CDX2, a highly sensitive and specific marker of adenocarcinomas of intestinal origin: an immunohistochemical survey of 476 primary and metastatic carcinomas. Am J Surg Pathol. 2003;27(3):303–10.
38. Golz R, Schubert GE. Prostatic specific antigen: immunoreactivity in urachal remnants. J Urol. 1989;141(6):1480–2.
39. Torenbeek R, Lagendijk JH, Van Diest PJ, Bril H, van de Molengraft FJ, Meijer CJ. Value of a panel of antibodies to identify the primary origin of adenocarcinomas presenting as bladder carcinoma. Histopathology. 1998;32(1):20–7.
40. Bates AW, Baithun SI. Secondary neoplasms of the bladder are histological mimics of nontransitional cell primary tumours: clinicopathological and histological features of 282 cases. Histopathology. 2000;36(1):32–40.
41. Grignon DJ, Ro JY, Ayala AG, Johnson DE, Ordonez NG. Primary adenocarcinoma of the urinary bladder. A clinicopathologic analysis of 72 cases. Cancer. 1991;67(8):2165–72.
42. Gopalan A, Sharp DS, Fine SW, et al. Urachal carcinoma: a clinicopathologic analysis of 24 cases with outcome correlation. Am J Surg Pathol. 2009;33(5):659–68.
43. Tamboli P, Mohsin SK, Hailemariam S, Amin MB. Colonic adenocarcinoma metastatic to the urinary tract versus primary tumors of the urinary tract with glandular differentiation: a report of 7 cases and investigation using a limited immunohistochemical panel. Arch Pathol Lab Med. 2002;126(9):1057–63.
44. Skinnider BF, Oliva E, Young RH, Amin MB. Expression of alpha-methylacyl-CoA racemase (P504S) in nephrogenic adenoma: a significant immunohistochemical pitfall compounding the differential diagnosis with prostatic adenocarcinoma. Am J Surg Pathol. 2004;28(6):701–5.
45. Xiao GQ, Burstein DE, Miller LK, Unger PD. Nephrogenic adenoma: immunohistochemical evaluation for its etiology and differentiation from prostatic adenocarcinoma. Arch Pathol Lab Med. 2006;130(6):805–10.
46. Gupta A, Wang HL, Policarpio-Nicolas ML, et al. Expression of alpha-methylacyl-coenzyme A racemase in nephrogenic adenoma. Am J Surg Pathol. 2004;28(9):1224–9.
47. Gilcrease MZ, Delgado R, Vuitch F, Albores-Saavedra J. Clear cell adenocarcinoma and nephrogenic adenoma of the urethra and urinary bladder: a histopathologic and immunohistochemical comparison. Hum Pathol. 1998;29(12):1451–6.
48. Sim SJ, Ro JY, Ordonez NG, Park YW, Kee KH, Ayala AG. Metastatic renal cell carcinoma to the bladder: a clinicopathologic and immunohistochemical study. Mod Pathol. 1999;12(4): 351–5.
49. Drew PA, Murphy WM, Civantos F, Speights VO. The histogenesis of clear cell adenocarcinoma of the lower urinary tract. Case series and review of the literature. Hum Pathol. 1996;27(3):248–52.
50. Tong GX, Weeden EM, Hamele-Bena D, et al. Expression of PAX8 in nephrogenic adenoma and clear cell adenocarcinoma of the lower urinary tract: evidence of related histogenesis? Am J Surg Pathol. 2008;32(9):1380–7.
51. Varma M, Morgan M, Amin MB, Wozniak S, Jasani B. High molecular weight cytokeratin antibody (clone 34betaE12): a sensitive marker for differentiation of high grade invasive urothelial carcinoma from prostate cancer. Histopathology. 2003;42(2):167–72.
52. Chuang AY, DeMarzo AM, Veltri RW, Sharma RB, Bieberich CJ, Epstein JI. Immunohistochemical differentiation of high-grade prostate carcinoma from urothelial carcinoma. Am J Surg Pathol. 2007;31(8):1246–55.
53. Emerson RE, Cheng L. Immunohistochemical markers in the evaluation of tumors of the urinary bladder: a review. Anal Quant Cytol Histol. 2005;27(6):301–16.
54. Kaimaktchiev V, Terracciano L, Tornillo L, et al. The homeobox intestinal differentiation factor CDX2 is selectively expressed in gastrointestinal adenocarcinomas. Mod Pathol. 2004;17(11): 1392–9.
55. Suh N, Yang XJ, Tretiakova MS, Humphrey PA, Wang HL. Value of CDX2, villin, and alpha-methylacyl coenzyme A racemase immunostains in the distinction between primary adenocarcinoma of the bladder and secondary colorectal adenocarcinoma. Mod Pathol. 2005;18(9):1217–22.
56. Lane Z, Hansel DE, Epstein JI. Immunohistochemical expression of prostatic antigens in adenocarcinoma and villous adenoma of the urinary bladder. Am J Surg Pathol. 2008;32(9):1322–6.
57. Epstein JI, Kuhajda FP, Lieberman PH. Prostate-specific acid phosphatase immunoreactivity in adenocarcinomas of the urinary bladder. Hum Pathol. 1986;17(9):939–42.
58. Riedel I, Liang FX, Deng FM, et al. Urothelial umbrella cells of human ureter are heterogeneous with respect to their uroplakin composition: different degrees of urothelial maturity in ureter and bladder? Eur J Cell Biol. 2005;84(2–3):393–405.
59. Wang X, Jones TD, Maclennan GT, et al. P53 expression in small cell carcinoma of the urinary bladder: biological and prognostic implications. Anticancer Res. 2005;25(3B):2001–4.
60. Blomjous CE, Vos W, De Voogt HJ, Van der Valk P, Meijer CJ. Small cell carcinoma of the urinary bladder. A clinicopathologic, morphometric, immunohistochemical, and ultrastructural study of 18 cases. Cancer. 1989;64(6):1347–57.
61. Mills SE, Wolfe 3rd JT, Weiss MA, et al. Small cell undifferentiated carcinoma of the urinary bladder. A light-microscopic, immunocytochemical, and ultrastructural study of 12 cases. Am J Surg Pathol. 1987;11(8):606–17.
62. Martignoni G, Eble JN. Carcinoid tumors of the urinary bladder. Immunohistochemical study of 2 cases and review of the literature. Arch Pathol Lab Med. 2003;127(1):e22–4.
63. Iczkowski KA, Shanks JH, Allsbrook WC, et al. Small cell carcinoma of urinary bladder is differentiated from urothelial carcinoma by chromogranin expression, absence of CD44 variant 6 expression, a unique pattern of cytokeratin expression, and more intense gamma-enolase expression. Histopathology. 1999;35(2): 150–6.
64. Jones TD, Kernek KM, Yang XJ, et al. Thyroid transcription factor 1 expression in small cell carcinoma of the urinary bladder: an immunohistochemical profile of 44 cases. Hum Pathol. 2005;36(7):718–23.
65. Abrahams NA, Moran C, Reyes AO, Siefker-Radtke A, Ayala AG. Small cell carcinoma of the bladder: a contemporary clinicopathological study of 51 cases. Histopathology. 2005;46(1):57–63.
66. Grignon DJ, Ro JY, Ayala AG, et al. Small cell carcinoma of the urinary bladder. A clinicopathologic analysis of 22 cases. Cancer. 1992;69(2):527–36.
67. Pan CX, Yang XJ, Lopez-Beltran A, et al. c-kit Expression in small cell carcinoma of the urinary bladder: prognostic and therapeutic implications. Mod Pathol. 2005;18(3):320–3.
68. Soriano P, Navarro S, Gil M, Llombart-Bosch A. Small-cell carcinoma of the urinary bladder. A clinico-pathological study of ten cases. Virchows Arch. 2004;445(3):292–7.
69. Iczkowski KA, Shanks JH, Bostwick DG. Loss of CD44 variant 6 expression differentiates small cell carcinoma of urinary bladder from urothelial (transitional cell) carcinoma. Histopathology. 1998;32(4):322–7.

70. Samaratunga H, Khoo K. Micropapillary variant of urothelial carcinoma of the urinary bladder; a clinicopathological and immunohistochemical study. Histopathology. 2004;45(1):55–64.
71. Lin O, Cardillo M, Dalbagni G, Linkov I, Hutchinson B, Reuter VE. Nested variant of urothelial carcinoma: a clinicopathologic and immunohistochemical study of 12 cases. Mod Pathol. 2003;16(12):1289–98.
72. Cintorino M, Del Vecchio MT, Bugnoli M, Petracca R, Leoncini P. Cytokeratin pattern in normal and pathological bladder urothelium: immunohistochemical investigation using monoclonal antibodies. J Urol. 1988;139(2):428–32.
73. Cheng L, Leibovich BC, Cheville JC, et al. Paraganglioma of the urinary bladder: can biologic potential be predicted? Cancer. 2000;88(4):844–52.
74. Kato H, Suzuki M, Mukai M, Aizawa S. Clinicopathological study of pheochromocytoma of the urinary bladder: immunohistochemical, flow cytometric and ultrastructural findings with review of the literature. Pathol Int. 1999;49(12):1093–9.
75. Kovacs K, Bell D, Gardiner GW, Honey RJ, Goguen J, Rotondo F. Malignant paraganglioma of the urinary bladder: immunohistochemical study of prognostic indicators. Endocr Pathol. 2005;16(4): 363–9.
76. Grignon DJ, Ro JY, Mackay B, et al. Paraganglioma of the urinary bladder: immunohistochemical, ultrastructural, and DNA flow cytometric studies. Hum Pathol. 1991;22(11):1162–9.
77. Moyana TN, Kontozoglou T. Urinary bladder paragangliomas. An immunohistochemical study. Arch Pathol Lab Med. 1988;112(1): 70–2.
78. Ikegami H, Iwasaki H, Ohjimi Y, Takeuchi T, Ariyoshi A, Kikuchi M. Sarcomatoid carcinoma of the urinary bladder: a clinicopathologic and immunohistochemical analysis of 14 patients. Hum Pathol. 2000;31(3):332–40.
79. Westfall DE, Folpe AL, Paner GP, et al. Utility of a comprehensive immunohistochemical panel in the differential diagnosis of spindle cell lesions of the urinary bladder. Am J Surg Pathol. 2009;33(1): 99–105.
80. Torenbeek R, Blomjous CE, de Bruin PC, Newling DW, Meijer CJ. Sarcomatoid carcinoma of the urinary bladder. Clinicopathologic analysis of 18 cases with immunohistochemical and electron microscopic findings. Am J Surg Pathol. 1994;18(3):241–9.
81. Jones EC, Young RH. Myxoid and sclerosing sarcomatoid transitional cell carcinoma of the urinary bladder: a clinicopathologic and immunohistochemical study of 25 cases. Mod Pathol. 1997;10(9): 908–16.

Chapter 20
Kidney

Fan Lin and Ximing J. Yang

Abstract This chapter provides a practical overview of frequently used markers in the diagnosis and differential diagnosis of both common and rare renal neoplasms, with a specific focus on renal epithelial tumors and their mimickers. The chapter contains 52 questions; each question is addressed with a table, concise note and representative pictures if applicable. In addition to the literature review, the authors have included their own experience and tested numerous antibodies reported in the literature. The most effective diagnostic panels of antibodies have been recommended for many entities, such as PAX8, RCCMa, and KIM-1 being suggested as the best diagnostic panel for identifying clear cell renal cell carcinoma. Furthermore, immunophenotypes of normal renal tissues have been described, which tends to be neglected in literature. Prognostic markers for renal cell carcinoma have been briefly mentioned.

Keywords Clear cell renal cell carcinoma • Chromophobe renal cell carcinoma • Papillary renal cell carcinoma • Oncocytoma • RCCMa • KIM-1 • PAX8 • CD10 • S100A1 • pVHL • CK7

FREQUENTLY ASKED QUESTIONS

Differential Diagnoses

F. Lin (✉)
Department of Pathology and Laboratory Medicine, Geisinger Medical Center, 100 N. Academy Ave, Danville, PA 17822, USA
e-mail: flin1@geisinger.edu

F. Lin and J. Prichard (eds.), *Handbook of Practical Immunohistochemistry: Frequently Asked Questions*, DOI 10.1007/978-1-4419-8062-5_20, © Springer Science+Business Media, LLC 2011

Table 20.1 Summary of frequently used antibodies

Markers	Localization (N, M, C)	Function	Application and pitfalls
CD10	M	Also called common acute lymphoblastic leukemia antigen (CALLA), a 100 kD zinc-dependent membrane metallopeptidase	Positive in CRCC and PRCC; also positive in glomeruli and many other nonrenal tumors
KIM-1	M+C	Kidney injury molecule-1, a type I transmembranous glycoprotein	Positive in nearly 100% PRCC and 80% of CRCC; also positive in acute tubular necrosis. But usually negative in ChRCC and oncocytoma.
RCCMa	M+C	200 kD glycoprotein	Positive in CRCC and PRCC
GST-alpha	C	Glutathione-transferase alpha, a super family of dimeric ubiquitous enzymes with function of biotransformation and detoxification of many xenobiotics	Positive in 80% CRCC, 10–20% of PRCC and oncocytoma; and usually negative in ChRCC
PAX2	N	Transcription factor in the paired box gene family	Positive in CRCC and oncocytoma, and some of PRCC and ChRCC
PAX8	N	Transcription factor in the paired box gene family	Similar to PAX2; but usually with stronger nuclear signal. Also positive in thyroid carcinoma and ovarian serous carcinoma.
CA IX	M+C	Carbonic anhydrase IX, an enzyme with function of maintaining intracellular and extracellular pH	Diffusely positive in CRCC and some PRCC; also positive in normal gastric mucosa and biliary ducts.
Vimentin	C	Intermediate filament	Positive in CRCC and PRCC, and negative in ChRCC and oncocytoma
EMA	M	Epithelial marker	Showing coexpression with vimentin in CRCC and collecting duct carcinoma
AE1/AE3	M	Epithelial marker	Approximately 10% of CRCC may be negative or only very focally positive
CK7	M+C	Epithelial marker	Positive in type I PRCC and ChRCC; usually only focally positive in oncocytoma and usually negative in CRCC and metanephric adenoma.
CK20	M+C	Epithelial marker	May be positive in type II PRCC

(continued)

Table 20.1 (continued)

Markers	Localization (N, M, C)	Function	Application and pitfalls
CK5/6	M+C	High molecular weight CK, epithelial marker	Positive in collecting duct carcinoma and urothelial carcinoma
CK903	M+C	A high molecular weight CK (34betaE12), epithelial marker	Positive in collecting duct carcinoma and urothelial carcinoma
CD117	M	Also called c-kit, protooncogene, activating mutation may promote cell proliferation and decrease apoptosis	Positive in ChRCC and oncocytoma; but usually negative in CRCC and PRCC.
Ron Oncogene	C	A protooncogene, encoding a receptor tyrosine kinase	Positive in both ChRCC and oncocytoma; also expressed in ovarian epithelial tumors and others.
WT1	N	Wilms' tumor gene 1, a tumor suppressor gene	Positive in Wilms' tumor and metanephric adenoma
Ber-EP4 (EpCAM)	M	Epithelial cell adhesion molecule, a glycosylated transmembrane cell surface protein	Diffusely positive in ChRCC, CDC, and some PRCC; usually negative or only focally positive in CRCC and oncocytoma.
Ksp-cad	M+C	Kidney-specific cadherin is a calcium-dependent cell adhesion molecule	Positive in both ChRCC and oncocytoma and about 30% of CRCC
Beta-defensin-1	M+C	A candidate tumor suppressor gene located in chromosome 8p23	Positive in both ChRCC and oncocytoma
Parvalbumin	M+C	Calcium-binding protein	Positive in both ChRCC and oncocytoma
Vinculin	M+C	A cytoskeletal protein, associated with membrane actin-filament-attachment sites of cell–cell and cell–matrix adherens-type junctions	Positive in both ChRCC and oncocytoma
P504S (AMACR)	C	Alpha-methylacryl CoA racemase with a role in the beta-oxidation of branched-chain fatty acid and derivatives	Positive in PRCC and some CRCC; usually negative in ChRCC and oncocytoma
S100	N+C	A low molecular weight, acidic, dimeric, calcium-binding protein, and high solubility in 100% ammonium sulfate	Positive in CRCC and oncocytoma and usually negative in ChRCC. The antibody works the best when using a rabbit polyclonal antibody (Dako, code no. Z0311).
S100A1	N+C	Belongs to the family of S100 calcium-binding proteins	Positive in CRCC and oncocytoma and usually negative in ChRCC. Similar to S100 but with more reproducible results
MUC1	M+C	A membrane-associated glycoprotein expressed in various tumor types	Positive in type I PRCC and negative in type II PRCC
HMB-45	M+C	Melanocytic marker	Positive in angiomyolipoma and some translocation renal cell carcinomas
TFE3	N	80 kD transcription factor 3, located in Xp11.2	Positive in translocation renal cell carcinomas
UEA1	C+M	Ulex europaeus agglutinin-1	Positive in collecting duct carcinoma
CD57	M+C	A natural killer cell-associated antigen	Positive in Wilms' tumor and metanephric adenoma
CD56	M+C	A natural killer cell-associated antigen	Positive in Wilms' tumor and metanephric adenoma
pVHL	M+C	Tumor suppressor gene	Positive in CRCC, PRCC, ChRCC, and oncocytoma; a relatively sensitive and specific marker for identifying metastatic RCC
Uroplakin III	C	Urothelial-specific transmembrane protein	Expressed in normal urothelium and urothelial neoplasm

Note: *N* nuclear staining, *M* membranous staining, *C* cytoplasmic staining, *CRCC* clear cell renal cell carcinoma, *ChRCC* chromophobe renal cell carcinoma, *CDC* collecting duct carcinoma, *PRCC* papillary renal cell carcinoma

References: [1–69]

Table 20.2 Summary of common immunostaining markers in renal epithelial neoplasms

Antibodies	CRCC	PRCC	ChRCC	Onco	CDC	MTSCC	UC
EMA	+	+	+	+	+	+	+
CK7	–	+	+	–	+	+	+
CK20	–	–	–	–	–	–	+/–
CK903	–	–	–	–	+	–	+
p63	–	–	–	–	–	–	+
CD10	+	+	–/+	–/+	–	–	–
KIM-1[a]	+	+	–	–	–	N/A	–

(continued)

Table 20.2 (continued)

Antibodies	CRCC	PRCC	ChRCC	Onco	CDC	MTSCC	UC
PAX2/PAX8	+	+	+/–	+	+	–	–
RCCMa	+	+	–/+	–	–	–	–
Vinculin	–	–	+	+	+	N/A	N/A
CD117	–	–	+	+	+	–	–
S100A1/S100	+	+/–	–	+	–	–	–
S100P	–	–	–	–	–	–	+
CD15	–	–	–	+/–	–	–	+/–
GST-alpha	+	–/+	–	–/+	N/A	–	N/A
Vimentin	+	+/–	–	–	+	–	–
Ksp-cad	–/+	–	+	+	–	–	–
P504S (AMACR)	–/+	+	–	–	–	+/–	–
CA IX	+	+	–	–	–/+	N/A	+
UEA1	–	–	–	–	+	–	+
pVHL	+	+	+	+	N/A	N/A	–

Note: "+" usually greater than 70% of cases are positive, "–" less than 5% of cases are positive, "+/–" usually more than 50% of cases are positive, "–/+" less than 50% of cases are positive, *N/A* data not available

CRCC clear cell renal cell carcinoma, *PRCC* papillary renal cell carcinoma, *ChRCC* chromophobe renal cell carcinoma, *Onco* oncocytoma, *CDC* collecting duct carcinoma, *MTSCC* mucinous tubular and spindle cell carcinoma, *UC* urothelial carcinoma

[a]KIM-1 is not commercially available yet

References: [1–4, 6–8, 10–72]

Table 20.3 Markers for proximal and distal normal tubules and glomeruli

Antibodies	Proximal tubules	Distal tubules	Glomeruli
CK7	0 (0/20)	100% (20/20)	0 (0/20)
CK20	0 (0/20)	0 (0/20)	0 (0/20)
EMA	0 (0/20)	100% (20/20)	0 (0/20)
Vimentin	0 (0/20)	0 (0/20)	100% (20/20)
E-cadherin	0 (0/20)	100% (20/20)	0 (0/20)
CD10	100% (20/20)	0 (0/20)	100% (20/20)
CK903	0 (0/20)	100% (20/20), F	0 (0/20)
CK19	100% (20/20)	100% (20/20)	0 (0/20)
P504S (AMACR)	100% (20/20)	100% (20/20), W	0 (0/20)
S100A1	100% (20/20)	100% (20/20), F	0 (0/20)
Villin	100% (20/20)	0 (0/20)	0 (0/20)
KIM-1	0 (0/20)	0 (0/20)	0 (0/20)
pVHL	100% (20/20)	100% (20/20)	0 (0/20)
GST-alpha	ND	ND	ND
RCCMa	100% (20/20)	0 (0/20)	0 (0/20)
Ksp-cad	100% (20/20)	100% (920/20)	0 (0/20)
PAX2	0 (0/20)	100% (20/20)	0 (0/20)
PAX8	10% (20/20), W	100% (20/20)	0 (0/20)
CA IX	100% (20/20),W	100% (20/20), W	0 (0/20)
CD117 (c-kit)	0 (0/20)	0 (0/20)	0 (0/20)
WT1	0 (0/20)	0 (0/20)	0 (0/20)
CD57	0 (0/20)	0 (0/20)	0 (0/20)
MUC1	0 (0/20)	100% (20/20)	0 (0/20)
Parvalbumin	0 (0/20)	100% (20/20)	0 (0/20)

Note: *W* weak, *F* focal

The results were based on GML data from 20 cases of normal renal tissues on TMA sections

S100A1 and parvalbumin show both nuclear and cytoplasmic staining pattern

From our experience, the RCC antibody (Vp-R150; clone: 66.4.C2; Vector Laboratory, Inc.) works well on the Ventana system but not in the Dako system

Stain for CA IX is very weak in our testing

S100A1 in distal tubular staining is very focal (1+ out of 4+)

PAX8 is a similar marker to PAX2, but it usually shows stronger nuclear staining and more reproducible results. The staining signal of PAX8 is much stronger in distal tubules than in proximal tubules

Table 20.4 Markers for clear cell renal cell carcinoma

Antibodies	Literature	GML data
CD10	+	90% (74/82)
PAX8	+	95% (89/94)
RCCMa	+	89% (72/81)
Vimentin	+	86% (76/88)
EMA	+	85% (17/20)
KIM-1	+	75% [a]
CA IX	+	91% (73/80)
pVHL	V	99% (76/77)
PAX2	+	84% (68/81)
P504S	–/+	44% (37/84)
S100	+	85% [a]
S100A1	+	80% (64/80)
GST-alpha	+	ND
CK7	–	11% (9/79)
CK20	–	0 (0/79)
CK19	+/–	58% (45/77)
CD117	–	5% (1/20)
Ksp-cad	–/+	40% (8/20)
Parvalbumin	–	2.5% (2/80)

Note: *V* variable, *ND* no data available

The results of S100 and KIM-1 are based on our previously published data

Representative markers are shown in Figs. 20.1–20.7, including KIM-1, pVHL, PAX8, CA IX, RCCMa, and CD10

[a] Based on the author's previously published data

References: [1–4, 6, 8, 15, 21–24, 26–33, 38, 41, 43, 46, 49, 51–53, 56, 73]

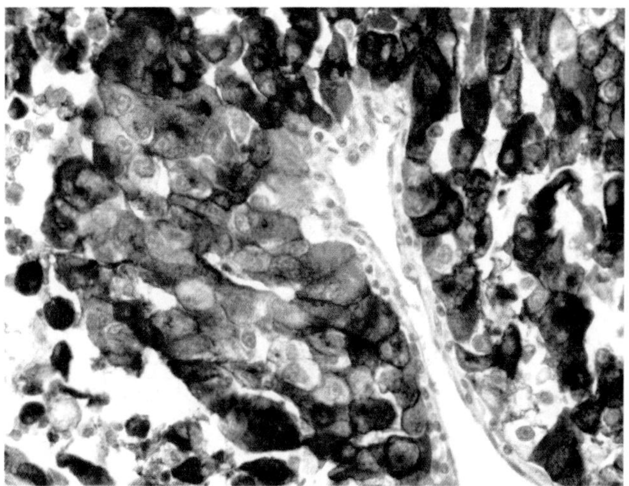

Fig. 20.2 Clear cell renal cell carcinoma positive for KIM-1

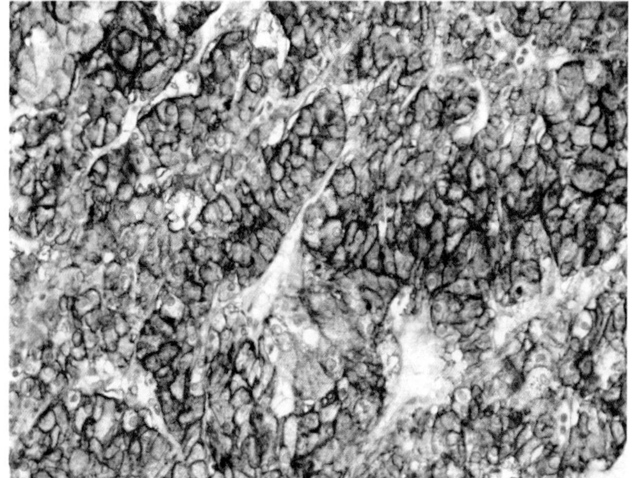

Fig. 20.3 Clear cell renal cell carcinoma positive for pVHL

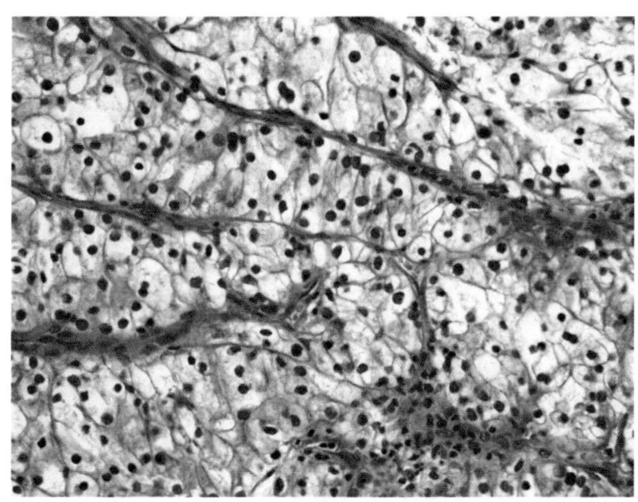

Fig. 20.1 Clear cell renal cell carcinoma on H&E stained slide

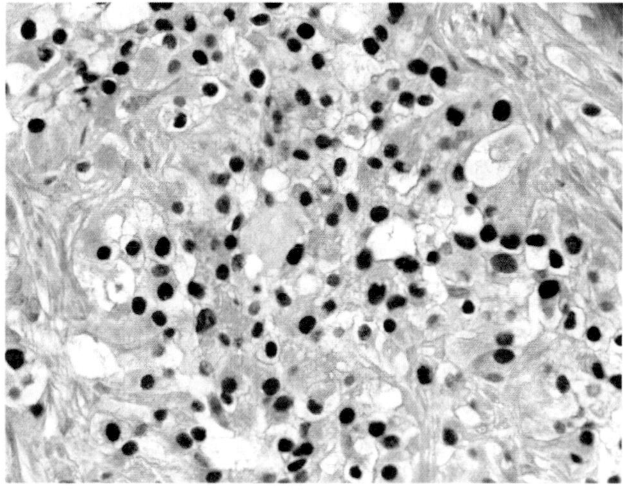

Fig. 20.4 Clear cell renal cell carcinoma positive for PAX8

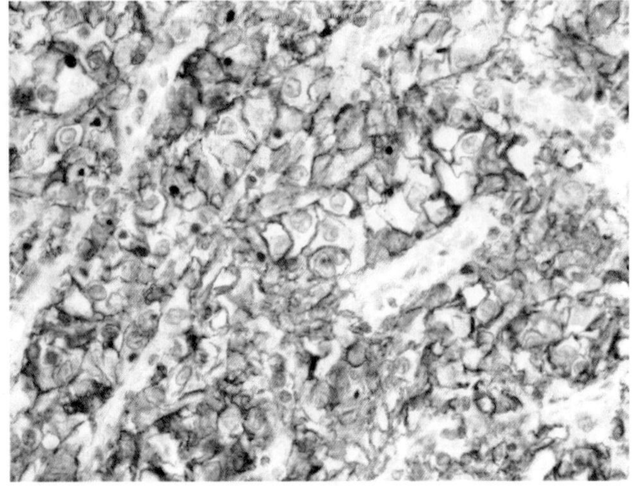

Fig. 20.5 Clear cell renal cell carcinoma positive for CAIX

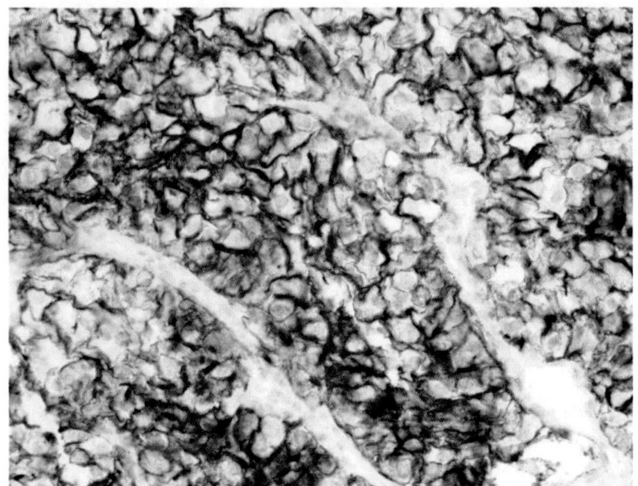

Fig. 20.7 Clear cell renal cell carcinoma positive for CD10

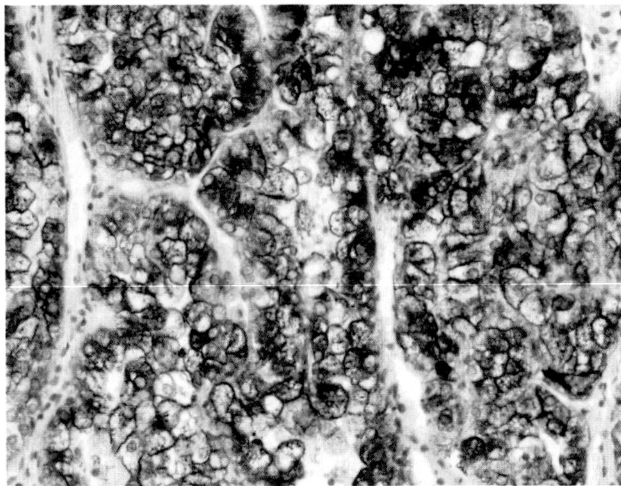

Fig. 20.6 Clear cell renal cell carcinoma positive for RCCMa

Table 20.5 Markers for papillary RCC

Antibodies	Literature	GML data
P504S (AMACR)	+	96% (22/23)
KIM-1	+	93%
pVHL	+	100% (25/25)
RCCMa	+	88% (22/25)
CK7	+	91% (21/23)
CD10	+	70% (16/23)
CK20	–	0 (0/25)
Vimentin	+/–	78% (18/23)
PAX2	+	57% (13/23)
PAX8	+	97% (65/67)
Ksp-cad	–	0 (0/10)
S100A1	ND	68% (17/25)

Note: *ND* no data available

Representative markers are shown in Fig. 20.8a–d, including pVHL, KIM-1, and P504S (AMACR)

References: [1–6, 8, 21–24, 33, 37–41, 54, 74]

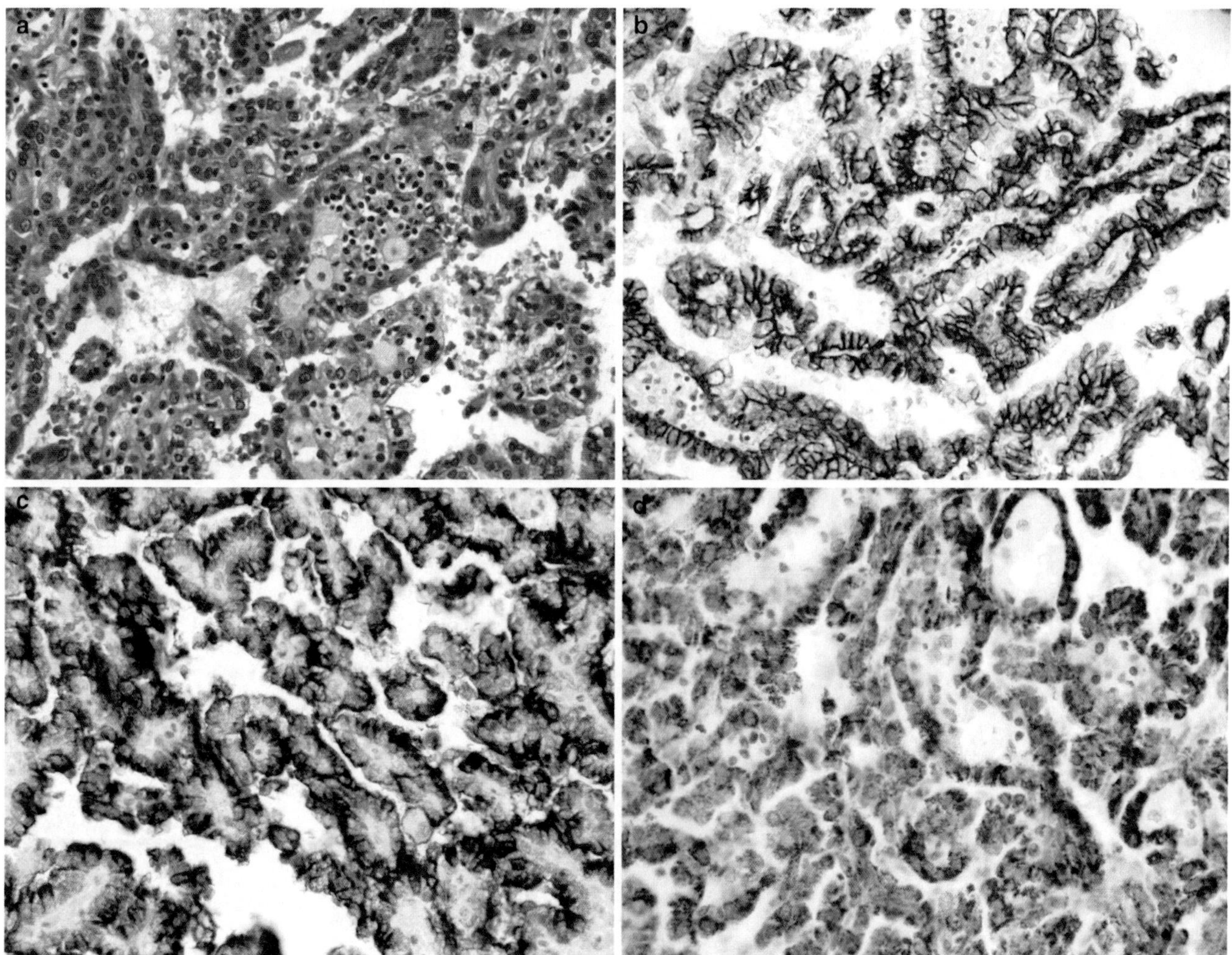

Fig. 20.8 Papillary renal cell carcinoma on H&E stained section (**a**), positive for pVHL (**b**), KIM-1 (**c**), and P504S (**d**)

Table 20.6 Markers for chromophobe RCC

Antibodies	Literature	GML data
CK7	+	100% (28/28)
Ber-EP4 (EpCAM)	+	100% (14/14)
CD117	+	71% (20/28)
S100A1	−	3.6% (1/28)
KIM-1	−	0 (0/28)
Claudin 7	+	ND
CD10	−/+	29% (8/28)
Ksp-cad	+	93% (26/28)
Vimentin	−	0 (0/28)
PAX2	+/−	29% (8/28)
PAX8	+/−	60% (6/10)
B-defensin-1	+	100% (14/14)
Parvalbumin	+	96% (27/28)
CK19	+	935 (14/15)
VHL	V	100% (28/28)
RCCMa	−	0 (0/20)
Ron Oncogene	+	100% (14/14)
CD15	−	8% (2/24)

Note: *ND* no data available, *V* variable

Our data show that all cases are positive for CK7, with 4 of 28 cases showing only focal positivity (<25% of tumor cells stained). The staining for PAX2 and PAX8 is weak compared with oncocytoma and CRCC. The staining for Ksp-cad and parvalbumin tends to be strong and diffuse (>50% of tumor cells stained)

Representative markers are shown in Fig. 20.9a–d to include CK7, Ber-EP4, and S100A1

References: [1–6, 8, 10, 12–18, 22, 26–28, 30–33, 38, 39, 41, 42, 44, 46, 49, 55, 57, 59, 60, 62, 65–68, 70, 74–80]

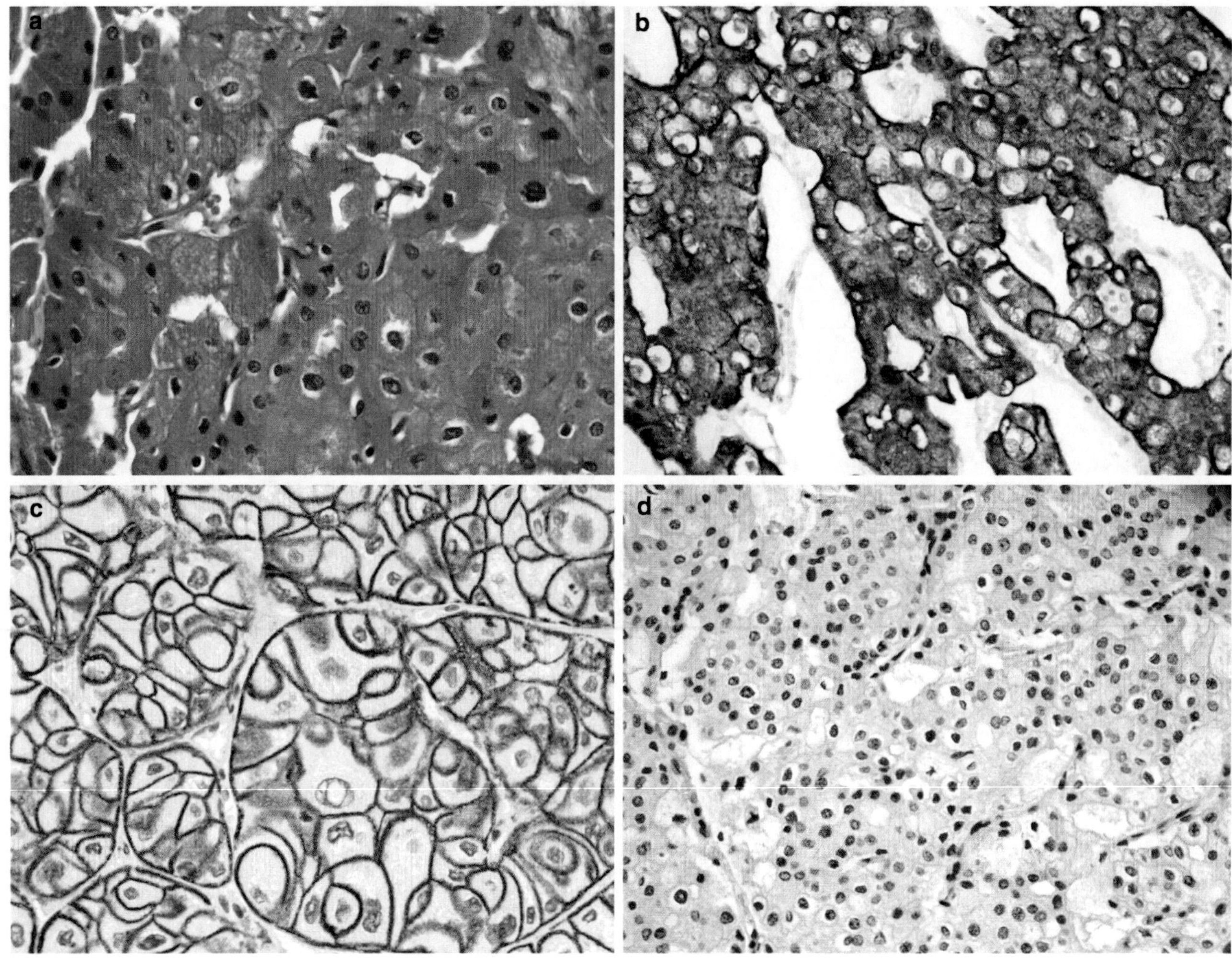

Fig. 20.9 Chromophobe renal cell carcinoma on H&E stained section (**a**), diffusely positive for CK7 (**b**) and EpCAM/BerEp4 (**c**), and negative for S100A1 (**d**)

Table 20.7 Markers for oncocytoma

Antibodies	Literature	GML data
CD117 (c-kit)	+	86% (18/21)
CK7	–/very focal +	33% (7/21), focal
S100A1	+	81% (17/21)
Parvalbumin	+	71% (15/21), focal
KIM-1	–	0 (0/21)
Ber-EP4 (EpCAM)	–	7% (1/14), focal
CD15	+/–	86% (18/21)
PAX2	V	86% (18/21)
PAX8	+	100% (15/15)
Ron oncogen	+	100% (5/5)
Ksp-cad	+	86% (18/21), focal
Beta-defensin-1	+	86% (18/21)
Vimentin	–	29% (6/21), focal
RCCMa	–	0 (0/21)
VHL	V	100% (21/21)

Note: *V* variable, *ND* no data available, focal – less than 25% tumor cells stained

The staining for both CK7 and Ber-EP4 (EpCAM) tends to be focal (<5% of the tumor cells in these cases); the nuclear and cytoplasmic staining for S100A1 tend to diffuse in the majority of cases, but it can be focal as well. Positivity for S100A1 is rarely seen in a chromophobe RCC. Staining for CD15 is seen in approximately 86% of cases; however, it is usually negative in a chromophobe RCC. Positive staining for Ksp-cad and parvalbumin tends to be focal (<25% of cells stained). PAX2 is positive in 86% of oncocytoma and only focally positive in 30% of ChRCC. The staining for both PAX2 and PAX8 is stronger and more diffuse than that in ChRCC

Representative markers are shown in Fig. 20.10a–e to include CK7, S100A1, Ber-EP4, and CD15

References: [1–6, 8, 10, 12–18, 22, 26–28, 30–33, 38, 39, 41, 42, 44, 46, 49, 55, 57, 59, 60, 62, 65–68, 70, 73, 75–79]

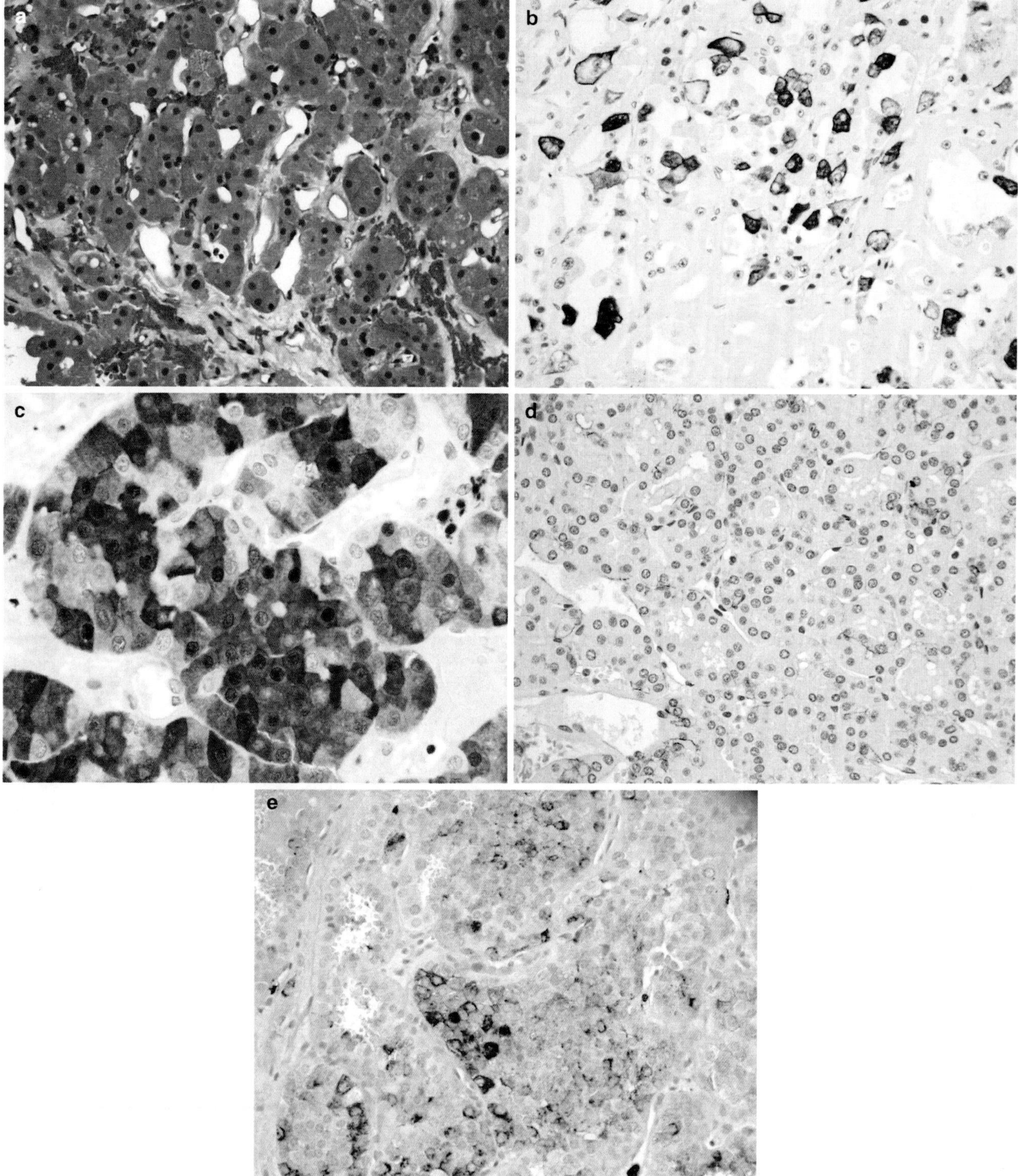

Fig. 20.10 Oncocytoma on H&E stained section (**a**), patchy positive for CK7 (**b**), S100A1 nuclear and cytoplasmic positivity (**c**), negative for EpCAM/BerEP4 (**d**), and focally positive for CD15 (**e**)

Table 20.8 Markers for collecting duct carcinoma

Antibodies	Literature
CK7	+
CK903	+
UEA1	+
CD10	–
p63	–
PAX8	+
KIM-1	–
Vinculin	+
E-cadherin	+
CD117 (c-kit)	+
CK19	+
CA IX	–/+
INI-1	+/–
HIG 2	+

Note: Complete loss of INI-1 expression was demonstrated in 20% of cases; in contrast, loss of expression of INI-1 has been reported in most medullary carcinomas of the kidney

Representative markers are shown in Fig. 20.11a–c to include PAX8 and p63

References: [1–6, 10, 14, 16, 21, 38, 69, 81–86]

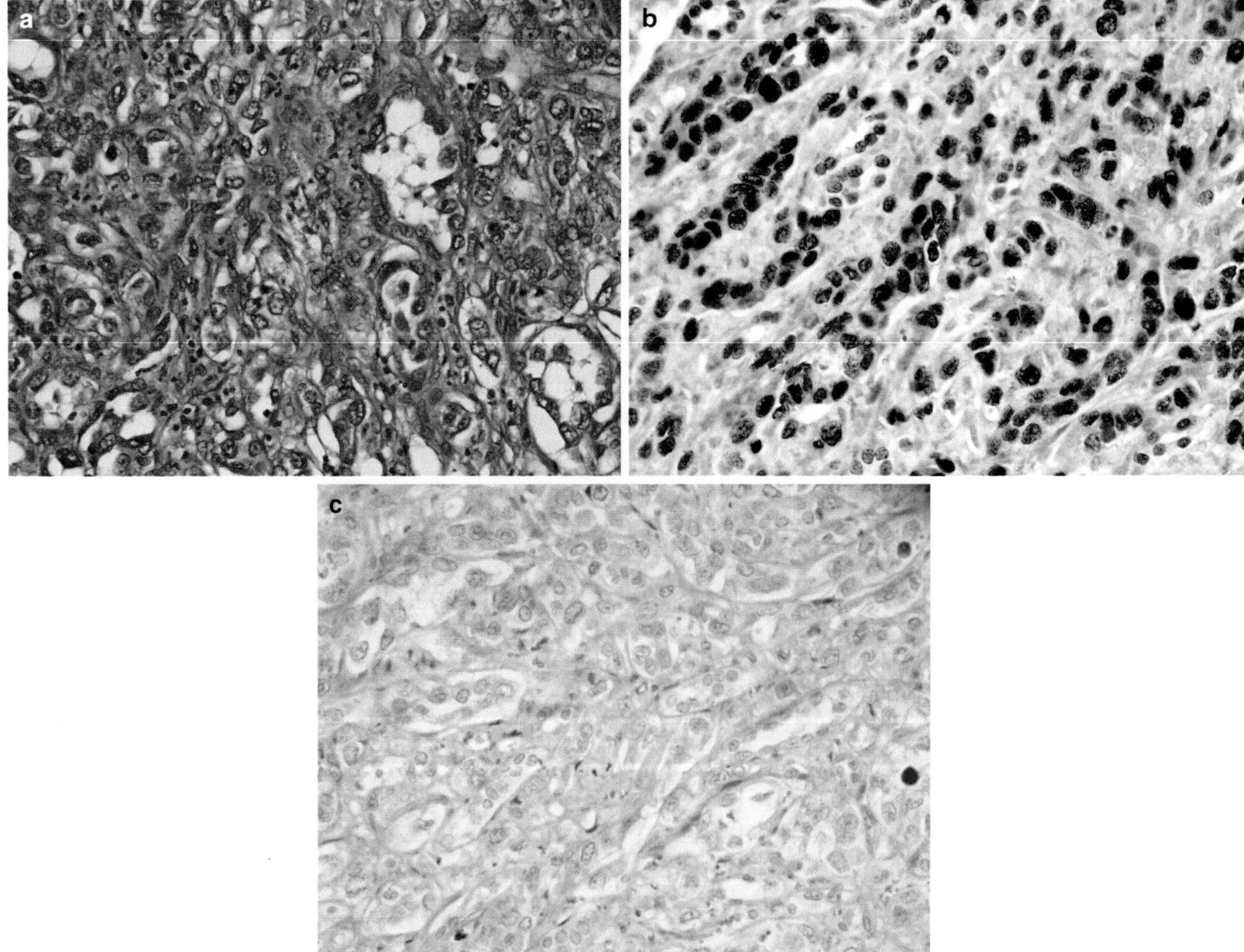

Fig. 20.11 Collecting duct carcinoma on H&E stained section (**a**) with positive for PAX8 (**b**) and nearly negative for p63 (**c**)

Table 20.9 Markers for medullary carcinoma of the kidney

Antibodies	Literature
AE1/AE3	+
CK7	+
CEA	+
UEA1	+
EMA	+
CK19	+
Topoisomerase IIa	+
INI-1	Loss of expression
KIM-1	–

References: [1–5, 83–88]

Table 20.10 Markers for urothelial carcinoma of the renal pelvis

Antibodies	Literature
CK7	+
CK5/6	+
CK903	+
CK20	+/–
Uroplakin III	+
S100P	+
p63	+
Thrombomodulin	+/–
UEA1	+
PAX8	–

References: [1–5, 74, 84]

Table 20.11 Markers for mucinous tubular and spindle cell carcinoma of the kidney

Antibodies	Literature
CK7	+
P504S (AMACR)	+
PAX8	+
HIG 2	+
EMA	+
CA IX	–/+
Ksp-cad	–/focal +
34betaE12	–/+
c-Kit (CD117)	–
CD10	–/focal +
RCCMa	–

Note: Focal – less than 25% of tumor cells stained

References: [1–5, 47, 48, 85]

Table 20.12 Markers for sarcomatoid RCC

Antibodies	Literature
AE1/AE3	+
EMA	+
Vimentin	+
KIM-1	+
pVHL	+
PAX8	+
CD10	+
RCCMa	–
P504S (AMACR)	ND

Note: *ND* no data

References: [1–5, 89, 90]

Table 20.13 Markers for unclassified RCC

Antibodies	Literature
EMA	+
AE1/AE3	+
CK7	–
Vimentin	–
CD10	+/–
P504S (AMACR)	–/+
PAX2	–/+
CA IX	+/–
TFE3	–
RCCMa	–

References: [1–5, 91]

Table 20.14 Markers for tubulocystic carcinoma

Antibodies	Literature
CD10	+
P504S (AMACR)	+
CK19	+
Parvalbumin	+
CK903	–/+
PAX2	–

Note: A representative case is shown in Fig. 20.12a, and positive staining for P504S in shown in Fig. 20.12b

References: [1–5, 29, 92]

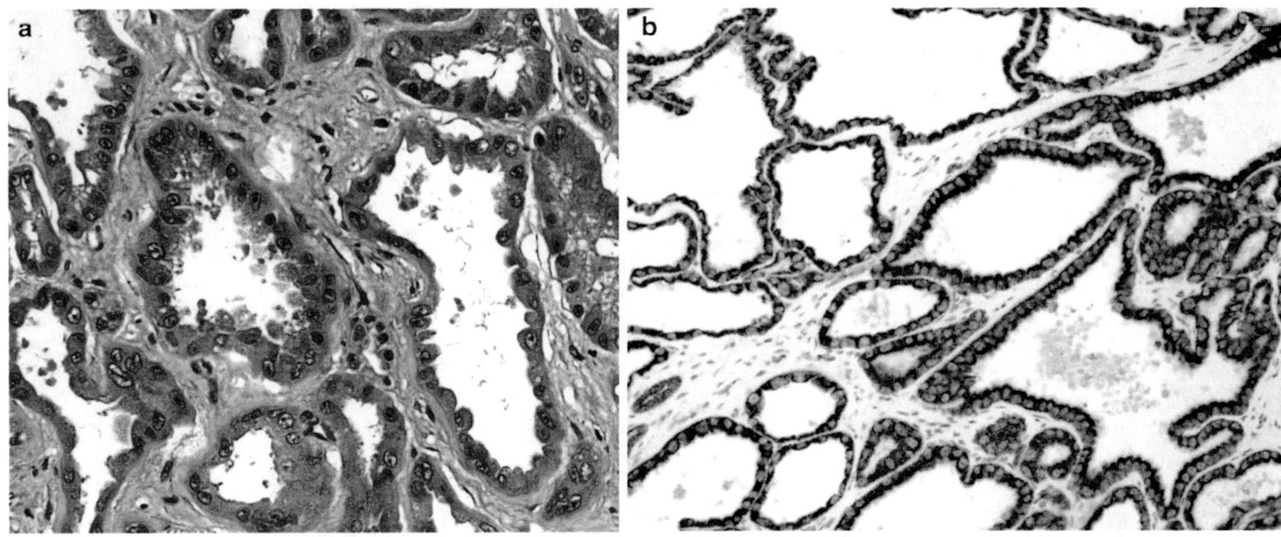

Fig. 20.12 Tubulocystic carcinoma on H&E stained section (**a**) and positive for P504S (**b**)

Table 20.15 Markers for XP11 translocation RCC

Antibodies	Literature
TFE3	+
HMB-45	Focal +
MART-1	Focal +
MiTF	–
EMA	Usually –
CAM 5.2	Usually –
Vimentin	Usually –
PAX2/PAX8	+
CA IX	–
HIF-1 alpha	+
Ksp-cad	–
Ber-EP4	–/+

Note: An example of translocation RCC was shown in Fig. 20.13a with positive staining for TEF3 (Fig. 20.13b)

References: [1–5, 37, 40, 93]

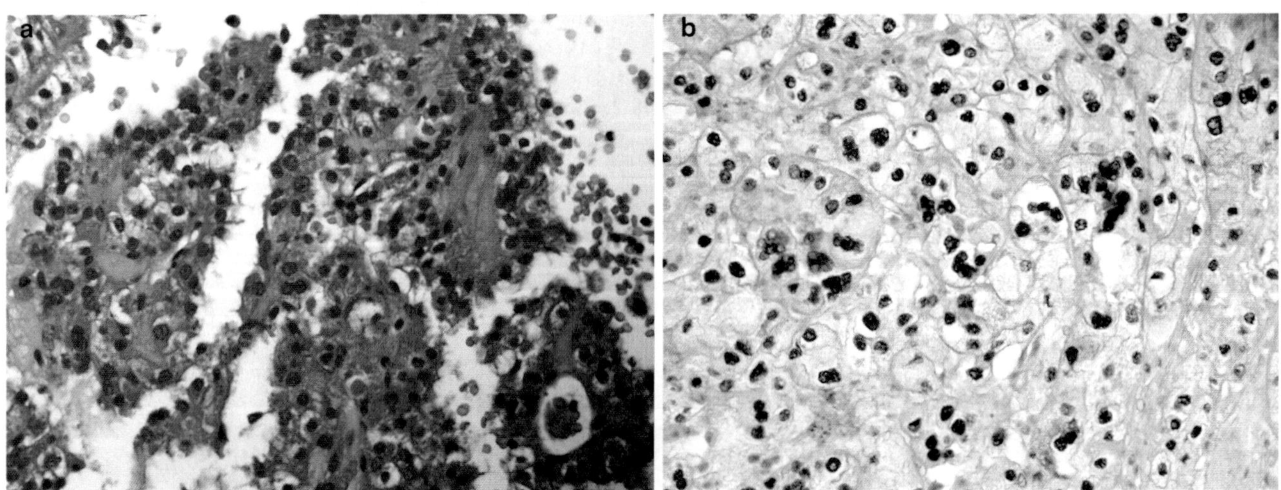

Fig. 20.13 XP11 translocation renal cell carcinoma on H&E stained section (**a**) and positive for TFE3 (**b**)

Table 20.16 Markers for angiomyolipoma

Antibodies	Literature
HMB-45	+
Cytokeratin	–
SMA	+
MART-1	+
EMA	–
S100	–

References: [1–5]

Table 20.17 Prognostic markers in renal cell carcinoma

Antibodies	Poor prognostic indicator
CA IX	Over expression
HIF-1 alpha	Over expression
IMP3	Over expression
Ki-67	High proliferative index
p53	Over expression
p27	Loss of expression
Ber-EP4	Over expression
VEGF/VEGF-R	Over expression
EGFR	Over expression
mTOR pathway/PTEN	Loss of expression
CRP	Over expression
S100A4	Over expression

Note: *CRP* C-reactive protein, *CA IX* carbonic anhydrase IX, *HIF-1* hypoxic-induced factor 1, *VEGF/VEGF-R* vascular endothelial growth factor and receptor, *Ber-EP4* epithelial cell adhesion molecule, *EGFR* epidermal growth factor receptor, *PTEN* phosphatase and tensin homolog deleted on chromosome 10

References: [1–5, 94–97]

Table 20.18 Markers for Wilms' tumor (epithelial component)

Antibodies	Literature
WT1	+
CD57	+
CK22	+
CK8	+
CK18	+
CD56	–/+

References: [1–5, 9]

Table 20.19 Markers for clear cell sarcoma of the kidney

Antibodies	Literature
Vimentin	+/–
Bcl-2	+/–
INI-1	+

Note: Cytokeratin, CD34, S100, CD99, desmin, and EMA are usually negative

References: [1–5]

Table 20.20 Markers for rhabdoid tumor of the kidney

Antibodies	Literature
Vimentin	Diffuse +
EMA	Focal +
INI-1	–
Cytokeratin	Focal +

Note: S100, CD99, NSE, and desmin are usually negative

References: [1–5]

Table 20.21 Markers for nephrogenic adenoma

Antibodies	Literature
AE1/AE3	+
P504S	+/–
CK7	+
PSA	–/focal +

References: [1–5]

Table 20.22 Markers for metanephric adenoma

Antibodies	Literature
CK7	–
CD57	+
WT1	+
EMA	–
S100	+
AE1/AE3	–
CD56	+
P504S	–

References: [1–5, 25]

Table 20.23 Markers for mesoblastic nephroma

Antibodies	Literature
Vimentin	+
WT1	–
Cytokeratin	–
CD34	–
Bcl-2	–
Desmin	+
Actin	+
S100	–

References: [1–5]

Table 20.24 Markers for juxtaglomerular cell tumor

Antibodies	Literature
Renin	+
SMA	+
MSA	+
CD31	+
S100	–
Desmin	–
Cytokeratin	–

References: [1–5]

Table 20.25 Papillary RCC vs. papillary urothelial carcinoma on biopsy samples

Antibodies	PRCC (N = 44)	Noninvasive PUC	Invasive PUC
S100P	0 (0/44)	91% (29/32)	68% (27/40)
pVHL	91% (40/44)	0 (0/32)	0 (0/40)
P504S	93% (41/44)	0 (0/32)	8% (3/40)
CK7	93% (41/44)	100% (32/32)	98% (39/40)
CK20	0 (0/44)	63% (20/32)	58% (23/40)
KIM-1	91% (40/44)	15% (4/26)	15% (6/40)

Note: *PRCC* papillary renal cell carcinoma, *PUC* papillary urothelial carcinoma

p63 also proved to be a good marker; it is usually positive in PUC and negative in PRCC

Reference: [98]

Table 20.26 Chromophobe RCC vs. oncocytoma

	ChRCC		Oncocytoma	
Antibodies	Literature	GML data	Literature	GML data
CK7	Diffuse +	100% (28/28)	–/focal +	33% (7/21)
Ber-EP4	Diffuse +	100% (14/14)	–/focal +	7% (1/14)
S100A1	–	3.6% (1/28)	+	81% (17/21)
CD15	–	8% (2/24)	+/–	86% (18/21)
Claudin 7	+	ND	–	ND
Claudin 8	M +	ND	C +	ND
PAX2	+	29% (8/28)	+	86% (18/21)
PAX8	+	60% (6/10)	+	100% (15/15)
Ksp-cad	+	93% (26/28)	+	86% (18/21)
Parvalbumin	+	96% (27/28)	+	71% (15/21)

Note: *ND* no data available, *M* membranous; *C* cytoplasmic

After testing many markers reported in the literature, we have identified the panel of 4 antibodies (CK7, Ber-EP4, S100A1, and CD15) to be the most useful panel in differentiating these two entities. The staining for CK7 tends to be diffuse (more than 50% of tumor cells stained) in ChRCC and focal and patchy (less than 10% of tumor cells stained) in oncocytoma. Our data showed only 4 of 28 ChRCCs demonstrated focal CK7 positivity; in contrast, 7 of 21 oncocytomas showed focal CK7 positivity (less than 5% of tumor cells stained). Figures 20.9a–d and 20.10a–e showed the utility of these markers. The nuclear and cytoplasmic staining for S100A1 in oncocytoma can be focal, but the staining is rarely observed in a chromophobe RCC, even a focal stain

Both Ksp-cad and parvalbumin are usually positive in ChRCC and oncocytoma; however, the positivity tends to be more diffuse (>50% of tumor cells stained) and stronger in ChRCC than that in oncocytoma

References: [1–6, 8, 14, 15, 20, 26–28, 30–33, 55, 57, 60, 73, 77, 80, 99]

Table 20.27 Clear cell RCC vs. chromophobe RCC

	CRCC		ChRCC	
Antibodies	Literature	GML data	Literature	GML data
CK7	–	11% (9/79)	+	100% (28/28)
CD117	–	5% (1/20)	+	71% (20/28)
B-definsin-1	–	ND	+	100% (14/14)
KIM-1[a]	+	75%	–	0
RCCMa	+	89% (72/81)	–	0 (0/20)
CA IX	+	91% (73/80)	–	ND
Vimentin	+	86% (76/88)	–	0 (0/28)
GST-alpha	+	ND	–	ND
Ksp-cad	–/+	40% (8/20)	+	93% (26/28)
PAX2	+	84% (68/81)	+	29% (8/28)
PAX8	+	95% (89/94)	+/–	60% (6/10)

Note: *ND* no data available

References: [1–6, 8, 10, 12, 15, 18, 22, 25–33, 46, 51–53, 55, 62, 73]

[a]Based on the author's previously published data

Table 20.28 Clear cell RCC vs. collecting duct carcinoma

Antibodies	CRCC	CDC
CK7	–/+	+
UEA1	–	+
CD10	+	–
RCCMa	+	–/+
CK903	–	+
CA IX	+	–/+
KIM-1	+	–

References: [1–6, 10, 14, 16, 21, 38, 69, 81]

Table 20.29 Clear cell RCC vs. urothelial carcinoma

Antibodies	CRCC	UC
CK7	–/focal +	+
CK20	–	+/–
p63	–	+
PAX8/PAX2	+	–
RCCMa	+	–
Vimentin	+	–/+

References: [1–5, 81]

Table 20.30 Papillary RCC vs. clear cell papillary RCC

Antibodies	Papillary RCC	Clear cell papillary RCC
PAX2	–	+
RCCMa	+	–
CD10	+	–/+
P504S (AMACR)	+	–/+
34betaE12	–	+
CA IX	+	+
CK7	+/–	+

References: [1–5, 100, 101]

Table 20.31 High-grade papillary RCC vs. collecting duct carcinoma

Antibodies	High-grade PRCC	Collecting duct carcinoma
P504S (AMACR)	+	–/+
CD10	+	–
RCCMa	+	–
CD117	–	+
UEA1	–	+
CK19	–	+
E-cadherin	–	+

References: [1–5]

Table 20.32 Type II papillary RCC vs. collecting duct carcinoma

Antibodies	Type II PRCC	Collecting duct carcinoma
P504S (AMACR)	+	–
CK7	–/+	+/–
CK20	+/–	–
CD10	+	–
CD117	–	+
UEA1	–	+
CK19	–	+
RCCMa	+	–

References: [1–5]

Table 20.33 Papillary RCC vs. mucinous tubular and spindle cell carcinoma (MTSC)

Antibodies	PRCC	MTSC
CK7	+	+
P504S (AMACR)	+	+
CD10	+	–
RCCMa	+	ND
CA IX	+	–

References: [1–5]

Table 20.34 Type I papillary RCC vs. type II papillary RCC

Markers	Type I PRCC	Type II PRCC
CK7	+	–/+
MUC1	+/–	–
CK20	–	+/–
E-cadherin	–	+/–
P504S (AMACR)	+	Strongly +

References: [1–5]

Table 20.35 Urothelial carcinoma vs. collecting duct carcinoma

Antibodies	Urothelial carcinoma	Collecting duct carcinoma
p63	+	–
CA IX	+	–/+
PAX8/PAX2	–	+/–
S100P	+	ND
CK20	+/–	–
CD10	+/–	–
Thrombomodulin	+	ND
Vimentin	–/focal +	+/–

Note: *ND* no data available

References: [1–5, 32, 81]

Table 20.36 Sarcomatoid RCC vs. sarcomatoid urothelial carcinoma

Antibodies	Sarcomatoid RCC	Sarcomatoid urothelial carcinoma
CK7	–/+	+/–
CK20	–	+/–
CK5/6	–	+/–
Thrombomodulin	–	+/–
S100P	–	+/–
pVHL	+/–	–
CD10	+/–	–
p63	–	+/–

References: [1–5]

Table 20.37 Multicystic RCC vs. benign renal cysts

Antibodies	Cystic RCC	Benign cyst
EMA	+	+
Vimentin	+	–
KIM-1	+	–
CD10	+	–
PAX2	+	–

References: [1–5, 102]

Table 20.38 Clear cell RCC vs. xanthogranulomatous pyelonephritis

Antibodies	CRCC	Pyelonephritis
EMA	+	–
Vimentin	+	–
CD68	–	+
PAX2/PAX8	+	–
CD10	+	–
RCCMa	+	–

References: [1–5]

Table 20.39 Papillary RCC vs. metanephric adenoma

Antibodies	Papillary RCC	Metanephric adenoma
CK7	+	–
P504S (AMACR)	+	–
WT1	–	+
CD56	–	+
CD57	–	+
S100	–	+

References: [1–5, 25]

Table 20.40 Metanephric adenoma vs. papillary adenoma

Antibodies	Metanephric adenoma	Papillary adenoma
CK7	–	+
CD57	+	–
WT1	+	–
P504S (AMACR)	–	+

References: [1–5]

Table 20.41 Metanephric adenoma vs. Wilms' tumor

Antibodies	Metanephric adenoma	Wilms' tumor
S100	+	–
AE1/AE3	–	+ (epithelial)
CD57	+	+
CD56	+	+
WT1	+	+

References: [1–5, 25]

Table 20.42 Wilms' tumor vs. neuroblastoma

Antibodies	Wilms' tumor	Neuroblastoma
WT1	+	–/very focal+
NB84	–/very focal +	+
GFAP	+/–	–

References: [1–5, 103]

Table 20.43 Epithelioid angiomyolipoma vs. renal cell carcinoma

Antibodies	Epithelioid angiomyolipoma	Renal cell carcinoma
AE1/AE3	–	+
HMB-45	+	–
S100	–	+/–
SMA	+	–
MART-1	+	–
CA IX	–	+
CD10	–	+
EMA	–	+
PAX2/PAX8	–	+
RCCMa	–	+

References: [1–5]

Table 20.44 Wilms' tumor vs. clear cell sarcoma

Antibodies	Wilms' tumor	Clear cell sarcoma
WT1	+	Usually –
CD57	+	–
AE1/AE3	+ (epithelial)	–
CD56	+	–
CK22	+/–	–
CK8	+/–	–
CK18	+/–	–

References: [1–5]

Table 20.45 Wilms' tumor vs. rhabdoid tumor

Antibodies	Wilms' tumor	Rhabdoid tumor
WT1	+	–
INI-1	+	–
EMA	– (stroma)	Focal +
CD57	+	–

References: [1–5]

Table 20.46 Cystic nephroblastoma vs. cystic nephroma

Antibodies	Cystic nephroblastoma	Cystic nephroma
WT1	+	–
CD57	+	–
CD56	+	–
CK	+/–	–

References: [1–5]

Table 20.47 Rhabdoid tumor vs. rhabdomyosarcoma

Antibodies	Rhabdoid tumor	Rhabdomyosarcoma
Vimentin	+	+
EMA	Focal +	–
Myogenin	–	+
Desmin	–	+

References: [1–5]

Table 20.48 Mesoblastic nephroma vs. stromal-rich Wilms' tumor

Antibodies	Mesoblastic nephroma	Stromal-rich Wilms' tumor
WT1	–	+
CK	–	+/–
CD34	–	–

References: [1–5]

Table 20.49 Nephrogenic adenoma vs. urothelial carcinoma

Antibodies	Nephrogenic adenoma	Urothelial carcinoma
CK20	–	+/–
P504S (AMACR)	+/–	–/+
S100P	–	+
CK7	+	+
PSA	Focal +	–
PSAP	Focal +	–
p63	ND	+

Note: *ND* no data available

References: [1–5]

Table 20.50 Metanephric adenoma vs. congenital mesoblastic nephroma

Antibodies	Metanephric adenoma	Mesoblastic nephroma
WT1	+	–
CD57	+	–
S100	+	–
CD56	+	–
CK	–	–

References: [1–5]

Table 20.51 Metanephric adenofibroma vs. Wilms' tumor

Antibodies	Metanephric adenofibroma	Wilms' tumor
CD34	+	–
AE1/AE3	–	+ (epithelial)
WT1	+	+

References: [1–5]

Table 20.52 Common metastases in the kidney

Antibodies	RCC	Lung	Melanoma	Breast	GI	Ovary
CK7	–	+	–	+	+	+
CK20	–	–	–	–	+/–	–
TTF-1	–	+	–	–	–	–
GCDFP-15	–	–	–	–/+	–	–
CDX2	–	–	–	–	+/–	–
WT1	–	–	–	–	–	+/–
S100	+/–	+/–	+	+/–	–	–
MART-1	–	–	+	–	–	–
ER	–	–	–	+	–	+/–
VHL	+	–	–	–	–	–[a]
KIM-1	+	–	–	–	–	–[a]
PAX8	+	–	–	–	–	+

Note: Both KIM-1 and VHL are frequently expressed in clear cell carcinoma of the ovary and uterus but usually negative in other types of adenocarcinoma

[a]Based on the author's previously published data

References: [1–5, 22, 104]

References

1. Eble JN, Sauter G, Epstein JI, Sesterhenn IA. WHO classifications of tumors, Pathology and genetics of tumours of the urinary system and male genital organs. Lyon, France: International Agency for Research on Cancer; 2004.
2. Murphy WM, Grignon DJ, Perlman EJ. Tumors of the kidney, bladder, and related urinary structures, Fascicle 1. 4th ed. Washington, DC: American Registry of Pathology; 2004.
3. Bostwick DG, Cheng L. Urologic surgical pathology. 2nd ed. Philadelphia, PA: Elsevier; 2008.
4. Chu PG, Weiss LM. Modern immunohistochemistry. New York, NY: Cambridge University Press; 2009.
5. Dabbs DJ. Diagnostic immunohistochemistry. 3rd ed. Philadelphia, PA: Churchill Livingstone Elsevier; 2010.
6. Kim MK, Kim S. Immunohistochemical profile of common epithelial neoplasms arising in the kidney. Appl Immunohistochem Mol Morphol. 2000;10(4):332–8.
7. Mertz KD, Demichelis F, Sboner A, et al. Association of cytokeratin 7 and 19 expression with genomic stability and favorable prognosis in clear cell renal cell cancer. Int J Cancer. 2008;123(3): 569–76.
8. Skinnider BF, Folpe AL, Hennigar RA, et al. Distribution of cytokeratins and vimentin in adult renal neoplasms and normal renal tissue: potential utility of a cytokeratin antibody panel in the differential diagnosis of renal tumors. Am J Surg Pathol. 2005;29(6):747–54.
9. Vasei M, Moch H, Mousavi A, Kajbafzadeh AM, Sauter G. Immunohistochemical profiling of Wilms tumor: a tissue microarray study. Appl Immunohistochem Mol Morphol. 2008;16(2): 128–34.
10. Kobayashi N, Matsuzaki O, Shirai S, Aoki I, Yao M, Nagashima Y. Collecting duct carcinoma of the kidney: an immunohistochemical evaluation of the use of antibodies for differential diagnosis. Hum Pathol. 2008;39(9):1350–9.
11. Haitel A, Susani M, Wick N, Mazal PR, Wrba F. c-kit overexpression in chromophobe renal cell carcinoma is not associated with c-kit mutation of exons 9 and 11. Am J Surg Pathol. 2005;29(6):842.
12. Huo L, Sugimura J, Tretiakova MS, et al. C-kit expression in renal oncocytomas and chromophobe renal cell carcinomas. Hum Pathol. 2005;36(3):262–8.
13. Kruger S, Sotlar K, Kausch I, Horny HP. Expression of KIT (CD117) in renal cell carcinoma and renal oncocytoma. Oncology. 2005;68(2–3):269–75.
14. Li G, Gentil-Perret A, Lambert C, Genin C, Tostain J. S100A1 and KIT gene expressions in common subtypes of renal tumours. Eur J Surg Oncol. 2005;31(3):299–303.
15. Memeo L, Jhang J, Assaad AM, et al. Immunohistochemical analysis for cytokeratin 7, KIT, and PAX2: value in the differential diagnosis of chromophobe cell carcinoma. Am J Clin Pathol. 2007;127(2):225–9.
16. Miettinen M, Lasota J. KIT (CD117): a review on expression in normal and neoplastic tissues, and mutations and their clinicopathologic correlation. Appl Immunohistochem Mol Morphol. 2005;13(3):205–20.
17. Pan CC, Chen PC, Chiang H. Overexpression of KIT (CD117) in chromophobe renal cell carcinoma and renal oncocytoma. Am J Clin Pathol. 2004;121(6):878–83.
18. Wang HY, Mills SE. KIT and RCC are useful in distinguishing chromophobe renal cell carcinoma from the granular variant of clear cell renal cell carcinoma. Am J Surg Pathol. 2005;29(5): 640–6.
19. Brunner A, Schaefer G, Veits L, Brunner B, Prelog M, Ensinger C. EpCAM overexpression is associated with high-grade urothelial carcinoma in the renal pelvis. Anticancer Res. 2008;28(1A):125–8.
20. Went P, Dirnhofer S, Salvisberg T, et al. Expression of epithelial cell adhesion molecule (EpCam) in renal epithelial tumors. Am J Surg Pathol. 2005;29(1):83–8.
21. Han WK, Alinani A, Wu CL, et al. Human kidney injury molecule-1 is a tissue and urinary tumor marker of renal cell carcinoma. J Am Soc Nephrol. 2005;16(4):1126–34.
22. Lin F, Zhang PL, Yang XJ, et al. Human kidney injury molecule-1 (hKIM-1): a useful immunohistochemical marker for diagnosing renal cell carcinoma and ovarian clear cell carcinoma. Am J Surg Pathol. 2007;31(3):371–81.
23. Jiang Z, Fanger GR, Woda BA, et al. Expression of alpha-methylacyl-CoA racemase (P504s) in various malignant neoplasms and normal tissues: a study of 761 cases. Hum Pathol. 2003;34(8): 792–6.
24. Lin F, Brown RE, Shen T, Yang XJ, Schuerch C. Immunohistochemical detection of P504S in primary and metastatic renal cell carcinomas. Appl Immunohistochem Mol Morphol. 2004;12(2):153–9.
25. Azabdaftari G, Alroy J, Banner BF, Ucci A, Bhan I, Cheville JC. S100 protein expression distinguishes metanephric adenomas from other renal neoplasms. Pathol Res Pract. 2008;204(10): 719–23.
26. Li G, Barthelemy A, Feng G, et al. S100A1: a powerful marker to differentiate chromophobe renal cell carcinoma from renal oncocytoma. Histopathology. 2007;50(5):642–7.
27. Lin F, Yang W, Betten M, Teh BT, Yang XJ, The French Kidney Cancer Study Group. Expression of S-100 protein in renal cell neoplasms. Hum Pathol. 2006;37(4):462–70.
28. Rocca PC, Brunelli M, Gobbo S, et al. Diagnostic utility of S100A1 expression in renal cell neoplasms: an immunohistochemical and quantitative RT-PCR study. Mod Pathol. 2007;20(7): 722–8.

29. Amin MB, MacLennan GT. Tubulocystic carcinoma of the kidney: clinicopathological analysis of 31 cases of a distinctive rate subtype of renal cell carcinoma. Am J Surg Pathol. 2008;33(3):384–392.
30. Daniel L, Lechevallier E, Giorgi R, et al. Pax-2 expression in adult renal tumors. Hum Pathol. 2001;32(3):282–7.
31. Gokden N, Gokden M, Phan DC, McKenney JK. The utility of PAX-2 in distinguishing metastatic clear cell renal cell carcinoma from its morphologic mimics: an immunohistochemical study with comparison to renal cell carcinoma marker. Am J Surg Pathol. 2008;32(10):1462–7.
32. Gupta R, Balzer B, Picken M, et al. Diagnostic implications of transcription factor Pax 2 protein and transmembrane enzyme complex carbonic anhydrase IX immunoreactivity in adult renal epithelial neoplasms. Am J Surg Pathol. 2009;33(2):241–7.
33. Mazal PR, Stichenwirth M, Koller A, Blach S, Haitel A, Susani M. Expression of aquaporins and PAX-2 compared to CD10 and cytokeratin 7 in renal neoplasms: a tissue microarray study. Mod Pathol. 2005;18(4):535–40.
34. Dorai T, Sawczuk IS, Pastorek J, Wiernik PH, Dutcher JP. The role of carbonic anhydrase IX overexpression in kidney cancer. Eur J Cancer. 2005;41(18):2935–47.
35. Leppert JT, Lam JS, Pantuck AJ, Figlin RA, Belldegrun AS. Carbonic anhydrase IX and the future of molecular markers in renal cell carcinoma. BJU Int. 2005;96(3):281–5.
36. Shuch B, Li Z, Belldegrun AS. Carbonic anhydrase IX and renal cell carcinoma: prognosis, response to systemic therapy, and future vaccine strategies. BJU Int. 2008;101 Suppl 4:25–30.
37. Argani P, Netto GJ, Parwani AV. Papillary renal cell carcinoma with low-grade spindle cell foci: a mimic of mucinous tubular and spindle cell carcinoma. Am J Surg Pathol. 2008;32(9):1353–9.
38. Avery AK, Beckstead J, Renshaw AA, Corless CL. Use of antibodies to RCC and CD10 in the differential diagnosis of renal neoplasms. Am J Surg Pathol. 2000;24(2):203–10.
39. Butnor KJ, Nicholson AG, Allred DC, et al. Expression of renal cell carcinoma-associated markers erythropoietin, CD10, and renal cell carcinoma marker in diffuse malignant mesothelioma and metastatic renal cell carcinoma. Arch Pathol Lab Med. 2006;130(6):823–7.
40. Camparo P, Vasiliu V, Molinie V, et al. Renal translocation carcinomas: clinicopathologic, immunohistochemical, and gene expression profiling analysis of 31 cases with a review of the literature. Am J Surg Pathol. 2008;32(5):656–70.
41. Chu P, Arber DA. Paraffin-section detection of CD10 in 505 nonhematopoietic neoplasms. Frequent expression in renal cell carcinoma and endometrial stromal sarcoma. Am J Clin Pathol. 2000;113(3):374–82.
42. Huang W, Kanehira K, Drew S, Pier T. Oncocytoma can be differentiated from its renal cell carcinoma mimics by a panel of markers: an automated tissue microarray study. Appl Immunohistochem Mol Morphol. 2009;17(1):12–7.
43. Langner C, Ratschek M, Rehak P, Schips L, Zigeuner R. CD10 is a diagnostic and prognostic marker in renal malignancies. Histopathology. 2004;45(5):460–7.
44. Martignoni G, Pea M, Brunelli M, et al. CD10 is expressed in a subset of chromophobe renal cell carcinomas. Mod Pathol. 2004;17(12):1455–63.
45. Mukhopadhyay S, Valente AL, de la Roza G. Cystic nephroma: a histologic and immunohistochemical study of 10 cases. Arch Pathol Lab Med. 2004;128(12):1404–11.
46. Pan CC, Chen PC, Ho DM. The diagnostic utility of MOC31, BerEP4, RCC marker and CD10 in the classification of renal cell carcinoma and renal oncocytoma: an immunohistochemical analysis of 328 cases. Histopathology. 2004;45(5):452–9.
47. Paner GP, Srigley JR, Radhakrishnan A, et al. Immunohistochemical analysis of mucinous tubular and spindle cell carcinoma and papillary renal cell carcinoma of the kidney: significant immunophenotypic overlap warrants diagnostic caution. Am J Surg Pathol. 2006;30(1):13–9.
48. Shen SS, Ro JY, Tamboli P, et al. Mucinous tubular and spindle cell carcinoma of kidney is probably a variant of papillary renal cell carcinoma with spindle cell features. Ann Diagn Pathol. 2007;11(1):13–21.
49. Skinnider BF, Amin MB. An immunohistochemical approach to the differential diagnosis of renal tumors. Semin Diagn Pathol. 2005;22(1):51–68.
50. Olgac S, Hutchinson B, Tickoo SK, Reuter VE. Alpha-methylacyl-CoA racemase as a marker in the differential diagnosis of metanephric adenoma. Mod Pathol. 2006;19(2):218–24.
51. Zhou M, Roma A, Magi-Galluzzi C. The usefulness of immunohistochemical markers in the differential diagnosis of renal neoplasms. Clin Lab Med. 2005;25(2):247–57.
52. McGregor DK, Khurana KK, Cao C, et al. Diagnosing primary and metastatic renal cell carcinoma: the use of the monoclonal antibody 'Renal Cell Carcinoma Marker'. Am J Surg Pathol. 2001;25(12):1485–92.
53. Chuang ST, Chu P, Sugimura J, et al. Overexpression of glutathi one s-transferase alpha in clear cell renal cell carcinoma. Am J Clin Pathol. 2005;123(3):421–9.
54. Wang KL, Weinrach DM, Luan C, et al. Renal papillary adenoma – a putative precursor of papillary renal cell carcinoma. Hum Pathol. 2007;38(2):239–46.
55. Liu L, Qian J, Singh H, Meiers I, Zhou X, Bostwick DG. Immunohistochemical analysis of chromophobe renal cell carcinoma, renal oncocytoma, and clear cell carcinoma: an optimal and practical panel for differential diagnosis. Arch Pathol Lab Med. 2007;131(8):1290–7.
56. Grignon DJ, Abdel-Malak M, Mertens WC, Sakr WA, Shepherd RR. Glutathione S-transferase expression in renal cell carcinoma: a new marker of differentiation. Mod Pathol. 1994;7(2):186–9.
57. Adley BP, Papavero V, Sugimura J, Teh BT, Yang XJ. Diagnostic value of cytokeratin 7 and parvalbumin in differentiating chromophobe renal cell carcinoma from renal oncocytoma. Anal Quant Cytol Histol. 2006;28(4):228–36.
58. Hes O, Brunelli M, Michal M, et al. Oncocytic papillary renal cell carcinoma: a clinicopathologic, immunohistochemical, ultrastructural, and interphase cytogenetic study of 12 cases. Ann Diagn Pathol. 2006;10(3):133–9.
59. Abrahams NA, MacLennan GT, Khoury JD, et al. Chromophobe renal cell carcinoma: a comparative study of histological, immunohistochemical and ultrastructural features using high throughput tissue microarray. Histopathology. 2004;45(6):593–602.
60. Martignoni G, Pea M, Chilosi M, et al. Parvalbumin is constantly expressed in chromophobe renal carcinoma. Mod Pathol. 2001;14(8):760–7.
61. Young AN, Amin MB, Moreno CS, et al. Expression profiling of renal epithelial neoplasms: a method for tumor classification and discovery of diagnostic molecular markers. Am J Pathol. 2001;158(5):1639–51.
62. Shen SS, Krishna B, Chirala R, Amato RJ, Truong LD. Kidney-specific cadherin, a specific marker for the distal portion of the nephron and related renal neoplasms. Mod Pathol. 2005;18(7):933–40.
63. Mazal PR, Exner M, Haitel A, et al. Expression of kidney-specific cadherin distinguishes chromophobe renal cell carcinoma from renal oncocytoma. Hum Pathol. 2005;36(1):22–8.
64. Thedieck C, Kuczyk M, Klingel K, Steiert I, Muller CA, Klein G. Expression of Ksp-cadherin during kidney development and in renal cell carcinoma. Br J Cancer. 2005;92(11):2010–7.

65. Young AN, de Oliveira Salles PG, Lim SD, et al. Beta defensin-1, parvalbumin, and vimentin: a panel of diagnostic immunohistochemical markers for renal tumors derived from gene expression profiling studies using cDNA microarrays. Am J Surg Pathol. 2003;27(2):199–205.
66. Sun CQ, Arnold R, Fernandez-Golarz C, et al. Human beta-defensin-1, a potential chromosome 8p tumor suppressor: control of transcription and induction of apoptosis in renal cell carcinoma. Cancer Res. 2006;66(17):8542–9.
67. Patton KT, Tretiakova MS, Yao JL, et al. Expression of RON proto-oncogene in renal oncocytoma and chromophobe renal cell carcinoma. Am J Surg Pathol. 2004;28(8):1045–50.
68. Rampino T, Gregorini M, Soccio G, et al. The Ron proto-oncogene product is a phenotypic marker of renal oncocytoma. Am J Surg Pathol. 2003;27(6):779–85.
69. Kuroda N, Naruse K, Miyazaki E, et al. Vinculin: Its possible use as a marker of normal collecting ducts and renal neoplasms with collecting duct system phenotype. Mod Pathol. 2000;13(10): 1109–14.
70. Donald CD, Sun CQ, Lim SD, et al. Cancer-specific loss of beta-defensin 1 in renal and prostatic carcinomas. Lab Invest. 2003;83(4):501–5.
71. Kamada M, Suzuki K, Kato Y, Okuda H, Shuin T. von Hippel-Lindau protein promotes the assembly of actin and vinculin and inhibits cell motility. Cancer Res. 2001;61(10):4184–9.
72. Otani M, Shimizu T, Serizawa H, Ebihara Y, Nagashima Y. Low-grade renal cell carcinoma arising from the lower nephron: a case report with immunohistochemical, histochemical and ultrastructural studies. Pathol Int. 2001;51(12):954–60.
73. Wasco MJ, Pu RT. Comparison of PAX-2, RCC antigen, and antiphosphorylated H2AX antibody (gamma-H2AX) in diagnosing metastatic renal cell carcinoma by fine-needle aspiration. Diagn Cytopathol. 2008;36(8):568–73.
74. Jadallah S et al. PAX8 expression in clear cell, papillary and chromphobe RCC and urothelial carcinoma of renal pelvis. Mod Pathol. 2009;22 Suppl 1:174A.
75. Roehrl MH, Selig MK, Nielsen GP, Dal Cin P, Oliva E. A renal cell carcinoma with components of both chromophobe and papillary carcinoma. Virchows Arch. 2007;450(1):93–101.
76. Murakami T, Sano F, Huang Y, et al. Identification and characterization of Birt-Hogg-Dube associated renal carcinoma. J Pathol. 2007;211(5):524–31.
77. Adley BP, Gupta A, Lin F, Luan C, Teh BT, Yang XJ. Expression of kidney-specific cadherin in chromophobe renal cell carcinoma and renal oncocytoma. Am J Clin Pathol. 2006;126(1):79–85.
78. Schuetz AN, Yin-Goen Q, Amin MB, et al. Molecular classification of renal tumors by gene expression profiling. J Mol Diagn. 2005;7(2):206–18.
79. Javed R, Zhai QJ, Shen SS, Krishman B, Roy JY, Truong L. PAX-8 Is a specific marker for renal neoplasms comparison with PAX-2, renal cell carcinoma marker antigen (RCCM) and kidney specific cadherin (KSP). Mod Pathol. 2009;22 Suppl 1:174A.
80. Eisengart LJ, Rohan SM, Parimi V, Wei JJ, Yang XJ. CK7 and Claudin 7 are superior to other markers in distinguishing oncocytoma from chromophobe renal cell carcinoma-automatic imaging analysis and hierarchical clustering analysis. Mod Pathol. 2010;23 Suppl 1:188A.
81. Carvalho JC, Thomas DG, McHugh JB, Shah RB, Kunju LP. p63 is useful in distinguishing collecting duct renal carcinoma from its morphologic mimics. Mod Pathol. 2010;23 Suppl 1:182A.
82. Elwood H, Schultz L, Illei, et al. Immunohistochemical Loss of INI-1 expression in collecting duct carcinoma (CDC) [USCAP abstract 834]. Mod Pathol. 2010;23 Suppl 1s:189A.
83. Vankalakunti M, Gown AM, Gupta R, et al. An analysis of INI1 nuclear expression in collecting duct carcinoma (CDC) and renal medullary carcinoma (RMC): Diagnostic and pathogenic implications. Mod Pathol. 2010;23 Suppl 1:225A.
84. Vankalakunti M, Westfall DE, Parakh RS, et al. Immunohistochemical (IHC) expression of ulex europaeus agglutinin-1 (UEA-1) in the spectrum of adult renal epithelial neoplasms-A study of 165 cases. Mod Pathol. 2010;23 Suppl 1:225A.
85. Baydar DE, Schultz L, Illei PB, et al. Pax8, HIG-2, KSP cadherin and CA-IX expression in papillary RCC collecting ducts RCC and MTSC. Mod Pathol. 2010;23 Suppl 1:179A.
86. Amin M, Shah RB, Vasco MW, et al. Utility of kidney injury molecule (KIM-1) staining in a wide spectrum of traditional and newly recognized renal epithelial neoplasms: Diagnostic and histogenic implications. Mod Pathol. 2009;22 Suppl 1:156A.
87. Watanabe IC, Billis A, Guimaraes MS, et al. Renal medullary carcinoma: report of seven cases from Brazil. Mod Pathol. 2007;20(9):914–20.
88. Cheng JX, Tretiakova M, Gong C, Mandal S, Krausz T, Taxy JB. Renal medullary carcinoma: Rhabdoid features and the absence of INI1 expression as markers of aggressive behavior. Mod Pathol. 2008;21(6):647–52.
89. Chang A, Montgomery E, Epstein JI. Immunohistochemical profile of sarcomatoid renal cell carcinoma. Mod Pathol. 2010;23 Suppl 1:183A.
90. Malhotra R, Zhang PL, Bonventre JV, et al. Kidney injury molecule-1 (KIM-1) expression in sarcomatoid differentiation in renal cell carcinoma (RCC): Implications for differential diagnosis of malignant spindle cell lesions of the kidney. Mod Pathol. 2009;22 Suppl 1:181A.
91. Shukla A, Carvalho J, Shah RB, Kunju LP. Unclassified renal cell carcinoma: Clinico-pathologic and immunohistochemical analysis. Mod Pathol. 2010;23 Suppl 1:219A.
92. Yang XJ, Zhou M, Hes O, et al. Tubulocystic carcinoma of the kidney: Clinicopathologic and molecular characterization. Am J Surg Pathol. 2008;32(2):177–87.
93. Argani P, Hicks J, De Marzo A, et al. XP11 translocation renal cell carcinoma (RCC): Extended immunohistochemical (IHC) profile emphasizing noval RCC markers. Mod Pathol. 2010;23 Suppl 1:175A.
94. Huang J, Elson P, Aydin H, et al. IMP-3 is an independent prognostic marker in clear cell renal cell carcinoma. Mod Pathol. 2010;23 Suppl 1:196A.
95. Kiremitci S, Kankaya D, Tulunay O, Baltaci S. Expression pattern of epidermal growth factor receptor (EGFR) in clear cell renal cell carcinoma (CRCC): Association with clinicopathological features and clinical outcomes. Mod Pathol. 2010;23 Suppl 1:200A.
96. Lin F, Wood C, Yang XJ, Yang W. Expression of S-100A4 protein in renal cell carcinoma associated with high tumor grade and metastasis. Mod Pathol. 2006;19 Suppl 1:147A.
97. Bandiera A, Melloni G, Freschi M, et al. Prognostic factors and analysis of S100a4 protein in resected pulmonary metastases from renal cell carcinoma. World J Surg. 2009;33(7):1414–1420.
98. Lin F, Shi J, Yang XJ, Zhang PL, Dupree W. A useful panel of immunohistochemical markers in differentiating papillary renal cell caricnoma from papillary urothelial carcinoma [USCAP abstract 756]. Mod Pathol. 2008;21 Suppl 1s:166A.
99. Kim SS, Choi C, Choi YD. Immunohistochemical stain for Cytokeratin 7, S100A1, and Claudin 8 is valuable in differential diagnosis of chromophone renal cell carcinoma from renal oncocytoma. Mod Pathol. 2009;22 Suppl 1:176A.
100. Westfall DE, Luthringer DJ, Alsabeh R, Parakh RS, Vankalakunti M, Amin MB. Detailed immunohistochemical (IHC) characterization of the recently described clear cell-papillary renal cell carcinoma of the kidney. Mod Pathol. 2010;23 Suppl 1:228A.

101. Lopez JI, Anton I, Onate JM, Garcia-Munoz H. Clear cell papillary renal cell carcinoma a histological study of 12 cases in patients under 40 years of age. Mod Pathol. 2010;23 Suppl 1:204A.
102. Shi J, Yang XJ, Zhang PL, et al. Evaluation of expression of human kidney injury molecule-1 (hKIM-1), P504S, S100, vimentin and EMA in renal cystic lesions. Mod Pathol. 2007;20 Suppl 1:176A.
103. Miettinen M, Chatten J, Paetau A, Stevenson A. Monoclonal antibody NB84 in the differential diagnosis of neuroblastoma and other small round cell tumors. Am J Surg Pathol. 1998;22(3):327–32.
104. Lin F, Shi J, Liu H, et al. Immunohistochemical detection of the von Hippel-Lindau gene product (pVHL) in human tissues and tumors: a useful marker for metastatic renal cell carcinoma and clear cell carcinoma of the ovary and uterus. Am J Clin Pathol. 2008;129(4):592–605.

Chapter 21
Testis and Paratesticular Tissues

Myra Wilkerson

Abstract The diagnosis of testicular neoplasms is often based solely on morphologic pattern recognition, but there are newer markers that can play a significant role in the identification of germ cell tumors such as SALL4 and OCT3/4. Similarly, GAL-3 and other newer markers can be helpful in the identification of sex cord/stromal tumors. Many of the markers used in the identification of testicular tumors may be present in normal testicular cells as well, but their expression patterns may change according to the life stage of the patient. This chapter attempts to address that question, although the literature is somewhat sparse. Markers of normal paratesticular epithelia are included, as well as markers in paratesticular tumors. Basic algorithms are provided to assist in the workup of testicular and paratesticular neoplasms.

Keywords Germ cell tumors • Sex cord/stromal tumors • Gonadoblastoma • Syncytiotrophoblast • Paratesticular neoplasms • Placental-like alkaline phosphatase • SALL4

FREQUENTLY ASKED QUESTIONS

M. Wilkerson (✉)
Department of Pathology and Laboratory Medicine, Geisinger Wyoming Valley Medical Center, 1000 East Mountain Blvd., Wilkes-Barre, PA 18711, USA
e-mail: mwilkerson@geisinger.edu

F. Lin and J. Prichard (eds.), *Handbook of Practical Immunohistochemistry: Frequently Asked Questions*,
DOI 10.1007/978-1-4419-8062-5_21, © Springer Science+Business Media, LLC 2011

Table 21.1 Antibodies frequently used in testicular and paratesticular neoplasms

Antibody	Localization	Function	Applications and pitfalls
AE1/AE3	C	Intermediate filament in cytoskeleton	Often in a punctate, perinuclear distribution in sex cord/stromal tumors. Typically does not stain germ cell tumors, but can be focal, often in a dot-like or globular pattern
AFP	C	Protein produced by fetal yolk sac, gastrointestinal epithelium and liver	Useful marker in germ cell tumors, but also present in hepatocellular carcinoma
Ber-EP4	M	Cell adhesion molecule	Adenocarcinoma-related marker. Has been reported in few cases of mesothelioma
CALRET	C; some N	Neuronal calcium binding protein	Mesothelioma-related marker. Also identifies Wolffian-derived structures/tumors and urothelial carcinoma
CAM 5.2	C	Intermediate filament in cytoskeleton	Typically does not stain germ cell tumors, but can be focal, often in a dot-like or globular pattern
CD30	M; C	Transmembrane glycoprotein	Useful in the diagnosis of embryonal carcinoma, but may be positive in anaplastic large cell lymphoma and Reed–Sternberg cells
CEA	C	Cell surface glycoprotein; produced by fetal gut epithelium; plays a role in cell adhesion	Adenocarcinoma-related marker
c-kit	M; C	Transmembrane glycoprotein receptor kinase	Commonly expressed in seminoma, but may also be seen in renal carcinoma
D2-40	C; M	Oncofetal transmembrane mucoprotein	Expressed by fetal germ cells and germ cell tumors. Will also stain lymphatic endothelium and mesothelial cells
GAL-3	C	Beta-galactoside binding lectin	Expressed in adult Sertoli and Leydig cells, but not in fetal or prepubertal stages. May be detected in thyroid, colon, pancreatic, and breast carcinomas
hCG	C	Glycoprotein produced by syncytiotrophoblast	
INHA	C	Inhibits release of follicle stimulating hormone	Useful in sex cord stromal tumors, and also produced by syncytiotrophoblast and adrenal neoplasms
Melan-a	D	Protein in melanosomes	Useful to identify Leydig cells, unless differential includes melanoma, testicular tumor of androgenital syndrome, or granulosa cell tumor
MOC31	C; M	Glycoprotein on cell surface and cytoplasm of epithelia	Adenocarcinoma-related marker. Can indicate Muellerian differentiation. Not expressed in squamous epithelium
NSE	C	Neuronal form of a glycolytic enzyme	Expressed in germ cell tumors, and also in tumors of neural and neuroendocrine origin
OCT4	N	Stem cell transcriptional regulator	Useful in germ cell tumors
PLAP	C; M	Enzyme produced by syncytiotrophoblast	Useful in germ cell tumors; however, also (+) in many carcinomas. Seminomas usually demonstrate membranous staining, but sometimes perinuclear. Embryonal carcinomas show focal staining, but often more intense than seminomas
SALL4	N	Regulates transcription of OCT4	Detected in all germ cell tumors, but not in any sex cord/stromal tumors
TAG 72	C	Tumor-associated glycoprotein	Adenocarcinoma-related marker
TM	M	Endothelial cell-associated cofactor for thrombin-mediated activator of protein C	Mesothelial-related marker, and also positive in urothelial carcinoma, squamous cell carcinoma, and vascular tumors
Vim	C	Intermediate filament in cytoskeleton	
WT1	C; N	Transcription factor involved in gonadal development	Mesothelial-related marker. Also confirms Muellerian differentiation

C cytoplasmic staining, *M* membranous staining, *N* nuclear staining

References: [1–19]

Table 21.2 Markers for normal testicular cells at different life stages

	FSC	PSC	ASC	FLC	PLC	ALC	FGC	PGC	AGC
GAL-3	–	–	+	–	–	+	–	–	–
ARP	–	–	+	+	+	+	–	–	– or +[a]
Vim	+	–	+	ND	+	+ or –	ND	ND	–
CALRET	ND	ND	+ Focal	ND	ND	+	ND	ND	–
INHA	ND	ND	+	ND	ND	+	ND	ND	ND
c-kit	ND	ND	–	ND	ND	+	ND	ND	+ or –[b]
ERalpha	ND	ND	–	ND	ND	– or +	ND	ND	–
ERbeta	ND	ND	– or +	ND	ND	+ or –	ND	ND	+ or –[c]
PR	ND	ND	–	ND	ND	–	ND	ND	– or +
OCT4	ND	ND	–	ND	ND	–	+	–	+ or –[d]
SALL4	ND	ND	–	ND	ND	–	ND	+ or –[e]	+ or –[e]
CK18	+	+	+ or –	ND	ND	–	ND	ND	–
CAM 5.2	+	+		–	–	ND	ND	ND	ND

Abbreviations: *F/P/A-SC* fetal/prepubertal/adult Sertoli cells, *F/P/A-LC* fetal/prepubertal/adult Leydig cells, *F/P/A-GC* fetal/prepubertal/adult germ cells

Notes:

[a](+) In germ cells except (–) in spermatogonia

[b](+) In spermatogonia and acrosomal granules of round spermatids; (–) in spermatocytes and elongating spermatids

[c](+) In spermatogonia, spermatocytes, and early spermatids; (–) in elongating spermatids

[d](–) In secondary spermatocytes, spermatids, spermatozoa

[e](+) In spermatogonia; (–) in secondary spermatocytes, spermatids, spermatozoa

References: [2, 4, 6, 9, 11, 20–40]

Table 21.3 Markers for germ cell tumors

	ITGCN	CS	SS	EC	YST	CC
PLAP	+	+	–	+	– or +	+ or –
c-kit	+	+	– or +	– or +	– or +	–
OCT4	+	+	–	+[a]	–	–
AE1/AE3	–	– or +	–	+	+	+[b]
EMA	ND	–	ND	–	–	– or +
AFP	–	–	–	– or +	+[c]	–
CD30	–	–	–	+	–	–
INHA	–	–	–	–	–	+[d]
Vim	ND	– or +	– or +	–	– or +	–
NSE	+	+	–	+ or –	+ or –	– or +
CK18	ND	ND	+	+	+	+[e]
p53	+	+	+	+	–	–
D2-40	+	+	ND	–	ND	ND
CEA	ND	–	–	– or +	– or +	+ or –[f]
hCG	–	–	–	–	–	+[g]
A-AT	ND	– or +	ND	– or +	+	– or +
SP1	ND	–	–	–	ND	+[h]
CD99	–	–	ND	–	– or +	–
HPL	ND	–	–	– or +	–	+[h]
CAM 5.2	–	– or +[i]	– or +[i]	+	+	+
Chrom	–	–	–	–	– or +	–
S100	–	–	–	– or +	–	–
Desmin	ND	– or +	–	–	ND	ND
SALL4	+	+	+	+	+	+
NANOG	+	+	–	+	–	–
CD10	ND	ND	ND	ND	ND	+[h]
SOX2	–	–	–	+	–	–

Abbreviations: *ITGCN* intratubular germ cell neoplasia, *CS* classic seminoma, *SS* spermatocytic seminoma, *EC* embryonal carcinoma, *YST* yolk sac tumor, *CC* choriocarcinoma

See Figs. 21.1–21.12

Notes: All tumors in this table are negative for LCA and calretinin

[a]Demonstrates both nuclear and cytoplasmic staining

[b](+) In syncytiotrophoblast, intermediate trophoblast, and cytotrophoblast

[c]Staining is often patchy and granular; columnar cells of Schiller–Duvall bodies are (–); hyaline globules are (–) but may stain around edge

[d](+) In cytotrophoblast and intermediate trophoblast

[e](+) In cytotrophoblast and syncytiotrophoblast

[f]May be (+) in syncytiotrophoblast

[g](+) In syncytiotrophoblast and intermediate trophoblast; (–) in cytotrophoblast

[h](+) In intermediate trophoblast and syncytiotrophoblast

[i]If (+), often shows a dot-like pattern in the cytoplasm

References: [2–4, 6, 7, 10, 12, 15–17, 19, 20, 22, 23, 38, 41–79]

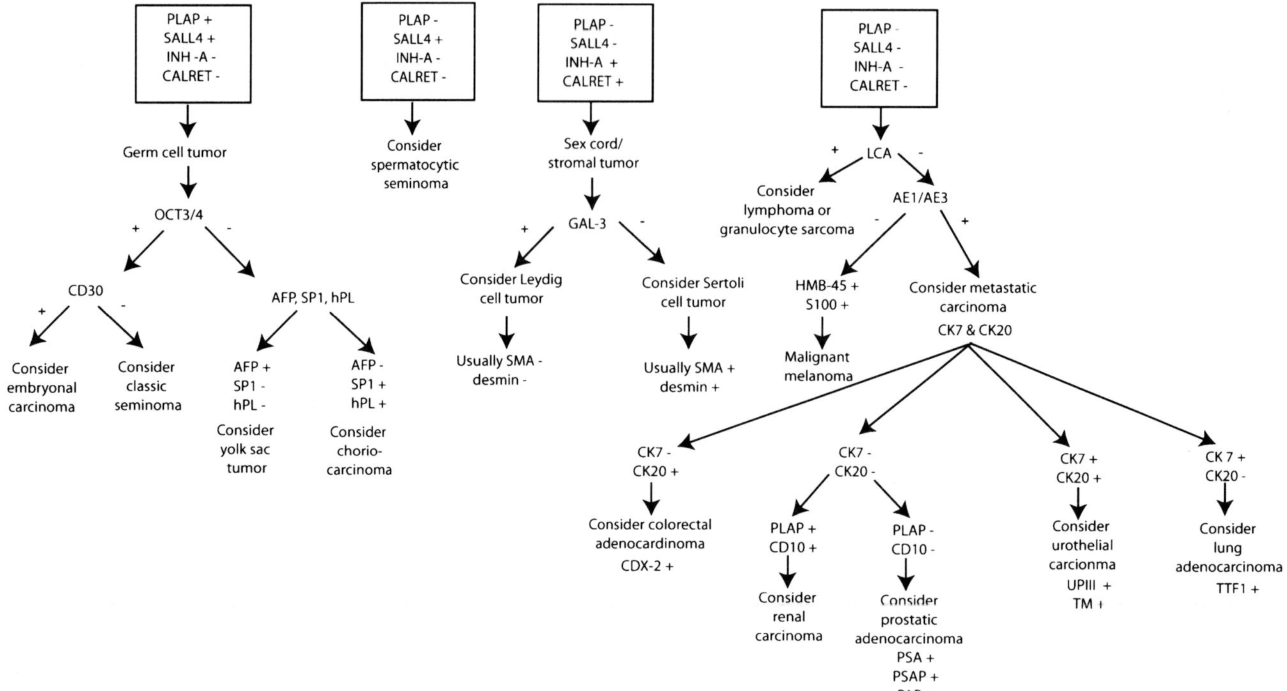

Fig. 21.1 Suggested algorithm for working up testicular neoplasms

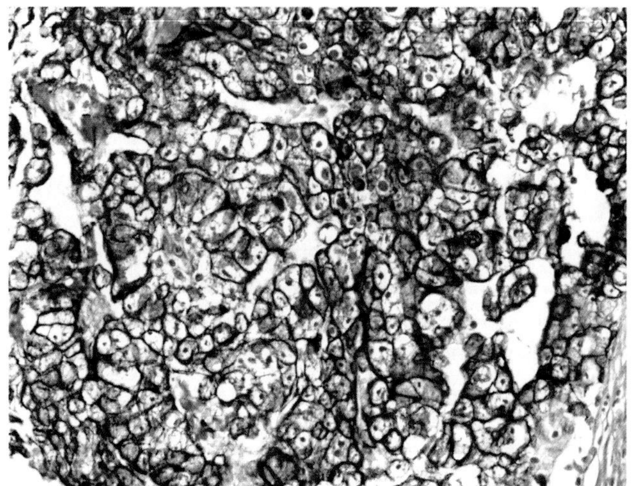

Fig. 21.2 Cytokeratin AE1/AE3 demonstrates strong diffuse cytoplasmic staining in embryonal carcinoma

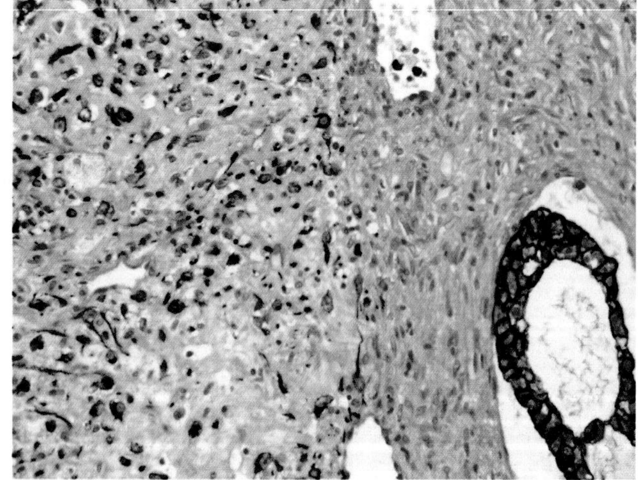

Fig. 21.3 In this case of choriocarcinoma, CAM 5.2 demonstrates both a dot-like cytoplasmic perinuclear pattern in the cells on the *left* and diffuse cytoplasmic staining in the gland-like structure on the *right*

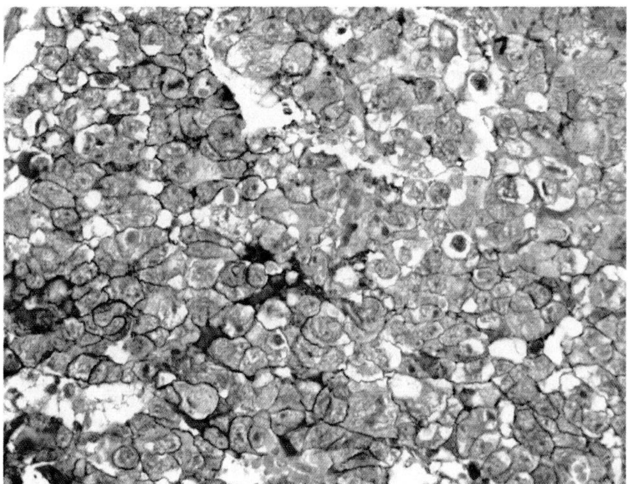

Fig. 21.4 CD30 staining in an embryonal carcinoma

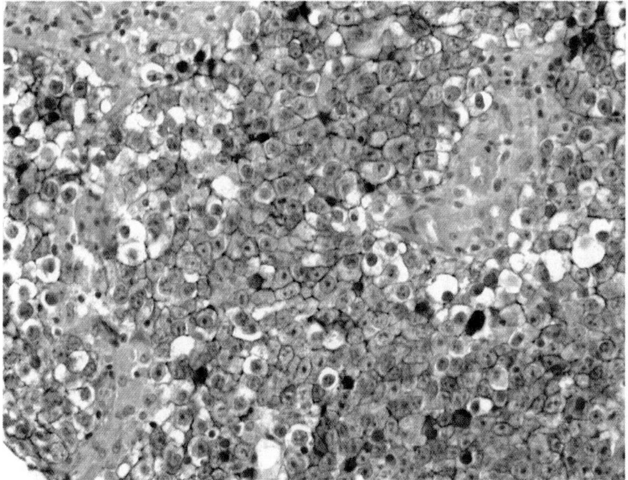

Fig. 21.5 c-kit may demonstrate both membranous and cytoplasmic staining as seen in this classic seminoma

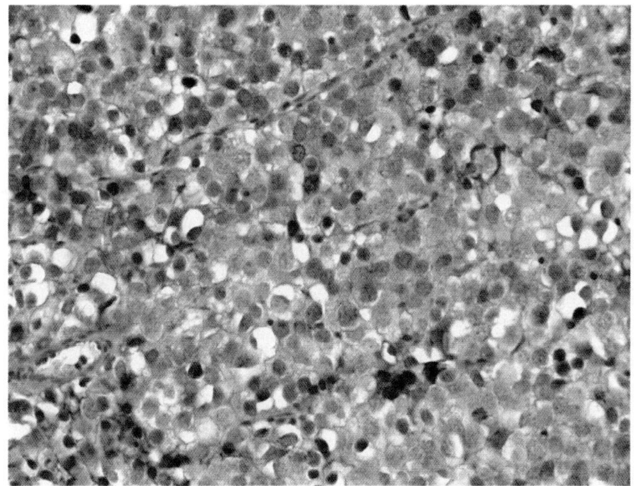

Fig. 21.6 c-kit may demonstrate membranous and cytoplasmic staining as seen in this spermatocytic seminoma

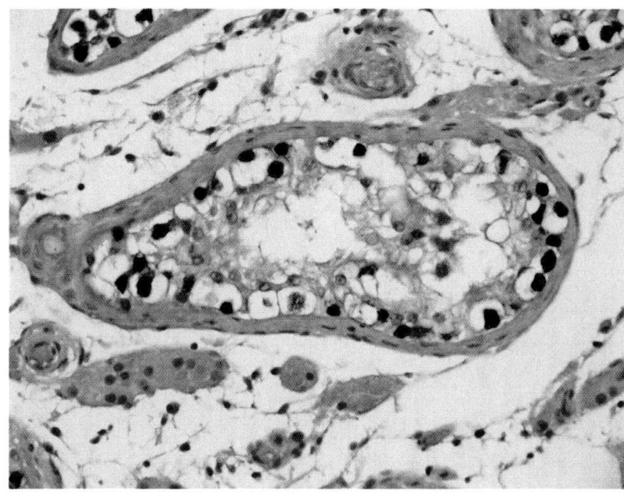

Fig. 21.7 OCT4 demonstrates strong nuclear staining of intratubular germ cell neoplasia, but does not stain the Sertoli cells within the seminiferous tubules or the Leydig cells in the interstitium

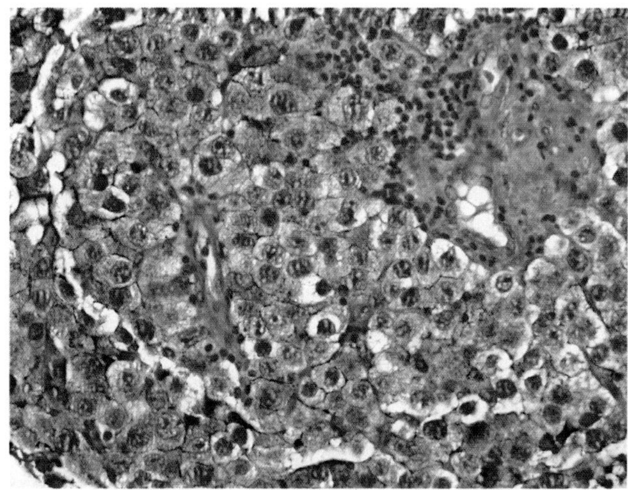

Fig. 21.8 PLAP demonstrates membranous staining in this classic seminoma

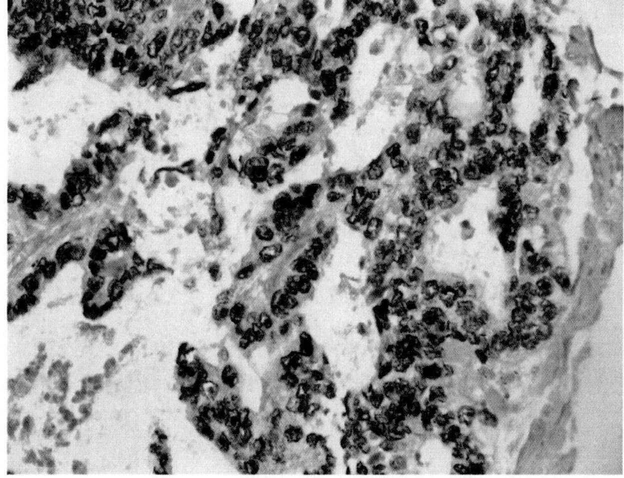

Fig. 21.9 SALL4 demonstrates nuclear staining in this embryonal carcinoma

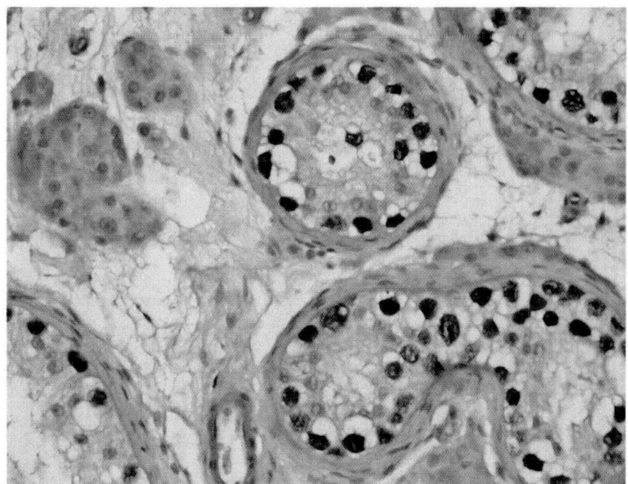

Fig. 21.10 SALL4 demonstrates strong nuclear staining of intratubular germ cell neoplasia, but does not stain the Sertoli cells within the seminiferous tubules or the Leydig cells in the interstitium

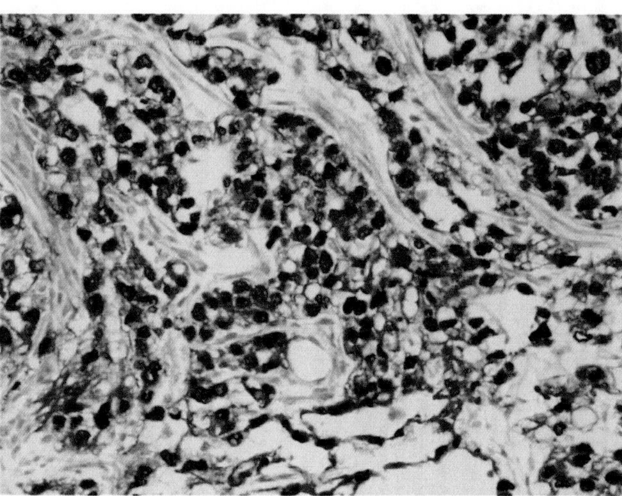

Fig. 21.12 This yolk sac tumor was stained for cytokeratin AE1/AE3 and SALL4. The tumor cells are positive for both, with the cytoplasm demonstrating a positive reaction for cytokeratin (*red* chromagen) and the nuclei staining for SALL4 (*brown* chromagen)

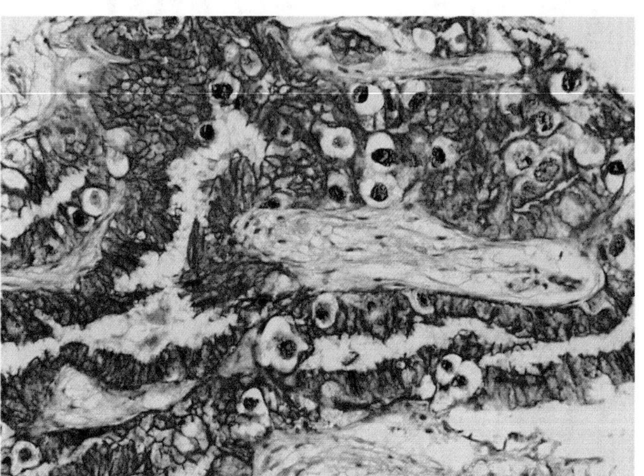

Fig. 21.11 Double-stained slide demonstrating extension of intratubular germ cell neoplasia into the rete testis. The neoplastic germ cells demonstrate nuclear staining (*brown* chromagen) for SALL4, but are negative for cytokeratin. The normal epithelium of the rete testis demonstrates cytoplasmic and membranous staining for CK AE1/AE3 (*red* chromagen), but are negative for SALL4

Table 21.4 Markers for sex cord/stromal tumors

	LCT	SCT	AdGCT	JuGCT	LCCSCT
Melan-a	+	+ or –	ND	ND	+
INHA	+	+ or –	+	+	+
CALRET	+	+	+	+	+
Vim	+	+	+	+	+
AE1/AE3	– or +[a]	– or +[a]	+ or –	+ or –	+ or –
CAM 5.2	– or +	+ or –	+ or –	+ or –	+ or –
CK7	– or +[a]	– or +[a]	ND	ND	ND
CK20	– or +[a]	– or +[a]	ND	ND	ND
EMA	– or +	– or +	–	–	–
S100	– or +	+ or –	– or +[b]	+ or –[b]	+
Synap	– or +	– or +	ND	ND	ND
Chrom	+ or –	+ or –	ND	–	ND
CD99	+ or –	– or +	+	+ or –	ND
GAL-3	+	–	ND	–	ND
PLAP	– or +	– or +	ND	–	–
SMA	–	+ or –	+	+ or –	ND
Desmin	– or +	+ or –	– or +	– or +	+
MIS	+	+	+	+	ND

Abbreviations: *LCT* Leydig cell tumor, *SCT* Sertoli cell tumor, *AdGCT* adult granulosa cell tumor, *JuGCT* juvenile granulosa cell tumor, *LCCSCT* large cell calcifying Sertoli cell tumor

Note: All tumors in this table are usually negative for AFP, hCG, LCA, OCT4, CEA, c-kit, SALL4, and NSE

See Fig. 21.13

[a]If (+), often in a punctate perinuclear pattern

[b]Stains nucleus

References: [9, 10, 14, 23, 24, 27–29, 33, 36–39, 41, 48, 74, 79–89]

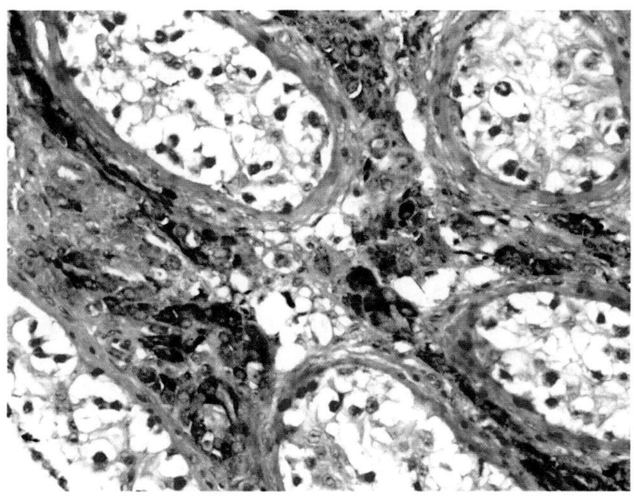

Fig. 21.13 Inhibin-alpha stains Leydig cells in the interstitium and rare Sertoli cells within the seminiferous tubules. It does not stain the intratubular germ cell neoplasia (the large clear cells)

Table 21.5 Markers for gonadoblastoma

	Sex cord cells	Germ cells
WT1	+	–
INHA	+	–
AE1/AE3	+	–
Vim	+	–
AMH	+	–
MIS	+	+
OCT4	–	+
PLAP	–	+
c-kit	–	+
p53	–	+

Note: Basement membrane-like hyaline material stains (+) for laminin

See Figs. 21.14–21.16

References: [13, 62, 90–92]

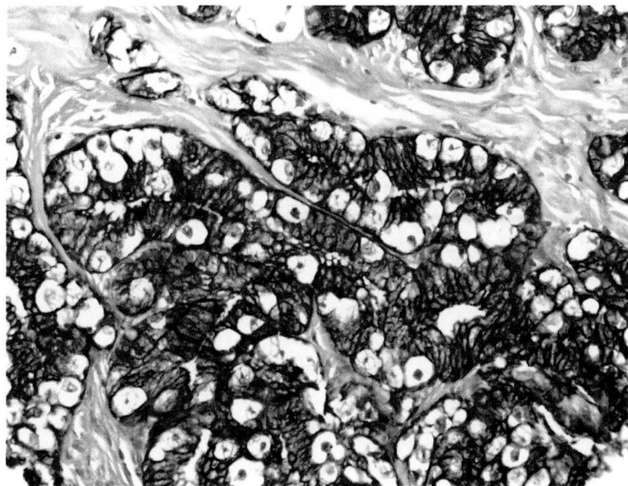

Fig. 21.14 Cytokeratin AE1/AE3 does not stain intratubular germ cell neoplasia (the large clear cells), but may demonstrate staining in Sertoli cells within the tubules as seen here

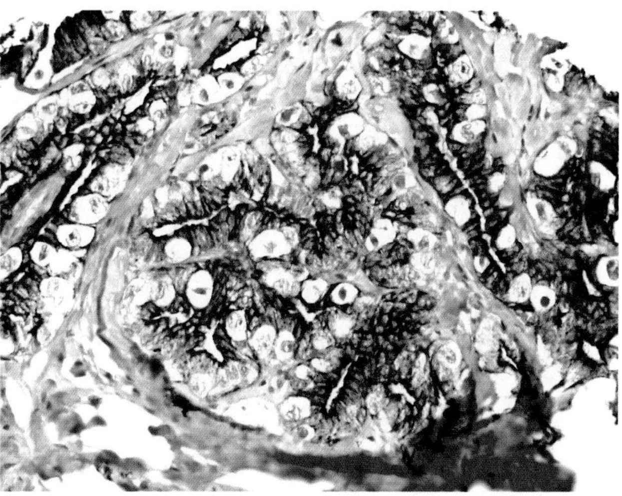

Fig. 21.15 CAM 5.2 does not stain intratubular germ cell neoplasia (the large clear cells), but may demonstrate staining in Sertoli cells within the tubules as seen here

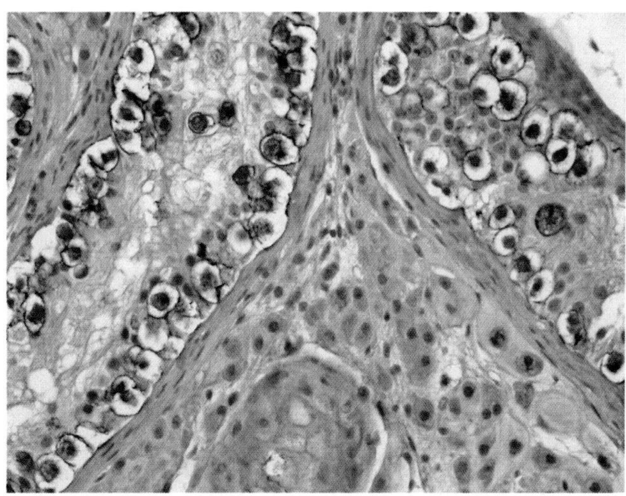

Fig. 21.16 c-kit demonstrates strong cytoplasmic staining of intratubular germ cell neoplasia, but does not stain the Sertoli cells within the tubules. The Leydig cells in the interstitium demonstrate weak, nonspecific cytoplasmic staining (they generally do not stain for c-kit) and no membranous staining

Table 21.6 Markers for syncytiotrophoblast in germ cell tumors

hCG	+
GPC3	+
HPL	+
SP1	+
CK8	+
CK18	+
CK19	+
EGFR	+
CD10	+
CEA	+ or –
PLAP	+ or –
INHA	+ or –
AE1/AE3	+ or –
SALL4	–
AFP	–

See Figs. 21.17 and 21.18

References: [3, 4, 10, 17, 44, 58, 61, 66, 67, 79, 93, 94]

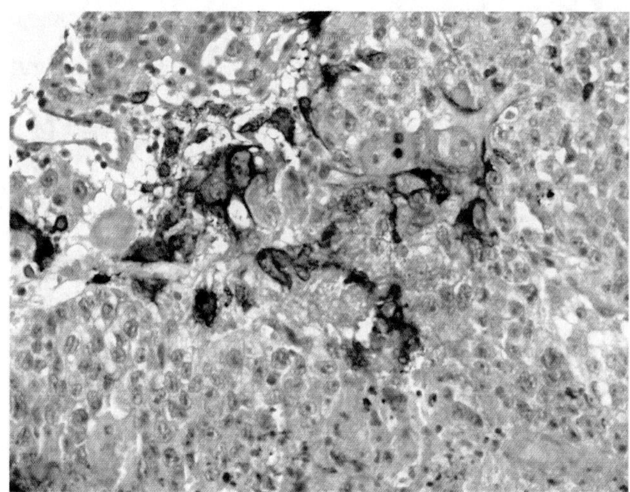

Fig. 21.17 CD10 highlights syncytiotrophoblast in an embryonal carcinoma

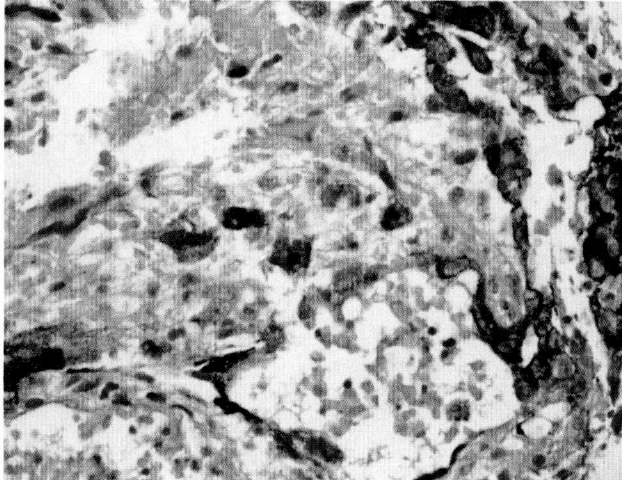

Fig. 21.18 Glypican-3 highlights syncytiotrophoblast in this mixed germ cell tumor

Table 21.7 Markers of testicular neoplasms in other tumors

	RCC	PrCa	ColCa	UCa	Mel	Lym
INHA	ND	ND	ND	ND	–	–
CD30	ND	ND	–	ND	–	See Chap. 27
PLAP	+	–	+	–	–	–
EMA	+	+	+	+	–	–
AE1/AE3	+	+	+	+	–	–
SALL4	ND	ND	ND	ND	ND	–
OCT4	–	–	ND	ND	–	–
CALRET	ND	–	ND	ND	–	–

Abbreviations: *RCC* renal carcinoma, *PrCa* prostatic adenocarcinoma, *ColCa* colonic adenocarcinoma, *UCa* urothelial carcinoma, *Mel* malignant melanoma, *Lym* lymphoma

References: [20, 27, 38, 48, 54, 56]

Table 21.8 Markers in normal paratesticular epithelia

	Rete testis	Epididymis	Ductus efferens	Ductus deferens	Seminal vesicles
CK7	+	+	+	+	+
CK8	+	+	+	+	+
CK18	+	+	+	+	+
CK19	+	+	+	+	+
CK5	ND	+	+	+	+
AE1/AE3	+	ND	ND	ND	ND
Vimentin	+ or –	ND	–	ND	ND
PR	ND	+	ND	ND	ND
ERalpha	ND	–	–	ND	ND
ERbeta	ND	–	+	ND	ND
Desmin	–	ND	–	ND	ND
SMA	–	ND	ND	ND	ND
S100	– or +	ND	ND	ND	ND
INHA	– or +	–	ND	ND	ND
CD99	–	–	ND	ND	ND
PLAP	–	–	ND	ND	ND
Chromogranin	– or +	– or +	ND	ND	ND
SALL4	–	–	ND	ND	ND
OCT4	–	–	ND	ND	ND
CALRET	– or +	–	ND	ND	ND

References: [4, 21, 26, 30, 32, 33, 38, 39]

Table 21.9 Markers in paratesticular tumors

	Rete testis ACa	Adenomatoid tumor	Malignant mesothelioma	Papillary cystadenoma	Papillary serous ACa	Epididymal ACa
AE1/AE3	+	+	+	ND	+	ND
CK903	ND	–	+ or –	ND	ND	ND
Pan-CK	ND	+	+	ND	ND	ND
CK5/6	–	ND	+	ND	ND	ND
CK7	+	ND	+	+	+	ND
CK20	ND	ND	–	ND	ND	ND
CAM 5.2	+	+	+	ND	ND	ND
EMA	+	+	– or +	ND	+	+
Vim	– or +	+	+	ND	– or +	ND
CALRET	– or +	+	+	ND	+ or –	+ or –
TM	+ or –	+	+ or –	ND	+ or –	+ or –
WT1	–	+	+	ND	+	–
D2-40	ND	ND	+	ND	ND	ND
CEA	– or +	–	–	ND	+ or –	+ or –
MOC31	ND	–	ND	+	+	ND
Ber-EP4	ND	–	–	ND	+	ND
TAG 72	ND	–	–	ND	+ or –	ND
HBME-1	ND	+	ND	ND	ND	ND
NSE	+	ND	ND	ND	ND	ND
S100	ND	ND	–	ND	+ or –	ND
Chrom	+	–	– or +	ND	ND	ND
Desmin	ND	ND	–	ND	ND	ND
CD30	ND	ND	– or +	ND	ND	ND
c-kit	ND	ND	–	ND	ND	ND
CD15	+ or –	–	–	+	+ or –	+ or –
FVIII	ND	–	–	ND	ND	ND
CD34	ND	–	ND	ND	ND	ND
p53	ND	–	ND	ND	ND	ND
CD10	+	ND	+ or –	ND	+ or –	+
CA-125	ND	ND	ND	ND	+	ND
CA19-9	+ or –	ND	ND	ND	ND	+
hCG	–	–	–	ND	–	ND
AFP	–	–	–	ND	–	ND
PLAP	–	–	–	ND	– or +	ND
OCT4	–	–	–	ND	ND	ND
INHA	–	–	–	ND	ND	ND
ER	ND	ND	ND	+	+	ND
PR	ND	ND	ND	+	+	ND
N-cad	ND	ND	+	ND	ND	ND
E-cad	ND	ND	– or +	ND	ND	ND

Abbreviation: *ACa* adenocarcinoma

See Fig. 21.19

References: [1, 8, 10, 38, 48, 95–103]

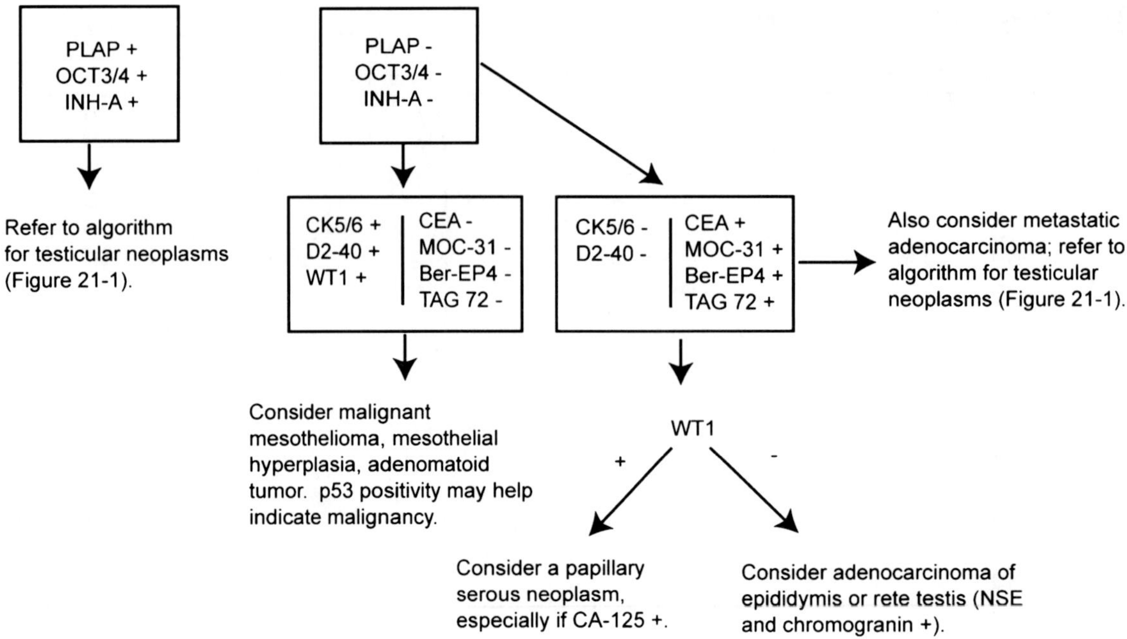

Fig. 21.19 Suggested algorithm for working up paratesticular neoplasms

Note for All Tables

Note: "+" – usually greater than 70% of cases are positive; "–" – less than 5% of cases are positive; "+ or –" – usually more than 50% of cases are positive; "– or +" – less than 50% of cases are positive.

References

1. Amin MB. Selected other problematic testicular and paratesticular lesions: rete testis neoplasms and pseudotumors, mesothelial lesions and secondary tumors. Mod Pathol. 2005;18 Suppl 2:S131–45.
2. Augusto D, Leteurtre E, De La Taille A, Gosselin B, Leroy X. Calretinin: a valuable marker of normal and neoplastic Leydig cells of the testis. Appl Immunohistochem Mol Morphol. 2002; 10(2):159–62.
3. Bahrami A, Ro JY, Ayala AG. An overview of testicular germ cell tumors. Arch Pathol Lab Med. 2007;131(8):1267–80.
4. Cao D, Li J, Guo CC, Allan RW, Humphrey PA. SALL4 is a novel diagnostic marker for testicular germ cell tumors. Am J Surg Pathol. 2009;33(7):1065–77.
5. Cheville JC, Rao S, Iczkowski KA, Lohse CM, Pankratz VS. Cytokeratin expression in seminoma of the human testis. Am J Clin Pathol. 2000;113(4):583–8.
6. de Jong J, Stoop H, Gillis AJ, et al. Differential expression of SOX17 and SOX2 in germ cells and stem cells has biological and clinical implications. J Pathol. 2008;215(1):21–30.
7. Dekker I, Rozeboom T, Delemarre J, Dam A, Oosterhuis JW. Placental-like alkaline phosphatase and DNA flow cytometry in spermatocytic seminoma. Cancer. 1992;69(4):993–6.
8. Delahunt B, Eble JN, King D, Bethwaite PB, Nacey JN, Thornton A. Immunohistochemical evidence for mesothelial origin of paratesticular adenomatoid tumour. Histopathology. 2000;36(2):109–15.
9. Devouassoux-Shisheboran M, Deschildre C, Mauduit C, et al. Expression of galectin-3 in gonads and gonadal sex cord stromal and germ cell tumors. Oncol Rep. 2006;16(2):335–40.
10. Emerson RE, Ulbright TM. The use of immunohistochemistry in the differential diagnosis of tumors of the testis and paratestis. Semin Diagn Pathol. 2005;22(1):33–50.
11. Comperat E, Tissier F, Boye K, De Pinieux G, Vieillefond A. Non-Leydig sex-cord tumors of the testis. The place of immunohistochemistry in diagnosis and prognosis. A study of twenty cases. Virchows Arch. 2004;444(6):567–71.
12. Gopalan A, Dhall D, Olgac S, et al. Testicular mixed germ cell tumors: a morphological and immunohistochemical study using stem cell markers, OCT3/4, SOX2 and GDF3, with emphasis on morphologically difficult-to-classify areas. Mod Pathol. 2009; 22(8):1066–74.
13. Hussong J, Crussi FG, Chou PM. Gonadoblastoma: immunohistochemical localization of Mullerian-inhibiting substance, inhibin, WT-1, and p53. Mod Pathol. 1997;10(11):1101–5.
14. Iczkowski KA, Bostwick DG, Roche PC, Cheville JC. Inhibin A is a sensitive and specific marker for testicular sex cord-stromal tumors. Mod Pathol. 1998;11(8):774–9.
15. Jones TD, Ulbright TM, Eble JN, Cheng L. OCT4: a sensitive and specific biomarker for intratubular germ cell neoplasia of the testis. Clin Cancer Res. 2004;10(24):8544–7.
16. Kang JL, Meyts ER, Skakkebaek NE. Immunoreactive neuron-specific enolase (NSE) is expressed in testicular carcinoma-in-situ. J Pathol. 1996;178(2):161–5.
17. Mostofi FK, Sesterhenn IA, Davis Jr CJ. Immunopathology of germ cell tumors of the testis. Semin Diagn Pathol. 1987;4(4): 320–41.
18. Unni SK, Modi DN, Pathak SG, Dhabalia JV, Bhartiya D. Stage-specific localization and expression of c-kit in the adult human testis. J Histochem Cytochem. 2009;57(9):861–9.
19. Tickoo SK, Hutchinson B, Bacik J, et al. Testicular seminoma: a clinicopathologic and immunohistochemical study of 105 cases with special reference to seminomas with atypical features. Int J Surg Pathol. 2002;10(1):23–32.

20. de Jong J, Stoop H, Dohle GR, et al. Diagnostic value of OCT3/4 for pre-invasive and invasive testicular germ cell tumours. J Pathol. 2005;206(2):242–9.
21. Feitz WF, Debruyne FM, Ramaekers FC. Intermediate filament proteins as tissue specific markers in normal and neoplastic testicular tissue. Int J Androl. 1987;10(1):51–6.
22. Donner J, Kliesch S, Brehm R, Bergmann M. From carcinoma in situ to testicular germ cell tumour. APMIS. 2004;112(2):79–88.
23. Gordon MD, Corless C, Renshaw AA, Beckstead J. CD99, keratin, and vimentin staining of sex cord-stromal tumors, normal ovary, and testis. Mod Pathol. 1998;11(8):769–73.
24. Groisman GM, Dische MR, Fine EM, Unger PD. Juvenile granulosa cell tumor of the testis: a comparative immunohistochemical study with normal infantile gonads. Pediatr Pathol. 1993;13(4):389–400.
25. Honecker F, Kersemaekers AM, Molier M, et al. Involvement of E-cadherin and beta-catenin in germ cell tumours and in normal male fetal germ cell development. J Pathol. 2004;204(2):167–74.
26. Luetjens CM, Didolkar A, Kliesch S, et al. Tissue expression of the nuclear progesterone receptor in male non-human primates and men. J Endocrinol. 2006;189(3):529–39.
27. McCluggage WG, Shanks JH, Whiteside C, Maxwell P, Banerjee SS, Biggart JD. Immunohistochemical study of testicular sex cord-stromal tumors, including staining with anti-inhibin antibody. Am J Surg Pathol. 1998;22(5):615–9.
28. McLaren K, Thomson D. Localization of S-100 protein in a Leydig and Sertoli cell tumour of testis. Histopathology. 1989;15(6):649–52.
29. Nielsen K, Jacobsen GK. Malignant Sertoli cell tumour of the testis. An immunohistochemical study and a review of the literature. APMIS. 1988;96(8):755–60.
30. Pelletier G, El-Alfy M. Immunocytochemical localization of estrogen receptors alpha and beta in the human reproductive organs. J Clin Endocrinol Metab. 2000;85(12):4835–40.
31. Pais V, Leav I, Lau KM, Jiang Z, Ho SM. Estrogen receptor-beta expression in human testicular germ cell tumors. Clin Cancer Res. 2003;9(12):4475–82.
32. Ramaekers F, Feitz W, Moesker O, et al. Antibodies to cytokeratin and vimentin in testicular tumour diagnosis. Virchows Arch A Pathol Anat Histopathol. 1985;408(2–3):127–42.
33. Renshaw AA, Gordon M, Corless CL. Immunohistochemistry of unclassified sex cord-stromal tumors of the testis with a predominance of spindle cells. Mod Pathol. 1997;10(7):693–700.
34. Bar-Shira Maymon B, Yavetz H, Schreiber L, Paz G. Immunohistochemistry in the evaluation of spermatogenesis and Sertoli cell's maturation status. Clin Chem Lab Med. 2002;40(3):217–20.
35. Romeo R, Marcello MF. Some considerations on the human Leydig cell (immunohistochemical observations). Arch Ital Urol Androl. 1999;71(3):143–8.
36. Sasano H, Nakashima N, Matsuzaki O, et al. Testicular sex cord-stromal lesions: immunohistochemical analysis of cytokeratin, vimentin and steroidogenic enzymes. Virchows Arch A Pathol Anat Histopathol. 1992;421(2):163–9.
37. Sato K, Ueda Y, Sakurai A, et al. Large cell calcifying Sertoli cell tumor of the testis: comparative immunohistochemical study with Leydig cell tumor. Pathol Int. 2005;55(6):366–71.
38. Kommoss F, Oliva E, Bittinger F, et al. Inhibin-alpha CD99, HEA125, PLAP, and chromogranin immunoreactivity in testicular neoplasms and the androgen insensitivity syndrome. Hum Pathol. 2000;31(9):1055–61.
39. Cao QJ, Jones JG, Li M. Expression of calretinin in human ovary, testis, and ovarian sex cord-stromal tumors. Int J Gynecol Pathol. 2001;20(4):346–52.
40. Carpino A, Rago V, Pezzi V, Carani C, Ando S. Detection of aromatase and estrogen receptors (ERalpha, ERbeta1, ERbeta2) in human Leydig cell tumor. Eur J Endocrinol. 2007;157(2):239–44.
41. Al-Agha OM, Axiotis CA. An in-depth look at Leydig cell tumor of the testis. Arch Pathol Lab Med. 2007;131(2):311–7.
42. Albores-Saavedra J, Huffman H, Alvarado-Cabrero I, Ayala AG. Anaplastic variant of spermatocytic seminoma. Hum Pathol. 1996;27(7):650–5.
43. Caillaud JM, Bellet D, Carlu C, Droz JP. Immunohistochemistry of germ cell tumors of the testis. Study of beta HCG and AFP. Prog Clin Biol Res. 1985;203:139–40.
44. Burke AP, Mostofi FK. Placental alkaline phosphatase immunohistochemistry of intratubular malignant germ cells and associated testicular germ cell tumors. Hum Pathol. 1988;19(6):663–70.
45. Bartkova J, Bartek J, Lukas J, et al. p53 protein alterations in human testicular cancer including pre-invasive intratubular germ-cell neoplasia. Int J Cancer. 1991;49(2):196–202.
46. Burke AP, Mostofi FK. Intratubular malignant germ cells in testicular biopsies: clinical course and identification by staining for placental alkaline phosphatase. Mod Pathol. 1988;1(6):475–9.
47. Bailey D, Marks A, Stratis M, Baumal R. Immunohistochemical staining of germ cell tumors and intratubular malignant germ cells of the testis using antibody to placental alkaline phosphatase and a monoclonal anti-seminoma antibody. Mod Pathol. 1991;4(2): 167–71.
48. Emerson RE, Ulbright TM. Morphological approach to tumours of the testis and paratestis. J Clin Pathol. 2007;60(8):866–80.
49. Bosman FT, Giard RW, Nieuwenhuijen Kruseman AC, Knijnenburg G, Spaander PJ. Human chorionic gonadotrophin and alpha-fetoprotein in testicular germ cell tumours: a retrospective immunohistochemical study. Histopathology. 1980;4(6):673–84.
50. Bomeisl PE, MacLennan GT. Spermatocytic seminoma. J Urol. 2007;177(2):734.
51. Battifora H, Sheibani K, Tubbs RR, Kopinski MI, Sun TT. Antikeratin antibodies in tumor diagnosis. Distinction between seminoma and embryonal carcinoma. Cancer. 1984;54(5):843–8.
52. Bartkova J, Rejthar A, Bartek J, Kovarik J. Differentiation patterns of testicular germ-cell tumours as revealed by a panel of monoclonal antibodies. Tumour Biol. 1987;8(1):45–56.
53. Wittekind C, Wichmann T, Von Kleist S. Immunohistological localization of AFP and HCG in uniformly classified testis tumors. Anticancer Res. 1983;3(5):327–30.
54. Wick MR, Swanson PE, Manivel JC. Placental-like alkaline phosphatase reactivity in human tumors: an immunohistochemical study of 520 cases. Hum Pathol. 1987;18(9):946–54.
55. Rajpert-De Meyts E, Kvist M, Skakkebaek NE. Heterogeneity of expression of immunohistochemical tumour markers in testicular carcinoma in situ: pathogenetic relevance. Virchows Arch. 1996;428(3):133–9.
56. Pallesen G, Hamilton-Dutoit SJ. Ki-1 (CD30) antigen is regularly expressed by tumor cells of embryonal carcinoma. Am J Pathol. 1988;133(3):446–50.
57. Niehans GA, Manivel JC, Copland GT, Scheithauer BW, Wick MR. Immunohistochemistry of germ cell and trophoblastic neoplasms. Cancer. 1988;62(6):1113–23.
58. Mostofi FK, Sesterhenn IA, Davis Jr CJ. Developments in histopathology of testicular germ cell tumors. Semin Urol. 1988;6(3): 171–88.
59. Miller JS, Lee TK, Epstein JI, Ulbright TM. The utility of microscopic findings and immunohistochemistry in the classification of necrotic testicular tumors: a study of 11 cases. Am J Surg Pathol. 2009;33(9):1293–8.
60. Miettinen M, Virtanen I, Talerman A. Intermediate filament proteins in human testis and testicular germ-cell tumors. Am J Pathol. 1985;120(3):402–10.
61. Manivel JC, Niehans G, Wick MR, Dehner LP. Intermediate trophoblast in germ cell neoplasms. Am J Surg Pathol. 1987;11(9): 693–701.
62. Manivel JCMD, Jessurun JMD, Wick MRMD, Dehner LPMD. Placental alkaline phosphatase immunoreactivity in testicular germ-cell neoplasms. Am J Surg Pathol. 1987;11(1):21–9.

63. Manivel JC, Simonton S, Wold LE, Dehner LP. Absence of intratubular germ cell neoplasia in testicular yolk sac tumors in children. A histochemical and immunohistochemical study. Arch Pathol Lab Med. 1988;112(6):641–5.
64. Lind HM, Haghighi P. Carcinoembryonic antigen staining in choriocarcinoma. Am J Clin Pathol. 1986;86(4):538–40.
65. Eglen DE, Ulbright TM. The differential diagnosis of yolk sac tumor and seminoma. Usefulness of cytokeratin, alpha-fetoprotein, and alpha-1-antitrypsin immunoperoxidase reactions. Am J Clin Pathol. 1987;88(3):328–32.
66. Fogel M, Lifschitz-Mercer B, Moll R, et al. Heterogeneity of intermediate filament expression in human testicular seminomas. Differentiation. 1990;45(3):242–9.
67. Lifschitz-Mercer B, Fogel M, Moll R, et al. Intermediate filament protein profiles of human testicular non-seminomatous germ cell tumors: correlation of cytokeratin synthesis to cell differentiation. Differentiation. 1991;48(3):191–8.
68. Leroy X, Augusto D, Leteurtre E, Gosselin B. CD30 and CD117 (c-kit) used in combination are useful for distinguishing embryonal carcinoma from seminoma. J Histochem Cytochem. 2002; 50(2):283–5.
69. Kraggerud SM, Berner A, Bryne M, Pettersen EO, Fossa SD. Spermatocytic seminoma as compared to classical seminoma: an immunohistochemical and DNA flow cytometric study. APMIS. 1999;107(3):297–302.
70. Koshida K, Wahren B. Placental-like alkaline phosphatase in seminoma. Urol Res. 1990;18(2):87–92.
71. Jorgensen N, Muller J, Jaubert F, Clausen OP, Skakkebaek NE. Heterogeneity of gonadoblastoma germ cells: similarities with immature germ cells, spermatogonia and testicular carcinoma in situ cells. Histopathology. 1997;30(2):177–86.
72. Cummings OW, Ulbright TM, Eble JN, Roth LM. Spermatocytic seminoma: an immunohistochemical study. Hum Pathol. 1994;25(1):54–9.
73. Ferreiro JA. Ber-H2 expression in testicular germ cell tumors. Hum Pathol. 1994;25(5):522–4.
74. Jimenez-Quintero LP, Ro JY, Zavala-Pompa A, et al. Granulosa cell tumor of the adult testis: a clinicopathologic study of seven cases and a review of the literature. Hum Pathol. 1993;24(10): 1120–5.
75. Jacobsen GK, Jacobsen M, Clausen PP. Distribution of tumor-associated antigens in the various histologic components of germ cell tumors of the testis. Am J Surg Pathol. 1981;5(3): 257–66.
76. Jacobsen GK, Norgaard-Pedersen B. Placental alkaline phosphatase in testicular germ cell tumours and in carcinoma-in-situ of the testis. An immunohistochemical study. Acta Pathol Microbiol Immunol Scand [A]. 1984;92(5):323–9.
77. Hustin J, Collette J, Franchimont P. Immunohistochemical demonstration of placental alkaline phosphatase in various states of testicular development and in germ cell tumours. Int J Androl. 1987;10(1):29–35.
78. Hittmair A, Rogatsch H, Hobisch A, Mikuz G, Feichtinger H. CD30 expression in seminoma. Hum Pathol. 1996;27(11):1166–71.
79. Kalhor N, Ramirez PT, Deavers MT, Malpica A, Silva EG. Immunohistochemical studies of trophoblastic tumors. Am J Surg Pathol. 2009;33(4):633–8. doi:10.1097/PAS.0b013e318191f2eb.
80. Al-Bozom IA, El-Faqih SR, Hassan SH, El-Tiraifi AE, Talic RF. Granulosa cell tumor of the adult type: a case report and review of the literature of a very rare testicular tumor. Arch Pathol Lab Med. 2000;124(10):1525–8.
81. Ventura T, Discepoli S, Coletti G, et al. Light microscopic, immunocytochemical and ultrastructural study of a case of Sertoli cell tumor of the testis. Tumori. 1987;73(6):649–53.
82. Perez-Atayde AR, Joste N, Mulhern H. Juvenile granulosa cell tumor of the infantile testis. Evidence of a dual epithelial-smooth muscle differentiation. Am J Surg Pathol. 1996;20(1):72–9.
83. Nistal M, Lazaro R, Garcia J, Paniagua R. Testicular granulosa cell tumor of the adult type. Arch Pathol Lab Med. 1992;116(3): 284–7.
84. Morgan DR, Brame KG. Granulosa cell tumour of the testis displaying immunoreactivity for inhibin. BJU Int. 1999;83(6): 731–2.
85. Matias-Guiu X, Pons C, Prat J. Mullerian inhibiting substance, alpha-inhibin, and CD99 expression in sex cord-stromal tumors and endometrioid ovarian carcinomas resembling sex cord-stromal tumors. Hum Pathol. 1998;29(8):840–5.
86. Kratzer SS, Ulbright TM, Talerman A, et al. Large cell calcifying Sertoli cell tumor of the testis: contrasting features of six malignant and six benign tumors and a review of the literature. Am J Surg Pathol. 1997;21(11):1271–80.
87. Henley JD, Young RH, Ulbright TM. Malignant Sertoli cell tumors of the testis: a study of 13 examples of a neoplasm frequently misinterpreted as seminoma. Am J Surg Pathol. 2002;26(5):541–50.
88. Harms D, Kock LR. Testicular juvenile granulosa cell and Sertoli cell tumours: a clinicopathological study of 29 cases from the Kiel Paediatric Tumour Registry. Virchows Arch. 1997;430(4):301–9.
89. Plata C, Algaba F, Andujar M, et al. Large cell calcifying Sertoli cell tumour of the testis. Histopathology. 1995;26(3):255–9.
90. Roth LM, Eglen DE. Gonadoblastoma. Immunohistochemical and ultrastructural observations. Int J Gynecol Pathol. 1989;8(1): 72–81.
91. Rey R, Sabourin JC, Venara M, et al. Anti-Mullerian hormone is a specific marker of sertoli- and granulosa-cell origin in gonadal tumors. Hum Pathol. 2000;31(10):1202–8.
92. Cools M, Stoop H, Kersemaekers AM, et al. Gonadoblastoma arising in undifferentiated gonadal tissue within dysgenetic gonads. J Clin Endocrinol Metab. 2006;91(6):2404–13. doi:10.1210/jc.2005-2554.
93. Hori K, Uematsu K, Yasoshima H, Yamada A, Sakurai K, Ohya M. Testicular seminoma with human chorionic gonadotropin production. Pathol Int. 1997;47(9):592–9.
94. Hechelhammer L, Storkel S, Odermatt B, Heitz PU, Jochum W. Epidermal growth factor receptor is a marker for syncytiotrophoblastic cells in testicular germ cell tumors. Virchows Arch. 2003;443(1):28–31.
95. Ballotta MR, Borghi L, Barucchello G. Adenocarcinoma of the rete testis. Report of two cases. Adv Clin Pathol. 2000;4(4): 169–73.
96. Detassis C, Pusiol T, Piscioli F, Luciani L. Adenomatoid tumor of the epididymis: immunohistochemical study of 8 cases. Urol Int. 1986;41(3):232–4.
97. Crisp-Lindgren N, Travers H, Wells MM, Cawley LP. Papillary adenocarcinoma of rete testis. Autopsy findings, histochemistry, immunohistochemistry, ultrastructure, and clinical correlations. Am J Surg Pathol. 1988;12(6):492–501.
98. Jones MA, Young RH, Srigley JR, Scully RE. Paratesticular serous papillary carcinoma. A report of six cases. Am J Surg Pathol. 1995;19(12):1359–65.
99. Kamiya M, Eimoto T. Malignant mesothelioma of the tunica vaginalis. Pathol Res Pract. 1990;186(5):680–4.
100. Menon PK, Vasudevarao, Sabhiki A, Kudesia S, Joshi DP, Mathur UB. A case of carcinoma rete testis: histomorphological, immunohistochemical and ultrastructural findings and review of literature. Indian J Cancer. 2002;39(3):106–11.
101. Perez-Ordonez B, Srigley JR. Mesothelial lesions of the paratesticular region. Semin Diagn Pathol. 2000;17(4):294–306.
102. Winstanley AM, Landon G, Berney D, Minhas S, Fisher C, Parkinson MC. The immunohistochemical profile of malignant mesotheliomas of the tunica vaginalis: a study of 20 cases. Am J Surg Pathol. 2006;30(1):1–6.
103. Chu AY, Litzky LA, Pasha TL, Acs G, Zhang PJ. Utility of D2-40, a novel mesothelial marker, in the diagnosis of malignant mesothelioma. Mod Pathol. 2005;18(1):105–10.

Chapter 22
Pancreas and Ampulla

Fan Lin and Hanlin L. Wang

Abstract This chapter provides a practical overview of frequently used markers in the diagnosis and differential diagnosis of both common and rare pancreatic and ampullary neoplasms, with a specific focus on pancreatic ductal adenocarcinoma and its mimickers. The chapter contains 40 questions; each question is addressed with a table, concise note and representative pictures if applicable. In addition to the literature review, the authors have included their own experience and tested numerous antibodies reported in the literature. The most effective diagnostic panels of antibodies have been recommended for many entities, such as pVHL, maspin, S100P and IMP-3 being suggested as the best diagnostic panel for identifying pancreatic ductal adenocarcinoma. Furthermore, immunophenotypes of normal pancreatic and ampullary tissues have been described, which tends to be neglected in the literature. Prognostic markers for pancreatic ductal adenocarcinoma and pancreatic endocrine neoplasm have been briefly mentioned.

Keywords Ductal adenocarcinoma • Pancreatic endocrine neoplasm • Acinar cell carcinoma • Solid-pseudopapillary neoplasm • Pancreatic endocrine neoplasm • pVHL • Maspin • S100P • IMP-3 • Beta-catenin • MUC1 • MUC2 • MUC5AC • CK17

FREQUENTLY ASKED QUESTIONS

Pancreas

F. Lin (✉)
Department of Pathology and Laboratory Medicine, Geisinger Medical Center, 100 N. Academy Ave, Danville, PA 17822, USA
e-mail: flin1@geisinger.edu

F. Lin and J. Prichard (eds.), *Handbook of Practical Immunohistochemistry: Frequently Asked Questions*,
DOI 10.1007/978-1-4419-8062-5_22,

Differential Diagnosis

Ampulla

Table 22.1 Summary of applications and limitations of useful markers

Antibodies	Staining pattern	Function	Key applications and pitfalls
CK7	M + C	Epithelial marker	Positive in DAC; usually negative in ACC and SPN
CK20	M + C	Epithelial marker	Positive in most CC and MCN and some DAC
CK17	M + C	Epithelial marker	Positive in DAC and usually negative in normal/reactive ducts
CK19	M + C	Epithelial marker	Positive in DAC; increasing malignant potential when positive in PEN
S100P	N + C	Belongs to the family of S100 calcium-binding proteins	N and C staining in most DAC; usually negative or cytoplasmic staining in normal/reactive ducts and other entities (PEN, ACC, and SPN)
S100A6	N + C	Belongs to the family of S100 calcium-binding proteins	N and C staining in most DAC and a small portion of reactive ducts
pVHL	M + C	Tumor suppressor gene	Positive in both normal ducts and acini; negative in DAC, ACC, mucinous tumors, and SPN
IMP-3 (KOC)	C	Encodes a protein with four K-homologous domains; regulation of tumor cell proliferation	Positive in DAC and PEN; usually negative in normal/reactive ducts
Annexin A8	C	A member of the annexin family of calcium-regulated membrane binding proteins	Positive in DAC; usually negative or weakly positive in normal ducts
Claudin 18	C	Component of tight junctions	Positive in DAC; usually negative or weakly positive in normal ducts
Claudin 4		Component of tight junctions	Positive in DAC; usually and also weakly positive in normal ducts
Claudin 5	M	Component of tight junctions	Positive in SPN; negative in ACC, PEN, and PB
Claudin 7	M	Component of tight junctions	Positive in ACC, PEN, and PB; negative or focal cytoplasmic positivity in SPN
Maspin	N + C	Related to the serpin family of protease inhibitors; plays a role in tumor invasion and metastasis	Positive in DAC; usually negative in normal/reactive ducts and acini
Mesothelin	M + C	A 40 kDa protein expressed in normal mesothelium and overexpressed in some cancers, such as mesothelioma, ovarian carcinoma, and DAC	Positive in DAC; usually negative in normal ducts and ACC
Prostate stem cell antigen (PSCA)	C	Glycosylphosphatidylinositol-anchored cell membrane glycoprotein; overexpressed in prostatic carcinoma, bladder and pancreatic carcinomas	Positive in DAC; may be positive in normal ducts and acini

(continued)

Table 22.1 (continued)

Antibodies	Staining pattern	Function	Key applications and pitfalls
CA19-9	C	Also called carbohydrate antigen 19-9 or sialylated Lewis (a) antigen; overexpressed in adenocarcinoma of colon and pancreas	Positive in DAC; also positive or weakly positive in normal ducts
MOC-31	M	Expressed in various adenocarcinomas and normal glandular epithelium; usually negative in mesothelioma	Positive in DAC; also positive or weakly positive in normal ducts and acini
Ber-EP4	M + C	Expressed in various adenocarcinomas and normal glandular epithelium; usually negative in mesothelioma	Positive in DAC; also positive or weakly positive in normal ducts
TAG 72 (B72.3)	M + C	Expressed in various adenocarcinomas and normal glandular epithelium	Positive in DAC; also positive or weakly positive in normal ducts
Carcinoembryonic antigen (CEA)	C	Expressed in various adenocarcinomas and normal glandular epithelium	Positive in DAC; usually negative in normal ducts
DPC4/SMAD4	N	Tumor suppressor gene	Loss of expression in most invasive mucinous carcinomas and about 60% of DACs; positive in normal ducts and ACC
p53	N	Tumor suppressor gene	Overexpression more frequently seen in DAC but can be seen in reactive conditions
CDX-2	N	A caudal-related homeobox transcription factor expressed in intestinal epithelium	Positive in IPMN, CC, some MCN, and about 10% of DAC
Beta-catenin	M or N + C	A subunit of the cadherin protein complex. Has been implicated as an integral component in the Wnt signaling pathway. Normally expressed in membrane of epithelial cells and is important for the function of E-cadherin. Mutation results in nuclear accumulation	N and M staining in >90% of SPN; N staining also reported in significant numbers of PB and some ACC; M staining in normal ducts, DAC and PEN
E-cadherin	M	An adhesion molecule expressed in epithelial lineage	Loss of expression in SPN and undifferentiated carcinoma, some ACC and PB; M staining in others
Chromogranin	C	Present in the cores of amine and peptide hormone and neurotransmitter dense-core secretory vesicles	Positive in PEN; rarely positive in SPN and ACC
Trypsin	C	An enzyme of pancreatic origin; catalyzes the hydrolysis of proteins to smaller polypeptide units	Positive in ACC and negative in SPN; background staining is a common problem
MUC1	C + M	A membrane-associated glycoprotein expressed in various tumor types	Positive in DAC; negative or infrequently positive in CC and IPMN
MUC2	C + M	A membrane-associated glycoprotein expressed in various tumor types	Positive in CC and frequently positive in IPMN but negative in DAC
MUC4	C + M	A membrane-associated glycoprotein expressed in various tumor types	Positive in DAC and usually negative in normal/reactive ducts
MUC5AC	C + M	A membrane-associated glycoprotein expressed in various tumor types	Positive in DAC, IPMN, and some MCN; usually negative in normal pancreatic ducts
MUC6	C	A membrane-associated glycoprotein expressed in various tumor types	Positive in CC, some IPMN, and normal ducts; usually negative in DAC

Note: *N* nuclear staining, *M* membranous staining, *C* cytoplasmic staining

DAC ductal adenocarcinoma, *SPN* solid pseudopapillary neoplasm, *PEN* pancreatic endocrine neoplasm, *IPMN* intraductal papillary mucinous neoplasm, *MCN* mucinous cystic neoplasm, *CC* colloid carcinoma, *ACC* acinar cell carcinoma, *PB* pancreatoblastoma. IMP-3 also known as K homology domain-containing protein overexpressed in cancer (KOC)

References: [1–58]

Table 22.2 Summary of useful markers in common tumors

Antibodies	DAC	ACC	PEN	SPN	PB
CK7	+	– or +	+ or –	–	+ or –
CK19	+	– or +	– or +	–	+ or –
Mesothelin	+	–	–	–	+ or –
S100P	+	–	–	–	+ or –
Maspin	+	–	–	–	+ or –
Beta-catenin	M	M or N + C	M	N + C	N + C, or M
E-cadherin	+	+	+	–	– or +
Chromogranin	–	–	+	–	– or +
CD10	–	–	+	+	– or +
IMP-3	+	–	+ or –	–	– or +
Trypsin	–	+	–	–	+
Claudin 5	ND	–	–	M+	–
Claudin 7	ND	M+	M+	– or focal C+	M+

Note: *ND* no data, *M* membranous staining, *N* nuclear staining, *C* cytoplasmic, *DAC* ductal adenocarcinoma, *ACC* acinar cell carcinoma, *PEN* pancreatic endocrine neoplasm, *SPN* solid-pseudopapillary neoplasm, *PB* pancreatoblastoma

The immunostaining results on PB are largely dependent upon the components in the tumor, such as acinar, squamous, ductal, or even endocrine component

References: [1–58]

Table 22.3 Markers for normal pancreatic ducts and acini

Antibodies	Pancreatic ducts	Pancreatic acini
CAM 5.2	+	+
CK7	+	+
CK20	–	–
CK19	Focal +	–
CK17	Usually –	–
S100P	– or cytoplasmic +	–
S100A6	– or weak cytoplasmic and nuclear staining	–
pVHL	+	Focal +
mCEA	– or weak + on luminal side	–
CA19-9	– or focal +	Weak +
Trypsin	–	+
MOC-31	+	+
Ber-EP4	+	+
TAG 72 (B72.3)	–	–
IMP-3	– or very focal +	–
Maspin	Usually –	–
Annexin A8	Weak +	Weak +
Claudin 4	Weak +	Weak +
Claudin 18	Focal +	+
PSCA	+	+
Mesothelin	Weak +	–
MUC1	Weak + on luminal side	–
MUC2	–	–
MUC4	–	–
MUC5AC	–	–
MUC6	+	–
DPC4/SMAD4	+	+
p53	– or very weakly +	–
CDX-2	– or +	– or +

Note: Focal – less than 10% of tissue stained

The table is from GML data based on 40 cases on TMA sections and routine sections; the stains are performed on both the Dako and Ventana Systems

Normal and reactive pancreatic ducts are usually negative for CK20, CK17, maspin, IMP3, S100P (nuclear staining), mCEA, trypsin, MUC2, MUC4, and MUC5AC

Approximately 10% of pancreatic ducts and acini are focally positive for CDX-2

Table 22.4 Markers for ductal adenocarcinoma of the pancreas

Antibodies	Literature	GML data (N = 70)
pVHL	–	100% negative
Maspin	+	100%
IMP-3	+	90%
S100P	+	96%
S100A6	+	96%
CAM 5.2	+	75%
CK7	+	96%
CK20	– or focal +	15%
CK17	+	60%
CK19	+	75%
Mesothelin	+	57%
mCEA	+	85%
MOC-31	+	97%
CA19-9	+	84%
Annexin A8	+	ND
MUC1	+	95%
MUC2	–	4%
MUC4	+	50%
MUC5AC	+	67%
MUC6	– or +	17%
Claudin 4	+	94%
Claudin 18	+	80%
PSCA	+ or –	56%
DPC4/SMAD4	+ or –	41%
p53	+ or –	60%
CDX-2	– or +	5%
Fascin	+	85%

Note: *ND* no data

GML data is based on TMA sections containing 50 cases and 20 cases of routine sections

Many markers have been reported in the literature. However, our experience shows that pVHL, maspin, S100P, and IMP-3 are the best panel of markers in the distinction of DAC from normal/reactive pancreatic ducts. Representative cases for these four markers are shown in Figs. 22.1–22.5. It should be noted that maspin is positive in both normal gastric mucosa and duodenal mucosa. Background staining for S100P sometimes is present. In this instance, S100A6 can be a good substitute, although weak nuclear and cytoplasmic staining for S100A6 can be seen in normal/reactive pancreatic ducts

Other markers including MUC1, MUC5AC, CA19-9, mesothelin, and p53 are shown in Figs. 22.6–22.10

Normal pancreatic ducts and acini are usually positive for MOC-31, PSCA, claudin 4, and claudin 18, which limits the application of these markers in the distinction between DAC and reactive ducts. Strong background staining is frequently seen in annexin A8 and fascin; in addition, many stromal cells and endothelial cells are positive for fascin

Among the group of cytokeratins being tested (CK7, CK20, CK17, CK19, and CAM 5.2), CK17 appears to be the only promising marker in differentiating adenocarcinoma from normal/reactive ducts since it usually lacks expression or is only very focally positive in normal ducts

Loss of DPC4/SMAD4 expression has been reported in approximately 60% of pancreatic ductal adenocarcinomas, which can be useful in differentiating pancreatic origin from other mucinous neoplasms, including an ovarian mucinous neoplasm. A metastatic carcinoma with the loss of DPC4/SMAD4 expression is suggestive of a pancreatic origin, although it is not absolutely specific (it has been reported in other tumors, including metastatic colonic adenocarcinomas). Examples of DAC negative and positive for DPC4/SMAD4 are shown in Figs. 22.11 and 22.12

References: [1–34, 37–39, 41–44, 58]

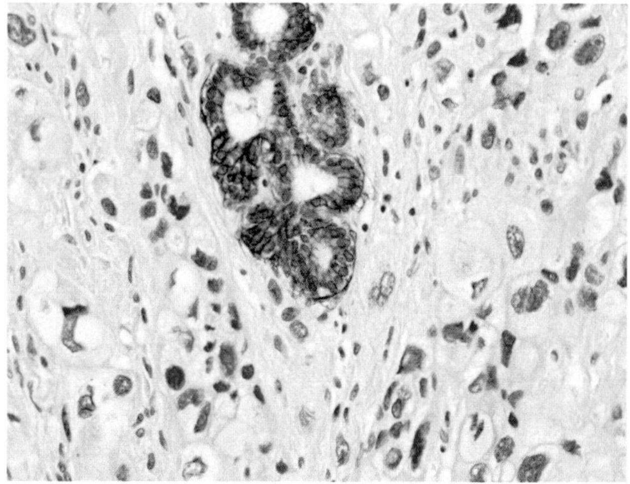

Fig. 22.1 Invasive ductal adenocarcinoma shows the loss of expression of pVHL, and normal ducts show membranous and cytoplasmic staining

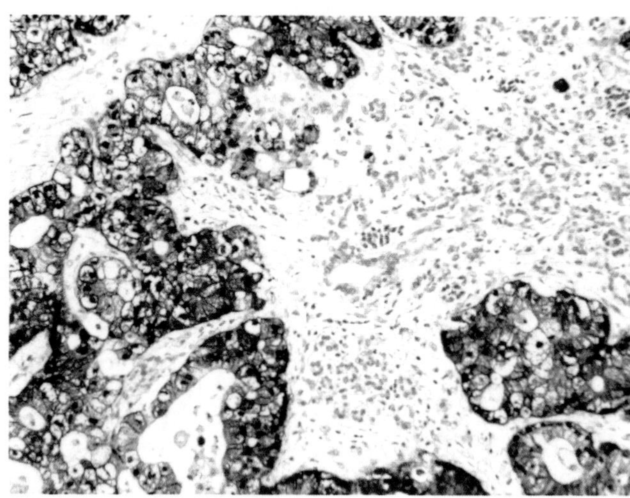

Fig. 22.3 Nuclear and cytoplasmic positivity of S100P in ductal adenocarcinoma, whereas the normal ducts are negative. Note that only nuclear staining or nuclear and cytoplasmic staining is regarded as positive

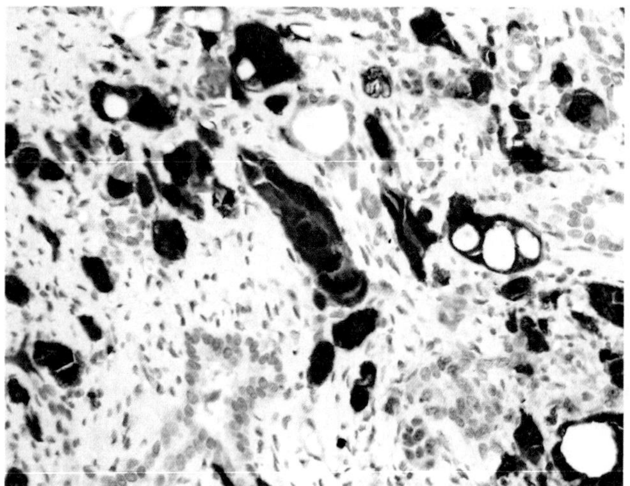

Fig. 22.2 High-grade adenocarcinoma shows nuclear and cytoplasmic staining for maspin

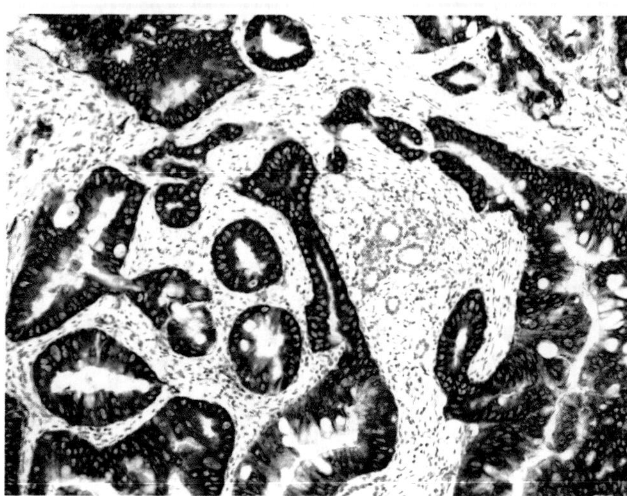

Fig. 22.4 Strong cytoplasmic staining for IMP-3 seen in ductal adenocarcinoma

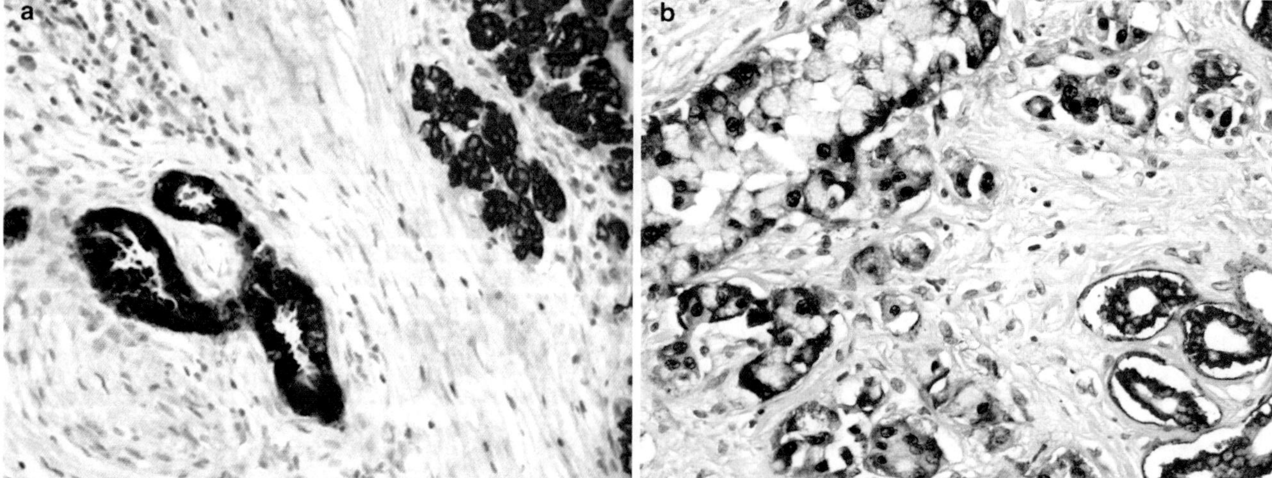

Fig. 22.5 Double-staining technique (**a**) showing carcinoma positive for maspin (*brown*) and normal ducts positive for pVHL (*purple*). Double-staining technique (**b**) showing carcinoma positive for S100P (*brown*) and normal ducts positive for pVHL (*purple*)

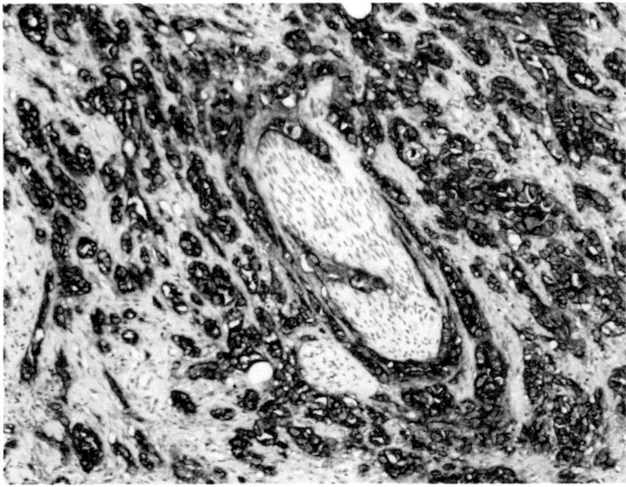

Fig. 22.6 Ductal adenocarcinoma shows strongly positive cytoplasmic staining for MUC1

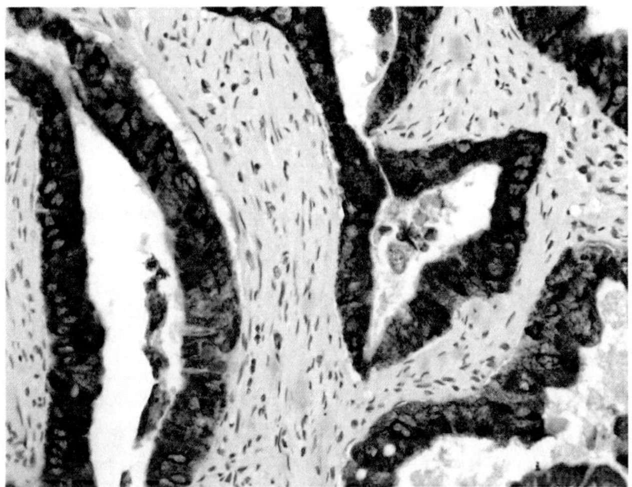

Fig. 22.7 Ductal adenocarcinoma shows strongly positive cytoplasmic staining for MUC5AC

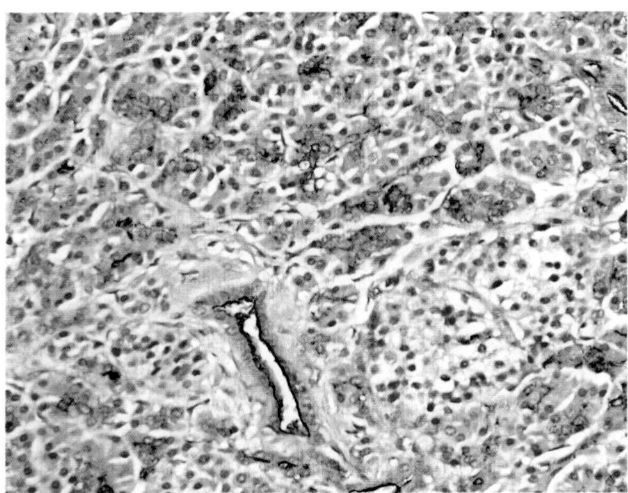

Fig. 22.8 CA19-9 is not a very useful marker since it is also expressed in normal ducts and acini

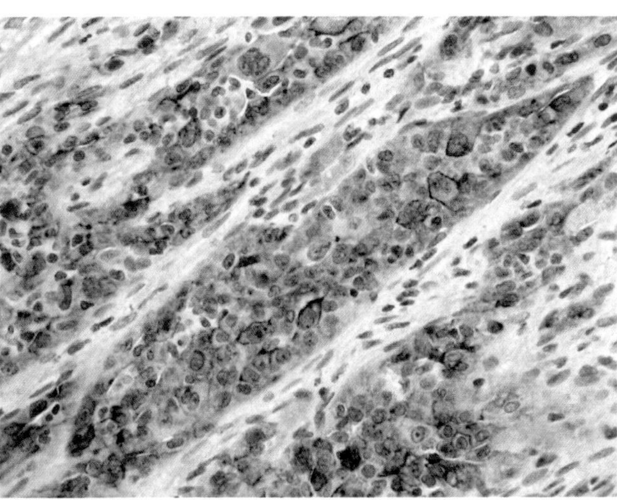

Fig. 22.9 Ductal adenocarcinoma showing membranous staining for mesothelin

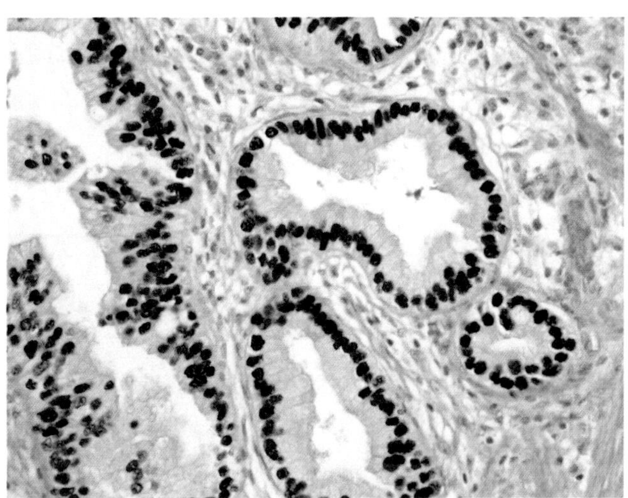

Fig. 22.10 Strong nuclear staining for p53 in ductal adenocarcinoma

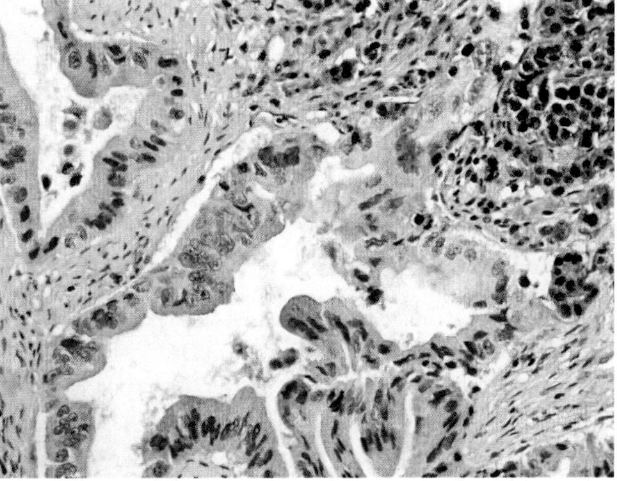

Fig. 22.11 Ductal adenocarcinoma showing the loss of expression of DPC4/SMAD4. Note that inflammatory cells and stromal cells show nuclear positivity as an internal positive control

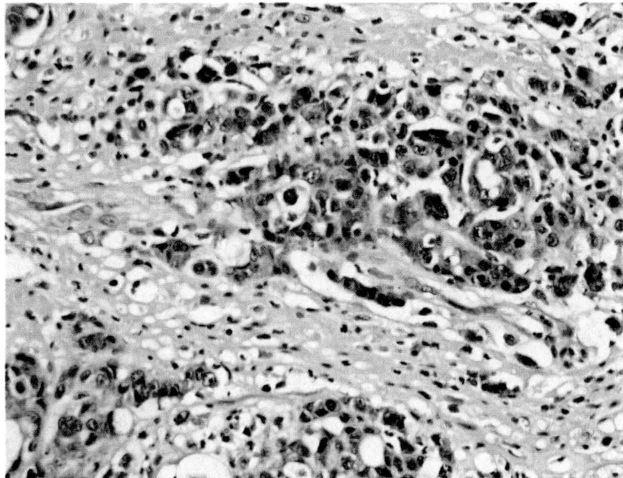

Fig. 22.12 Ductal adenocarcinoma showing positive staining for DPC4/SMAD4. Note that inflammatory cells and stromal cells show nuclear positivity as an internal positive control

Table 22.5 Markers for adenosquamous carcinoma of the pancreas

Antibodies	Literature
CK7	+
CK19	+
CEA	+
CA19-9	+
CK5/6	+
CK903	+
p63	+

Note: Adenosquamous carcinoma can be seen in both the gallbladder and ampulla

References: [1–3]

Table 22.6 Markers for colloid carcinoma of the pancreas

Antibodies	Literature
MUC1	– or +
MUC2	+
CDX-2	+
CK7	+
CK20	+ or –
CA19-9	+
CEA	+
pVHL	–
S100P	+
IMP-3	+
Maspin	+

Note: MUC2 and CDX-2 are usually positive in CC, which is useful in differentiating it from DAC. A case of CC with MUC2 and CDX-2 positivity is shown in Fig. 22.13

In contrast, DAC tends to be positive for MUC1 and negative for MUC2 and CDX-2. Other markers including S100P, pVHL, IMP-3, and maspin have limited value in the distinction of these two entities

Colloid carcinoma (noncystic mucinous adenocarcinoma) can be seen in both the gallbladder and ampulla

References: [1–3, 59]

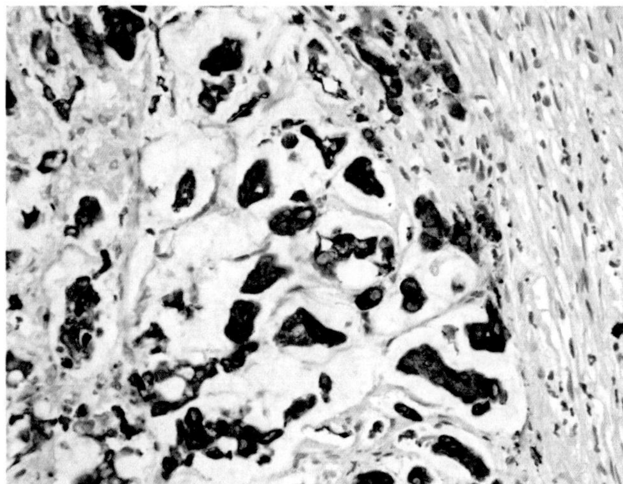

Fig. 22.13 MUC2 is frequently positive in colloid carcinoma and negative in ductal adenocarcinoma

Table 22.7 Markers for medullary carcinoma of the pancreas

Antibodies	Literature
CK7	+
CK20	–
CEA	+ or –
CA19-9	+ or –
MLH1	+ or –
MSH2	+ or –
MSH6	+ or –
PMS2	+ or –
E-cadherin	+

Note: Approximately 30% of reported cases demonstrate microsatellite instability (MSI) with the loss of expression of either MLH1/PMS2 or MSH2/MSH6. Most reported cases show the loss of expression of MLH1. K-ras mutation is an infrequent finding in medullary carcinoma compared with DAC. A representative case with the loss of expression of MSH2 is shown in Figs. 22.14 and 22.15

References: [1, 2, 60–62]

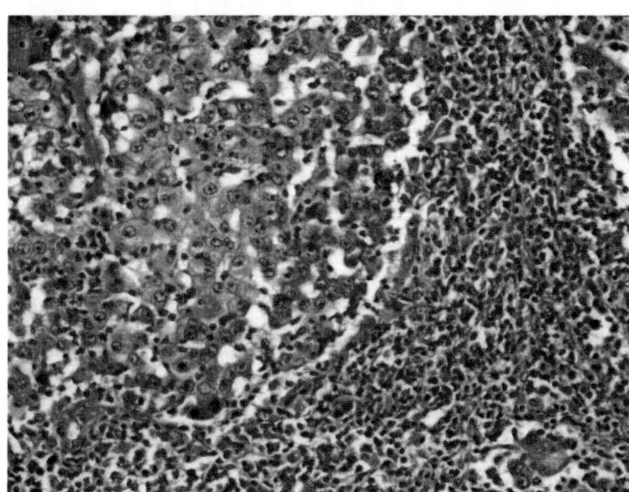

Fig. 22.14 Medullary carcinoma on H&E-stained slide

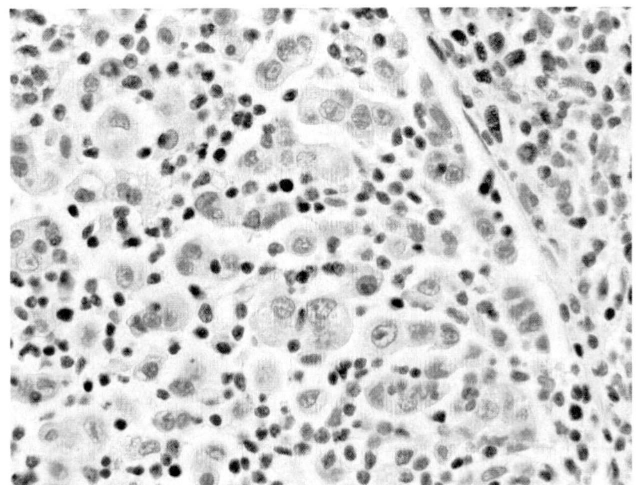

Fig. 22.15 Medullary carcinoma on the loss of expression of microsatellite instability marker MSH2. Note that the lymphoid cells serve as an internal positive control

Table 22.8 Markers for undifferentiated carcinoma of the pancreas

Antibody	Literature
CK7	+ or –
CK19	+ or –
CEA	+ or –
MUC1	+ or –
CA19-9	+ or –
Vimentin	+ or –
CK20	–
E-cadherin	–
MSI markers	+

Note: Loss of expression of E-cadherin in this tumor is a characteristic finding. Immunostaining for the other markers can vary depending on the degree of differentiation of the tumor. The tumor is positive for MSI (microsatellite instability) markers (MLH1, MSH2, MSH6, and PMS2), which can be useful in distinction from medullary carcinoma of the pancreas since both tumors present with poorly differentiated histomorphology

References: [1, 63]

Table 22.9 Markers for hepatoid carcinoma of the pancreas

Antibodies	Literature
Hep Par 1	+
Polyclonal CEA	Canalicular +
CD10	Canalicular +
AFP	+ or –
CK7	+ or –
Bile stain	+ or –

Note: Bile stain – a histochemical stain

Hepatoid carcinoma can also be seen in both the gallbladder and ampulla

References: [1, 64]

Table 22.10 Markers for signet ring cell carcinoma of the pancreas

Antibodies	Literature
CK7	+
CK20	+ or –
CEA	+
MOC-31	+
CDX-2	+ or –
CA19-9	+ or –

Note: Signet ring cell carcinoma can also be seen in both gallbladder and ampulla

Reference: [1]

Table 22.11 Markers for undifferentiated carcinoma with osteoclast-like giant cells

Antibodies	Malignant mononuclear cells	Benign giant cells
AE1/AE3	+ or –	–
CK7	+ or –	–
CK20	–	–
CD68	–	+

References: [1–3]

Table 22.12 Markers for acinar cell carcinoma

Antibodies	Literature
CK7	– or focal +
Mesothelin	–
Trypsin	+
S100P	–
AE1/AE3	+
CK19	– or focal +
CK20	–
CEA	+ or –
MOC-31	+ or –
Beta-catenin	M or M + N
pVHL	–
Vimentin	+ or –

Note: Approximately 25% of ACCs may show both nuclear and membranous positivity for beta-catenin. A histochemical stain of PAS-D is usually positive in acinar cell carcinoma. Trypsin is usually positive but may give a strong background staining

Chromogranin and synaptophysin are usually negative or show only scattered positivity in endocrine cells. When greater than 25% of tumor cells are positive for endocrine markers, the tumor would be regarded as mixed acinar and endocrine carcinoma

References: [1, 5, 7, 25–28, 33, 46, 47, 55]

Table 22.13 Markers for pancreatic endocrine neoplasm

Antibodies	Literature	GML data (N = 16)
Synaptophysin	+	100% (16/16)
Chromogranin	+	100% (16/16)
NSE	+	100% (16/16)
Beta-catenin	M+	100% (16/16)
CD56	+	44% (7/16)
PR	– or +	56% (9/16)
ER	–	0 (0/16)
CAM 5.2	+	100% (16/16)
CK7	+ or –	0 (0/16)
CK20	–	6% (1/16)
Vimentin	–	38% (6/16)
CDX-2	V	6% (1/16)
Insulin	V	13% (2/16)
CK19	+ or –	25% (4/16)

Note: *M*+ membranous positivity, *V* variable

Our study of a small number of cases (N = 16) shows that one case is positive for beta-catenin with both nuclear and cytoplasmic staining. CK7 and CK20 are negative in all cases except one case with focal (5%) CK20 immunoreactivity. Nine of 16 cases are diffusely and strongly positive for progesterone receptor (PR)

A representative case with vacuolated cytoplasm (lipid-rich pancreatic endocrine neoplasm) is shown in Figs. 22.16 and 22.17 with positive staining for chromogranin, synaptophysin, and CD56. CD56 is the most sensitive but relatively nonspecific marker for neuroendocrine differentiation; however, in our study, only 44% of cases were positive for CD56

CK19 positivity in PEN may be associated with a more aggressive clinical behavior

Reference: [1]

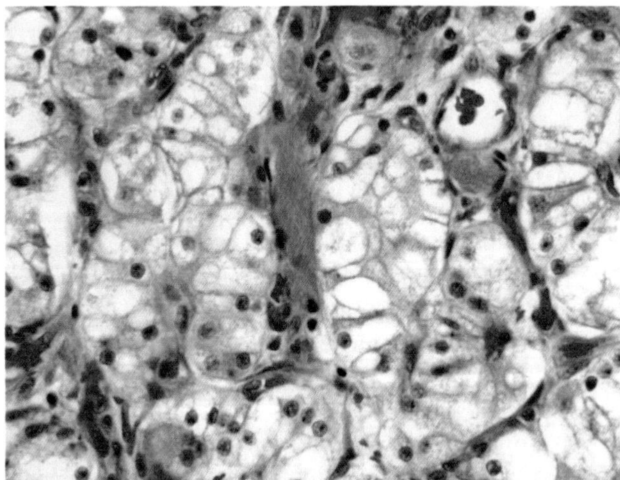

Fig. 22.16 Lipid-rich variant of pancreatic endocrine neoplasm

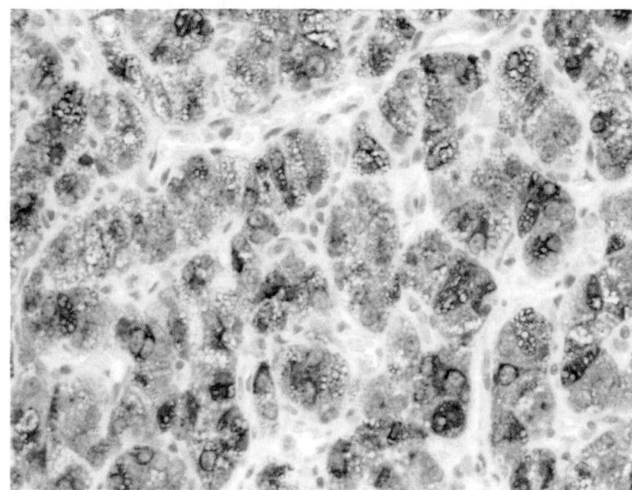

Fig. 22.17 Lipid-rich variant of pancreatic endocrine neoplasm positive for chromogranin

Table 22.14 Markers for solid-pseudopapillary neoplasm of the pancreas

Antibodies	Literature
Beta-catenin	N + C positive
E-cadherin	–
Chromogranin	–
CD10	+
AE1/AE3	Focal + or –
CK7	–
Vimentin	+
Trypsin	–
Alpha-1 antitrypsin	+
CD56	+
NSE	+ or –
Synaptophysin	– or +
Claudin 5	M+
Claudin 7	– or focal cytoplasmic +
Progesterone receptors (PR)	+ or –
Estrogen receptors (ER)	–

Note: N + C positive – both nuclear and cytoplasmic positivity; M+ – membranous positivity

Beta-catenin, E-cadherin, CD10, and chromogranin are the effective panel of antibodies to confirm the diagnosis of solid and pseudopapillary neoplasm of the pancreas. Over 90% of SPTs show both nuclear and membranous staining for beta-catenin. A representative case is shown in Figs. 22.18 and 22.19

References: [1, 5, 37, 45–52]

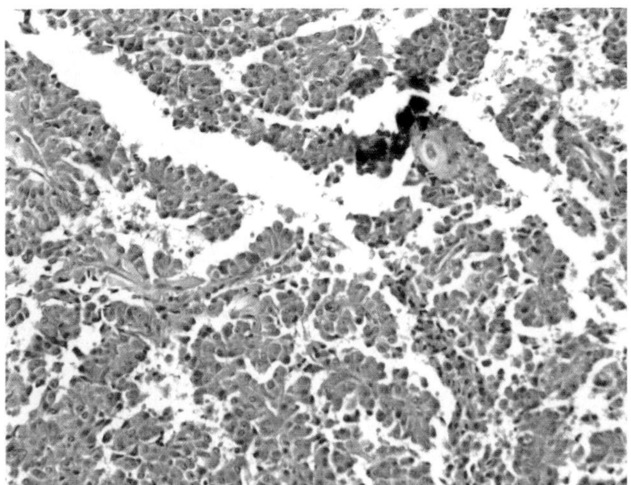

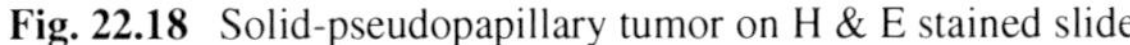

Fig. 22.18 Solid-pseudopapillary tumor on H & E stained slide

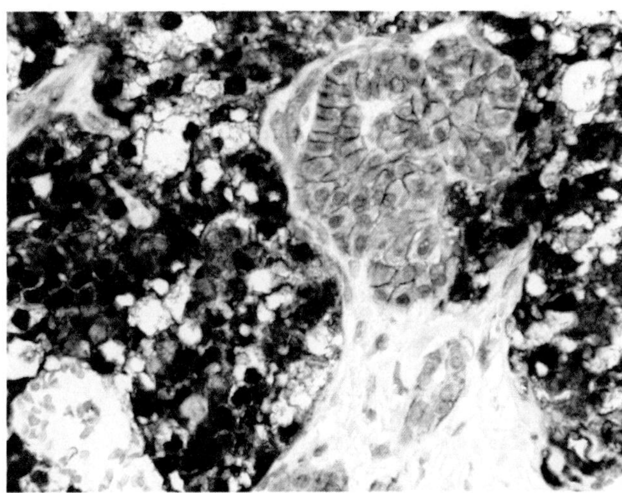

Fig. 22.19 Solid-pseudopapillary tumor showing nuclear and cytoplasmic staining for beta-catenin. Note that normal pancreatic duct shows membranous staining

Table 22.15 Markers for pancreatoblastoma

Antibodies	Acinar	Endocrine	Ductal
CK7	+	−	+
CK19	+	−	+
CAM 5.2	+	+	+
Trypsin	+	−	−
NSE	−	+	−
Synaptophysin	−	+	−
Chromogranin	−	+	−
CEA	−	−	+
TAG 72 (B72.3)	−	−	+

Note: Most pancreatoblastomas consist of both acinar and squamous components; some may also contain endocrine and ductal components. The immunostaining results are largely dependent upon the components in the tumor. Nuclear staining of beta-catenin has been reported in a significant percentage of cases, which is similar to the findings in SPN and acinar cell carcinoma. The "squamous component" usually lacks the typical squamous phenotype; i.e., positive for CK5/6, CK14, and CK17. Instead, it is usually positive for EMA, CK8, CK18, and CK19 but negative for CK7

Alpha-fetoprotein may be positive in some cases, which is in keeping with the primitive nature of this neoplasm

References: [1, 5, 7, 53, 54, 56, 57]

Table 22.16 Markers for serous cystadenoma

Antibodies	Literature	GML data (N = 13)
pVHL	+	100% (13/13)
MUC6	+ or −	92% (12/13)
Inhibin-alpha	+	92% (12/13)
NSE	+	54% (7/13)
CK7	+	100% (13/13)
CK20	−	0 (0/13)
S100P	−	0 (0/13)
Synaptophysin	−	0 (0/13)
Chromogranin	−	0 (0/13)
TAG 72 (B72.3)	−	0 (0/13)
CEA	−	0 (0/13)
CA19-9	− or +	31% (4/13)
MOC-31	−	70% (9/13)
aPAS	+	100% (13/13)
aMucicarmine	−	0 (0/13)

Note: aPAS for glycogen is usually positive, and mucicarmine for mucin is usually negative. Both pVHL and MUC6 tend to show diffuse and strong cytoplasmic and membranous staining; in contrast, both NSE and inhibin-alpha more frequently show focal and weak staining. One should be aware that a significant number of cases may be positive for MOC-31 and CA19-9, which are also positive in a high percentage of pancreatic mucin-producing neoplasms and ductal carcinomas

An example of tumor diffusely and strongly positive for pVHL, MUC6, and inhibin-alpha is shown in Figs. 22.20–22.23

References: [1, 2, 65]

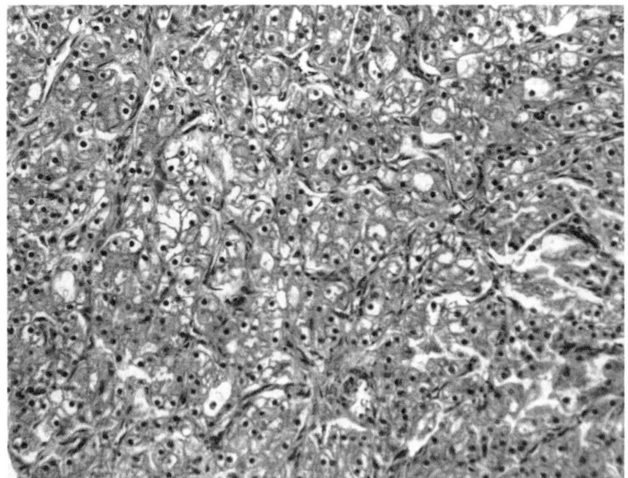

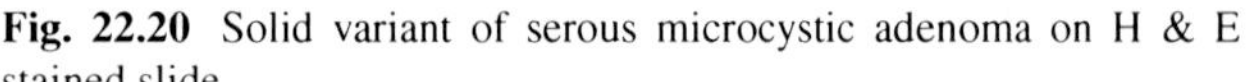

Fig. 22.20 Solid variant of serous microcystic adenoma on H & E stained slide

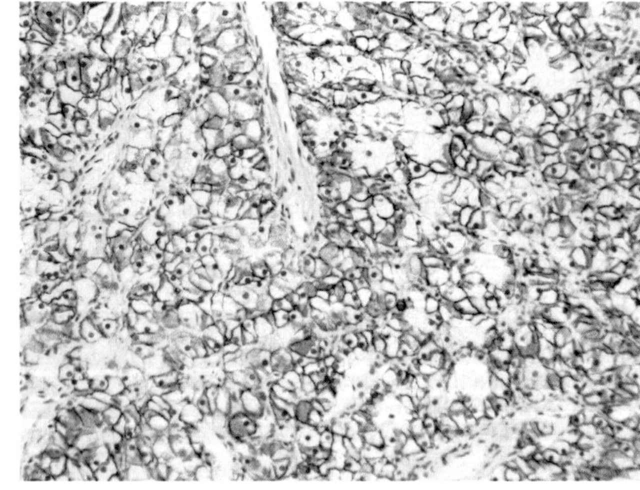

Fig. 22.21 Solid variant of serous microcystic adenoma positive for pVHL

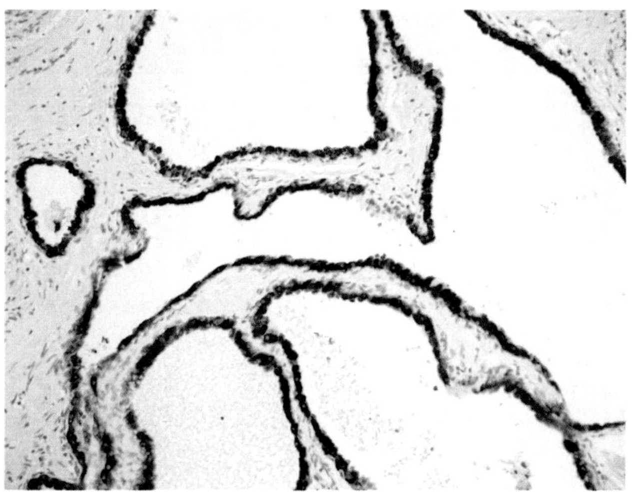

Fig. 22.22 Serous microcystic adenoma positive for MUC6

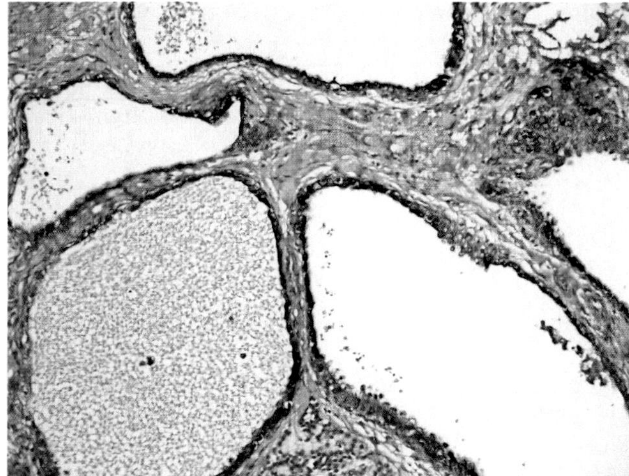

Fig. 22.23 Serous microcystic adenoma positive for inhibin-alpha

Table 22.17 Markers for mucinous cystic neoplasm

Antibodies	Literature	GML data (N = 12)
CK7	+	100% (12/12)
S100P	+	67% (8/12)
pVHL	−	33% (4/12)
CD10	+	33% (4/12)
Estrogen receptor (ER)	+	25% (3/12)
Inhibin-alpha	+ or −	67% (8/12)
Progesterone receptor (PR)	+ or −	50% (6/12)
CK20	− or +	33% (4/12)
CAM 5.2	+	100% (12/12)
CEA	+	100% (12/12)
CA19-9	+	92% (11/12)
CDX-2	−	25% (3/12)
MUC1	−	17% (2/12)
MUC2	− or +	0 (0/12)
MUC5AC	+	67% (8/12)
MUC6	−	50% (6/12)
DPC4/SMAD4	+	100% (12/12)

Note: The ovarian type stroma in MCN is usually positive for ER, PR, CD10, and inhibin-alpha. Expression of different types of mucins is not very useful in differentiating MCN from IPMN. MUC2 is frequently expressed in goblet cells of MCN

Our data showed all four S100P-negative cases were positive for pVHL; CDX-2 was only focally positive; CD10 was also expressed on the lining mucinous epithelium in two cases. The staining for ER, PR, and inhibin-alpha tended to be focal (less than 10% of the tumor stained) and weak. The positivity rate for ER was lower than reported in the literature, which may be due the inadequate fixation in formalin since the majority of specimens were grossed in a fresh status

References: [1, 2, 66]

Table 22.18 Markers for intraductal papillary mucinous neoplasm

Antibodies	Literature	GML data (N = 18)
CK7	+	100% (18/18)
S100P	+	18/18 (100%)
pVHL	–	0 (0/18)
CK19	+	75% (12/16)
CK20	– or +	62.5% (10/16)
CDX-2	+ or –	37.5% (6/16)
CEA	+	100% (18/18)
CA19-9	+	62.5% (10/16)
MUC1	V	50% (9/18)
MUC2	V	44% (8/18)
MUC5AC	+	100% (18/18)
MUC6	ND	78% (14/18)
DPC4/SMAD4	+	100% (18/18)

Note: *ND* no data, *V* variable

Intestinal-type IPMN is usually positive for MUC2, CDX-2, and CK20

Gastric foveolar-type IPMN is usually negative for both MUC1 and MUC2. Pancreatobiliary-type IPMN is usually positive for MUC1 and negative for MUC2 and CDX-2

Expression of S100P and loss of expression of pVHL are present in all types of IPMN. Expression of DPC4/SMAD4 was present in all tested cases. MUC6 tends to be expressed in the basal layer of epithelial cells; the papillary structures projecting into the cystic space are frequently negative for MUC6

References: [1, 2, 40, 66, 67]

Table 22.19 Markers for intraductal oncocytic papillary neoplasm

Antibodies	Literature
TAG 72 (B72.3)	+
Mesothelin	+
Hep Par 1	+
MUC1	+
CEA	+ or –
CA19-9	+ or –
CDX-2	–
Claudin 4	–
pVHL	–
S100P	+

References: [1, 33]

Table 22.20 Markers for pancreatic intraepithelial neoplasia 1 and 2

Antibodies	Literature
S100P	+
pVHL	–
p53	– or +
Maspin	+ or –
IMP-3	+ or –
Annexin A8	– or +
Mesothelin	– or +
Claudin 18	– or +

References: [1, 6, 10–13, 17, 19–22, 26–30, 33–35, 42, 43]

Table 22.21 Markers for pancreatic intraepithelial neoplasia 3

Antibodies	Literature
pVHL	–
S100P	+
Maspin	+
IMP-3	+
MUC1	+
MUC2	–
MUC4	+
MUC5AC	+
MUC6	+
DPC4/SMAD4	+
p53	+ or –
Claudin 18	+
Annexin A8	+
Mesothelin	+

References: [1, 6, 10–13, 17, 19–22, 26–30, 33–35, 42, 43]

Table 22.22 Markers for intraductal tubular neoplasm of the pancreas

Antibodies	Literature
CK7	+
CK20	–
CK19	+
CEA	+
CA19-9	+
MUC5AC	+
MUC6	+
MUC1	– or +
MUC2	–
Ki-67	Low
Mucicarmine	+

Reference: [1]

Table 22.23 Markers for chronic pancreatitis

Antibodies	Literature	GML data
S100P	– or cytoplasmic only	– or cytoplasmic only
pVHL	+	+
Maspin	–	–
IMP-3	–	–
Mesothelin	–	Weak +
PSCA	–	+
Annexin A8	–	Weak +
Claudin 18	–	Weak +
mCEA	+ or –	Weak + on luminal side
MOC-31	+	+
CA19-9	+	+

Note: Our experience showed 100% of benign and reactive pancreatic ductal cells are positive for pVHL; in contrast, ductal carcinomas are negative for pVHL in nearly 100% of cases. Non-neoplastic ducts are usually negative for S100P, IMP-3, and maspin

References: [1, 9–13, 17, 19–22, 26–29, 32, 34, 35]

Table 22.24 Ductal adenocarcinoma vs. chronic pancreatitis

Antibodies	DAC	Pancreatitis
Maspin	+	–
pVHL	–	+
S100P	+	– or cytoplasmic + only
IMP-3	+	–
CK17	+ or –	Usually –
p53	+ or –	– or very weak +
mCEA	+	Usually – or focal +
Mesothelin	+	–
MUC1	+	+ or –
Annexin A8	+	–
Claudin 18	+	– or weak +

Note: It has been demonstrated that 100% of benign and reactive pancreatic ductal cells are positive for pVHL; in contrast, ductal carcinoma is negative for pVHL in nearly 100% of cases. Our experience showed maspin, IMP-3, and S100P are the three best positive markers for identifying adenocarcinoma. Very weak positivity in non-neoplastic ducts can be seen in maspin and IMP-3 stains. Reactive ducts may show cytoplasmic staining for S100P. Markers such as TAG 72 (B72.3), MOC-31, and Ber-EP4 are usually positive in adenocarcinoma, but they are frequently positive or weakly positive in normal or reactive ducts as well

References: [1, 9–13, 17, 19–22, 26–29, 32–35, 38, 39, 42–44]

Table 22.25 Pancreatic endocrine neoplasm vs. solid pseudopapillary neoplasm

Antibodies	PEN	SPN
Beta-catenin	M+	N + C
E-cadherin	+	–
Chromogranin	+	–
Cytokeratin	+	–
Vimentin	–	+
PR	– or +	+ or –
CD10	–	+
Claudin 5	–	M+
Claudin 7	M+	– or focal cytoplasmic +

Note: *M* membranous, *N* nuclear, *C* cytoplasmic, *PEN* pancreatic endocrine neoplasm, *SPN* solid pseudopapillary neoplasm

Over 90% of SPN show nuclear and cytoplasmic positivity for beta-catenin and loss expression of E-cadherin. Expression of chromogranin in SPN has not been reported. Our study shows PR is positive in 56% of PEN cases ($N = 16$)

References: [1, 2, 45–52]

Table 22.26 Pancreatic endocrine neoplasm vs. acinar cell carcinoma

Antibodies	PEN	ACC
Chromogranin	+	Usually –
CK7	+ or –	– or focal +
Trypsin	–	+
Beta-catenin	M+	M or N + C
E-cadherin	+	+ or –

Note: *PEN* pancreatic endocrine neoplasm, *ACC* acinar cell carcinoma

References: [1, 55]

Table 22.27 Pancreatic endocrine neoplasm vs. pancreatoblastoma

Antibodies	PEN	PB
Beta-catenin	M+	Usually N + C
E-cadherin	+	Usually –
Chromogranin	+	Usually –
CK7	+ or –	– or +

Note: *PEN* pancreatic endocrine neoplasm, *PB* pancreatoblastoma

This panel of immunostaining markers is very useful for a PB mainly composed of acinar and squamous components. In a PB case with additional ductal and endocrine components, the staining results would be more complicated. In general, nuclear positivity and loss of E-cadherin expression are highly suggestive of PB after the exclusion of acinar cell carcinoma and SPN

References: [1, 53, 54, 56, 57]

Table 22.28 Acinar cell carcinoma vs. solid pseudopapillary neoplasm

Antibodies	ACC	SPN
CD10	–	+
Beta-catenin	M or N + C	N + C
Trypsin	+	–
E-cadherin	+	–
AE1/AE3	+	– or focal +
PR	–	+ or –
Bcl-6	+	–
Claudin 5	–	M+
Claudin 7	M+	– or focal cytoplasmic +
CEA	+ or –	–
Alpha-1 antitrypsin	–	+

Note: *ACC* acinar cell carcinoma, *SPN* solid pseudopapillary neoplasm. Interpretation of trypsin and alpha-1 antitrypsin may be difficult due to the presence of background staining

Up to 30% of ACCs may show both nuclear and cytoplasmic staining for beta-catenin

References: [1, 45–52, 54]

Table 22.29 Acinar cell carcinoma vs. ductal adenocarcinoma

Antibodies	ACC	DAC
CK7	– or very focal +	+
Mesothelin	–	+ or –
S100P	–	+
Trypsin	+	–
IMP-3	–	+
Vimentin	+ or –	–
CK19	– or focal +	+ or –
DPC4/SMAD4	+	+ or –

Note: *ACC* acinar cell carcinoma, *DAC* ductal adenocarcinoma

References: [1, 25–29, 31, 32, 54]

Table 22.30 Acinar cell carcinoma vs. pancreatoblastoma

Antibody	ACC	PB
Beta-catenin	M or N + C	N + C, or M
E-cadherin	M	– or M
CK7	– or focal +	Focal +
Trypsin	+	+

Note: *ACC* acinar cell carcinoma, *PB* pancreatoblastoma

Identification of squamous component/squamous differentiation is the key to making a distinction between these entities. However, the "squamous component" usually lacks the typical squamous phenotype, i.e., positive for CK5/6 and other high molecular weight cytokeratins. Approximately 30% of ACCs may show nuclear beta-catenin staining and loss of expression of E-cadherin; in contrast, over 90% of PBs show nuclear and cytoplasmic beta-catenin positivity and loss expression of membranous E-cadherin

References: [1, 53–57]

Table 22.31 Solid pseudopapillary neoplasm vs. pancreatoblastoma

Antibody	SPN	PB
Claudin 5	M+	–
Claudin 7	– or focal cytoplasmic +	M+
PR	+ or –	–
CD10	+	Usually –
Trypsin	–	+
Cytokeratin	– or focal +	+
CK7	–	– or focal +
Beta-catenin	N + C	N + C or M+
E-cadherin	–	– or +
Alpha-1 antitrypsin	+	–

Note: *SPN* solid pseudopapillary neoplasm, *PB* pancreatobiliary blastoma

Interpretation of trypsin and alpha-1 antitrypsin may be difficult due to the presence of background staining

Expression of beta-catenin and E-cadherin has a limited value in the distinction between SPN and PB

References: [1, 45–57]

Table 22.32 Markers for hematopoietic malignancies in the pancreas

Markers	B-cell lymphoma	Myeloid sarcoma	Plasmacytoma/ MM	Hodgkin's lymphoma
CD3	–	+ or –	–	–
CD20	+	–	–	–
CD15	–	–	–	+
CD30	– or +	–	–	+
CD38	–	–	+	–
CD138	–	–	+	–
CD117	–	+	–	–
CD34	–	+	–	–
CD43	+ or –	+	–	–
EMA	–	–	+ or –	–

Note: *MM* multiple myeloma

CD43 is a sensitive but not specific marker for myeloid sarcoma (granulocytic sarcoma); CD138 is a sensitive but not specific marker for MM/plasmacytoma; MM is frequently positive for both CD138 and EMA, which may mislead one to call it epithelial neoplasm

References: [1, 68]

Table 22.33 Metastases in the pancreas

Markers	PDC	Kidney	Lung-A	Melanoma	Stomach	Lung-S	Colon	Breast
CK7	+	–	+	–	+	+ or –	–	+
CK20	–	–	–	–	+ or –	–	+	–
S100	–	–	+ or –	+	–	–	–	– or +
MOC-31	+	–	+	–	+	+ or –	+	+
TTF1	–	–	+	–	–	+	–	–
CDX-2	–	–	–	–	+ or –	–	+	–
KIM-1	–	+	–	–	–	–	–	–
CD10	–	+	–	–	–	–	–	–
ER	–	–	–	–	–	–	–	+
Synap	–	–	–	–	–	+	–	–
DPC4/SMAD4	– or +	+	+	+	+	+	+	+

Note: *PDC* pancreatic ductal carcinoma, *Lung-A* lung adenocarcinoma, *Lung-S* lung small cell carcinoma, *Synap* synaptophysin, *ER* estrogen receptors

Mucinous adenocarcinomas of the lung are frequently positive for CDX-2 and negative for TTF1; in addition, a small percentage of lung adenocarcinomas can be positive for ER

S100 is a highly sensitive (98%) but not specific marker for screening melanoma. Caution should be taken if the sample is fixed in alcohol, since the S100 antigen is not preserved well after alcohol fixation. If melanoma is suspected, then other markers including MART-1 and HMB-45 should be done

Some metastatic small cell carcinomas of the lung can be negative for both synaptophysin and chromogranin, but they are very infrequently negative for CD56. Ki-67 proliferative index tends to be very high (>50%); it would be extremely unusual to have a small cell carcinoma with a low Ki-67 index

The majority (>90%) of the metastatic colonic adenocarcinomas are positive for both CK20 and CDX-2; however, it should be noted that medullary carcinoma of the colon with microsatellite instability (MSI) frequently shows the loss of expression of both CDX-2 and CK20. In this case, the tumor cells would demonstrate the loss of expression of either MLH1/PMS2 or MSH2/MSH6, and rarely loss either PMS2 or MSH6 only

References: [1–3, 5–8, 58, 69, 70]

Table 22.34 Prognostic markers in pancreatic adenocarcinoma

Markers	Literature	Association
DNMT1	Overexpression	Advanced stage
HDAC1	Overexpression	Advanced stage
uPAR	Gene amplification	Poor prognosis
Dkk-3	Low expression	Poor prognosis
MicroRNAs	Overexpression of 155, 203, 210, and 222	Poor prognosis
ALCAM/CD166	Overexpression	Poor prognosis
DPC4/SMAD4	Loss expression	Poor prognosis
S100A6	Nuclear positivity	Poor prognosis

Note: *DNMT1* DNA methyltransferase 1, *HDAC1* histone deacetylase-1, *uPAR* urokinase-type plasminogen activator receptor, *ALCAM* activated leukocyte cell adhesion molecule, *Dkk-3* Dickkopf-related protein 3

References: [1, 71–74]

Table 22.35 Predictive markers for pancreatic endocrine neoplasm

Markers	Literature	Association
CK19 (RCK 108 antibody)	+	Poor prognosis
Ki-67	>5%	Metastatic disease
67-kDa laminin receptors	+	Metastatic disease
CD44 isoforms (v6 and v9)	+	Good prognosis
Topoisomerase II alpha	Overexpression	Malignant
CD99	Loss expression	Poor prognosis
Survivin	Nuclear +	Poor prognosis

References: [1, 75–81]

Table 22.36 Markers for normal ampulla of Vater

Antibodies	GML data (N = 20)
CK7	80% (16/20)
CK20	100% (20/20)
CK17	0 (0/20)
CK19	100% (20/20)
MUC1	0 (0/20)
MUC2	100% (20/20)
pVHL	60% (12/20)
S100P	50% (10/20)
Maspin	95% (19/20)
IMP-3	40% (8/20), focal
Villin	90% (18/20)
CDX-2	100% (20/20)
Hep Par1	85% (17/20)
CEA	100% (20/20)
Ber-EP4	100% (20/20)
MOC-31	100% (20/20)

Note: The data is from GML based on 20 cases of ampullary biopsy specimens

Focal - less than 10% stained

pVHL, maspin, IMP-3, and S100P are a panel of very useful markers in the distinction of normal pancreatic ducts from pancreatic ductal adenocarcinoma. The frequent expression of these four markers makes them less useful in the diagnosis of ampullary adenocarcinoma

Table 22.37 Markers for ampullary adenocarcinoma – intestinal type

Antibodies	Literature
CK7	– or +
CK20	+
CDX-2	+
Hep Par 1	+
Villin	+
MUC2	+
CK7	– or +
CK17	–
MUC1	–
MUC5AC	–

References: [2, 8, 33, 82, 83]

Table 22.38 Markers for ampullary adenocarcinoma – pancreatobiliary type

Antibodies	Literature
S100P	+
pVHL	–
CK17	+
CK7	+ or –
CK20	–
CDX-2	–
Hep Par 1	–
MUC2	–
Villin	+ or –
MUC1	+
MUC5AC	+

References: [8, 33, 82, 83]

Table 22.39 Ampullary adenocarcinoma, intestinal type vs. pancreatobiliary type

Antibodies	Pancreatobiliary type	Intestinal type
MUC1	+	–
MUC2	–	+
CK20	–	+
CDX-2	–	+
Hep Par 1	–	+
CK17	+	–
CK7	+ or –	– or +
S100P	+	N/A
MUC5AC	+	–
Villin	V	+

Note: *V* variable

References: [2, 8, 33, 82, 83]

Table 22.40 Ampullary adenocarcinoma vs. pancreatic adenocarcinoma

Antibodies	ADCI	ADCP	DAC
CK7	+	+	+
CK20	+	–	– or +
CDX-2	+	–	–
Mesothelin	NA	NA	+
IMP-3	NA	NA	+
Hep Par 1	+	–	–
MUC1	–	+	+
MUC2	+	–	–

Note: *ADCI* ampullary adenocarcinoma intestinal type, *ADCP* ampullary adenocarcinoma pancreatobiliary type, *DAC* ductal adenocarcinoma of the pancreas, *NA* not available

References: [1, 2, 8, 33, 82]

Note for All Tables

Note: "+" – usually greater than 70% of cases are positive; "–" – less than 5% of cases are positive; "+ or –" – usually more than 50% of cases are positive; "– or +" – less than 50% of cases are positive.

References

1. Hruban RH, Pitman MB, Klimstra DS. AFIP atlast of tumor pathology, Tumors of the pancreas, vol. 4. Fascicle 6 ed. Washington, DC: American Registry of Pathology; 2007.
2. Chu PG, Weiss LM. Modern immunohistochemistry. New York, NY: Cambridge University Press; 2009.
3. Dabbs DJ. Diagnostic immunohistochemistry. 3rd ed. Philadelphia, PA: Churchill Livingstone Elsevier; 2010.
4. Taylor C, Cote R. Immunomicroscopy: a diagnostic tool for the surgical pathologist, Major problems in pathology. 3rd ed. Philadelphia, PA: Saunders Elsevier; 2006.
5. Goldstein NS, Bassi D. Cytokeratins 7, 17, and 20 reactivity in pancreatic and ampulla of vater adenocarcinomas. Percentage of positivity and distribution is affected by the cut-point threshold. Am J Clin Pathol. 2001;115(5):695–702.
6. Hornick JL, Lauwers GY, Odze RD. Immunohistochemistry can help distinguish metastatic pancreatic adenocarcinomas from bile duct adenomas and hamartomas of the liver. Am J Surg Pathol. 2005;29(3):381–9.
7. Chu P, Wu E, Weiss LM. Cytokeratin 7 and cytokeratin 20 expression in epithelial neoplasms: a survey of 435 cases. Mod Pathol. 2000;13(9):962–72.
8. Chu PG, Schwarz RE, Lau SK, Yen Y, Weiss LM. Immunohistochemical staining in the diagnosis of pancreatobiliary and ampulla of Vater adenocarcinoma: application of CDX2, CK17, MUC1, and MUC2. Am J Surg Pathol. 2005;29(3):359–67.
9. Lau SK, Prakash S, Geller SA, Alsabeh R. Comparative immunohistochemical profile of hepatocellular carcinoma, cholangiocarcinoma, and metastatic adenocarcinoma. Hum Pathol. 2002;33(12):1175–81.
10. Bhardwaj A, Marsh Jr WL, Nash JW, Barbacioru CC, Jones S, Frankel WL. Double immunohistochemical staining with MUC4/p53 is useful in the distinction of pancreatic adenocarcinoma from chronic pancreatitis: a tissue microarray-based study. Arch Pathol Lab Med. 2007;131(4):556–62.
11. Coppola D, Lu L, Fruehauf JP, et al. Analysis of p53, p21WAF1, and TGF-beta1 in human ductal adenocarcinoma of the pancreas: TGF-beta1 protein expression predicts longer survival. Am J Clin Pathol. 1998;110(1):16–23.
12. Apple SK, Hecht JR, Lewin DN, Jahromi SA, Grody WW, Nieberg RK. Immunohistochemical evaluation of K-ras, p53, and HER-2/neu expression in hyperplastic, dysplastic, and carcinomatous lesions of the pancreas: evidence for multistep carcinogenesis. Hum Pathol. 1999;30(2):123–9.
13. DiGiuseppe JA, Hruban RH, Goodman SN, et al. Overexpression of p53 protein in adenocarcinoma of the pancreas. Am J Clin Pathol. 1994;101(6):684–8.
14. Werling RW, Yaziji H, Bacchi CE, Gown AM. CDX2, a highly sensitive and specific marker of adenocarcinomas of intestinal origin: an immunohistochemical survey of 476 primary and metastatic carcinomas. Am J Surg Pathol. 2003;27(3):303–10.
15. Moskaluk CA, Zhang H, Powell SM, Cerilli LA, Hampton GM, Frierson Jr HF. Cdx2 protein expression in normal and malignant human tissues: an immunohistochemical survey using tissue microarrays. Mod Pathol. 2003;16(9):913–9.
16. De Lott LB, Morrison C, Suster S, Cohn DE, Frankel WL. CDX2 is a useful marker of intestinal-type differentiation: a tissue microarray-based study of 629 tumors from various sites. Arch Pathol Lab Med. 2005;129(9):1100–5.
17. Yantiss RK, Woda BA, Fanger GR, et al. KOC (K homology domain containing protein overexpressed in cancer): a novel molecular marker that distinguishes between benign and malignant lesions of the pancreas. Am J Surg Pathol. 2005;29(2):188–95.
18. Zhao H, Mandich D, Cartun RW, Ligato S. Expression of K homology domain containing protein overexpressed in cancer in pancreatic FNA for diagnosing adenocarcinoma of pancreas. Diagn Cytopathol. 2007;35(11):700–4.
19. Kashima K, Ohike N, Mukai S, Sato M, Takahashi M, Morohoshi T. Expression of the tumor suppressor gene maspin and its significance in intraductal papillary mucinous neoplasms of the pancreas. Hepatobiliary Pancreat Dis Int. 2008;7(1):86–90.
20. Agarwal B, Ludwig OJ, Collins BT, Cortese C. Immunostaining as an adjunct to cytology for diagnosis of pancreatic adenocarcinoma. Clin Gastroenterol Hepatol. 2008;6(12):1425–31.
21. Ohike N, Maass N, Mundhenke C, et al. Clinicopathological significance and molecular regulation of maspin expression in ductal adenocarcinoma of the pancreas. Cancer Lett. 2003;199(2):193–200.
22. Cao D, Zhang Q, Wu LS, et al. Prognostic significance of maspin in pancreatic ductal adenocarcinoma: tissue microarray analysis of 223 surgically resected cases. Mod Pathol. 2007;20(5):570–8.
23. Wente MN, Jain A, Kono E, et al. Prostate stem cell antigen is a putative target for immunotherapy in pancreatic cancer. Pancreas. 2005;31(2):119–25.
24. Argani P, Rosty C, Reiter RE, et al. Discovery of new markers of cancer through serial analysis of gene expression: prostate stem cell antigen is overexpressed in pancreatic adenocarcinoma. Cancer Res. 2001;61(11):4320–4.
25. McCarthy DM, Maitra A, Argani P, et al. Novel markers of pancreatic adenocarcinoma in fine-needle aspiration: mesothelin and prostate stem cell antigen labeling increases accuracy in cytologically borderline cases. Appl Immunohistochem Mol Morphol. 2003;11(3):238–43.
26. Ordonez NG. Application of mesothelin immunostaining in tumor diagnosis. Am J Surg Pathol. 2003;27(11):1418–28.
27. Hassan R, Laszik ZG, Lerner M, Raffeld M, Postier R, Brackett D. Mesothelin is overexpressed in pancreaticobiliary adenocarcinomas but not in normal pancreas and chronic pancreatitis. Am J Clin Pathol. 2005;124(6):838–45.
28. Frierson Jr HF, Moskaluk CA, Powell SM, et al. Large-scale molecular and tissue microarray analysis of mesothelin expression in common human carcinomas. Hum Pathol. 2003;34(6):605–9.
29. Swierczynski SL, Maitra A, Abraham SC, et al. Analysis of novel tumor markers in pancreatic and biliary carcinomas using tissue microarrays. Hum Pathol. 2004;35(3):357–66.
30. Baruch AC, Wang H, Staerkel GA, Evans DB, Hwang RF, Krishnamurthy S. Immunocytochemical study of the expression of mesothelin in fine-needle aspiration biopsy specimens of pancreatic adenocarcinoma. Diagn Cytopathol. 2007;35(3):143–7.
31. Jhala N, Jhala D, Vickers SM, et al. Biomarkers in diagnosis of pancreatic carcinoma in fine-needle aspirates. Am J Clin Pathol. 2006;126(4):572–9.
32. Cao D, Maitra A, Saavedra JA, Klimstra DS, Adsay NV, Hruban RH. Expression of novel markers of pancreatic ductal adenocarcinoma in pancreatic nonductal neoplasms: additional evidence of different genetic pathways. Mod Pathol. 2005;18(6):752–61.
33. Lin F, Shi J, Liu H, et al. Diagnostic utility of S100P and von Hippel-Lindau gene product (pVHL) in pancreatic adenocarcinoma-with

implication of their roles in early tumorigenesis. Am J Surg Pathol. 2008;32(1):78–91.
34. Karanjawala ZE, Illei PB, Ashfaq R, et al. New markers of pancreatic cancer identified through differential gene expression analyses: claudin 18 and annexin A8. Am J Surg Pathol. 2008;32(2):188–96.
35. Sato N, Fukushima N, Maitra A, et al. Gene expression profiling identifies genes associated with invasive intraductal papillary mucinous neoplasms of the pancreas. Am J Pathol. 2004;164(3):903–14.
36. Tsukahara M, Nagai H, Kamiakito T, et al. Distinct expression patterns of claudin-1 and claudin-4 in intraductal papillary-mucinous tumors of the pancreas. Pathol Int. 2005;55(2):63–9.
37. Hewitt KJ, Agarwal R, Morin PJ. The claudin gene family: expression in normal and neoplastic tissues. BMC Cancer. 2006;6:186.
38. Chhieng DC, Benson E, Eltoum I, et al. MUC1 and MUC2 expression in pancreatic ductal carcinoma obtained by fine-needle aspiration. Cancer. 2003;99(6):365–71.
39. Giorgadze TA, Peterman H, Baloch ZW, et al. Diagnostic utility of mucin profile in fine-needle aspiration specimens of the pancreas: an immunohistochemical study with surgical pathology correlation. Cancer. 2006;108(3):186–97.
40. Luttges J, Zamboni G, Longnecker D, Kloppel G. The immunohistochemical mucin expression pattern distinguishes different types of intraductal papillary mucinous neoplasms of the pancreas and determines their relationship to mucinous noncystic carcinoma and ductal adenocarcinoma. Am J Surg Pathol. 2001;25(7):942–8.
41. Deng H, Shi J, Wilkerson M, Meschter S, Dupree W, Lin F. Usefulness of S100P in diagnosis of adenocarcinoma of pancreas on fine-needle aspiration biopsy specimens. Am J Clin Pathol. 2008;129(1):81–8.
42. Dowen SE, Crnogorac-Jurcevic T, Gangeswaran R, et al. Expression of S100P and its novel binding partner S100PBPR in early pancreatic cancer. Am J Pathol. 2005;166(1):81–92.
43. Sato N, Fukushima N, Matsubayashi H, Goggins M. Identification of maspin and S100P as novel hypomethylation targets in pancreatic cancer using global gene expression profiling. Oncogene. 2004;23(8):1531–8.
44. Yamaguchi H, Inoue T, Eguchi T, et al. Fascin overexpression in intraductal papillary mucinous neoplasms (adenomas, borderline neoplasms, and carcinomas) of the pancreas, correlated with increased histological grade. Mod Pathol. 2007;20(5):552–61.
45. Notohara K, Hamazaki S, Tsukayama C, et al. Solid-pseudopapillary tumor of the pancreas: immunohistochemical localization of neuroendocrine markers and CD10. Am J Surg Pathol. 2000;24(10): 1361–71.
46. Abraham SC, Klimstra DS, Wilentz RE, et al. Solid-pseudopapillary tumors of the pancreas are genetically distinct from pancreatic ductal adenocarcinomas and almost always harbor beta-catenin mutations. Am J Pathol. 2002;160(4):1361–9.
47. Tanaka Y, Kato K, Notohara K, et al. Frequent beta-catenin mutation and cytoplasmic/nuclear accumulation in pancreatic solid-pseudopapillary neoplasm. Cancer Res. 2001;61(23):8401–4.
48. Audard V, Cavard C, Richa H, et al. Impaired E-cadherin expression and glutamine synthetase overexpression in solid pseudopapillary neoplasm of the pancreas. Pancreas. 2008;36(1):80–3.
49. Chetty R, Serra S. Membrane loss and aberrant nuclear localization of E-cadherin are consistent features of solid pseudopapillary tumour of the pancreas. An immunohistochemical study using two antibodies recognizing different domains of the E-cadherin molecule. Histopathology. 2008;52(3):325–30.
50. El-Bahrawy MA, Rowan A, Horncastle D, et al. E-cadherin/catenin complex status in solid pseudopapillary tumor of the pancreas. Am J Surg Pathol. 2008;32(1):1–7.
51. Comper F, Antonello D, Beghelli S, et al. Expression pattern of claudins 5 and 7 distinguishes solid-pseudopapillary from pancreatoblastoma, acinar cell and endocrine tumors of the pancreas. Am J Surg Pathol. 2009;33(5):768–74.
52. Pettinato G, Manivel JC, Ravetto C, et al. Papillary cystic tumor of the pancreas. A clinicopathologic study of 20 cases with cytologic, immunohistochemical, ultrastructural, and flow cytometric observations, and a review of the literature. Am J Clin Pathol. 1992;98(5):478–88 [see comment] [erratum appears in Am J Clin Pathol 1993;99(6):764].
53. Klimstra DS, Wenig BM, Adair CF, Heffess CS. Pancreatoblastoma. A clinicopathologic study and review of the literature. Am J Surg Pathol. 1995;19(12):1371–89.
54. Abraham SC, Wu TT, Klimstra DS, et al. Distinctive molecular genetic alterations in sporadic and familial adenomatous polyposis-associated pancreatoblastomas: frequent alterations in the APC/beta-catenin pathway and chromosome 11p. Am J Pathol. 2001;159(5):1619–27.
55. Abraham SC, Wu TT, Hruban RH, et al. Genetic and immunohistochemical analysis of pancreatic acinar cell carcinoma: frequent allelic loss on chromosome 11p and alterations in the APC/beta-catenin pathway. Am J Pathol. 2002;160(3):953–62.
56. Kerr NJ, Chun YH, Yun K, Heathcott RW, Reeve AE, Sullivan MJ. Pancreatoblastoma is associated with chromosome 11p loss of heterozygosity and IGF2 overexpression. Med Pediatr Oncol. 2002;39(1):52–4.
57. Tanaka Y, Kato K, Notohara K, et al. Significance of aberrant (cytoplasmic/nuclear) expression of beta-catenin in pancreatoblastoma. J Pathol. 2003;199(2):185–90.
58. van Heek T, Rader AE, Offerhaus GJ, et al. K-ras, p53, and DPC4 (MAD4) alterations in fine-needle aspirates of the pancreas: a molecular panel correlates with and supplements cytologic diagnosis. Am J Clin Pathol. 2002;117(5):755–65.
59. Adsay NV, Pierson C, Sarkar F, et al. Colloid (mucinous noncystic) carcinoma of the pancreas. Am J Surg Pathol. 2001;25(1):26–42.
60. Wilentz RE, Goggins M, Redston M, et al. Genetic, immunohistochemical, and clinical features of medullary carcinoma of the pancreas: a newly described and characterized entity. Am J Pathol. 2000;156(5):1641–51.
61. Banville N, Geraghty R, Fox E, et al. Medullary carcinoma of the pancreas in a man with hereditary nonpolyposis colorectal cancer due to a mutation of the MSH2 mismatch repair gene. Hum Pathol. 2006;37(11):1498–502.
62. Nakata B, Wang YQ, Yashiro M, et al. Negative hMSH2 protein expression in pancreatic carcinoma may predict a better prognosis of patients. Oncol Rep. 2003;10(4):997–1000.
63. Winter JM, Ting AH, Vilardell F, et al. Absence of E-cadherin expression distinguishes noncohesive from cohesive pancreatic cancer. Clin Cancer Res. 2008;14(2):412–8.
64. Hameed O, Xu H, Saddeghi S, Maluf H. Hepatoid carcinoma of the pancreas: a case report and literature review of a heterogeneous group of tumors. Am J Surg Pathol. 2007;31(1):146–52.
65. Kosmahl M, Wagner J, Peters K, Sipos B, Kloppel G. Serous cystic neoplasms of the pancreas: an immunohistochemical analysis revealing alpha-inhibin, neuron-specific enolase, and MUC6 as new markers. Am J Surg Pathol. 2004;28(3):339–46.
66. Handra-Luca A, Flejou JF, Rufat P, et al. Human pancreatic mucinous cystadenoma is characterized by distinct mucin, cytokeratin and CD10 expression compared with intraductal papillary-mucinous adenoma. Histopathology. 2006;48(7):813–21.
67. Ueda M, Miura Y, Kunihiro O, et al. MUC1 overexpression is the most reliable marker of invasive carcinoma in intraductal papillary-mucinous tumor (IPMT). Hepatogastroenterology. 2005;52(62):398–403.
68. Swerdlow H, Campo E, Harris N, et al. WHO classification of tumours of haematopoietic and lymphoid tissues. 4th ed. Lyon, France: International Agency for Research on Cancer; 2008. p. 439. Accessed 10/1/2009.
69. Chu P, Arber DA. Paraffin-section detection of CD10 in 505 nonhematopoietic neoplasms. Frequent expression in renal cell carcinoma and endometrial stromal sarcoma. Am J Clin Pathol. 2000;113(3): 374–82.

70. Lin F, Zhang PL, Yang XJ, et al. Human kidney injury molecule-1 (hKIM-1): a useful immunohistochemical marker for diagnosing renal cell carcinoma and ovarian clear cell carcinoma. Am J Surg Pathol. 2007;31(3):371–81.
71. Wang W, Gao J, Man XH, Li ZS, Gong YF. Significance of DNA methyltransferase-1 and histone deacetylase-1 in pancreatic cancer. Oncol Rep. 2009;21(6):1439–47.
72. Hildenbrand R, Niedergethmann M, Marx A, et al. Amplification of the urokinase-type plasminogen activator receptor (uPAR) gene in ductal pancreatic carcinomas identifies a clinically high-risk group. Am J Pathol. 2009;174(6):2246–53.
73. Fong D, Hermann M, Untergasser G, et al. Dkk-3 expression in the tumor endothelium: a novel prognostic marker of pancreatic adenocarcinomas. Cancer Sci. 2009;100(8):1414–20.
74. Kahlert C, Weber H, Mogler C, et al. Increased expression of ALCAM/CD166 in pancreatic cancer is an independent prognostic marker for poor survival and early tumour relapse. Br J Cancer. 2009;101(3):457–64.
75. Ali A, Serra S, Asa SL, Chetty R. The predictive value of CK19 and CD99 in pancreatic endocrine tumors. Am J Surg Pathol. 2006;30(12):1588–94.
76. Pelosi G, Pasini F, Bresaola E, et al. High-affinity monomeric 67-kD laminin receptors and prognosis in pancreatic endocrine tumours. J Pathol. 1997;183(1):62–9.
77. Imam H, Eriksson B, Oberg K. Expression of CD44 variant isoforms and association to the benign form of endocrine pancreatic tumours. Ann Oncol. 2000;11(3):295–300.
78. Ohike N, Morohoshi T. Pathological assessment of pancreatic endocrine tumors for metastatic potential and clinical prognosis. Endocr Pathol. 2005;16(1):33–40.
79. Diaz-Rubio JL, Duarte-Rojo A, Saqui-Salces M, Gamboa-Dominguez A, Robles-Diaz G. Cellular proliferative fraction measured with topoisomerase IIalpha predicts malignancy in endocrine pancreatic tumors. Arch Pathol Lab Med. 2004;128(4):426–9.
80. Goto A, Niki T, Terado Y, Fukushima J, Fukayama M. Prevalence of CD99 protein expression in pancreatic endocrine tumours (PETs). Histopathology. 2004;45(4):384–92.
81. Grabowski P, Griss S, Arnold CN, et al. Nuclear survivin is a powerful novel prognostic marker in gastroenteropancreatic neuroendocrine tumor disease. Neuroendocrinology. 2005;81(1):1–9.
82. Zhou H, Schaefer N, Wolff M, Fischer HP. Carcinoma of the ampulla of Vater: comparative histologic/immunohistochemical classification and follow-up. Am J Surg Pathol. 2004;28(7):875–82.
83. Schirmacher P, Buchler MW. Ampullary adenocarcinoma – differentiation matters. BMC Cancer. 2008;8:251.

Chapter 23
Liver, Bile Ducts, and Gallbladder

Jeffrey Prichard and Fan Lin

Abstract The liver is a common site for metastatic tumors, so differentiation of primary from metastatic lesions and identification of site of origin of metastatic tumors are frequent questions faced by pathologists. This chapter focuses on the application of immunohistochemical markers to these questions of hepatic and biliary tumor pathology. Staining profiles are presented for differentiating primary hepatocellular carcinomas, adenoma, and dysplastic nodules. Prognostic markers of hepatocellular adenoma subtypes are described. Challenges of distinguishing intrahepatic cholangiocarcinoma from metastatic mimics are addressed. A unique combination of complimentary markers useful in discriminating reactive from neoplastic epithelium in the gallbladder is shown. A process is defined utilizing an initial screening panel and subsequent confirmatory markers for unknown primary tumors in liver. Photomicrographs illustrate characteristic staining patterns.

Keywords Liver • Gallbladder • Hepatocellular • Canalicular • Biliary • Cholangiocarcinoma • HepPar-1 • AFP • Glypican-3 • Alpha-1antitrypsin • pVHL • Maspin • IMP3 (KOC)

FREQUENTLY ASKED QUESTIONS

J. Prichard (✉)
Department of Pathology and Laboratory Medicine, Geisinger Medical Center, 100 North Academy Avenue, Danville, PA 17822, USA
e-mail: jwprichard@geisinger.edu

Non-neoplastic Markers

Hepatocellular Tumor Markers

Bile Ducts and Gallbladder

Differential Diagnoses

F. Lin and J. Prichard (eds.), *Handbook of Practical Immunohistochemistry: Frequently Asked Questions*, DOI 10.1007/978-1-4419-8062-5_23, © Springer Science+Business Media, LLC 2011

21. Reactive biliary epithelium vs. dysplasia/adenocarcinoma of the common bile duct (Table 23.21) (p. 401)
22. Differential diagnosis of biliary tract/pancreas adenocarcinoma (Fig. 23.29, Table 23.22) (p. 402)
23. Initial four marker screening IHC panel for unknown primary tumor in liver (Table 23.23) (p. 403)
24. Confirmatory markers of unknown primary tumors of liver (Table 23.24) (p. 404)

Table 23.1 Summary of common markers in hepatobiliary pathology

Antibodies	Staining pattern	Function	Key applications and pitfalls
HepPar-1	C	General hepatocellular marker	Sensitive and specific when diffuse for both reactive and neoplastic hepatocellular lesions; exception is metastatic hepatoid adenocarcinomas; sensitivity drops in high-grade HCC
TTF-1 (8G7G3/1 clone) cytoplasmic	C	General hepatocellular marker	Cytoplasmic staining of hepatocellular cells; sensitivity parallels HepPar-1; TTF-1 SPT24 clone lacks staining
Alpha fetoprotein	C	HCC marker	Specific but not sensitive marker of HCC. Can also stain hepatoid carcinoma and yolk sac tumors
Glypican-3	C + M	HCC marker	Strong diffuse staining favors HCC over benign hepatic lesions, strongest in high-grade HCC; negative staining not helpful; not specific to hepatocellular tumors
Heat shock protein 70 (HSP70)	C	HCC marker	Used in combination with glypican-3 and glutamine synthetase to differentiate low-grade HCC from dysplastic nodules; not specific to hepatocellular tumors
Glutamine synthetase	C + M	HCC marker	Strong diffuse staining favors HCC over benign hepatic lesions; also positive in HA and DN
Beta-catenin (nuclear)	M + N	HCC marker	Nuclear expression in HA increased risk of progression to HCC
pCEA	M + C	Canalicular marker	Most sensitive for demonstrating canalicular staining pattern of hepatocellular lesions, better in low-grade HCC
CD10	M + C	Canalicular marker	Less sensitive marker for canalicular differentiation of hepatocellular lesions, only canalicular staining pattern is specific
Villin	M + C	Canalicular marker	Least sensitive marker for canalicular differentiation of hepatocellular lesions; also positive in many MAC
CD34	C	Endothelial marker	Diffusely positive in sinusoidal cells in HCC, but only focally in cirrhosis. Also positive in EH
MOC-31	M	Adenocarcinoma marker	Very sensitive marker for CC and MAC; HCC are negative or very weak in 95% of cases
CK7	C	Adenocarcinoma marker	Very sensitive marker for CC and MAC; negative in colorectal MAC and HCC and HB; some high-grade HCC show focal positivity
CK19	C	Adenocarcinoma marker	Very sensitive marker for CC and MAC; negative in colorectal MAC and HCC and HB; some high-grade HCC show focal positivity
CK20	C	Metastatic marker	Positive in colorectal MAC and hepatoid MAC and negative in CC
CAM5.2	C	Carcinoma marker	Positive in HCC, CC and MAC; not specific
CKAE1/3	C	Carcinoma marker	Positive in HCC, CC and MAC; not specific
Alpha-1 antitrypsin	C	Marker of alpha-1 antitrypsin disease	Identify alpha-1 antitrypsin accumulation
S100P	N + C	Belongs to the family of S100 calcium-binding proteins	Usually negative or cytoplasmic staining in normal/reactive gallbladder mucosa
pVHL	M + C	Tumor suppressor gene	Positive in normal and reactive gallbladder mucosa
IMP3 (KOC)	C	Encodes a protein withfour K-homologous domains; regulationof tumor cell proliferation	Usually negative in gallbladder mucosa
Maspin	C + N	Related to the serpinfamily of protease inhibitors; plays rolein tumor invasionand metastasis	Usually negative or weakly positive in normal gallbladder mucosa

Note: *N* nuclear staining, *M* membranous staining, *C* cytoplasmic staining, *HA* hepatic adenoma, *DN* dysplastic nodule, *HCC* hepatocellular carcinoma, *FLV* hepatocellular carcinoma, fibrolamellar variant, *HB* hepatoblastoma, *BDA* bile duct adenoma, *CC* cholangiocarcinoma, *MAC* metastatic adenocarcinomas, *EH* epithelioid hemangioendothelioma

References: [1–14, 16–43]

Table 23.2 Summary of common markers in common lesions

Antibodies	HCC	CC	MAC
HepPar-1	+	–	–
AFP	–/+	–	–/+
Glypican-3	+/–	–	–/+
pCEA	+ (Canalicular)	+	+
mCEA	–	+/–	+/–
CD10	+/– (Canalicular)	–	–/+
Villin	–/+ (Canalicular)	–/+	–/+
CD34	+ (Sinusoidal)	–	–/+
MOC-31	–/+	+	+
CK7	–/+	+	–/+
CK19	–	+	–/+
CK20	–	–/+	–/+
CAM5.2	+	+	+
CKAE1/3	–/+	+	+
S-100	–	–	–/+
HMB-45	–	–	–/+
Vimentin	–	–/+	–/+
ER	–	–	–/+
PR	–/+	–	–/+
S100P	–/+	–/+	–/+
pVHL	–/+	+	–
IMP3 (KOC)	–/+	–/+	+/–
Maspin	–	–/+	+/–

Note: *ND* no data, *M* membranous staining, *N* nuclear staining, *C* cytoplasmic

References: [1–11, 16–40, 44–54]

Table 23.3 Markers in normal hepatocytes and bile ducts

Antibodies	Hepatocytes, GML data (N = 28)	Bile ducts, GML data (N = 28)
AE1/AE3	–/+	+
AFP	–/+	–
B72.3	–	–
B-catenin	+	+
BerEP4	–	+
CA19-9	–	+
CAM5.2	+	+
CD10	+	–
CD15	–	–
CD31	–	–
CD34	–	–
CD56	–	–
CDX2	–	–
Chromogranin	–	–
CK7	–	+
CK5/6	–	–
CK17	–	–
CK19	–	+/–
CK20	–	–
CK903	–	–/+
EMA	–	+
ER	–	–
Glypican-3	–	–
HepPar-1	+	–
KOC (IMP3)	–	–
Maspin	–	–
mCEA	–	–
MOC31	–	+
MUC1	–	–
MUC2	–	–
MUC4	–	–
MUC5AC	–	–
MUC6	–	+
p16	–	–
p53	–	–
p63	–	–
pCEA	+	
PR	–	–
S100	–	–
S100A6	–	+/–
S100P	–	–/+
TTF-1 (8G7G31)	–/+	–
VHL	–	+
Villin	–	–/+
Vimentin	–	–

Note: Normal and neoplastic hepatocytes have a characteristic staining with HepPar-1 showing strongly large cytoplasmic granules (Fig. 23.1). There is a reported cross reaction of a clone of TTF-1 (8G7G31) with staining that parallels HepPar-1, though is not very common in our experience with the clone. AFP and is negative in normal hepatocytes, but can focally stain hepatocytes in cirrhosis. CK7 is negative in normal hepatocytes but is present in periportal hepatocytes in reactive conditions. CAM5.2 shows a much stronger periportal hepatocyte pattern even in normal liver than CK7 (Fig. 23.2). Normal bile ducts and ductules stain strongly for CK7 and AE1/AE3 (Figs. 23.3 and 23.4). Beta-catenin staining is membranous in normal hepatocytes, though can show nuclear translocation in neoplasia (Fig. 23.5).The canalicular architecture formed by adjoining hepatocytes can be clearly demonstrate with CD10 and pCEA (Figs. 23.6 and 23.7). In the normal liver, vimentin will highlight sinusoidal endothelial cells as well as Kupffer and stellate cells, none of which are stained by typical endothelial markers CD34 and CD31 (Fig. 23.8). In reactive conditions and cirrhosis, CD34 shows periportal sinusoidal staining involving a minority of the lobule

References: [1–6, 17, 18, 24, 28–32, 36, 55]

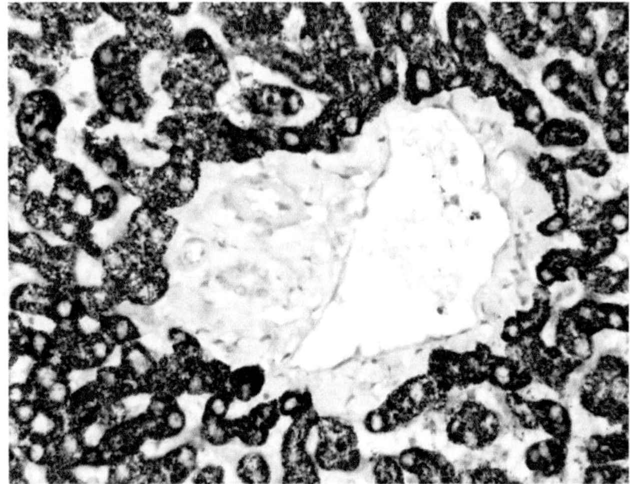

Fig. 23.1 Normal liver, HepPar-1, shows characteristic strong, coarsely granular cytoplasmic staining of normal hepatocytes

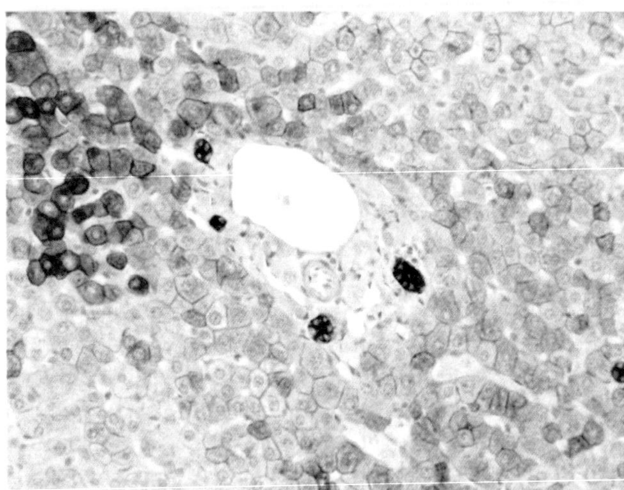

Fig. 23.2 Normal liver, CAM5.2, shows periportal accentuation in hepatocyte cytoplasm and strong staining of portal biliary structures

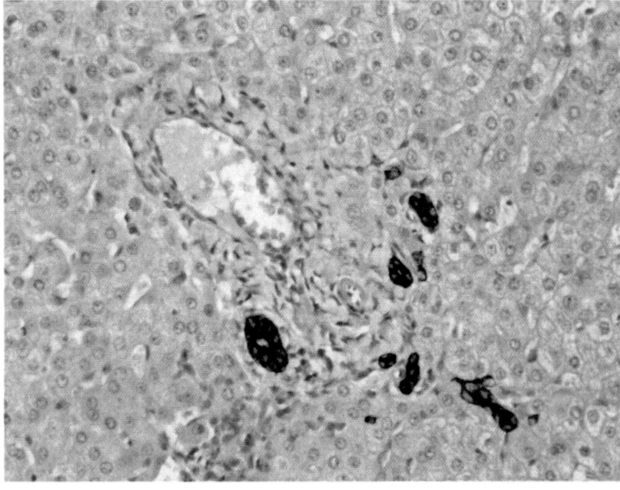

Fig. 23.3 Normal liver, CK7, only stains biliary structures. Interface hepatocyte may express CK7 in reactive conditions of cirrhosis

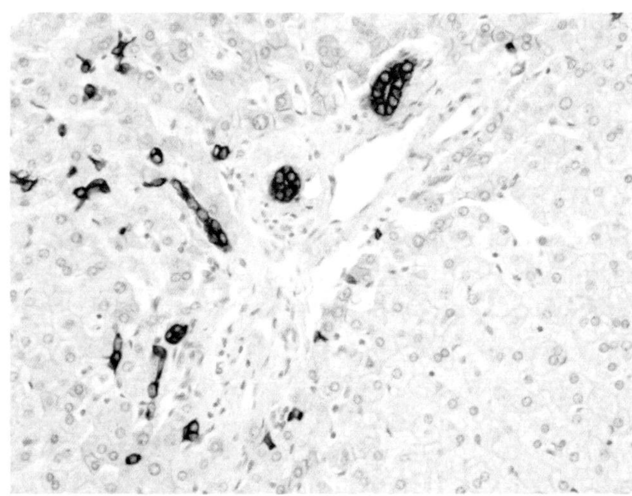

Fig. 23.4 Normal liver, AE1/AE3, shows similar staining pattern to CK7 highlighting biliary structures

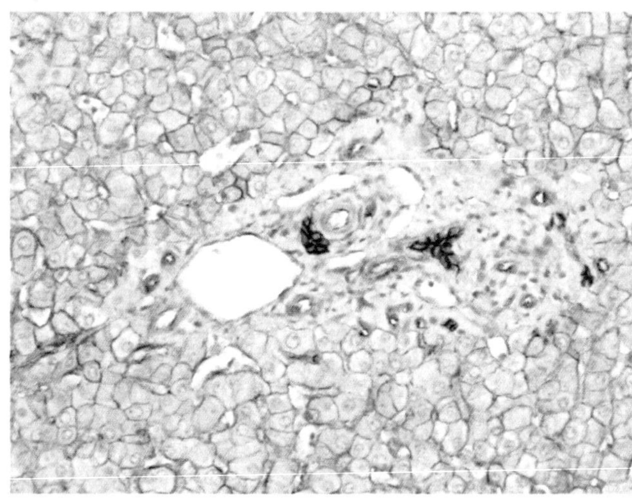

Fig. 23.5 Normal liver, beta-catenin, shows membranous staining of both ducts and hepatocytes. Nuclear staining is lacking and in the normal liver

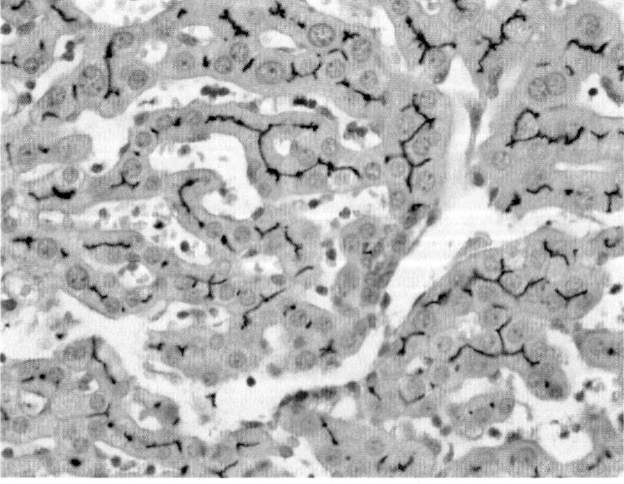

Fig. 23.6 Normal liver, CD10, staining the bile canaliculi

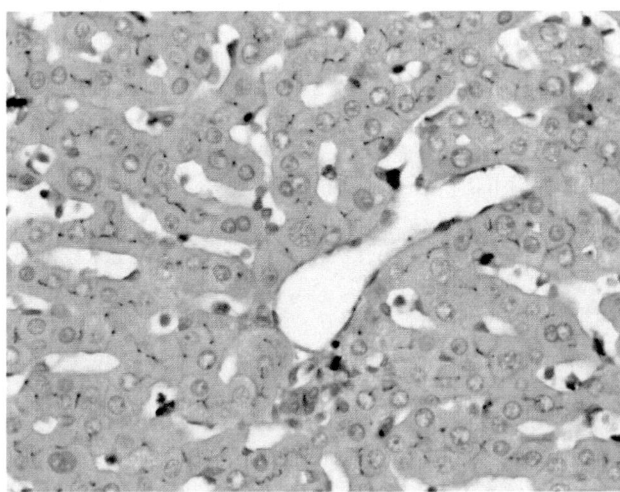

Fig. 23.7 Normal liver, pCEA, staining the bile canaliculi and sinusoidal Kupffer cells

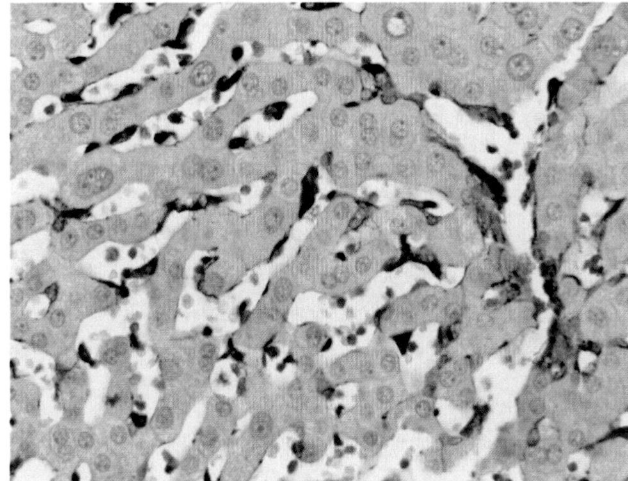

Fig. 23.8 Normal liver, vimentin, highlighting sinusoidal endothelium and sinusoidal Kupffer cells

Table 23.4 Markers of arterial and venous endothelium

Antibodies	Literature
CD10	+
CD31	+
CD34	+
Factor VIII	+

References: [1–10, 36]

Table 23.5 Markers of sinusoidal endothelium

Antibodies	Literature
CD10	+
CD31	+/–
CD34	+/–
Factor VIII	–/+
Vimentin	–/+
CD4	+
CD14	+
CD16	+
CDw32	+
ICAM-1	+
D2-40	–

Note: Sinusoidal endothelial cells stain with CD31 and CD34 only at the periphery of regenerative or cirrhotic nodules, but stain slightly more in HA and diffusely in HCC

References: [1–10, 36]

Table 23.6 Markers of Kupffer cells

Antibody	Literature
CK7, 19, 10	–
CD68 KP-1	+
CD68 PGM1	+
Vimentin	+

References: [1–6, 36]

Table 23.7 Markers of sinusoidal stellate cells

Antibodies	Literature
Vimentin	+
Desmin	+/–
SMA	+/–
CD68	–
GFAP	+/–
N-CAM	+
Synaptophysin	–/+

Note: Stellate cells express smooth muscle actin and desmin when activated in inflammatory and neoplastic processes

References: [1–6, 56–62]

Table 23.8 Markers for benign/reactive epithelium of the gallbladder

Antibodies	GML data (N = 20)
S100P	5/20 Cytoplasmic +
pVHL	20/20
IMP3 (KOC)	5/20 (1+)
Maspin	10/20 1+ Weak
MUC1	2/20
MUC2	1/20
MUC6	19/20
p53	17/20, Weak

Note: *ND* no data, *M* membranous, *C* cytoplasmic, *Focal* less than 25% tumor cells stained

References: [1–3]

Table 23.9 Markers of hepatocellular adenoma

Antibodies	Literature
HepPar-1	+
ER/PR	+/−
CK7	+/− (Patchy)
B-catenin (nuclear)	+ (Beta-catenin type)
Glutamine synthetase	+ (Beta-catenin type)+ (Inflammatory type)
LFABP	+ (Inflammatory type)− (HNF1a type)
Serum amyloid A	+ (Inflammatory type)− (HNF1a type)

Note: *LFABP* liver fatty acid binding protein, *HNF1* HNF1-alpha-mutated subtype characterized by steatosis, *beta-catenin* beta-catenin-mutated subtype characterized by nuclear atypia in males are at greater risk of malignant transformation, *inflammatory* inflammatory/telangiectatic subtype characterized by gp130 mutation and inflammation, sinusoidal dilatation and thick-walled arteries

References: [1–6, 51, 63–76]

Table 23.10 Markers of hepatocellular carcinoma, conventional

Antibodies	Literature	GML data % (*N*)
AE1/AE3	−/+	17 (18)
AFP	−/+	33 (18)
B72.3	−	0 (18)
B-catenin	+/−	100 (18)
BerEP4	−/+	17 (18)
CAM5.2	+	89 (18)
CD10	+/−	61 (18)
CD31	+	100 (18)
CD34	+	100 (18)
CDX2	ND	0 (18)
CK7	−/+	6 (18)
CK17	ND	0 (18)
CK19	−	6 (18)
CK20	−	0 (18)
E-cadherin	ND	94 (18)
EMA	−	0 (18)
Glypican-3	+	72 (18)
HepPar-1	+	94 (18)
KOC (IMP3)	ND	17 (18)
Maspin	ND	0 (18)
MOC31	−/+	22 (18)
mCEA	−	0 (18)
MUC1	ND	0 (18)
MUC2	−	0 (18)
MUC4	ND	0 (18)
MUC5AC	−	0 (18)
MUC6	ND	0 (18)
pCEA	+	94 (18)
RCC	−	11 (18)
S100	−	0 (18)
S100P	ND	11 (18)
TTF-1 (8G7G31)	+/−	11 (18)
VHL	ND	17 (18)
Vimentin	−	0 (18)

(continued)

Table 23.10 (continued)

Note: HepPar-1 and AFP are the markers most characteristic of HCC (Fig. 23.9). A clone of TTF-1 (8G7G31) can focally stain similar to HepPar-1, though as frequently of as strongly in our experience (Fig. 23.10). More recently, Glypican-3 has been noted to be strongly positive in HCC, though this in not entirely specific. CK7 staining of HCC is patchy when present. Beta-catenin showed nuclear staining in two of the 18 HCC (Fig. 23.11). Vimentin and vascular markers CD31 and CD34 show diffuse sinusoidal staining of endothelial cells and do not stain the hepatocellular tumor cells. CD10 and pCEA show canalicular staining pattern

References: [1–14, 16–27, 30–34, 36, 37, 39, 40, 43, 55, 70, 77–81]

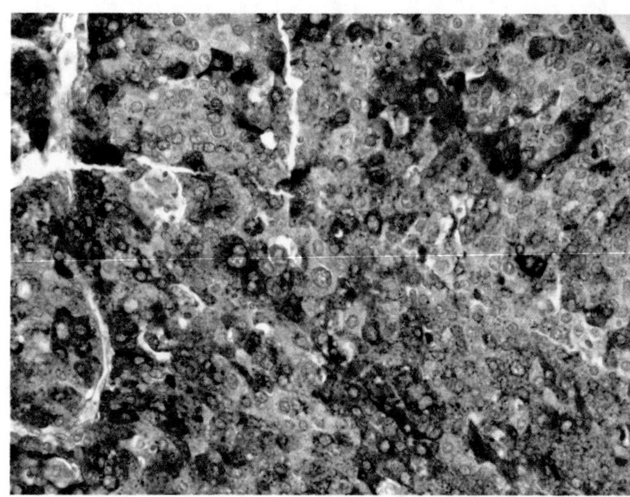

Fig. 23.9 Hepatocellular carcinoma diffuses strong cytoplasmic AFP expression

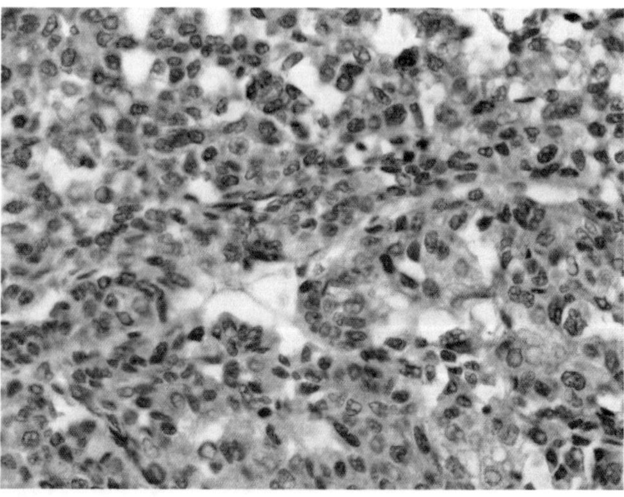

Fig. 23.10 Hepatocellular carcinoma, focal granular hepatocellular staining with TTF-1 clone 8G7G31. It is important to be aware of the expected nuclear pattern of staining that is associated with pulmonary and thyroid tumor to avoid misinterpreting this cytoplasmic finding

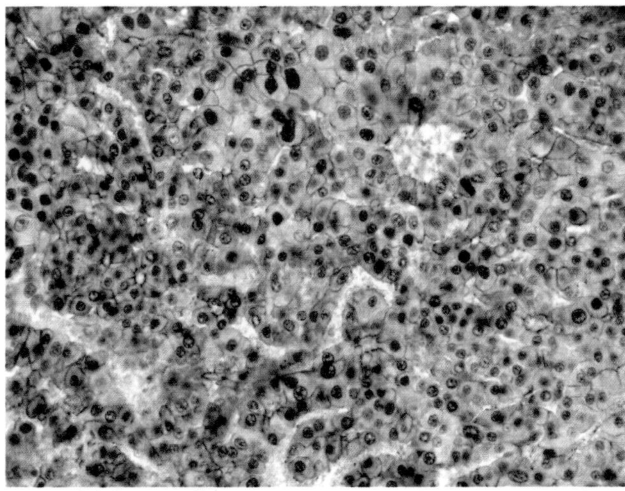

Fig. 23.11 Hepatocellular carcinoma, beta-catenin, is colocalized to the cytoplasmic membranes and the nucleus. Nuclear translocation of beta-catenin is the evidence of neoplasia in a hepatocellular proliferation

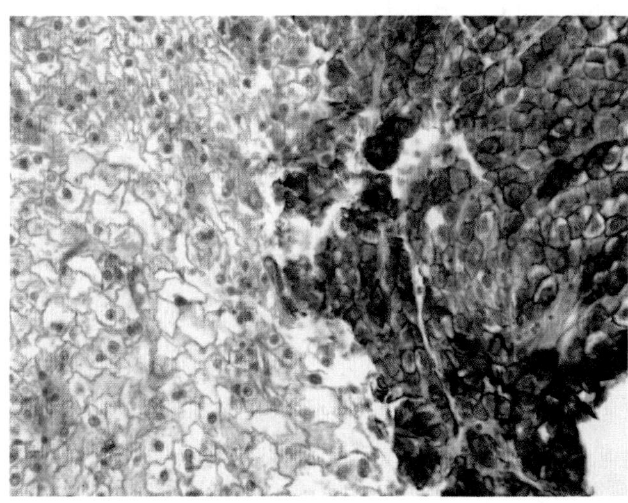

Fig. 23.12 Hepatocellular carcinoma with conventional area on the *right* strongly expressing CAM5.2 with a sharp transition to an area of clear cell variant on the *left* lacking CAM5.2 staining

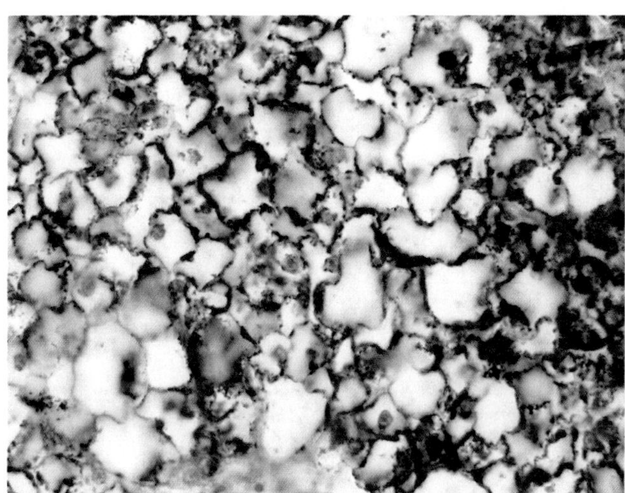

Fig. 23.13 Hepatocellular carcinoma, clear cell variant. The morphologic appearance can be concerning for renal or adrenal carcinomas, but fortunately it maintains the coarse granularity of HepPar-1 characteristic of hepatocellular carcinoma

Table 23.11 Markers of hepatocellular carcinoma variants

Antibodies	HCC	HCC-FL	HCC-clear	HCC-sarc
HepPar-1	+	+	+	+/–
AFP	–/+	–/+	–/+	–/+
Glypican-3	+	–/+	+	+
Synaptophysin	–	+	–	ND
CK7	–/+	+	–/+	+/–
Vimentin	–	–	–	–/+
mCEA	–	–/+	ND	ND
EMA	–/+	+	–	ND

Note: *HCC* conventional HCC, *HCC-FL* fibrolamellar variant of HCC, *HCC-clear* clear cell variant HCC, *HCC-sarc* sarcomatoid variant of HCC

When compared with conventional HCC, clear cell variant of HCC lacks CMA5.2 (Fig. 23.12) and glypican-3 staining, but maintains strong HepPar-1 staining of cytoplasm (Fig. 23.13) and canalicular staining with CD10

References: [1–6, 12, 17, 24, 80, 82–85]

Table 23.12 Markers of hepatoblastoma

Antibodies	Literature
HerPar1	+
AFP	+/–
CK18	+
CK19	+
AE1/AE3	+
Vimentin	+
EMA	+

References: [1–6, 37, 86–92]

Table 23.13 Markers for intrahepatic cholangiocarcinoma

Antibodies	Literature	GML data % (*N*)
AE1/AE3	+	100 (11)
AFP	–/+	0 (11)
B72.3	–/+	18 (11)
B-catenin		100 (11)
BerEP4	+	91 (11)
CAM5.2	+	100 (11)
CD10	–	0 (11)
CD31	–	0 (11)
CD34	–	0 (11)
CDX2	–/+	0 (11)
CK5/6	–/+	9 (11)
CK7	+	100 (11)
CK17	+/–	18 (11)
CK19	+	91 (11)
CK20	–/+	18 (11)
CK903	–/+	18 (11)
E-cadherin	+	100 (11)
EMA	+	73 (11)
ER	–	0 (11)
Glypican-3	–	0 (11)
HepPar-1	–	0 (11)
HMB-45	–	0 (11)
KIM-1	ND	0 (11)
KOC (IMP3)	ND	18 (11)
Maspin	ND	27 (11)
mCEA	+	55 (11)
MOC31	+	100 (11)
MUC1	+	55 (11)
MUC2	–/+	0 (11)
MUC4	–/+	9 (11)
MUC5AC	+/–	0 (11)
MUC6	–/+	9 (11)
NapsinA	ND	0 (11)
P504S	ND	36 (11)
P53	–/+	0 (11)
P63	–/+	9 (11)
pCEA	+	100 (11)
PR	–/+	0 (11)
RCC	ND	0 (11)
S100	ND	0 (11)
S100A6	ND	5 (11)
S100P	ND	10 (10)
TTF-1	ND	0 (11)
VHL	ND	80 (10)
Villin	–/+	9 (11)
Vimentin	ND	18 (11)

Note: *HCC* hepatocellular carcinoma, *CC* cholangiocarcinoma

Intrahepatic CC largely shares the immunophenotype of other upper gastrointestinal and pancreaticobiliary adenocarcinomas. Characteristically, cholangiocarcinoma is associated with sense sclerotic stroma (Fig. 23.14). Immunohistochemically, MOC31 positive and HepPar-1 negative distinguishing it from HCC (Fig. 23.15). There are specific markers of differentiation available for a few of the metastatic adenocarcinomas that share the differential

(continued)

Table 23.13 (continued)

cytokeratin pattern of CK7+, CK20– typical of CC. Unfortunately, the sensitivity of specific markers of metastatic adenocarcinomas is often lacking. In these instances, IHC cannot be definitive and the diagnosis of CC must be made by excluding metastatic adenocarcinoma on clinical and imaging grounds. Beta-catenin staining is membranous in cholangiocarcinoma. The CK20 staining found in rare cholangiocarcinomas is weak. There is some nonspecific background staining in the AFP slides

References: [1–6, 13, 16, 19, 20, 26, 39, 40, 44–51, 55, 81]

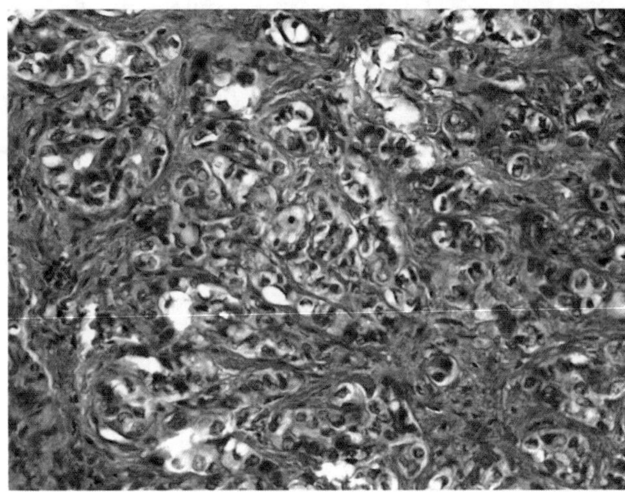

Fig. 23.14 Cholangiocarcinoma, hematoxylin and eosin, staining with the classic appearance of infiltrating small glands with closed lumens in a background of fibrotic stroma

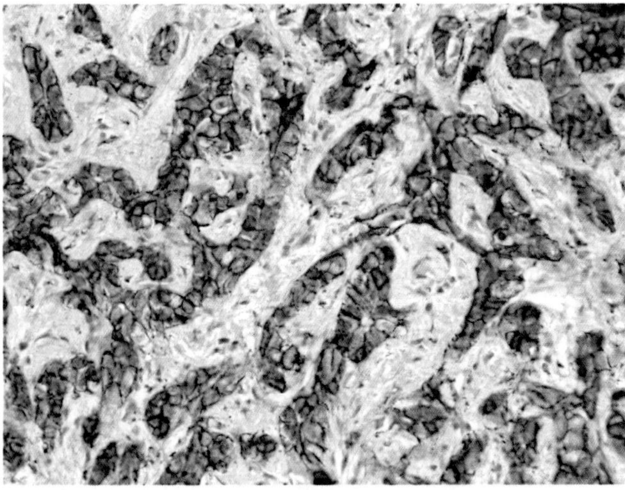

Fig. 23.15 Cholangiocarcinoma with strong membranous pattern of MOC31, which is a very sensitive, but not specific, marker of many types of adenocarcinoma including cholangiocarcinoma

Table 23.14 Markers for adenoma/dysplasia of the gallbladder

Antibodies	Literature
CK7	+
MUC1	v
MUC2	v
MUC5AC	– or +
MUC6	v
Beta-catenin	+ or –
Estrogen receptor	+ or –
pVHL	–
S100P	+
IMP3 (KOC)	+
Maspin	+
p53	+ or –

Note: *MUC1* usually positive in pyloric-type adenoma, *MUC2* usually positive in intestinal-type adenoma, *MUC6* usually positive in pyloric-type or biliary-type adenomas

p53 is usually positive in flat dysplasia but negative in adenoma; approximately 50% of adenomas are positive for ER and demonstrates nuclear positivity for beta-catenin

Our preliminary data show high-grade dysplasia usually demonstrates a loss of pVHL expression and overexpression of S100P, IMP3 (KOC), and maspin

References: [2, 93–96]

Table 23.15 Markers for adenocarcinoma of the gallbladder

Antibodies	Literature
CK7	+
CK20	+ or –
CK19	+
S100P	+
IMP3 (KOC)	+
Maspin	+
pVHL	–
p53	+
CEA	+
CA19-9	+
MUC1	+
MUC5AC	+

References: [2, 94–96]

Table 23.16 Differential diagnosis of tumors with hepatocellular morphology

Antibodies	HCC	HA	FNH	MAC-hepatoid
HepPar-1	+	+	+	–
AFP	–/+	–/+	–/+	+/–
pCEA	+ Canalicular	+ Canalicular	+ Canalicular	+ Canalicular
CK7	–/+	–/+ (Focal hepatocyte)	+ (Bile ductules)	–
CD34	+ Diffuse sinusoidal	+ Focal sinusoidal	+ Limited to periseptal sinusoids	–
ER		–/+		–
MOC31	–	–	–	+
Ber-EP4	–	–	–	+
SALL4	–	ND	ND	+/–
CK20	–	–	–	+/–
Glypican-3	+	–/+	–	+/–

Note: *HA* hepatic adenoma, *DN* dysplastic nodule, *HCC* hepatocellular carcinoma, *FLV* hepatocellular carcinoma, fibrolamellar variant, *HB* hepatoblastoma, *MAC* metastatic adenocarcinomas, *FNH* focal nodular hyperplasia

There are very few markers that can distinguish hepatic adenoma from dysplastic nodule. Fortunately, the presence of cirrhosis indicates a macroregenerative or dysplastic nodule, whereas hepatic adenomas occur in non-cirrhotic livers

References: [1–10, 16–27, 36–40, 73, 74, 91, 97, 98]

Table 23.17 Panel for differential diagnosis of hepatocellular nodules in cirrhosis

Antibodies	Localization	RN/LGDN	HGDN	WD-HCC
Glypican-3	C	–	–/+	+
HSP70	N, C	–	–/+	+
GT	C	–	–/+	+

Note: *RN* regenerative nodule, *LGDN* low-grade dysplastic nodule, *HGDN* high-grade dysplastic nodule, *WD-HCC* well-differentiated HCC, *HSP70* heat shock protein 70, glypican-3, and *GT* glutamine synthetase

Using this three-marker panel, when at least two of them, regardless which, were positive, the sensitivity and specificity for the detection of eHCC-G1 were, respectively, 72 and 100%; the most sensitive combination was HSP70+/GPC3+ (59%) when a two-marker panel was used (Fig. 23.16)

References: [16–19, 99–103]

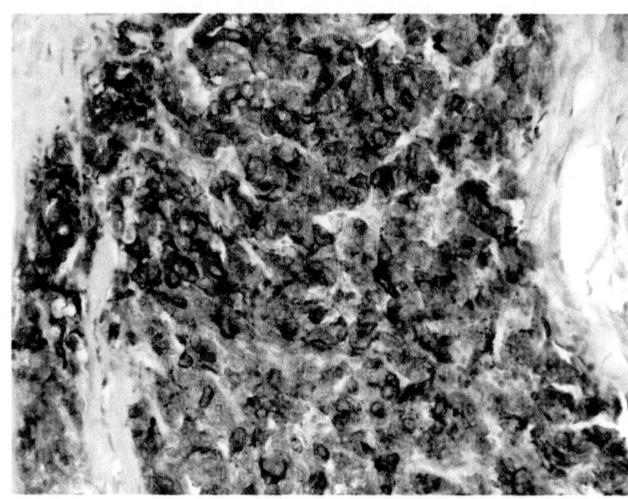

Fig. 23.16 Hepatocellular carcinoma, glypican-3, staining strongly and diffusely staining the cytoplasm is a good indication of high-grade neoplasia in hepatocellular proliferations

Table 23.18 Polygonal and clear cell tumors of the liver

	HCC	RCC	ACC	MEL	SQCC	NEC	LEI	AML	GIST
HepPar-1	+	–	–	–	–	–	–	–	–
pCEA	+	–	–	–	–	–	–	–	–
CD34	+	–	–	–	–	–	–	–/+	–/+
RCC	–	+	–	–	–	–	–	–	–
Inhibin	–	–	+	–	–	–	–	–	–
Vimentin	–	+	+	+	–/+	–/+	+	+	+
HMB-45	–	–	–	+	–	–	–	+	–
Melan-A	–	–	+	+	–	–	–	+	–
CK5	–	–	–	–	+	–	–	+	–
Desmin	–	–	–	–	–	–	+	+	–/+
Chromo	–	–	–	–	–	+	–	–	–
Synap	–	–	+/–	–	–	+	–	–	–
TTF-1[a]	–	–	–	–	–	–	–	–	–
S100	–	+/–	–	+	–/+	–/+	–	–	–/+
EMA	–	+/–	–	–	+	–/+	–/+	–	–
CD117	–/+	–/+[b]	–/+	–/+	–/+	–/+	–/+	–/+	+

Note: *HCC* hepatocellular carcinoma, *RCC* renal cell carcinoma, *ACC* adrenal cortical carcinoma, *MEL* melanoma, *SQCC* squamous cell carcinoma, *NEC* neuroendocrine tumor, *LEI*, epithelioid leiomyosarcoma, *AML* angiomyolipoma, *GIST* gastrointestinal stromal tumor

[a]TTF-1 may show cytoplasmic positivity in HCC

[b]CD117 is usually positive in both renal oncocytoma and chromophobe renal cell carcinoma. May tumors metastatic to the liver can exhibit similar clear cell morphology including HCC (Figs. 23.17–23.19) such as renal cell and adrenal cortical carcinoma. Since clear cell HCC maintains some of its hepatic markers, immunophenotyping should resolve these dilemmas

References: [1–12, 20–27, 36–40, 104, 105]

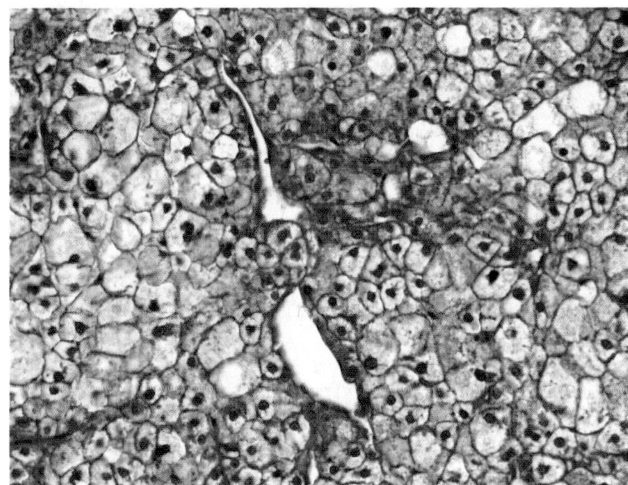

Fig. 23.17 Hepatocellular carcinoma, clear cell variant, hematoxylin and eosin staining with the nonspecific morphology of expanding sheet of polygonal cells with cleared cytoplasm and prominent nucleoli

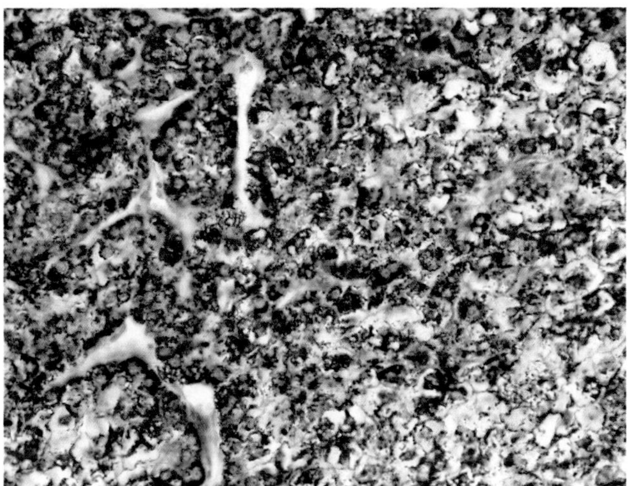

Fig. 23.18 Hepatocellular carcinoma, clear cell variant, with coarse granular HepPar-1 cytoplasmic staining

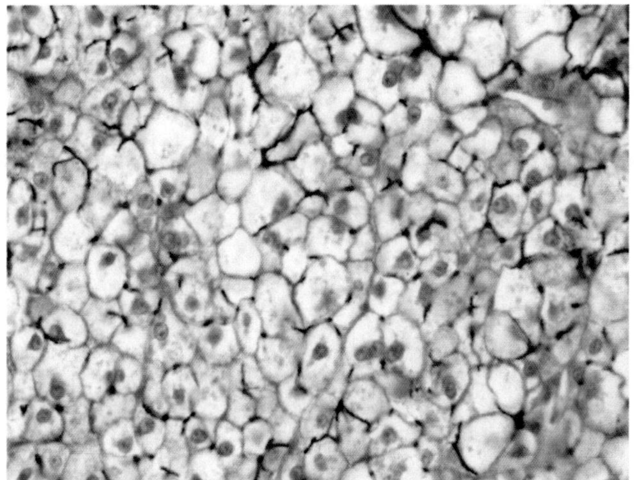

Fig. 23.19 Hepatocellular carcinoma, clear cell variant, demonstrating hepatic origin with canalicular pattern of CD10 staining

Table 23.19 Hepatocellular carcinoma vs. cholangiocarcinoma

Antibodies	HCC	CC
HepPar-1	+	–
AFP	–/+	–
pCEA	+	+
Glypican-3	+	–
CD10	+	–/+
MOC31	–/+	+
CK7	–/+	+
CK19	–	+

Note: pCEA and CD10 show canalicular staining in HCC. Staining with CK7 or MOC31 is not sufficient to diagnose a combine HCC-CC tumor without mixed morphologic features

HCC can show striking pseudoglandular formation simulation the glandular spaces of adenocarcinoma (Fig. 23.20). Fortunately, the clear cell variant of HCC retains diagnostic findings including canalicular architecture by CD10 and pCEA, which demonstrate that the pseudoglandular spaces of HCC are dilated canaliculi (Fig. 23.21). CD34 and CD31 will still demonstrate the "capillarized" transformation of the hepatic sinusoidal endothelial cells rimming the trabeculae of HCC (Fig. 23.22)

References: [1–6, 16–27]

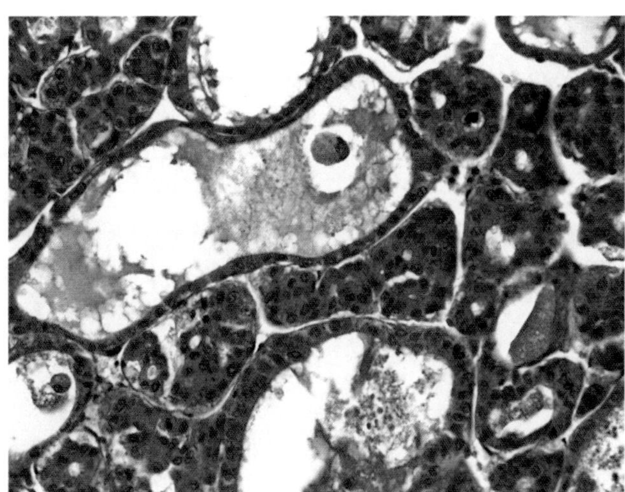

Fig. 23.20 Hepatocellular carcinoma with exaggerated pseudoglandular structures mimicking an adenocarcinoma. Bile is present in some canaliculi given a clue to the true origin

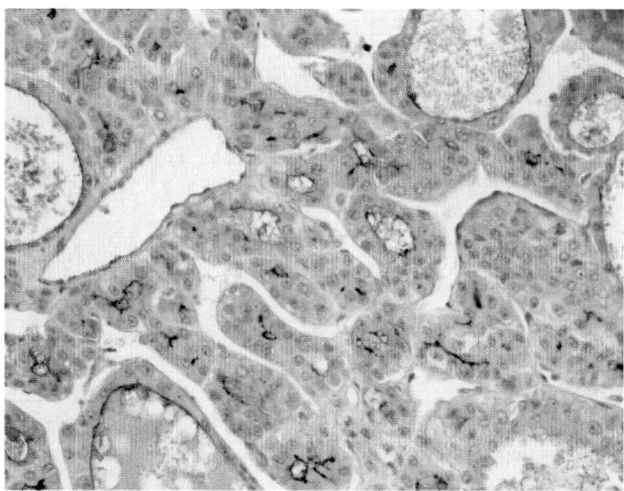

Fig. 23.21 The same hepatocellular carcinoma as in the previous figure stained with pCEA to highlight the canalicular structures including the dilated canalicular spaces mimicking glands

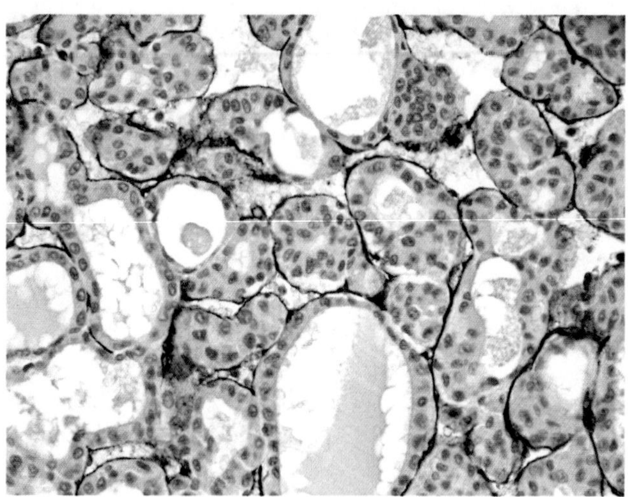

Fig. 23.22 Another section of the pseudoglandular hepatocellular carcinoma with CD31 providing sharp endothelial staining surrounding the expanded hepatocellular nests. The diffuse, complete endothelial lining is very characteristic of hepatocellular carcinoma. CD34 will provide the same pattern of staining

Table 23.20 Reactive epithelial atypia vs. dysplasia/adenocarcinoma of the gallbladder

Antibodies	Dysplasia/ adenocarcinoma	Reactive atypia
S100P	+	–
pVHL	–	+
IMP3 (KOC)	+	–
S100A6	+	–
S100A4	+	–
p53	+	– or focal +
Maspin	+	–
CEA	Cytoplasmic +	Apical surface+

Note: An example of expression of pVHL in normal gallbladder mucosa is shown in Figs. 23.23 and 23.24. In contrast, the loss of expression of pVHL and overexpression of maspin, S100P, and IMP3 typical of adenocarcinoma are demonstrated in Figs. 23.25–23.28 also contrast the benign normal mucosa

References: [2, 94–96]

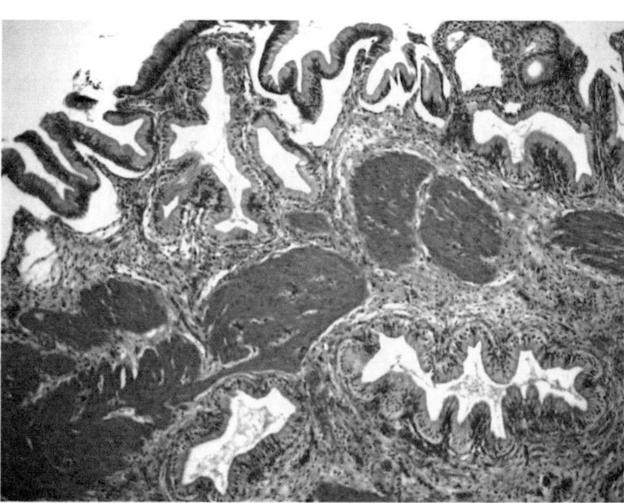

Fig. 23.23 Benign gallbladder with hematoxylin and eosin staining

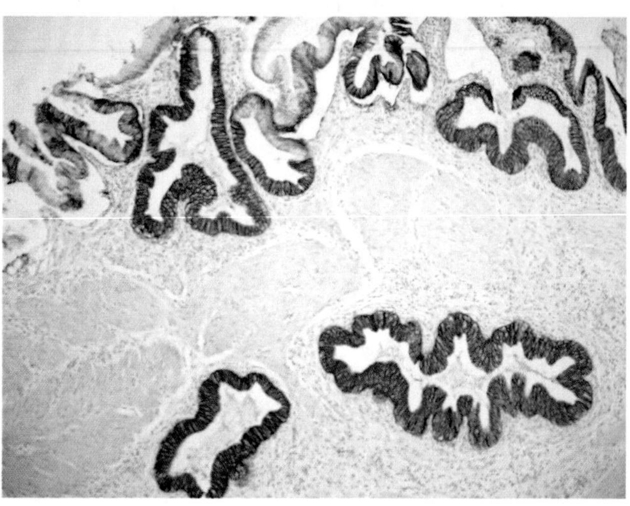

Fig. 23.24 Corresponding section of the benign gallbladder block stained with pVHL demonstrating strong complete staining of glandular epithelium of the benign mucosa

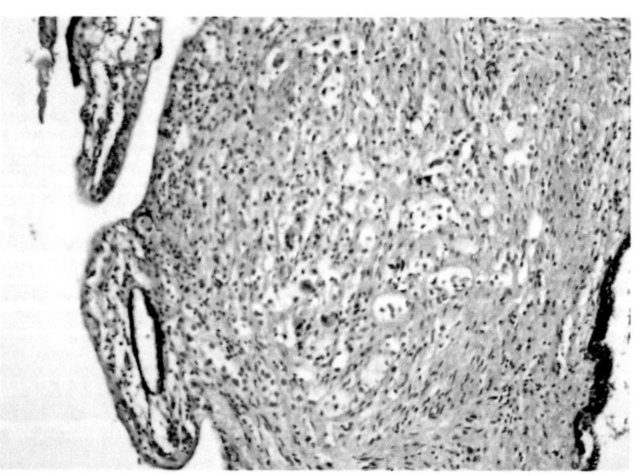

Fig. 23.25 Gallbladder adenocarcinoma, pVHL, highlights the benign surface epithelium, but there is a complete lack of staining of the small invasive tumor nests in the intervening stroma

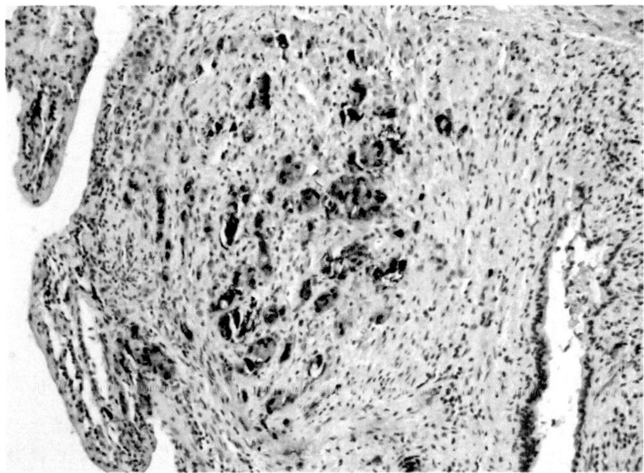

Fig. 23.26 Gallbladder adenocarcinoma, S100P, demonstrates an opposite but complimentary immunoreactivity compared with pVHL. The S100P assay does not stain the benign surface glandular epithelium of the gallbladder section, but does strongly mark the small nest of adenocarcinoma

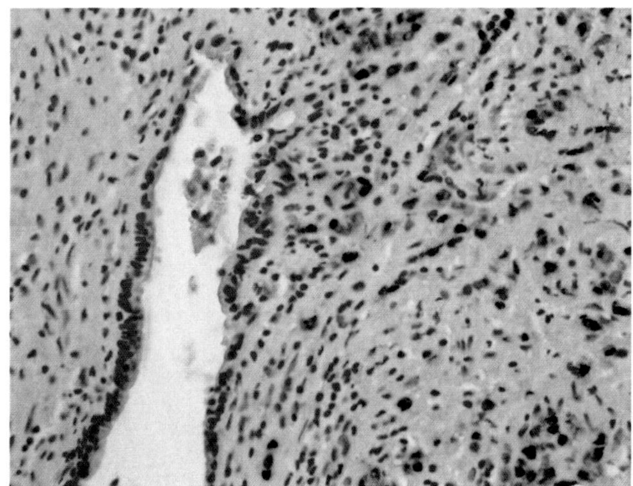

Fig. 23.27 Gallbladder adenocarcinoma, maspin staining performs much like the S100P in this slide by reveal in the small nests and single tumor cells infiltrating adjacent to this unmarked benign epithelium

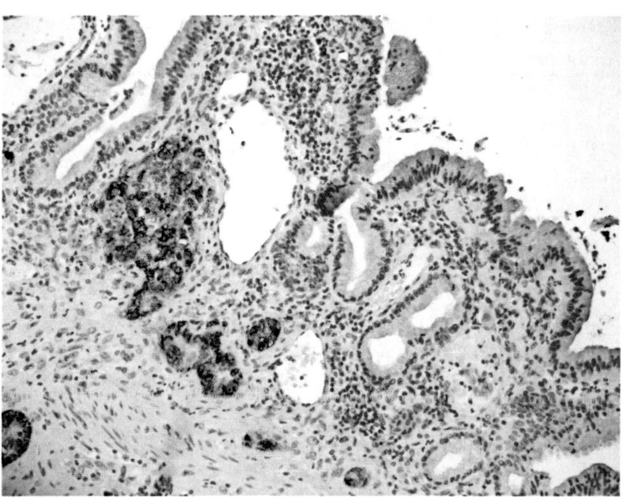

Fig. 23.28 Gallbladder adenocarcinoma, IMP3 (KOC), is another marker capable of differentially staining positively for gallbladder adenocarcinoma while not staining associated benign reactive epithelium

Table 23.21 Reactive biliary epithelium vs. dysplasia/adenocarcinoma of the common bile duct

Antibodies	Reactive atypia	Dysplasia/adenocarcinoma
S100P	– or cytoplasmic	+
pVHL	+	–
IMP3 (KOC)	–	+
Maspin	–	+
CEA	Apical	Cytoplasmic +
p53	– or focal weak	+ or –
Dpc4/SMAD4	+	– or +

References: [2, 106–109]

Table 23.22 Differential diagnosis of biliary tract/pancreas adenocarcinoma

Antibodies	IHCCA GML% (*N*)	PADC	AADC (intestinal)	AADC (pan)	CBADC	GBADC GML% (*N*)
CK17	18 (11)	+	ND	+	+/–	ND
MUC5AC	0 (11)	+	–	+	+/–	+
VHL	80 (10)	–	ND	– or +	–	0 (23)
Maspin	27 (11)	+	ND	+ or –	+	100 (23)
MUC2	0 (11)	–	+	+ or –	–	–
S100P	10 (10)	+	ND	+ or –	+	85 (20)
IMP3	18 (11)	+	ND	+ or –	+	78 (23)
Villin	0 (11)	–	+	+ or –	–/+	ND
CDX2	0 (11)	–	+	–	–/+	ND
CK7	100 (11)	+	– or +	+ or –	+	+
CK20	18 (11)	–	+	–	–	–
HepPar-1	0 (11)	–	+	–	–	–

Note: Our small study series ($N = 11$) of intrahepatic cholangiocarcinomas shows a nearly opposite expression profile in intrahepatic cholangioCA compared with other biliary tract carcinomas (pancreas, common bile duct and ampullary ADC, biliary type), in which pVHL is expressed and the loss of expression of maspin and S100P is noted. An example of this staining in intrahepatic cholangioCA is demonstrated in Fig. 23.29. This may provide a method to differentiate primary intrahepatic cholangiocarcinoma from metastatic adenocarcinoma to the liver

The percentages are based on the data from Geisinger Medical Laboratory (GML)

IHCCA intrahepatic cholangiocarcinoma, *PADC* pancreatic adenocarcinoma, *AADC (intestinal type)* ampullary adenocarcinoma, intestinal type, *AADC (pan)* ampullary adenocarcinoma, biliary type, *CBADC* common bile duct adenocarcinoma, *GBADC* gallbladder adenocarcinoma

References: [1–3, 106–110]

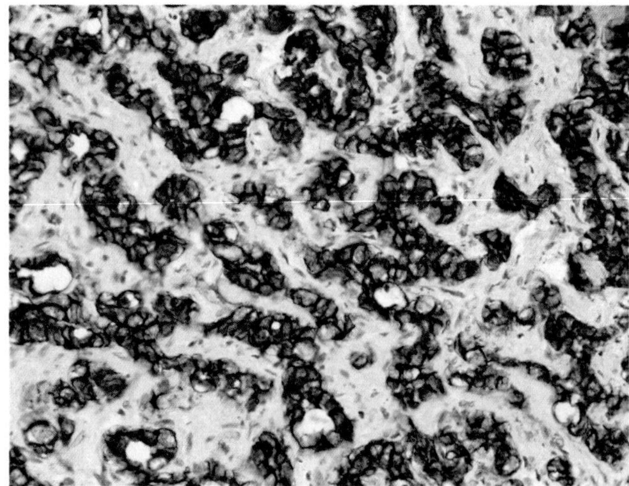

Fig. 23.29 Intrahepatic cholangiocarcinoma; in extrahepatic biliary adenocarcinoma, there is consistent negative staining with pVHL and complementary positive staining of maspin, S100P, and IMP3 (KOC). Surprisingly, the immunoreactivities are reversed with intrahepatic cholangiocarcinomas with strong staining for pVHL and as seen in this figure and lack of staining for these other antibodies

Table 23.23 Initial four marker screening IHC panel for unknown primary tumor in liver

GROUP	Diagnoses	HepPar-1	MOC-31	CK7	CK20
Group 1	Hepatocellular carcinoma	+	–	–/+	–
Group 2	Metastatic hepatoid carcinoma	+	+	–	+
Group 3	Breast adenocarcinoma	+	+	+	–
	Lung adenocarcinoma				
Group 4	Cholangiocarcinoma	–	+	+	–
	Breast adenocarcinoma				
	Lung adenocarcinoma				
	Upper GI adenocarcinoma				
	Pancreaticobiliary adenocarcinoma				
	Endocervical adenocarcinoma				
	Urothelial carcinoma				
	Neuroendocrine turnor				
Group 5	Cholangiocarcinoma	–	+	+	+
	Neuroendocrine tumor				
	Upper GI adenocarcinoma				
	Pancreaticobiliary adenocarcinoma				
	Mucinous lung adenocarcinoma				
	Urothelial carcinoma				
Group 6	Colorectal adeno-carcinoma	–	+	–	+
	Appendiceal adenocarcinoma				
	Small intestinal adenocarcinoma				
	Merkel cell carcinoma				
Group 7	Squamous cell carcinoma	–	+	–	–
	Renal cell carcinoma				
	Medullary colorectal adenocarcinoma				
	Neuroendocrine carcinoma				
	Adernal corticalcinoma				
	Prostate adenocarcinoma				
	Germ cell tumor				
Group 8	Mesothelioma	–	–	+	–
Group 9	Sarcoma	–	–	–	–
	Angiomyolipoma				
	Hematopoietic tumor				
	Melanoma				
	Poorly differentiated carcinoma				

Note: An initial screening panel for tumor or unknown origin in the liver could include HepPar-1, MOC-31, CK7, and CK20. The findings from this group of stains should lead to a more limited differential diagnosis for which specific confirmatory stains can be chosen from the next table. It is not always possible to determine the origin of a tumor, in which case, excluded sites and a group of possible site of origin can be included in the report

References: [1–6, 20–41, 51, 75, 76, 91, 92, 98, 104, 105, 112–116]

Table 23.24 Confirmatory markers of unknown primary tumors of liver

Tumors	Antibodies
Renal cell carcinoma	RCC, VHL, PAX8, CD10, KIM-1
Hepatocellular carcinoma	Glypican-3, CD34 (sinusoidal), CD10/pCEA canalicular
Melanoma	S100, HMB-45, Melan-A, Mart-1
Breast adenocarcinoma	GCDFP-15, mammaglobin, ER, PR
Medullary colorectal carcinoma	Negative MSI markers, MSH2, MSH6, MLH1, PMS2
Lung adenocarcinoma	NapsinA, TTF-1, surfactant
Upper GI adenocarcinoma	CDX-2
Endocervical adenocarcinoma	HPV ISH, p16, mCEA
Metastatic hepatoid carcinoma	SALL4
Neuroendocrine carcinoma	Chromogranin, synaptophysin, CD56
Mesothelioma	Calretinin, CK5/6, WT1
Prostate adenocarcinoma	PSA, PAP, P504S
Urothelial carcinoma	CK5/6, p63, thrombomodulin, Uroplakin III

Note: Once the results of the initial screening IHC panel have narrowed down the differential diagnosis, choose confirmatory stains based on the morphology ad clinical setting. Immunoreactivity for these confirmatory stains should further characterize the tumor. Some tumors may not express a differentiated immunoprofile by IHC, and the differential will rely on clinical findings. For additional markers related to tumors of unknown primary, refer to Chap. 7

References: [1–6, 16–40, 42, 43, 51, 55, 75, 76, 91, 98]

Note for All Tables

Note: "+" – usually greater than 70% of cases are positive; "–" – less than 5% of cases are positive; "+ or –" – usually more than 50% of cases are positive; "– or +" – less than 50% of cases are positive.

References

1. Chu PG, Weiss LM. Modern immunohistochemistry. New York, NY: Cambridge University Press; 2009.
2. Dabbs DJ. Diagnostic immunohistochemistry. 3rd ed. Philadelphia, PA: Churchill Livingstone Elsevier; 2010.
3. Taylor C, Cote R. Immunomicroscopy a diagnostic tool for the surgical pathologist, Major problems in pathology. 3rd ed. Philadelphia, PA: Saunders Elsevier; 2006.
4. Geller SA, Dhall D, Alsabeh R. Application of immunohistochemistry to liver and gastrointestinal neoplasms: liver, stomach, colon, and pancreas. Arch Pathol Lab Med. 2008;132(3):490–9.
5. Mills SE. Histology for pathologists. 3rd ed. Philadelphia: Lippincott Williams & Wilkins; 2007. p. 696–7.
6. Burt AD, Portmann BC, Ferrell LD. MacSween's pathology of the liver. 5th ed. Philadelphia: Churchill Livingstone Elsevier; 2007. p. 20–45.
7. De Young BR, Frierson Jr HF, Ly MN, Smith D, Swanson PE. CD31 immunoreactivity in carcinomas and mesotheliomas. Am J Clin Pathol. 1998;110(3):374–7.
8. de Boer WB, Segal A, Frost FA, Sterrett GF. Can CD34 discriminate between benign and malignant hepatocytic lesions in fine-needle aspirates and thin core biopsies? Cancer. 2000;90(5):273–8.
9. Gottschalk-Sabag S, Ron N, Glick T. Use of CD34 and factor VIII to diagnose hepatocellular carcinoma on fine needle aspirates. Acta Cytol. 1998;42(3):691–6.
10. Coston WM, Loera S, Lau SK, Ishizawa S, Jiang Z, Wu CL, et al. Distinction of hepatocellular carcinoma from benign hepatic mimickers using Glypican-3 and CD34 immunohistochemistry. Am J Surg Pathol. 2008;32(3):433–44.
11. Lin F, Shi J, Liu H, et al. Immunohistochemical detection of the von Hippel–Lindau gene product (pVHL) in human tissues and tumors: a useful marker for metastatic renal cell carcinoma and clear cell carcinoma of the ovary and uterus. Am J Clin Pathol. 2008;129(4):592–605.
12. Shah S, Gupta S, Shet T, Maheshwari A, Wuntkal R, Mohandas KM. Metastatic clear cell variant of hepatocellular carcinoma with an occult hepatic primary. Hepatobiliary Pancreat Dis Int. 2005;4(2):306–7.
13. Maeda T, Kajiyama K, Adachi E, Takenaka K, Sugimachi K, Tsuneyoshi M. The expression of cytokeratins 7, 19, and 20 in primary and metastatic carcinomas of the liver. Mod Pathol. 1996;9(9):901–9.
14. Rullier A, Le Bail B, Fawaz R, Blanc JF, Saric J, Bioulac-Sage P. Cytokeratin 7 and 20 expression in cholangiocarcinomas varies along the biliary tract but still differs from that in colorectal carcinoma metastasis. Am J Surg Pathol. 2000;24(6):870–6.
15. Harder J, Waiz O, Otto F, Geissler M, Olschewski M, Weinhold B, et al. EGFR and HER2 expression in advanced biliary tract cancer. World J Gastroenterol. 2009;15(36):4511–7.
16. Kandil DH, Cooper K. Glypican-3: a novel diagnostic marker for hepatocellular carcinoma and more. Adv Anat Pathol. 2009;16(2):125–9.
17. Shafizadeh N, Ferrell LD, Kakar S. Utility and limitations of glypican-3 expression for the diagnosis of hepatocellular carcinoma at both ends of the differentiation spectrum. Mod Pathol. 2008;21(8):1011–8. Epub 6 Jun 2008.
18. Wang HL, Anatelli F, Zhai QJ, Adley B, Chuang ST, Yang XJ. Glypican-3 as a useful diagnostic marker that distinguishes hepatocellular carcinoma from benign hepatocellular mass lesions. Arch Pathol Lab Med. 2008;132(11):1723–8.
19. Yamauchi N, Watanabe A, Hishinuma M, Ohashi K, Midorikawa Y, Morishita Y, et al. The glypican 3 oncofetal protein is a promising diagnostic marker for hepatocellular carcinoma. Mod Pathol. 2005;18(12):1591–8.
20. Christensen WN, Boitnott JK, Kuhajda FP. Immunoperoxidase staining as a diagnostic aid for hepatocellular carcinoma. Mod Pathol. 1989;2(1):8–12.

21. Varma V, Cohen C. Immunohistochemical and molecular markers in the diagnosis of hepatocellular carcinoma. Adv Anat Pathol. 2004;11(5):239–49.
22. Haratake J, Hashimoto H. An immunohistochemical analysis of 13 cases with combined hepatocellular and cholangiocellular carcinoma. Liver. 1995;15(1):9–15.
23. Fanni D, Nemolato S, Ganga R, Senes G, Gerosa C, Van Eyken P, et al. Cytokeratin 20-positive hepatocellular carcinoma. Eur J Histochem. 2009;53(4):269–73.
24. Kakar S, Gown AM, Goodman ZD, Ferrell LD. Best practices in diagnostic immunohistochemistry: hepatocellular carcinoma versus metastatic neoplasms. Arch Pathol Lab Med. 2007;131(11):1648–54.
25. Krishna M. Diagnosis of metastatic neoplasms: an immunohistochemical approach. Arch Pathol Lab Med. 2010;134(2):207–15.
26. Lau SK, Prakash S, Geller SA, Alsabeh R. Comparative immunohistochemical profile of hepatocellular carcinoma, cholangiocarcinoma, and metastatic adenocarcinoma. Hum Pathol. 2002;33(12):1175–81.
27. Wieczorek TJ, Pinkus JL, Glickman JN, Pinkus GS. Comparison of thyroid transcription factor-1 and hepatocyte antigen immunohistochemical analysis in the differential diagnosis of hepatocellular carcinoma, metastatic adenocarcinoma, renal cell carcinoma, and adrenal cortical carcinoma. Am J Clin Pathol. 2002;118:911–21.
28. Van Eyken P. Cytokeratin immunohistochemistry in liver histopatology. Adv Clin Pathol. 2000;4(4):201–11.
29. Zatloukal K, Stumptner C, Fuchsbichler A, Fickert P, Lackner C, Trauner M, et al. The keratin cytoskeleton in liver diseases. J Pathol. 2004;204(4):367–76.
30. Yang XR, Xu Y, Shi GM, Fan J, Zhou J, Ji Y, et al. Cytokeratin 10 and cytokeratin 19: predictive markers for poor prognosis in hepatocellular carcinoma patients after curative resection. Clin Cancer Res. 2008;14(12):3850–9.
31. Yong X-R, Xu Y, Shi G-M, Fan J, Zhou J, Ji Y, et al. Cytokeratin 10 and cytokeratin 19: predictive markers for poor prognosis in hepatocellular carcinoma patients after curative resection. Clin Cancer Res. 2008;14(12):3850–9.
32. Lackner C, Gogg-Kamerer M, Zatloukal K, Stumptner C, Brunt EM, Denk H. Ballooned hepatocytes in steatohepatitis: the value of keratin immunohistochemistry for diagnosis. J Hepatol. 2008;48(5):821–8. Epub 22 Feb 2008.
33. Lee MJ, Lee HS, Kim WH, Choi Y, Yang M. Expression of mucins and cytokeratins in primary carcinomas of the digestive system. Mod Pathol. 2003;16(5):403–10.
34. Listrom MB, Dalton LW. Comparison of keratin monoclonal antibodies MAK-6, AE1:AE3, and CAM-5.2. Am J Clin Pathol. 1987;88(3):297–301.
35. Jain R, Fischer S, Serra S, Chetty R. The use of cytokeratin 19 (CK19) immunohistochemistry in lesions of the pancreas, gastrointestinal tract, and liver. Appl Immunohistochem Mol Morphol. 2010;18(1):9–15.
36. Lefkowitch JH. Special stains in diagnostic liver pathology. Semin Diagn Pathol. 2006;23(3–4):190–8.
37. Fan Z, van de Rijn M, Montgomery K, Rouse RV. Hep par 1 antibody stain for the differential diagnosis of hepatocellular carcinoma: 676 tumors tested using tissue microarrays and conventional tissue sections. Mod Pathol. 2003;16(2):137–44.
38. Roskams T. The role of immunohistochemistry in diagnosis. Clin Liver Dis. 2002;6(2):571–89.
39. Morrison C, Marsh Jr W, Frankel WL. A comparison of CD10 to pCEA, MOC-31, and hepatocyte for the distinction of malignant tumors in the liver. Mod Pathol. 2002;15(12):1279–87.
40. Porcell AI, De Young BR, Proca DM, Frankel WL. Immunohistochemical analysis of hepatocellular and adenocarcinoma in the liver: MOC31 compares favorably with other putative markers. Mod Pathol. 2000;13(7):773–8.
41. Weinreb I, Cunningham KS, Perez-Ordoñez B, Hwang DM. CD10 is expressed in most epithelioid hemangioendotheliomas: a potential diagnostic pitfall. Arch Pathol Lab Med. 2009;133(12):1965–8.
42. Gu K, Shah V, Ma C, Zhang L, Yang M. Cytoplasmic immunoreactivity of thyroid transcription factor-1 (clone 8G7G3/1) in hepatocytes: true positivity or cross-reaction? Am J Clin Pathol. 2007;128(3):382–8.
43. Pan C-C, Chen PC-H, Tsay S-H, Chiang H. Cytoplasmic immunoreactivity for thyroid transcription factor-1 in hepatocellular carcinoma. A comparative immunohistochemical analysis of four commercial antibodies using a tissue array technique. Am J Clin Pathol. 2004;121:343–9.
44. Batheja N, Suriawinata A, Saxena R, Ionescu G, Schwartz M, Thung SN. Expression of p53 and PCNA in cholangiocarcinoma and primary sclerosing cholangitis. Mod Pathol. 2000;13(12):1265–8.
45. Kanamoto M, Yoshizumi T, Ikegami T, Imura S, Morine Y, Ikemoto T, et al. Cholangiolocellular carcinoma containing hepatocellular carcinoma and cholangiocellular carcinoma, extremely rare tumor of the liver: a case report. J Med Invest. 2008;55(1–2):161–5.
46. Kang YK, Kim WH, Jang JJ. Expression of G1-S modulators (p53, p16, p27, cyclin D1, Rb) and Smad4/Dpc4 in intrahepatic cholangiocarcinoma. Hum Pathol. 2002;33(9):877–83.
47. Mosnier JF, Kandel C, Cazals-Hatem D, Bou-Hanna C, Gournay J, Jarry A, et al. N-cadherin serves as diagnostic biomarker in intrahepatic and perihilar cholangiocarcinomas. Mod Pathol. 2009;22(2):182–90. Epub 11 Jul 2008.
48. Nakanuma Y, Harada K, Ishikawa A, Zen Y, Sasaki M. Anatomic and molecular pathology of intrahepatic cholangiocarcinoma. J Hepatobiliary Pancreat Surg. 2003;10(4):265–81.
49. Rizzi PM, Ryder SD, Portmann B, Ramage JK, Naoumov NV, Williams R. p53 Protein overexpression in cholangiocarcinoma arising in primary sclerosing cholangitis. Gut. 1996;38(2):265–8.
50. Röcken C, Pross M, Brucks U, Ridwelski K, Roessner A. Cholangiocarcinoma occurring in a liver with multiple bile duct hamartomas (von Meyenburg complexes). Arch Pathol Lab Med. 2000;124(11):1704–6.
51. Nash JW, Morrison C, Frankel WL. The utility of estrogen receptor and progesterone receptor immunohistochemistry in the distinction of metastatic breast carcinoma from other tumors in the liver. Arch Pathol Lab Med. 2003;127(12):1591–5.
52. Esheba GE, Longacre TA, Atkins KA, Higgins JP. Expression of the urothelial differentiation markers GATA3 and placental S100 (S100P) in female genital tract transitional cell proliferations. Am J Surg Pathol. 2009;33(3):347–53.
53. Findeis-Hosey JJ, Yang Q, Spaulding BO, Wang HL, Xu H. IMP3 expression is correlated with histologic grade of lung adenocarcinoma. Human Pathol. 2010;41(4):477–84. Epub 11 Dec 2009.
54. Lu D, Vohra P, Chu PG, Woda B, Rock KL, Jiang Z. An oncofetal protein IMP3: a new molecular marker for the detection of esophageal adenocarcinoma and high-grade dysplasia. Am J Surg Pathol. 2009;33(4):521–5.
55. Werling RW, Yaziji H, Bacchi CE, Gown AM. CDX2, a highly sensitive and specific marker of adenocarcinomas of intestinal origin: an immunohistochemical survey of 476 primary and metastatic carcinomas. Am J Surg Pathol. 2003;27(3):303–10.
56. Jarmay K, Gallai M, Karacsony G, et al. Decorin and actin expression and distribution in patients with chronic hepatitis C following interferon-alpha-2b-treatment. J Hepatol. 2000;32:993–1002.
57. Knittel T, Kobold D, Saile B, et al. Rat liver myofibroblasts and hepatic stellate cells: different cell populations of the fibroblast lineage with fibrogenic potential. Gastroenterology. 1999;117:1205–21.
58. Moreira RK. Hepatic stellate cells and liver fibrosis. Arch Pathol Lab Med. 2007;131(11):1728–34.

59. Okabe H, Beppu T, Hayashi H, Horino K, Masuda T, Komori H, et al. Hepatic stellate cells may relate to progression of intrahepatic cholangiocarcinoma. Ann Surg Oncol. 2009;16(9):2555–64. Epub 23 Jun 2009.
60. Snover D. Immunohistochemical analysis in steatohepatitis: does it have a role in diagnosis and management? Am J Clin Pathol. 2005;123(4):491–3.
61. Svegliati Baroni G, D'Ambrosio L, Ferretti G, et al. Fibrogenic effect of oxidative stress on rat hepatic stellate cells. J Hepatol. 1999;30:868–75.
62. Tomanovic NR, Boricic IV, Brasanac DC, Stojsic ZM, Delic DS, Brmbolic BJ. Activated liver stellate cells in chronic viral C hepatitis: histopathological and immunohistochemical study. J Gastrointestin Liver Dis. 2009;18(2):163–7.
63. Bioulac-Sage P, Balabaud C, Bedossa P, et al. Pathological diagnosis of liver cell adenoma and focal nodular hyperplasia: Bordeaux update. J Hepatol. 2007;46:521–7.
64. Bioulac-Sage P, Balabaud C, Zucman-Rossi J. Subtype classification of hepatocellular adenoma. Dig Surg. 2010;27(1):39–45. Epub 1 Apr 2010.
65. Bioulac-Sage P, Blanc JF, Rebouissou S, Balabaud C, Zucman-Rossi J. Genotype phenotype classification of hepatocellular adenoma. World J Gastroenterol. 2007;13(19):2649–54.
66. Bioulac-Sage P, Laumonier H, Couchy G, Le Bail B, Sa Cunha A, Rullier A, et al. Hepatocellular adenoma management and phenotypic classification: the Bordeaux experience. Hepatology. 2009;50(2):481–9.
67. Bioulac-Sage P, Laumonier H, Laurent C, Zucman-Rossi J, Balabaud C. Hepatocellular adenoma: what is new in 2008. Hepatol Int. 2008;2(3):316–21. Epub 1 May 2008.
68. Chen ZM, Crone KG, Watson MA, Pfeifer JD, Wang HL. Identification of a unique gene expression signature that differentiates hepatocellular adenoma from well-differentiated hepatocellular carcinoma. Am J Surg Pathol. 2005;29:1600–8.
69. Cohen C, Lawson D, DeRose PB. Sex and androgenic steroid receptor expression in hepatic adenomas. Human Pathology. 1998;29(12):1428–32.
70. Micchelli ST, Vivekanandan P, Boitnott JK, Pawlik TM, Choti MA, Torbenson M. Malignant transformation of hepatic adenomas. Mod Pathol. 2008;21:491–7.
71. Torbenson M, Lee JH, Choti M, et al. Hepatic adenomas: analysis of sex steroid receptor status and the Wnt signaling pathway. Mod Pathol. 2002;15(3):189–96.
72. Zucman-Rossi J, Jeannot E, Tran Van Nhieu J, et al. Genotype–phenotype correlation in hepatocellular adenoma: new classification and relationship with HCC. Hepatology. 2006;43:515–24.
73. Ahmad I, Iyer A, Marginean CE, Yeh MM, Ferrell L, Qin L, et al. Diagnostic use of cytokeratins, CD34, and neuronal cell adhesion molecule staining in focal nodular hyperplasia and hepatic adenoma. Hum Pathol. 2009;40(5):726–34. Epub 20 Jan 2009.
74. Rebouissou S, Bioulac-Sage P, Zucman-Rossi J. Molecular pathogenesis of focal nodular hyperplasia and hepatocellular adenoma. J Hepatol. 2008;48(1):163–70.
75. Masood S, West AB, Barwick KW. Expression of steroid hormone receptors in benign hepatic tumors. An immunocytochemical study. Arch Pathol Lab Med. 1992;116(12):1355–9.
76. Yamamoto M, Nakajo S, Tahara E. Immunohistochemical analysis of estrogen receptors in human gallbladder. Acta Pathol Jpn. 1990;40(1):14–21.
77. Chen Ban K, Singh H, Krishnan R, Fong Seow H. Comparison of the expression of beta-catenin in hepatocellular carcinoma in areas with high and low levels of exposure to aflatoxin B1. J Surg Oncol. 2004;86(3):157–63.
78. Torbenson M, Kannangai R, Abraham S, Sahin F, Choti M, Wang J. Concurrent evaluation of p53, beta-catenin, and alpha-fetoprotein expression in human hepatocellular carcinoma. Am J Clin Pathol. 2004;122:377–82.
79. Peroukides S, Bravou V, Alexopoulos A, Varakis J, Kalofonos H, Papadaki H. Survivin overexpression in HCC and liver cirrhosis differentially correlates with p-STAT3 and E-cadherin. Histol Histopathol. 2010;25(3):299–307.
80. Malouf G, Falissard B, Azoulay D, Callea F, Ferrell LD, Goodman ZD, et al. Is histological diagnosis of primary liver carcinomas with fibrous stroma reproducible among experts? J Clin Pathol. 2009;62(6):519–24. Epub 20 Jan 2009.
81. Lau SK, Weiss LM, Chu PG. Differential expression of MUC1, MUC2, and MUC5AC in carcinomas of various sites: an immunohistochemical study. Am J Clin Pathol. 2004;122(1):61–9.
82. Cho MS, Lee SN, Sung SH, Han WS. Sarcomatoid hepatocellular carcinoma with hepatoblastoma-like features in an adult. Pathol Int. 2004;54(6):446–50.
83. Fu Y, Kobayashi S, Kushida Y, Saoo K, Haba R, Mori S, et al. Sarcomatoid hepatocellular carcinoma with chondroid variant: case report with immunohistochemical findings. Pathol Int. 2000;50(11):919–22.
84. Górnicka B, Ziarkiewicz-Wróblewska B, Wróblewski T, Wilczynski GM, Koperski L, Krawczyk M, et al. Carcinoma, a fibrolamellar variant–immunohistochemical analysis of 4 cases. Hepatogastroenterology. 2005;52(62):519–23.
85. Ward SC, Huang J, Tickoo SK, Thung SN, Ladanyi M, Klimstra DS. Fibrolamellar carcinoma of the liver exhibits immunohistochemical evidence of both hepatocyte and bile duct differentiation. Mod Pathol. 2010;23(9):1180–90.
86. Abenoza P, Manivel JC, Wick MR, Hagen K, Dehner LP. Hepatoblastoma: an immunohistochemical and ultrastructural study. Hum Pathol. 1987;18(10):1025–35.
87. Cajaiba MM, Neves JI, Casarotti FF, de Camargo B, ChapChap P, Sredni ST, et al. Hepatoblastomas and liver development: a study of cytokeratin immunoexpression in twenty-nine hepatoblastomas. Pediatr Dev Pathol. 2006;9(3):196–202.
88. López-Terrada D, Gunaratne PH, Adesina AM, Pulliam J, Hoang DM, Nguyen Y, et al. Histologic subtypes of hepatoblastoma are characterized by differential canonical Wnt and Notch pathway activation in DLK+ precursors. Hum Pathol. 2009;40(6):783–94. Epub 5 Feb 2009.
89. Stocker JT. Hepatoblastoma. Semin Diagn Pathol. 1994;11(2): 136–43.
90. Warfel KA, Hull MT. Hepatoblastomas: an ultrastructural and immunohistochemical study. Ultrastruct Pathol. 1992;16(4): 451–61.
91. Ushiku T, Shinozaki A, Shibhara J, et al. SALL4 represents fetal gut differentiation of gastric cancer, and is diagnostically useful in distinguishing hepatoid gastric carcinoma from hepatocellular carcinoma. Am J Surg Pathol. 2010;34:533–40.
92. Machado I, Noguera R, Santonja N, Donat J, Fernandez-Delgado R, Acevedo A, et al. Immunohistochemical study as a tool in differential diagnosis of pediatric malignant rhabdoid tumor. Appl Immunohistochem Mol Morphol. 2010;18(2):150–8.
93. Lin F, Liu H, Shi J, Xu Y, Zhang J, Wang HL. Diagnostic utility of von Hipple–Lindau gene product (pVHL) and S100P in adenocarcinoma and dysplasia of the gallbladder. Abstract presentation in CAP 2009.
94. Lin F, Shi J, Wang HL, Liu H. Diagnostic utility of von Hipple–Lindau gene product (pVHL), maspin, KOC, and S100P in adenocarcinoma of the gallbladder. Accepted for poster presentation in the coming USCAP meeting, 2010 in Washington, DC.
95. Nagata S et al. Co-expression of gastric and biliary. Oncol Rep. 2007;17:721–9.
96. Shibahara H et al. Pathologic features of mucin. Am J Surg Pathol. 2004;28:327–38.

97. Yang GC, Yang GY, Tao LC. Distinguishing well-differentiated hepatocellular carcinoma from benign liver by the physical features of fine-needle aspirates. Mod Pathol. 2004;17(7):798–802.
98. Terracciano LM, Glatz K, Mhawech P, et al. Hepatoid adenocarcinoma with liver metastasis mimicking hepatocellular carcinoma. Am J Surg Pathol. 2003;27:1302–12.
99. Di Tommaso L, Destro A, Seok JY, Balladore E, Terracciano L, Sangiovanni A, et al. The application of markers (HSP70 GPC3 and GS) in liver biopsies is useful for detection of hepatocellular carcinoma. J Hepatol. 2009;50(4):746–54. Epub 25 Dec 2008.
100. Di Tommaso L, Franchi G, Park YN, Fiamengo B, Destro A, Morenghi E, et al. Diagnostic value of HSP70, glypican 3, and glutamine synthetase in hepatocellular nodules in cirrhosis. Hepatology. 2007;45(3):725–34.
101. Hytiroglou P, Theise ND. Differential diagnosis of hepatocellular nodular lesions. Semin Diagn Pathol. 1998;15(4):285–99.
102. Libbrecht L, Severi T, Cassiman D, et al. Glycipan-3 expression distinguishes small hepatocellular carcinomas from cirrhosis, dysplastic nodules, and focal nodular hyperplasia-like nodules. Am J Surg Pathol. 2006;30:1405–11.
103. Roskams T, Kojiro M. Pathology of early hepatocellular carcinoma: conventional and molecular diagnosis. Semin Liver Dis. 2010;30(1):17–25. Epub 19 Feb 2010.
104. Hornick JL, Fletcher CD. PEComa: what do we know so far? Histopathology. 2006;48(1):75–82.
105. Tryggvason G, Blöndal S, Goldin RD, Albrechtsen J, Björnsson J, Jónasson JG. Epithelioid angiomyolipoma of the liver: case report and review of the literature. APMIS. 2004;112(9):612–6.
106. Chu PG, Schwarz RE, Lau SK, Yen Y, Weiss LM. Immunohistochemical staining in the diagnosis of pancreatobiliary and ampulla of Vater adenocarcinoma: application of CDX2, CK17, MUC1, and MUC2. Am J Surg Pathol. 2005;29(3):359–67.
107. Hruban RH, Pitman MB, Klimstra DS. AFIP Atlast of Tumor Pathology, Tumors of the Pancreas, vol. 4. 6th ed. Washington, DC: American Registry of Pathology; 2007.
108. Levy M, Lin F, Xu H, Dhall D, Spaulding BO, Wang HL. S100P, von Hippel-Lindau gene product, and IMP3 serve as a useful immunohistochemical panel in the diagnosis of adenocarcinoma on endoscopic bile duct biopsy. Hum Pathol. 2010;41(9): 1210–9.
109. Lin F, Shi J, Liu H, et al. Diagnostic utility of S100P and von Hippel–Lindau gene product (pVHL) in pancreatic adenocarcinoma – with implication of their roles in early tumorigenesis. Am J Surg Pathol. 2008;32(1):78–91.
110. Zhou H, Schaefer N, Wolff M, Fischer HP. Carcinoma of the ampulla of Vater: comparative histologic/immunohistochemical classification and follow-up. Am J Surg Pathol. 2004;28(7): 875–82.
111. Yesim G, Gupse T, Zafer U, Ahmet A. Mesenchymal hamartoma of the liver in adulthood: immunohistochemical profiles, clinical and histopathological features in two patients. J Hepatobiliary Pancreat Surg. 2005;12(6):502–7.
112. Doi H, Horiike N, Hiraoka A, Koizumi Y, Yamamoto Y, Hasebe A, et al. Primary hepatic marginal zone B cell lymphoma of mucosa-associated lymphoma of mucosa-associated lymphoid tissue type: case report and review of the literature. Int J Hematol. 2008;88:418–23. Epub 23 Sep 2008.
113. Anagnostopoulos G, Sakorafas GH, Grigoriadis K, Kostopoulos P. Malignant fibrous histiocytoma of the liver: a case report and review of the literature. Mt Sinai J Med. 2005;72(1):50–2.
114. Fujita S, Lauwers GY. Primary hepatic malignant fibrous histiocytoma: report of a case and review of the literature. Pathol Int. 1998;48(3):225–9.
115. Yuri T, Danbara N, Shikata N, Fujimoto S, Nakano T, Sakaida N, et al. Malignant rhabdoid tumor of the liver: case report and literature review. Pathol Int. 2004;54(8):623–9.
116. Guglielmi A, Frameglia M, Iuzzolino P, Martignoni G, De Manzoni G, Laterza E, et al. Solitary fibrous tumor of the liver with CD 34 positivity and hypoglycemia. J Hepatobiliary Pancreat Surg. 1998;5(2):212–6.
117. Zhang MF, Zhang ZY, Fu J, Yang YF, Yun JP. Correlation between expression of p53, p21/WAF1, and MDM2 proteins and their prognostic significance in primary hepatocellular carcinoma. J Transl Med. 2009;22(7):110.

Chapter 24
Upper Gastrointestinal Tract

Jinhong Li and Fan Lin

Abstract The application of immunohistochemistry in the diagnostic gastrointestinal pathology is similar to many other organ systems. The most commonly used markers are epithelial cell markers such as cytokeratin AE1/3, cytokeratin 7 and cytokeratin 20, and markers for common mesenchymal tumors such as CD117, CD34, S100, desmin, etc. Tumors of neuroendocrine origin are probably more commonly seen in the digestive and pulmonary systems. A synaptophysin and chromogranin immunostain generally can confirm their neuroendocrine nature. Use of immunohistochemical studies to evaluate dysplasia in Barrett's esophagus is still investigational, although many have found p53 overexpression helpful in confirming dysplasia, particularly in high-grade dysplasia. The use of immunohistochemical studies in nonneoplastic diseases of the gastrointestinal tract is limited. Finally, immunohistochemistry, like GCDFP-15 immunostain, may play a critical role in differentiating certain metastases, such as lobular carcinoma of the breast, from primary tumors, including gastric signet ring cell carcinoma.

Keywords Dysplasia • Carcinoma • GIST • Neuroendocrine • Metastasis • Keratin • CD117 • Synaptophysin

FREQUENTLY ASKED QUESTIONS

Esophagus and Esophagogastric Junction

Stomach

F. Lin (✉)
Department of Pathology and Laboratory Medicine, Geisinger Medical Center, 100 N. Academy Ave, Danville, PA 17822, USA
e-mail: flin1@geisinger.edu

F. Lin and J. Prichard (eds.), *Handbook of Practical Immunohistochemistry: Frequently Asked Questions*,
DOI 10.1007/978-1-4419-8062-5_24,

Small Intestine

23. Markers used in differentiating intestinal adenocarcinoma from adenocarcinoma of ampullary/biliary origin (Table 24.23) (p. 417)
24. Markers used in differentiating carcinomas of small and large intestines (Table 24.24) (p. 417)
25. Markers used in differentiating carcinoid tumor, gangliocytic paraganglioma, and gastric glomus tumor (Table 24.25, Fig. 24.8a, b) (pp. 417–418)
26. Common hormones secreted by GI tract carcinoid tumors (Table 24.26) (p. 418)
27. Markers used in the mesenchymal tumors of the small intestine (Table 24.27) (p. 418)
28. Markers used in celiac disease (Table 24.28) (p. 418)
29. Markers used in microvillous inclusion disease (Table 24.29) (p. 419)
30. GI tract lymphoma. (Please refer to Lymphoma chapter 27)

Table 24.1 Antibodies frequently used in gastrointestinal tract diseases

Antibodies	Staining pattern	Function	Key applications and pitfalls
Pankeratin	C+M	A family of fibrous structural proteins. Keratin monomers assemble into bundles to form intermediate filaments.	To confirm epithelial origin of the neoplasm, certain sarcomas such as synovial sarcoma, epithelioid angiosarcoma, and epithelioid sarcoma could be positive for keratin; necrotic cells of nonepithelial origin may show positive stain.
AE1/AE3	C+M		Similar to pankeratin
CK5/6	C		Most commonly in squamous cell carcinoma and mesothelioma
CK903 (HMWK)	C		Also called high molecular weight cytokeratin or 34betaE12. Positive in squamous cell carcinoma and urothelial carcinoma.
CK20	C+M		Most commonly used in combination with CK7 in tumors of upper and lower GI tracts, lung and breast origin.
			Could be positive for certain tumors of upper GI tract, pancreatobiliary, ovarian, and urothelial origin
CK7	C		Most commonly used in combination with CK20; could be positive for certain tumors of lower GI tract such as adenocarcinoma of anal gland origin.
			Most carcinomas of pulmonary, breast, urothelial, and pancreatobiliary origin are positive for CK7.
CK19	C+M		Usually positive for gastric adenocarcinoma
CAM 5.2			Reactive against CK8 and CK18, and usually positive for adenocarcinoma and also squamous cell carcinoma
CDX-2	N	A protein encoded by the CDX-2 gene; functions as homeobox transcription factor	Mostly used to confirm intestinal epithelial origin, usually strongly positive for colorectal carcinoma.
			Certain intestinal type carcinomas of non-GI tract origin such as nasal, pulmonary, and female genital organs may show positive reactivity for CDX-2.
Synaptophysin	C	A synaptic vesicle glycoprotein, present in neuroendocrine cells and in virtually all neurons	Most common marker for tumors of neuroendocrine origin such as carcinoid tumor.
			Could also be positive for certain tumors of unclear lineage such as desmoplastic small round cell tumor and solid pseudopapillary tumor of the pancreas, etc.
			More sensitive and less specific than chromogranin
Chromogranin-A	C	A member of the chromogranin family in secretory vesicles of neurons and endocrine cells.	Usually used in combination with synaptophysin in tumors of neuroendocrine origin

References: [1–12]

Table 24.2 Markers expressed in normal gastrointestinal tract tissue

Markers	Cells/tissue
Pankeratin	Mucosal and serosal epithelial cells of GI tract; enteroendocrine cells and Paneth cells
AE1/AE3	Mucosal and serosal epithelial cells of GI tract; enteroendocrine cells and Paneth cells
CK5/6	Squamous epithelium of the esophagus and anal skin, serosal mesothelial cells
p63	Squamous epithelium of the esophagus and anal skin (nuclear stain)
CK20	Lower GI tract mucosal epithelium and portion of upper GI tract glandular epithelium (stomach and small intestine); Merkel cells in anal squamous zone
CK7	Upper GI tract, anal glands, biliary epithelium and squamous epithelium
Desmin	Smooth muscle
Alpha-SMA	Smooth muscle and myofibroblasts
S100	Nerve, myoepithelial cells, and melanocytes of the esophagus and perianal skin
CD117	Gastrointestinal pacemaker cells known as interstitial cells of Cajal and mast cells in lamina propria
CD34	Endothelial cells and most stromal fibroblasts (dendritic interstitial cells) of the GI tract, and interstitial cells of Cajal
CD31	Endothelial cells
CDX-2	Small and large intestinal epithelial cells (nuclear stain, stronger in lower GI tract)
Synaptophysin	Neuroendocrine cells in crypts
Chromogranin	Neuroendocrine cells in crypts (Fig. 24.1)
Gastrin	G cells in gastric antrum and duodenum
MUC2	Intestinal type secretory mucin
MUC5AC	Gastric surface type secretory mucin
MUC6	Gastric pyloric gland type secretory mucin
MLH1, MSH2, MSH6, and PMS2	Mismatch repair proteins expressed in normal tissue cells (nuclear stain)
Calretinin	Neuronal cells and mesothelial cells
NSE	Enteric ganglia, enteroendocrine cells
CEA	Enterocyte
Villin	Enterocyte with brush-border accentuation
CD3	Intraepithelial and lamina propria T lymphocytes
CD68	Macrophages and muciphages
Defensin HD5	Paneth cells

References: [13, 14]

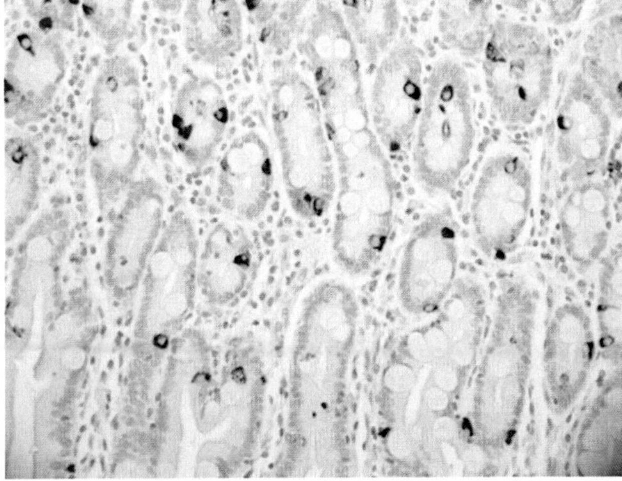

Fig. 24.1 Enteroendocrine cells. Chromogranin A immunostain highlights scattered enteroendocrine cells in normal duodenum mucosa

Table 24.3 Markers for normal small intestinal mucosa

	Small intestine (ileum)		Duodenum		
Antibody	Surface epithelium	Deep glands	Surface epithelium	Deep glands	Brunner's glands
AE1/AE3	20/20	20/20	20/20	20/20	10/10, W
CK7	0/20	0/20	20/20	20/20	10/10, W
CK20	20/20	20/20, W	20/20	20/20	0/10
MUC1	0/20	0/20	0/20	0/20	0/10
MUC2	20/20, GC	20/20, GC	20/20, GC	20/20, GC	0/10
MUC4	2/20	14/20, GC	0/20	3/20	0/10
MUC5AC	0/20	0/20	2/20	0/20	0/10
MUC6	0/20	0/20	0/20	0/20	10/10
CDX-2	20/20	20/20	20/20	20/20	0/10
CEA	10/20, W,	10/20, W, AP	0/20	0/20	0/10
CA19-9	3/20	0/20	0/20	0/20	0/10
TAG 72 (B72.3)	20/20, GC	20/20, GC	0/20	20/20, GC	0/10
MOC-31	20/20	20/20	20/20	20/20	10/10, W
Ber-EP4	20/20	20/20	20/20	20/20	10/10, W
CD15	20/20, GC	20/20, GC	20/20, GC	20/20, GC	5/10
P504S	20/20, W	20/20, W	20/20, W	20/20, W	0/10
Beta-catenin	20/20, M	20/20, M	20/20, M	20/20, M	10/10, M
Hep Par1	20/20	20/20	20/20	20/20	0/10
Villin	20/20	20/20, AP	20/20	20/20, AP	0/10
CD10	20/20	20/20, AP	20/20	20/20, AP	0/10

Note: *M* membranous staining, *W* weak, *GC* goblet cells, *AP* apical side

Table 24.4 Markers for normal gastric mucosa

	Gastric body		Gastric antrum	
Antibody	Surface epithelium	Deep glands	Surface epithelium	Deep glands
AE1/AE3	20/20	20/20, weaker	22/20	22/20
CK7	8/20, W, F	6/20, focal	3/20	15/20, F
CK20	19/19	0/19	20/20	0/20
CAM 5.2	20/20, S	20/20, S	22/22	22/22
MUC1	0/20	3/20, F	0/20	0/20
MUC2	0/20	0/20	0/20	0/20
MUC4	5/20	0/20	7/20	3/20
MUC5AC	20/20, D, S	0/20	20/20	20/20
MUC6	0/20	8/20, F	0/20	20/20
CEA	20/20, W, F	0/20	16/20	0/20
CA19-9	0/20	0/20	0/20	0/20
TAG 72 (B72.3)	0/20	0/20	0/20	0/20
MOC-31	0/20	20/20, W, F	20/20, W	20/20
Ber-EP4	0/20	20/20, W, F	3/20	20/20
CD15	20/20	20/20, S, D	0/20	20/20
p53	0/20	0/20	0/20	0/20
CDX-2	0/20	0/20	0/20	0/20
Beta-catenin	20/20, M	20/20, M	20/20, M	20/20, M
Hep Par1	0/20	0/20	0/20	0/20
Villin	0/20	0/20	0/20	0/20
CD10	0/20	0/20	2/20	2/20

Note: *W* weak, *F* focal (<10%), *D* diffuse (>50%), *S* strong, *M* membranous staining

Table 24.5 Markers for esophageal adenocarcinoma

Antibodies	GML data (%) (N = 30)
AE1/AE3	100 (30/30)
CK7	83 (25/30)
CK20	37 (11/30)
CAM 5.2	100 (30/30)
MUC1	27 (8/30)
MUC2	7 (2/30), focal
MUC4	37 (11/30)
MUC5AC	43 (13/30)
MUC6	40 (12/30)
ER/PR	0 (0/30)
GCDFP-15	0 (0/30)
S100P	73 (22/30)
IMP-3 (KOC)	57 (17/30)
Maspin	100 (30/30)
CDX-2	43 (13/30)
TTF1	0 (0/30)
CEA	83 (25/30)
MOC-31	100 (30/30)
Ber-EP4	100 (30/30)
TAG 72 (B72.3)	30 (9/30)
Napsin A	17 (5/30)
Hep Par1	33 (10/30)
P504S	73 (22/30)

Note: Examples of immunoreactivity for maspin and Hep Par1 are shown in Fig. 24.2a, b

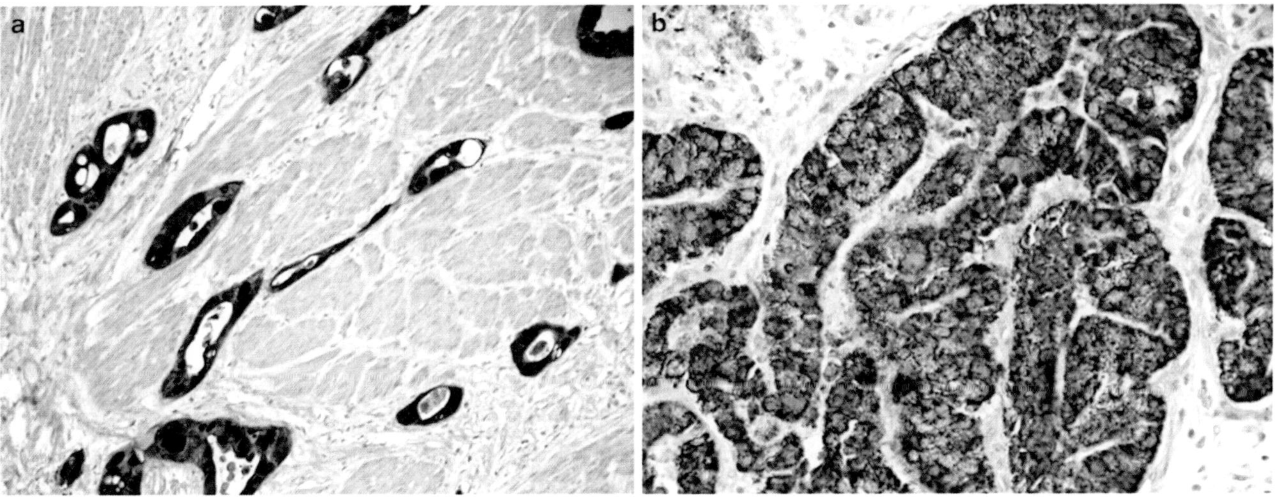

Fig. 24.2 (a, b) Esophageal adenocarcinoma. Note that immunoreactivity for maspin and Hep Par1 is shown in (a) and (b)

Table 24.6 Markers used in the differential diagnosis of esophageal granular cell tumors

Antibody	Granular cell tumor	Leiomyoma	Neurofibroma
S100	+	–	+
CD57	+/–	–	+/–
Desmin	–	+	–
SMA	–	+	–
CD68	+	–	
Inhibin	+	–	–

Note: Granular cell tumors usually cause pseudoepitheliomatous hyperplasia of overlying squamous epithelium, which should not be misdiagnosed as squamous cell carcinoma. An example is shown in Fig. 24.3a, b

References: [15–17]

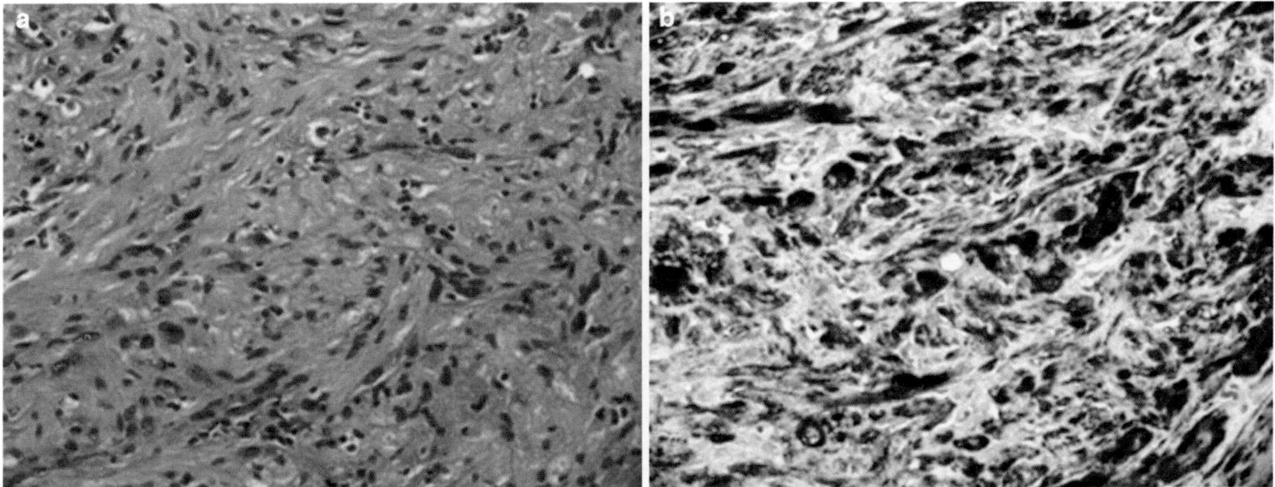

Fig. 24.3 (a, b) A granular cell tumor arising in distal esophagus. (a) H&E tissue section reveals relatively bland tumor cells with abundant granular eosinophilic cytoplasm. (b) The tumor cells exhibit strong positive immunoreactivity for S100 protein

Table 24.7 Markers used in the differential diagnosis of esophageal squamous cell carcinoma

Antibody	Squamous cell carcinoma	Melanoma	Esophageal small cell carcinoma
AE1/AE3	+	–	+
p63	+	–	–
CK903	+	–	–/+
CK5/6	+	–	–
S100	–	+	–
Melan A	–	+	–
HMB-45	–	+	–
Chromogranin	–	–	+
Synaptophysin	–	–/+	+
TTF1	–	–	–/+
CAM 5.2	+	–	–/+

Note: Small cell carcinoma of esophageal origin is considered indistinguishable from that of pulmonary origin according to histological and immunohistochemical features as well as clinical behavior. Small cell carcinoma of the lung has a much higher percentage of TTF1 positivity (approximately 90%)

References: [18–25]

Table 24.8 Markers used in the differential diagnosis of poorly differentiated squamous cell carcinoma, adenocarcinoma, and thymic carcinoma

Antibody	PDSCC	PDAC	Thymic carcinoma
CK5/6	+	–	+
p63	+	–	+
CK903	+	–	+
CK20	–	–/+	–
CK7	–/+	+	+/–
CD5	–	–	+/–

Note: *PDSCC* poorly differentiated squamous cell carcinoma, *PDAC* poorly differentiated adenocarcinoma

References: [26–33]

Table 24.9 Markers used in the differential diagnosis of esophageal mesenchymal tumors

Antibody	Leiomyoma/ leiomyosarcoma	GIST	Schwannoma
Desmin	+	–/+	–
CD117	–/+	+	–
CD34	–	+	–/+
S100	–	–	+
DOG1	–	+	–
PDGFR-alpha	–	+	–

GIST gastrointestinal stromal tumor

Note: GISTs with Kit mutation in exon 11 are more sensitive to tyrosine kinase inhibitor treatment than GISTs with Kit mutation in exon 9 and GISTs without Kit mutation. After a diagnosis of GIST is established, a molecular study for Kit mutation analysis might be performed

References: [34–40]

Table 24.10 Markers used in differentiating esophageal basaloid carcinoma, adenoid cystic carcinoma, and high-grade neuroendocrine carcinoma

Antibody	BC	ACC	HGNEC
CK5/6	+	+	–
p63	+	+	–
CK7	–/+	+	+
CK19	+	+	–
CAM 5.2	–	+	+
CEA	–/+	+	+
Chromogranin	–	–	+
Synaptophysin	–	–	+
S100	–	+	–
CD117	–	+	–

Note: *BC* basaloid carcinoma, *ACC* adenoid cystic carcinoma, *HGNEC* high-grade neuroendocrine carcinoma

The peripheral rim of palisading cells in basaloid carcinoma could be positive for S100 and SMA. In ACC, S100 also stains basaloid type cells

References: [41–47]

Table 24.11 Markers used in the esophageal intestinal metaplasia (Barrett's)

Antibody	Gastric cardia mucosa	Barrett's esophagus
CDX-2	–	+
CK7	–	+
Das1+	–	+
Hep Par1	–	+
Villin	–/+	+

Note: The use of immunohistochemistry to diagnose Barrett's esophagus is still investigational. Identifying goblet cells in H&E sections is still the key; these markers and Alcian blue stain are helpful in equivocal cases

References: [48–56]

Table 24.12 Markers used in differentiating reactive atypia from dysplasia in Barrett's

Antibody	Reactive atypia	Dysplasia
p53	+/−	Overexpression
P504S	−	+
IMP-3 (KOC)	−/+	Overexpression

Note: The use of immunohistochemistry to diagnose dysplasia in Barrett's esophagus is also investigational. It is more reliable in high-grade dysplasia with increased intensity of the above stainings and should not be used as the sole criteria to diagnose dysplasia. Architectural and cytologic atypia should still be the key in the evaluation of dysplasia. These markers may be used in difficult cases such as cases with ulceration and active inflammation with marked reactive atypia. Other markers under investigation also include p16 and Ki-67.

An example of p53 staining in the high-grade dysplasia is shown in Fig. 24.4

References: [57–63]

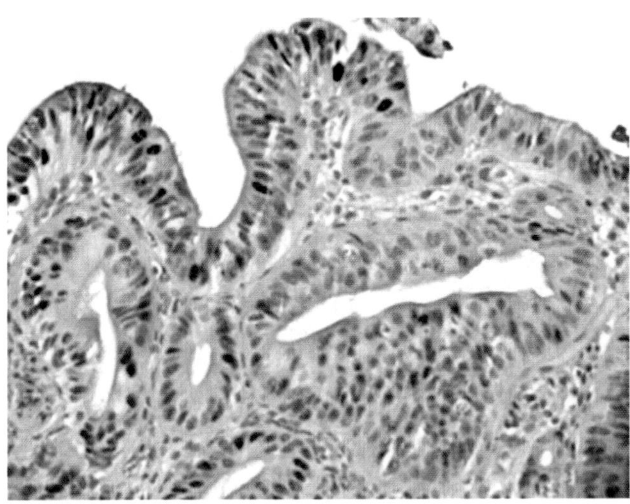

Fig. 24.4 Increased p53 staining in high-grade dysplasia at GE junction. There is strong diffuse p53 nuclear immunoreactivity in the high-grade dysplasia arising within a Barrett's esophagus

Table 24.13 Markers for gastric adenocarcinoma

Antibody	GML data (%) (*N*)
AE1/AE3	100 (18)
CK7	83 (18)
CK20	61 (18)
CK5/6	0 (18)
CK903	6 (18)
MUC1	13 (22)
MUC2	17 (18)
MUC4	22 (18)
MUC5AC	0 (18)
MUC6	0 (18)
ER/PR	0 (18)
GCDFP-15	0 (18)
S100P	67 (18)
IMP-3 (KOC)	56 (18)
Maspin	67 (18)
VHL	0 (18)
CA19-9	39 (18)
CDX-2	39 (18)
TTF1	0 (18)
MOC-31	67 (18)
Ber-EP4	67 (18)
CD10	28 (18)

Table 24.14 Gastric adenocarcinoma and carcinoid tumors

Antibody	Gastric adenocarcinoma	Carcinoid tumors
AE1/AE3	+	+
CAM 5.2	+	+
CK18/19	+	+
CK7	+ /−	−/+
CK20	−/+	−/+
CDX-2	−/+	−/+
Synaptophysin	−/rare focal +	+
Chromogranin	−	+
MOC-31	+	+
CEA	+	+/−

References: [64–66]

Table 24.15 Gastric adenocarcinoma with unusual differentiation

Antibody	Hepatoid variant	Yolk-sac variant	Choriocarcinoma
Hep Par1	+	N/A	N/A
AFP	N/A	+	N/A
Beta-hCG	N/A	N/A	+

Note: The diagnosis of these rare variants of gastric adenocarcinoma requires morphological correlation, as these markers may also stain some of the typical types of gastric adenocarcinomas

References: [67–72]

Table 24.16 Markers used in the differential diagnosis of gastric carcinoma and common metastases of other origins

Antibody	GAC	MBAC	MPAC	SQCC
CK7	+/−	+	+	−/+
CK20	−/+	−	−	−/+
CDX-2	−/+	−	−/+	−
GCDFP	−	+/−	−	−
TTF1	−	−	+/−	−
Surfactant A	−	−	+	−
ER	−/+	+/−	−/+	−
p63	−	−	−	+
CK5/6	−	−	−	+

Note: *GAC* gastric adenocarcinoma, *MBAC* metastatic breast adenocarcinoma, *MPAC* metastatic pulmonary adenocarcinoma, *SQCC* squamous cell carcinoma

The most common metastatic tumors to the stomach are from the breast, lung, and melanoma. Less frequent sites include the ovary, kidney, liver, and colon, etc.

References: [65, 73, 74]

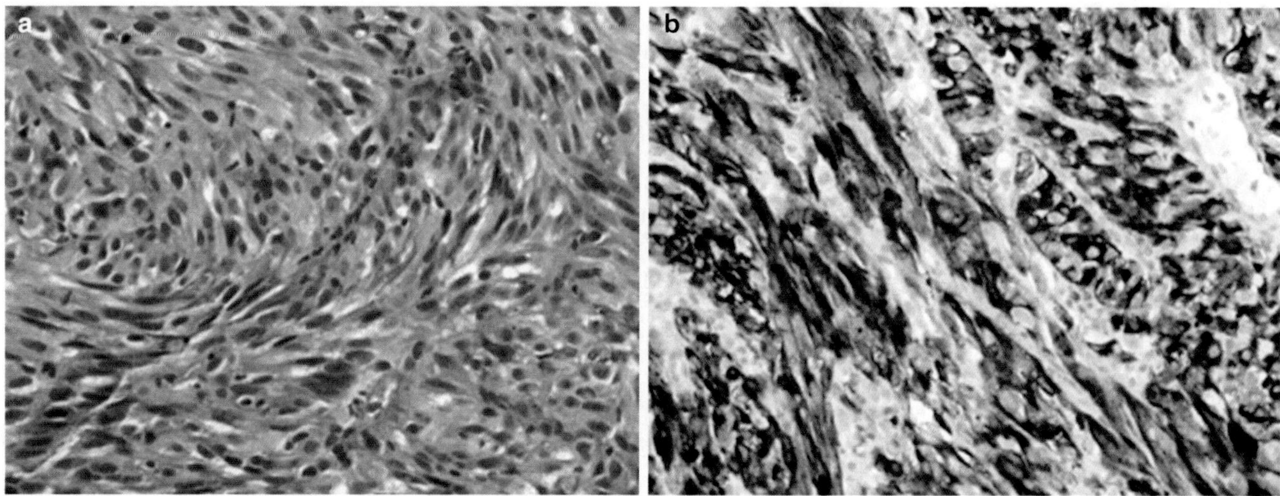

Fig. 24.5 (**a**, **b**) Metastatic melanoma in stomach. (**a**) H&E section shows a spindle cell tumor mimicking GIST in a patient presenting with a gastric mass. (**b**) The tumor cells are strongly positive for Melan A. Tumor cells are also positive for S100 protein and HMB-45 (photos not shown)

Table 24.17 Prognostic markers in gastric adenocarcinoma (may be suggestive of poorer prognosis)

Makers	Immunoreactivity/expression
Ki-67	High proliferative index/overexpression
CD34	Overexpression
Bcl-2	Expression
E-cadherin	Loss of expression
p53	Overexpression
Cyclin D1	Overexpression
IGF-IR	Overexpression
Her-2/neu	Amplified/overexpression
CDX-2	Expression

Note: An example of gastric signet ring cell carcinoma with decreased E-cadherin expression is shown in Fig. 24.6

References: [75–83]

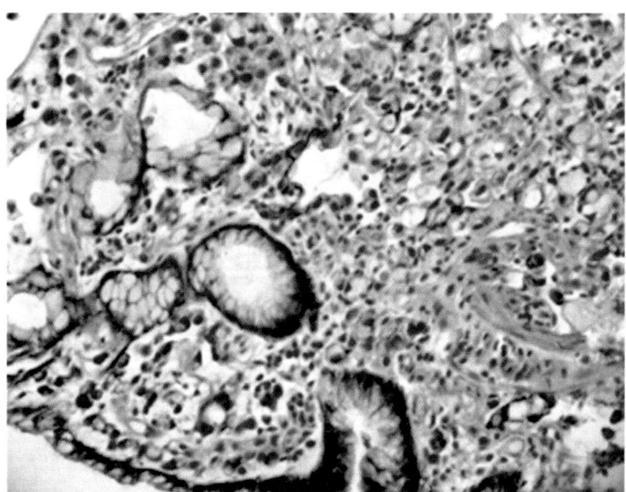

Fig. 24.6 Gastric signet ring cell carcinoma. Decrease or loss of E-cadherin expression could be seen in a small portion of gastric signet ring cell carcinomas, in particular in those arising in younger patients with mutation of the E-cadherin (CDH1) gene

Table 24.18 Gastrointestinal stromal tumors and their major differential diagnosis

Antibody	GIST	Leiomyoma/ leiomyosarcoma	Schwannoma	Metastatic melanoma
Desmin	–/+	+	–	–
CD117	+	–/+	–	–
CD34	+	–	–/+	–
S100	–	–	+	+
DOG1	+	–	–	–
PDGFR-alpha	+	–	–	–
HMB-45	–	–	–	+
Melan A	–	–	–	+

Note: *GIST* gastrointestinal stromal tumor

An example of GIST positive for CD117 is shown in Fig. 24.7

References: [84, 85]

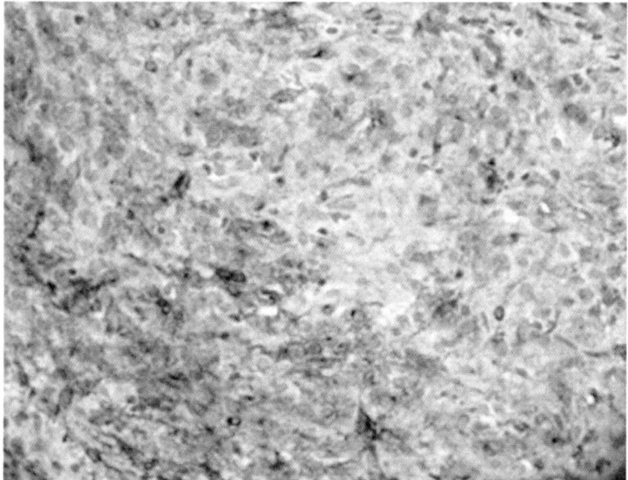

Fig. 24.7 Gastrointestinal stroma tumor (GIST). Positive CD117 immunoreactivity typically seen in the vast majority of gastrointestinal stroma tumors

Table 24.19 Markers used in gastric xanthelasma

Antibody	Gastric xanthelasma	Signet ring cell Ca
CD68	+	–
Factor XIIIa	+	–
AE1/AE3	–	+
Vimentin	+	–

References: [86–88]

Table 24.20 Markers used in inflammatory fibroid polyp

Antibody	Inflammatory fibroid polyp
CD34	+
CD35	+
MSA	+ (~20%)
CD68	+ (~37%)
Cyclin D1	–/+
PDGFR-alpha	+/–
SMA	+ (~26%)
Calponin	+
Fascin	+

References: [89–92]

Table 24.21 Markers used in Menetrier's disease

Antibody	Menetrier's disease
TGF-alpha	Overexpression

References: [93, 94]

Table 24.22 Markers used in infectious disease

Antibody	Stain pattern	Common application
CMV	Nuclear stain in CMV-infected cells	Suspected CMV esophagitis and enteritis
HSV I and HSV II	Nuclear and cytoplasmic stain in HSV-infected cells	Suspected HSV esophagitis and enteritis
Helicobacter pylori	Highlights the *H. pylori* organism	Suspected *H. pylori* gastritis and *H. pylori* infection status post therapy

Note: *CMV* cytomegalovirus, *HSV* herpes simplex virus

These antibodies are useful for confirmation when H&E tissue sections are suspicious for viral inclusions and *H. pylori*-like organisms

References: [95–99]

Table 24.23 Markers used in differentiating intestinal adenocarcinoma from adenocarcinoma of ampullary/biliary origin

Antibody	Small intestinal adenocarcinoma	Adenocarcinoma of biliary origin
MUC2	+/–	+/–
CDX-2	+/–	+/–
Hep Par1	–/+	–
CK20	+/–	–/+
CK17	–/+	+
MUC1	+/–	+/–
CK18, 19	+	+
CK7	+	+

Note: The immunophenotype overlap between these two groups of tumors is substantial

References: [100–103]

Table 24.24 Markers used in differentiating the carcinomas of small and large intestines

Antibody	Carcinoma of upper GI tract	Colorectal carcinoma
CK20	+/–	+, rare –
CK7	+/–	–
CDX-2	+/–	+, rare –
P504S	–, rare +	+/–

References: [104–106]

Table 24.25 Markers used in differentiating carcinoid tumor, gangliocytic paraganglioma, and gastric glomus tumor

Antibody	CT	GP	Glomus tumor
AE1/AE3	+	–/+	–
S100	–	+, sustentacular cells	–
Synaptophysin	+	+	–
Chromogranin	+	+	–
SMA	–	–	+
Calponin	–	–	+

Note: *CT* carcinoid tumor, *GP* gangliocytic paraganglioma

S100 immunostain highlights the peripheral sustentacular cells in a gangliocytic paraganglioma is shown in Fig. 24.8a, b

References: [107–113]

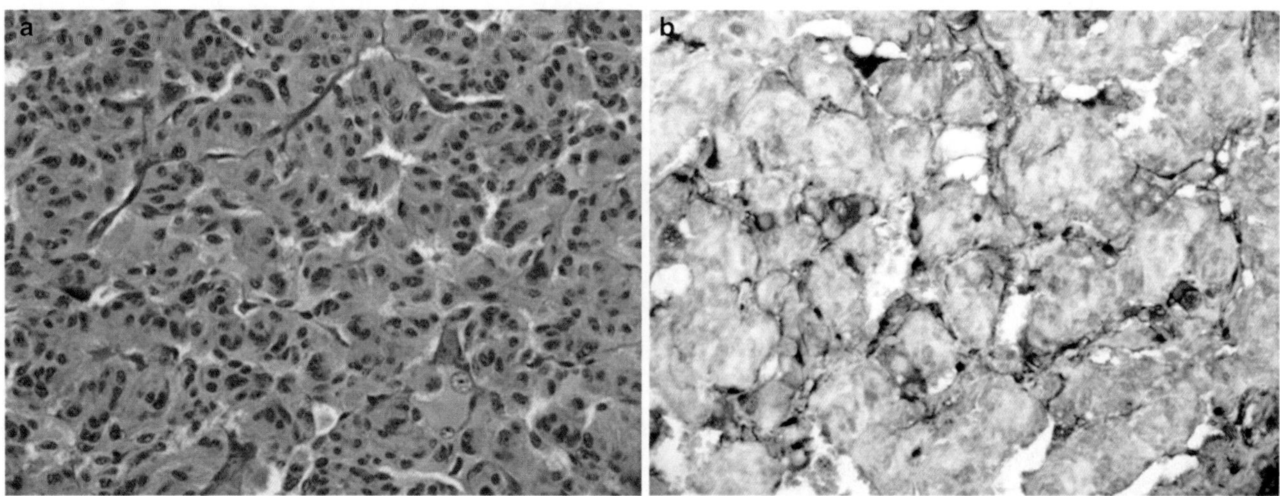

Fig. 24.8 (**a**, **b**) Duodenal gangliocytic paraganglioma. (**a**) H&E section shows a tumor exhibiting an organoid growth pattern. (**b**) S100 protein immunostain highlights the peripheral sustentacular cells in the tumor

Table 24.26 Common hormones secreted by GI tract carcinoid tumors

Primacy site	Hormone likely secreted	Comment
Stomach	Gastrin, histamine, and rarely serotonin	Three subtypes, I, II, and III; type III, the sporadic type, is usually larger in size and has a more aggressive behavior.
Proximal duodenum	Usually gastrin	Gastrin-producing tumors account for most duodenal carcinoid tumors.
Duodenum, near papilla of Vater	Usually somatostatin	Approximately 20% of duodenal carcinoid tumors produce somatostatin.
Distal small intestine and appendix	Usually serotonin	Carcinoid tumors of appendix may show unusual morphology such as seen in goblet cell carcinoid tumors.

Note: Some carcinoid tumors may also produce calcitonin, insulin, glucagon, and ACTH, etc.

References: [112, 114–116]

Table 24.27 Markers used in the mesenchymal tumors of the small intestine

Antibody	GIST	LMS	LS	SN	SFT	IMT	DT
Desmin	–	+	–	–	–	–/+	–/+
SMA	–/+	+	–	–	–	+/–	–/+
CD117	+	–	–	–	–	–	–/+
CD34	+	–	–	–	+	–/+	–
S100	–	–	+	+	–	–	–
Beta-catenin	–	–	–	–	–	–	+
CD99	–	–	–	–	+/–	–/+	–
Bcl-2	–	–	–	–	–/+	–/+	–
ALK1	–	–	–	–	–	–/+	–
MDM2	–	–	+	–	–	+	–/+

Note: *GIST* gastrointestinal stroma tumor, *LMS* leiomyosarcoma, *LS* liposarcoma, *SN* schwannoma, *SFT* solitary fibrous tumor, *IMT* inflammatory myofibroblastic tumor, *DT* desmoid tumor

References: [117–125]

Table 24.28 Markers used in celiac disease

Antibody	Literature
CD3	+
CD4	–
CD8	+

Note: Diagnosis of celiac disease generally relies on the morphological findings (intraepithelial lymphocytosis, villous blunting, increase in lamina propria lymphoplasmacytic cells, and crypt hyperplasia); when IEL is equivocal, immunostain for CD3 might be helpful

Loss of CD8 expression in lymphocytes in celiac disease is considered suggestive of higher possibility to progress to refractory sprue and enteropathy-associated T cell lymphoma

References: [126, 127]

Table 24.29 Markers used in microvillous inclusion disease

Antibody	MVID	Normal
CD10	Intracytoplasmic CD10 positivity in surface enterocytes	Linear brush-border stain
CEA	Intracytoplasmic positivity	Linear brush-border stain
Alkaline phosphatase	Intracytoplasmic positivity	Linear brush-border stain

References: [128–131]

References

1. Lee MJ, Lee HS, Kim WH, Choi Y, Yang M. Expression of mucins and cytokeratins in primary carcinomas of the digestive system. Mod Pathol. 2003;16(5):403–10.
2. Zhou Q, Toivola DM, Feng N, Greenberg HB, Franke WW, Omary MB. Keratin 20 helps maintain intermediate filament organization in intestinal epithelia. Mol Biol Cell. 2003;14(7):2959–71.
3. Chu P, Wu E, Weiss LM. Cytokeratin 7 and cytokeratin 20 expression in epithelial neoplasms: a survey of 435 cases. Mod Pathol. 2000;13(9):962–72.
4. Kende AI, Carr NJ, Sobin LH. Expression of cytokeratins 7 and 20 in carcinomas of the gastrointestinal tract. Histopathology. 2003;42(2):137–40.
5. Chu PG, Weiss LM. Expression of cytokeratin 5/6 in epithelial neoplasms: an immunohistochemical study of 509 cases. Mod Pathol. 2002;15(1):6–10.
6. Werling RW, Yaziji H, Bacchi CE, Gown AM. CDX2, a highly sensitive and specific marker of adenocarcinomas of intestinal origin: an immunohistochemical survey of 476 primary and metastatic carcinomas. Am J Surg Pathol. 2003;27(3):303–10.
7. Portela-Gomes GM, Stridsberg M. Chromogranin A in the human gastrointestinal tract: an immunocytochemical study with region-specific antibodies. J Histochem Cytochem. 2002;50(11):1487–92.
8. Yang A, Kaghad M, Wang Y, et al. p63, a p53 homolog at 3q27-29, encodes multiple products with transactivating, death-inducing, and dominant-negative activities. Mol Cell. 1998;2(3):305–16.
9. Di Como CJ, Urist MJ, Babayan I, et al. p63 expression profiles in human normal and tumor tissues. Clin Cancer Res. 2002;8(2):494–501.
10. Kaufmann O, Fietze E, Mengs J, Dietel M. Value of p63 and cytokeratin 5/6 as immunohistochemical markers for the differential diagnosis of poorly differentiated and undifferentiated carcinomas. Am J Clin Pathol. 2001;116(6):823–30.
11. Willert K, Nusse R. Beta-catenin: a key mediator of Wnt signaling. Curr Opin Genet Dev. 1998;8(1):95–102.
12. Krasinskas AM, Goldsmith JD. Immunohistology of the gastrointestinal tract. In: Dabbs DJ, editor. Diagnostic immunohistochemistry. 3rd ed. Philadelphia: Churchill Livingstone Elsevier; 2010. p. 500–40.
13. Bacchi CE, Gown AM. Distribution and pattern of expression of villin, a gastrointestinal-associated cytoskeletal protein, in human carcinomas: a study employing paraffin-embedded tissue. Lab Invest. 1991;64(3):418–24.
14. Dahl J, Greenson JK, Gramlich TL, Petras RE, Fenger C. Histology of small intestine, colon and anal canal. In: Mills SE, editor. Histology for pathologists. 3rd ed. Philadelphia: Lippincott Williams & Williams; 2006. p. 601–83.
15. Goldblum JR, Rice TW, Zuccaro G, Richter JE. Granular cell tumors of the esophagus: a clinical and pathologic study of 13 cases. Ann Thorac Surg. 1996;62(3):860–5.
16. John BK, Dang NC, Hussain SA, et al. Multifocal granular cell tumor presenting as an esophageal stricture. J Gastrointest Cancer. 2008;39(1–4):107–13.
17. David O, Jakate S. Multifocal granular cell tumor of the esophagus and proximal stomach with infiltrative pattern: a case report and review of the literature. Arch Pathol Lab Med. 1999;123(10):967–73.
18. Yamamoto J, Ohshima K, Ikeda S, Iwashita A, Kikuchi M. Primary esophageal small cell carcinoma with concomitant invasive squamous cell carcinoma or carcinoma in situ. Hum Pathol. 2003;34(11):1108–15.
19. Takahashi Y, Noguchi T, Takeno S, Kimura Y, Okubo M, Kawahara K. Reduced expression of p63 has prognostic implications for patients with esophageal squamous cell carcinoma. Oncol Rep. 2006;15(2):323–8.
20. Yun JP, Zhang MF, Hou JH, et al. Primary small cell carcinoma of the esophagus: clinicopathological and immunohistochemical features of 21 cases. BMC Cancer. 2007;7:38.
21. Lam KY, Law S, Wong J. Malignant melanoma of the oesophagus: clinicopathological features, lack of p53 expression and steroid receptors and a review of the literature. Eur J Surg Oncol. 1999;25(2):168–72.
22. Cheuk W, Chan JK. Thyroid transcription factor-1 is of limited value in practical distinction between pulmonary and extrapulmonary small cell carcinomas. Am J Surg Pathol. 2001;25(4):545–6.
23. Takubo K, Nakamura K, Sawabe M, et al. Primary undifferentiated small cell carcinoma of the esophagus. Hum Pathol. 1999;30(2):216–21.
24. Lohmann CM, Hwu WJ, Iversen K, Jungbluth AA, Busam KJ. Primary malignant melanoma of the oesophagus: a clinical and pathological study with emphasis on the immunophenotype of the tumours for melanocyte differentiation markers and cancer/testis antigens. Melanoma Res. 2003;13(6):595–601.
25. Lu J, Xue LY, Lu N, Zou SM, Liu XY, Wen P. Superficial primary small cell carcinoma of the esophagus: clinicopathological and immunohistochemical analysis of 15 cases. Dis Esophagus. 2010;23(2):153–9.
26. Makino T, Yamasaki M, Takeno A, et al. Cytokeratins 18 and 8 are poor prognostic markers in patients with squamous cell carcinoma of the oesophagus. Br J Cancer. 2009;101(8):1298–306.
27. Sengpiel C, Konig IR, Rades D, et al. p53 Mutations in carcinoma of the esophagus and gastroesophageal junction. Cancer Invest. 2009;27(1):96–104.
28. Brown JG, Familiari U, Papotti M, Rosai J. Thymic basaloid carcinoma: a clinicopathologic study of 12 cases, with a general discussion of basaloid carcinoma and its relationship with adenoid cystic carcinoma. Am J Surg Pathol. 2009;33(8):1113–24.
29. Truong LD, Mody DR, Cagle PT, Jackson-York GL, Schwartz MR, Wheeler TM. Thymic carcinoma. A clinicopathologic study of 13 cases. Am J Surg Pathol. 1990;14(2):151–66.
30. Suster S. Thymic carcinoma: update of current diagnostic criteria and histologic types. Semin Diagn Pathol. 2005;22(3):198–212.
31. Kuo TT, Chan JK. Thymic carcinoma arising in thymoma is associated with alterations in immunohistochemical profile. Am J Surg Pathol. 1998;22(12):1474–81.
32. Dorfman DM, Shahsafaei A, Chan JK. Thymic carcinomas, but not thymomas and carcinomas of other sites, show CD5 immunoreactivity. Am J Surg Pathol. 1997;21(8):936–40.
33. Tateyama H, Eimoto T, Tada T, Hattori H, Murase T, Takino H. Immunoreactivity of a new CD5 antibody with normal epithelium and malignant tumors including thymic carcinoma. Am J Clin Pathol. 1999;111(2):235–40.

34. Wong NA, Pawade J. Mast cell-rich leiomyomas should not be mistaken for gastrointestinal stromal tumours. Histopathology. 2007;51(2):273–5.
35. Zhang X, Rong TH, Wu QL, et al. Differential diagnosis and treatment of esophageal stromal tumors and smooth muscle tumors [in Chinese]. Ai Zheng. 2006;25(7):901–5.
36. Miettinen M, Sarlomo-Rikala M, Sobin LH, Lasota J. Esophageal stromal tumors: a clinicopathologic, immunohistochemical, and molecular genetic study of 17 cases and comparison with esophageal leiomyomas and leiomyosarcomas. Am J Surg Pathol. 2000;24(2):211–22.
37. Miettinen M, Sarlomo-Rikala M, Lasota J. Gastrointestinal stromal tumors: recent advances in understanding of their biology. Hum Pathol. 1999;30(10):1213–20.
38. Debiec-Rychter M, Sciot R, Le Cesne A, et al. KIT mutations and dose selection for imatinib in patients with advanced gastrointestinal stromal tumours. Eur J Cancer. 2006;42(8):1093–103.
39. West RB, Corless CL, Chen X, et al. The novel marker, DOG1, is expressed ubiquitously in gastrointestinal stromal tumors irrespective of KIT or PDGFRA mutation status. Am J Pathol. 2004;165(1):107–13.
40. Espinosa I, Lee CH, Kim MK, et al. A novel monoclonal antibody against DOG1 is a sensitive and specific marker for gastrointestinal stromal tumors. Am J Surg Pathol. 2008;32(2):210–8.
41. Li TJ, Zhang YX, Wen J, Cowan DF, Hart J, Xiao SY. Basaloid squamous cell carcinoma of the esophagus with or without adenoid cystic features. Arch Pathol Lab Med. 2004;128(10): 1124–30.
42. Sarbia M, Verreet P, Bittinger F, et al. Basaloid squamous cell carcinoma of the esophagus: diagnosis and prognosis. Cancer. 1997;79(10):1871–8.
43. Tsubochi H, Suzuki T, Suzuki S, et al. Immunohistochemical study of basaloid squamous cell carcinoma, adenoid cystic and mucoepidermoid carcinoma in the upper aerodigestive tract. Anticancer Res. 2000;20(2B):1205–11.
44. Serrano MF, El-Mofty SK, Gnepp DR, Lewis Jr JS. Utility of high molecular weight cytokeratins, but not p63, in the differential diagnosis of neuroendocrine and basaloid carcinomas of the head and neck. Hum Pathol. 2008;39(4):591–8.
45. Emanuel P, Wang B, Wu M, Burstein DE. p63 Immunohistochemistry in the distinction of adenoid cystic carcinoma from basaloid squamous cell carcinoma. Mod Pathol. 2005;18(5):645–50.
46. Mino M, Pilch BZ, Faquin WC. Expression of KIT (CD117) in neoplasms of the head and neck: an ancillary marker for adenoid cystic carcinoma. Mod Pathol. 2003;16(12):1224–31.
47. Owonikoko T, Loberg C, Gabbert HE, Sarbia M. Comparative analysis of basaloid and typical squamous cell carcinoma of the oesophagus: a molecular biological and immunohistochemical study. J Pathol. 2001;193(2):155–61.
48. Chu PG, Jiang Z, Weiss LM. Hepatocyte antigen as a marker of intestinal metaplasia. Am J Surg Pathol. 2003;27(7):952–9.
49. Shi XY, Bhagwandeen B, Leong AS. CDX2 and villin are useful markers of intestinal metaplasia in the diagnosis of Barrett esophagus. Am J Clin Pathol. 2008;129(4):571–7.
50. Groisman GM, Amar M, Meir A. Expression of the intestinal marker Cdx2 in the columnar-lined esophagus with and without intestinal (Barrett's) metaplasia. Mod Pathol. 2004;17(10): 1282–8.
51. Glickman JN, Wang H, Das KM, et al. Phenotype of Barrett's esophagus and intestinal metaplasia of the distal esophagus and gastroesophageal junction: an immunohistochemical study of cytokeratins 7 and 20, Das-1 and 45 MI. Am J Surg Pathol. 2001;25(1):87–94.
52. Sarbia M, Donner A, Franke C, Gabbert HE. Distinction between intestinal metaplasia in the cardia and in Barrett's esophagus: the role of histology and immunohistochemistry. Hum Pathol. 2004;35(3):371–6.
53. Ormsby AH, Goldblum JR, Rice TW, et al. Cytokeratin subsets can reliably distinguish Barrett's esophagus from intestinal metaplasia of the stomach. Hum Pathol. 1999;30(3):288–94.
54. Shearer C, Going J, Neilson L, Mackay C, Stuart RC. Cytokeratin 7 and 20 expression in intestinal metaplasia of the distal oesophagus: relationship to gastro-oesophageal reflux disease. Histopathology. 2005;47(3):268–75.
55. Wang J, Qin R, Ma Y, et al. Differential gene expression in normal esophagus and Barrett's esophagus. J Gastroenterol. 2009;44(9): 897–911.
56. Flucke U, Steinborn E, Dries V, et al. Immunoreactivity of cytokeratins (CK7, CK20) and mucin peptide core antigens (MUC1, MUC2, MUC5AC) in adenocarcinomas, normal and metaplastic tissues of the distal oesophagus, oesophago-gastric junction and proximal stomach. Histopathology. 2003;43(2):127–34.
57. Lu D, Vohra P, Chu PG, Woda B, Rock KL, Jiang Z. An oncofetal protein IMP3: a new molecular marker for the detection of esophageal adenocarcinoma and high-grade dysplasia. Am J Surg Pathol. 2009;33(4):521–5.
58. Odze RD. Update on the diagnosis and treatment of Barrett esophagus and related neoplastic precursor lesions. Arch Pathol Lab Med. 2008;132(10):1577–85.
59. Shi XY, Bhagwandeen B, Leong AS. p16, cyclin D1, Ki-67, and AMACR as markers for dysplasia in Barrett esophagus. Appl Immunohistochem Mol Morphol. 2008;16(5):447–52.
60. Dorer R, Odze RD. AMACR immunostaining is useful in detecting dysplastic epithelium in Barrett's esophagus, ulcerative colitis, and Crohn's disease. Am J Surg Pathol. 2006;30(7):871–7.
61. Hanas JS, Lerner MR, Lightfoot SA, et al. Expression of the cyclin-dependent kinase inhibitor p21(WAF1/CIP1) and p53 tumor suppressor in dysplastic progression and adenocarcinoma in Barrett esophagus. Cancer. 1999;86(5):756–63.
62. Moskaluk CA, Heitmiller R, Zahurak M, Schwab D, Sidransky D, Hamilton SR. p53 and p21(WAF1/CIP1/SDI1) gene products in Barrett esophagus and adenocarcinoma of the esophagus and esophagogastric junction. Hum Pathol. 1996;27(11):1211–20.
63. Ireland AP, Clark GW, DeMeester TR. Barrett's esophagus. The significance of p53 in clinical practice. Ann Surg. 1997;225(1):17–30.
64. Al-Khafaji B, Noffsinger AE, Miller MA, DeVoe G, Stemmermann GN, Fenoglio-Preiser C. Immunohistologic analysis of gastrointestinal and pulmonary carcinoid tumors. Hum Pathol. 1998;29(9):992–9.
65. Park SY, Kim BH, Kim JH, Lee S, Kang GH. Panels of immunohistochemical markers help determine primary sites of metastatic adenocarcinoma. Arch Pathol Lab Med. 2007;131(10):1561–7.
66. Kim MA, Lee HS, Yang HK, Kim WH. Cytokeratin expression profile in gastric carcinomas. Hum Pathol. 2004;35(5):576–81.
67. Roberts CC, Colby TV, Batts KP. Carcinoma of the stomach with hepatocyte differentiation (hepatoid adenocarcinoma). Mayo Clin Proc. 1997;72(12):1154–60.
68. Louhimo J, Nordling S, Alfthan H, von Boguslawski K, Stenman UH, Haglund C. Specific staining of human chorionic gonadotropin beta in benign and malignant gastrointestinal tissues with monoclonal antibodies. Histopathology. 2001;38(5):418–24.
69. Plaza JA, Vitellas K, Frankel WL. Hepatoid adenocarcinoma of the stomach. Ann Diagn Pathol. 2004;8(3):137–41.
70. Villari D, Caruso R, Grosso M, Vitarelli E, Righi M, Barresi G. Hep Par 1 in gastric and bowel carcinomas: an immunohistochemical study. Pathology. 2002;34(5):423–6.
71. Jan YJ, Chen JT, Ho WL, Wu CC, Yeh DC. Primary coexistent adenocarcinoma and choriocarcinoma of the stomach. A case report and review of the literature. J Clin Gastroenterol. 1997;25(3):550–4.
72. Saigo PE, Brigati DJ, Sternberg SS, Rosen PP, Turnbull AD. Primary gastric choriocarcinoma. An immunohistological study. Am J Surg Pathol. 1981;5(4):333–42.

73. O'Connell FP, Wang HH, Odze RD. Utility of immunohistochemistry in distinguishing primary adenocarcinomas from metastatic breast carcinomas in the gastrointestinal tract. Arch Pathol Lab Med. 2005;129(3):338–47.
74. van Velthuysen ML, Taal BG, van der Hoeven JJ, Peterse JL. Expression of oestrogen receptor and loss of E-cadherin are diagnostic for gastric metastasis of breast carcinoma. Histopathology. 2005;46(2):153–7.
75. Park DI, Yun JW, Park JH, et al. HER-2/neu amplification is an independent prognostic factor in gastric cancer. Dig Dis Sci. 2006;51(8):1371–9.
76. Matsubara J, Yamada Y, Hirashima Y, et al. Impact of insulin-like growth factor type 1 receptor, epidermal growth factor receptor, and HER2 expressions on outcomes of patients with gastric cancer. Clin Cancer Res. 2008;14(10):3022–9.
77. Kim JH, Kim MA, Lee HS, Kim WH. Comparative analysis of protein expressions in primary and metastatic gastric carcinomas. Hum Pathol. 2009;40(3):314–22.
78. Chen L, Li X, Wang GL, Wang Y, Zhu YY, Zhu J. Clinicopathological significance of overexpression of TSPAN1, Ki67 and CD34 in gastric carcinoma. Tumori. 2008;94(4):531–8.
79. Feakins RM, Nickols CD, Bidd H, Walton SJ. Abnormal expression of pRb, p16, and cyclin D1 in gastric adenocarcinoma and its lymph node metastases: relationship with pathological features and survival. Hum Pathol. 2003;34(12):1276–82.
80. Kopp R, Diebold J, Dreier I, et al. Prognostic relevance of p53 and bcl-2 immunoreactivity for early invasive pT1/pT2 gastric carcinomas: indicators for limited gastric resections? Surg Endosc. 2005;19(11):1507–12.
81. Chen HC, Chu RY, Hsu PN, et al. Loss of E-cadherin expression correlates with poor differentiation and invasion into adjacent organs in gastric adenocarcinomas. Cancer Lett. 2003;201(1):97–106.
82. Mizoshita T, Tsukamoto T, Nakanishi H, et al. Expression of Cdx2 and the phenotype of advanced gastric cancers: relationship with prognosis. J Cancer Res Clin Oncol. 2003;129(12):727–34.
83. Lee HS, Lee HK, Kim HS, Yang HK, Kim YI, Kim WH. MUC1, MUC2, MUC5AC, and MUC6 expressions in gastric carcinomas: their roles as prognostic indicators. Cancer. 2001;92(6):1427–34.
84. Rubin BP, Singer S, Tsao C, et al. KIT activation is a ubiquitous feature of gastrointestinal stromal tumors. Cancer Res. 2001;61(22):8118–21.
85. Taniguchi M, Nishida T, Hirota S, et al. Effect of c-kit mutation on prognosis of gastrointestinal stromal tumors. Cancer Res. 1999;59(17):4297–300.
86. Kaiserling E, Heinle H, Itabe H, Takano T, Remmele W. Lipid islands in human gastric mucosa: morphological and immunohistochemical findings. Gastroenterology. 1996;110(2):369–74.
87. Ludvikova M, Michal M, Datkova D. Gastric xanthelasma associated with diffuse signet ring carcinoma. A potential diagnostic problem. Histopathology. 1994;25(6):581–2.
88. Nakasono M, Hirokawa M, Muguruma N, et al. Colorectal xanthomas with polypoid lesion: report of 25 cases. APMIS. 2004;112(1):3–10.
89. Lasota J, Wang ZF, Sobin LH, Miettinen M. Gain-of-function mutations, earlier reported in gastrointestinal stromal tumors, are common in small intestinal inflammatory fibroid polyps. A study of 60 cases. Mod Pathol. 2009;22(8):1049–56.
90. Pantanowitz L, Antonioli DA, Pinkus GS, Shahsafaei A, Odze RD. Inflammatory fibroid polyps of the gastrointestinal tract: evidence for a dendritic cell origin. Am J Surg Pathol. 2004;28(1):107–14.
91. Kim MK, Higgins J, Cho EY, Ko YH, Oh YL. Expression of CD34, bcl-2, and kit in inflammatory fibroid polyps of the gastrointestinal tract. Appl Immunohistochem Mol Morphol. 2000;8(2):147–53.
92. Hasegawa T, Yang P, Kagawa N, Hirose T, Sano T. CD34 expression by inflammatory fibroid polyps of the stomach. Mod Pathol. 1997;10(5):451–6.
93. Bluth RF, Carpenter HA, Pittelkow MR, Page DL, Coffey RJ. Immunolocalization of transforming growth factor-alpha in normal and diseased human gastric mucosa. Hum Pathol. 1995;26(12):1333–40.
94. Dempsey PJ, Goldenring JR, Soroka CJ, et al. Possible role of transforming growth factor alpha in the pathogenesis of Menetrier's disease: supportive evidence form humans and transgenic mice. Gastroenterology. 1992;103(6):1950–63.
95. Rimsza LM, Vela EE, Frutiger YM, et al. Rapid automated combined in situ hybridization and immunohistochemistry for sensitive detection of cytomegalovirus in paraffin-embedded tissue biopsies. Am J Clin Pathol. 1996;106(4):544–8.
96. Spano LC, Lima Pereira FE, Gomes da Silva Basso N, Mercon-de-Vargas PR. Human cytomegalovirus infection and abortion: an immunohistochemical study. Med Sci Monit. 2002;8(6):BR230–5.
97. Feiden W, Borchard F, Burrig KF, Pfitzer P. Herpes oesophagitis. I. Light microscopical and immunohistochemical investigations. Virchows Arch A Pathol Anat Histopathol. 1984;404(2):167–76.
98. Cao J, Li ZQ, Borch K, Petersson F, Mardh S. Detection of spiral and coccoid forms of *Helicobacter pylori* using a murine monoclonal antibody. Clin Chim Acta. 1997;267(2):183–96.
99. Rotimi O, Cairns A, Gray S, Moayyedi P, Dixon MF. Histological identification of *Helicobacter pylori*: comparison of staining methods. J Clin Pathol. 2000;53(10):756–9.
100. Chu PG, Schwarz RE, Lau SK, Yen Y, Weiss LM. Immunohistochemical staining in the diagnosis of pancreatobiliary and ampulla of Vater adenocarcinoma: application of CDX2, CK17, MUC1, and MUC2. Am J Surg Pathol. 2005;29(3):359–67.
101. Goldstein NS, Bassi D. Cytokeratins 7, 17, and 20 reactivity in pancreatic and ampulla of vater adenocarcinomas. Percentage of positivity and distribution is affected by the cut-point threshold. Am J Clin Pathol. 2001;115(5):695–702.
102. Zhou H, Schaefer N, Wolff M, Fischer HP. Carcinoma of the ampulla of Vater: comparative histologic/immunohistochemical classification and follow-up. Am J Surg Pathol. 2004;28(7):875–82.
103. Sarbia M, Fritze F, Geddert H, von Weyhern C, Rosenberg R, Gellert K. Differentiation between pancreaticobiliary and upper gastrointestinal adenocarcinomas: is analysis of cytokeratin 17 expression helpful? Am J Clin Pathol. 2007;128(2):255–9.
104. Vang R, Gown AM, Barry TS, et al. Cytokeratins 7 and 20 in primary and secondary mucinous tumors of the ovary: analysis of coordinate immunohistochemical expression profiles and staining distribution in 179 cases. Am J Surg Pathol. 2006;30(9):1130–9.
105. Chen ZM, Ritter JH, Wang HL. Differential expression of alpha-methylacyl coenzyme A racemase in adenocarcinomas of the small and large intestines. Am J Surg Pathol. 2005;29(7):890–6.
106. Lin A, Weiser MR, Klimstra DS, et al. Differential expression of alpha-methylacyl-coenzyme A racemase in colorectal carcinoma bears clinical and pathologic significance. Hum Pathol. 2007;38(6):850–6.
107. Weinrach DM, Wang KL, Blum MG, Yeldandi AV, Laskin WB. Multifocal presentation of gangliocytic paraganglioma in the mediastinum and esophagus. Hum Pathol. 2004;35(10):1288–91.
108. Hironaka M, Fukayama M, Takayashiki N, Saito K, Sohara Y, Funata N. Pulmonary gangliocytic paraganglioma: case report and comparative immunohistochemical study of related neuroendocrine neoplasms. Am J Surg Pathol. 2001;25(5):688–93.
109. Burke AP, Helwig EB. Gangliocytic paraganglioma. Am J Clin Pathol. 1989;92(1):1–9.
110. Perrone T, Sibley RK, Rosai J. Duodenal gangliocytic paraganglioma. An immunohistochemical and ultrastructural study and a hypothesis concerning its origin. Am J Surg Pathol. 1985;9(1):31–41.
111. Srivastava A, Hornick JL. Immunohistochemical staining for CDX-2, PDX-1, NESP-55, and TTF-1 can help distinguish gastrointestinal carcinoid tumors from pancreatic endocrine and pulmonary carcinoid tumors. Am J Surg Pathol. 2009;33(4):626–32.

112. Bornstein-Quevedo L, Gamboa-Dominguez A. Carcinoid tumors of the duodenum and ampulla of vater: a clinicomorphologic, immunohistochemical, and cell kinetic comparison. Hum Pathol. 2001;32(11):1252–6.
113. Barbareschi M, Roldo C, Zamboni G, et al. CDX-2 homeobox gene product expression in neuroendocrine tumors: its role as a marker of intestinal neuroendocrine tumors. Am J Surg Pathol. 2004;28(9):1169–76.
114. Capella C, Solcia E, Sobin LH, Arnold R. Endocrine tumors of the small intestine. In: Hamilton SR, Aaltonen LA, editors. WHO classification of tumours, volume 2, Pathology & genetics: tumours of the digestive system. Lyon, France: IARC press; 2000. p. 77–82.
115. Makhlouf HR, Burke AP, Sobin LH. Carcinoid tumors of the ampulla of Vater: a comparison with duodenal carcinoid tumors. Cancer. 1999;85(6):1241–9.
116. Jaffee IM, Rahmani M, Singhal MG, Younes M. Expression of the intestinal transcription factor CDX2 in carcinoid tumors is a marker of midgut origin. Arch Pathol Lab Med. 2006;130(10):1522–6.
117. Miettinen M, Sobin LH, Sarlomo-Rikala M. Immunohistochemical spectrum of GISTs at different sites and their differential diagnosis with a reference to CD117 (KIT). Mod Pathol. 2000;13(10):1134–42.
118. Dow N, Giblen G, Sobin LH, Miettinen M. Gastrointestinal stromal tumors: differential diagnosis. Semin Diagn Pathol. 2006;23(2):111–9.
119. Sarlomo-Rikala M, Kovatich AJ, Barusevicius A, Miettinen M. CD117: a sensitive marker for gastrointestinal stromal tumors that is more specific than CD34. Mod Pathol. 1998;11(8):728–34.
120. Miettinen M, Virolainen M, Maarit-Sarlomo-Rikala. Gastrointestinal stromal tumors – value of CD34 antigen in their identification and separation from true leiomyomas and schwannomas. Am J Surg Pathol. 1995;19(2):207–16.
121. Greenson JK. Gastrointestinal stromal tumors and other mesenchymal lesions of the gut. Mod Pathol. 2003;16(4):366–75.
122. Brimo F, Dion D, Huwait H, Turcotte R, Nahal A. The utility of MDM2 and CDK4 immunohistochemistry in needle biopsy interpretation of lipomatous tumours: a study of 21 Tru-Cut biopsy cases. Histopathology. 2008;52(7):892–5.
123. Carlson JW, Fletcher CD. Immunohistochemistry for beta-catenin in the differential diagnosis of spindle cell lesions: analysis of a series and review of the literature. Histopathology. 2007;51(4):509–14.
124. Montgomery E, Torbenson MS, Kaushal M, Fisher C, Abraham SC. Beta-catenin immunohistochemistry separates mesenteric fibromatosis from gastrointestinal stromal tumor and sclerosing mesenteritis. Am J Surg Pathol. 2002;26(10):1296–301.
125. Bhattacharya B, Dilworth HP, Iacobuzio-Donahue C, et al. Nuclear beta-catenin expression distinguishes deep fibromatosis from other benign and malignant fibroblastic and myofibroblastic lesions. Am J Surg Pathol. 2005;29(5):653–9.
126. Ho-Yen C, Chang F, van der Walt J, Mitchell T, Ciclitira P. Recent advances in refractory coeliac disease: a review. Histopathology. 2009;54(7):783–95.
127. Robert ME. Gluten sensitive enteropathy and other causes of small intestinal lymphocytosis. Semin Diagn Pathol. 2005;22(4): 284–94.
128. Groisman GM, Amar M, Livne E. CD10: a valuable tool for the light microscopic diagnosis of microvillous inclusion disease (familial microvillous atrophy). Am J Surg Pathol. 2002;26(7): 902–7.
129. Groisman GM, Ben-Izhak O, Schwersenz A, Berant M, Fyfe B. The value of polyclonal carcinoembryonic antigen immunostaining in the diagnosis of microvillous inclusion disease. Hum Pathol. 1993;24(11):1232–7.
130. Raafat F, Green NJ, Nathavitharana KA, Booth IW. Intestinal microvillous dystrophy: a variant of microvillous inclusion disease or a new entity? Hum Pathol. 1994;25(11):1243–8.
131. Russo P. GI tract enteropathies of infancy and childhood. In: Odze RD, Goldblum JR, editors. Surgical pathology of the GI tract, liver, biliary tract and pancreas. Philadelphia, PA: Saunders; 2008. p. 169–83.

Chapter 25
Lower Gastrointestinal Tract and Microsatellite Instability

Jinhong Li and Fan Lin

Abstract Use of immunohistochemistry in the diagnostic gastrointestinal pathology of the lower GI tract is similar to that of the upper GI tract. CK20, CK7, and CDX-2 are probably the most commonly used markers and can identify the histogenesis of the vast majority of lower GI tract carcinomas. Tumors of neuroendocrine origin are also common in the lower GI tract, and for these, CDX-2, synaptophysin, and chromogranin immunostains are very helpful. Diagnosis of tumors of mesenchymal origin is generally straightforward based on tumor histology with the help of immunohistochemistry. The differential diagnosis between appendiceal mucinous tumors and ovarian mucinous tumors occasionally could be challenging because the two share significant similarities in both tumor histology and immunophenotype. As microsatellite instability (MSI) is thought to play a role not only in tumorigenesis but also in prognosis and response to adjuvant chemotherapy regimens, MSI testing is becoming popular. In general, immunohistochemistry and PCR-based tests for MSI correlate very well. Immunohistochemical studies are approximately 90–95% sensitive for hereditary nonpolyposis colorectal cancer (HNPCC) syndrome. Finally, in conjunction with immunohistochemistry, molecular pathology may broaden its use in pathology practice as demonstrated by K-ras and BRAF mutation test in colorectal carcinomas.

Keywords Carcinoma • Neuroendocrine tumor • CK20 • CK7 • CDX-2 • MSI • K-ras • BRAF

F. Lin (✉)
Department of Pathology and Laboratory Medicine, Assistant Professor, Pathology and Laboratory Medicine, Temple Univeristy, Geisinger Medical Center, Danville, PA 17822, USA
e-mail: flin1@geisinger.edu

FREQUENTLY ASKED QUESTIONS

Appendix, Colon, and Rectum

Frequently used antibodies in lower GI tract. (Please refer to the upper GI Chap. 24.)

Anus

F. Lin and J. Prichard (eds.), *Handbook of Practical Immunohistochemistry: Frequently Asked Questions*,
DOI 10.1007/978-1-4419-8062-5_25,

Microsatellite Instability Test (p. 428)

17. What is microsatellite instability? (p. 428)
18. What is the diagnostic accuracy of the immunohistochemical stains? (p. 428)
19. What is the clinical significance of MSI? (p. 428)
20. What are the 2004 revised Bethesda guidelines for MSI testing? (p. 428)
21. What are the general recommendations for the detection of MSI? (p. 429)
22. What is the recommended panel of MSI markers? (p. 429)
23. What is the significance for a surgical pathologist regarding MSI? (pp. 429–430)
24. How to interpret immunohistochemical staining results (p. 429)

Table 25.1 Markers for normal colonic mucosa

Antibody	GML data (*N* = 20)
AE1/AE3	100% (20/20)
CK7	0 (0/20)
CK20	100% (20/20)
CAM 5.2	100% (20/20)
CK17	0 (0/20)
CK19	100% (20/20)
EMA	10% (2/20)
Vimentin	0 (0/20)
TAG 72 (B72.3)	0 (0/20)
MOC-31	100% (20/20)
Ber-EP4	100% (20/20)
CEA	100% (20/20)
CA19-9	15% (3/20)
CD15	100% (20/20)
Villin	100% (20/20, weak)
CD56	0 (0/20)
Chromogranin	100% (20/20, scattered cells)
CD10	0 (0/20)
Beta-catenin	100% (20/20)
MUC1[a]	25% (5/20)
MUC2[b]	100% (20/20)
MUC4[c]	100% (20/20)
MUC5AC	0 (0/20)
MUC6	0 (0/20)
CDX-2	100% (20/20)
p53	0 (0/20)
Hep Par 1	0 (0/20)

Note: CK20 staining is much stronger in the surface epithelium than in the deeper colonic glands. MUC4 positivity is very weak, and immunoreactivity for MUC1 is only focal (less than 25% of the tissues stained). CK19 reactivity is weak and only on the surface colonic epithelium. MUC2 is positive only in goblet cells. MOC-31, Ber-EP4, and CEA are positive in all cases, but TAG 72 (B72.3) is negative. Chromogranin reveals scattered positively stained enteroendocrine cells. Beta-catenin shows membranous staining in all cases

Table 25.2 Markers for colorectal adenocarcinoma

Antibodies	GML data (*N* = 38)
AE1/AE3	97% (37/38)
CK7	3% (1/38)
CK20	97% (37/38)
CK17	0 (0/38)
CK19	16% (6/38), weak
CAM 5.2	100% (38/38)
MUC1	16% (6/38)
MUC2	55% (21/38)
MUC4	74% (28/38)
MUC5AC	26% (10/38)
MUC6	8% (3/38)
ER	0 (0/38)
PR	0 (0/38)
GCDFP-15	0 (0/38)
S100P	55% (21/38)
IMP-3 (KOC)	50% (19/38)
Maspin	89% (34/38)
VHL	16% (6/38)
CA19-9	55% (21/38)
CDX-2	95% (36/38)
TTF1	0 (0/38)
CEA	100% (38/38)
MOC-31	100% (38/38)
Ber-EP4	100% (38/38)
CD10	16% (6/38)
Vimentin	0 (0/38)
Beta-catenin	63% (24/38)
Villin	82% (31/38)
Napsin A	29% (11/38)
Hep Par 1	11% (4/38)
P504S	90% (33/38)

Note: Based on GML TMA data. Focal positivity (<25% of the tumor cells stained) for VHL, napsin A, and Hep Par 1 is noted in 6, 11, and 4 cases, respectively. CD10 positivity is seen on the luminal surface. The positivity for MUC5AC and CK7 are focal (<10% of the tumor cells). Two CK20-positive and CDX-2-positive cases demonstrate very focal staining (<5% of the tumor cells)

Table 25.3 Appendiceal/colorectal adenocarcinoma vs. primary ovarian carcinoma

Antibody	Appendiceal/colorectal	Ovarian
CK7	– or +	+
CK20	+	+ or –
CDX-2	+	– or +
MDM2	–	+
WT1	–	+
MUC2	+	– or +
MUC5AC	+	+
Beta-catenin	Nuclear and membranous +	Membranous +

Note: CK7 is usually diffusely positive in both serous and mucinous ovarian carcinoma. CK20 and CDX-2 are usually "patchy" positive in mucinous ovarian tumor and negative in serous carcinoma. In contrast, both CDX-2 and CK20 are diffusely positive in appendiceal and colorectal adenocarcinoma

The differential diagnosis between appendiceal and ovarian adenocarcinoma could be difficult in certain cases due to the significant overlap between both tumor histology and immunophenotype

References: [1–8]

Table 25.4 Appendiceal carcinoid tumors

Antibody	Appendiceal carcinoid tumor
Synaptophysin	+
Chromogranin	+
CK7	– or +
CK20	– or +
CDX-2	+ or –
AE1/AE3	+

Note: Appendiceal carcinoid tumors may show unusual histology, such as in tubular and in goblet cell subtypes. Their immunophenotype is similar regarding the different morphology. The most common hormone secreted by appendiceal carcinoid tumor is serotonin. An example is shown in Fig. 25.1a–d

References: [9–12]

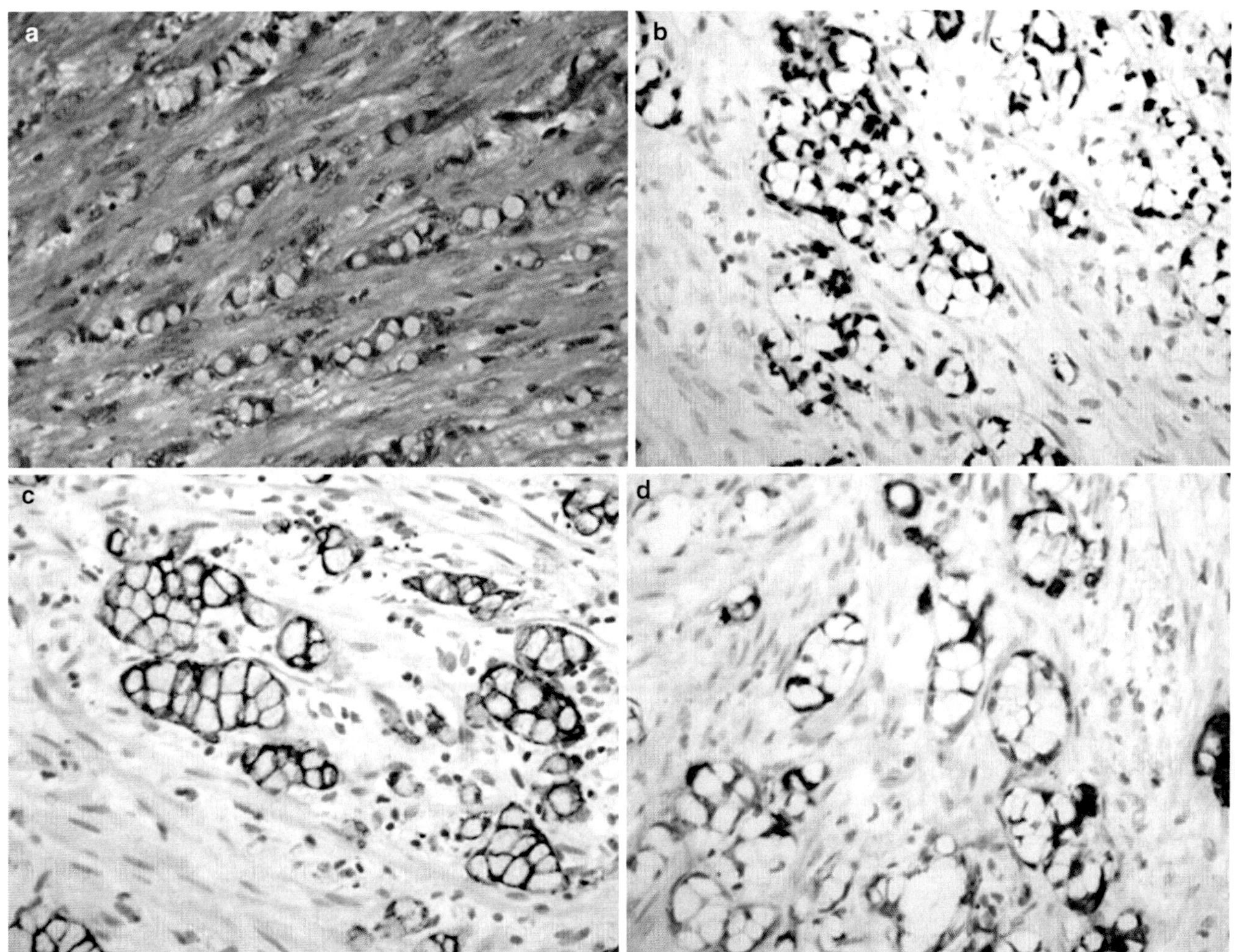

Fig. 25.1 (**a–d**) Goblet cell carcinoid tumor of the appendix. H&E tissue section shows the tumor cells with goblet cell morphology infiltrating appendiceal wall (**a**). The tumor cells demonstrate positive immunoreactivity for CDX-2 (**b**), CK20 (**c**) and CK7 (**d**). The tumor cells are also positive for synaptophysin and chromogranin (not shown)

Table 25.5 MSI-associated mucinous adenocarcinoma and medullary carcinoma

Antibody	MSI-positive mucinous carcinoma	Medullary adenocarcinoma	Poorly differentiated colonic carcinoma
CDX-2	– or +	– or +	+
CK7	+ or –	– or focal +	–
CK20	– or +	– or +	+
AE1/AE3	+	+	+
MSI	Present	Present in >50% cases	Usually absent
Calretinin	–	+ or –	– or +

Note: MSI may lead to aberrant expression of CDX-2, CK7, and CK20 in a subset of colonic adenocarcinomas. Loss of or markedly reduced expression of CK20 and CDX-2 is a frequent finding in medullary carcinoma of the colon with evidence of MSI. To complicate this matter further, some of cases with absence of expression CK20 and CDX-2 may also focally express CK7

References: [13–17]

Table 25.6 Colorectal adenocarcinoma and common metastatic adenocarcinomas

Antibody	CRC	MBAC	MUC	MPAC	MLAC
CK7	–	+	+	– or +	+
CK20	+	–	+	– or +	–
CDX-2	+	–	–	–	– or +
GCDFP-15	–	– or +	–	–	–
TTF1	–	–	–	–	+
PSA	–	–	–	+	–
PSAP	–	–	–	+	–
p63	–	–	+	–	–

Note: *CRC* colorectal adenocarcinoma, *MBAC* metastatic breast adenocarcinoma, *MUC* metastatic urothelial adenocarcinoma, *MPAC* metastatic prostatic adenocarcinoma, *MLAC* metastatic lung adenocarcinoma

References: [3, 18–24]

Table 25.7 Markers used in differentiating colonic adenocarcinoma from peritoneal mesothelioma

Antibody	Adenocarcinoma	Mesothelioma
Calretinin	–	+
CK5/6	–	+
WT1	–	+
CEA	+	–
MOC-31	+	–
CDX-2	+	–
AE1/AE3	+	+

References: [25–27]

Table 25.8 Prognostic markers in colorectal adenocarcinoma

Antigens/genes	Poor prognosis
p53	Overexpression
Beta-catenin	Decrease (membranous and cytoplasmic)
K-ras	Mutation
BRAF	Mutation

Note: The presence of K-ras or BRAF mutations may lead to a resistance to anti-EGFR therapy

References: [28–33]

Table 25.9 Rectal carcinoid tumor vs. prostatic adenocarcinoma

Antibody	Rectal carcinoid tumor	Prostatic adenocarcinoma
AE1/AE3	+	+
PSAP	+	+
PSA	–	+
Synaptophysin	+	–
Chromogranin	+	–
P504S	– or +	+

References: [34, 35]

Table 25.10 Markers used in mesenchymal tumors of the large intestine

Marker	GIST	Leiomyosarcoma	Schwannoma	Kaposi sarcoma	SFT	Ganglioneuroma
Desmin	–/+	+	–	–	–	–
SMA	–/+	+	–	+/–	–	–
CD117	+	–	–	–/+	–	–
CD34	+	–	–	+	+	–
S100	–	–	+	–	–	+
NSE	–	–	+/–	–	–	+
HHV8	–	–	–	+	–	–
CD99	–	–	–	–	+	–
Bcl-2	–	–	–	+/–	+/–	–

GIST gastrointestinal stromal tumor, *SFT* solitary fibrous tumor

References: [36–41]

Table 25.11 Markers used in dysplasia in inflammatory bowel disease (IBD)

Antibody	Reactive atypia	Dysplasia
p53	–/+	++
P504S	–/+	++

References: [42–46]

Table 25.12 Markers used in Hirschsprung's disease

Antibody	Interpretation
NSE	Helpful in highlighting ganglion cells
Calretinin	Hypertrophied nerve fibers in Hirschsprung's disease patients usually lose calretinin immunoreactivity
Acetylcholine esterase	Need frozen tissue/section to perform this immunostain, which displays increased acetylcholine-esterase-positive nerve fibers in muscularis mucosae and lamina propria

Note: An example of immunostaining for calretinin is demonstrated in Fig. 25.2a, b

The key to diagnosing Hirschsprung's disease depends on thorough examination of H&E sections to ensure that there is an absence of ganglion cell in an adequate specimen

References: [47–49]

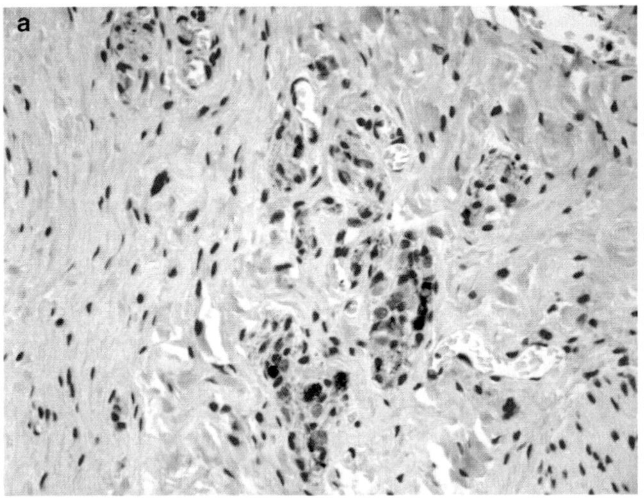

Fig. 25.2 (**a**, **b**) Loss of calretinin immunoreactivity in hypertrophied nerve bundles in Hirschsprung's disease. Nerves and ganglia show positive immunoreactivity for calretinin in normal control (**a**). In addition to absence of ganglion cells, the thick nerve bundles in Hirschsprung's disease exhibit loss of calretinin immunoreactivity (**b**)

Table 25.13 Colorectal adenocarcinoma and adenocarcinoma of anal gland origin

Markers	Colorectal carcinoma	Anal gland adenocarcinoma
AE1/AE3	+	+
CK7	−	+
CK20	+	−
CDX-2	+	−

References: [50, 51]

Table 25.14 Markers for anal Paget's disease vs. melanoma is situ

Antibody	Anal Paget's disease associated with colorectal carcinoma	Primary anal Paget's disease (not associated with underlying carcinoma)	Melanoma in situ
CK7	+	+	−
CK20	+	−	−
GCDFP-15	−	+	−
Mucin	+	+	−
Melan-A	−	−	+
S100	−	−	+

References: [52–56]

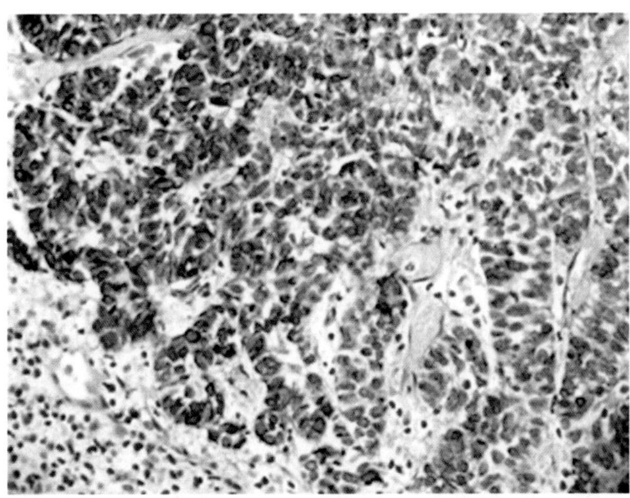

Fig. 25.3 Anal gland adenocarcinoma. The tumor cells exhibit positive CK7 immunoreactivity

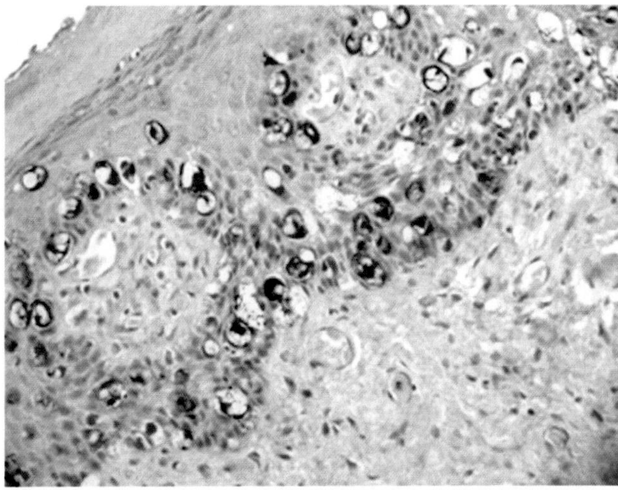

Fig. 25.4 Anal Paget's disease with underlying mucinous adenocarcinoma. The tumor cells involve the overlying epidermis with a pagetoid spreading and exhibit positive CK20 immunoreactivity

Table 25.15 Anal squamous cell carcinoma vs. melanoma

Antibody	Squamous cell carcinoma	Melanoma
AE1/AE3	+	–
p63	+	–
CK903	+	–
CK5/6	+	–
S100	–	+
Melan-A	–	+
HMB-45	–	+

References: [57–62]

Table 25.16 Markers for the differential diagnosis of anorectal granular cell tumor

Antibody	Granular cell tumor	Leiomyoma	Carcinoid tumor	Nevi
S100	+	–	–	+
CD57	+/–	–	–/+	–/+
Desmin	–	+	–	–
SMA	–	+	–	–
Melan-A	–	–	–	+
CAM 5.2	–	–	+	–
Synaptophysin	–	–	+	–/+

References: [63, 64]

25.2 Microsatellite Instability Test

25.2.1 What Is Microsatellite Instability?

Microsatellite instability (MSI) is a condition usually characterized by mutations, either an addition or a deletion of bases within nucleotide repeats known as microsatellite regions. MSI has been reported in up to 15% of colorectal adenocarcinomas. Microsatellite loci contain a repetitive sequence of one to six nucleotides in length. MSI was first reported in colorectal adenocarcinomas of patients with hereditary nonpolyposis colorectal cancer (HNPCC), also known as Lynch syndrome. This status of high-frequency mutagenesis is due to the mutations in one or more of the main DNA mismatch repair (MMR) genes. At the molecular level, defects in several DNA MMR proteins have been identified to underlie HNPCC, most often affecting MLH1 and MSH2 and less frequently involving MSH6, PMS1, or PMS2. In sporadic colorectal adenocarcinomas, loss of expression of MLH1 protein is frequently due to hypermethylation of the promoter gene for MLH1. In contrast, in HNPCC germline mutations of one of the genes for MMR proteins, especially MSH2, is the most common finding. These proteins can be detected by immunohistochemistry in addition to molecular testing.

References: [65–69]

25.2.2 What Is the Diagnostic Accuracy of the Immunohistochemical Stains?

In general, PCR-based tests for MSI and immunohistochemistry correlate very well, but there are rare (<3%) examples of germline mutations producing a detectable protein yet still causing MSI. Immunohistochemical studies are approximately 90–95% sensitive for HNPCC syndrome compared to the PCR-based MSI analysis. Loss of protein expression for any of the mismatch repair genes indicates a genetic defect or epigenetic alteration but does not differentiate between acquired/somatic vs. germline defects.

It should be mentioned that even a PCR-based test revealing the absence of MSI does not entirely exclude HNPCC, because approximately 10% of HNPCC carcinomas and 33% of HNPCC adenomas do not have MSI, particularly small adenomas (<1 cm).

References: [17, 70–73]

25.2.3 What Is the Clinical Significance of MSI?

Approximately 90% of HNPCCs and approximately 10–15% of sporadic colorectal cancers, which are far more common, have MSI. The presence of high MSI in the adenoma further increases the possibility of a germline mutation in one of the mismatch repair genes associated with HNPCC.

In general, microsatellite instability-high frequency (MSI-H) independently predicts improved overall survival.

Although the literature continues to evolve, there is evidence to suggest that high MSI, regardless of whether it involves a sporadic or HNPCC carcinoma (stage II, T3N0M0), may also predict a worse response to adjuvant chemotherapy regimens.

References: [71, 74]

25.2.4 What Are the 2004 Revised Bethesda Guidelines for MSI Testing?

1. Patient diagnosed with colorectal cancer (CRC) before the age of 50 years.
2. Patient diagnosed with adenomatous polyp before the age of 40 years.
3. Presence of synchronous or metachronous colorectal or other HNPCC-related tumors (stomach, urinary bladder, ureter and renal pelvis, biliary tract, brain [glioblastoma],

sebaceous gland adenomas, keratoacanthomas, and small bowel cancer), regardless of age.

4. CRCs diagnosed before the age of 60 years with morphology suggestive of MSI-H (including the presence of tumor-infiltrating lymphocytes, Crohn-like lymphocytic reaction, mucinous or signet ring cell differentiation, or medullary growth pattern).
5. CRC in a patient with one or more first-degree relatives with CRC or other HNPCC-related tumors (one of the cancers must have been diagnosed before the age of 50 years, and adenomas must have been diagnosed before the age of 40 years).
6. CRC in a patient with two or more relatives with CRC or other HNPCC-related tumors, regardless of age.

References: [75–79]

25.2.5 What Are the General Recommendations for the Detection of MSI?

1. Patient screening – following the 2004 revised Bethesda guidelines.
2. If immunohistochemical studies show detectable MMR proteins (MLH1, MSH2, MSH6, and PMS2), the patient is unlikely (5% or less) to have an MMR deficiency. In general, no further test is required for this patient.
3. If immunohistochemical stains reveal loss expression of one or more of the MMR proteins (MLH1, MSH2, MSH6, and PMS2), a PCR-based test for MSI should be considered.
4. If a germline gene alteration is identified, an appropriate genetic counseling to see if there are any familial implications should be considered.

References: [70, 71, 75, 80]

25.2.6 What Is the Recommended Panel of MSI Markers?

Immunohistochemical stains for four DNA mismatch repair proteins (MLH1, MSH2, MSH6, and PMS2) are typically recommended as a screening panel. In the DNA mismatch repair complex formation, MLH1 is required to form MLH1/PMS2 complex, and MSH2 is required to form MSH2/MSH6 complex. Loss of expression of MLH1 will result in the absence of PMS2. The same holds true for MSH2 and its binding partner MSH6. Based on this, some data also suggest that MSH6 and PMS2 can be used as the initial screening markers. If PMS2 and MSH6 are present, then MLH1 and MSH2 should be expressed as well. In contrast, while either PMS2 or MSH6 is lost, the status of expression of MLH1 and MSH2 is uncertain. Therefore, additional immunostains for assessing the expression of MLH1 and MSH2 would be needed. The studies from Shia et al. demonstrated the patterns of immunohistochemical staining results for MSI markers as follow: concurrent loss of MLH1/PMS2 – 65%; concurrent loss of MSH2/MSH6 – 18%; PMS2 loss only – 9%; and MSH6 loss only – 7%.

References: [70–73, 81]

25.2.7 What Is the Significance for a Surgical Pathologist Regarding MSI?

A colorectal carcinoma with MSI frequently demonstrates aberrant expression of cytokeratin 20 and CDX-2. In a medullary carcinoma of the colon with MSI, approximately 80% of cases show complete loss of expression or significantly reduced expression of CK20 and CDX-2 as shown in Fig. 25.5a–f. Other histological types of colorectal carcinoma with MSI also show complete or partial loss of expression of CK20 and CDX-2 in approximately 50% of cases. To complicate this matter further, CK7 can be expressed in a small portion of colorectal carcinomas, including carcinoma with MSI. It is important to be aware of this finding since CK20 and CDX-2 have been widely accepted as the diagnostic markers in identifying a colorectal primary while working on tumor of unknown origin. Loss of expression or only focal expression of CK20 and CDX-2 does not entirely exclude the possibility of a colorectal primary. If a colorectal primary is suspected, MSI markers (MLH1, MSH2, MSH6, and PMS2) should be included in the working panel.

References: [14–16, 82]

25.2.8 How to Interpret Immunohistochemical Staining Results

Optimization and validation of MSI antibodies need to be carried out in each individual laboratory. The staining for MSI antibodies can be variable from run to run. Therefore, in addition to positive and negative controls, a complete absence of nuclear staining for one or more MSI antibodies with a

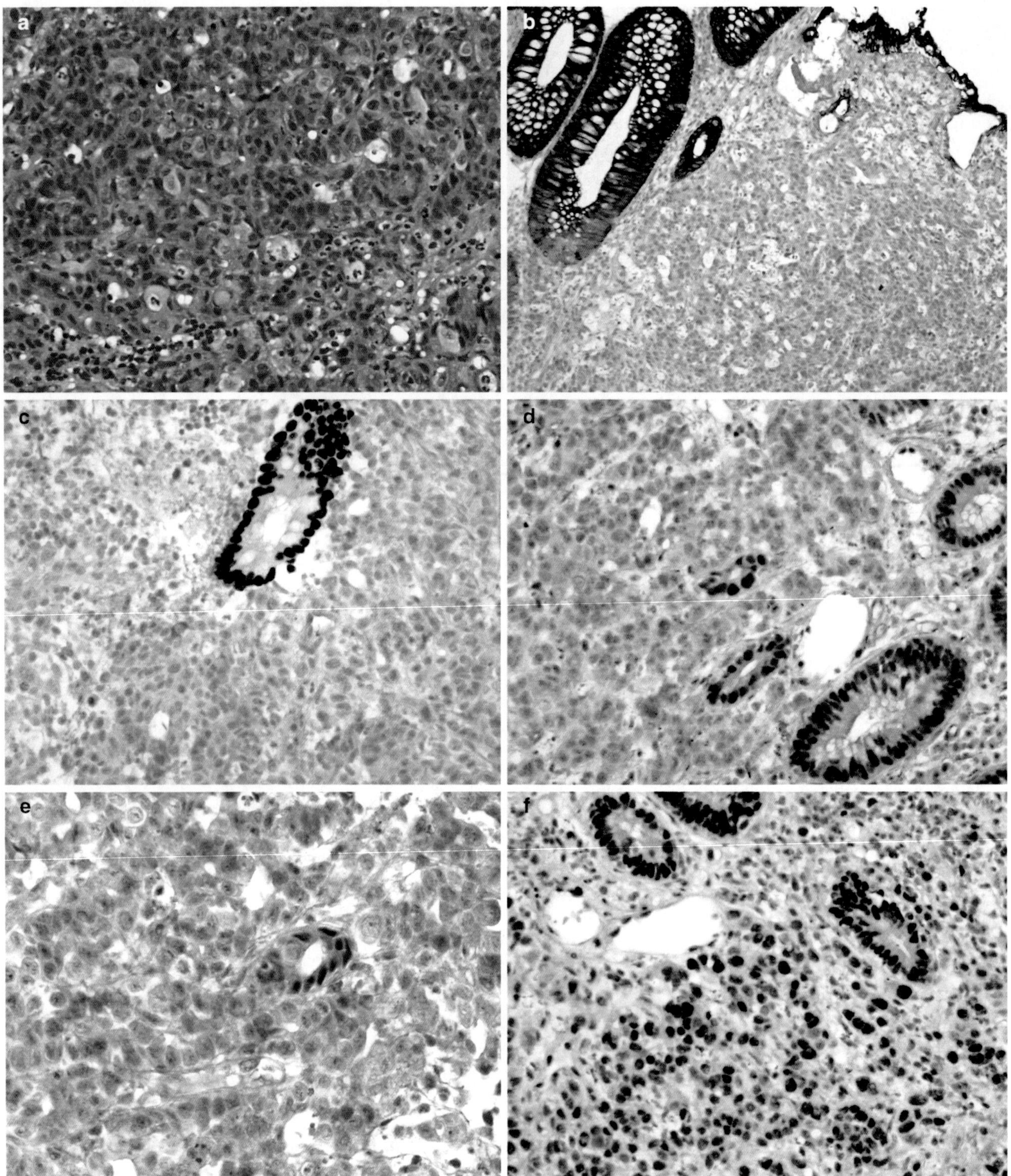

Fig. 25.5 (**a**–**f**) A case of medullary carcinoma of the colon demonstrated on H&E section (**a**). Note that the tumor cells have complete loss of expression of CK20 (**b**) and CDX-2 (**c**), no immunoreactivity for either MLH1 (**d**) or PMS2 (**e**), with strong positive internal control of trapped normal glands and inflammatory cells, and retain the expression of MSH2 (**f**) and MSH6 (not shown)

satisfactory internal positive control is essential for rendering "evidence of MSI." Lymphoid cells and crypts of normal glandular epithelium are good internal positive controls. Caution should be taken if the internal positive control is weak.

References: [70, 71, 73]

References

1. Vang R, Gown AM, Wu LS, et al. Immunohistochemical expression of CDX2 in primary ovarian mucinous tumors and metastatic mucinous carcinomas involving the ovary: comparison with CK20 and correlation with coordinate expression of CK7. Mod Pathol. 2006;19(11):1421–8.
2. Fraggetta F, Pelosi G, Cafici A, Scollo P, Nuciforo P, Viale G. CDX2 immunoreactivity in primary and metastatic ovarian mucinous tumours. Virchows Arch. 2003;443(6):782–6.
3. Vang R, Gown AM, Barry TS, et al. Cytokeratins 7 and 20 in primary and secondary mucinous tumors of the ovary: analysis of coordinate immunohistochemical expression profiles and staining distribution in 179 cases. Am J Surg Pathol. 2006;30(9):1130–9.
4. Lee MJ, Lee HS, Kim WH, Choi Y, Yang M. Expression of mucins and cytokeratins in primary carcinomas of the digestive system. Mod Pathol. 2003;16(5):403–10.
5. Goldstein NS, Bassi D, Uzieblo A. WT1 is an integral component of an antibody panel to distinguish pancreaticobiliary and some ovarian epithelial neoplasms. Am J Clin Pathol. 2001;116(2):246–52.
6. Guerrieri C, Franlund B, Fristedt S, Gillooley JF, Boeryd B. Mucinous tumors of the vermiform appendix and ovary, and pseudomyxoma peritonei: histogenetic implications of cytokeratin 7 expression. Hum Pathol. 1997;28(9):1039–45.
7. Ronnett BM, Kurman RJ, Shmookler BM, Sugarbaker PH, Young RH. The morphologic spectrum of ovarian metastases of appendiceal adenocarcinomas: a clinicopathologic and immunohistochemical analysis of tumors often misinterpreted as primary ovarian tumors or metastatic tumors from other gastrointestinal sites. Am J Surg Pathol. 1997;21(10):1144–55.
8. Seidman JD, Elsayed AM, Sobin LH, Tavassoli FA. Association of mucinous tumors of the ovary and appendix. A clinicopathologic study of 25 cases. Am J Surg Pathol. 1993;17(1):22–34.
9. Cai YC, Banner B, Glickman J, Odze RD. Cytokeratin 7 and 20 and thyroid transcription factor 1 can help distinguish pulmonary from gastrointestinal carcinoid and pancreatic endocrine tumors. Hum Pathol. 2001;32(10):1087–93.
10. Barbareschi M, Roldo C, Zamboni G, et al. CDX-2 homeobox gene product expression in neuroendocrine tumors: its role as a marker of intestinal neuroendocrine tumors. Am J Surg Pathol. 2004;28(9): 1169–76.
11. Alsaad KO, Serra S, Schmitt A, Perren A, Chetty R. Cytokeratins 7 and 20 immunoexpression profile in goblet cell and classical carcinoids of appendix. Endocr Pathol. 2007;18(1):16–22.
12. Burke AP, Sobin LH, Federspiel BH, Shekitka KM. Appendiceal carcinoids: correlation of histology and immunohistochemistry. Mod Pathol. 1989;2(6):630–7.
13. Winn B, Tavares R, Fanion J, et al. Differentiating the undifferentiated: immunohistochemical profile of medullary carcinoma of the colon with an emphasis on intestinal differentiation. Hum Pathol. 2009;40(3):398–404.
14. Lugli A, Tzankov A, Zlobec I, Terracciano LM. Differential diagnostic and functional role of the multi-marker phenotype CDX2/CK20/CK7 in colorectal cancer stratified by mismatch repair status. Mod Pathol. 2008;21(11):1403–12.
15. Hinoi T, Tani M, Lucas PC, et al. Loss of CDX2 expression and microsatellite instability are prominent features of large cell minimally differentiated carcinomas of the colon. Am J Pathol. 2001;159(6):2239–48.
16. McGregor DK, Wu TT, Rashid A, Luthra R, Hamilton SR. Reduced expression of cytokeratin 20 in colorectal carcinomas with high levels of microsatellite instability. Am J Surg Pathol. 2004;28(6): 712–8.
17. Wright CL, Stewart ID. Histopathology and mismatch repair status of 458 consecutive colorectal carcinomas. Am J Surg Pathol. 2003;27(11):1393–406.
18. Suh N, Yang XJ, Tretiakova MS, Humphrey PA, Wang HL. Value of CDX2, villin, and alpha-methylacyl coenzyme A racemase immunostains in the distinction between primary adenocarcinoma of the bladder and secondary colorectal adenocarcinoma. Mod Pathol. 2005;18(9):1217–22.
19. Wang HL, Lu DW, Yerian LM, et al. Immunohistochemical distinction between primary adenocarcinoma of the bladder and secondary colorectal adenocarcinoma. Am J Surg Pathol. 2001;25(11): 1380–7.
20. Cathro HP, Stoler MH. Expression of cytokeratins 7 and 20 in ovarian neoplasia. Am J Clin Pathol. 2002;117(6):944–51.
21. Nishizuka S, Chen ST, Gwadry FG, et al. Diagnostic markers that distinguish colon and ovarian adenocarcinomas: identification by genomic, proteomic, and tissue array profiling. Cancer Res. 2003;63(17):5243–50.
22. Inamura K, Satoh Y, Okumura S, et al. Pulmonary adenocarcinomas with enteric differentiation: histologic and immunohistochemical characteristics compared with metastatic colorectal cancers and usual pulmonary adenocarcinomas. Am J Surg Pathol. 2005;29(5):660–5.
23. Tan J, Sidhu G, Greco MA, Ballard H, Wieczorek R. Villin, cytokeratin 7, and cytokeratin 20 expression in pulmonary adenocarcinoma with ultrastructural evidence of microvilli with rootlets. Hum Pathol. 1998;29(4):390–6.
24. Yatabe Y, Koga T, Mitsudomi T, Takahashi T. CK20 expression, CDX2 expression, K-ras mutation, and goblet cell morphology in a subset of lung adenocarcinomas. J Pathol. 2004;203(2):645–52.
25. Chu AY, Litzky LA, Pasha TL, Acs G, Zhang PJ. Utility of D2-40, a novel mesothelial marker, in the diagnosis of malignant mesothelioma. Mod Pathol. 2005;18(1):105–10.
26. Ordonez NG. Immunohistochemical diagnosis of epithelioid mesothelioma: an update. Arch Pathol Lab Med. 2005;129(11): 1407–14.
27. Ordonez NG. Value of cytokeratin 5/6 immunostaining in distinguishing epithelial mesothelioma of the pleura from lung adenocarcinoma. Am J Surg Pathol. 1998;22(10):1215–21.
28. Pancione M, Forte N, Fucci A, et al. Prognostic role of beta-catenin and p53 expression in the metastatic progression of sporadic colorectal cancer. Hum Pathol. 2010;41(6):867–76.
29. Pancione M, Forte N, Sabatino L, et al. Reduced beta-catenin and peroxisome proliferator-activated receptor-gamma expression levels are associated with colorectal cancer metastatic progression: correlation with tumor-associated macrophages, cyclooxygenase 2, and patient outcome. Hum Pathol. 2009;40(5):714–25.
30. Xie D, Sham JS, Zeng WF, et al. Heterogeneous expression and association of beta-catenin, p16 and c-myc in multistage colorectal tumorigenesis and progression detected by tissue microarray. Int J Cancer. 2003;107(6):896–902.
31. De Roock W, Piessevaux H, De Schutter J, et al. KRAS wild-type state predicts survival and is associated to early radiological response in metastatic colorectal cancer treated with cetuximab. Ann Oncol. 2008;19(3):508–15.
32. Lievre A, Bachet JB, Boige V, et al. KRAS mutations as an independent prognostic factor in patients with advanced colorectal cancer treated with cetuximab. J Clin Oncol. 2008;26(3):374–9.

33. Loupakis F, Ruzzo A, Cremolini C, et al. KRAS codon 61, 146 and BRAF mutations predict resistance to cetuximab plus irinotecan in KRAS codon 12 and 13 wild-type metastatic colorectal cancer. Br J Cancer. 2009;101(4):715–21.
34. Azumi N, Traweek ST, Battifora H. Prostatic acid phosphatase in carcinoid tumors. Immunohistochemical and immunoblot studies. Am J Surg Pathol. 1991;15(8):785–90.
35. Sobin LH, Hjermstad BM, Sesterhenn IA, Helwig EB. Prostatic acid phosphatase activity in carcinoid tumors. Cancer. 1986;58(1):136–8.
36. Miettinen M, Sobin LH, Sarlomo-Rikala M. Immunohistochemical spectrum of GISTs at different sites and their differential diagnosis with a reference to CD117 (KIT). Mod Pathol. 2000;13(10):1134–42.
37. Miettinen M, Furlong M, Sarlomo-Rikala M, Burke A, Sobin LH, Lasota J. Gastrointestinal stromal tumors, intramural leiomyomas, and leiomyosarcomas in the rectum and anus: a clinicopathologic, immunohistochemical, and molecular genetic study of 144 cases. Am J Surg Pathol. 2001;25(9):1121–33.
38. Ramos da Silva S, Bacchi MM, Bacchi CE, Elgui de Oliveira D. Human bcl-2 expression, cleaved caspase-3, and KSHV LANA-1 in Kaposi sarcoma lesions. Am J Clin Pathol. 2007;128(5):794–802.
39. Shekitka KM, Sobin LH. Ganglioneuromas of the gastrointestinal tract. Relation to Von Recklinghausen disease and other multiple tumor syndromes. Am J Surg Pathol. 1994;18(3):250–7.
40. Parfitt JR, Rodriguez-Justo M, Feakins R, Novelli MR. Gastrointestinal Kaposi's sarcoma: CD117 expression and the potential for misdiagnosis as gastrointestinal stromal tumour. Histopathology. 2008;52(7):816–23.
41. Shidham VB, Chivukula M, Gupta D, Rao RN, Komorowski R. Immunohistochemical comparison of gastrointestinal stromal tumor and solitary fibrous tumor. Arch Pathol Lab Med. 2002;126(10): 1189–92.
42. Marx A, Wandrey T, Simon P, et al. Combined alpha-methylacyl coenzyme A racemase/p53 analysis to identify dysplasia in inflammatory bowel disease. Hum Pathol. 2009;40(2):166–73.
43. Dorer R, Odze RD. AMACR immunostaining is useful in detecting dysplastic epithelium in Barrett's esophagus, ulcerative colitis, and Crohn's disease. Am J Surg Pathol. 2006;30(7):871–7.
44. Wong NA, Mayer NJ, MacKell S, Gilmour HM, Harrison DJ. Immunohistochemical assessment of Ki67 and p53 expression assists the diagnosis and grading of ulcerative colitis-related dysplasia. Histopathology. 2000;37(2):108–14.
45. Harpaz N, Peck AL, Yin J, et al. p53 protein expression in ulcerative colitis-associated colorectal dysplasia and carcinoma. Hum Pathol. 1994;25(10):1069–74.
46. Bruwer M, Schmid KW, Senninger N, Schurmann G. Immunohistochemical expression of P53 and oncogenes in ulcerative colitis-associated colorectal carcinoma. World J Surg. 2002;26(3):390–6.
47. Kapur RP, Reed RC, Finn L, et al. Calretinin immunohistochemisty versus acetylcholinersterase histochemistry in the elevation of suction rectal biopsies for Hirschsprung disease. Pediatr Dev Pathol. 2009;12(1):6–15.
48. Monforte-Munoz H, Gonzalez-Gomez I, Rowland JM, Landing BH. Increased submucosal nerve trunk caliber in aganglionosis: a "positive" and objective finding in suction biopsies and segmental resections in Hirschsprung's disease. Arch Pathol Lab Med. 1998;122(8):721–5.
49. MacKenzie JM, Dixon MF. An immunohistochemical study of the enteric neural plexi in Hirschsprung's disease. Histopathology. 1987;11(10):1055–66.
50. Hobbs CM, Lowry MA, Owen D, Sobin LH. Anal gland carcinoma. Cancer. 2001;92(8):2045–9.
51. Lisovsky M, Patel K, Cymes K, Chase D, Bhuiya T, Morgenstern N. Immunophenotypic characterization of anal gland carcinoma: loss of p63 and cytokeratin 5/6. Arch Pathol Lab Med. 2007;131(8):1304–11.
52. Nowak MA, Guerriere-Kovach P, Pathan A, Campbell TE, Deppisch LM. Perianal Paget's disease: distinguishing primary and secondary lesions using immunohistochemical studies including gross cystic disease fluid protein-15 and cytokeratin 20 expression. Arch Pathol Lab Med. 1998;122(12):1077–81.
53. Goldblum JR, Hart WR. Perianal Paget's disease: a histologic and immunohistochemical study of 11 cases with and without associated rectal adenocarcinoma. Am J Surg Pathol. 1998;22(2):170–9.
54. Battles OE, Page DL, Johnson JE. Cytokeratins, CEA, and mucin histochemistry in the diagnosis and characterization of extramammary Paget's disease. Am J Clin Pathol. 1997;108(1):6–12.
55. Smith KJ, Tuur S, Corvette D, Lupton GP, Skelton HG. Cytokeratin 7 staining in mammary and extramammary Paget's disease. Mod Pathol. 1997;10(11):1069–74.
56. Ohnishi T, Watanabe S. The use of cytokeratins 7 and 20 in the diagnosis of primary and secondary extramammary Paget's disease. Br J Dermatol. 2000;142(2):243–7.
57. Balachandra B, Marcus V, Jass JR. Poorly differentiated tumours of the anal canal: a diagnostic strategy for the surgical pathologist. Histopathology. 2007;50(1):163–74.
58. Kaufmann O, Fietze E, Mengs J, Dietel M. Value of p63 and cytokeratin 5/6 as immunohistochemical markers for the differential diagnosis of poorly differentiated and undifferentiated carcinomas. Am J Clin Pathol. 2001;116(6):823–30.
59. Stelow EB, Moskaluk CA, Mills SE. The mismatch repair protein status of colorectal small cell neuroendocrine carcinomas. Am J Surg Pathol. 2006;30(11):1401–4.
60. Longacre TA, Kong CS, Welton ML. Diagnostic problems in anal pathology. Adv Anat Pathol. 2008;15(5):263–78.
61. Owens SR, Greenson JK. Immunohistochemical staining for p63 is useful in the diagnosis of anal squamous cell carcinomas. Am J Surg Pathol. 2007;31(2):285–90.
62. Chute DJ, Cousar JB, Mills SE. Anorectal malignant melanoma: morphologic and immunohistochemical features. Am J Clin Pathol. 2006;126(1):93–100.
63. Ryan P, Nguyen VH, Gholoum S, et al. Polypoid PEComa in the rectum of a 15-year-old girl: case report and review of PEComa in the gastrointestinal tract. Am J Surg Pathol. 2009;33(3): 475–82.
64. Walsh SN, Hurt MA. Cutaneous fetal rhabdomyoma: a case report and historical review of the literature. Am J Surg Pathol. 2008;32(3):485–91.
65. Umar A. Lynch syndrome (HNPCC) and microsatellite instability. Dis Markers. 2004;20(4–5):179–80.
66. Samowitz WS, Curtin K, Ma KN, et al. Microsatellite instability in sporadic colon cancer is associated with an improved prognosis at the population level. Cancer Epidemiol Biomarkers Prev. 2001;10(9):917–23.
67. Peltomaki P. Deficient DNA mismatch repair: a common etiologic factor for colon cancer. Hum Mol Genet. 2001;10(7):735–40.
68. Lynch HT, Lanspa SJ, Boman BM, et al. Hereditary nonpolyposis colorectal cancer – Lynch syndromes I and II. Gastroenterol Clin North Am. 1988;17(4):679–712.
69. Alexander J, Watanabe T, Wu TT, Rashid A, Li S, Hamilton SR. Histopathological identification of colon cancer with microsatellite instability. Am J Pathol. 2001;158(2):527–35.
70. Dabbs DJ. Diagnostic immunohistochemistry: theranostic and genomic applications. 3rd ed. Philadelphia, PA: Saunders Elsevier; 2010.
71. Odze RD, Goldblum JR, editors. Surgical pathology of the GI tract, liver, biliary tract and pancreas. Philadelphia, PA: Saunders Elsevier; 2009.
72. Greenson JK, Huang SC, Herron C, et al. Pathologic predictors of microsatellite instability in colorectal cancer. Am J Surg Pathol. 2009;33(1):126–33.

73. Jover R, Paya A, Alenda C, et al. Defective mismatch-repair colorectal cancer: clinicopathologic characteristics and usefulness of immunohistochemical analysis for diagnosis. Am J Clin Pathol. 2004;122(3):389–94.
74. Brueckl WM, Moesch C, Brabletz T, et al. Relationship between microsatellite instability, response and survival in palliative patients with colorectal cancer undergoing first-line chemotherapy. Anticancer Res. 2003;23(2C):1773–7.
75. Boland CR, Thibodeau SN, Hamilton SR, et al. A National Cancer Institute Workshop on Microsatellite Instability for cancer detection and familial predisposition: development of international criteria for the determination of microsatellite instability in colorectal cancer. Cancer Res. 1998;58(22):5248–57.
76. Umar A, Boland CR, Terdiman JP, et al. Revised Bethesda Guidelines for hereditary nonpolyposis colorectal cancer (Lynch syndrome) and microsatellite instability. J Natl Cancer Inst. 2004;96(4):261–8.
77. Umar A, Risinger JI, Hawk ET, Barrett JC. Testing guidelines for hereditary non-polyposis colorectal cancer. Nat Rev Cancer. 2004;4(2):153–8.
78. Gologan A, Krasinskas A, Hunt J, Thull DL, Farkas L, Sepulveda AR. Performance of the revised Bethesda guidelines for identification of colorectal carcinomas with a high level of microsatellite instability. Arch Pathol Lab Med. 2005;129(11):1390–7.
79. Greenson JK, Bonner JD, Ben-Yzhak O, et al. Phenotype of microsatellite unstable colorectal carcinomas: well-differentiated and focally mucinous tumors and the absence of dirty necrosis correlate with microsatellite instability. Am J Surg Pathol. 2003;27(5):563–70.
80. Gologan A, Sepulveda AR. Microsatellite instability and DNA mismatch repair deficiency testing in hereditary and sporadic gastrointestinal cancers. Clin Lab Med. 2005;25(1):179–96.
81. Shia J, Tang LH, Vakiani E, et al. Immunohistochemistry as first-line screening for detecting colorectal cancer patients at risk for hereditary nonpolyposis colorectal cancer syndrome: a 2-antibody panel may be as predictive as a 4-antibody panel. Am J Surg Pathol. 2009;33(11):1639–45.
82. Zhu SB, Schuerch C, Lin F. Absent or low expression of CK20 and CDX2 associated with microsatellite instability in poorly differentiated colorectal carcinomas (PDCC) [USCAP abstract 567]. Mod Pathol. 2005;18(Suppl 4a):124A.

Chapter 26
Soft Tissue and Bone Tumors

Shaobo Zhu and Markku Miettinen

Abstract Immunohistochemistry is a powerful adjunctive technique for the pathologic diagnosis of soft tissue and bone tumors, although some tumors still lack specific markers. This chapter includes the questions about the immunohistochemical markers for normal soft tissue and bone, soft tissue and bone tumors, and their utility for differentiation. The questions are answered in the form of tables. The photos of selected markers are also included. New markers such as MDM2, TLS/EWS-CHOP chimeric oncoproteins, HHV8, TFE3, and TLE1, as well as other commonly used markers, are discussed.

Keywords Immunohistochemistry • Soft tissue • Bone • Tumor • Sarcoma • Immunohistochemical markers • Pathologic diagnosis • MDM2 • CDK4 • HHV8 LANA • TLS/EWS-CHOP • TFE3 • TLE1

FREQUENTLY ASKED QUESTIONS

Adipocytic Tumors

S. Zhu (✉)
Department of Pathology and Laboratory Medicine, Geisinger Medical Center, 100 N. Academy Ave, Danville, PA 17822, USA
e-mail: szhu1@geisinger.edu

Fibroblastic and Fibrohistiocytic Tumors

Fibrohistiocytic Tumors

F. Lin and J. Prichard (eds.), *Handbook of Practical Immunohistochemistry: Frequently Asked Questions*,
DOI 10.1007/978-1-4419-8062-5_26,

Table 26.1 Summary of applications and limitations of useful markers

Antibody	Staining pattern	Function	Key applications and pitfalls
AE1/AE3	C	Epithelial marker; cocktail acidic (AE1) and basic keratins (AE3), including high and low molecular weight keratins, numbers 1–8, 9–17, and 19	Positive in epithelioid sarcoma, synovial sarcoma, extrarenal rhabdoid tumor, and other soft tissue tumors with epithelial differentiation, some angiosarcomas and leiomyosarcomas, and sporadically other sarcomas
ALK-1	C + N	A tyrosine kinase receptor for the growth factor pleiotrophin	Positive in anaplastic large cell lymphoma, some large B-cell lymphomas, inflammatory myofibroblastic tumor, and possibly some rhabdomyosarcomas
Bcl-2	M + C + N	A mitochondrial and microsomal protein and an inhibitor of apoptosis. Normally expressed by small B lymphocytes of the mantle and marginal zones and by T cells	Positive in follicular derived B-cell lymphomas. Present in normal T-cell and B-cell subsets and many soft tissue tumors, such as solitary fibrous tumor, synovial sarcoma, and GIST
Ber-BP4	M	A cell surface glycoprotein broadly distributed in epithelial cells. Expressed in all epithelial cells, except for superficial layers of squamous epithelium, hepatocytes, and gastric parietal cells	Positive in carcinomas, biphasic synovial sarcoma, and some desmoplastic small round cell tumors
Beta-catenin	M + C + N	A component of cell–cell adhesion and Wnt signal transduction pathway	Nuclear positivity in desmoid fibromatosis (80%), variable. Widespread cytoplasmic expression in epithelial and mesenchymal cells
Brachyury	N	A transcription factor encoded by the T gene and is essential for *mesoderm* formation and *cellular differentiation*	A diagnostic marker for chordoma
CD1a	M	MHC-related glycoprotein. Expressed in immature T cells, interdigitating reticulum cells, and Langerhans cells	Positive in lymphoblastic lymphoma and Langerhans cell histiocytosis
Calponin	C	Calcium binding protein; inhibits smooth muscle ATPase	Marker for smooth muscle, myofibroblasts, and myoepithelial cells. Also positive in synovial sarcoma

(continued)

Table 26.1 (continued)

Antibody	Staining pattern	Function	Key applications and pitfalls
Calretinin	C or N + C	Calcium binding protein	Positive in mesothelial cells, adipocytes, mast cells, neural cells, and sex cord tumors
CD10	M	A zinc-dependent cell membrane metalloprotein, also known as common acute lymphoblastic leukemia antigen	Positive in follicular center cells, acute lymphocytic leukemia, some renal cell carcinomas, melanoma, rhabdomyosarcoma, and many fibroblastic tumors
CD31	M + C	A membrane glycoprotein found at endothelial cell junctions and on the surface of platelets	Very sensitive and specific endothelial marker. Positive in vascular tumors. Also expressed in intratumoral macrophages
CD34	C + M	A transmembrane glycoprotein; marker for endothelial and hematopoietic progenitor cell	Positive in vascular tumors, spindle cell lipoma, many fibroblastic tumors, DFSP, neurofibroma, some smooth muscle tumors, epithelioid sarcoma, less specific and sensitive marker for vascular tumors than CD31
CD56	M + C	A cell adhesion molecule, marker for neuroendocrine differentiation	Positive in neuroendocrine tumors and a variety of sarcomas, including neuroblastoma, rhabdomyosarcoma, synovial sarcoma, and mesenchymal chondrosarcoma
CD57 (Leu7)	M	A myelin-associated glycoprotein	Marker for NK cells, T-cell subset, neuroendocrine tumors, and nerve sheath tumors. Also positive in neuroblastoma, EW/PNET, granular cell tumors, synovial sarcoma, leiomyosarcoma, and some carcinomas
CD68	C + M	A glycoprotein associated with lysosomes	Marker for lysosomes. Positive for histiocytes/monocytes, benign and malignant fibrous histiocytoma, granular cell tumors, and other sarcomas, melanomas, and carcinomas
CDK4	N	A catalytic subunit of the protein kinase complex that is important for cell cycle G1 phase progression	Positive in variety of tumors. A marker to differentiate liposarcoma from lipoma and to separate dedifferentiated liposarcoma from poorly differentiated sarcomas
CD99	M	A cell surface glycoprotein	Positive in EW/PNET and lymphoblastic lymphoma (almost 100% membrane positivity), often in synovial sarcoma, MPNST, mesenchymal chondrosarcoma, hemangiopericytoma, and some other soft tissue tumors
CD163	M	A transmembrane protein mediating the endocytosis of haptoglobin–hemoglobin complexes	A specific marker for monocytes and macrophages; positive in histiocytes except for many multinucleated forms
CD207 (Langerin)	M	A type II membrane-associated C-type lectin known to be expressed exclusively by Langerhans cells	A marker for Langerhans cell histocytosis
Claudin1		Marker for epithelial and perineurial cells	Positive in perineurioma. Variable expression in synovial sarcoma, epithelioid sarcoma, and ES/PNET
Chromogranin A	C	An acidic glycoprotein located in neurosecretory granules	Positive in epithelial neuroendocrine tumors (carcinoid/carcinomas), and paraganglioma
CK5/6	M + C	Basic keratins, an epithelial marker	Squamous and basal cells, squamous or basal cell differentiation in carcinoma
CK7	M + C	Basic, low molecular weight keratin, an epithelial marker	Positive in many carcinomas and epithelial elements of synovial sarcoma
CK8 (CAM5.2)	C	Low molecular weight keratin, an epithelial marker	Positive in most carcinomas and synovial and epithelioid sarcoma
CK14	C	Low molecular weight keratin, an epithelial marker	Positive in carcinoma with stratified epithelial differentiation and biphasic synovial sarcoma

(continued)

Table 26.1 (continued)

Antibody	Staining pattern	Function	Key applications and pitfalls
CK17	C	Acidic type I cytokeratin, an epithelial marker	Positive in some carcinomas and adamantinoma, and focally in biphasic synovial sarcoma
CK19	C	Low molecular weight keratin, an epithelial marker	Positive in most carcinomas and synovial and epithelioid sarcoma
CK20	M + C	Low molecular weight keratin, an epithelial marker	Positive in most GI carcinomas and other carcinomas
D2-40 (podoplanin)	M, C	A transmembrane sialoglycoprotein	Positive in mesothelial cells, lymphatic endothelial cells, seminomas, and many carcinomas
Desmin	C	Intermediate filament related to the sarcomere	Very sensitive marker for smooth muscle and striated muscle tumors. Also positive in myoid cells and some reticulum cells of the lymph node, submesothelial fibroblasts, desmoid tumors, DSRCT, and tumors with heterologous myoid differentiation (MPNST, rhabdoid tumor)
EBNA-1	N	EBV nuclear antigen	Positive in EBV-associated smooth muscle tumors or some lymphomas
E-cadherin	M	The major calcium-dependent cell adhesion molecule of epithelial cells	Expression by carcinomas is inversely proportional to the degree of differentiation, positive in sarcoma with epithelioid differentiation, such as synovial sarcoma
EMA (MUC1)	M + C	One of human milk fat globule proteins, a epithelial marker	Positive in carcinomas, synovial sarcoma, epithelioid sarcoma, perineurioma, chordoma, and angiomatoid fibrous histiocytomas
ER	N	Estrogen receptor	Positive in breast carcinoma, cellular angiofibroma, angiomyofibroblastoma, and female deep smooth muscle tumors
Factor XIIIa	C	Subunit of plasma clotting factor XII; a marker for dermal dendrocyte	Positive in intratumoral histiocytes, present in greater quantity in benign fibrous histiocytoma than in DFSP
FGF23	C	A member of the *fibroblast growth factor* (FGF) family which is responsible for *phosphate* metabolism	Positive in phosphaturic mesenchymal tumor. Information on specificity is limited
FLI-1	N	Nuclear transcription factor, an endothelial marker	Positive in vascular tumors and Ewing Sarcoma/PNET, and lymphoblastic lymphoma
GFAP	C	One of the major types of intermediate filament, a marker of astrocytes	Positive in some nerve sheath tumors (especially schwannomas), sustentacular cells of paragangliomas, and myoepithelial tumors
GLUT1	C + M	Major glucose transporter at epithelial and endothelial tissue	Positive in perineurioma and infantile hemangiomas but absent in other pediatric vascular tumors including vascular malformations
h-Caldesmon	C	A cytoskeleton-associated protein which regulates cellular contraction	Positive in smooth muscle tumors, glomus tumors, GIST, and myopericytomas
HHV8 LANA	N	Latent nuclear antigen of human herpes virus type 8	Positive in Kaposi's sarcoma, primary effusion lymphoma, and Castleman disease
HMB45	C	Recognizes the antigen gp100 on melanosomes	Positive in melanoma, cellular blue nevus, and PEComas, including angiomyolipoma
INI-1	N	A member of the SWI/SWF chromatin-remodeling complex, encoded by a putative tumor suppressor gene. Normally expresses in all tissues.	Loss of nuclear expression in epithelioid sarcoma, rhabdoid tumor, and atypical teratoid/rhabdoid tumor

(continued)

Table 26.1 (continued)

Antibody	Staining pattern	Function	Key applications and pitfalls
Ki-67 (MIB-1)	N	Nuclear proliferation marker; expression in cells in the G1, M, G2, and S phase of the cell cycle except G0 phase	Marker for proliferation index. Ki-67 index (the number of Ki-67-positive tumor cells/10 HPF) positively correlated with mitotic count, cellularity, and the histological grade. Threshold values vary by tumor.
MDM2	N	Functions both as an *E3 ubiquitin ligase* that recognizes the *N-terminal trans*-activation domain (TAD) of the *p53* tumor suppressor and an inhibitor of *p53* transcriptional activation	Positive in variety of tumors. A marker to differentiate atypical lipomatous tumor/ well-differentiated liposarcoma from lipoma and to separate dedifferentiated liposarcoma from other poorly differentiated sarcomas
Melan A (MART-1)	C	Marker for melanosomes	Positive for melanoma and PEComas (variable)
MITF	N	Transcription factor involved in the development of melanocytes and regulation of melanin synthesis, a nuclear melanocytic marker	Positive in melanoma, clear cell sarcoma, and most PEComas, histiocytes including osteoclasts
MOC31	M	A glycoprotein in epithelium, but absent on mesothelial tissues	Marker for adenocarcinoma and other carcinomas negative for mesothelium, and positive for DSRCT
MSA	C	Actin subsets. Contractile microfilament proteins	Marker for smooth muscle and striated muscle tumors, and myofibroblastic and myoepithelial differentiation
MyoD1	N	Protein which regulates muscle differentiation	Present in immature skeletal muscle cells. Specific marker for rhabdomyosarcoma. Only nuclear staining is specific for skeletal muscle differentiation. Also positive in tumors with rhabdomyoblastic differentiation. Cytoplasmic staining has no diagnostic significance
Myogenin	N	Transcription factor, member of the MyoD family involved in skeletal muscle development and repair	Present in immature skeletal muscle cells. Specific marker for rhabdomyosarcoma. Cytoplasmic staining is not specific for skeletal muscle differentiation. Also positive in other tumors with rhabdomyoblastic differentiation
NB84	C	An antibody raised against an antigen from human neuroblastoma tissue	A highly sensitive marker for neuroblastoma. Up to 25% of ES/PNET react with NB84, rare rhabdomyosarcomas, esthesisoneuroblastomas, DRCT, and Wilms's tumor are positive for this marker. NB 84 is more sensitive but less specific than synaptophysin for the diagnosis of neuroblastoma
NFP	C	Neurofilament protein, a marker for neurons and axonal processes except for olfactory sensory neurons	Positive for neuroblastic tumors. NF68 is more prevalent than medium (NF160) and high (NF200) molecular weight neurofilament proteins.
NSE	C	Neuron specific enolase, a marker for neuronal cells and cells with neuroendocrine differentiation	Low specificity. Also reacts with smooth muscle cells. Additional markers are always needed to support a diagnosis of neuroendocrine or neural tumor
Osteocalcin	C	A noncollugenous protein in the bone. It is secreted by osteoblasts only	A specific marker for osteoblastic differentiation. Positive in osteosarcoma and mesenchymal chondrosarcoma
Protein gene product 9.5 (PGP 9.5)		A member of the ubiquitin hydrolase family of proteins, expressed in neural and neuroendocrine cells	A sensitive neural/nerve sheath marker, but specificity is low
PR	N	Progesterone receptor	Positive in breast carcinoma, cellular angiofibroma, angiomyofibroblastomas vulval nerve sheath tumor, aggressive angiomyxoma, and female deep smooth muscle tumors

(continued)

Table 26.1 (continued)

Antibody	Staining pattern	Function	Key applications and pitfalls
S100	N, C	A calcium binding protein. Marker for Langerhans cells, myoepithelial cells, melanocytes, chondrocytes, Schwann cells, and adipocytes	Positive in benign and malignant nerve sheath tumors, melanoma, some adipocytic tumors, chondrocytic tumors, ossifying fibromyxoid tumor, and some chordomas
SMM-HC	C	Smooth muscle myosin heavy chain, a cytoplasmic structural protein and a major component of the contractile apparatus in smooth muscle cells	Smooth muscle, myofibroblasts, and myoepithelial cells
SOX9	N	A transcription factor functions during chondrocyte differentiation	Sensitive marker for cartilaginous differentiation. Also in cartilage elements of mesenchymal chondrosarcoma. Information on specificity is limited
Synaptophysin	C	Synaptic vesicle membrane protein	Present in small neurosecretory vesicles of neuroendocrine and neural cells
TFE3	N	Product of ASPL-TFE3 gene fusion due to unbalanced translocation, der(17)t(X;17)(p11.2;q25)	A sensitive and specific marker for alveolar soft part sarcoma. Also positive in translocation-type renal cell carcinoma, granular cell tumors, and some PEComas. Only nuclear staining is diagnostic
TLS/EWS-CHOP chimeric oncoproteins	N	Fusion oncoproteins of *t(12;22)(q13;q11-12)* and *t(12;22)(q13;q12)* translocations	A marker for myxoid/round cell liposarcoma
TLE1	N	A transcriptional corepressor that inhibit Wnt signaling and other cell fate determination signals, and have an established role in repressing differentiation	A highly sensitive and relatively specific marker for synovial sarcoma, occasionally positive in other soft tissue tumors
Type IV collagen	C	A type of *collagen* found primarily in the *basal lamina*	Pericellular expression in glomus tumor
Vimentin	C	Intermediate filament of cytoskeleton expressed in all mesenchymal cells	Positive in most sarcoma, melanoma, some carcinomas and lymphoma, but negative in alveolar soft part sarcoma and perivascular epithelioid cell neoplasms
vWF	C	A large *glycoprotein* synthesized by endothelial cells and megakaryocytes and involves in *hemostasis*	Positive for vascular tumors, such as hemangioma and hemangioendotheliomas. Low sensitivity in poorly differentiated vascular tumors. Can be found in zones of tumor necrosis and hemorrhage
VEGFR3	M	Vascular endothelial growth factor 3, a receptor tyrosine kinase, formerly known as FLT4	Specific marker for lymphatic endothelial cells. Positive in a variety of vascular tumors, including Kaposi's sarcoma and kaposiform, and Dabska-type hemangioendotheliomas, and many angiosarcomas
WT-1	N	A zinc finger transcription factor essential for correct mammalian urogenital development	Marker for DSRCT and mesothelial cells. Expressed in serous carcinoma of ovarian and extraovarian origin, mullerian smooth muscle tumors, mesothelioma, and desmoplastic small round cell tumor (note cariboxyterminus only present in the latter)

Note: *C* cytoplasmic staining; *M* membranous staining; *N* nuclear staining; *DFSP* dermatofibrosarcoma protuberans; *DSRCT* desmoplastic small round cell tumor; *EW/PNET* Ewing's sarcoma/primitive neuroectodermal tumor; *GIST* gastrointestinal stomal tumor; *MPNST* malignant peripheral nerve sheath tumor; *PEComas* perivascular epithelioid cell tumors

References: [1–4]

Table 26.2 Markers positive for normal soft tissue and bone

Tissue	Markers positive
Adipocytes	Vimentin, S100 (variable), calretinin
Chondrocyte	S100, SOX9
Endothelium	Vimentin, CD31, CD34, vWF, FLI-1, CK8, CK18, thrombomodulin, UEAI, D2-40 (lymphatic endothelium)
Fibroblasts	Vimentin, CD10, CD99
Langerhans cell	S100, CD1a, CD207
Myofibroblast	Desmin, MSA, vimentin (varies)
notochord	EMA, keratins, S100 (varies)
Osteoblast	CD56, vimentin
Osteoclast	CD68, MITF, vimentin
Perineurial cell	Claudin1, GLUT1, EMA
Smooth muscle	Desmin, NSE, SMA, MSA
Skeletal muscle	Vimentin, desmin, myoglobin, CD56, GFAP
Schwann cell	Vimentin, CD56, CD57, S100
Synovial cell	CD68, clusterin
Nerve	CD34, vimentin (fibroblasts), S100 (Schwann cells), EMA (perineurial cells)

Table 26.3 Markers for spindle cell lipoma/pleomorphic lipoma

Antibody	Literature
Vimentin	+
CD34	+
Bcl-2	+
S100	– or +
MDM2	– or + (atypical examples may show nuclear positivity)
CDK4	– or + (atypical examples may show nuclear positivity)

Note: *ND* no data; *M* membranous staining; *N* nuclear staining

S100 is expressed in mature lipocytes and not expressed in spindle cells and floret-like giant cells

Figure 26.1

References: [5–10]

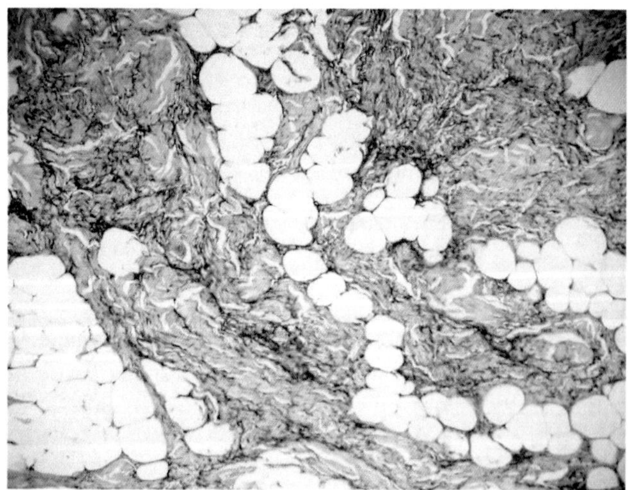

Fig. 26.1 Spindle cell lipoma shows CD34 positivity in spindled tumor cells

Table 26.4 Markers for well differentiated liposarcoma/dedifferentiated liposarcoma

Antibody	Literature
Vimentin	+
CD34	+ variable
MDM2	+ nuclear positivity in varying numbers of cells
CDK4	+
S100	+ variable

Note: CD34 is focally positive in spindle cells and negative in lipoblasts

MDM2 and CDK4 are positive in both lipogenic and non-lipogenic components

S100 is positive in lipogenic component

Figures 26.2–26.4

References: [8, 11–13]

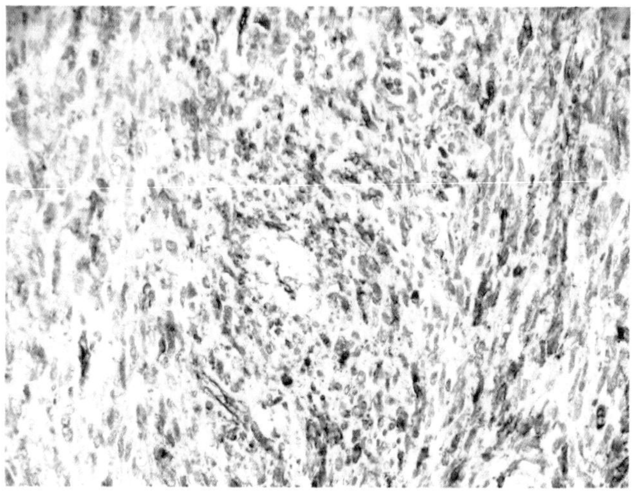

Fig. 26.2 Liposarcoma demonstrates immunoreactivity for CD34

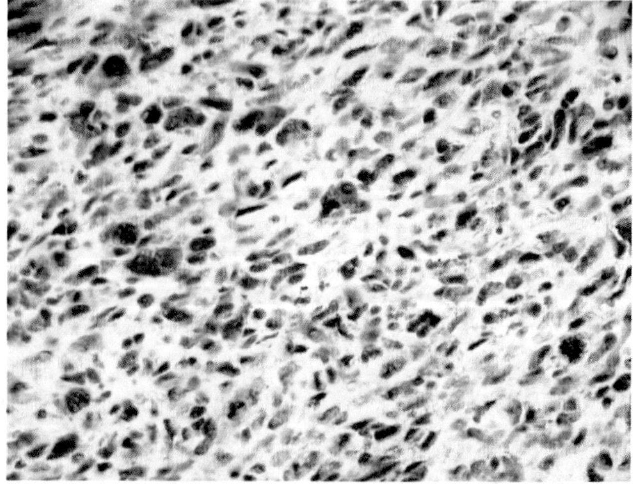

Fig. 26.3 Poorly differentiated liposarcoma shows intense immunostaining for CDK4

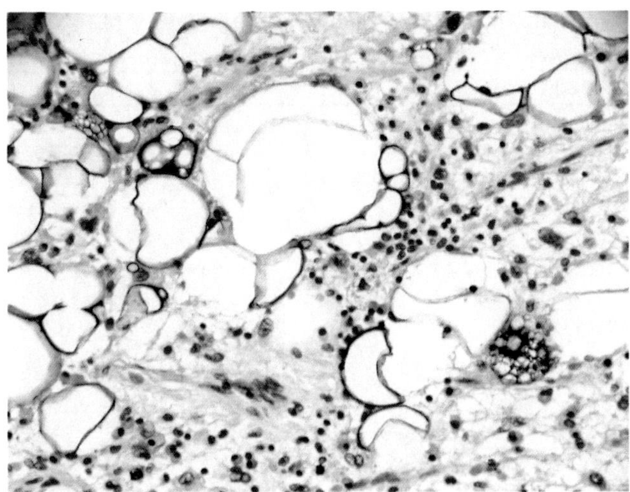

Fig. 26.4 Well-differentiated liposarcoma is positive for S100

Table 26.5 Markers for myxoid/round cell liposarcoma

Antibody	Literature
TLS/EWS-CHOP chimeric oncoproteins	+
S100	+
CDK4	–
MDM2	–
CD34	–

References: [14–16]

Table 26.6 Markers for nodular fasciitis

Antibody	Literature
SMA	+
MSA	+
Calponin	+
CD68	+
Desmin	–
h-Caldesmon	–
S100	–

Note: CD68 is expressed in the histiocytes and osteoclast-like giant cells, occasionally in the spindle cells

References: [3, 17]

Table 26.7 Markers for palmar and plantar (superficial) fibromatosis

Antibody	Literature
Vimentin	+
SMA	+ focal
Desmin	+ focal
Beta-catenin	– or + rare nuclear positivity
CD34	–
Keratins	–
EMA	–
S100	–

Note: Beta-catenin expression shows cytoplasm and/or nuclear staining, only nuclear staining is specific

References: [1, 2, 4, 18]

Table 26.8 Markers for deep fibromatosis

Antibody	Literature
SMA	+
Desmin	+
Beta-catenin 1	+
CD34	–
S100	–
Keratins	–
EMA	–
CD117	–

References: [19, 20]

Table 26.9 Markers for inflammatory myofibroblastic tumor/inflammatory fibrosarcoma

Antibody	Literature
Vimentin	+
MSA	+
SMA	+
Calponin	+
Desmin	+
ALK-1	+ or –
Keratins	– or +
CD68	– or +
Myogenin	–
h-Caldesmon	–
S100	–
CD117	–

Note: Keratin is expressed in 70–90% of lesions of genitourinary tract

Figure 26.5

References: [21–26]

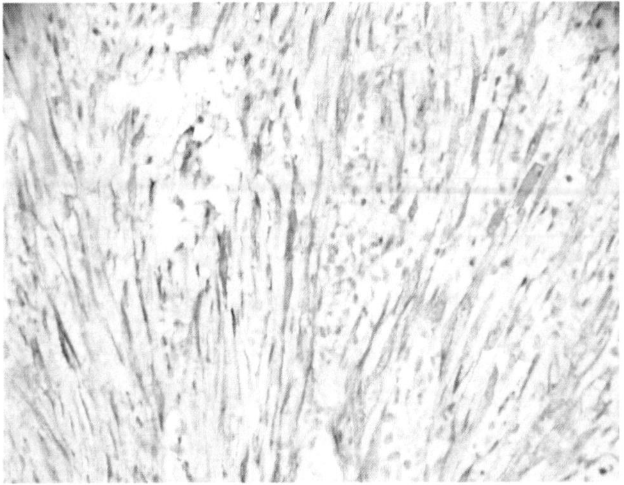

Fig. 26.5 ALK-1 expression in inflammatory myofibroblastic tumor

Table 26.10 Markers of myofibroma/myofibromatosis

Antibody	Literature
Vimentin	+ (all cells)
SMA	+ (myofibroblastic elements)
MSA	+ (myofibroblastic elements)
S100	–
EMA	–
Keratin	–
Desmin	–

References: [3, 27, 28]

Table 26.11 Markers for angiomyofibroblastoma

Antibody	Literature
Vimentin	+
Desmin	+
ER	+
PR	+
CD34	– or +
SMA	–
Keratin	–
S100	–

Note: In postmenopausal women, desmin staining may be reduced or absent

References: [29–33]

Table 26.12 Markers for cellular angiofibroma

Antibody	Literature
Vimentin	+
ER	+
PR	+
Desmin	+ or –
CD34	+ or –
SMA	– or +
S100	–
EMA	–
Keratin	–

Note: ER/PR are expressed more often in female than in male

References: [3, 34]

Table 26.13 Markers of mammary-type myofibroblastoma

Antibody	Literature
Desmin	+
CD34	+
CD10	+
CD99	+
Bcl-2	+
ER	+
PR	+
AR	+
SMA	– or +

References: [3, 35]

Table 26.14 Markers for myxoinflammatory fibroblastic tumor

Antibody	Literature
Vimentin	+
Keratin	– or +
CD68	– or +
CD34	– or +
Myogenin	–
S100	–
CD30	–
CD15	–
SMA	–
CD20	–
CD3	–

References: [3, 28]

Table 26.15 Markers for low-grade myofibroblastic sarcoma

Antibody	Literature
Desmin	+ or –
SMA	+ or –
HHF35	– or +
Fibronectin	– or +
S100	–
Keratin	–
h-Caldesmon	–

References: [3, 36]

Table 26.16 Markers for low-grade fibromyxoid sarcoma, including spindle cell tumor with giant rosettes

Antibody	Literature
Vimentin	+
MSA	– or +
SMA	– or +
EMA	– or +
Desmin	–
S100	–
Beta-catenin	–

References: [37, 38]

Table 26.17 Markers for myxofibrosarcoma

Antibody	Literature
Vimentin	+
MSA	– or + focal
SMA	– or + focal
Desmin	–
S100	–
CD34	–
CD68	–

References: [36, 39]

Table 26.18 Markers for benign fibrous histiocytoma

Antibody	Literature
CD163	+
CD68	+
Factor XIIIa	+
SMA	+ or –
Desmin	–
Keratin	–
S100	–
CD34	–

Note: CD68 and factor XIIIa are expressed in histiocytes

References: [1–4]

Table 26.19 Markers for juvenile xanthogranuloma and reticulohistiocytoma

Antibody	Literature
CD31	+
CD68	+
CD163	+
Factor XIIIa	+
CD1a	–
S100	–

Note: Histiocytes are negative for factor XIIIa in multicentric reticulohistiocytosis

References: [40, 41]

Table 26.20 Markers for atypical fibroxanthoma

Antibody	Literature
CD10	+
CD99	+
CD168	+
CD68	+ or –
P63	– or +
Factor XIIIa	– or +
SMA	– or +
S100	– or +
Desmin	–
CD34	–
Keratin	–
EMA	–

References: [42, 43]

Table 26.21 Markers for dermatofibrosarcoma protuberans/giant cell fibroblastoma

Antibody	Literature
CD34	+
CD31	–
Factor XIIIa	–
Desmin	–
S100	–
EMA	–

References: [20, 44, 45]

Table 26.22 Markers for angiomatoid fibrous histiocytoma

Antibody	Literature
EMA	+
CD68	+
Desmin	+ or –
Myogenin/MyoD1	–
CD31	–
CD34	–

References: [1–4]

Table 26.23 Markers for plexiform fibrohistiocytic tumor

Antibody	Literature
Vimentin	+
SMA	+
CD68	+
Desmin	–
CD34	–
S100	–
NKI/C3	–

Note: CD68 – positive for multinucleated giant cells and histiocyte-like cells

SMA – positive for spindle cells

References: [46–48]

Table 26.24 Markers for soft tissue giant cell tumor

Antibody	Literature
Vimentin	+
CD68	+
CD163	+
SMA	+ variable
Desmin	–
CD34	–
CD31	–
Cytokeratin	–
S100	–

Note: Both mononuclear cells and multinucleated giant cells are positive for CD68; only mononuclear cells are positive for CD163

References: [3, 49]

Table 26.25 Markers for undifferentiated pleomorphic sarcoma (pleomorphic malignant fibrous histiocytoma)

Antibody	Literature
Vimentin	+
MDM2	+
CDK4	+
SMA	– or +
Desmin	– or focally +
Keratins	–
S100	–
h-Caldesmon	–
CD45	–
CD20	–
CD30	–

References: [50–53]

Table 26.26 Markers for leiomyoma and leiomyosarcoma

Antibody	Literature
Desmin	+
SMA	+
MSA	+
Calponin	+
h-Caldesmon	+
SMM-HC	+
PR	+
ER	+ or –
S100	–
Keratin	–
EMA	–
CD34	–

Note: ER and PR positive in leiomyoma of deep soft tissue (Müllerian type tumors) and vulva in female

Figures 26.6 and 26.7

References: [54–56]

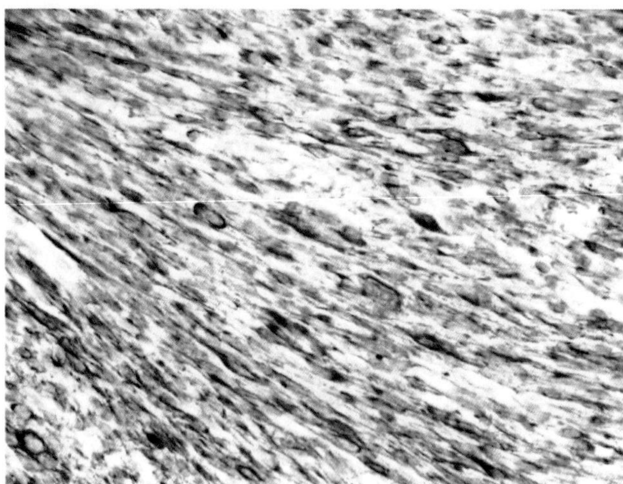

Fig. 26.6 Leiomyosarcoma shows diffuse and strong immunoreactivity for desmin

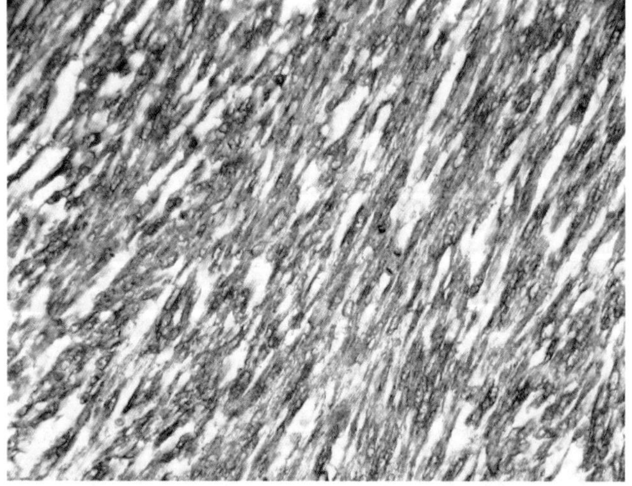

Fig. 26.7 Leiomyosarcoma shows diffuse and strong immunoreactivity for SMA

Table 26.27 Markers for EBV-associated leiomyosarcoma

Antibody	Literature
Desmin	+
SMA	+
MSA	+
Calponin	+
h-Caldesmon	+
SMM-HC	+
EBNA-1	+
EBER (in situ hybridization)	+ (nuclear)
S100	–
Keratin	–
EMA	–
CD34	–

References: [3, 57]

Table 26.28 Markers for rhabdomyoma

Antibody	Literature
Desmin	+
MSA	+
Myoglobin	+
Vimentin	– or +
SMA	–
S100	–
GFAP	–
Keratin	–
EMA	–
CD68	–

References: [42, 58]

Table 26.29 Markers for rhabdomyosarcoma

Antibody	Literature
Desmin	+
MSA	+
Myogenin	+ variable
MyoD1	+ variable
Myoglobin	– or +
SMA	– or +
NSE	– or +
Keratin	– or + (focal)
FLI-1	–
CD45	–

Note: Desmin – negative in undifferentiated cells

MyoD1/myogenin – only nuclear staining is specific

SMA/NSE/keratin – focal or rare positivity

Figures 26.8 and 26.9

References: [26, 59–62]

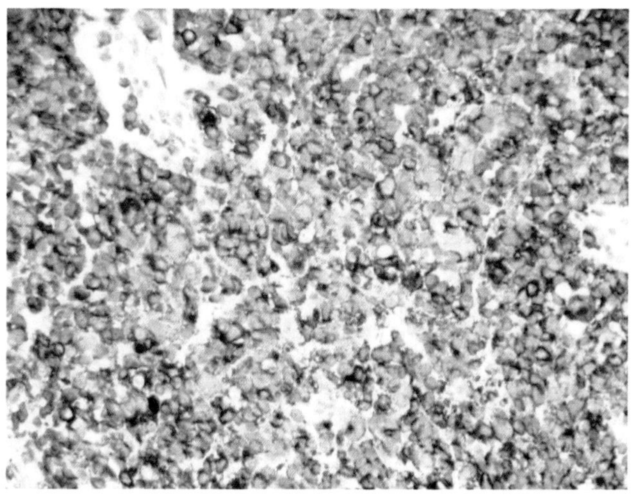

Fig. 26.8 Rhabdomyosarcoma shows diffuse and strong staining for desmin

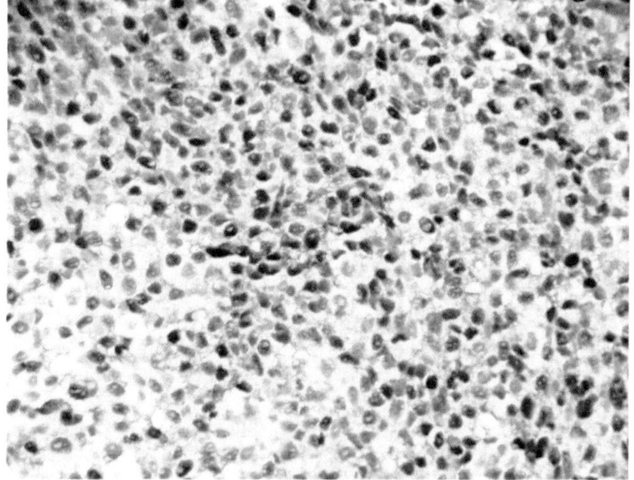

Fig. 26.9 Rhabdomyosarcoma shows strong nuclear staining for myogenin

Table 26.30 Markers for hemangiopericytoma (HPC)/solitary fibrous tumor (SFT) of soft tissue

Antibody	Literature
Vimentin	+
CD34	+
CD99	+
CD10	+ or –
Bcl-2	+ or –
Beta-catenin	– or +
EMA	– or +
SMA	– or +
CD31	–
Keratin	–
Desmin	–
CD117	–
S100	–

Figures 26.10 and 26.11

References: [15, 48, 63–65]

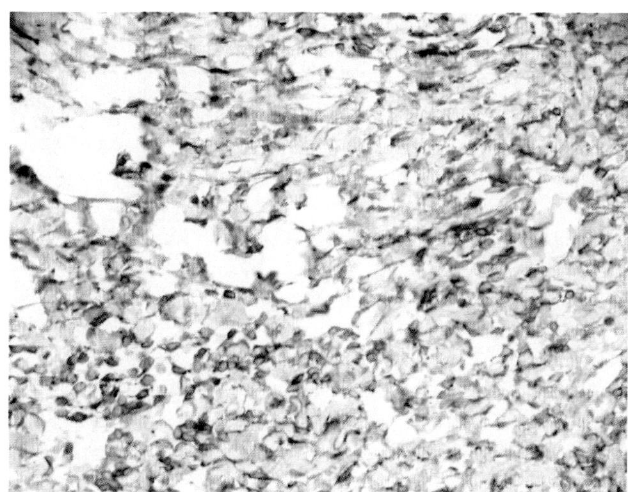

Fig. 26.10 Solitary fibrous tumor shows diffuse and strong positive staining for Bcl-2

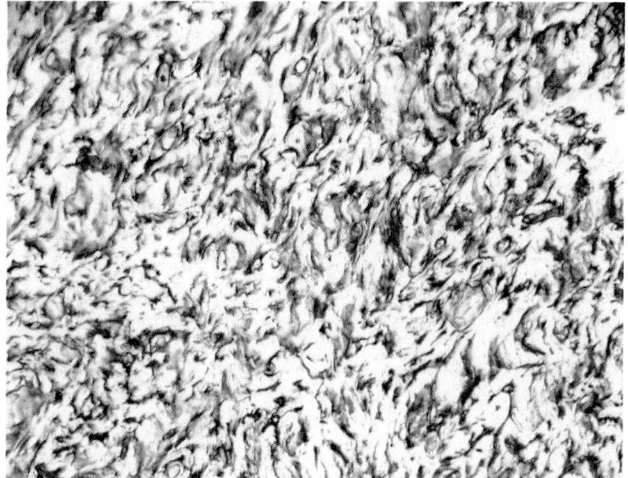

Fig. 26.11 Solitary fibrous tumor shows diffuse and strong positive staining for CD34

Table 26.31 Markers for myopericytoma family of tumors (infantile myofibromatosis, solitary myofibroma, infantile hemangiopericytoma myopericytoma, and glomangiopericytoma)

Antibody	Literature
SMA	+
CD34	–
Desmin	–

References: [3, 66]

Table 26.32 Markers for glomus tumors

Antibody	Literature
SMA	+
Type IV collagen	+
h-Caldesmon	+
Keratin	–
S100	–
Desmin	–
CD34	–

References: [3, 67]

Table 26.33 Markers for kaposiform hemangioendothelioma

Antibody	Literature
CD31	+
CD34	+
FLI-1	+
VEGFR3	+
vWF	–
GLUT1	–
HHV8 LANA	–

References: [18, 68–71]

Table 26.34 Markers for capillary hemangioma

Antibody	Literature
CD31	+
CD34	+
FLI-1	+
vWF	+
GLUT1	+ (juvenile type only)

References: [3, 69]

Table 26.35 Markers for epithelioid hemangioma

Antibody	Literature
CD31	+
CD34	+
FLI-1	+
VEGFR3	+
vWF	+
Keratin	+ or –

References: [8, 69]

Table 26.36 Markers for spindle cell hemangioma

Antibody	Literature
CD31	+
CD34	+
FLI-1	+
VEGFR3	+
vWF	+
SMA	+
HHV8 LANA	–

Note: Vacuolated endothelial cell – positive for CD31, CD34, FLI-1, and vWF; spindle cells – positive for SMA

References: [3, 69]

Table 26.37 Markers for Dabska-type and retiform hemangioendothelioma

Antibody	Literature
CD31	+
CD34	+
FLI-1	+
VEGFR3	+
D2-40	+
vWF	+
Keratin	–
EMA	–
S100	–
Desmin	–

References: [69, 72–75]

Table 26.38 Markers for epithelioid hemangioendothelioma

Antibody	Literature
CD31	+
CD34	+
FLI-1	+
vWF	+
VEGFR3	+
Keratin	– or +
SMA	– or +
EMA	–

References: [8, 69, 71, 76]

Table 26.39 Markers for angiosarcoma

Antibody	Literature
Vimentin	+
VEGFR3	+ varies
CD31	+
CD34	+ varies (50%)
FLI-1	+
Keratin	+ (varies, more often in epithelioid type)
vWF	– or + (well differentiated mostly)
EMA	–
S100	–

Figure 26.12

References: [26, 69, 77]

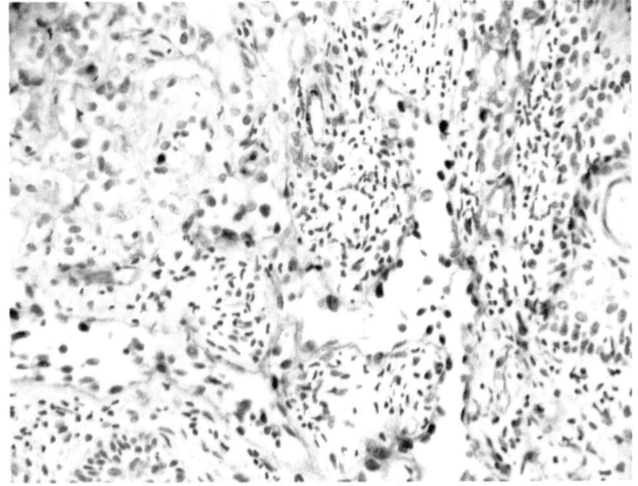

Fig. 26.12 Angiosarcoma shows immunoreactivity for CD31

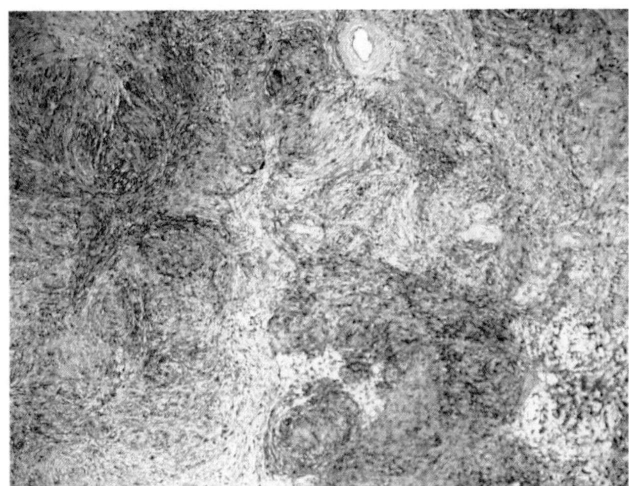

Fig. 26.13 Schwannoma shows strong positivity for S100

Table 26.40 Markers for Kaposi sarcoma

Antibody	Literature
CD31	+
CD34	+
FLI-1	+
vWF	+
HHV8 LANA	+
D2-40	+
VEGFR3	+
vWF	–

Note: HHV8 LANA is a highly sensitive and specific marker for Kaposi sarcoma

References: [69, 78]

Table 26.41 Markers for neurofibroma

Antibody	Literature
S100	+ (Schwann cells)
CD34	+ (fibroblasts)
EMA	+ (perineurial cells)
NFP	+ (axons)
Calretinin	+

References: [1–4]

Table 26.42 Markers for schwannoma/nerve sheath myxoma

Antibody	Literature
S100	+
CD56	+
CD57	+
Calretinin	+
CD34	–
EMA	–
NFP	–

Figure 26.13

References: [1–4]

Table 26.43 Markers for psammomatous melanotic schwannoma

Antibody	Literature
S100	+ diffuse
GFAP	+
HMB45	+
MelanA	+

References: [1–4]

Table 26.44 Markers for malignant peripheral nerve sheath tumor (MPNST)

Antibody	Literature
S100	+ or – variable, often residual Schwann cells only
CD56	+ or –
CD57	+ or –
Desmin	– or +
Keratin	–
HMB45	–
MART1	–

Note: S100 – focally positive in spindled MPNST, diffusely and strongly positive in epithelioid MPNST

Desmin: positive in some spindle cell MPNST

References: [79, 80]

Table 26.45 Markers for granular cell tumor

Antibody	Literature
Vimentin	+
NSE	+
calretinin	+
S100	+
CD68	+
Inhibin	+
Protein gene product 9.5 (PGP9.5)	+

Note: Inhibin: only positive in benign granular tumors

S100/NSE: negative in congenital granular cell tumor

Figure 26.14

References: [3, 81]

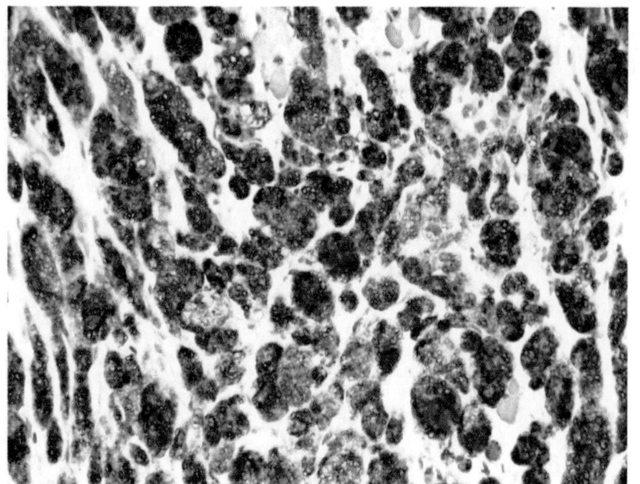

Fig. 26.14 Granular cell tumor shows diffuse nuclear and cytoplasmic immunostaining for S100

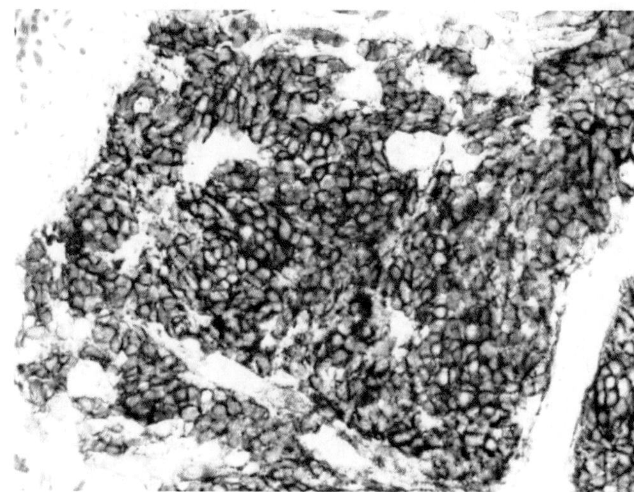

Fig. 26.15 Neuroblastoma. Immunoperoxidase stain shows strong positive CD56 staining of membranes and cytoplasm of the tumor cells

Table 26.46 Markers for neurothekeomas

Antibody	Literature
Vimentin	+
NKI/C3	+
CD10	+
Protein gene product 9.5	+
CD68	– or +
SMA	– or +
S100	–
GFAP	–
MelanA	–

References: [82, 83]

Table 26.47 Markers for perineurioma

Antibody	Literature
EMA	+
Claudin1	+
GLUT1	+
S100	– or +

Note: S100: only positive in intraneural involvement
References: [3, 84]

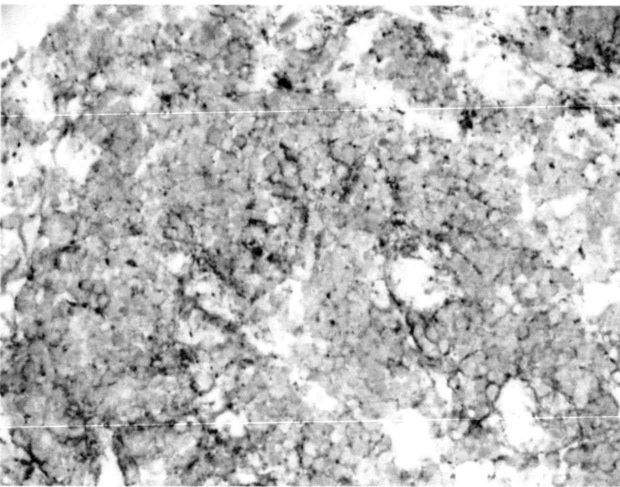

Fig. 26.16 Synaptophysin staining in neuroblastoma

Table 26.48 Markers for neuroblastoma

Antibody	Literature
NB84	+
Neurofilament	+
Synaptophysin	+
NSE	+
Protein gene product 9.5	+
TrkA	+
Chromogranin	+ or –
Myogenin	–
Desmin	–
Keratin	–
TdT	–
CD99	–

Figures 26.15 and 26.16
References: [3, 85, 86]

Table 26.49 Markers for clear cell sarcoma of soft parts

Antibody	Literature
S100	+
HMB45	+
MiTF	+
MelanA	+ or –
Synaptophysin	– or +
CD56	– or +
EMA	– or +
C-kit	– or +
CD34	– or +
Keratin	– or +
SMA	–
Desmin	–
CAM5.2	–

References: [87, 88]

Table 26.50 Markers for myxoma

Antibody	Literature
Vimentin	+
SMA	– or +
CD34	– or +
Desmin	– or +
S100	–

References: [1–4]

Table 26.51 Markers for aggressive angiomyxoma

Antibody	Literature
Desmin	+
Vimentin	+
MSA	+
ER	+
PR	+
CD34	+ or –
SMA	– or +
S100	–
Keratin	–

References: [33, 89]

Table 26.52 Markers for ossifying fibromyxoid tumor of soft parts

Antibody	Literature
Vimentin	+
S100	+
Keratin	– or +
SMA	– or +
Desmin	– or +
CD57	– or +
NSE	– or +
GFAP	– or +
EMA	–

Note: S100 is positive in 70% of typical tumor and 30% of malignant tumor

References: [3, 90]

Table 26.53 Markers for mixed tumor/myoepithelioma/parachordoma

Antibody	Literature
Vimentin	+
S100	+
Keratin	+ variable
Calponin	+
EMA	+ or –
SMA	– or +
CD57	– or +
NSE	– or +
GFAP	– or +
P63	– or +
Desmin	–

References: [3, 91]

Table 26.54 Markers for pleomorphic hyalinizing angiectatic tumor

Antibody	Literature
CD34	+
Vimentin	+
EMA	– or +
S100	–
Desmin	–
Keratin	–
CD31	–

References: [1–4]

Table 26.55 Markers for phosphaturic mesenchymal tumor

Antibody	Literature
FGF23	+
Vimentin	+
CD31	–
CD34	–
S100	–

References: [3, 92]

Table 26.56 Markers for perivascular epithelioid cell neoplasms (angiomyolipoma of the kidney or other organs, clear cell sugar tumor of the lung, lymphangioleiomyomatosis, and clear cell myomelanocytic tumor of the falciform ligament/ligamentum teres)

Antibody	Literature
CD1a	+
HMB45	+
MelanA	+
Calponin	+
MSA	+
SMA	+
S100	– or +
Desmin	– or +
Keratin	–
CD34	–

References: [3, 5]

Table 26.57 Markers for epithelioid sarcoma

Antibody	Literature
Vimentin	+
CK8	+
CK19	+
EMA	+
CD34	+ or –
p63	– or +
INI-1	– or + typically lacks nuclear positivity
MSA	– or +
CK14	–
CK5/6	–
CK20	–
CD31	–

References: [93, 94]

Table 26.58 Markers for alveolar soft part sarcoma

Antibody	Literature
TFE3	+
NSE	– or +
Vimentin	– or +
S100	– or +
NSE	– or +
CD34	– or +
CK	–
EMA	–
Synaptophysin	–
Myogenin	–
MelanA	–

Note: Nuclear staining for TFE3 is highly sensitive and specific

References: [2, 95, 96]

Table 26.59 Markers for Ewing sarcoma and primitive neuroectodermal tumor (ES/PNET)

Antibody	Literature
CD99	+
FLI-1	+
Vimentin	+ or –
Synaptophysin	– or +
NSE	– or +
Keratin	– or +
CD117	– or +
S100	– or +
TdT	–
Desmin	–
CD45	–
CD56	–
Synaptophysin	–

Figure 26.17

References: [1, 97, 98]

Table 26.60 Markers for synovial sarcoma

Antibody	Literature
TLE1	+
EMA	+ epithelial of biphasic tumors, focal in monophasic examples
Bcl-2	+
CK7	+
CK19	+
Calponin	+
CD99	+ varies
CK AE1/AE3	+ or –
E-Cadherin	+ or –
Beta-catenin	– or +
S100	– or +
SMA	– or +
CD117	– or +
Desmin	–
CD34	–
h-Caldesmon	–

Note: Cytokeratin expression is focal in monophasic synovial sarcoma and poorly differentiated synovial sarcoma

TLE1 is rarely positive in MPNST

Figures 26.18–26.20

References: [63, 99–103]

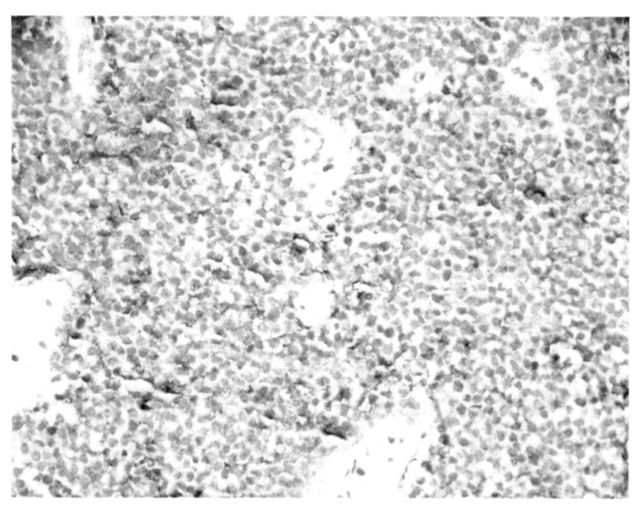

Fig. 26.17 Ewing sarcoma shows CD99 immunostaining on the membranes of the tumor cells

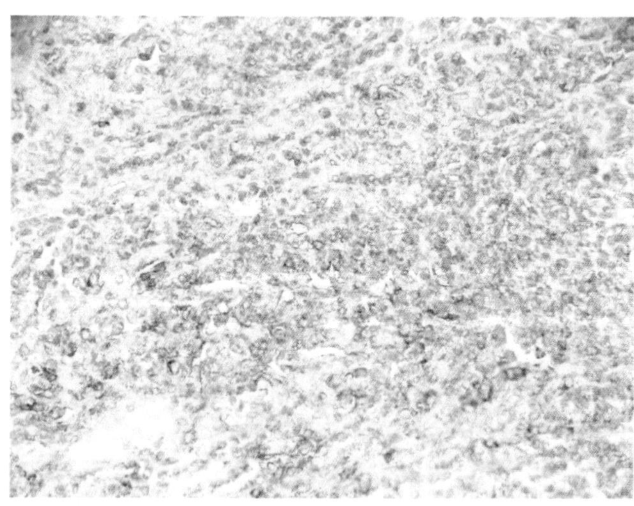

Fig. 26.18 Synovial sarcoma shows focal positivity for EMA

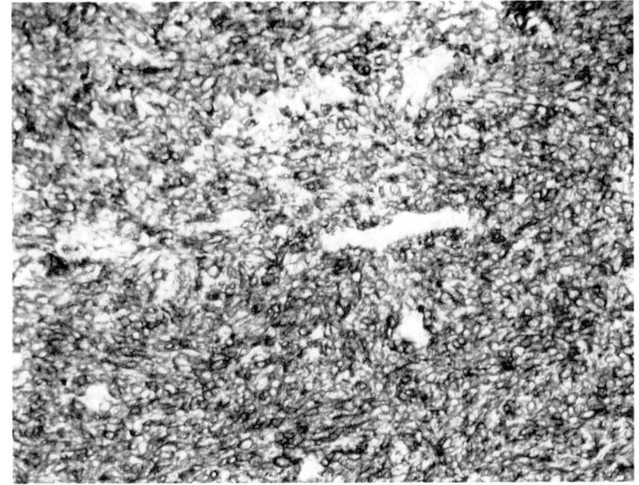

Fig. 26.19 Synovial sarcoma shows diffuse and strong staining for Bcl-2

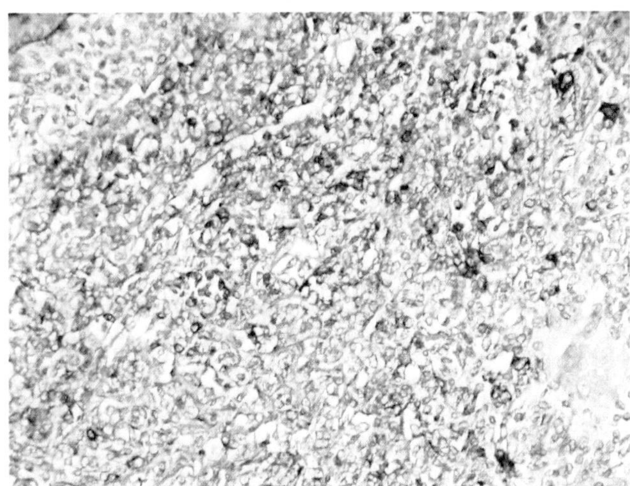

Fig. 26.20 Synovial sarcoma is focally positive for CK AE1/AE3

Table 26.61 Markers for desmoplastic small round cell tumor

Antibody	Literature
Vimentin	+
Desmin	+
CK AE1/AE3/CAM5.2	+
EMA	+
Ber-Ep4	+
WT-1	+
MOC31	+
NSE	+ or –
CD15	+ or –
CD99	– or +
Synaptophysin	– or +
MSA	– or +
SMA	– or +
Calretinin	–
CK5/6	–
CK20	–
Chromogranin	–
Neurofilament	–
S100	–
MyoD1	–
Myogenin	–

References: [104, 105]

Table 26.62 Markers for malignant extrarenal rhabdoid tumor

Antibody	Literature
Vimentin	+
CD99	+
Synaptophysin	+ or –
CD57	+ or –
NSE	+ or –
Pancytokeratin	+ or –
CAM5.2	+ or –
EMA	+ or –
S100	– or +
MSA	– or +
SMA	– or +
HMB45	–
Chromogranin	–
Desmin	–
Myoglobin	–
CD34	–
Beta-catenin	–
GFAP	–
INI-1	–

References: [106, 107]

Table 26.63 Markers for mesenchymal chondrosarcoma

Antibody	Literature
SOX9	+
S100	+
Vimentin	+
CD99	+
NSE	+ or 3–
Desmin	– or +
SMA	– or +
Myogenin	–
CK AE1/AE3	–
HMB45	–
Myoglobin	–
EMA	–
Synaptophysin	–

Note: S100: positive in chondrocytes only

CD99: positive in small cells strongly, staining absent or focal and weak in cartilaginous areas

Desmin: usually focally positive in small cells

References: [108–112]

Table 26.64 Markers for chordoma

Antibody	Literature
Vimentin	+
Brachyury	+
CK8	+
CK18	+
CK19	+
EMA	+
CEA	+
S100	+ or –

References: [110, 113, 114]

Table 26.65 Markers for adamantinoma

Antibody	Literature
Vimentin	+
EMA	+
CKAE 1/3	+
CK14	+
CK19	+
CK5	+ or –
CK17	+ or –
CK7	– or +
CK13	– or +
CK8	–
CK18	–
S100	–

References: [14, 115–117]

Table 26.66 Markers for Langerhans cell histiocytosis

Antibody	Literature
S100	+
CD1a	+
CD207 (Langerin)	+
CD68	+
CD45	–
Keratin	–
EMA	–
CD15	–
CD30	–

References: [118, 119]

Table 26.67 Inflammatory myofibroblastic tumor (IMT)/inflammatory fibrosarcoma (IF) vs. dendritic reticulum cell tumor (DCT)

Antibody	DCT	IMT/IF
CD21	+	–
CD35	+	–
ALK-1	–	+ or –
S100	+	–

References: [1–4]

Table 26.68 Inflammatory myofibroblastic tumor (IMT)/inflammatory fibrosarcoma (IF) vs. sarcomatoid urothelial carcinoma (SUC)

Antibody	SUC	IMT/IF
p63	+	–
EMA	+	–
SMA	–	+
ALK-1	–	+ or –

References: [1–4]

Table 26.69 Myxoinflammatory fibroblastic sarcoma (MFS) vs. Hodgkin's lymphoma (HL)

Antibody	MFS	HL
CD15	–	+
CD30	–	+

References: [1–4]

Table 26.70 Fibrosarcoma (CF) vs. monomorphic synovial sarcoma (MSS) vs. malignant peripheral nerve sheath tumor (MPNST) vs. spindle cell carcinoma (SCC) vs. spindle cell melanoma (SCM) vs. dermatofibrosarcoma protuberans (DFSP) vs. spindle cell rhabdomyosarcoma (SCR) vs. leiomyosarcoma (LMS) vs. spindle cell angiosarcoma (SCA)

Antibody	CF	MSS	MPNST	SCC	SCM	DFSP	SCR	LMS	SCA
Desmin	–	–	– or +	–	–	–	+	+	–
Myogenin	–	–	–	–	–	–	+	–	–
SMA	–	– or +	–	–	–	–	–	+	–
EMA	–	+	–	+	–	–	–	–	–
Keratins	–	+	–	+	–	–	–	– or +	–
S100	–	–	+ or –	–	+	–	–	–	–
CD34	–	+ or –	+ or –	–	–	+	–	–	+
MelanA	–	–	–	–	+	–	–	–	–

References: [1–4]

Table 26.71 Low-grade fibromyxoid sarcoma (LGFS) vs. neurofibroma/perineurioma vs. desmoid tumors

Antibody	LGFS	Neurofibroma/perineurioma	Desmoid tumors
S100	–	+	–
EMA	–	+	–
SMA	–	–	+
Desmin	–	–	+

References: [1–4]

Table 26.72 Juvenile xanthogranuloma (JXG)/reticulohistiocytoma (RC) vs. Langerhans cell histiocytosis (LCH)

Antibody	JXG/RC	LCH
CD1a	–	+
S100	–	+
CD68	+	–
CD31	+	–
CD163	+	– or + only in some mononuclear histiocytes

References: [1–4]

Table 26.73 Dermatofibroma protuberans (DFSP) vs. dermatofibroma (DF) vs. fibrosarcoma arising in DFSP

Antibody	DF	DFSP	Fibrosarcoma in DFSP
CD34	– or + positive in deep lesion	+ diffuse	– or +
Factor XIIIa	+ diffuse	– focal and weak	–

References: [1–4]

Table 26.74 Rhabdomyosarcoma (RMS) vs. Ewing sarcoma/PNET (ES/PNET) vs. neuroblastoma (NB) vs. desmoplastic small round cell tumor (DSRCT) vs. synovial sarcoma (SS) vs. lymphoma

Antibody	RMS	ES/PNET	NB	DSRCT	SS	Lymphoma
Myogenin	+	–	–	–	–	–
MyoD1	+	–	–	–	–	–
Desmin	+		–	+	–	–
CD99	–	+	–	– or +	– or +	–
CD45	–	–	–	–	–	+
Keratins	–	– or +	–	+	+	–
Synaptophysin	–	+ or –	+	–	–	–
Neurofilament	–	–	+	–	–	–

References: [1–4]

Table 26.75 Leiomyoma vs. GIST vs. schwannoma

Antibody	Leiomyoma	GIST	Schwannoma
SMA	+	– or + variable	–
CD117	–	+	–
CD34	–	+ variable	–
S100	–	– or + especially in intestinal ones	+

References: [1–4]

Table 26.76 Glomus tumors (GT) vs. hemangiopericytoma (HPC)/solitary fibrous tumor (SFT) of soft tissue

Antibody	GT	HPC/SFT
SMA	+	–
CD34	–	+

References: [1–4]

Table 26.77 Kaposiform hemangioendothelioma (KH) vs. juvenile capillary hemangioma (CH)

Antibody	KH	CH
CD31	+	+
CD34	+	+
FLI-1	+	+
vWF	–	+
GLUT1	–	+

References: [1–4]

Table 26.78 Neurofibroma vs. schwannoma vs. perineurioma

Antibody	Neurofibroma	Schwannoma	Perineurioma
S100	+ (Schwann cells)	+ (all cells)	–
CD34	+ (fibroblasts)	– or + capsular and degenerative areas	–
EMA	+ (focal)	– or + capsular area	+
NFP	+	–	–
Claudin1	–	–	+
GLUT1	–	–	+

References: [1–4]

Table 26.79 ES/PNET vs. lymphoblastic lymphoma (LL)

Antibody	ES/PNET	LL
CD99	+	+
FLI-1	+	+
CD45	–	+
TdT	–	+
CD10	–	+
CD43	–	+

References: [1–4]

Table 26.80 ES/PNET vs. neuroblastoma

Antibody	ES/PNET	Neuroblastoma
CD99	+	–
FLI-1	+	–
CD56	–	+

References: [1–4]

Table 26.81 Chordoma vs. chondrosarcoma

Antibody	Chordoma	Chondrosarcoma
Keratins	+	–
EMA	+	–
Brachyury	+	–
S100	+	+
D2-40	–	+

References: [1–4]

Table 26.82 Chordoma vs. renal cell carcinoma

Antibody	Chordoma	Renal cell carcinoma
Keratins	+	+
EMA	+	+
Brachyury	+	–
S100	+	–
RCC	–	+
KIM1	–	+

References: [1–4]

Table 26.83 Langerhans cell histiocytosis (LCH) vs. Hodgkin lymphoma (HL)

Antibody	LCH	HL
S100	+	–
CD1a	+	–
CD207	+	–
CD15	–	+
CD30	–	+

References: [1–4]

Table 26.84 Epithelioid sarcoma (ES) vs. epithelioid angiosarcoma (EA) vs. epithelioid malignant peripheral nerve sheath tumor (EPNST) vs. epithelioid leiomyosarcoma (ELMS) vs. sclerosing epithelioid fibrosarcoma (SEF) vs. epithelioid osteosarcoma (EO)

Antibody	ES	EA	EPNST	ELMS	SEF	EO
Vimentin	+	+	+	+	+	+
SMA	– or +	–	–	+	–	–
Desmin	– or +	–	– or +	+	–	–
S100	–	–	+ or –	– or +	–	–
CD31	–	+	–	–	–	–
Keratins	+	– or +	– or +	+	–	–
Osteocalcin	–	–	–	–	–	+

References: [1–4]

Table 26.85 Rhabdomyoma vs. granular cell tumor

Antibody	Rhabdomyoma	Granular cell tumor
CD68	–	+
S100	–	+
MSA	+	–
Desmin	+	–
Myoglobin	+	–

References: [1–4]

Table 26.86 Rhabdomyosarcoma vs. leiomyosarcoma

Antibody	Rhabdomyosarcoma	Leiomyosarcoma
Desmin	+	+
MSA	+	+
Myogenin	+	–
MyoD1	+	–
SMA	–	+
h-Caldesmon	–	+
SMMHC	–	+

References: [1–4]

Note for All Tables

Note: "+" – usually greater than 70% of cases are positive; "–" – less than 5% of cases are positive; "+ or –" – usually more than 50% of cases are positive; "– or +" – less than 50% of cases are positive.

References

1. Dabbs DJ. Diagnostic immunohistochemistry. 3rd ed. Philadelphia, PA: Churchill Livingstone Elsevier; 2010. Accessed 14 Apr 2010.
2. Fletcher CD, Unni KK, Mertens F. WHO classification of tumours: pathology & genetics: tumours of soft tissue and bone. Lyon, France: IARC Press (International Agency for Research on Cancer); 2002. p. 427.
3. Folpe AL, Inwards CY. Foundations in diagnostic pathology: bone and soft tissue pathology. Philadelphia, PA: Saunders Elsevier; 2010. p. 462.
4. Weiss SW, Goldblum JR. Enzinger and Weiss's soft tissue tumors. 5th ed. Philadelphia, PA: Mosby Elsevier; 2008. p. 1257. Accessed 21 May 2010.
5. Adachi Y, Horie Y, Kitamura Y, et al. CD1a expression in PEComas. Pathol Int. 2008;58(3):169–73.
6. Albritton KH, Randall RL. Prospects for targeted therapy of synovial sarcoma. J Pediatr Hematol Oncol. 2005;27(4):219–22.
7. de Vreeze RS, de Jong D, Tielen IH, et al. Primary retroperitoneal myxoid/round cell liposarcoma is a nonexisting disease: an immunohistochemical and molecular biological analysis. Mod Pathol. 2009;22:223–31.
8. Haimoto H, Kato K, Suzuki F, Nagura H. The ultrastructural changes of S-100 protein localization during lipolysis in adipocytes. An immunoelectron-microscopic study. Am J Pathol. 1985;121(2):185–91.
9. Suster S, Fisher C. Immunoreactivity for the human hematopoietic progenitor cell antigen (CD34) in lipomatous tumors. Am J Surg Pathol. 1997;21(2):195–200.
10. Templeton SF, Solomon Jr AR. Spindle cell lipoma is strongly CD34 positive. An immunohistochemical study. J Cutan Pathol. 1996;23(6):546–50.
11. Binh MB, Garau XS, Guillou L, Aurias A, Coindre JM. Reproducibility of MDM2 and CDK4 staining in soft tissue tumors. Am J Clin Pathol. 2006;125(5):693–7.
12. Binh MB, Sastre-Garau X, Guillou L, et al. MDM2 and CDK4 immunostainings are useful adjuncts in diagnosing well-differentiated and dedifferentiated liposarcoma subtypes: a comparative analysis of 559 soft tissue neoplasms with genetic data. Am J Surg Pathol. 2005;29(10):1340–7.
13. Hostein I, Pelmus M, Aurias A, Pedeutour F, Mathoulin-Pelissier S, Coindre JM. Evaluation of MDM2 and CDK4 amplification by real-time PCR on paraffin wax-embedded material: a potential tool for the diagnosis of atypical lipomatous tumours/well-differentiated liposarcomas. J Pathol. 2004;202(1):95–102.
14. Benassi MS, Campanacci L, Gamberi G, et al. Cytokeratin expression and distribution in adamantinoma of the long bones and osteofibrous dysplasia of tibia and fibula. An immunohistochemical study correlated to histogenesis. Histopathology. 1994;25(1):71–6.
15. Hisaoka M, Tsuji S, Morimitsu Y, et al. Detection of TLS/FUS-CHOP fusion transcripts in myxoid and round cell liposarcomas by nested reverse transcription-polymerase chain reaction using archival paraffin-embedded tissues. Diagn Mol Pathol. 1998;7(2):96–101.
16. Oikawa K, Ishida T, Imamura T, et al. Generation of the novel monoclonal antibody against TLS/EWS-CHOP chimeric oncoproteins that is applicable to one of the most sensitive assays for myxoid and round cell liposarcomas. Am J Surg Pathol. 2006;30(3):351–6.
17. Montgomery EA, Meis JM. Nodular fasciitis. Its morphologic spectrum and immunohistochemical profile. Am J Surg Pathol. 1991;15(10):942–8.
18. Folpe AL, Veikkola T, Valtola R, Weiss SW. Vascular endothelial growth factor receptor-3 (VEGFR-3): a marker of vascular tumors with presumed lymphatic differentiation, including Kaposi's sarcoma, kaposiform and Dabska-type hemangioendotheliomas, and a subset of angiosarcomas. Mod Pathol. 2000; 13(2):180–5.
19. Bhattacharya B, Dilworth HP, Iacobuzio-Donahue C, et al. Nuclear beta-catenin expression distinguishes deep fibromatosis from other benign and malignant fibroblastic and myofibroblastic lesions. Am J Surg Pathol. 2005;29(5):653–9.
20. Carlson JW, Fletcher CD. Immunohistochemistry for beta-catenin in the differential diagnosis of spindle cell lesions: analysis of a series and review of the literature. Histopathology. 2007;51(4):509–14.
21. Ceballos KM, Nielsen GP, Selig MK, O'Connell JX. Is anti-h-caldesmon useful for distinguishing smooth muscle and myofibroblastic tumors? An immunohistochemical study. Am J Clin Pathol. 2000;114(5):746–53.
22. Coffin CM, Hornick JL, Fletcher CD. Inflammatory myofibroblastic tumor: comparison of clinicopathologic, histologic, and immunohistochemical features including ALK expression in atypical and aggressive cases. Am J Surg Pathol. 2007;31(4):509–20.
23. Coffin CM, Watterson J, Priest JR, Dehner LP. Extrapulmonary inflammatory myofibroblastic tumor (inflammatory pseudotumor). A clinicopathologic and immunohistochemical study of 84 cases. Am J Surg Pathol. 1995;19(8):859–72.
24. Cook JR, Dehner LP, Collins MH, et al. Anaplastic lymphoma kinase (ALK) expression in the inflammatory myofibroblastic tumor: a comparative immunohistochemical study. Am J Surg Pathol. 2001;25(11):1364–71.
25. Harik LR, Merino C, Coindre JM, Amin MB, Pedeutour F, Weiss SW. Pseudosarcomatous myofibroblastic proliferations of the bladder: a clinicopathologic study of 42 cases. Am J Surg Pathol. 2006;30(7):787–94.
26. Miettinen M, Rapola J. Immunohistochemical spectrum of rhabdomyosarcoma and rhabdomyosarcoma-like tumors. Expression of cytokeratin and the 68-kD neurofilament protein. Am J Surg Pathol. 1989;13(2):120–32.
27. Daimaru Y, Hashimoto H, Enjoji M. Myofibromatosis in adults (adult counterpart of infantile myofibromatosis). Am J Surg Pathol. 1989;13(10):859–65.
28. Meis-Kindblom JM, Kindblom LG. Acral myxoinflammatory fibroblastic sarcoma: a low-grade tumor of the hands and feet. Am J Surg Pathol. 1998;22(8):911–24.
29. Fletcher CD, Tsang WY, Fisher C, Lee KC, Chan JK. Angiomyofibroblastoma of the vulva. A benign neoplasm distinct from aggressive angiomyxoma. Am J Surg Pathol. 1992;16(4):373–82.
30. Laskin WB, Fetsch JF, Mostofi FK. Angiomyofibroblastomalike tumor of the male genital tract: analysis of 11 cases with comparison to female angiomyofibroblastoma and spindle cell lipoma. Am J Surg Pathol. 1998;22(1):6–16.
31. Laskin WB, Fetsch JF, Tavassoli FA. Angiomyofibroblastoma of the female genital tract: analysis of 17 cases including a lipomatous variant. Hum Pathol. 1997;28(9):1046–55.

32. Nielsen GP, Rosenberg AE, Young RH, Dickersin GR, Clement PB, Scully RE. Angiomyofibroblastoma of the vulva and vagina. Mod Pathol. 1996;9(3):284–91.
33. Ockner DM, Sayadi H, Swanson PE, Ritter JH, Wick MR. Genital angiomyofibroblastoma. Comparison with aggressive angiomyxoma and other myxoid neoplasms of skin and soft tissue. Am J Clin Pathol. 1997;107(1):36–44.
34. Iwasa Y, Fletcher CD. Cellular angiofibroma: clinicopathologic and immunohistochemical analysis of 51 cases. Am J Surg Pathol. 2004;28(11):1426–35.
35. Lee AH, Sworn MJ, Theaker JM, Fletcher CD. Myofibroblastoma of breast: an immunohistochemical study. Histopathology. 1993;22(1):75–8.
36. Mentzel T, Calonje E, Wadden C, et al. Myxofibrosarcoma. Clinicopathologic analysis of 75 cases with emphasis on the low-grade variant. Am J Surg Pathol. 1996;20(4):391–405.
37. Goodlad JR, Mentzel T, Fletcher CD. Low grade fibromyxoid sarcoma: clinicopathological analysis of eleven new cases in support of a distinct entity. Histopathology. 1995;26(3):229–37.
38. Lane KL, Shannon RJ, Weiss SW. Hyalinizing spindle cell tumor with giant rosettes: a distinctive tumor closely resembling low-grade fibromyxoid sarcoma. Am J Surg Pathol. 1997;21(12):1481–8.
39. Fukunaga M, Fukunaga N. Low-grade myxofibrosarcoma: progression in recurrence. Pathol Int. 1997;47(2–3):161–5.
40. Nascimento AG. A clinicopathologic and immunohistochemical comparative study of cutaneous and intramuscular forms of juvenile xanthogranuloma. Am J Surg Pathol. 1997;21(6):645–52.
41. Sonoda T, Hashimoto H, Enjoji M. Juvenile xanthogranuloma. Clinicopathologic analysis and immunohistochemical study of 57 patients. Cancer. 1985;56(9):2280–6.
42. Kanner WA, Brill II LB, Patterson JW, Wick MR. CD10, p63 and CD99 expression in the differential diagnosis of atypical fibroxanthoma, spindle cell squamous cell carcinoma and desmoplastic melanoma. J Cutan Pathol. 2010;37:744–50.
43. Longacre TA, Smoller BR, Rouse RV. Atypical fibroxanthoma. Multiple immunohistologic profiles. Am J Surg Pathol. 1993; 17(12):1199–209.
44. Altman DA, Nickoloff BJ, Fivenson DP. Differential expression of factor XIIIa and CD34 in cutaneous mesenchymal tumors. J Cutan Pathol. 1993;20(2):154–8.
45. Goldblum JR, Reith JD, Weiss SW. Sarcomas arising in dermatofibrosarcoma protuberans: a reappraisal of biologic behavior in eighteen cases treated by wide local excision with extended clinical follow up. Am J Surg Pathol. 2000;24(8):1125–30.
46. Hollowood K, Holley MP, Fletcher CD. Plexiform fibrohistiocytic tumour: clinicopathological, immunohistochemical and ultrastructural analysis in favour of a myofibroblastic lesion. Histopathology. 1991;19(6):503–13.
47. Moosavi C, Jha P, Fanburg-Smith JC. An update on plexiform fibrohistiocytic tumor and addition of 66 new cases from the Armed Forces Institute of Pathology, in honor of Franz M. Enzinger, MD. Ann Diagn Pathol. 2007;11(5):313–9.
48. Remstein ED, Arndt CA, Nascimento AG. Plexiform fibrohistiocytic tumor: clinicopathologic analysis of 22 cases. Am J Surg Pathol. 1999;23(6):662–70.
49. O'Connell JX, Wehrli BM, Nielsen GP, Rosenberg AE. Giant cell tumors of soft tissue: a clinicopathologic study of 18 benign and malignant tumors. Am J Surg Pathol. 2000;24(3):386–95.
50. Coindre JM, Hostein I, Maire G, et al. Inflammatory malignant fibrous histiocytomas and dedifferentiated liposarcomas: histological review, genomic profile, and MDM2 and CDK4 status favour a single entity. J Pathol. 2004;203(3):822–30.
51. Fanburg-Smith JC, Miettinen M. Angiomatoid "malignant" fibrous histiocytoma: a clinicopathologic study of 158 cases and further exploration of the myoid phenotype. Hum Pathol. 1999;30(11): 1336–43.
52. Fletcher CD, Gustafson P, Rydholm A, Willen H, Akerman M. Clinicopathologic re-evaluation of 100 malignant fibrous histiocytomas: prognostic relevance of subclassification. J Clin Oncol. 2001;19(12):3045–50.
53. Khalidi HS, Singleton TP, Weiss SW. Inflammatory malignant fibrous histiocytoma: distinction from Hodgkin's disease and non-Hodgkin's lymphoma by a panel of leukocyte markers. Mod Pathol. 1997;10(5):438–42.
54. Nielsen GP, Rosenberg AE, Koerner FC, Young RH, Scully RE. Smooth-muscle tumors of the vulva. A clinicopathological study of 25 cases and review of the literature. Am J Surg Pathol. 1996;20(7):779–93.
55. Paal E, Miettinen M. Retroperitoneal leiomyomas: a clinicopathologic and immunohistochemical study of 56 cases with a comparison to retroperitoneal leiomyosarcomas. Am J Surg Pathol. 2001;25(11):1355–63.
56. Perez-Montiel MD, Plaza JA, Dominguez-Malagon H, Suster S. Differential expression of smooth muscle myosin, smooth muscle actin, h-caldesmon, and calponin in the diagnosis of myofibroblastic and smooth muscle lesions of skin and soft tissue. Am J Dermatopathol. 2006;28(2):105–11.
57. Jenson HB, Montalvo EA, McClain KL, et al. Characterization of natural Epstein–Barr virus infection and replication in smooth muscle cells from a leiomyosarcoma. J Med Virol. 1999;57(1):36–46.
58. Kapadia SB, Meis JM, Frisman DM, Ellis GL, Heffner DK. Fetal rhabdomyoma of the head and neck: a clinicopathologic and immunophenotypic study of 24 cases. Hum Pathol. 1993;24(7):754–65.
59. Folpe AL. MyoD1 and myogenin expression in human neoplasia: a review and update. Adv Anat Pathol. 2002;9(3):198–203.
60. Parham DM, Webber B, Holt H, Williams WK, Maurer H. Immunohistochemical study of childhood rhabdomyosarcomas and related neoplasms. Results of an Intergroup Rhabdomyosarcoma study project. Cancer. 1991;67(12):3072–80.
61. Wexler LH, Ladanyi M. Diagnosing alveolar rhabdomyosarcoma: morphology must be coupled with fusion confirmation. J Clin Oncol. 2010;28(13):2126–8.
62. Williamson D, Missiaglia E, de Reynies A, et al. Fusion gene-negative alveolar rhabdomyosarcoma is clinically and molecularly indistinguishable from embryonal rhabdomyosarcoma. J Clin Oncol. 2010;28(13):2151–8.
63. Renshaw AA. O13 (CD99) in spindle cell tumors. Reactivity with hemangiopericytoma, solitary fibrous tumor, synovial sarcoma, and meningioma but rarely with sarcomatoid mesothelioma. Appl Immunohistochem. 1995;3:250–6.
64. Tihan T, Viglione M, Rosenblum MK, Olivi A, Burger PC. Solitary fibrous tumors in the central nervous system. A clinicopathologic review of 18 cases and comparison to meningeal hemangiopericytomas. Arch Pathol Lab Med. 2003;127(4):432–9.
65. van de Rijn M, Lombard CM, Rouse RV. Expression of CD34 by solitary fibrous tumors of the pleura, mediastinum, and lung. Am J Surg Pathol. 1994;18(8):814–20.
66. Shidham VB, Chivukula M, Gupta D, Rao RN, Komorowski R. Immunohistochemical comparison of gastrointestinal stromal tumor and solitary fibrous tumor. Arch Pathol Lab Med. 2002;126(10):1189–92.
67. Nuovo M, Grimes M, Knowles D. Glomus tumors: a clinicopathologic and immunohistochemical analysis of forty cases. Surg Pathol. 1990;3:31–45.
68. Fletcher CD, Beham A, Schmid C. Spindle cell haemangioendothelioma: a clinicopathological and immunohistochemical study indicative of a non-neoplastic lesion. Histopathology. 1991;18(4):291–301.
69. Folpe AL, Chand EM, Goldblum JR, Weiss SW. Expression of Fli-1, a nuclear transcription factor, distinguishes vascular

neoplasms from potential mimics. Am J Surg Pathol. 2001;25(8):1061–6.

70. Mentzel T, Mazzoleni G, Dei Tos AP, Fletcher CD. Kaposiform hemangioendothelioma in adults. Clinicopathologic and immunohistochemical analysis of three cases. Am J Clin Pathol. 1997;108(4):450–55.
71. Middleton LP, Duray PH, Merino MJ. The histological spectrum of hemangiopericytoma: application of immunohistochemical analysis including proliferative markers to facilitate diagnosis and predict prognosis. Hum Pathol. 1998;29(6):636–40.
72. Calonje E, Fletcher CD, Wilson-Jones E, Rosai J. Retiform hemangioendothelioma. A distinctive form of low-grade angiosarcoma delineated in a series of 15 cases. Am J Surg Pathol. 1994;18(2):115–25.
73. Dabska M. Malignant endovascular papillary angioendothelioma of the skin in childhood. Clinicopathologic study of 6 cases. Cancer. 1969;24(3):503–10.
74. Duke D, Dvorak A, Harris TJ, Cohen LM. Multiple retiform hemangioendotheliomas. A low-grade angiosarcoma. Am J Dermatopathol. 1996;18(6):606–10.
75. Fanburg-Smith JC, Michal M, Partanen TA, Alitalo K, Miettinen M. Papillary intralymphatic angioendothelioma (PILA): a report of twelve cases of a distinctive vascular tumor with phenotypic features of lymphatic vessels. Am J Surg Pathol. 1999;23(9):1004–10.
76. Mentzel T, Beham A, Calonje E, Katenkamp D, Fletcher CD. Epithelioid hemangioendothelioma of skin and soft tissues: clinicopathologic and immunohistochemical study of 30 cases. Am J Surg Pathol. 1997;21(4):363–74.
77. Fletcher CD, Beham A, Bekir S, Clarke AM, Marley NJ. Epithelioid angiosarcoma of deep soft tissue: a distinctive tumor readily mistaken for an epithelial neoplasm. Am J Surg Pathol. 1991;15(10):915–24.
78. Hammock L, Reisenauer A, Wang W, Cohen C, Birdsong G, Folpe AL. Latency-associated nuclear antigen expression and human herpesvirus-8 polymerase chain reaction in the evaluation of Kaposi sarcoma and other vascular tumors in HIV-positive patients. Mod Pathol. 2005;18(4):463–8.
79. Weiss SW, Langloss JM, Enzinger FM. Value of S-100 protein in the diagnosis of soft tissue tumors with particular reference to benign and malignant Schwann cell tumors. Lab Invest. 1983;49(3):299–308.
80. Wick MR, Swanson PE, Scheithauer BW, Manivel JC. Malignant peripheral nerve sheath tumor. An immunohistochemical study of 62 cases. Am J Clin Pathol. 1987;87(4):425–33.
81. Le BH, Boyer PJ, Lewis JE, Kapadia SB. Granular cell tumor: immunohistochemical assessment of inhibin-alpha, protein gene product 9.5, S100 protein, CD68, and Ki-67 proliferative index with clinical correlation. Arch Pathol Lab Med. 2004;128(7):771–5.
82. Fetsch JF, Laskin WB, Hallman JR, Lupton GP, Miettinen M. Neurothekeoma: an analysis of 178 tumors with detailed immunohistochemical data and long-term patient follow-up information. Am J Surg Pathol. 2007;31(7):1103–14.
83. Laskin WB, Fetsch JF, Miettinen M. The "neurothekeoma": immunohistochemical analysis distinguishes the true nerve sheath myxoma from its mimics. Hum Pathol. 2000;31(10):1230–41.
84. Rankine AJ, Filion PR, Platten MA, Spagnolo DV. Perineurioma: a clinicopathological study of eight cases. Pathology. 2004;36(4):309–15.
85. Miettinen M, Chatten J, Paetau A, Stevenson A. Monoclonal antibody NB84 in the differential diagnosis of neuroblastoma and other small round cell tumors. Am J Surg Pathol. 1998;22(3): 327–32.
86. Wirnsberger GH, Becker H, Ziervogel K, Hofler H. Diagnostic immunohistochemistry of neuroblastic tumors. Am J Surg Pathol. 1992;16(1):49–57.
87. Hisaoka M, Ishida T, Kuo TT, et al. Clear cell sarcoma of soft tissue: a clinicopathologic, immunohistochemical, and molecular analysis of 33 cases. Am J Surg Pathol. 2008;32(3):452–60.
88. Meis-Kindblom JM. Clear cell sarcoma of tendons and aponeuroses: a historical perspective and tribute to the man behind the entity. Adv Anat Pathol. 2006;13(6):286–92.
89. Fetsch JF, Laskin WB, Lefkowitz M, Kindblom LG, Meis-Kindblom JM. Aggressive angiomyxoma: a clinicopathologic study of 29 female patients. Cancer. 1996;78(1):79–90.
90. Miettinen M, Finnell V, Fetsch JF. Ossifying fibromyxoid tumor of soft parts – a clinicopathologic and immunohistochemical study of 104 cases with long-term follow-up and a critical review of the literature. Am J Surg Pathol. 2008;32(7):996–1005.
91. Hornick JL, Fletcher CD. Myoepithelial tumors of soft tissue: a clinicopathologic and immunohistochemical study of 101 cases with evaluation of prognostic parameters. Am J Surg Pathol. 2003;27(9):1183–96.
92. Shimada T, Mizutani S, Muto T, et al. Cloning and characterization of FGF23 as a causative factor of tumor-induced osteomalacia. Proc Natl Acad Sci U S A. 2001;98(11):6500–5.
93. Laskin WB, Miettinen M. Epithelioid sarcoma: new insights based on an extended immunohistochemical analysis. Arch Pathol Lab Med. 2003;127(9):1161–8.
94. Miettinen M, Fanburg-Smith JC, Virolainen M, Shmookler BM, Fetsch JF. Epithelioid sarcoma: an immunohistochemical analysis of 112 classical and variant cases and a discussion of the differential diagnosis. Hum Pathol. 1999;30(8):934–42.
95. Argani P, Lal P, Hutchinson B, Lui MY, Reuter VE, Ladanyi M. Aberrant nuclear immunoreactivity for TFE3 in neoplasms with TFE3 gene fusions: a sensitive and specific immunohistochemical assay. Am J Surg Pathol. 2003;27(6):750–61.
96. Ladanyi M, Argani P, Hutchinson B, Jhanwar VE. Prominent nuclear immunoreactivity for TF3 as a specific marker for alveolar soft part sarcoma and pediatric renal tumors containing TFE3 gene fusions. Mod Pathol. 2002;15:312A.
97. Folpe AL, Goldblum JR, Rubin BP, et al. Morphologic and immunophenotypic diversity in Ewing family tumors: a study of 66 genetically confirmed cases. Am J Surg Pathol. 2005;29(8):1025–33.
98. Folpe AL, Hill CE, Parham DM, O'Shea PA, Weiss SW. Immunohistochemical detection of FLI-1 protein expression: a study of 132 round cell tumors with emphasis on CD99-positive mimics of Ewing's sarcoma/primitive neuroectodermal tumor. Am J Surg Pathol. 2000;24(12):1657–62.
99. Jagdis A, Rubin BP, Tubbs RR, Pacheco M, Nielsen TO. Prospective evaluation of TLE1 as a diagnostic immunohistochemical marker in synovial sarcoma. Am J Surg Pathol. 2009;33(12):1743–51.
100. Knosel T, Heretsch S, Altendorf-Hofmann A, et al. TLE1 is a robust diagnostic biomarker for synovial sarcomas and correlates with t(X;18): analysis of 319 cases. Eur J Cancer. 2010;46(6):1170.
101. Kosemehmetoglu K, Vrana JA, Folpe AL. TLE1 expression is not specific for synovial sarcoma: a whole section study of 163 soft tissue and bone neoplasms. Mod Pathol. 2009;22(7):872–8.
102. Pelmus M, Guillou L, Hostein I, Sierankowski G, Lussan C, Coindre JM. Monophasic fibrous and poorly differentiated synovial sarcoma: immunohistochemical reassessment of 60 t(X;18)(SYT-SSX)-positive cases. Am J Surg Pathol. 2002;26(11):1434–40.
103. Terry J, Saito T, Subramanian S, et al. TLE1 as a diagnostic immunohistochemical marker for synovial sarcoma emerging from gene expression profiling studies. Am J Surg Pathol. 2007;31(2):240–6.
104. Ordonez NG. Desmoplastic small round cell tumor. I: A histopathologic study of 39 cases with emphasis on unusual histological patterns. Am J Surg Pathol. 1998;22(11):1303–13.
105. Ordonez NG. Desmoplastic small round cell tumor. II: An ultrastructural and immunohistochemical study with emphasis on

new immunohistochemical markers. Am J Surg Pathol. 1998;22(11):1314–27.

106. Fanburg-Smith JC, Hengge M, Hengge UR, Smith Jr JS, Miettinen M. Extrarenal rhabdoid tumors of soft tissue: a clinicopathologic and immunohistochemical study of 18 cases. Ann Diagn Pathol. 1998;2(6):351–62.

107. Hoot AC, Russo P, Judkins AR, Perlman EJ, Biegel JA. Immunohistochemical analysis of hSNF5/INI1 distinguishes renal and extra-renal malignant rhabdoid tumors from other pediatric soft tissue tumors. Am J Surg Pathol. 2004;28(11):1485–91.

108. Granter SR, Renshaw AA, Fletcher CD, Bhan AK, Rosenberg AE. CD99 reactivity in mesenchymal chondrosarcoma. Hum Pathol. 1996;27(12):1273–6.

109. Hoang MP, Suarez PA, Donner LR, et al. Mesenchymal chondrosarcoma: a small cell neoplasm with polyphenotypic differentiation. Int J Surg Pathol. 2000;8(4):291.

110. Oakley GJ, Fuhrer K, Seethala RR. Brachyury, SOX-9, and podoplanin, new markers in the skull base chordoma vs chondrosarcoma differential: a tissue microarray-based comparative analysis. Mod Pathol. 2008;21(12):1461–9.

111. Swanson PE, Lillemoe TJ, Manivel JC, Wick MR. Mesenchymal chondrosarcoma. An immunohistochemical study. Arch Pathol Lab Med. 1990;114(9):943–8.

112. Wehrli BM, Huang W, De Crombrugghe B, Ayala AG, Czerniak B. Sox9, a master regulator of chondrogenesis, distinguishes mesenchymal chondrosarcoma from other small blue round cell tumors. Hum Pathol. 2003;34(3):263–9.

113. Rosenberg AE, Brown GA, Bhan AK, Lee JM. Chondroid chordoma – a variant of chordoma. A morphologic and immunohistochemical study. Am J Clin Pathol. 1994;101(1):36–41.

114. Tirabosco R, Mangham DC, Rosenberg AE, et al. Brachyury expression in extra-axial skeletal and soft tissue chordomas: a marker that distinguishes chordoma from mixed tumor/myoepithelioma/parachordoma in soft tissue. Am J Surg Pathol. 2008;32(4):572–80.

115. Hazelbag HM, Fleuren GJ, vd Broek LJ, Taminiau AH, Hogendoorn PC. Adamantinoma of the long bones: keratin subclass immunoreactivity pattern with reference to its histogenesis. Am J Surg Pathol. 1993;17(12):1225–33.

116. Jain D, Jain VK, Vasishta RK, et al. Adamantinoma: a clinicopathological review and update. Diagn Pathol. 2008;3:8.

117. Jundt G, Remberger K, Roessner A, Schulz A, Bohndorf K. Adamantinoma of long bones. A histopathological and immunohistochemical study of 23 cases. Pathol Res Pract. 1995;191(2):112–20.

118. Kenn W, Eck M, Allolio B, et al. Erdheim–Chester disease: evidence for a disease entity different from Langerhans cell histiocytosis? Three cases with detailed radiological and immunohistochemical analysis. Hum Pathol. 2000;31(6):734–9.

119. Lau SK, Chu PG, Weiss LM. Immunohistochemical expression of Langerin in Langerhans cell histiocytosis and non-Langerhans cell histiocytic disorders. Am J Surg Pathol. 2008;32(4):615–9.

Chapter 27
Lymph Node

Xiaohong (Mary) Zhang and Nadine S. Aguilera

Abstract This chapter provides information about immunohistochemical (IHC) studies used in diagnosing specific hematolymphoid neoplasms in an up-to-date and easy-to-use format for the busy pathologist. It lists the most useful IHC markers of lymphoid and histiocytic/dendritic neoplasms based on new WHO classification of tumors of hematopoietic and lymphoid tissue (2008). Most recent general information about IHC markers used in hematopoietic neoplasms is listed in Table 1. When a lymph node biopsy is suspected to have a hematopoietic neoplasm, the frequently used markers are presented in Table 2. Tables 3 to 5 illustrate the IHC markers used for the differential diagnoses of mature B-cell lymphomas, mature T-cell lymphomas and lymphoid neoplasms with blastic morphology. IHC markers helpful in lymphomas may also be expressed in non-hematopoietic neoplasms; these are explained in Table 6. Other tables focus on the IHC markers used for specific lymphoid or histiocytic/dendritic neoplasms. We hope that this chapter will be useful in diagnosing and the differential of hematopoietic neoplasms.

Keywords B-cell lymphoma • T-cell lymphoma • NK-cell lymphoma • Histiocytic and dendritic cell neoplasm • Immunodeficiency-associated lymphoproliferative disorders

FREQUENTLY ASKED QUESTIONS

X.M. Zhang (✉)
Department of Pathology and Laboratory Medicine, Geisinger Wyoming Valley Medical Center, 1000 East Mountain Blvd., Wilkes-Barre, PA 18711, USA
e-mail: xmzhang1@geisinger.edu

F. Lin and J. Prichard (eds.), *Handbook of Practical Immunohistochemistry: Frequently Asked Questions*,
DOI 10.1007/978-1-4419-8062-5_27, © Springer Science+Business Media, LLC 2011

Mature T- and NK-Cell Neoplasms

Hodgkin Lymphoma

Immunodeficiency-Associated Lymphoproliferative Disorders

Histiocytic and Dendritic Cell Neoplasms

Table 27.1 Summary of applications and limitations of useful markers

Antibodies	Staining pattern	Function	Key applications and pitfalls
ALK	C, N, M	A tyrosine kinase receptor belongs to the insulin receptor superfamily, normally silent in lymphocytes	Positive in ALCL (Fig. 27.13) and some DLBCL; correlated with t(2;5) or variant translocations
Annexin A1	C	Ca^{2+}-dependent phospholipid-binding protein that inhibits NF-κB signal transduction and avoid apoptosis	Positive in HCL and negative in other B-cell lymphomas. Need to be used with CD20 since myeloid cells and some T cells also express it.
BCL-1 (cyclin D1)	N	Cyclin regulating cyclin-dependent kinase in G1 cell cycle, related to t(11;14)(q13;q32)	Positive in mantle cells, HCL, some plasma cell neoplasms
BCL-2	M, C	Protein in mitochondrion and inhibiting apoptosis	Positive in T- and B-cell lymphomas, especially useful in FL (positive) and BL (negative)
BCL-6	N	Proto-oncogene; marker for follicular center B/T cells, CD30+ perifollicular cells, rare T-cell subset	Positive in some B-cell lymphomas, such as FL, BL, and DLBCL (Fig. 27.8)
βF1	M	One TCR antibody	Positive in αβT cells, less affected by Michel's solution, identify some unusual CD3 negative T-cell lymphoma
BOB.1	N, C	Coactivator of OCT-2	Positive in B cells, lost in HRS cells of CHL
CD1a	M	MHC-related glycoprotein (Chr 1q22-23)[a]; marker for immature T cells and Langerhans cells	Positive in lymphoblastic lymphoma and Langerhans proliferative disorders (Fig. 27.20)
CD2	M	E rosette receptor, member of the Ig superfamily (Chr 1p13.1); marker for T cells and NK cells	Pan-T-cell marker; positive in NK-cell lymphoma and in neoplastic mast cells
CD3	M, C	Member of Ig superfamily (Chr 11q23); marker for T cells and NK cells	Best pan-T-cell marker (Fig. 27.1); positive in T-cell (M) and some NK-cell lymphomas (C)
CD4	M	MHC class II co-receptor, HIV receptor (Chr 12pter-p12); marker for T helper/inducer cells, macrophages, monocytes, Langerhans cells, and histiocytes	Positive in MF, SS, BPDC, HS; evaluation of T-cell neoplasms, histiocytic neoplasms, and Langerhans cell histiocytosis
CD5	M	CD72 receptor, TCR/BCR signaling, T–B interaction (Chr 11q13); marker for T cells and B-cell subset	Classification of mature B-cell lymphomas; evaluation of T-cell lymphomas (often lost)
CD7	M	Member of Ig superfamily (Chr 17q25.2-3); marker for T cells	Evaluation of T-cell lymphomas (often lost) and acute leukemia
CD8	M	MHC class I co-receptor, member of Ig superfamily (Chr 2p12); marker for T-cell subset (T cytotoxic/suppressor cells) and NK cells	Evaluation of T-cell lymphomas (positive in HSTL and SPTCL often), also stains normal splenic sinuses
CD10	M	Cell membrane metallopeptidase (Chr 3q21-27); marker for precursor B cells, follicular center B/T cells, granulocytes, and nonhematolymphoid tissue such as myoepithelium, endometrial stroma, brush border of GI, and kidney	Evaluation of follicular lymphomas, pre-B-ALL, BL, AITL, MDS
CD11b	M	Integrin family, binds CD54, ECM, iC3b (Chr 16p11-13); marker for granulocytes, monocytes, macrophages, and follicular dendritic cells	Positive in acute myeloid leukemia [AML-M1, M2, M3 (35–70%), M4, and M5], HCL, sinus histiocytosis with massive lymphadenopathy
CD11c	M	Integrin family, binds CD54, fibrinogen, iC3b (Chr 16p11-13); marker for myeloid cells, NK cells, dendritic cells	Positive in HCL, B-CLL, MZL
CD13	M, C	Aminopeptidase (Chr 15); marker for granulocytes and macrophages	Classification for myeloid leukemia (CD33 is more specific)
CD14	M	Receptor for LPS (Chr 5); marker for monocytes	Mostly useful in monocytic neoplasm and MDS in flow cytometry study
CD15	M, C	Carbohydrate adhesion molecule (not a protein, Chr 11); marker for granulocytes, eosinophils, monocytes	Positive in HRS cells of CHL (Fig. 27.14), acute myeloid leukemia, some adenocarcinoma
CD16	M	Fc γRIII (Chr 1q23); marker for NK cells, granulocytes, and T-cell subset	Positive in some NK/T-cell lymphomas

(continued)

Table 27.1 (continued)

Antibodies	Staining pattern	Function	Key applications and pitfalls
CD19	M	Co-receptor with CD21 (Chr 16); marker for B cells, first B-cell antigen after HLA-DR	Good pan-B-cell markers, especially in flow cytometry study
CD20	M	Marker for B cells from pre-pre B to memory B cells (Chr 11), initially expressed on B cells after CD19/CD10 and before CD21/CD22	Best pan-B-cell marker, target for Rutoxin and other anti-CD20 antibodies
CD21	M	C3d/EBV/HHV8 receptor (CR2), BCR co-receptor (Chr 1); marker for follicular dendritic cells and mature B cells	Detection of residual follicles, positive in follicular cell neoplasm, HCL, MZL, MCL
CD22	M, C	B-mono/B–T interaction, SIGLEC family, and Ig superfamily (Chr 9); marker for B cells	Positive in some B-cell lymphomas, HCL, and B-ALL
CD23	M	IgE receptor (Chr 19); marker for B-cell subset, activated macrophages, eosinophils, follicular dendritic cells	Classification of mature B-cell lymphomas, positive in follicular dendritic network
CD25	M, C	IL-2α receptor (Chr 10p15.1); marker for activated T and B cells, macrophages, some thymocytes, and myeloid precursors	Evaluation of HCL and T-cell lymphoma for target anti-CD25 therapy, positive in neoplastic mast cells
CD27	M	Member of the TNF receptor superfamily, required for generation and long-term maintenance of T-cell immunity	Positive in memory T cells
CD30	M, C, G	Member of the TNF family, CD153 receptor, lymphocyte activation antigen (Chr 1); marker for activated T and B cells, HRS cells of CHL	Positive in immunoblasts (Fig. 27.11), anaplastic large cell lymphoma (Fig. 27.12), HRS cells (Fig. 27.15), and EC
CD34	M, C	CD62L receptor (Chr 1); marker for myeloblasts, lymphoblasts, stromal cells, endothelial cells	Positive in some lymphoblastic lymphomas and myeloid sarcoma and some nonhematopoietic neoplasms, such as GIST, angiosarcoma, solitary fibrous tumor
CD35	M	C3b/C4b receptor (Chr 1); marker for follicular dendritic cells, erythrocytes, B-cell/T-cell subsets, granulocytes	Positive in follicular dendritic cell sarcoma, MZL
CD38	M	Multifunctional enzyme (Chr 4); marker for plasma cells, immature T and B cells, NK cells, and erythroid/myeloid precursors	Plasma cell marker, positive in LPL, plasma cell neoplasm, and worse prognostic marker for CLL
CD43	M	Sialophorin (Chr 16); marker for T cells, monocytes, and granulocytes	Positive in T-cell lymphomas, aberrant expression in some mature B-cell lymphomas, histiocytic and monocytic neoplasms, myeloid sarcoma
CD45	M, C	Protein tyrosine phosphatase, receptor type, C (PTPRC) (Chr 1); leukocyte common antigen; marker for leukocytes	Positive in hematopoietic neoplasms, but may be negative in poorly differentiated ones
CD45RA	M, C	Isoform of CD45; marker for naïve lymphocytes, granulocytes, and monocytes	Positive in T- and B-cell lymphomas
CD45RB	M, C	Isoform of CD45; marker for lymphocytes, granulocytes, monocytes, and macrophages	Positive in T- and B-cell lymphomas (Fig. 27.7)
CD45RO	M, C	Isoform of CD45; marker for activated/memory lymphocytes, monocytes, and granulocytes	Positive in lymphoma, histiocytic sarcoma, and myeloid sarcoma
CD52	M	GPI-anchored antigen on all mature lymphocytes (Chr 1p36); marker for T-, B-cells, monocytes, macrophages, dendritic cells	Evaluation of T-cell lymphoma for target anti-CD52 therapy
CD56	M	NCAM (Chr 11); marker for NK cells, T-cell subset, neural cell adhesion molecule (NCAM)	Positive in NK/T-cell lymphomas, some plasma cell neoplasms, neuroendocrine tumors

(continued)

Table 27.1 (continued)

Antibodies	Staining pattern	Function	Key applications and pitfalls
CD57	M	Protein of glucuronyltransferase gene family (Chr 11); marker for NK cells, T-cell subset, and neuroendocrine cells	Positive in some NK/T-cell lymphomas, neuroendocrine tumors, and other nonhematopoietic tumors
CD61	M	Integrin beta-3 encoded by the ITGB3 gene, along with the alpha IIb chain in platelets, participate in cell adhesion as well as cell-surface-mediated signaling	Positive in thrombocytes
CD68 (PGM1, KP1)	C, M	Glycoprotein mainly located in lysosomes (Chr 17); marker for macrophages, monocytes, histiocytes, and granulocytes	Best marker for macrophages and histiocytes (Fig. 27.16) (PGM1 more specific than KP1, KP1 also stains myeloid sarcoma)
CD79a	M	Component of BCR (Chr 19q13); marker for B cells and plasma cells	B-cell lymphoma and plasma cell neoplasm (Fig. 27.6)
CD79b	M	Component of BCR (Chr 17q23); marker for B cells and plasma cells	Absent in CLL, HCL
CD99	M, C	MIC2 gene product (Chr X); marker for all leukocytes but highest on immature T cells, also on nonhematopoietic cells	Positive in lymphoblastic lymphoma, myeloid sarcoma (Fig. 27.19), Ewing sarcoma/PNET
CD103	C	Mucosal integrin (Chr 17p13); marker for intestinal intraepithelial lymphocytes	Positive in EATL, HCL
CD117	C , M	c-kit; marker for mast cells, granulocytic precursors, Cajal cells of the gastrointestinal tract	Positive in myeloid sarcoma, mastocytosis, GIST
CD123	M	IL-3α-chain receptor (Chr Xp22.3 and Yp11.3); marker for plasmacytoid dendritic cells	Positive in blastoid plasmacytoid dendritic cell neoplasm, HCL
CD138	M	Syndecan-1 (Chr 2); marker for plasma cells, some B cells, and epithelial cells	Positive in plasma cell neoplasms (Fig. 27.3), PEL
CD163	M, C	Glycoprotein endocytic scavenger receptor haptoglobin–hemoglobin complex (Chr 12); marker for some histiocytes	Positive in histiocytic sarcoma
CD207	M, C	Langerin (Chr 2); marker for Langerhans cells	Positive in Langerhans cell histiocytosis
Clusterin	M, C, N	Normal expression in follicular dendritic cells	Positive in anaplastic large cell lymphoma, follicular dendritic cell tumor
CXCL13	C, M	Cytokine of CXC chemokine family; markers for follicular center Th cells	Positive in AITL
CyclinD2 and D3	C	Members of highly conserved cyclin family, cyclins function as regulators of cyclin-dependent kinases	Worse prognostic markers in DLBCL
DBA.44	C, M	B-cell antigen	Detection of HCL (>95% +), some B-cell lymphomas
EBV			
EBER	N	EBV-encoded early RNA	Most sensitive marker for EBV
EBNA-2	N	Nuclear protein, main viral transactivator	Present in both latent and lytic stages of EBV
LMP-1	M	Latent membrane protein	Present in latent stage of EBV
EMA (MUC-1)	C, M	Episialin–glycoprotein	Positive in some anaplastic large cell lymphoma, NLPHL, plasma cell neoplasm
Fascin	C	Actin bundling protein; marker for follicular dendritic cells, histiocytes, and EBV-infected immunoblasts	Positive in HRS cells of CHL, EBV positive T- and B-cell lymphoma, follicular dendritic sarcoma
FLIP	C	CASP8 and FADD-like apoptosis regulator, also called FLICE-like inhibitory protein (FLIP)	Worse prognostic marker for DLBCL
FOXP1	N	Forkhead Box P1 (FOXP1) is a member of the FOX family of transcription factors	Overexpression related to the poor prognosis in DLBCL
Granzyme A, B, and M	C	Neutral serine proteases inside granules of Tc cells and NK cells	Positive in some T-cell lymphoma, histiocytic sarcoma
HHV8	C	Kaposi's sarcoma-associated herpesvirus, formal name – human herpesvirus type 8	Positive in PEL, LBCL arising in HHV8-associated MCD

(continued)

Table 27.1 (continued)

Antibodies	Staining pattern	Function	Key applications and pitfalls
HLA-DR	M	Major histocompatibility complex, MHC class II, cell surface receptor	Worse prognostic marker for DLBCL
ICAM (CD54)	M	Intercellular adhesion molecule present in the membranes of leukocytes and endothelial cells. It is a ligand for LFA-1 (integrin).	Worse prognostic marker for DLBCL
IgHs	M, C	Heavy immunoglobulin chains, M in B cells, C in plasma cells	Detection of monoclonal population
IgA	M, C		Positive in some plasma cell neoplasms, alpha HCD
IgG	M, C		Positive in some plasma cell neoplasms, gamma HCD
IgM	M, C		Positive in LPL, Mu HCD
IgD	M, C		Positive in MCL
IgLs	M, C	Light immunoglobulin chains, M in B cells, C in plasma cells	Detection of monotypic population
Kappa	M, C		Positive in B-cell lymphomas and plasma cell neoplasms (Fig. 27.4)
Lambda	M, C		Positive in B-cell lymphomas, plasma cell neoplasms, more often in LHCDD, LBCL arising in HHV8-associated MCD (Fig. 27.5)
LMO2	N	The LMO2 protein has a central and crucial role in hematopoietic development and is highly conserved	Positive in DLBCL, indicate better prognosis
Lysosome	C	Organelles containing enzymes	Positive in histiocyte (Fig. 27.17), HS and myeloid sarcoma (Fig. 27.18)
Mast cell tryptase	C	Serine protease; marker of mast cells	Detection of mast cell neoplasm
MIB-1 (Ki-67)	N	Nuclear proliferation antigens	Proliferation index (Fig. 27.10)
MUM-1	N, C	Present in plasma cells, some germinal center B cells, some activated T cells	Positive in plasma cell neoplasm, LPL, DLBCL, some T-cell lymphomas, CHL
Myeloperoxidase	C	Peroxidase enzyme, most abundantly present in granulocytes	Positive in myeloid sarcoma, detect extramedullary hematopoiesis
OCT-2	N	Transcription factor of IgH; present in B cells, plasma cells	Positive in B cells, lost in HRS cells of CHL
P53	N	a tumor suppressor protein that in humans is encoded by the *TP53* gene	Positive in some DLBCL (Fig. 27.9)
PAX-5/BSAP	N	B-cell-specific activator protein	Positive in B cells, especially in activated B cells, B-cell lymphoma (Fig. 27.2), weak in HRS cells of CHL
PD-1	M	Programmed Death 1, a member of the extended CD28/CTLA-4 family of T-cell regulators, PD-1 and its ligands negatively regulate immune responses	CD3+/PD-1+ T cells ring LP cells in NLPHD but not RS cells in CHL
Perforin	C	One of the cytotoxic granules in Tc and NK cells	Positive in some T-cell and NK-cell lymphomas
PKC-β	C	Protein kinase C is a family of enzymes that are involved in controlling the function of other proteins through the phosphorylation of these proteins	Worse prognostic marker for DLBCL
REL	N	Rel proto-oncogene protein encoded by the *REL* gene, it is a member of the NF-κB family of transcription factors	The REL gene is amplified or mutated in several B-cell lymphomas, including DLBCL, PMBL, HL
S-100	C, M	Low molecular weight protein, present in cells derived from the neural crest	Positive in Langerhans cell tumor (Fig. 27.21), interdigitating dendritic cell sarcoma, Rosai Dorfman disease
TCL1	M	Proto-oncogene at 14q32	Positive in TPL, blastic plasmacytoid cell neoplasm
TCRδ1	M	One component of TCR, positive in γδT cells	Positive in PCGD-TCL, most HSTL
TdT	N	Terminal deoxytransferase; marker of T- and B-lymphoblsts	Positive in some lymphoblastic lymphomas/ leukemias, some AML (M0, M1)
TIA	C	One of the cytotoxic granules in Tc and NK cells	Positive in some T- and NK-cell lymphomas

(continued)

Table 27.1 (continued)

Antibodies	Staining pattern	Function	Key applications and pitfalls
TRAF1	M, C	TNF receptor-associated factor 1, the protein complex formed by this protein and TRAF2 mediates the antiapoptotic signals from TNF receptors. The expression of this protein can be induced by Epstein–Barr virus (EBV).	Positive in PMBL
TRAP	C	Tartrate-resistant acid phosphatase, a glycosylated monomeric metalloenzyme, highly expressed by osteoclasts, activated macrophages, neurons	Positive in HCL, Gaucher's disease, HIV-induced encephalopathy, and bone diseases
XIAP	C	X-linked inhibitor of apoptosis protein (XIAP) is a member of the inhibitor of apoptosis family of proteins	High proportions of XIAP may function as a tumor marker and worse prognostic marker for DLBCL
ZAP70	M	Zeta-chain-associated protein kinase 70, a member of protein tyrosine kinase family, express normally in T cells and NK cells and play a critical role in T-cell signaling	Prognostic marker for B-CLL

Note: [a]All chromosome (Chr) locations of the markers are from Wikipedia, the free encyclopedia. http://en.wikipedia.org

N nuclear staining; *M* membranous staining; *C* cytoplasmic staining; *G* Golgi accentuation pattern; *AITL* angioimmunoblastic T-cell lymphoma; *ALCL* anaplastic large cell lymphoma; *ALK* anaplastic lymphoma kinase; *ALL* acute lymphoblastic leukemia; *AML* acute myeloid leukemia; *BCR* B-cell receptor; *BL* Burkitt lymphoma; *BPDC* blastic plasmacytoid dendritic cell neoplasm; *CD* cluster of differentiation; *CHL* classical Hodgkin lymphoma; *CLL* chronic lymphocytic leukemia; *DLBCL* diffuse large B-cell lymphoma; *EATL* enteropathy-associated T-cell lymphoma; *EBV* Epstein–Barr virus; *EC* embryonal carcinoma; *EMA* epithelial membrane antigen; *FL* follicular lymphoma; *GIST* gastrointestinal stromal tumor; *HCD* heavy chain disease; *HCL* hairy cell leukemia; *HRS* Hodgkin and Reed–Sternberg cell; *HS* histiocytic sarcoma; *HSTL* hepatosplenic T-cell lymphoma; *IgH* immunoglobulin heavy chains; *IgL* immunoglobulin light chains; *LBCL* large B-cell lymphoma; *LP* lymphocyte predominant cells; *LPL* lymphoplasmacytic lymphoma; *MCD* multicentric Castleman disease; *MCL* mantle cell lymphoma; *MF* mycosis fungoides; *MDS* myelodysplastic syndrome; *MZL* marginal zone lymphoma; *NCAM* neural cell adhesion molecule; *NLPHL* nodular lymphocyte predominant Hodgkin lymphoma; *NK* nature killer cell; *PCGD-TCL* primary cutaneous γδ T-cell lymphoma; *PEL* pleural effusion lymphoma; *PMBL* primary mediastinal (thymic) large B-cell lymphoma; *PNET* primitive neuroectodermal tumor; *PTL* peripheral T-cell lymphoma; *RS* Reed–Sternberg cells; *SPTCL* subcutaneous panniculitis-like T-cell lymphoma; *SS* Sezary syndrome; *TCL1* T-cell leukemia/lymphoma protein 1; *TCR* T-cell receptor; *TPL* T-cell prolymphocytic leukemia

References: [1–3]

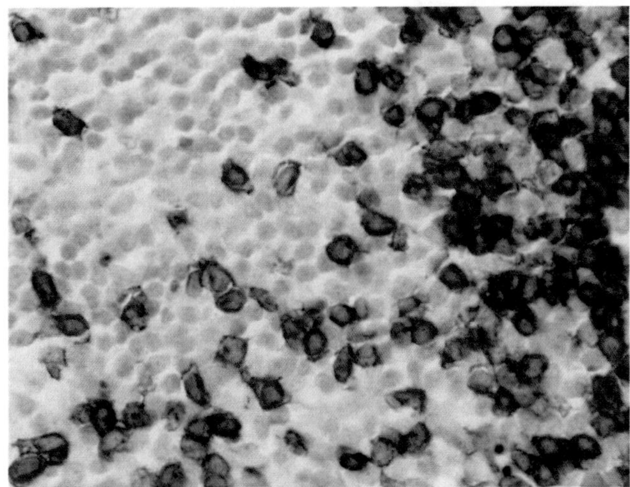

Fig. 27.1 CD3 highlights T cells in normal lymph node

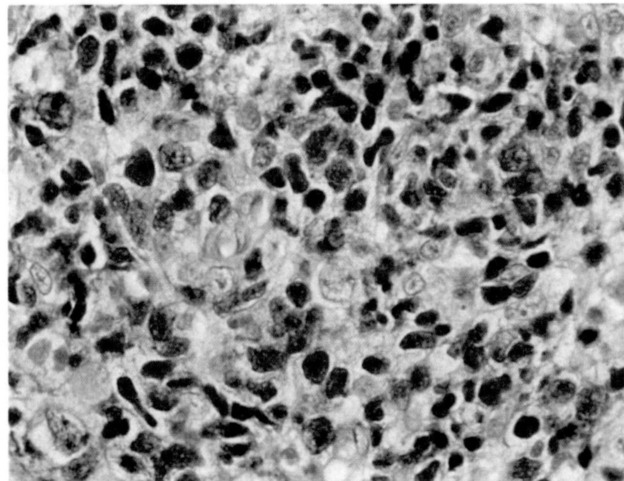

Fig. 27.2 PAX-5 in diffuse large B-cell lymphoma

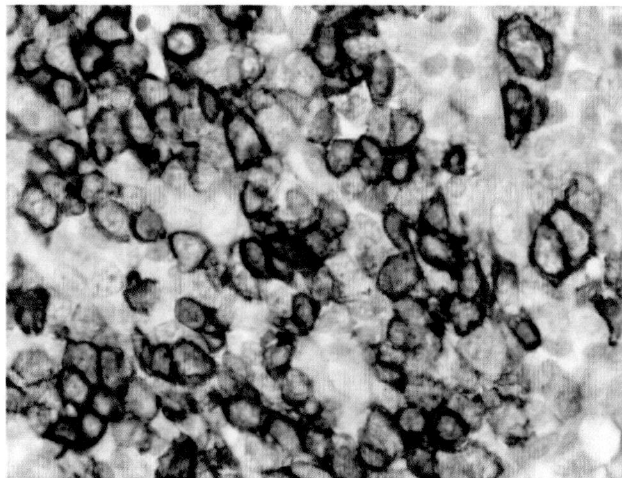

Fig. 27.3 CD138 in plasma cell myeloma

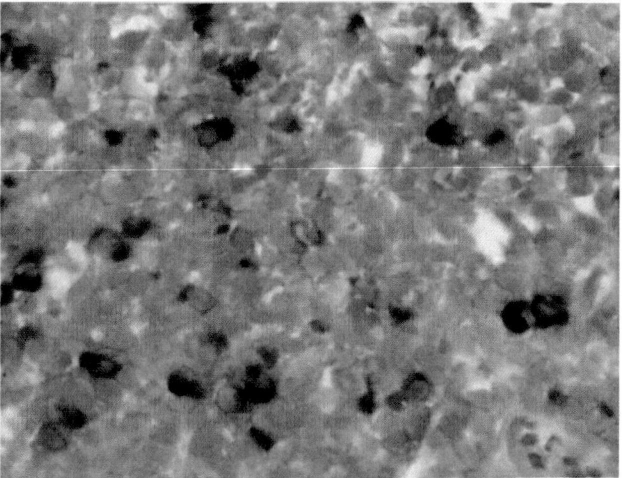

Fig. 27.4 Kappa light chain (in situ hybridization)

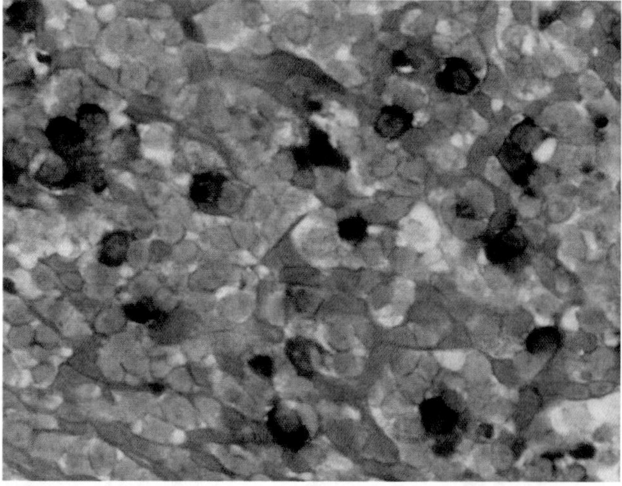

Fig. 27.5 Lambda light chain (in situ hybridization)

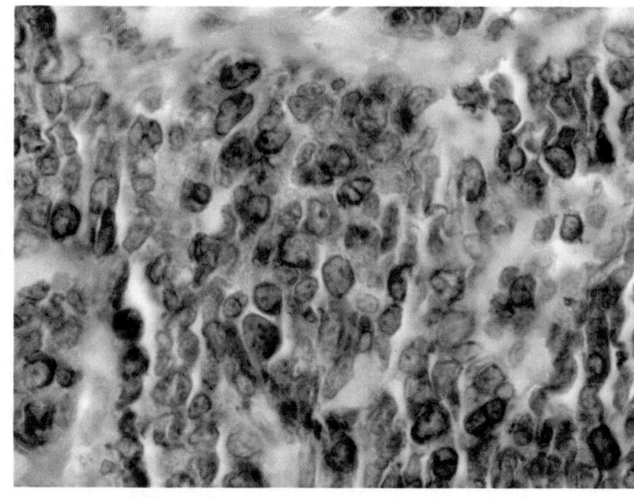

Fig. 27.6 CD79a in diffuse large B-cell lymphoma

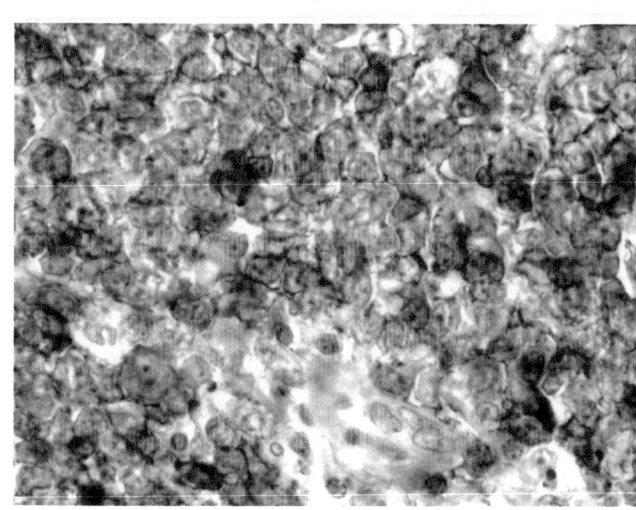

Fig. 27.7 CD45RB in diffuse large B-cell lymphoma

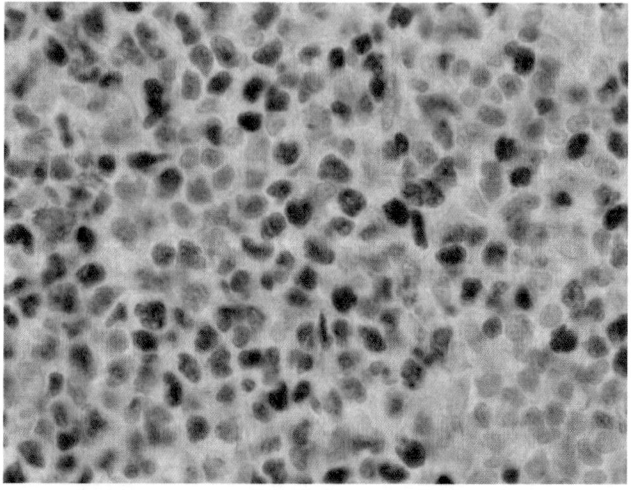

Fig. 27.8 BCL-6 in diffuse large B cell lymphoma

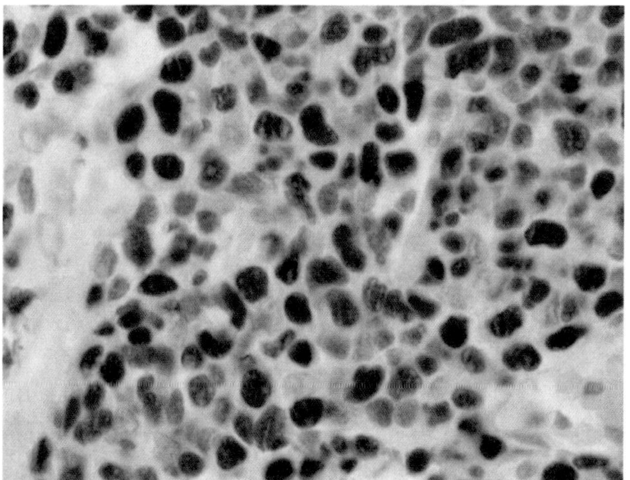

Fig. 27.9 P53 in diffuse large B-cell lymphoma

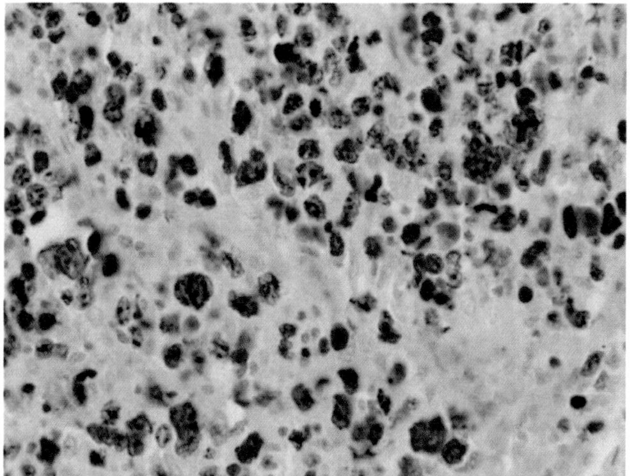

Fig. 27.10 Ki-67 stains proliferative cells in diffuse large B-cell lymphoma

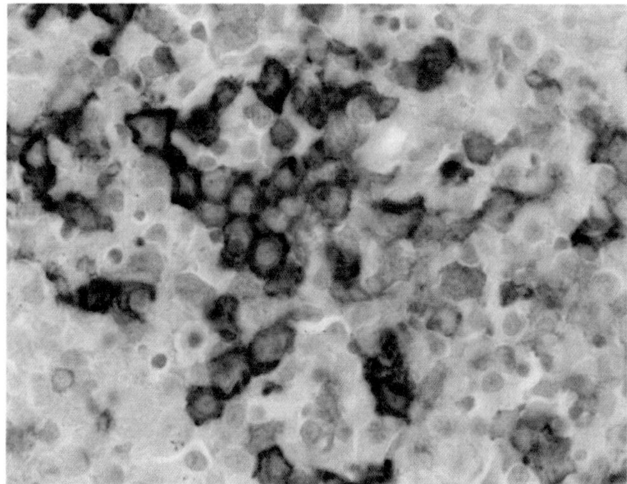

Fig. 27.11 CD30 in diffuse large B-cell lymphoma

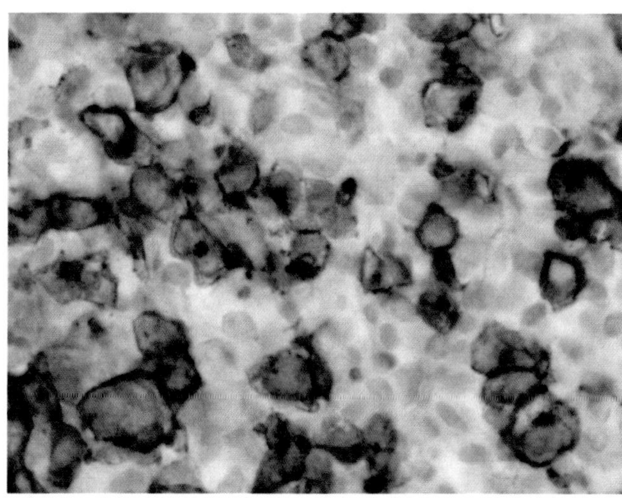

Fig. 27.12 CD30 in anaplastic large cell lymphoma

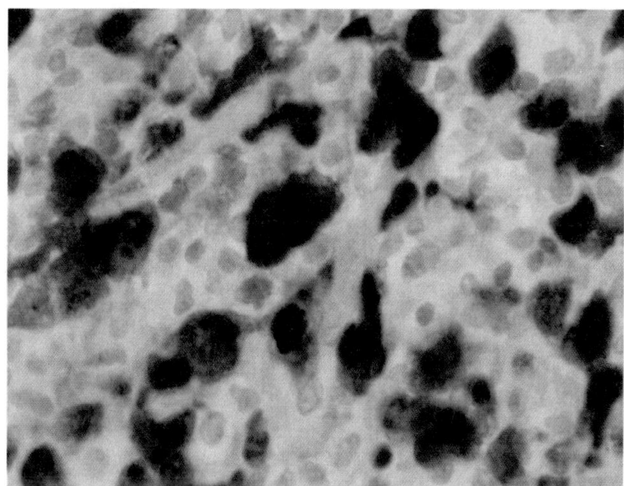

Fig. 27.13 ALK-1 in anaplastic large cell lymphoma

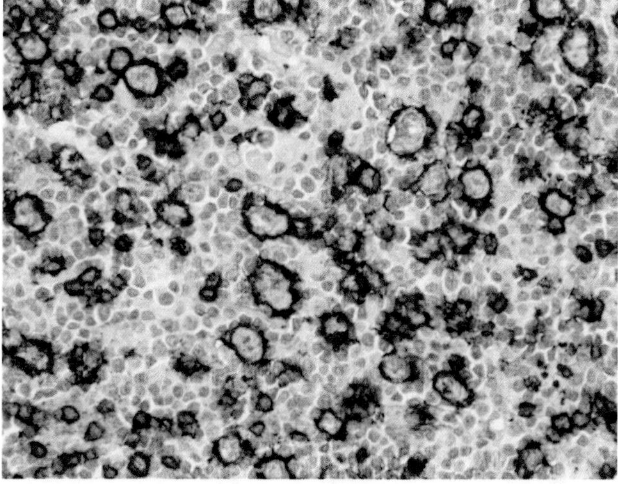

Fig. 27.14 CD15 in classical Hodgkin lymphoma

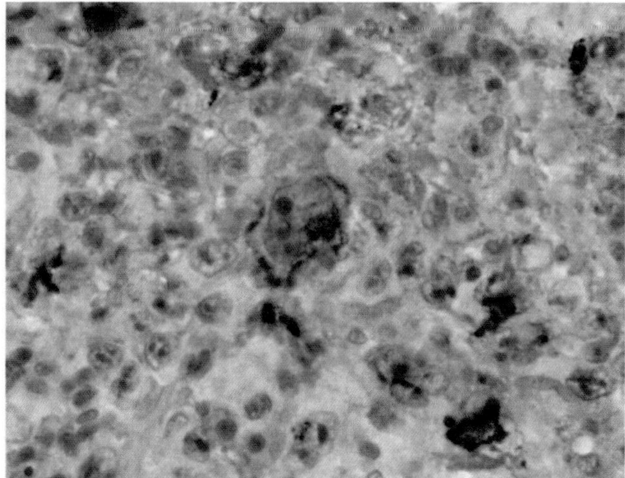

Fig. 27.15 CD30 in classical Hodgkin lymphoma

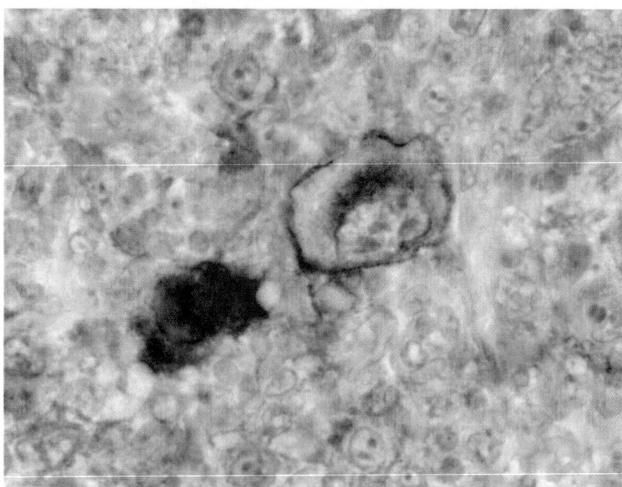

Fig. 27.16 CD68 highlights the histiocytes in histiocytic sarcoma

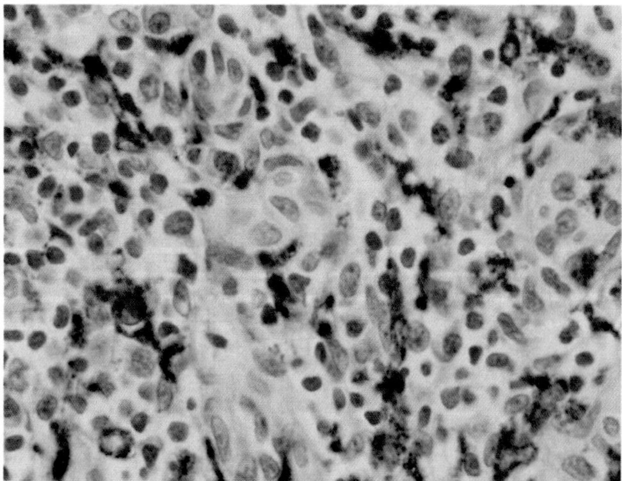

Fig. 27.17 Lysozyme in histiocytes of normal lymph node

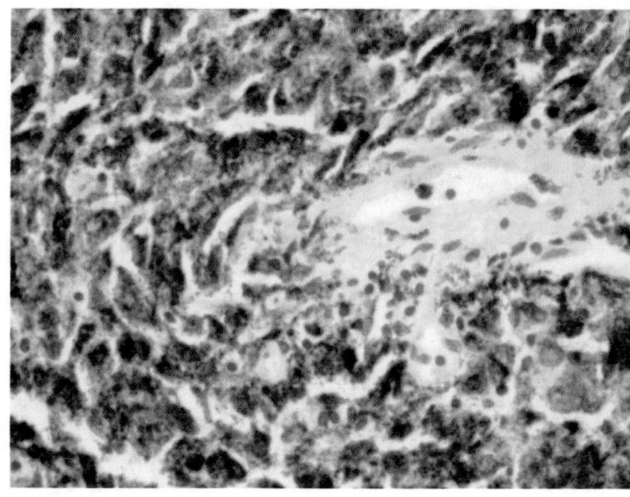

Fig. 27.18 Lysozyme in myeloid sarcoma

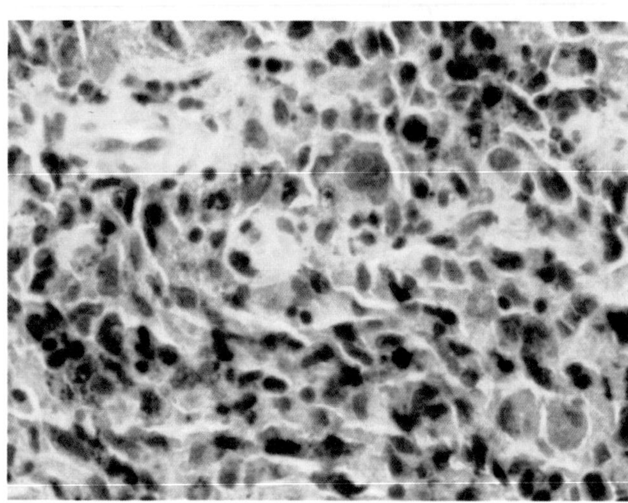

Fig. 27.19 CD99 in myeloid sarcoma

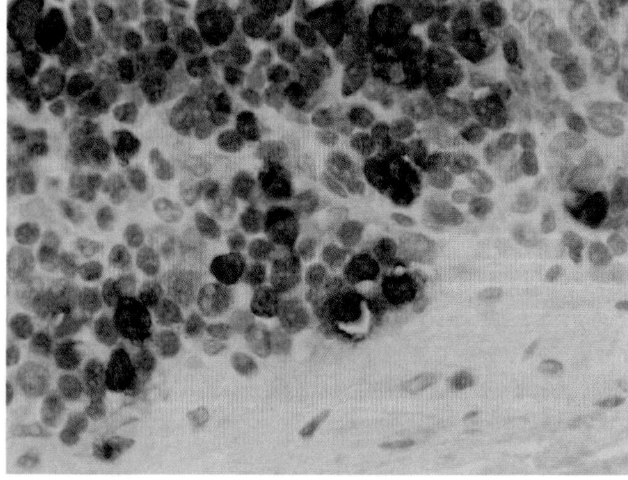

Fig. 27.20 CD1a in Langerhans cell histiocytosis

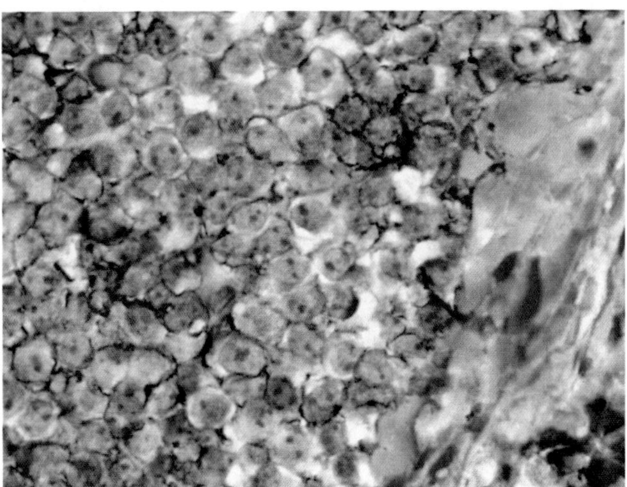

Fig. 27.21 S-100 in Langerhans cell histiocytosis

Table 27.2 Frequently used markers in lymphoid and histiocytic neoplasm

Markers	B-ALL	T-ALL	Mature BCN	Mature T/NKN	CHL	HDCN
CD3	–	+	–	+	–	–
CD20	+ or –	–	+	–	–	–
CD79a	+ or –	–	+	–	–	–
PAX-5	+ or –	–	+	–	+ weak	–
CD5	–	+ or –	+*	+*	–	–
CD23	–	–	+*	–	–	–
CD10	+	+ or –	+*	–	–	N/A
CD2	–	+ or –	–	+*	–	–
CD4	–	+ or –	–	+*	–	+
CD8	–	+*	–	+*	–	–
CD7	–	+*	–	+*	–	–
CD34	+	+	–	–	–	–
TdT	+	+	–	–	–	–
CD99	+	+	–	–	N/A	–
CD15	N/A	N/A	–	–	+	–
CD30	N/A	N/A	+*	+*	+	–
CD68	N/A	N/A	–	–	–	+*
S-100	N/A	N/A	–	–	N/A	+*
CD1a	–	+	–	–	N/A	+*
CD123	N/A	N/A	–	–	N/A	+*
CD163	N/A	N/A	–	–	N/A	+*
MIB (Ki-67)	+	+	+	+	N/A	N/A

Note: *B-ALL* B-cell acute lymphoblastic leukemia/lymphoma (B-lymphoblastic leukemia/lymphoma); *T-ALL* T-cell acute lymphoblastic leukemia/lymphoma (T-lymphoblastic leukemia/lymphoma); *BCN* B-cell neoplasms; *T/NKCN* T/NK-cell neoplasms; *HL* Hodgkin lymphoma; *HDCN* histocytic and dendritic cell neoplasms; N/A no data available

*Please see mostly used markers for neoplasm of blastic morphology in Table 27.5 (B-ALL, T-ALL), for mature BCN in Table 27.3, for mature TCN in Table 27.4, for CHL in Tables 27.55 and 27.56, and for HDCN in Tables 27.61–27.65

References: [1, 2]

Table 27.3 Markers for mature B-lymphocytic neoplasms

	CLL/SLL	MCL	FL	MZL	LPL/WM	HCL	PLL
CD3	–	–	–	–	–	–	–
CD5	+	+	–	–	–	–	–
CD10	–	–	+	–	– or +	– or +	–
CD20	+	+	+	+	+	+	+
CD23	+	–	+ or –	– or +	– or +	– or +	–
BCL-1	–	+	–	–	–	+	–
BCL-2	+	+	+	+	+	+	+
BCL-6	–	–	+	–	–	–	–
MIB	+*	+*	+*	+*	+*	+*	+*
Kappa/lambda	Monotypic	Monotypic	Monotypic	Monotypic	Monotypic	Monotypic	Monotypic

Note: Reactive lymphadenopathy shows mixed CD3+ T cells and CD20+ B cells with CD10+/BCL-2– germinal centers and polytypic kappa and lambda light chains

CLL/SLL chronic lymphocytic leukemia/small lymphocytic lymphoma; *MCL* mantle cell lymphoma; *FL* follicular lymphoma; *MZL* marginal zone lymphoma; *LPL/WM* lymphoplasmacytic lymphoma, Waldenstrom macroglobulinemia (WM) is found in a significant subset of LPL and defined as LPL with bone marrow involvement and an IgM monoclonal gammopathy; *HCL* hairy cell leukemia; *PLL* prolymphocytic leukemia; *Variable

References: [1, 2]

Table 27.4 Markers for mature T-lymphocytic and NK-cell neoplasms

	TPLL	TLGL	ATLL	EATL	HSTL	SPTCL	MF/SS	AITL	ALCL	PTCL	ENK/T, nasal
CD2	+	+	+	+	+	+	+	+	+ or –	+	+
CD3	+	+	+	+	+	+	+	+	+ or –	+	–*
CD4	+	–	+	–	–	–	+	+	+ or –	+ or –	–
CD8	+ or –	+	–	– or +	+ or –	+	– or +	–	– or +	– or+	– or +
CD5	+	– or +	+	–	–	+	+ or –	+	+ or –	– or +	–
CD7	+	– or +	–	+	+	+	– or +	+	– or +	– or +	–
TIA	–	+	–	+	+	+	–	–	+	–	+
GrB	–	+	–	+	–	+	–	–	+	–	+
CD25	–	+	+	– or +	–	N/A	–	–	+	–	–
CD30	–	–	– or +	– or +	–	–	–	–	+	– or +	–
CD56	–	–	–	– or +	+	–	–	–	+ or –	–	+
CD57	–	+	–	–	–	–	–	–	–	–	–
EBV	–	–	–	–	–	–	–	–	–	–	+
CD20	–	–	–	–	–	–	–	–	–	–	–

Note: "N/A" no data available. "–*" negative in membrane stain, may be positive in cytoplasmic stain

AITL angioimmunoblastic T-cell lymphoma; *ALCL* anaplastic large cell lymphoma; *ATLL* adult T-cell leukemia/lymphoma; *EATL* enteropathy-associated T-cell lymphoma; *ENK/T, nasal* extranodal NK/T-cell lymphoma, nasal type; GrB granzyme B *HSTL* hepatosplenic T-cell lymphoma; *MF/SS* mycosis fungoides/Sezary syndrome; *PTCL* peripheral T-cell lymphoma; *SPTCL* subcutaneous panniculitis-like T-cell lymphoma; *TLGL* T-cell large granular lymphocytic leukemia; *TPLL* T-cell prolymphocytic leukemia

All T-cell lymphomas are positive for CD2 and CD3, except that ALCL may be negative for either of them. NK-cell neoplasms may have cytoplasmic CD3

References: [1, 2]

Table 27.5 Markers for neoplasms with blastic morphology

	B-ALL/LBL	T-ALL/LBL	Agg. NKL	BL	MCL-B	MS
CD2	–	+	+ or –	–	–	– or +
CD3	–	+	+*	–	–	–
CD20	– or +	–	–	+	+	–
CD79a	+	– or +	–	+	+	– or +
PAX-5	+	–	–	+	+	– or +
CD4	–	+ or –	+ or –	–	–	+ or –
CD5	–	+	–	–	+	–
CD10	+	+ or –	–	+	–	–
CD34	+	+	–	–	–	+ or –
TdT	+	+	–	–	–	– or +
CD56	–	– or +	+	–	–	– or +
EBV	–	–	+	+	–	–

Note: *Agg. NKL* aggressive NK-cell leukemia; *B-ALL/LBL* precursor B-cell acute lymphoblastic leukemia/lymphoma; *BL* Burkitt lymphoma; *MCL-B* mantle cell lymphoma, blastoid variant; *MS* myeloid sarcoma; *NK* nature killer cell; *T-ALL/LBL* precursor T-cell acute lymphoblastic leukemia/lymphoma; *Cytoplasmic stain

References: [1, 2]

Table 27.6 Markers for both lymphomas and nonhematopoietic neoplasms

	Lymphomas	Nonhematopoietic neoplasms
CD10	pre-B-ALL, FL, BL, AITL	RCC, HCC, endometrial stromal sarcoma, rhabdomyosarcoma
CD15	CHL	Adenocarcinoma
CD25	HCL, ATLL, most B-cell lymphomas, mast cell neoplasm	Neuroblastoma
CD30	ALCL, DLBCL, CHL, PEL	Embryonal carcinoma
CD34	ALL, some AML	GIST, myofibroblastic tumors, DFSP, NF, angiosarcoma, KS, epithelioid hemangioendothelioma, solitary fibrous tumor
CD56	Aggressive NK-cell leukemia, extranodal NK/T-cell lymphoma, EATL type II, primary cutaneous γd TCL, blastic plasmacytoid dendritic cell neoplasm	Neuroblastoma, neuroendocrine tumor, pheochromocytoma
CD57	NK/T-cell neoplasms	Neuroblastoma, glioma, NF, neuroendocrine tumor, nerve sheath tumor, leiomyosarcoma, rhabdomyosarcoma, synovial sarcoma, some prostate carcinoma
CD68	HS, LCH, JXG	Neurothekeoma, melanoma, schwannoma, granular cell tumor, RCC
CD99	ALL	Neuroblastoma, Ewing's sarcoma/PNET, synovial sarcoma, granulosa cell tumor, Sertoli–Leydig cell tumor, malignant rhabdoid tumor, GIST
CD117	Myeloid sarcoma, mast cell tumor	GIST, dysgerminoma, seminoma, intratubular germ cell neoplasia, small cell carcinoma of lung, adenoid cystic carcinoma
CD138	Plasma cell neoplasm, PEL	SCC, TCC (92%), RCC (63%), HCC (60%), colonic adenocarcinoma (90%), BCC (70%)
BCL-2	FL, MZL, MCL, SLL, T-cell lymphomas	Adenoid cystic carcinoma, medullary carcinoma of thyroid, synovial sarcoma

AITL angioimmunoblastic T-cell lymphoma; *ALCL* anaplastic large cell lymphoma; *ALL* acute lymphoblastic leukemia/lymphoma; *AML* acute myeloid leukemia; *ATLL* adult T-cell leukemia/lymphoma; *BCC* basal cell carcinoma; *BL* Burkitt lymphoma; *CHL* classical Hodgkin lymphoma; *DFSP* dermatofibrosarcoma protuberans; *DLBC* diffuse large B-cell lymphoma; *EATL* enteropathy-associated T-cell lymphoma; *KS* Kaposi's sarcoma; *FL* follicular lymphoma; *GIST* gastrointestinal stromal tumor; *HCC* hepatocellular carcinoma; *HCL* hairy cell leukemia; *HS* histiocytic sarcoma; *JXG* juvenile xanthogranuloma; *LCH* Langerhans cell histiocytosis; *MCL* mantle cell lymphoma; *MZL* marginal zone lymphoma; *NF* neurofibroma; *RCC* renal cell carcinoma; *PEL* pleural effusion lymphoma; *PNET* primitive neuroectodermal tumor; *PTL* peripheral T-cell lymphoma; *SCC* squamous cell carcinoma; *SLL* small lymphocytic lymphoma; *TCC* transitional cell carcinoma; *TCL* T-cell lymphoma

References: [1, 4]

Table 27.7 Markers for B-cell chronic lymphocytic leukemia/small lymphocytic lymphoma (CLL/SLL)

Antibodies	Result	Comment
CD19	+	
CD20	+	
CD22	+	
CD79a	+	
PAX-5	+	
CD5	+	
CD23	+	
CD43	+	
CD11c	+	Weak
BCL-2	+	
CD10	–	
BCL-1	–	
CD79b	–	
FMC-7	–	
CD38	+ or –	Prognostic marker, + in worse prognosis
ZAP70	+ or –	Prognostic marker associated with an IgHv unmutated CLL genotype, 20% discordant; + in worse prognosis

Note: Postulated normal counterpart: antigen experienced B cell

Reference: [5]

Table 27.8 Markers for B-cell prolymphocytic leukemia (BPLL)

Antibodies	Result	Comment
IgM	+	
CD19	+	
CD20	+	
CD22	+	
CD79a	+	
CD79b	+	
FMC-7	+	
CD5	–	+ in 20–30% cases
CD23	–	+ in 10–20% cases
CD38	–	+ in 46% cases
ZAP70	+	

Note: Postulated normal counterpart: unknown mature B cell

Reference: [6]

Table 27.9 Markers for splenic B-cell marginal zone lymphoma (SMZL)

Antibodies	Result	Comment
IgD	+	
CD20	+	
CD79a	+	
CD5	–	
CD10	–	
CD23	–	
CD43	–	
BCL-1	–	
BCL-2	+	
BCL-6	–	

Note: Postulated normal counterpart: B cell of unknown differentiation

Reference: [7]

Table 27.10 Markers for hairy cell leukemia (HCL)

Antibodies	Result	Comment
CD19	+	
CD20	+	
CD22	+	Experimental therapy with anti-CD22 antibody
CD25	+	Experimental therapy with anti-CD25 antibody
CD11c	+	
CD103	+	
CD123	+	
Annexin A1 (ANX1)	+	Only in hairy cell lymphoma not in other B-cell lymphomas, must compare to CD20
DBA.44	+	
FMC-7	+	
T-bet	+	Weak
TRAP	+	
BCL-1	+	Weak
CD5	–	
CD10	–	Approximate 14% HCL positive for CD10
CD23	–	Approximate 17% HCL positive for CD23

Note: Postulated normal counterpart: memory B cell

References: [8, 9]

Table 27.11 Markers for splenic B-cell lymphoma/leukemia, unclassifiable – splenic diffuse red pulp small B-cell lymphoma

Antibodies	Result
IgG	+
IgD	–
CD20	+
DBA.44	+
ANXA1	–
CD5	–
CD10	–
CD11c	–[a]
CD23	–
CD25	–
CD103	–[a]
CD123	–

Note: Postulated normal counterpart: unknown peripheral blood B cell

References: [10, 11]

[a] Some are positive

Table 27.12 Markers for splenic B-cell lymphoma/leukemia, unclassifiable – hairy cell leukemia-variant (HCL-v)

Antibodies	Result
DBA.44	+
CD11c	+
CD20	+
IgG	+
CD103	+
FMC-7	+
CD25	–
ANXA1	–
TRAP	–
CD123	–
HC2	–

Note: It has many immunophenotypic features of HCL, but lacks some markers

Postulated normal counterpart: activated B cell at late stage of maturation

Reference: [10]

Table 27.13 Markers for lymphoplasmacytic lymphoma (LPL)

Antibodies	Result	Comment
IgM	+	Usually
IgG	+	Sometimes
IgA	+	Rare
IgD	–	
CD19	+	
CD20	+	
CD22	+	
CD79a	+	
CD38	+	
CD138	+	Plasma cells
CD5	–	
CD10	–	
CD23	–	
CD103	–	

Note: Postulated normal counterpart: probable postfollicular B cell that differentiates to plasma cellReference: [12]

Table 27.14 Markers for heavy chain disease (HCD)

Antibodies	Result	Comment
CD20	+	Lymphocytes
CD79a	+	Lymphocytes
CD138	+	Plasma cells
CD5	–	
CD10	–	
IgM	+	Mu HCD. Bence Jones light chains are commonly found in the urine particularly kappa chains, but they are not assembled with heavy chain.
IgA	+	Alpha HCD

Note: Postulated normal counterpart: postgerminal center B cell with the ability to differentiate to a plasma cell but with a defective gamma heavy chain gene

Reference: [13]

Table 27.15 Markers for plasma cell neoplasms

Antibodies	Result	Comment
CD79a	+	
CD38	+	
CD138	+	
CD19	–	
CD56	+	67–79%
BCL-1	+	Some
CD117	+ or –	
CD20	+ or –	
CD52	+ or –	
CD10	+ or –	
CD45	+ or –	

Note: Postulated normal counterpart: postgerminal center long-lived plasma cell with somatic hypermutation and class switch *Monoclonal gammopathy of undetermined significance (MGUS)* with clonal IgM paraprotein may progress to lymphoplasmacytic lymphoma and/or Waldenstrom macroglobulinemia; non-IgM MGUS (IgG or IgA) to malignant plasma cell neoplasm

Postulated normal counterpart: IgG and IgA MGUS from postgerminal center plasma cell with somatic hypermutation and class switch; IgM MGUS from B lymphocyte with somatic hypermutation but without class switch

Extraosseous plasmacytoma expresses markers of plasma cell neoplasm with gamma chain in most of cases

Monoclonal immunoglobulin deposition diseases:

Primary amyloidosis: positive for amyloid P component with lambda light chain predominant

Monoclonal light and heavy chain deposition diseases: expressing kappa light chain in 80% of cases

Osteosclerotic myeloma (POEMS syndrome): IgG or IgA with lambda light chain in almost all cases

Reference: [14]

Table 27.16 Markers for extranodal marginal zone lymphoma of mucosa-associated lymphoid tissue (MALT lymphoma)

Antibodies	Result	Comment
IgM	+	Most, IgA or IgG less often
CD20	+	
CD79a	+	
CD21	+	Stain the expanded follicular dendritic network
CD35	+	Stain the expanded follicular dendritic network
CD43	+ or –	
CD11c	+ or –	Weak
CD5	–	
CD10	–	
CD23	–	
BCL-1	–	

Note: Postulated normal counterpart: postgerminal center marginal zone B cell

Reference: [15]

Table 27.17 Markers for nodal marginal zone lymphoma (NMZL)

Antibodies	Result	Comment
CD20	+	
CD79a	+	
CD43	+	Approximately 50%
BCL-2	+	
IgD	–	A few of cases positive
CD5	–	
CD10	–	
CD23	–	
BCL-1	–	
BCL-6	–	

Note: Postulated normal counterpart: postgerminal center marginal zone B cell

Reference: [16]

Table 27.18 Markers for follicular lymphoma (FL)

Antibodies	Result	Comment
CD19	+	Most
CD20	+	
CD22	+	
CD79a	+	
CD10	+	Grade 3B may be CD10–
BCL-2	+	
BCL-6	+	
CD21	+	Weak
CD23	+	
CD5	–	
CD43	–	
BCL-1	–	
IRF4/MUM-1	–	Grade 3B may be IRF4/MUM-1+
Ki-67	+	<20% in grade 1–2, >20% in grade 3. If >20% in grade 1–2, clinical behavior is more aggressive and similar to grade 3.

Note: Postulated normal counterpart: germinal center B cell

Follicular lymphoma variant:

Pediatric FL: increased proportion of BCL-2 negative grade 3 FL (BCL-2 positive FL shows worse outcome than BCL-2 negative FL)

Primary intestinal FL: similar immunohistochemical markers

Other extranodal FL: similar immunohistochemical markers

Intrafollicular neoplasm/in situ FL: similar immunohistochemical markers

Reference: [17]

Table 27.19 Markers for primary cutaneous follicle center lymphoma (PCFCL)

Antibodies	Result	Comment
CD20	+	
CD79a	+	
CD10	+	
BCL-2	–	Strong bcl-2 expression suspects systemic involvement or a nodal FL involving the skin secondarily
BCL-6	+	
IRF4/MUM-1	–	
FOXP1	–	
CD5	–	
CD43	–	

Note: Postulated normal counterpart: mature germinal center derived B cell

Reference: [18]

Table 27.20 Markers for mantle cell lymphoma (MCL)

Antibodies	Result	Comment
IgM	+	
IgD	+	
CD20	+	
CD79a	+	
CD5	+	
CD43	+	
FMC-7	+	
BCL-1	+ (nuclear)	
BCL-2	+	
CD10	–	Blastoid/pleomorphic variants may have aberrant phenotypes of CD5–, CD10+, BCL-6+
BCL-6	–	

Note: Postulated normal counterpart: peripheral B cell of inner mantle zone, mostly of naïve pregerminal center type

Reference: [19]

Table 27.21a Markers for diffuse large B-cell lymphoma (DLBCL), not otherwise specified

Antibodies	Result	Comment
CD19	+	Most
CD20	+	
CD22	+	
CD79a	+	
CD30	+	In anaplastic variant
CD5	–	+ in 10% of cases
CD10	+	In 30–60% of cases
BCL-6	+	In 60–90% of cases
IRF4/MUM-1	+	In 35–65% of cases
FOXP1	+	
P53	+	In 20–60% of cases
BCL-1	–	
Ki-67	+	>40% of tumor cells

Note: *Common morphologic variant*:

Centroblastic variant: similar immunohistochemical markers

Immunoblastic variant: similar immunohistochemical markers

Anaplastic variant: similar immunohistochemical markers

Rare morphologic variant: similar immunohistochemical markers

Table 27.21b Markers for subgrouping DLBCL, NOS by immunophenotyping

Antibodies	Germinal center-like	Nongerminal center-like
CD10	+	–
BCL-2	+	–
BCL-6	+	–
IRF4/MUM-1	–	+
Cyclin D2	–	+

Table 27.21c Markers for prognosis and predictive factors of DLBCL

Adverse prognosis	Favorable outcome
BCL-2	BCL-6
X-linked inhibitor of apoptosis protein (XIAP)	CD10
IRF4/MUM-1	LMO2
Cyclin D2	
Cyclin D3	
P53	
CD5	
FOXP1	
PKC-β	
ICAM1	
HLA-DR	
c-FLIP	
EBV	
Ki-67 high index	

Note: Treatment with anti-CD20 antibody (rituximab) eliminates the negative impact of BCL-2 and positive impact of BCL-6. Postulated normal counterpart: peripheral B cell of either germinal center or postgerminal center (activated) type

Reference: [20]

Table 27.22 Markers for T-cell/histiocyte-rich large B-cell lymphoma (THRLBCL)

Antibodies	Result	Comment
CD20	+	
CD79a	+	
BCL-2	+	Variable
BCL-6	+	
EMA	+	
CD15	–	
CD30	–	
CD138	–	

Note: Background of T cells: CD3+, CD5+, CD8+, TIA1+; histiocytes: CD68+. Postulated normal counterpart: germinal center B cell

Reference: [21]

Table 27.23 Markers for primary diffuse large B-cell lymphoma of the CNS (CNS DLBCL)

Antibodies	Result	Comment
CD20	+	
CD22	+	
CD79a	+	
CD10	+	10–20% of cases
BCL-6	+	60–80% of cases
IRF4/MUM-1	+	90% of cases
BCL-2	+	Frequent, not related to t(14;18)(q32;q21)

Note: Postulated normal counterpart: activated (late germinal center) B cell

Reference: [22]

Table 27.24 Markers for primary cutaneous DLBCL, leg type

Antibodies	Result	Comment
CD20	+	
CD79a	+	
BCL-2	+	10% of cases negative
BCL-6	+	
IRF4/MUM-1	+	10% of cases negative
FOXP1	+	
CD10	–	

Note: Postulated normal counterpart: peripheral B cell of postgerminal center type

Reference: [23]

Table 27.25 Markers for EBV positive diffuse large B-cell lymphoma of the elderly

Antibodies	Result	Comment
CD20	+	Most
CD79a	+	
IRF4/MUM-1	+	
CD10	–	
BCL-6	–	
CD15	–	
CD30	+	Variable
LMP-1	+	94% of cases
EBNA-2	+	28% of cases

Note: It is an EBV+ clonal B-cell lymphoid proliferation that occurs in patients older than 50 years and without any known immunodeficiency or prior lymphoma

Plasmablastic feature may lack CD20

Postulated normal counterpart: mature B cell transformed by EBV

Reference: [24]

Table 27.26 Markers for DLBCL associated with chronic inflammation

Antibodies	Result	Comment
CD20	+	
CD79a	+	
IRF4/MUM-1	+	With loss of B-cell markers and showing plasma cell differentiation
CD138	+	
CD30	+	
T-cell markers	+	One or more, i.e., CD2, CD3, CD4, and/or CD7
EBV	+	Most cases (EBER, type III LMP+/EBNA-2+ latency profile)

Note: Most cases express CD20 and CD79a. A proportion of cases may show plasmacytic differentiation with loss of CD20 and expression of CD138

Postulated normal counterpart: EBV transformed late germinal center/postgerminal center B cell

Reference: [25]

Table 27.27 Markers for lymphomatoid granulomatosis (LYG)

Antibodies	Result	Comment
EBV	+	Most
CD20	+	
CD30	+	
CD15	–	

Note: It is usually polyclonal, rare cases monoclonal with cytoplasmic immunoglobulin in a background of CD3+ T cells with CD4+ > CD8+ cells. The early lesion may resemble a T-cell-rich B-cell lymphoma. Malignant cells can resemble Hodgkin cellsPostulated normal counterpart: mature B cell transformed by EBV

Reference: [26]

Table 27.28 Markers for primary mediastinal (thymic) large B-cell lymphoma (PMBL)

Antibodies	Result	Comment
CD19	+	Most
CD20	+	
CD22	+	
CD79a	+	
CD30	+	In 80% cases, weak and heterogeneous
CD15	–	Occasional +
IRF4/MUM-1	+	In 75% cases
CD23	+	In 70% cases
BCL-2	+	In 55–80% cases
BCL-6	+	In 45–100% cases
CD10	–	8–32% cases positive
CD54 (ICAM)	+	
CD95	+	
TRAF1	+	
Nuclear REL	+	
Immunoglobulin	–	

Note: Postulated normal counterpart: thymic medullary, asteroid (AID-positive) B cell

Reference: [27]

Table 27.29 Markers for intravascular large B-cell lymphoma (IVLBCL)

Antibodies	Result	Comment
CD19	+	Most
CD20	+	
CD22	+	
CD79a	+	
CD5	–	38% cases positive
CD10	–	13% cases positive
IRF4/MUM-1	+	87% cases
CD29[a]	–	β1 integrin
CD54[a]	–	ICAM1

Note: [a]Lack of the homing receptors may be related to the intravascular growth pattern

Postulated normal counterpart: transformed peripheral B cell

Reference: [28]

Table 27.30 Markers for ALK-positive large B-cell lymphoma (ALK-positive LBCL)

Antibodies	Result	Comment
T-, B-cell markers	–	CD3, CD20, CD79a
ALK	+	Strongly
EMA	+	Strongly
CD138	+	Strongly
CD38	+	Strongly
CD45	–	
CD30	–	*Different from ALCL*
Cytoplasmic Ig	+	Usually IgA, rare IgG
Cytokeratin	–	Occasional cases positive
CD4	–	Occasional cases positive
CD57	–	Occasional cases positive
CD43	–	Focally positive
IRF4/MUM-1	–	Occasional cases positive
Perforin	–	Focally positive

Note: *ALCL* anaplastic large cell lymphoma

Postulated normal counterpart: postgerminal center B cell with plasma cell differentiation

Reference: [29]

Table 27.31 Markers for plasmablastic lymphoma (PBL)

Antibodies	Result	Comment
CD138	+	
CD38	+	
IRF4/MUM-1	+	
CD45	– or weak +	
CD20	–	
PAX-5	–	
CD79a	+	50–85% cases
Cytoplasmic Ig	+	50–70% cases, most IgG with either κ or λ
CD56	–	CD56+ suspicious for plasma cell myeloma
EMA	+	
CD30	+	
Ki-67	+	>90% of tumor cells
EBV[a]	+	60–75% cases, 100% in the oral mucosal type and in association with HIV infection
HHV8	–	

Postulated normal counterpart: plasmablast – blastic proliferating B cell switching to plasma cell gene expression

Note: [a] EBER in situ hybridization is positive but LMP-1 is rarely positive

Reference: [30]

Table 27.32 Markers for large B-cell lymphoma arising in HHV8-associated multicentric Castleman disease (HHV8 MCD)

Antibodies	Result	Comment
HHV8	+	
LANA-1[a]	+	
Viral-λ IL-6[b]	+	
cIgM	+	
Lambda chain	+	
CD20	+ or –	
CD79a	–	
CD138	–	
CD38	– or +	
CD27	–	
EBV	–	

Notes:

[a]The latency-associated nuclear antigen (LANA) is a large nuclear protein that plays a role in the establishment and maintenance of latent Kaposi sarcoma-associated herpesvirus (KSHV) (HHV8) episome in the nucleus of infected cells

[b]Kaposi sarcoma-associated herpesvirus-encoded interleukin-6

Postulated normal counterpart: naïve B cell

References: [31, 32]

Table 27.33 Markers for primary effusion lymphoma (PEL)

Antibodies	Result	Comment
CD45	+	
Pan-B-cell markers	–	CD19, CD20, CD79a
Immunoglobulin	–	
BCL-6	–	
HLA-DR	+	
CD30	+	
CD38	+	
CD138	+	
EMA	+	
LANA	+	
HHV8	+	
EBV (EBER)	+	LMP-1 negative

Note: Postulated normal counterpart: postgerminal center B cell

Reference: [33]

Table 27.34 Markers for Burkitt lymphoma (BL)

Antibodies	Result	Comment
CD19	+	
CD20	+	
CD22	+	
CD10	+	
CD38	+	
CD43	+	
CD77	+	
BCL-6	+	
BCL-2	–	
Ki-67	+	In 100% of tumor cells

Note: Postulated normal counterpart: germinal center or postgerminal center B cell

Reference: [34]

Table 27.35 Markers for B-cell lymphoma, unclassifiable, with features intermediate between diffuse large B-cell lymphoma and Burkitt lymphoma

Antibodies	Result	Comment
CD19	+	
CD20	+	
CD22	+	
CD79a	+	
CD10	+	
BCL-2	+	
BCL-6	+	
IRF4/MUM-1	– or weak	
Ki-67	+	50–100% of tumor cells
c-*MYC*	+	*MYC* rearrangement is positive in BL and commonly positive in this lymphoma

Note: Postulated normal counterpart: B cell, most cases related to a germinal center stage

Reference: [35]

Table 27.36 Markers for B-cell lymphoma, unclassifiable, with features intermediate between diffuse large B-cell lymphoma and classical Hodgkin lymphoma

Antibodies	Result	Comment
CD45	+ or –	Variable
CD15	+	
CD30	+	
CD20	+	
CD79a	+	
PAX-5	+	
OCT-2	+	
BOB.1	+	
BCL-6	+	
CD10	–	
ALK	–	
P53	+	Majority cases

Note: Postulated normal counterpart: thymic B cell in mediastinum; alternative B cell in peripheral lymph node

Reference: [36]

Table 27.37 Markers for T-cell prolymphocytic leukemia (TPLL)

Antibodies	Result	Comment
CD2	+	
CD3	+	
CD7	+	
CD52	+	High intensity, target for antibody therapy
CD1a	–	Differentiate from T-ALL
TdT	–	Differentiate from T-ALL
CD4	+	60% cases CD4+/CD8–
CD8	+	25%: CD4+/CD8+, 15%: CD4–/CD8–
TCL1	+	Detecting residual TPLL on BM section after therapy

Note: Postulated normal counterpart: unknown T cell, probable at an intermediate stage of differentiation between cortical thymocyte and mature T lymphocyte

Reference: [37]

Table 27.38 Markers for T-cell large granular lymphocytic leukemia (TLGL)

Antibodies	Result	Comment
CD2	+	
CD3	+	
CD8	+	Most TCR αβ+
CD4	–	Uncommon CD4+, CD4+/CD8+, or CD4–/CD8–
CD5	–	
CD7	–	
CD57	+	80% of cases
CD16	+	80% of cases
CD94/NKG2	+	50% of cases
Cytotoxic effector proteins	+	Including TIA1, granzyme B, granzyme M, and perforin

Note: Immunostains of CD8 and cytotoxic effector proteins can be used to detected bone marrow involvement in bone marrow biopsy specimen

It is a heterogeneous disorder with a persistent (longer than 6 months) increase of large granular lymphocytes (>2 × 10^9/L) in peripheral blood without a clearly identified cause

Postulated normal counterpart: CD8-positive T cell

Reference: [38]

Table 27.39 Markers for chronic lymphoproliferative disorders of NK cells (CLPD-NK)

Antibodies	Result	Comment
CD3 surface	–	
CD3ε cytoplasm	+	
CD16	+	
CD56	+	
Cytotoxic effector proteins	+	Including TIA1, granzyme B, granzyme M
CD2	–	
CD7	–	
CD57	–	
CD5	+	Aberrant expression
CD8	+	
CD94/NKG2A	+	
CD161		Decreased

Note: It is a heterogeneous disorder with a persistent (longer than 6 months) increase of NK cells (>2 × 10^9/L) in peripheral blood without a clearly identified cause

KIR family of NK-cell receptor is abnormal in CLPD-NK, including either restricted expression or a complete lack of KIR expression

Postulated normal counterpart: mature NK cell

Reference: [39]

Table 27.40 Markers for aggressive NK-cell leukemia

Antibodies	Result	Comment
CD2	+	
CD3 surface	–	
CD3ε cytoplasm	+	
CD56	+	
Cytotoxic effector proteins	+	Including TIA1, granzyme B, granzyme M, and perforin
CD16	+	75%
CD57	–	
FAS ligand	+	Expressed on the surface of neoplastic cells and in the serum of affected patients

Note: Postulated normal counterpart: NK cell

Reference: [40]

Table 27.41 Markers for EBV positive T-cell lymphoproliferative disorders of childhood

Antibodies	Result	Comment
CD2	+	
CD3	+	
TIA	+	
CD56	–	
CD8	+	Most cases second to acute primary EBV infection
CD4	+	Severe chronic active EBV infection, rare cases are CD4+/CD8+
EBER	+	

Note: Postulated normal counterpart: cytotoxic CD8+ T cell or activated CD4+ T cell

Reference: [41]

Table 27.42 Markers for adult T-cell leukemia/lymphoma (ATLL)

Antibodies	Result	Comment
CD2	+	
CD3	+	
CD5	+	
CD7	–	
CD4	+	Most cases are CD4+/CD8–
CD8	–	A few cases: CD4–/CD8+ or CD4+/CD8+
CD25	+	Strongly + in nearly all cases
CD30	+	
ALK	–	
Chemokine receptor	+	Including CCR4, FOXP3 – a feature of regulatory T cells

Note: Postulated normal counterpart: peripheral CD4+ T cell, probable CD4+ CD25+ FOXP3+ regulatory T cell

Reference: [42]

Table 27.43 Markers for extranodal NK/T-cell lymphoma, nasal type

Antibodies	Result	Comment
CD2	+	
CD3 surface	–	
CD3ε cytoplasm	+	
CD56	+	A highly useful marker for NK cells, but not specific for ENK/TL, and can be positive in PTCL, particularly γδT cells
Cytotoxic effector proteins	+	Including TIA1, granzyme B, perforin
CD4	–	
CD5	–	
CD8	–	
TCRδ	–	
βF1	–	
CD16	–	
CD57	–	
CD43	+	
CD45RO	+	
CD25	+	
FAS/FASL	+	
CD7	–	Occasional positive
CD30	+	

Note: Lymphomas with CD3ε+, CD56–, EBV+, and cytotoxic molecules+ are classified as extranodal NK/T-cell lymphoma; those with CD3+, CD56–, negative for EBV and cytotoxic molecules are diagnosed as peripheral T-cell lymphoma, unspecified. EBER is the most reliable way to demonstrate the presence of EBV; LMP-1 stain is variable and inconsistent

Postulated normal counterpart: activated NK cell and, less commonly, cytotoxic T cell

Reference: [43]

Table 27.44 Markers for enteropathy-associated T-cell lymphoma (EATL)

Antibodies	EATL	Type II EATL[a]
CD3	+	+
CD5	–	–
CD7	+	+
CD8	–	+
CD4	–	–
CD56	–	+
CD103	+	
TCRβ	+	+
CD30	+	
Cytotoxic effector proteins	+	+

Note: Intraepithelial lymphocytes in adjacent enteropathic mucosa of the lymphoma may be CD3+, CD5–, CD8–, and CD4–, identical to that of lymphoma

Postulated normal counterpart: intraepithelial T cell of the intestine

[a]The monomorphic form of EATL (type II EATL) shows neoplastic T cells to be CD3+, CD4–, CD8+, CD56+, and TCRβ+. Both EATLs have a similar clinical course

Reference: [44]

Table 27.45 Markers for hepatosplenic T-cell lymphoma (HSTL)

Antibodies	Result	Comment
CD3	+	
TCRδ1	+	Most γδT cells express the Vδ1 epitope
TCRαβ	–	A minority of cases are αβT cells, considered as a variant
CD56	+ or –	
CD4	–	
CD8	– or +	
CD5	–	
Cytotoxic effector proteins	+	TIA1 and granzyme M+, but granzyme B and perforin negative
KIR[a]	+	Aberrant expression
CD94[b]	– or dim	

Notes:

[a]KIR: Killer immunoglobulin-like receptors are transmembrane glycoproteins expressed by natural killer cells and subsets of T cells

[b]CD94, also known as killer cell lectin-like receptor subfamily D, is a lectin and a receptor involving in cell signaling and normally expressing on the surface of natural killer cells

Postulated normal counterpart: peripheral γδ, or less commonly αβ, cytotoxic T cell of the innate immune system

Reference: [45]

Table 27.46 Markers for subcutaneous panniculitis-like T-cell lymphoma (SPTCL)

Antibodies	Result	Comment
CD3	+	
CD8	+	
CD4	–	
Cytotoxic effector proteins	+	Including TIA1, granzyme B, perforin
βF1	+	Differentiate from cutaneous γδT-cell lymphoma
CD56	–	

Note: Postulated normal counterpart: mature cytotoxic T cell

Reference: [46]

Table 27.47 Markers for mycosis fungoides (MF)

Antibodies	Result	Comment
CD2	+	
CD3	+	
TCRαβ	+	
CD5	+	
CD4	+	
CD8	–	Rare cases may be CD8+, more common in pediatric MF
CD7	–	
CLA	+	Associated with lymphocytes homing to the skin
Cytotoxic effector proteins	–	Only rarely positive in the early lesion, may be positive in some advanced tumors

Note: *CLA* cutaneous lymphocyte antigen

Postulated normal counterpart: mature skin-homing CD4+ T cell

Reference: [47]

Table 27.48 Markers for Sezary syndrome (SS)

Antibodies	Result	Comment
CD2	+	
CD3	+	
CD5	+	
TCRβ	+	
CD4	+	Most cases
CD8	–	Rare cases CD8+
CLA	+	
CCR4	+	
CD7	–	
CD26	–	

Note: CCR4: skin-homing receptor; CD26: also known as dipeptidyl peptidase-4 (DPP4) or adenosine deaminase complexing protein 2, is an enzyme expressed on the surface of most cell types and is associated with immune regulation, signal transduction and apoptosis; *CLA* cutaneous lymphocyte antigen.

Postulated normal counterpart: mature epidermotropic skin-homing CD4+ T cell

Reference: [48]

Table 27.49 Markers for primary cutaneous CD30 positive T-cell lymphoproliferative disorders

Table 27.49a Markers for primary cutaneous anaplastic large cell lymphoma (C-ALCL)

Antibodies	Result	Comment
CD3	+	
CD4	+	
CD5	+	
CD2	– or +	
Cytotoxic effector proteins	+	Including TIA1, granzyme B, perforin
CD8	–	<5% of cases CD8+
CD30	+	
CLA	+	
ALK	–	Different from systemic ALCL
EMA	–	
CD15	–	
CD56	–	Rare cases positive

Note: Postulated normal counterpart: transformed/activated skin-homing T cell

Table 27.49b Markers for lymphomatoid papulosis (LyP):

Antibodies	Type A	Type B	Type C
CD3	+	+	+
CD4	+	+	+
CD8	–	–	–
CD30	+	–	+

Note: There are *three histologic subtypes*, which represent a spectrum with overlapping features

Type A: scattered or small clusters of large or RS-like CD30+ cells intermingled with numerous inflammatory cells

Type B: epidermotropic infiltration of small atypical cells with cerebriform nuclei similar to that of MF

Type C: monotonous population or large clusters of large CD30+ T cells with relatively few admixed inflammatory cells

Postulated normal counterpart: activated skin-homing T cell

Reference: [49]

Table 27.50 Markers for primary cutaneous peripheral T-cell lymphoma (PTCL), rare subtype

Table 27.50a Markers for primary cutaneous gamma-delta T-cell lymphoma

Antibodies	Result	Comment
CD2	+	
CD3	+	
TCRδ	+	Strongly
βF1	–	
CD5	–	
CD7	+ or –	
CD56	+	
Cytotoxic effector proteins	+	Including TIA1, granzyme B, perforin
CD4	–	
CD8	–	Some cases CD8+

Note: Postulated normal counterpart: functionally mature and activated cytotoxic γδ T cell of the innate immune system

Table 27.50b Markers for primary cutaneous CD8-positive aggressive epidermotropic cytotoxic T-cell lymphoma

Antibodies	Result	Comment
CD3	+	
CD8	+	
βF1	+	
Cytotoxic effector proteins	+	Including TIA1, granzyme B, perforin
CD45RA	+ or –	
CD45RO	–	
CD2	– or +	
CD4	–	
CD5	–	
CD7	+ or –	

Note: Postulated normal counterpart: skin-homing CD8+ cytotoxic T cell

Table 27.50c Markers for primary cutaneous CD4-positive small/medium T-cell lymphoma

CD3	+	
CD4	+	
CD8	–	
CD30	–	
Cytotoxic effector proteins	–	Including TIA1, granzyme B, perforin

Note: Sometimes, primary cutaneous CD4-positive small/medium T-cell lymphoma loss of pan-T-cell markers; admixed polyclonal plasma cells and B cells may be present, which make distinction from a reactive process difficult

Postulated normal counterpart: skin-homing CD4+ T cell

Reference: [50]

Table 27.51 Markers for peripheral T-cell lymphoma, not otherwise specified

Antibodies	Result	Comment
CD2	+	
CD3	+	
CD5	–	
CD7	–	
βF1	+	
CD52	+	In 60% of cases
CD30	–	Rarely positive

Note: CD4+/CD8– predominant in nodal cases; some cases show CD4+/CD8+, CD4–/CD8–, or CD4–/CD8+/CD56+/cytotoxic granules+

Aberrant expression of B-cell markers, CD20 or CD79a, is occasionally seen

Follicular/perifollicular variant may have follicular T helper phenotype: CD10+, BCL-6+, PD-1+, and CXCL13+

Proliferation rate is usually high; Ki-67 index exceeding 70% is associated with a worse prognosis

Postulated normal counterpart: activated mature T cell, mostly CD4+ central memory type of adaptive immune system

Variants:

– Lymphoepithelioid (Lennert lymphoma)

Neoplastic cell – CD8+ T cells

– Follicular

– T-zone

Neoplastic cells – CD3+, CD4+, and CD5– or CD7–

References: [51, 52]

Table 27.52 Markers for angioimmuoblastic T-cell lymphoma (AITL)

Antibodies	Result	Comment
CD2	+	
CD3	+	
CD5	+	
CD4	+	Background of numerous reactive CD8+ T cells
CD10	+	60–100% of cases
BCL-6	+	60–100% of cases
PD-1	+	60–100% of cases
CXCL13	+	60–100% of cases

Note: Follicular dendritic cell meshworks, highlighting by CD21, CD23, and CD35, are expanded and usually surround the high endothelial venules

EBV-positive B cells are nearly always present; they may become DLBCL or HL

Postulated normal counterpart: CD4+ follicular helper T cells

Reference: [53]

Table 27.53 Markers for anaplastic large cell lymphoma (ALCL), ALK positive

Antibodies	Result	Comment
CD30	+	Strongly +, often cluster around blood vessels
ALK	+	Monoclonal Ab are better, polyclonal Ab may have false + stain
EMA	+	Some cases may be focally +
CD3	–	One or more T-cell markers +, some cases are all T cell markers negative – null cell phenotype
CD2	+	70% of cases
CD5	+	70% of cases
CD4	+	70% of cases
Cytotoxic effector proteins	+	Including TIA1, granzyme B, perforin
CD8	–	Rare CD8+ cases
CD43	+	2/3 cases positive
CD25	+	
CD15	+	Rare, only present focally
CD68	–	KP1+, PGM1–
BCL-2	–	
EBV	–	Both EBER and LMP-1

Note: Postulated normal counterpart: activated mature cytotoxic T cells

Reference: [54]

Table 27.54 Markers for anaplastic large cell lymphoma (ALCL), ALK negative

Antibodies	Result	Comment
CD30	+	Strongly and diffusely +
ALK	–	
EMA	+	Some cases may be focally +
CD3	+	One or more T-cell markers + in ½ cases
CD2	+	
CD5	–	
CD43	+	
CD4	+	Most cases
CD8	–	Rare cases +
Cytotoxic effector proteins	+	Including TIA1, granzyme B, perforin
EMA	–	Minority cases + focally, different from ALCL, ALK-positive
EBV	–	Both EBER and LMP-1
Clusterin	+	Nonspecific

Note: Postulated normal counterpart: activated mature cytotoxic T cells

Reference: [55]

Table 27.55 Markers for nodular lymphocyte predominant Hodgkin lymphoma (NLPHL)

Antibodies	Result	Comment
CD20	+	Fig. 27.22
CD79a	+	
CD75	+	
BCL-6	+	
CD45	+	
EMA	+	>50% cases
OCT-2	+	
BOB.1	+	
AID[a]	+	
IgD	+	9–27% cases, more common in young males
CD15	–	
CD30	–	

Note: [a]AID – activation induced deaminase, it causes mutations that produce antibody diversity in B cells and function as a B-cell marker

Most of LP cells are ringed by CD3+, LP-1+ T cells and, to a lesser extent, by CD57+ T cells. Background lymphocytes include B cells, CD4+/CD57+ T cells, LP-1+ T cells, CD4+/CD8+ T cells, but not CD8+/TIA+ T cells

CD21 can be used to detect follicular dendritic cell-formed nodules

Postulated normal counterpart: germinal center B cells at the centroblastic stage of differentiation

Reference: [56]

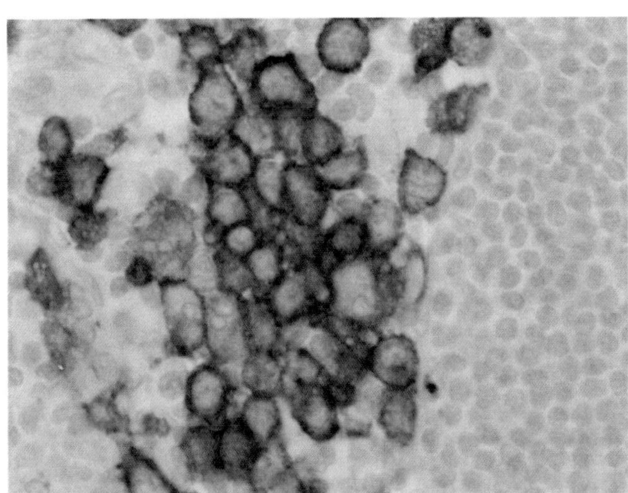

Fig. 27.22 CD20 in nodular lymphocyte predominant Hodgkin lymphoma

Table 27.56 Markers for classical Hodgkin lymphoma (CHL)

Antibodies	Result	Comment
CD15	+	75–85% cases, may be focally or only in Golgi area (Fig. 27.14)
CD30	+	Nearly all cases (Fig. 27.15)
CD45	–	
CD75	–	
CD68 (PGM)	–	
CD20	–	
CD79a	–	
PAX-5	+	Weakly
OCT-2	–	Both or either OCT-2 and BOB.1 negative
BOB.1	–	
IRF4/MUM-1	+	
CD138	–	
EBV	+	10–40% NS, 75% MC cases
EMA	–	Rare cases weakly +
PU.1	–	Transcription factor PU.1 is a protein that activates gene expression during myeloid and B-lymphoid cell development

Note: Most of HRS cells are Ki-67+

Four histological subtypes: nodular sclerosis, mixed cellularity, lymphocyte rich, and lymphocyte depleted. They are different in prognosis, but not an important predictive factor with modern radiation and chemotherapy

Postulated normal counterpart: 98% of cases from mature B cells at the germinal center stage of differentiation; rare cases from postthymic T cells

Reference: [57]

Table 27.57 Markers for lymphoproliferative diseases (LPD) associated with primary immune disorders (PID)

Table 27.57a Markers for non-neoplastic lymphoproliferative disorders (autoimmune lymphoproliferative syndrome, ALPS)

Antibodies	Result	Comment
CD3	+	Expansion of naïve T cells in PB and BM
CD4	–	
CD8	–	
CD45RA	+	
CD45RO	–	
CD57	+	
CD25	–	
EBV	+	

Note: Iatrogenic immunodeficiency-associated lymphoproliferative disorders have similar histological features as LPD. Non-neoplastic lymphoproliferative disorders include many diseases based on pathogenesis. Only ALPS is listed here

Markers for neoplastic lymphoproliferative disorders:

B-cell lymphoma: EBV+ with EBER (LMP-1 may be expressed); B-cell antigens may be decreased or lost

T-cell lymphoma: same markers as T-cell lymphoma

HL: same markers as Hodgkin lymphoma (Table 27.56)

References: [58, 59]

Table 27.58 Markers for lymphomas associated with HIV infection

Lymphomas also occurring in immunocompetent patients

Burkitt lymphoma (Table 27.34) – 30% of all HIV-associated lymphomas

- 1/3 cases showing BL features, EBV+ in 30%
- 2/3 cases showing plasmacytoid differentiation that is unique to AIDS patients, EBV+ in 50–70%

Diffuse large B-cell lymphoma (Table 27.21a) – 25–30% of HIV-associated lymphomas

- EBV+ in 30% cases
- Immunoblastic type in late course of HIV disease and primary central nervous system lymphoma, EBV+ in 90% of cases

Hodgkin lymphoma (Table 27.56)

- Most cases are mixed cellularity or lymphocyte depleted; some cases are nodular sclerosis
- EBV+ in nearly all cases, both EBER+ and LMP-1+

Other lymphomas – rare cases

- MALT lymphoma occurs in both adult and pediatric patients
- Peripheral T-cell and NK-cell lymphomas

Lymphomas occurring more specific in HIV+ patients

- Primary effusion lymphoma (Table 27.33)
- Plasmablastic lymphoma (Table 27.31)
- Lymphomas arising in HHV8-associated multicentric Castleman disease (Table 27.32)

Lymphomas occurring in other immunodeficient status

- Polymorphic lymphoid proliferations – resembling PTLD, but much less common than in posttransplant setting, representing less than 5% of HIV-associated lymphomas, CD30+, EBV+ (some EBV−)

Reference: [60]

Table 27.59 Markers for posttransplant lymphoproliferative disorders (PTLD)

Early lesions: plasmacytic hyperplasia and infectious mononucleosis-like PTLD

- Admixture of polyclonal B cells, plasma cells, and T cells without phenotypic aberrancy
- EBV+ in many but not in all cases; EBER+/LMP+ in infectious mononucleosis-like cases

Polymorphic PTLD

- B cells with or without light chain restriction in a background of heterogeneous T cells
- Light chain restriction or clonality may be focally present
- EBV+ (EBER+) – useful tool in differentiation from rejection
- Focal DLBCL-like lesions
- RS-like cells – CD30+, CD20+, CD15−

Monomorphic PTLD

Monomorphic T/NK-cell PTLD

- B-cells-associated markers positive: CD19, CD20, and CD79a
- Monoclonality – often γ or α heavy chains in 50% of cases
- CD30+
- EBV+ (EBER+) cases – usually with a late germinal center/postgerminal center phenotype: CD10−, BCL-6+/−, IRF4/MUM+
- EBV negative cases – usually with a germinal center phenotype: CD10+/−, BCL-6+, IRF4/MUM−, CD138−

Monomorphic T/NK-cell PTLD

Antibodies	Result	Comment
CD4	+ or −	
CD8	+ or −	
CD30	+	
ALK	+	
EBV	+	

Note: Pan-T-cell and sometimes NK-cell-associated markers are positive

Classical Hodgkin lymphoma type PTLD

- EBV+
- Same markers as CHL: CD15+, CD30+, CD3−, CD20−, CD45− (Table 27.56)

Reference: [61]

Table 27.60 Markers for histiocytic sarcoma

Antibodies	Result	Comment
CD4	+	
CD68	+	Fig. 27.23
CD163	+	
Lysozyme	+	Fig. 27.16
CD1a	–	Langerhans cell marker
Langerin	–	Langerhans cell marker
CD21	–	Follicular dendritic cell markers
CD35	–	Follicular dendritic cell markers
CD13	–	Myeloid marker
CD33	–	Myeloid marker
MPO	–	Myeloid marker
CD45	+	
CD45RO	+	
HLA-DR	+	
S-100	+	Weak and focal

Note: Negative for specific T cell, B cell, epithelial markers. Ki-67 proliferation rate is variable

Postulated normal counterpart: mature tissue histiocyte

Reference: [62]

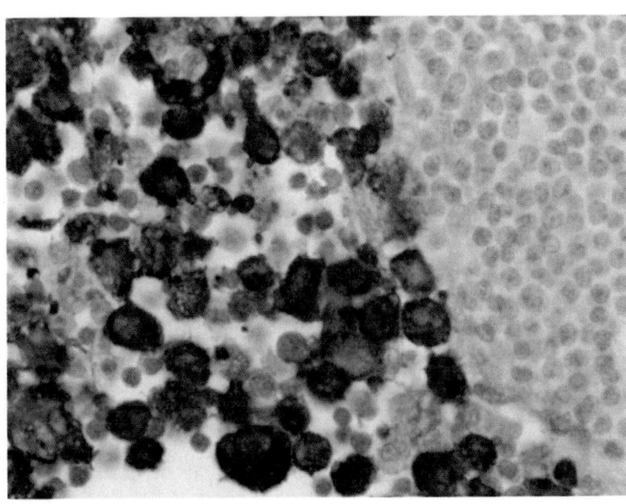

Fig. 27.23 CD68 in histiocytic sarcoma

Table 27.61 Markers for tumor derived from Langerhans cells

Antibodies	Result	Comment
CD1a	+	Fig. 27.20
Langerin	+	Malignant Langerhan cells may loss it occasionally
S-100	+	Fig. 27.21
CD68	+	
HLA-DR	+	
CD45	+	Low
CD30	–	

Note: Negative for specific T cell, B cell, follicular dendritic, epithelial markers. Ki-67 proliferation rate is variable-Postulated normal counterpart: mature Langerhans cell

Reference: [63]

Table 27.62 Markers for interdigitating dendritic cell (IDC) sarcoma

Antibodies	Result	Comment
S-100	+	
Fascin	+	
CD1a	–	
Langerin	–	
CD68	+	Weakly and variably
Lysozyme	+	Weakly and variably
CD45	–	Weakly and variably
P53	+	Strongly
CD34	–	
MPO	–	
CD30	–	

Note: It is negative for specific T cell, B cell, follicular dendritic, epithelial markers. Ki-67 proliferation rate is 10–20%. The negative markers are pertinent because the diagnosis is made by exclusion plus positive S-100 and Fascin. Postulated normal counterpart: interdigitating dendritic cell

Reference: [64]

Table 27.63 Markers for follicular dendritic cell (FDC) sarcoma

Antibodies	Result	Comment
CD21	+	FDC marker
CD23	+	FDC marker
CD35	+	FDC marker
CAN.42	+	FDC marker
KiM4P	+	FDC marker
D2-40	+	Stain lymphatic endothelium and follicular dendritic cells
Clusterin	+	Strongly, usually – or weakly + in other dendritic cell tumors
Desmoplakin	+	Protein associated with desmosomes that are intercellular junctions that tightly link adjacent cells
Fascin	+	
EGFR	+	Epidermal growth factor receptor
HLA-DR	+	
EMA	+	
S-100	+	
CD68	+	
CD1a	–	
Lysozyme	–	
MPO	–	
CD34	–	
CD3	–	
CD79a	–	
CD30	–	
HMB45	–	

Note: Cytokeratin, CD20, and CD45 may be focally expressed. Ki-67 proliferation rate is 1–25%. Postulated normal counterpart: follicular dendritic cell of the lymphoid follicles

Reference: [65]

Table 27.64 Markers for other rare dendritic cell tumors

Antibodies	Result	Comment
(a) Markers for fibroblastic reticular cell tumors		
SMA	+	
Desmin	+	
Cytokeratin	+	In a dendritic pattern
CD68	+	
(b) Markers for indeterminate dendritic cell tumors		
S-100	+	
CD1a	+	
Langerin	–	
CD30	–	

Note: Negative for specific T cell, B cell, histiocytic, follicular dendritic, epithelial markers. Variably positive for CD45, CD68, lysozyme, and CD4. Ki-67 proliferation rate is highly variable

Reference: [66]

Table 27.65 Markers for disseminated juvenile xanthogranuloma (JXG)

Antibodies	Result	Comment
CD14	+	Membrane
CD68 (PGM1)	+	Coarse granular pattern
CD168	+	Membrane and cytoplasmic
Stabilin-1	+	Transmembrane receptor protein that may function in angiogenesis, lymphocyte homing, cell adhesion, or receptor scavenging
Factor XIIIa	+	Positive in dermal/interstitial dendritic cells
Fascin	+	
S-100	+	In <20% of cases
CD1a	–	
Langerin	–	

Note: None of the markers are specific for DJX. The markers are common with macrophages. Postulated normal counterpart: the cell of origin is debated. It has both macrophage and dermal/interstitial dendritic cell phenotype

Reference: [67]

Note for All Tables

Note: "+" – usually greater than 70% of cases are positive; "–" – less than 5% of cases are positive; "+ or –" – usually more than 50% of cases are positive; "– or +" – less than 50% of cases are positive.

References

1. Lester SC. Special studies. Manual surgical pathology. 2nd ed. New York, NY: Elsevier Inc.; 2006. pp. 128.
2. Higgins RA, Blankenship JE, Kinney MC. Application of immunohistochemistry in the diagnosis of non-Hodgkin and Hodgkin lymphoma. Arch Pathol Lab Med. 2008;132:441–61.
3. Chaiwatanatorn K, Stamaratis G, Opeskin K, Firkin F, Nandurkar H. Protein kinase C-beta II expression in diffuse large B-cell lymphoma predicts for inferior outcome of anthracycline-based chemotherapy with and without rituximab. Leuk Lymphoma. 2009;50(10):1666–75.
4. Dabbs DJ. Diagnostic immunohistochemistry. 3rd ed. Philadelphia: Saunders Elsevier; 2010. pp. 274, 308, 405.
5. Muller-Hermelink HK, Montserrat E, Catovsky D, Campo E, Harris NL, Stein H. Chronic lymphocytic leukemia/small lymphocytic lymphoma. In: Swerdlow SH, Campo E, Harris NL, Jaffe ES, Pileri SA, Stein H, Thiele J and Vardiman JW. WHO classification of tumours of haematopoietic and lymphoid tissues. 4th ed. Lyon, France: International Agency for Research on Cancer; 2008. pp. 180.
6. Campo E, Catovsky D, Montserrat E, Muller-Hermelink HK, Harris NL, Stein H. B-cell prolymphocytic leukemia. In: Swerdlow SH, Campo E, Harris NL, Jaffe ES, Pileri SA, Stein H, Thiele J and Vardiman JW. WHO classification of tumours of haematopoietic and lymphoid tissues. 4th ed. Lyon, France: International Agency for Research on Cancer; 2008. pp. 183.
7. Isaacson PG, Piris MA, Berger F, Swerdlow SH. Splenic B-cell marginal zone lymphoma. In: Swerdlow SH, Campo E, Harris NL, Jaffe ES, Pileri SA, Stein H, Thiele J and Vardiman JW. WHO Classification of tumours of haematopoietic and lymphoid tissues. 4th ed. Lyon, France: International Agency for Research on Cancer; 2008. pp. 185.
8. Foucar K, Falini B, Catovsky D, Stein H. Hairy cell leukaemia. In: Swerdlow SH, Campo E, Harris NL, Jaffe ES, Pileri SA, Stein H, Thiele J and Vardiman JW. WHO classification of tumours of haematopoietic and lymphoid tissues. 4th ed. Lyon, France: International Agency for Research on Cancer; 2008. pp. 188.
9. Chen YH, Tallman MS, Goolsby C, Peterson L. Immunophenotypic variations in hairy cell leukemia. Am J Clin Pathol. 2006;125:251–9.
10. Piris M, Foucar K, Mollejo M, Campo E, Falini B. Splenic B-cell lymphoma/leukemia, unclassifiable. In: Swerdlow SH, Campo E, Harris NL, Jaffe ES, Pileri SA, Stein H, Thiele J and Vardiman JW. WHO classification of tumours of haematopoietic and lymphoid tissues. 4th ed. Lyon, France: International Agency for Research on Cancer; 2008. pp. 191.
11. Traverse-Glehen A, Baseggio L, Bauchu EC, Morel D, Gazzo S, Ffrench M, et al. Splenic red pulp lymphoma with numerous basophilic villous lymphocytes: a distinct clinicopathologic and molecular entity? Blood. 2008;111(4):2253–60.
12. Swerdlow SH, Berger F, Pileri SA, Harris NL, Jaffe ES, Stein H. Lymphoplasmacytic lymphoma. In: Swerdlow SH, Campo E, Harris NL, Jaffe ES, Pileri SA, Stein H, Thiele J and Vardiman JW. WHO classification of tumours of haematopoietic and lymphoid tissues. 4th ed. Lyon, France: International Agency for Research on Cancer; 2008. pp. 194.
13. Harris NL, Issacson PG, Grogan TM, Jaffe ES. Heavy chain disease. In: Swerdlow SH, Campo E, Harris NL, Jaffe ES, Pileri SA, Stein H, Thiele J and Vardiman JW. WHO classification of tumours of haematopoietic and lymphoid tissues. 4th ed. Lyon, France: International Agency for Research on Cancer; 2008. pp. 196.
14. McKenna RW, Kyle RA, Kuehl WM, Grogan TM, Harris NL, Coupland RW. Plasma cell neoplasms. In: Swerdlow SH, Campo E, Harris NL, Jaffe ES, Pileri SA, Stein H, Thiele J and Vardiman JW. WHO classification of tumours of haematopoietic and lymphoid tissues. 4th ed. Lyon, France: International Agency for Research on Cancer; 2008. pp. 200.
15. Isaacson PG, Chott A, Nakamura S, Muller-Hermelink HK, Harris NL, Swerdlow SH. Extranodal marginal zone lymphoma of mucosa-associated lymphoid tissue (MALT lymphoma). In: Swerdlow SH, Campo E, Harris NL, Jaffe ES, Pileri SA, Stein H, Thiele J and Vardiman JW. WHO classification of tumours of haematopoietic

and lymphoid tissues. 4th ed. Lyon, France: International Agency for Research on Cancer; 2008. pp. 214.

16. Campo E, Pileri SA, Jaffe ES, Muller-Hermelink HK, Nathwani BN. Nodal marginal zone lymphoma. In: Swerdlow SH, Campo E, Harris NL, Jaffe ES, Pileri SA, Stein H, Thiele J and Vardiman JW. WHO classification of tumours of haematopoietic and lymphoid tissues. 4th ed. Lyon, France: International Agency for Research on Cancer; 2008. pp. 218.
17. Harris NL, Swerdlow SH, Jaffe ES, Ott G. Follicular lymphoma. In: Swerdlow SH, Campo E, Harris NL, Jaffe ES, Pileri SA, Stein H, Thiele J and Vardiman JW. WHO classification of tumours of haematopoietic and lymphoid tissues. 4th ed. Lyon, France: International Agency for Research on Cancer; 2008. pp. 220.
18. Willemze R, Swerdlow SH, Harris NL, Vergier B. Primary cutaneous follicle center lymphoma. In: Swerdlow SH, Campo E, Harris NL, Jaffe ES, Pileri SA, Stein H, Thiele J and Vardiman JW. WHO classification of tumours of haematopoietic and lymphoid tissues. 4th ed. Lyon, France: International Agency for Research on Cancer; 2008. pp. 227.
19. Swerdlow SH, Campo E, Seto M, Muller-Hermelink HK. Mantle cell lymphoma. In: Swerdlow SH, Campo E, Harris NL, Jaffe ES, Pileri SA, Stein H, Thiele J and Vardiman JW. WHO classification of tumours of haematopoietic and lymphoid tissues. 4th ed. Lyon, France: International Agency for Research on Cancer; 2008. pp. 229.
20. Sein H, Warnke RA, Chan WC, Jaffe ES, Chang JKC, Gatter KC, et al. Diffuse large B-cell lymphoma, not otherwise specified. In: Swerdlow SH, Campo E, Harris NL, Jaffe ES, Pileri SA, Stein H, Thiele J and Vardiman JW. WHO classification of tumours of haematopoietic and lymphoid tissues. 4th ed. Lyon, France: International Agency for Research on Cancer; 2008. pp. 233.
21. De Wolf-Peeters C, Delabie J, Campo E, Jaffe ES, Delsol G. T cell/ histiocyte-rich large B cell lymphoma. In: Swerdlow SH, Campo E, Harris NL, Jaffe ES, Pileri SA, Stein H, Thiele J and Vardiman JW. WHO classification of tumours of haematopoietic and lymphoid tissues. 4th ed. Lyon, France: International Agency for Research on Cancer; 2008. pp. 238.
22. Kluin PM, Deckert M, Ferry JA. Primary diffuse large B-cell lymphoma of the CNS. In: Swerdlow SH, Campo E, Harris NL, Jaffe ES, Pileri SA, Stein H, Thiele J and Vardiman JW. WHO classification of tumours of haematopoietic and lymphoid tissues. 4th ed. Lyon, France: International Agency for Research on Cancer; 2008. pp. 240.
23. Meijer CJL, Vergier B, Duncan LM, Willemze R. Primary cutaneous DLBCL, leg type. In: Swerdlow SH, Campo E, Harris NL, Jaffe ES, Pileri SA, Stein H, Thiele J and Vardiman JW. WHO classification of tumours of haematopoietic and lymphoid tissues. 4th ed. Lyon, France: International Agency for Research on Cancer; 2008. pp. 242.
24. Nakamura S, Jaffe ES, Swerdlow SH. EBV positive diffuse large B-cell lymphoma of the elderly. In: Swerdlow SH, Campo E, Harris NL, Jaffe ES, Pileri SA, Stein H, Thiele J and Vardiman JW. WHO classification of tumours of haematopoietic and lymphoid tissues. 4th ed. Lyon, France: International Agency for Research on Cancer; 2008. pp. 243.
25. Chan JKC, Aozasa K, Gaulard P. DLBCL associated with chronic inflammation. In: Swerdlow SH, Campo E, Harris NL, Jaffe ES, Pileri SA, Stein H, Thiele J and Vardiman JW. WHO classification of tumours of haematopoietic and lymphoid tissues. 4th ed. Lyon, France: International Agency for Research on Cancer; 2008. pp. 245.
26. Pittaluga S, Wilson WH, Jaffe ES. Lymphomatoid granulomatosis. In: Swerdlow SH, Campo E, Harris NL, Jaffe ES, Pileri SA, Stein H, Thiele J and Vardiman JW. WHO classification of tumours of haematopoietic and lymphoid tissues. 4th ed. Lyon, France: International Agency for Research on Cancer; 2008. pp. 247.
27. Gaulard P, Harris NL, Pileri SA, Kutok JL, Stein KAM, Jaffe ES, et al. Primary mediastinal (thymic) large B-cell lymphoma. In: Swerdlow SH, Campo E, Harris NL, Jaffe ES, Pileri SA, Stein H, Thiele J and Vardiman JW. WHO classification of tumours of haematopoietic and lymphoid tissues. 4th ed. Lyon, France: International Agency for Research on Cancer; 2008. pp. 250.
28. Nakamura S, Ponzoni M, Campo E. Intravascular large B-cell lymphoma. In: Swerdlow SH, Campo E, Harris NL, Jaffe ES, Pileri SA, Stein H, Thiele J and Vardiman JW. WHO classification of tumours of haematopoietic and lymphoid tissues. 4th ed. Lyon, France: International Agency for Research on Cancer; 2008. pp. 252.
29. Delssol G, Campo E, Gascoyne RD. ALK-positive large B-cell lymphoma. In: Swerdlow SH, Campo E, Harris NL, Jaffe ES, Pileri SA, Stein H, Thiele J and Vardiman JW. WHO classification of tumours of haematopoietic and lymphoid tissues. 4th ed. Lyon, France: International Agency for Research on Cancer; 2008. pp. 254.
30. Stein H, Harris NL, Campo E. Plasmablastic lymphoma. In: Swerdlow SH, Campo E, Harris NL, Jaffe ES, Pileri SA, Stein H, Thiele J and Vardiman JW. WHO classification of tumours of haematopoietic and lymphoid tissues. 4th ed. Lyon, France: International Agency for Research on Cancer; 2008. pp. 256.
31. Isaacson PG, Campo E, Harris NL. Large B-cell lymphoma arising in HHV8-associated multicentric Castleman disease. In: Swerdlow SH, Campo E, Harris NL, Jaffe ES, Pileri SA, Stein H, Thiele J and Vardiman JW. WHO classification of tumours of haematopoietic and lymphoid tissues. 4th ed. Lyon, France: International Agency for Research on Cancer; 2008. pp. 258.
32. Burbelo PD, Issa AT, Ching KH, Wyvill KM, Little RF, Iadarola MJ, et al. Distinct profiles of antibodies to Kaposi sarcoma-associated herpesvirus antigens in patients with Kaposi sarcoma, multicentric Castleman disease, and primary effusion lymphoma. J Infect Dis. 2010;201(12):1919–22.
33. Said J, Cesarman E. Primary effusion lymphoma. In: Swerdlow SH, Campo E, Harris NL, Jaffe ES, Pileri SA, Stein H, Thiele J and Vardiman JW. WHO classification of tumours of haematopoietic and lymphoid tissues. 4th ed. Lyon, France: International Agency for Research on Cancer; 2008. pp. 260.
34. Leoncini L, Raphael M, Stein H, Harris NL, Jaffe ES, Kluin PM. Burkitt lymphoma. In: Swerdlow SH, Campo E, Harris NL, Jaffe ES, Pileri SA, Stein H, Thiele J and Vardiman JW. WHO classification of tumours of haematopoietic and lymphoid tissues. 4th ed. Lyon, France: International Agency for Research on Cancer; 2008. pp. 262.
35. Kluin PM, Harris NL, Stein H, Leoncini L. B-cell lymphoma, unclassifiable, with features intermediate between diffuse large B-cell lymphoma and Burkitt lymphoma. In: Swerdlow SH, Campo E, Harris NL, Jaffe ES, Pileri SA, Stein H, Thiele J and Vardiman JW. WHO classification of tumours of haematopoietic and lymphoid tissues. 4th ed. Lyon, France: International Agency for Research on Cancer; 2008. pp. 265.
36. Jaffe ES, Stein H, Swerdlow SH, Campo E, Pileri SA, Harris NL. B-cell lymphoma, unclassifiable, with features intermediate between diffuse large B-cell lymphoma and classical Hodgkin lymphoma. In: Swerdlow SH, Campo E, Harris NL, Jaffe ES, Pileri SA, Stein H, Thiele J and Vardiman JW. WHO classification of tumours of haematopoietic and lymphoid tissues. 4th ed. Lyon, France: International Agency for Research on Cancer; 2008. pp. 267.
37. Catovsky D, Muller-Hermelink HK, Ralfkiaer E. T-cell prolymphocytic leukemia. In: Swerdlow SH, Campo E, Harris NL, Jaffe ES, Pileri SA, Stein H, Thiele J and Vardiman JW. WHO classification of tumours of haematopoietic and lymphoid tissues. 4th ed. Lyon, France: International Agency for Research on Cancer; 2008. pp. 270.
38. Chan WC, Foucar K, Morice WG, Catovsky D. T-cell large granular lymphocytic leukemia. In: Swerdlow SH, Campo E, Harris NL, Jaffe ES, Pileri SA, Stein H, Thiele J and Vardiman JW. WHO classification of tumours of haematopoietic and lymphoid tissues. 4th

ed. Lyon, France: International Agency for Research on Cancer; 2008. pp. 272.

39. Villamor N, Morice WG, Chan WC, Foucar K. Chronic lymphoproliferative disorders of NK cells. In: Swerdlow SH, Campo E, Harris NL, Jaffe ES, Pileri SA, Stein H, Thiele J and Vardiman JW. WHO classification of tumours of haematopoietic and lymphoid tissues. 4th ed. Lyon, France: International Agency for Research on Cancer; 2008. pp. 274.
40. Chan JKC, Jaffe ES, Ralfiaer E, Ko YH. Aggressive NK-cell leukemia. In: Swerdlow SH, Campo E, Harris NL, Jaffe ES, Pileri SA, Stein H, Thiele J and Vardiman JW. WHO classification of tumours of haematopoietic and lymphoid tissues. 4th ed. Lyon, France: International Agency for Research on Cancer; 2008. pp. 276.
41. Quintanilla-Martines L, Kimura H, Jaffe ES. EBV-positive T-cell lymphoproliferative disorders of childhood. In: Swerdlow SH, Campo E, Harris NL, Jaffe ES, Pileri SA, Stein H, Thiele J and Vardiman JW. WHO classification of tumours of haematopoietic and lymphoid tissues. 4th ed. Lyon, France: International Agency for Research on Cancer; 2008. pp. 278.
42. Ohshima K, Jaffe ES, Kikuchi M. Adult T-cell leukemia/lymphoma. In: Swerdlow SH, Campo E, Harris NL, Jaffe ES, Pileri SA, Stein H, Thiele J and Vardiman JW. WHO classification of tumours of haematopoietic and lymphoid tissues. 4th ed. Lyon, France: International Agency for Research on Cancer; 2008. pp. 281.
43. Chan JKC, Quintanilla-Martines L, Ferry JA, Peh SC. Extranodal NK/T-cell lymphoma. In: Swerdlow SH, Campo E, Harris NL, Jaffe ES, Pileri SA, Stein H, Thiele J and Vardiman JW. WHO classification of tumours of haematopoietic and lymphoid tissues. 4th ed. Lyon, France: International Agency for Research on Cancer; 2008. pp. 285.
44. Isaacson PG, Chott A, Ott G, Stein H. Enteropathy-associated T-cell lymphoma. In: Swerdlow SH, Campo E, Harris NL, Jaffe ES, Pileri SA, Stein H, Thiele J and Vardiman JW. WHO classification of tumours of haematopoietic and lymphoid tissues. 4th ed. Lyon, France: International Agency for Research on Cancer; 2008. pp. 289.
45. Gaulard P, Jaffe ES, Krenacs L, Macon WR. Hepatosplenic T-cell lymphoma. In: Swerdlow SH, Campo E, Harris NL, Jaffe ES, Pileri SA, Stein H, Thiele J and Vardiman JW. WHO classification of tumours of haematopoietic and lymphoid tissues. 4th ed. Lyon, France: International Agency for Research on Cancer; 2008. pp. 292.
46. Jaffe ES, Gaulard P, Rafkiaer E, Cerroni L, Meiher CJLM. Subcutaneous panniculitis-like T-cell lymphoma. In: Swerdlow SH, Campo E, Harris NL, Jaffe ES, Pileri SA, Stein H, Thiele J and Vardiman JW. WHO classification of tumours of haematopoietic and lymphoid tissues. 4th ed. Lyon, France: International Agency for Research on Cancer; 2008. pp. 294.
47. Rafkiaer E, Cerroni L, Sander CA, Smoller BR, Willemze R. Mycosis fungoides. In: Swerdlow SH, Campo E, Harris NL, Jaffe ES, Pileri SA, Stein H, Thiele J and Vardiman JW. WHO classification of tumours of haematopoietic and lymphoid tissues. 4th ed. Lyon, France: International Agency for Research on Cancer; 2008. pp. 296.
48. Ralfkiaer E, Willemze R, Whittaker SJ. Sezary syndrome. In: Swerdlow SH, Campo E, Harris NL, Jaffe ES, Pileri SA, Stein H, Thiele J and Vardiman JW. WHO classification of tumours of haematopoietic and lymphoid tissues. 4th ed. Lyon, France: International Agency for Research on Cancer; 2008. pp. 299.
49. Ralfkiaer E, Willemze R, Pauli M, Kadin ME. Primary cutaneous CD30-positive T-cell lymphoproliferative disorders. In: Swerdlow SH, Campo E, Harris NL, Jaffe ES, Pileri SA, Stein H, Thiele J and Vardiman JW. WHO classification of tumours of haematopoietic and lymphoid tissues. 4th ed. Lyon, France: International Agency for Research on Cancer; 2008. pp. 300.
50. Gaulard P, Berti E, Willemze R, Jaffe ES. Primary cutaneous peripheral T-cell lymphoma, rare subtype. In: Swerdlow SH, Campo E, Harris NL, Jaffe ES, Pileri SA, Stein H, Thiele J and Vardiman JW. WHO classification of tumours of haematopoietic and lymphoid tissues. 4th ed. Lyon, France: International Agency for Research on Cancer; 2008. pp. 302.
51. Pilrei SA, Weisenburger DD, Sng I, Jaffe ES. Periperal T-cell lymphoma, not otherwise specified. In: Swerdlow SH, Campo E, Harris NL, Jaffe ES, Pileri SA, Stein H, Thiele J and Vardiman JW. WHO classification of tumours of haematopoietic and lymphoid tissues. 4th ed. Lyon, France: International Agency for Research on Cancer; 2008. pp. 306.
52. Went P, Agostinelli C, Gallamini A, Piccaluga PP, Ascani S, Sabattini E, et al. Marker expression in peripheral T-cell lymphoma: a proposed clinical-pathologic prognostic score. J Clin Oncol. 2006;24(16):2472–9.
53. Dogan A, Gaulard P, Jaffe ES, Ralfkiaer E, Muller-Hermelink HK. Angioimmunoblastic T-cell lymphoma. In: Swerdlow SH, Campo E, Harris NL, Jaffe ES, Pileri SA, Stein H, Thiele J and Vardiman JW. WHO classification of tumours of haematopoietic and lymphoid tissues. 4th ed. Lyon, France: International Agency for Research on Cancer; 2008. pp. 309.
54. Delsol G, Falini B, Muller-Hermelink HK, Campo E, Jaffe ES, Gsacoyne RD, et al. Anaplastic large cell lymphoma (ALCL), ALK-positive. In: Swerdlow SH, Campo E, Harris NL, Jaffe ES, Pileri SA, Stein H, Thiele J and Vardiman JW. WHO classification of tumours of haematopoietic and lymphoid tissues. 4th ed. Lyon, France: International Agency for Research on Cancer; 2008. pp. 312.
55. Mason DY, Harris NL, Delsol G, Stein H, Campo E, Kinney MC, et al. Anaplastic large cell lymphoma (ALCL), ALK-negative. In: Swerdlow SH, Campo E, Harris NL, Jaffe ES, Pileri SA, Stein H, Thiele J and Vardiman JW. WHO classification of tumours of haematopoietic and lymphoid tissues. 4th ed. Lyon, France: International Agency for Research on Cancer; 2008. pp. 317.
56. Poppema S, Delsol G, Pileri SA, Stein H, Swerdlow SH, Warnke RA, et al. Nodular lymphocyte predominant Hodgkin lymphoma. In: Swerdlow SH, Campo E, Harris NL, Jaffe ES, Pileri SA, Stein H, Thiele J and Vardiman JW. WHO classification of tumours of haematopoietic and lymphoid tissues. 4th ed. Lyon, France: International Agency for Research on Cancer; 2008. pp. 323.
57. Stein H, Delsol G, Pileri SA, Weiss LM, Poppema S, Jaffe ES. Classical Hodgkin lymphoma. In: Swerdlow SH, Campo E, Harris NL, Jaffe ES, Pileri SA, Stein H, Thiele J and Vardiman JW. WHO classification of tumours of haematopoietic and lymphoid tissues. 4th ed. Lyon, France: International Agency for Research on Cancer; 2008. pp. 326.
58. Van Krieken JH, Onciu M, Elenitoba-Johnson KSJ, Jaffe ES. Immunodeficiency-associated lymphoproliferative disorders. In: Swerdlow SH, Campo E, Harris NL, Jaffe ES, Pileri SA, Stein H, Thiele J and Vardiman JW. WHO classification of tumours of haematopoietic and lymphoid tissues. 4th ed. Lyon, France: International Agency for Research on Cancer; 2008. pp. 336.
59. Gaulard P, Swerdlow SH, Harris NL, Jaffe ES, Sundstrom C. Other iatrogenic immunodeficiency-associated lymphoproliferative disorders. In: Swerdlow SH, Campo E, Harris NL, Jaffe ES, Pileri SA, Stein H, Thiele J and Vardiman JW. WHO classification of tumours of haematopoietic and lymphoid tissues. 4th ed. Lyon, France: International Agency for Research on Cancer; 2008. pp. 350.
60. Raphael M, Said J, Borisch CE, Harris NL. Lymphomas associated with HIV infection. In: Swerdlow SH, Campo E, Harris NL, Jaffe ES, Pileri SA, Stein H, Thiele J and Vardiman JW. WHO classification of tumours of haematopoietic and lymphoid tissues. 4th ed. Lyon, France: International Agency for Research on Cancer; 2008. pp. 340.

61. Swerdlow SH, Webber SA, Chadburn A, Ferry JA. Post-transplant lymphoproliferative disorders. In: Swerdlow SH, Campo E, Harris NL, Jaffe ES, Pileri SA, Stein H, Thiele J and Vardiman JW. WHO classification of tumours of haematopoietic and lymphoid tissues. 4th ed. Lyon, France: International Agency for Research on Cancer; 2008. pp. 343.
62. Grogan TM, Pileri SA, Chan JKC, Weiss LM, Fletcher CDM. Histiocytic sarcoma. In: Swerdlow SH, Campo E, Harris NL, Jaffe ES, Pileri SA, Stein H, Thiele J and Vardiman JW. WHO classification of tumours of haematopoietic and lymphoid tissues. 4th ed. Lyon, France: International Agency for Research on Cancer; 2008. pp. 356.
63. Jaffe R, Weiss LM, Facchetti F. Tumor derived from Langerhans cells. In: Swerdlow SH, Campo E, Harris NL, Jaffe ES, Pileri SA, Stein H, Thiele J and Vardiman JW. WHO classification of tumours of haematopoietic and lymphoid tissues. 4th ed. Lyon, France: International Agency for Research on Cancer; 2008. pp. 358.
64. Weiss LM, Grogan TM, Chan JKC. Interdigitating dendritic cell sarcoma. In: Swerdlow SH, Campo E, Harris NL, Jaffe ES, Pileri SA, Stein H, Thiele J and Vardiman JW. WHO classification of tumours of haematopoietic and lymphoid tissues. 4th ed. Lyon, France: International Agency for Research on Cancer; 2008. pp. 361.
65. Chan JKC, Pileri SA, Delsol G, Fletcher CDM, Weiss LM, Grogan TM. Follicular dendritic cell sarcoma. In: Swerdlow SH, Campo E, Harris NL, Jaffe ES, Pileri SA, Stein H, Thiele J and Vardiman JW. WHO classification of tumours of haematopoietic and lymphoid tissues. 4th ed. Lyon, France: International Agency for Research on Cancer; 2008. pp. 363.
66. Weiss LM, Chan JKC, Fletcher CDM. Other rare dendritic cell sarcoma. In: Swerdlow SH, Campo E, Harris NL, Jaffe ES, Pileri SA, Stein H, Thiele J and Vardiman JW. WHO classification of tumours of haematopoietic and lymphoid tissues. 4th ed. Lyon, France: International Agency for Research on Cancer; 2008. pp. 365.
67. Jaffe R, Burgdorf W, Fletcher CDM. Disseminated juvenile xanthogranuloma. In: Swerdlow SH, Campo E, Harris NL, Jaffe ES, Pileri SA, Stein H, Thiele J and Vardiman JW. WHO classification of tumours of haematopoietic and lymphoid tissues. 4th ed. Lyon, France: International Agency for Research on Cancer; 2008. pp. 366.

Chapter 28
Bone Marrow

R. Patrick Dorion and Xiaohong (Mary) Zhang

Abstract This chapter provides an overview of immunohistochemical markers used frequently in assessing bone marrow diseases. These disease entities include lymphoid and myeloid leukemias, both acute and chronic, lymphoproliferative disorders, T and B cell neoplasms/lymphomas, myeloproliferative neoplasms, myelodysplastic syndromes, mast cell disease, plasma cell dyscrasias, and metastatic tumors to the bone marrow.

There is quite a bit of overlap between the markers used in the bone marrow workup for lymphoid diseases and lymphoma (Chap. 27), thus a review of that chapter might be helpful in the workup of lymphoproliferative disorders.

Also the marrow can be the site for metastatic tumors. The workup of metastatic disease to the marrow is the same as in any other site (Chap. 7) with the exception of markers that are rendered useless by the decalcification process.

Keywords Bone marrow • T and B cells • Blast • Acute lymphoblastic leukemia • Acute myelogenous leukemia • Myeloproliferative neoplasms • Myelodysplastic syndromes • Lymphoma • Chronic

FREQUENTLY ASKED QUESTIONS

Bone Marrow

1. Markers for bone marrow biopsies (Figs. 28.1–28.5, Table 28.1) (pp. 494–495)
2. Markers for acute leukemia (Figs. 28.1, 28.2, 28.6–28.10, Table 28.2) (p. 495)
3. Markers for myelodysplastic syndrome (Table 28.3) (p. 495)
4. Markers for myeloproliferative disorders (Table 28.4) (p. 496)
5. Markers for plasma cell disorders (Figs. 28.11–28.13, Table 28.5) (p. 496)

Markers for mature B and T cell neoplasms – please see Chap. 27

6. Markers for benign from malignant lymphoid aggregates in marrow biopsies (Fig. 28.14, Table 28.6) (p. 497)
7. Markers for mast cell disease (Table 28.7) (p. 497)

Markers for hairy cell leukemia and chronic lymphocytic leukemia – please see Chap. 27

8. Markers for metastatic tumors similar to workup of unknown primary elsewhere (Table 28.8) (p. 497)

R.P. Dorion (✉)
Department of Pathology and Laboratory Medicine, Geisinger Medical Center, 100 N. Academy Avenue, Danville, PA 17822, USA
e-mail: pdorion@geisinger.edu

F. Lin and J. Prichard (eds.), *Handbook of Practical Immunohistochemistry: Frequently Asked Questions*, DOI 10.1007/978-1-4419-8062-5_28, © Springer Science+Business Media, LLC 2011

Table 28.1 Markers for frequently used in bone marrows biopsies

Antibodies		Localization
CD3	Good Pan T cell marker	C and M
CD20	Good Pan B cell marker might become negative after rituximab therapy	C and M
CD15	Positive in Reed Sternberg cells and mature myeloid cells	C and M
CD30	Positive in Reed Sternberg cells. Anaplastic large cell lymphoma (Ki 1 Lymphoma)	M (Fig. 28.3)
CD5	T cell marker. Positive in CLL and some mature B cell lymphomas	M
CD10	Positive in B cells, follicular center cells and blasts in B cell ALL	M
CD34	Positive in primitive blasts both myeloid and lymphoid negative in (M3) acute promyelocytic leukemia	C and M
CD79a	B cell marker. Positive in plasma cells	M
CD117	aka C-kit positive in mast cells	C and M
CD138	Positive in plasma cells	M
CD38	Positive in plasma cells	M
CD123	Positive in plasmacytoid dendritic cells and myeloproliferative neoplasms	M
MPO	Positive in myeloid neoplasms with some differentiation	C
PAX5	Positive in B cells	N
Cyclin D1	Positive in B cells. aka BCL-1 indicates t(11;14) Positive in mantle cell lymphoma	N (Fig. 28.4)
Lysozyme	Useful in monocytoid and myeloid differentiation	C
Kappa CISH	Useful in determining clonality in B cells and plasma cells	C
Lambda CISH	Useful in determining clonality in B cells and plasma cells	C
CD11b	Positive in hairy cell leukemia (HCL), marginal zone lymphomas (MZL) and in monocytes, granulocytes, and histiocytes	M
CD11c	Positive in HCL and MZL	M
CD23	Marker for B cells, usually mature B cells and follicular lymphoma	M
CD45	Positive in leukocytes and lymphomas aka leukocyte common antigen	C and M
CD68 (KP1)	Strongly expressed in monocytes and macrophages. Also stains dendritic cells, neutrophils, basophils, mast cells, and activated T cells. Weak in some B cells and B cell ALL	C (granular)
CD103	Positive in HCL	C
Ki67 (MIB)	Positive in proliferating cells. Not too useful in bone marrows since the marrow is normally an active proliferative site. Some tumors like CLL have a low proliferative index (lower than a normal marrow)	N
TDT	Positive in primitive lymphoid and myeloid blasts. Negative in Burkitt's lymphoma	N
CD99	Positive in lymphoblastic lymphoma and Ewing's sarcoma	C and M
Glycophorin A	Positive in erythroid precursors	C
Hemoglobin A	Positive in erythroid precursors	C
Factor VIII, related antigen (von Willebrand factor)	Positive in megakaryocytes, platelets and endothelial cells	C
CD61	Positive in megakaryocytes	C
CD31 (PECAM)	Positive in endothelial cells megakaryocytes, monocytes, and granulocytes	C and M
Mast cell tryptase	Stains mast cells both benign and malignant	C
Parvovirus B19	Positive in parvovirus infected cells	N
CD2	T cell marker that is also positive in neoplastic mast cells	M (Fig. 28.5)
CD25	Marker for activated T and B cells. Positive in hairy cell leukemia and neoplastic mast cells	C and M
CD117 (C-kit)	Positive in early myeloid cells Acute megakaryoblastic leukemia (M7), mast cells, and neoplastic plasma cells, negative in acute erythroid leukemia (M6)	C

Fixation: All bone marrow biopsies should be fixed prior to decalcifying and processing. 10% neutral-buffered formalin is adequate for most biopsies. We currently use B Plus, a commercial proprietary formulation with no mercury

Decalcification: All bone marrow biopsies require some degree of decalcification before sectioning. The procedure routinely uses harsh chemicals, such as hydrochloric acid. This affects some of the epitopes. The time the biopsy spends in the decalcifying solution is crucial to the quality of the IHC stains. Some of the antigens are able to be retrieved after the decalcification procedure. In some cases, such as Her-2/neu (when trying to determine the origin of a metastatic tumor), it is not possible to retrieve the antigen

Clot sections when available and of good quality (particles present, not just red cells) are quite helpful since the marrow particles are not subjected to decalcification

Miscellaneous notes on markers for bone marrow biopsies

MPO myeloperoxidase is positive in acute myelogenous leukemias (M1, M2, M3, and M4) and variable staining in monocytic and monoblastic leukemias. If there is only partial involvement with leukemia in the marrow biopsy, caution should be used in interpreting since normal residual myeloblasts will be MPO positive (Fig. 28.1)

(continued)

Table 28.1 (continued)

HLA-DR is negative in acute promyelocytic leukemias (APL-M3)

CD117 can be used in biopsies with partial leukemic involvement since the positivity is stronger in the leukemic cells. MPO and CD117 do not always correlate well

Lysozyme and KP1 are present in normal neutrophils

CD34 is positive in acute myelogenous leukemias, however, it may not correlate well with flow cytometry since flow cytometry is evaluating surface antigenic activity and IHC picks up both surface and cytoplasmic activity

CD34 is positive in acute megakaryocytic leukemia (M7)

CD45ra is positive in acute myelogenous leukemia, however, it might not correlate well with flow cytometry as it is a surface marker (Fig. 28.2)

HgbA (aka CD235a) Hemoglobin A and glycophorin A are positive in acute erythroid leukemia (M6)

TDT is mostly negative in acute myelogenous leukemia. Can be positive in biphenotypic leukemias or in some subtypes such as when t(8;21) is present

Vimentin is positive in many acute myelogenous leukemias but is negative in acute megakaryocytic leukemias (M7)

Ki67 (aka MIB1) used in determining the proliferative index. In the marrow it is normally high. In acute myelogenous leukemias it is higher. The proliferative index in AML is higher than in ALL

Table 28.2 Markers for acute leukemia

Antibodies	Myeloid	Lymphoid	Localization
MPO	+	–	C (Fig. 28.1)
CD34	+	+ (primitive marker)	M or cytoplasmic vacuoles
CD117	+	–	M
F8a (Factor VIII)	+ (in megakaryocytic leukemia)	–	C and M
PAX5	–	+ (in B cell ALL)	N (Fig. 28.6)
CD10	–	+ (– in T cell ALL)	M (Fig. 28.7)
CD79a	+ (in megakaryocytes and t(8;21) AML)	+ (in B cells)	C and M (Fig. 28.8)
CD20	–	+	M (Fig. 28.9)
CD3	–	+ (in T cells)	M
CD45 (LCA)	+	+	M (Fig. 28.2)
(Other stains with low specificity)CD68	+ (in monocytes)	Weak + in 50% B cell ALL and mature B cell disorders	C
Lysozyme	+	–	C
CD15	+ (in matured myeloid cells)	–	C (Fig. 28.10)
CD123	+ (MPD as well)	–	C and M
CD99	+ (in some AML's)	+ (in some ALL's and Ewing's)	M
CD31	Nonspecific, + in megakaryocytes	–	M, C in megakaryocytes
CD61	+ In megakaryocytes	–	C and M

C cytoplasmic, *M* membrane, *N* nuclear

Note: The diagnosis of acute leukemia subtypes in bone marrow examinations is best made with flow cytometry. In cases of a "dry tap," peripheral blood can be submitted for flow cytometry if blasts are present. There are instances in which a marrow aspirate is not available, thus IHC in bone marrow biopsies can be helpful such as when there is a "dry tap," cluster or uneven distribution of immature cells, when flow cytometry does not pick up the abnormal population of cells and after chemotherapy when only a small population of malignant or early precursors are present. Also keep in mind that fixation and decalcification in bone marrow biopsies play a major role in how the special stains perform

Table 28.3 Markers for myelodysplastic syndrome (MDS)

Antibodies		Localization
CD34	Highlights blasts	M or cytoplasmic vacuoles
CD117	Highlights blasts	M
CD61 (42b)	+ In megakaryocytes and megakaryoblasts	C and M
Mast cell tryptase	+ In mast cells	C
Others:MPO	Not too useful since all myeloid cells will stain, useful in differentiating myeloid from lymphoid lines	C
Parvo B19	Useful in the differential diagnosis of erythrocytopenia with abnormal nucleated RBCs	N
HgbA	Useful in staining erythroblasts and nucleated RBCs	C

C cytoplasmic, *M* membrane, *N* nuclear

Note: IHC can be useful in determining the distribution of blasts and immature cells in MDS or myeloproliferative neoplasms (MPN)

"Normal" blasts are usually found around the bony trabecula. They are abnormal, distributed if found in the marrow cavity

Table 28.4 Markers for myeloproliferative neoplasms

Antibodies		Localization
CD34	Highlights blasts	M or cytoplasmic vacuoles
MPO	Highlights blasts	C
CD61	Highlights megakaryocytes and megakaryocyte precursors (e.g., essential thrombocytopenia, myelofibrosis)	C and M
HgbA	Highlights erythroid precursors	C
Others:CD33	Highlights myeloid cells	C and M
Mast cell tryptase	Useful in fibrotic marrows to exclude mastocytosis	C
CD117	Useful in mastocytosis	M
TDT	Picks up early lymphoid neoplasms	N
CD3	Picks up T cells	M
CD20	Picks up B cells	M
PAX5	Picks up B cells	N
Jak2	Molecular test important in polycythemia vera and essential thrombocythemia not available as a stain	N/A

C cytoplasmic, *M* membrane, *N* nuclear

Note: Myeloproliferative neoplasms (MPN) can have many overlapping features. At one point in their life cycle they all can have a similar morphologic appearance. Cytogenetic and molecular marker studies are a crucial component in the diagnosis of MPN (e.g., JAK2, Philadelphia Chromosome). IHC can be useful but they are not as helpful as in other entities. Morphology is still the best method.

Polycythemia vera (PV):

CD34 – Useful in determining the blast population in the background

MPO – Highlights myeloid precursors

Chronic myelogenous leukemia (CML):

CD34 – Highlights early myeloid precursors

MPO – Highlights myeloid precursors and mature granulocytes

Essential thrombocythemia (ET):

CD34 – Highlights megakaryocytes

CD99 – In conjunction with CD34 highlights megakaryocytes

CD61 – Stains megakaryocytes. Usually not needed since they are evident on H&E

Primary myelofibrosis, agnogenic myeloid metaplasia, idiopathic myelofibrosis:

Same markers as for ET

Chronic myelomonocytic leukemia (CMML):

CD68 (KP1) – Highlights monocytes and macrophages

CD123 – Highlights plasmacytoid monocytes

CD117 – Highlights blasts

CD34 – Highlights blasts

IHC does not have a major role in chronic neutrophilic leukemias, chronic eosinophilic leukemias, or paroxysmal nocturnal hemoglobinuria

Table 28.5 Markers for plasma cell disorders

Antibodies		Localization
CD138	+ In plasma cells, both benign and malignant	M (Fig. 28.11)
CD38	+ In plasma cells, both benign and malignant	N
Kappa CISH, lambda CISH	Both useful in determining clonality of plasma cells, Kappa and Lambda by IHC are not too useful due to background staining	C (Figs. 28.12 and 28.13)
CD45	+ In hematopoietic cells	M
CD56	Stains plasma cells, mostly in multiple myeloma, MGUS is weakly +, leukemic myelomas loose CD56	M
CD20	+ In B cells including plasma cells	M
Others:Ki67	Normal bone marrow has a high proliferative index 60–90%, tumors of plasma cells usually have a lower proliferative index	N
EBV	Useful in EBV-associated neoplasms	N
IgM, IgG, IgA, IgD, IgE	Some advocate these stains, the preferable method is immunofixation of serum to determine the type of clonal paraprotein present	–
PAX5	Negative in plasma cell malignancies	N
CD117	Marker for neoplastic and atypical plasma cells, it is negative in IgM myeloma	M

C cytoplasmic, *M* membrane, *N* nuclear

Table 28.6 Markers for differentiating benign from malignant lymphoid aggregates in bone marrow biopsies

Antibodies	Localization	
CD3	M	T cell marker
CD20	M	B cell marker
CD10	M	B cell marker – positive follicular lymphomas
CD79a	M	B cell marker
Kappa CISH	C	Plus H&E morphology
Lambda CISH	C	Plus H&E morphology
CD5	M	T cell marker. Useful in chronic lymphocytic leukemia where it is positive
Bcl-2	N and M	Positive in 90% of follicular lymphomas, lack of staining with BCL-2 suggests a benign aggregate (Fig. 28.14)

C cytoplasmic, *M* membrane, *N* nuclear

Note: Elderly females frequently have lymphoid aggregates of no consequence in the bone marrow

Often in bone marrow biopsies the sample is limited so there may not be enough tissue to run a panel. Shallow sections (do not cut into the block) are needed. CD3 and CD20 are recommended to start with

Malignant: Usually paratrabecular except CLL uniform pattern. Close to surface of bone, predominance of B or T cells

Benign: Central or perivascular, may have partial germinal centers. Deep in marrow mixed T and B cell infiltrate

Table 28.7 Markers for mast cell disease

Antibody	Localization	
CD117	M	Also known as C-kit mutated in systemic mastocytosis
Mast cell tryptase	C	+ In mast cells
CD5	C and M	Negative neoplastic mast cells
CD2	M	T cell marker that stains neoplastic mast cells
CD25	C and M	Positive in Hairy cell leukemia but also a good marker for neoplastic mast cells

C cytoplasmic, *M* membrane, *N* nuclear

Notes:

1. Megakaryoblastic leukemias stain positive for CD117; will not differentiate between benign and malignant mast cells, need morphologic correlation

2. Mast cell disease in the marrow can present as "myelofibrosis." Mast cell tryptase and CD117 can be used to determine whether it is myelofibrosis or mast cell disease presenting as a fibrotic marrow

3. An increase in marrow mast cells should be viewed with caution since multiple myeloma, lymphoproliferative disorders, and reactive pictures can also have an increase in mast cells

Table 28.8 Markers for metastatic tumors similar to workup of tumors of unknown primary elsewhere

Antibodies	Literature
CK A1, A3	Stains cytokeratin
CK7/CK20	See chart below
S100	Useful in tumors with neural origin or differentiation
SMA	Stains smooth muscle
MelanA	Useful in melanoma
HMB45	Useful in melanoma
Vimentin	Positive in sarcomas, AML
CK7/CK20 positive	Transitional cell, pancreatic and ovarian mucinous carcinomas
CK7 positive/CK20 negative	Breast, lung (nonsmall cell), ovarian serous, endometrial carcinomas, and mesothelioma (epithelial) and thymoma
CK7 negative/CK20 positive	Colorectal carcinoma
CK7/CK20 negative	Hepatocellular, renal cell, prostatic adenocarcinoma, squamous cell, and small cell neuroendocrine (NE) carcinomas

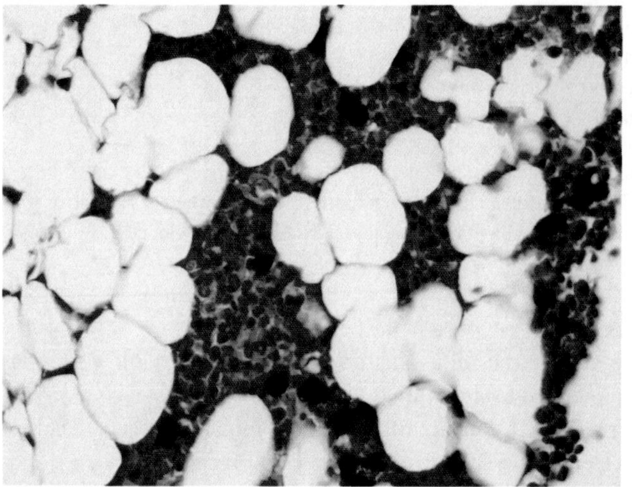

Fig. 28.1 MPO – myeloperoxidase in normal marrow

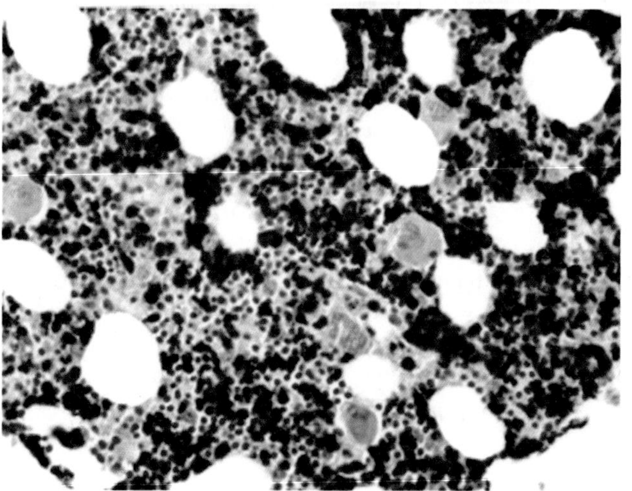

Fig. 28.2 CD45rb (LCA) – lymphoproliferative disorder in marrow

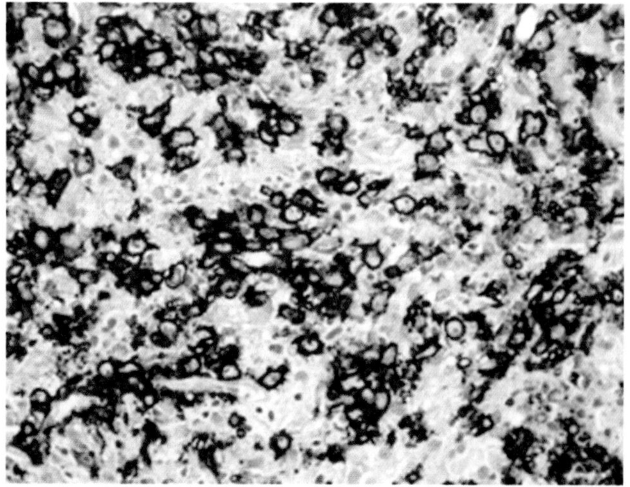

Fig. 28.3 CD30 – anaplastic lymphoma in marrow

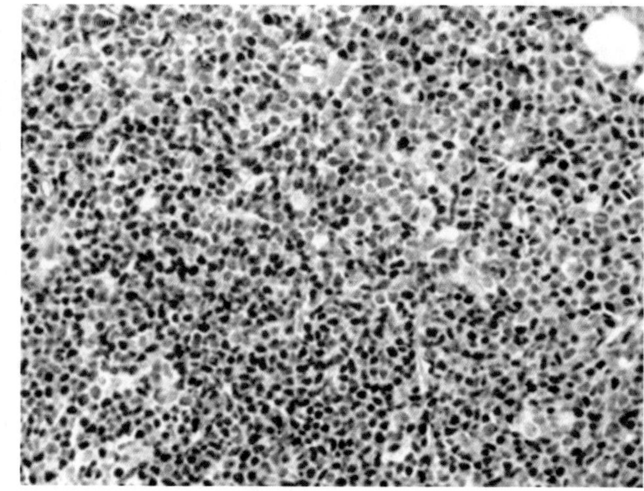

Fig. 28.4 Cyclin D1 – mantle cell lymphoma in marrow

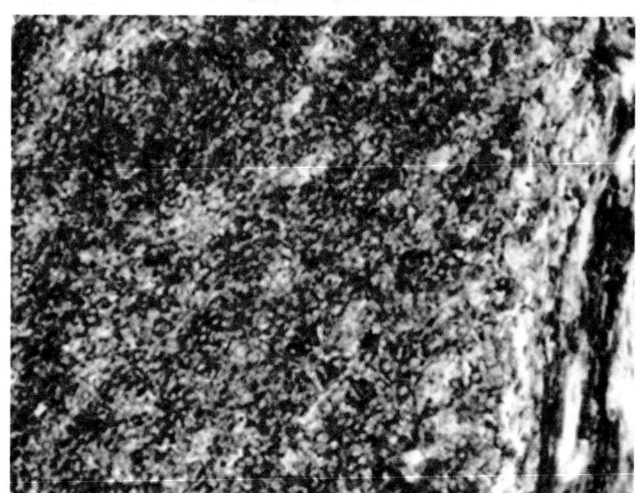

Fig. 28.5 CD2 – highlights T cells in marrow

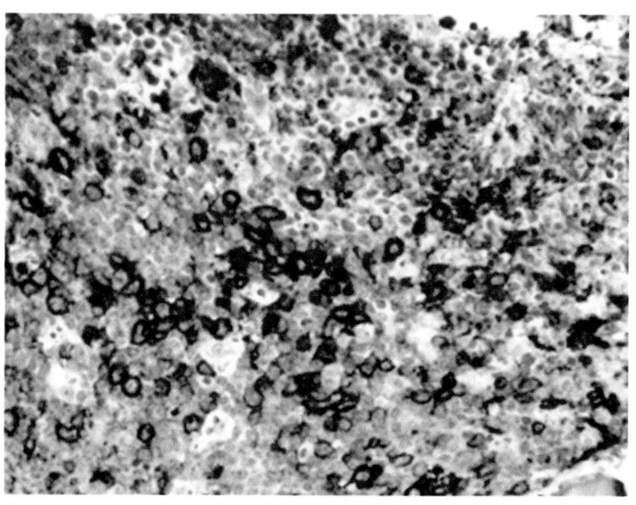

Fig. 28.6 PAX5 – B cell lymphoma in marrow

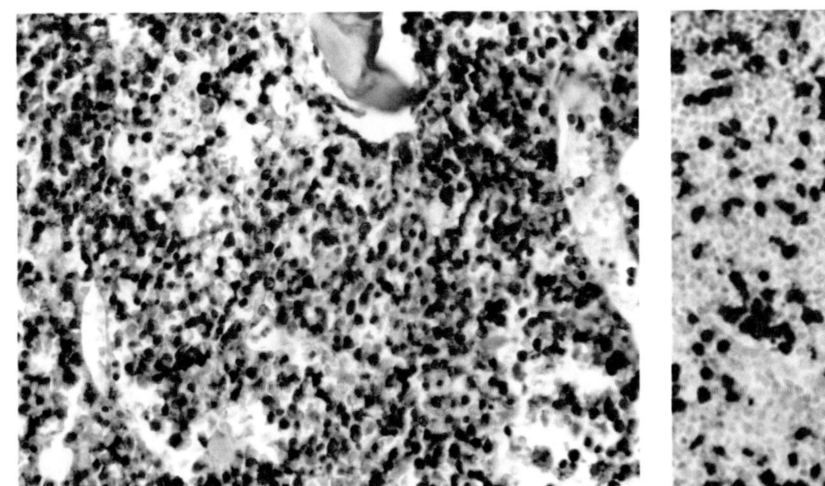

Fig. 28.7 CD10 – acute lymphoblastic leukemia

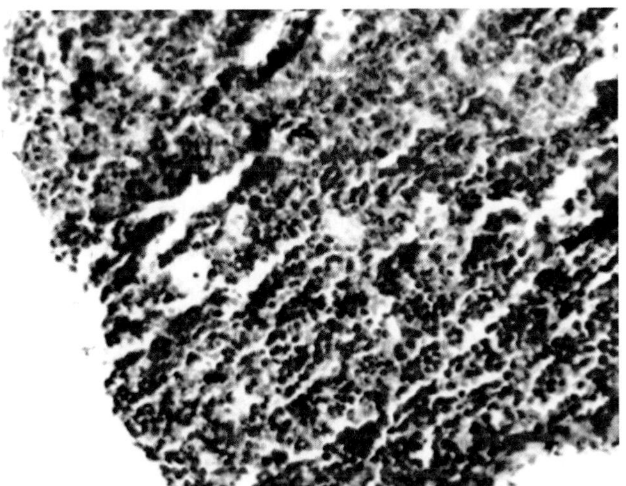

Fig. 28.8 CD79a – B cell lymphoma in marrow

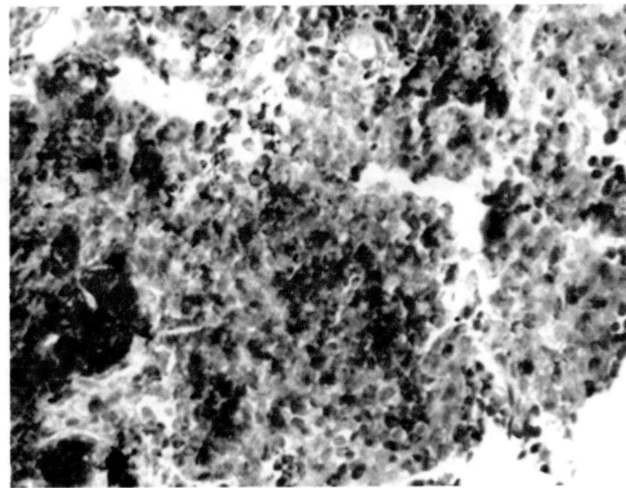

Fig. 28.9 CD20 – large B cell lymphoma in marrow

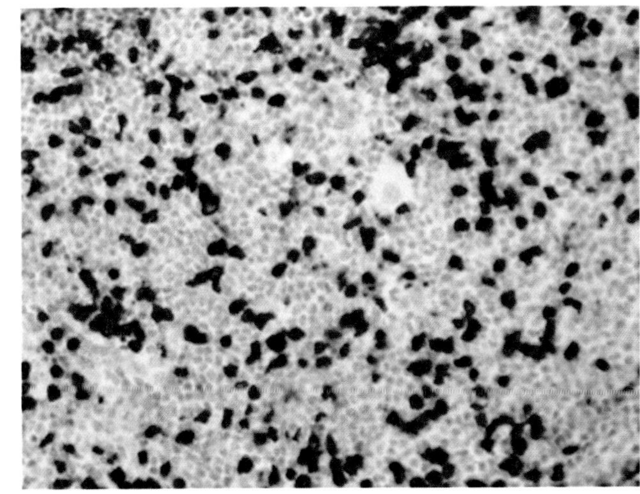

Fig. 28.10 CD15 – granulocytes in marrow

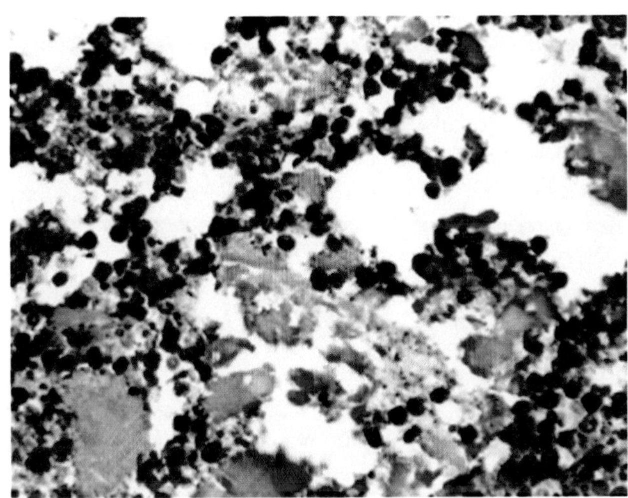

Fig. 28.11 CD138 – plasma cells in bone marrow

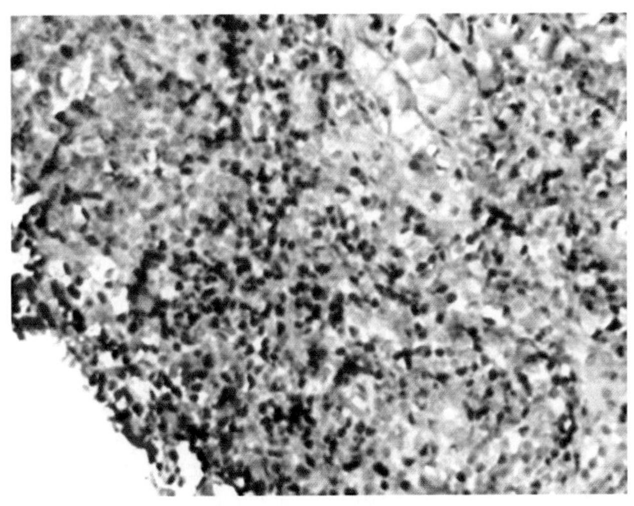

Fig. 28.12 Kappa CISH – kappa-restricted plasma cells in marrow

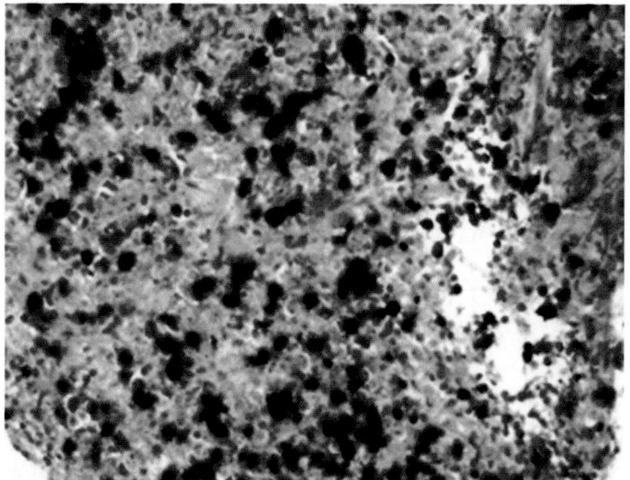

Fig. 28.13 Lambda CISH – lambda-restricted plasma cells in marrow

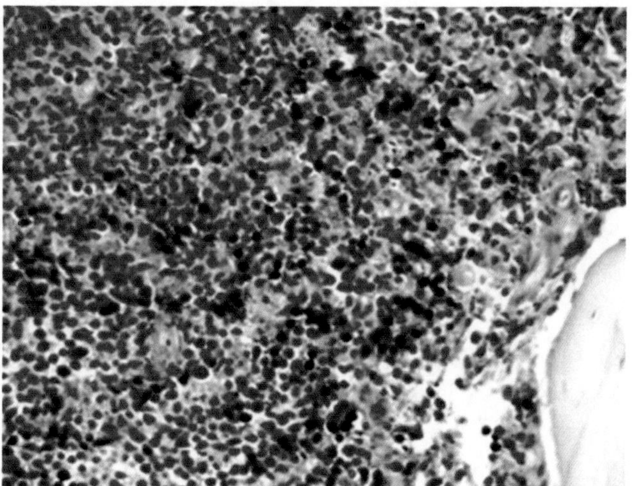

Fig. 28.14 Bcl-2 – follicular lymphoma in marrow

Note for All Tables

Note: "+" – usually greater than 70% of cases are positive; "–" – less than 5% of cases are positive; "+ or –" – usually more than 50% of cases are positive; "– or +" – less than 50% of cases are positive.

References

1. Arber DA, Jenkins KA. Paraffin section immunophenotyping of acute leukemias in bone marrow specimens. Am J Clin Pathol. 1996;106(4):462–8.
2. Beck RC, Tubbs RR, Hussein M, Pettay J, Hsi ED. Automated colorimetric in situ hybridization (CISH) detection of immunoglobulin (Ig) light chain mRNA expression in plasma cell (PC) dyscrasias and non-Hodgkin lymphoma. Diagn Mol Pathol. 2003;12(1):14–20.
3. Bene MC. Immunophenotyping of acute leukaemias. Immunol Lett. 2005;98(1):9–21.
4. Ben-Ezra JM, King BE, Harris AC, Todd WM, Kornstein MJ. Staining for Bcl-2 protein helps to distinguish benign from malignant lymphoid aggregates in bone marrow biopsies. Mod Pathol. 1994;7(5):560–4.
5. Dunphy CH, O'Malley DP, Perkins SL, Chang CC. Analysis of immunohistochemical markers in bone marrow sections to evaluate for myelodysplastic syndromes and acute myeloid leukemias. Appl Immunohistochem Mol Morphol. 2007;15(2):154–9.
6. Hans CP, Finn WG, Singleton TP, Schnitzer B, Ross CW. Usefulness of anti-CD117 in the flow cytometric analysis of acute leukemia. Am J Clin Pathol. 2002;117(2):301–5.
7. Horny HP, Campbell M, Steinke B, Kaiserling E. Acute myeloid leukemia: immunohistologic findings in paraffin-embedded bone marrow biopsy specimens. Hum Pathol. 1990;21(6):648–55.
8. Horny HP, Sotlar K, Valent P. Diagnostic value of histology and immunohistochemistry in myelodysplastic syndromes. Leuk Res. 2007;31(12):1609–16.
9. Krishnan C, George TI, Arber DA. Bone marrow metastases: a survey of nonhematologic metastases with immunohistochemical study of metastatic carcinomas. Appl Immunohistochem Mol Morphol. 2007;15(1):1–7.
10. Krober SM, Greschniok A, Kaiserling E, Horny HP. Acute lymphoblastic leukaemia: correlation between morphological/immunohistochemical and molecular biological findings in bone marrow biopsy specimens. Mol Pathol. 2000;53(2):83–7.
11. Kubic VL, Brunning RD. Immunohistochemical evaluation of neoplasms in bone marrow biopsies using monoclonal antibodies reactive in paraffin-embedded tissue. Mod Pathol. 1989;2(6):618–29.
12. Loyson SA, Rademakers LH, Joling P, Vroom TM, van den Tweel JG. Immunohistochemical analysis of decalcified paraffin-embedded human bone marrow biopsies with emphasis on MHC class I and CD34 expression. Histopathology. 1997;31(5):412–9.
13. Ngo N, Lampert IA, Naresh KN. Bone marrow trephine findings in acute myeloid leukaemia with multilineage dysplasia. Br J Haematol. 2008;140(3):279–86.
14. Pileri SA, Ascani S, Milani M, et al. Acute leukaemia immunophenotyping in bone-marrow routine sections. Br J Haematol. 1999;105(2):394–401.
15. Swerdlow H, Campo E, Harris N, et al. WHO classification of tumours of haematopoietic and lymphoid tissues. 4th ed. Lyon, France: International Agency for Research on Cancer; 2008. p. 439. Accessed 10/1/2009.
16. Takahashi Y, Murai C, Shibata S, et al. Human parvovirus B19 as a causative agent for rheumatoid arthritis. Proc Natl Acad Sci USA. 1998;95(14):8227–32.
17. Thiele J, Zirbes TK, Kvasnicka HM, Fischer R. Focal lymphoid aggregates (nodules) in bone marrow biopsies: differentiation between benign hyperplasia and malignant lymphoma – a practical guideline. J Clin Pathol. 1999;52(4):294–300.
18. Torlakovic EE, Naresh KN, Brunning RD. Bone marrow IHC. Chicago, IL: American Society for Clinical Pathology Press; 2009. p. 274. Accessed 10/26/2009.
19. Toth B, Wehrmann M, Kaiserling E, Horny HP. Immunophenotyping of acute lymphoblastic leukaemia in routinely processed bone marrow biopsy specimens. J Clin Pathol. 1999;52(9):688–92.
20. West KP, Warford A, Fray L, Allen M, Campbell AC, Lauder I. The demonstration of B-cell, T-cell and myeloid antigens in paraffin sections. J Pathol. 1986;150(2):89–101.

Chapter 29
Infectious Diseases

Dirk M. Elston, Lawrence E. Gibson, and Heinz Kutzner

Abstract Detection and identification of infectious microorganisms involve the use of conventional immunohistochemistry in addition to many other techniques, including culture, serology, histochemistry, in situ hybridization, polymerase chain reaction, and direct fluorescence antibody assays. This chapter takes into consideration all of these techniques while answering questions about bacterial, mycobacterial viral, fungal, and protozoan testing. The best techniques and testing conditions are described for dozens of the most clinically relevant microorganisms. The role of immunohistochemistry versus alternative techniques is clearly presented. Photomicrographs present the characteristic feature of optimized staining techniques. Topics for each organism including the sensitivity and specificity of the tests, how fixation and retrieval affect the results, when protease should be considered in an assay, and how these tests could be incorporated into your clinical practice are discussed.

Keywords Bacteria • *Bacillus anthracis* • *Bartonella henselae* • *Brucella melitensis* • *Francisella tularensis* • *Helicobacter pylori* • Leptospirosis • Lyme disease • *Rickettsia rickettsii* • Rocky Mountain spotted fever • *Treponema pallidum* • *Yersinia pestis* • *Pseudomonas aeruginosa* • Mycobacteria • Bacille Calmette-Guerin (BCG) • *Mycobacterium avium* • Paratuberculosis • *Mycobacterium tuberculosis* • *Mycobacterium bovis* • Virus • Cytomegalovirus • Epstein–Barr virus • Hepatitis C virus • Human herpes virus type 6 • Human herpes virus type 8 • Human papillomavirus • Herpes simplex virus • Influenza A virus • Ljungan virus • Parvovirus B19 • Rabies • Small pox • Variola • Varicella-Zoster virus • Viral Hemorrhagic Fevers • West Nile virus • Fungus • Protozoan • *Aspergillus* • Blastomyces • *Coccidioides immitis* • *Cryptococcus neoformans* • *Histoplasma capsulatum* • *Pneumocystis carinii* • Leishmaniasis

D.M. Elston (✉)
Department of Dermatology and Pathology,
Geisinger Medical Center, 100 North Academy Avenue,
Danville, PA 17822, USA
e-mail: dmelston@geisinger.edu

FREQUENTLY ASKED QUESTIONS

29.1 What Tests Are Available to Detect Bacteria?

For most bacteria, isolation in culture remains the gold standard for diagnosis. Serologic studies, in situ hybridization (ISH), polymerase chain reaction (PCR), and direct fluorescent antibody (DFA) assay are available. Although immunohistochemistry (IHC) is commonly used in veterinary medicine, it has become standard only for the detection of *Treponema pallidum* (*T. pallidum*) in humans. It is also used in some laboratories for the detection of *Rickettsia* [1].

29.1.1 *Bacillus anthracis*

Colorimetric IHC assays using a multistep indirect immunoalkaline phosphatase method with anti-*B. anthracis* cell wall (EAII-6G6-2-3) and *anti-B. anthracis* capsule (FDF-1B9) monoclonal antibodies have been developed, but are not in widespread use [2]. PCR assays show considerable promise in this setting, but IHC has been used in clinical practice.

29.1.1.1 How Sensitive Are the Tests?

During the bioterrorism scare of 2001, 117 skin biopsy samples were tested by the Infectious Disease Pathology Activity (IDPA) of the Centers for Disease Control and Prevention

F. Lin and J. Prichard (eds.), *Handbook of Practical Immunohistochemistry: Frequently Asked Questions*,
DOI 10.1007/978-1-4419-8062-5_29, © Springer Science+Business Media LLC 2011

(CDC). Of these, eight were positive for *B. anthracis* by IHC [3]. One advantage is that IHC assays can demonstrate bacilli, bacillary fragments, or granular bacterial fragments in formalin-fixed tissues even after 10 days of antibiotic treatment [4].

29.1.1.2 How Specific Are the Tests?

Limited data are available.

29.1.1.3 What Can Affect the Test?

The type of specimen is critical. The diagnosis of cutaneous anthrax should be made with skin biopsies from both the center and periphery of the eschar. For inhalational anthrax, pleural effusion cell blocks, pleural biopsies, and mediastinal lymph nodes demonstrate the largest number of bacilli.

29.1.2 *Bartonella henselae*

As microbiologic detection of *B. henselae* is problematic and molecular testing is not widely available, IHC assays are promising.

29.1.2.1 How Sensitive Is the Test?

A study of 24 samples of cat scratch lymphadenitis and 14 control specimens compared IHC based on a monoclonal antibody (mAB) with silver staining, PCR detection, and serologic testing for *B. henselae*. Sensitivity was as follows: mAB 6 (25%) detected, Steiner silver stain 11 (46%), and PCR 9 (38%). Interestingly, only two cases (8%) were positive for all three studies [5].

29.1.2.2 How Specific Are the Tests?

Control tissue was consistently negative with both IHC and PCR, while sensitivity is low, specificity appears high.

29.1.2.3 Does Fixation Affect the Test?

Testing can be performed on formalin-fixed, paraffin-embedded tissue, but optimal retrieval methods remain to be defined.

29.1.3 *Brucella melitensis*

B. melitensis, a widespread zoonotic pathogen, is a significant cause of abortion in farm animals and a cause of human sepsis.

29.1.3.1 How Sensitive Are the Tests?

In a study of 110 naturally occurring aborted sheep fetuses, *B. melitensis* antigens were detected by IHC in 33 of 110 fetuses (30%). Breakdown by tissue included lung (22.7%), liver (19%), spleen (11.8%), and kidney (5.4%) [6].

29.1.3.2 How Specific Are the Tests?

Limited data are available.

29.1.4 *Francisella tularensis*

Both IHC and DFA have been used to demonstrate the bacteria in formalin-fixed tissues [7].

29.1.4.1 How Sensitive Are the Tests?

Limited data are available.

29.1.4.2 How Specific Are the Tests?

Limited data are available. MAb T14 has demonstrated no cross-reactivity with *Yersinia pestis*, *Y. pseudotuberculosis*, *Y. enterocolitica*, *V. cholera*, *E. coli*, *S. typhimurium*, *Fr. novicida*, *Br. melitensis*, *Br. abortus*, *Br. suis*, *Br. ovis*, or *Br. neotomae*. MAb FB11 has demonstrated no cross-reactivity with *Fr. novicida*, *Br. abortus*, *Br. suis*, *Br. melitensis*, *Br. ovis*, *Y. pestis*, *Y. enterocolitica*, *Y. pseudotuberculosis*, *E. coli*, or *V. cholerae*. These antibodies are largely used for enzyme immunoassay (EIA), immunofluorescence.

29.1.5 *Helicobacter pylori*

29.1.5.1 How Sensitive Are the Tests?

IHC has proved superior to routine histochemistry, but results have varied. In a study of 48 cases, *H. pylori* was demonstrated by both techniques in 27. In two cases, the immunostain could not demonstrate the bacteria but they were identified with a modified Giemsa stain. In five cases, the bacteria were identified by the immunostain but not with the modified Giemsa stain [8]. In another study, bacteria were detected in 66% of tissue sections stained with the antibody. This compared favorably to silver stains and PCR [9]. In other studies, PCR and ISH have proved superior [10].

29.1.5.2 How Specific Are the Tests?

Using culture as the gold standard, specificity was 90% and sensitivity was 83.8%, compared with 53.8 and 90%, respectively for modified Geimsa and 82.5 and 70%, respectively for a Warthin–Starry stain [11].

29.1.5.3 Does Fixation Affect the Test?

Depending upon the fixation method and the staining system employed, optimal incubation conditions may vary. Formalin-fixed paraffin-embedded tissue sections require high temperature antigen unmasking in 10 mM citrate buffer, at pH 6.0, although this may vary with antibody system.

29.1.6 Leptospirosis

29.1.6.1 How Sensitive Are the Tests?

Some data suggest that IHC does not enhance sensitivity compared to silver staining, but it improved the ease of diagnosis [12]. One study demonstrated 78% sensitivity [13].

29.1.6.2 How Specific Are the Tests?

Specificity appears as high as 100%.

29.1.6.3 Does Fixation Affect the Test?

Some antibody systems require sections to be treated with trypsin. Antigen retrieval may be performed on slides preheated to 37°C by microwaving for 1.5 min at 630 W followed by 5 min at 180 W in Tris (pH 10) buffer, although the product insert should be consulted for the antibody system used.

29.1.7 Lyme Disease

29.1.7.1 How Sensitive and Specific Are the Tests?

IHC has demonstrated sensitivity as high as 96% with specificity of 99.4%, compared to 45.5% sensitivity and 100% specificity for PCR run on the same tissue. Other authors have found a sensitivity of only 39% and suggested that because the density of *B. burgdorferi* in human tissue is very low, the method is not useful in a clinical setting [14].

29.1.7.2 Does Fixation Affect the Test?

Some antibody systems require trypsin.

29.1.8 Rickettsia rickettsii/Rocky Mountain Spotted Fever

29.1.8.1 How Sensitive Are the Tests?

In one study, both immunoperoxidase staining and immunofluorescence detected the organism in nine of ten specimens [15]. Antibodies are available to detect spotted fever group and typhus group organisms.

29.1.8.2 How Specific Are the Tests?

It may not be possible to distinguish between spotted fever group organisms.

29.1.8.3 Does Fixation Affect the Test?

Antigen retrieval varies by antibody system.

29.1.9 Treponema pallidum

29.1.9.1 How Sensitive Are the Tests?

In one study, IHC testing was positive in 17/35 cases, compared with 9/35 for Dieterle staining and 14/36 for PCR [16]. Other studies have shown from 71 to 91% sensitivity in patients with secondary compared with 41% using a silver stain [17, 18].

29.1.9.2 How Specific Are the Tests?

Specificity is higher than with silver staining, but more data are needed regarding cross reaction with other spirochetes.

29.1.9.3 Does Fixation Affect the Test?

The effect of fixation on IHC may be pH sensitive. Both IHC and PCR require neutrally buffered formalin. Acid destroys DNA and epitopes.

29.1.10 *Yersinia pestis*

Culture remains the gold standard. Identification of the bacilli in formalin-fixed tissues can be performed using IHC, DFA, and PCR assays [19].

29.1.10.1 How Sensitive and Specific Are the Tests?

Limited data are available.

29.1.10.2 Does Fixation Affect the Test?

Choice of fixation has not shown a significant effect on results to date.

29.1.11 *Pseudomonas aeruginosa*

Culture remains the gold standard. Identification of the bacilli in formalin-fixed tissues can be performed using IHC and PCR assays [20]. In addition to specific monoclonal antibody staining, the anti-BCG stain has been used.

29.1.11.1 How Sensitive and Specific Are the Tests?

Limited data are available.

29.1.11.2 Does Fixation Affect the Test?

Choice of fixation has not shown a significant effect on results to date.

29.1.12 How Should I Incorporate These Tests into My Practice?

IHC has become standard for the detection of *T. pallidum*. It still suffers from limited sensitivity, and silver stains should be performed if there is a high degree of suspicion and the immunostain is negative. IHC is being used in some laboratories for the detection of *Rickettsia*. Testing for anthrax and other bioterrorism agents is likely to be performed by the CDC. Silver staining remains the most sensitive test for *B. henselae*, but is the least specific. IHC staining suffers from low sensitivity, but is useful for the confirmation of the diagnosis because of its high specificity. PCR remains helpful as a second-line test for IHC negative cases. Although culture remains the gold standard for the detection of *B. melitensis*, IHC can be used to demonstrate the presence of *B. melitensis* antigens in tissue sections (Figs. 29.1–29.3, Table 29.1).

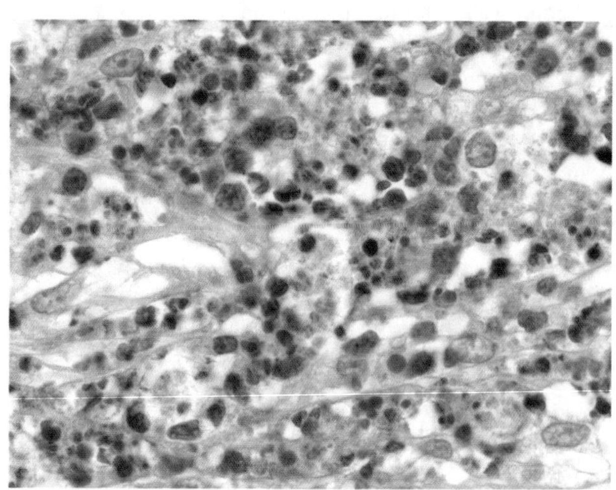

Fig. 29.1 Bacillary angiomatosis (*Bartonella henselae*) IHC ×200

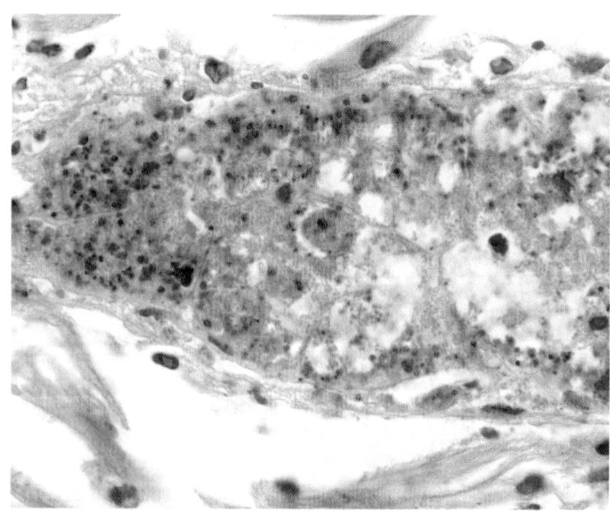

Fig. 29.2 Ecthyma gangrenosum (*Pseudomonas* sepsis) anti-BCG stain IHC ×400

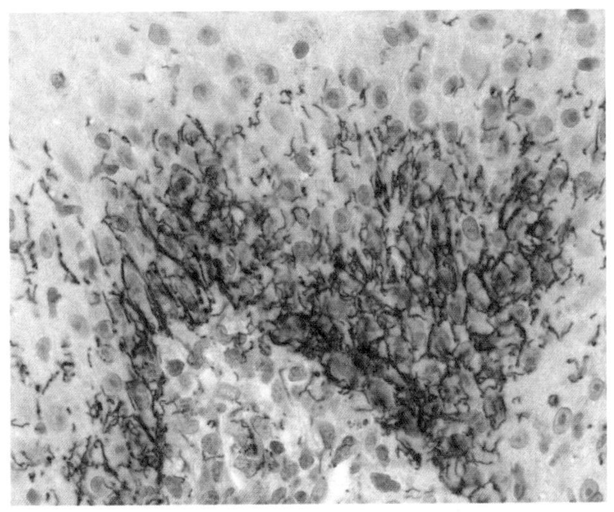

Fig. 29.3 Syphilis (*Treponema pallidum*) ×400

Table 29.1 Commonly used immunohistochemical stains for the detection of bacteria

Stain	Comment
B. henselae	Perform silver stain if negative and clinical suspicion high
Rickettsia	Immunostains for spotted fever and typhus groups
Treponema pallidum	Perform silver stain if negative and clinical suspicion high

29.2 What Tests Are Available to Detect Mycobacteria?

Culture, cutaneous tuberculin testing, and interferon gamma release assays remain the gold standards in the diagnosis of tuberculosis. Auramine–rhodamine staining is extremely sensitive, but requires a fluorescent microscope. For this reason, routine histochemical staining is still commonly performed and IHC has a place in the diagnostic armamentarium.

29.2.1 Anti-Bacille Calmette-Guerin Antibody Immunostain

29.2.1.1 How Sensitive Are the Tests?

Strong or moderate positive reactions are almost always observed for fungi. A wide variety of bacterial and protozoan species are positive. In one study, four protozoan and 12 bacterial species, including *Leptospira* and *Mycoplasma* were negative. Overall, IHC showed similar sensitivity to bacteriological culture and was more sensitive than routine histochemistry [21]. It has been used to detect atypical mycobacteria to include *M. abscessus* [22]. In the setting of leprosy, it has proved more sensitive than routine histochemical staining.

29.2.1.2 How Specific Are the Tests?

In the setting of early leprosy, false-positive staining was noted in 16% of patients [23]. IHC testing for anti-bacille Calmette-Guerin (BCG) is quite nonspecific in regard to the identity of the organism, as the antibody reacts with many bacteria, fungi, and protozoa in formalin-fixed paraffin-embedded tissue samples.

29.2.1.3 Does Fixation Affect the Test?

Heating of the sections in a microwave oven is generally the most effective method.

29.2.2 Mycobacterium avium subsp. paratuberculosis

29.2.2.1 How Sensitive Are the Tests?

Sensitivity of some antibodies may be as low as 5% compared to culture, while others may achieve 93% sensitivity [24, 25].

29.2.2.2 How Specific Are the Tests?

Limited data are available.

29.2.2.3 Does Fixation Affect the Test?

Limited data are available.

29.2.3 Mycobacterium tuberculosis and M. bovis

IHC has been used to detect tuberculosis organisms in tissue. One antibody targets the secreted mycobacterial antigen MPT64, and has been used in formalin-fixed tissue biopsies [26].

29.2.3.1 How Sensitive and Specific Are the Tests?

With IHC and PCR respectively, 64% (35/55) and 60% (33/55) of cases granulomatous lymphadenitis were positive in one study. Compared to PCR, IHC demonstrated sensitivity, specificity, positive, and negative predictive values of 90, 83, 86, and 88%, respectively [27]. In another study, acid fast bacilli were observed in only 36.1% of tuberculous granulomas with routine histochemical staining, while immuno-histochemical staining was positive in 100% with no false positives [28].

29.2.3.2 Does Fixation Affect the Test?

Limited data are available.

29.2.4 How Should I Incorporate These Tests into My Practice?

The BCG antibody is very useful as a screening method to detect a wide variety of pathogens, and is especially useful when pathological features suggest an infection, but no microorganism can be cultured or only formalin-fixed tissue samples are available. Specific IHC testing for mycobacteria is not yet in widespread clinical use. A cocktail of mycobacterial and cross-reacting antibodies developed by Cristina Riera from Barcelona includes anti-*M. bovis* BCG, anti-*M. tuberculosis*, and anti-leishmaniasis antibodies. It is currently receiving good reviews from some laboratories (Figs. 29.4–29.6, Table 29.2).

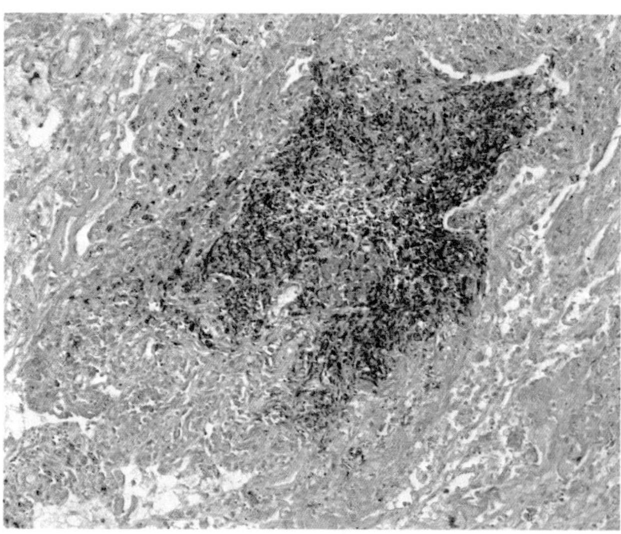

Fig. 29.4 Tuberculosis, lung IHC ×100

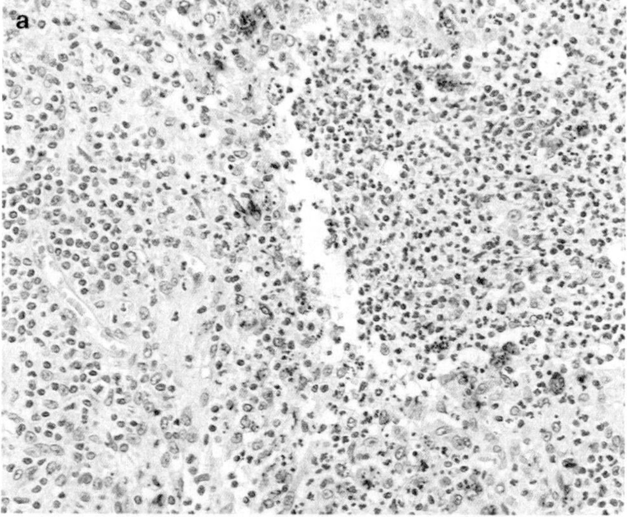

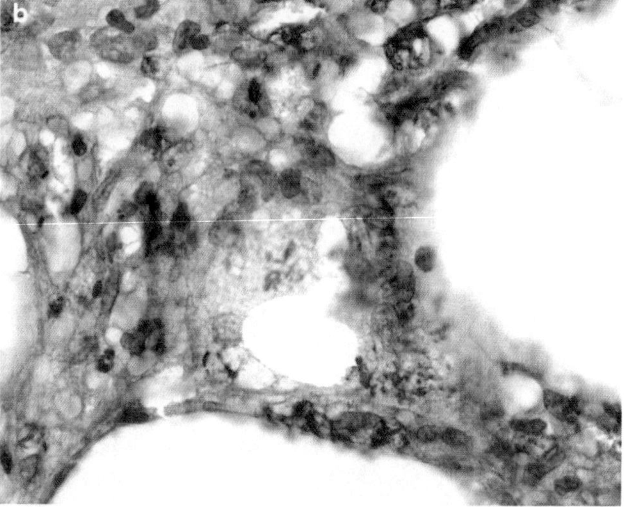

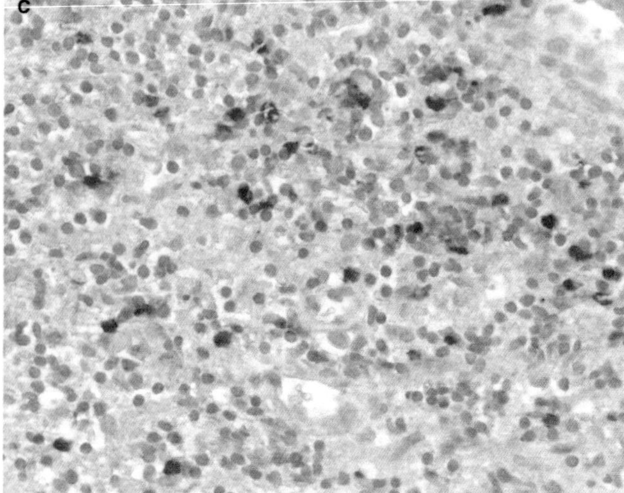

Fig. 29.5 (**a**) Atypical mycobacterial panniculitis IHC ×100. (**b**) Atypical mycobacterial panniculitis IHC ×400. (**c**) *Mycobacterium avium silvaticum* IHC ×100

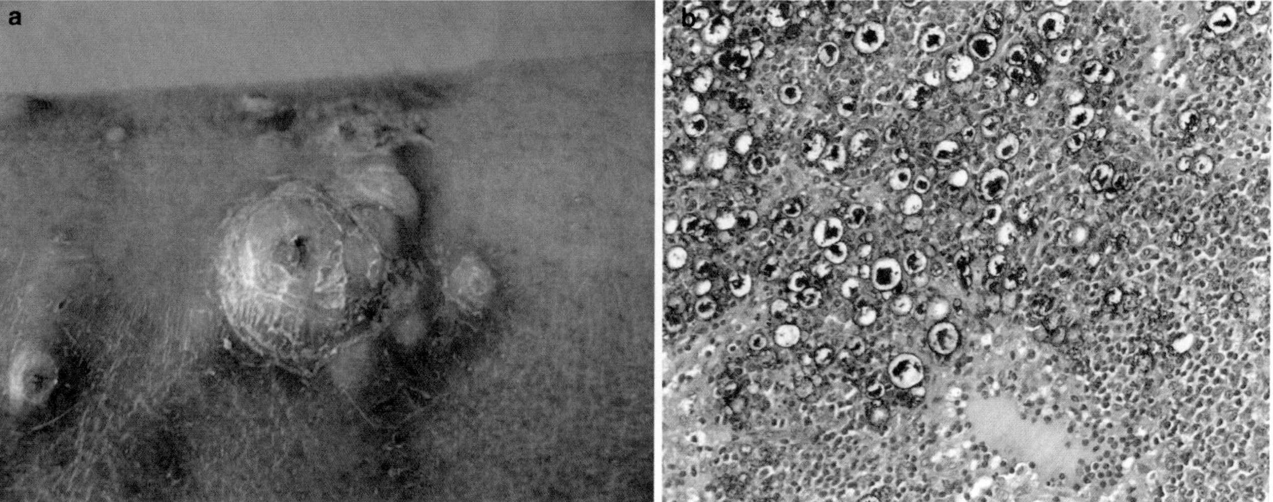

Fig. 29.6 (**a**) Lepromatous leprosy. (**b**) Lepromatous leprosy IHC ×100

Table 29.2 Commonly used immunohistochemical stains for the detection of mycobacteria

Stain	Comment
Anti-*BCG*	Broad screen for many mycobacteria, bacteria, and fungi
Mycobacterium avium subsp. *paratuberculosis*	Culture remains the gold standard
Mycobacterium tuberculosis and *M. bovis*	Culture, tuberculin testing, and interferon gamma release assays remain the gold standard

29.3 What Tests Are Available to Detect Viruses?

Serologic studies, such as ISH, PCR, and DFA, widely used for the diagnosis of viral diseases are available. IHC used to detect a number of viruses in veterinary medicine, but it has become standard only for a few in humans.

29.3.1 Cytomegalovirus

29.3.1.1 How Sensitive and Specific Are the Tests?

In one study, IHC detected the virus in only five of nine patients [29]. Another study showed the detection of virus in 23 of 36 tissue samples, number comparable to that seen with ISH. PCR is superior to both methods if fresh tissue is available [30, 31]. With newer methods, IHC achieves sensitivities of 75.7% with a specificity of 100% [32].

29.3.1.2 Does Fixation Affect the Test?

Formalin fixation decreases the sensitivity of IHC, but may have an even greater influence on PCR results.

29.3.2 Epstein–Barr Virus

ISH remains the gold standard for Epstein–Barr virus (EBV) detection in tissue, but IHC has also been used [33].

29.3.2.1 How Sensitive and Specific Are the Tests?

In one study, automated IHC had a sensitivity of 44% and specificity of 93%. In comparison, ISH achieved a sensitivity and specificity of 94 and 69%, respectively [34]. In some settings, PCR testing can produce results similar to ISH [35]. Some authors have cautioned that PCR detection may be problematic as much of the population has been infected and a positive result may not correspond to causation of the lesion being studied.

29.3.2.2 Does Fixation Affect the Test?

Data are limited.

29.3.3 Hepatitis C

29.3.3.1 How Sensitive and Specific Are the Tests?

Compared to the serology, 83 and 67% of the cases were positive with IHC and in situ RT-PCR, respectively [36]. In another study, 16 of 20 serum antibody-positive cases were detected with IHC, compared with 18 with RT-PCR and 19 with ISH [37]. Using a five-step peroxidase–antiperoxidase method, hepatitis C virus core and four nonstructural antigens were detected in 71 and 57% of patients, respectively [38]. Although IHC testing lacks sensitivity compared to other methods, it has the advantage of localizing the virus in tissue.

29.3.3.2 Does Fixation Affect the Test?

Data are limited.

29.3.4 Human Herpes Virus Type 6

29.3.4.1 How Sensitive Are the Tests?

With a modified avidin–biotin complex (ABC) method, staining for human herpes virus type 6 (HHV-6) was noted in six of eight patients [39].

29.3.4.2 How Specific Are the Tests?

Data are limited.

29.3.4.3 Does Fixation Affect the Test?

Data are limited.

29.3.5 Human Herpes Virus Type 8

29.3.5.1 How Sensitive and Specific Are the Tests?

IHC using a monoclonal antibody to human herpes virus 8 latent nuclear antigen-1, achieves sensitivity and specificity as high as 100% in paraffin-embedded tissue sections of Kaposi sarcoma [40].

29.3.5.2 Does Fixation Affect the Test?

The test works reliably in formalin-fixed tissue.

29.3.6 Human Papillomavirus

ISH is used more commonly in this setting and PCR with sequencing is also used.

29.3.6.1 How Sensitive Are the Tests?

HPV-L1 (human papillomavirus) capsid antibody can be helpful but does not detect nuclear HPV DNA. However, there are anti-HPV16 antibodies available for IHC.

29.3.6.2 How Specific and Sensitive Are the Tests?

Monoclonal antibodies to specific HPV types are available, and some have shown excellent sensitivity and specificity [41]. HPV 6 and 11 are the predominant viruses associated with condyloma and tend to remain benign. Other HPV types (e.g., 16/18/31/33/35/39/45/51/52/56/58/66) are more closely associated with cervical cancer. ISH may be of help if morphologic changes of viral infection are present or suspected and positive identification is clinically relevant for risk management or priority of treatment. A negative test does not rule out the presence of HPV as many HPV types are not detected by these tests to date. IHC for p16(INK4a), a marker of cell cycle dysregulation, is used as a surrogate marker for HPV in cervical dysplasias and carcinomas associated with high risk (HR-HPV) infections. As a surrogate marker, it shows greater specificity than sensitivity and is best used as a screening tool [42]. While p16 expression is commonly used in cervix, it plays little role in the evaluation of skin specimens.

29.3.6.3 Does Fixation Affect the Test?

The tests work well in formalin-fixed tissue.

29.3.7 Herpes Simplex Virus

DFA, culture and serologic assays are used much more commonly than IHC. ISH tests have also been developed for the examination of formalin-fixed, paraffin-embedded tissue.

29.3.7.1 How Sensitive Are the Tests?

DFA and ISH have high sensitivity and specificity. PCR is more sensitive than IHC for the detection of herpes simplex virus (HSV). In one study, the former was positive in approximately 90% of patients and the latter in approximately 50% [43].

29.3.7.2 How Specific Are the Tests?

IHC studies are used less often, but some antibodies produce very reproducible results in the laboratory. ISH is highly specific if viral genome is present.

29.3.7.3 Does Fixation Affect the Test?

Data are limited. ISH likely performs better in tissue fixed 24 h or less in formalin.

29.3.8 *Influenza A Virus*

Worldwide outbreaks of H1N1 swine influenza and H5N1 avian influenza have highlighted the need to develop better tests for the detection of influenza A virus in tissue. The H5-specific monoclonal antibody 7H10 has been used for immunohistochemical staining in formalin-fixed tissue. DFA and ELISA assays are also used.

29.3.8.1 How Sensitive Are the Tests?

IHC using 7H10 detected 28 of the 29 H5 virus strains tested, and the eight-residue-long linear epitope, FFWTILKP, allowed 7H10 to detect >98.3% of H5 subtypes reported before 2007 [44].

29.3.8.2 How Specific Are the Tests?

None of non-H5 strains were detected by 7H10.

29.3.8.3 Does Fixation Affect the Test?

Data are limited.

29.3.9 *Ljungan Virus*

Ljungan virus (LV), a viral pathogen implicated in fetal death, can be detected by IHC and PCR.

29.3.9.1 How Sensitive Are the Tests?

LV was demonstrated in five of five cases by IHC and confirmed three of five by real-time RT-PCR [45].

29.3.9.2 How Specific Are the Tests?

Only 1 of 18 control specimens was positive by IHC.

29.3.9.3 Does Fixation Affect the Test?

Can be performed on formalin-fixed tissue, but optimal retrieval methods remain to be determined.

29.3.10 *Parvovirus B19*

Parvovirus B19 infection is implicated in fifth disease, purpuric gloves and socks syndrome, adult arthritis syndrome, aplastic crisis, dilated cardiomyopathy, and fetal death from hydrops fetalis. Serologic assays, IHC, PCR, and ISH are often used to confirm the presence of the virus.

29.3.10.1 How Sensitive and Specific Are the Tests?

Compared to PCR results, the sensitivity of anti-B19V IHC in the setting of dilated cardiomyopathy was 80.0%, and the specificity was 86.0% [46].

29.3.10.2 Does Fixation Affect the Test?

Data are limited.

29.3.11 *Rabies*

Fluorescent and PCR assays are used more commonly than IHC.

29.3.11.1 How Sensitive Are the Tests?

An indirect immunoperoxidase technique (VNT-IIP) showed high sensitivity (92.8%) and specificity (87.0%) when compared with the fluorescent antibody virus neutralization test [47]. A direct rapid immunohistochemical test (dRIT) demonstrated 100% sensitivity and specificity compared to the direct fluorescent antibody test in field testing [48].

29.3.11.2 How Specific Are the Tests?

Antibodies against rabies may cross react with Duvenhage virus, Mokola virus ,and European bat lyssavirus-1 [49].

29.3.11.3 Does Fixation Affect the Test?

For analysis, a piece of fresh brain tissue should preferably be stored no longer than 24 h in formalin before embedding [50].

29.3.12 Small Pox (Variola)

Although both IHC and DFA have demonstrated the virus in a variety of tissues, including skin, liver, and fibroconnective tissue, fluorescent assays are used almost exclusively.

29.3.12.1 How Sensitive Are the Tests?

Fluorescent assays have shown excellent sensitivity and specificity. A rapid, sensitive real-time assay to detect *Variola* was developed using the *Vaccinia* virus as a target [51].

29.3.12.2 Does Fixation Affect the Test?

Data are limited.

29.3.13 Varicella-Zoster Virus

As with HSV, DFA is used much more commonly than IHC. ISH is also available for Varicella-Zoster virus (VZV).

29.3.13.1 How Sensitive and Specific Are the Tests?

In one study, IHC achieved a type-specific virus diagnostic accuracy of between 86.7 and 100% on smears, and 92.3% in skin sections [52]. Shell vial immunoperoxidase has demonstrated 87.6% sensitivity and 100% specificity when compared with cell culture [53].

ISH specificity is 100% if viral genome is present in the tissue.

29.3.13.2 Does Fixation Affect the Test?

Limited data are available but ISH performs better in tissue fixed in formalin for 24 h or less.

29.3.14 Viral Hemorrhagic Fevers

Hemorrhagic fever viruses include the *Filoviridae* (Ebola and Marburg viruses) and the *Arenaviridae* (Junin, Machupo, Guanarito, and Lassa viruses). These can be detected using PCR, IHC, or electron microscopy. During outbreaks of Ebola hemorrhagic fever in Africa, IHC was used successfully on skin punch biopsy samples in large numbers of fatal cases [54]. These tests are not generally available.

29.3.15 West Nile Virus

The diagnosis is usually made via serologic studies. A variety of antibodies are available including a rabbit-polyclonal anti-WNV (West Nile virus) antibody and a monoclonal antibody directed against an epitope on Domain III of the E protein of WNV.

29.3.15.1 How Sensitive Are the Tests?

In studies on the kidney, liver, lung, spleen, and small intestine of infected crows, the sensitivity of the monoclonal antibody-based IHC staining was only 72%, compared to 100% with the polyclonal antibody [55]. In human tissue, the concordance between IHC and serology was 41%, while the concordance between RT-PCR and serology was 63% [56].

29.3.15.2 How Specific Are the Tests?

Data are limited.

29.3.15.3 Does Fixation Affect the Test?

Data are limited.

29.3.16 How Should I Incorporate These Tests into My Practice?

IHC is commonly used for the detection of human herpes virus type 8 (HHV-8), and is also used for cytomegalovirus (CMV). Other techniques, such as DFA are widely used for other herpes viruses. ISH studies are commonly performed for HPV. Detection of HSV or VZV vial changes can most often be done morphologically on routinely stained sections. However, in cases with atypical presentations or where specific rapid differentiation is required for therapeutic purposes, ISH may play a role due to its specificity. Specialized laboratories, such as those at the CDC will perform a wider range of testing, including IHC for exotic viruses and those likely to be used as biological weapons (Figs. 29.7–29.12, Table 29.3).

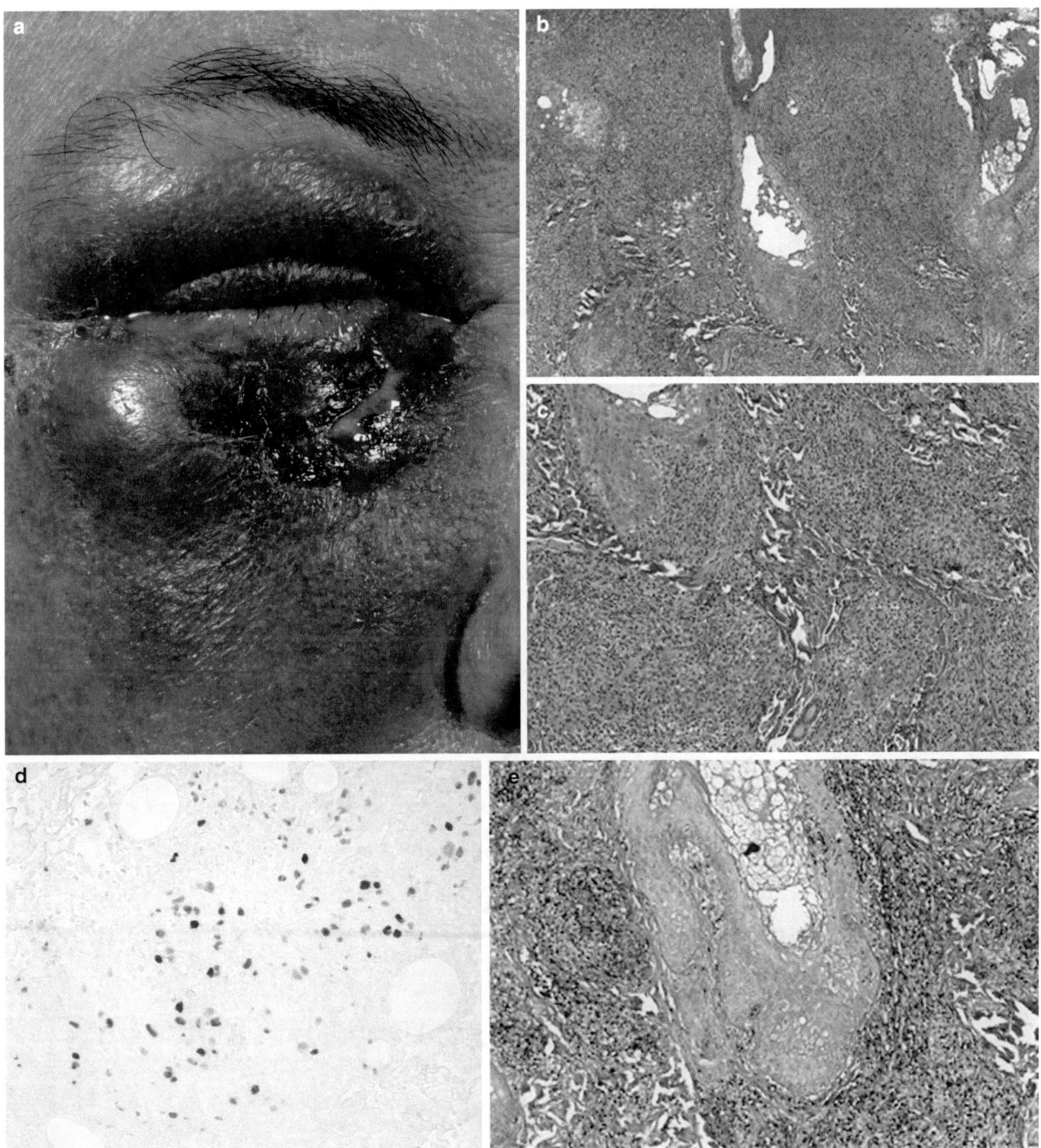

Fig. 29.7 (**a**) Epstein–Barr virus (EBV). (**b**) Epstein–Barr virus (EBV) H&E ×40. (**c**) Epstein–Barr virus (EBV) H&E ×80. (**d**) Epstein–Barr virus (EBV) ISH ×40. (**e**) Epstein–Barr virus (EBV) ISH ×100

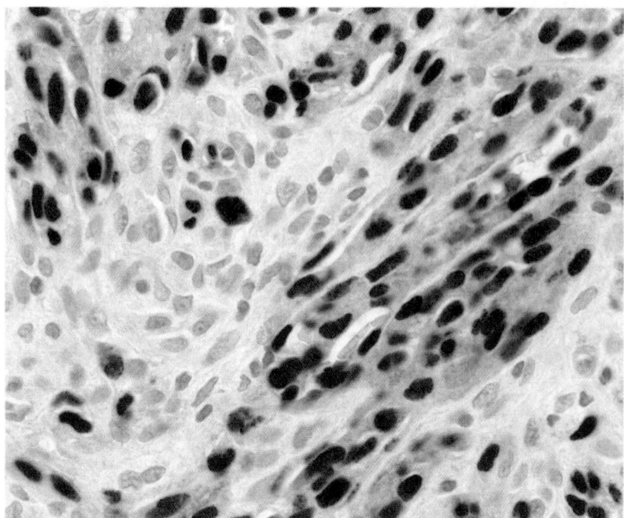

Fig. 29.8 Human herpes virus 8 (HHV8) IHC ×400

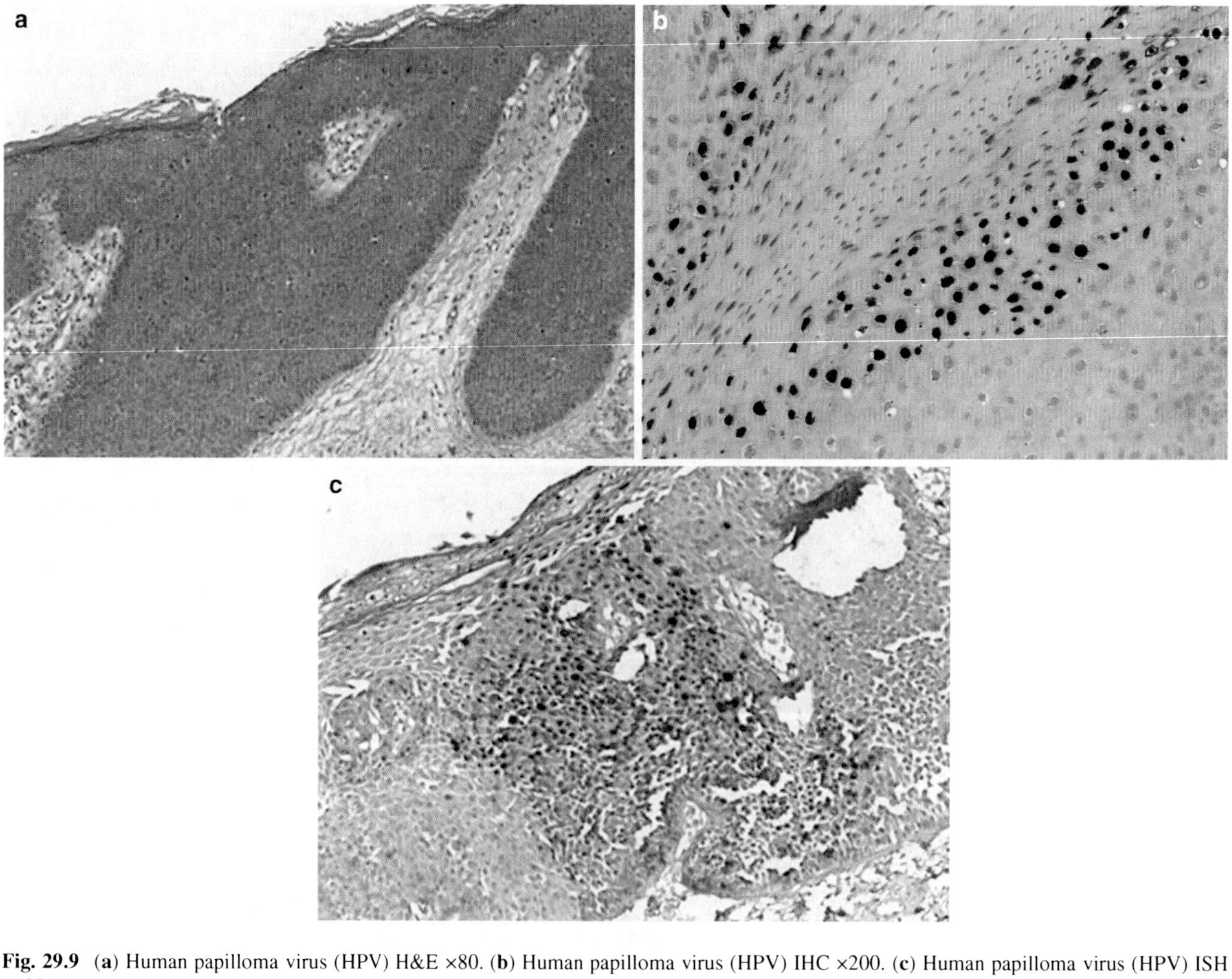

Fig. 29.9 (**a**) Human papilloma virus (HPV) H&E ×80. (**b**) Human papilloma virus (HPV) IHC ×200. (**c**) Human papilloma virus (HPV) ISH ×100

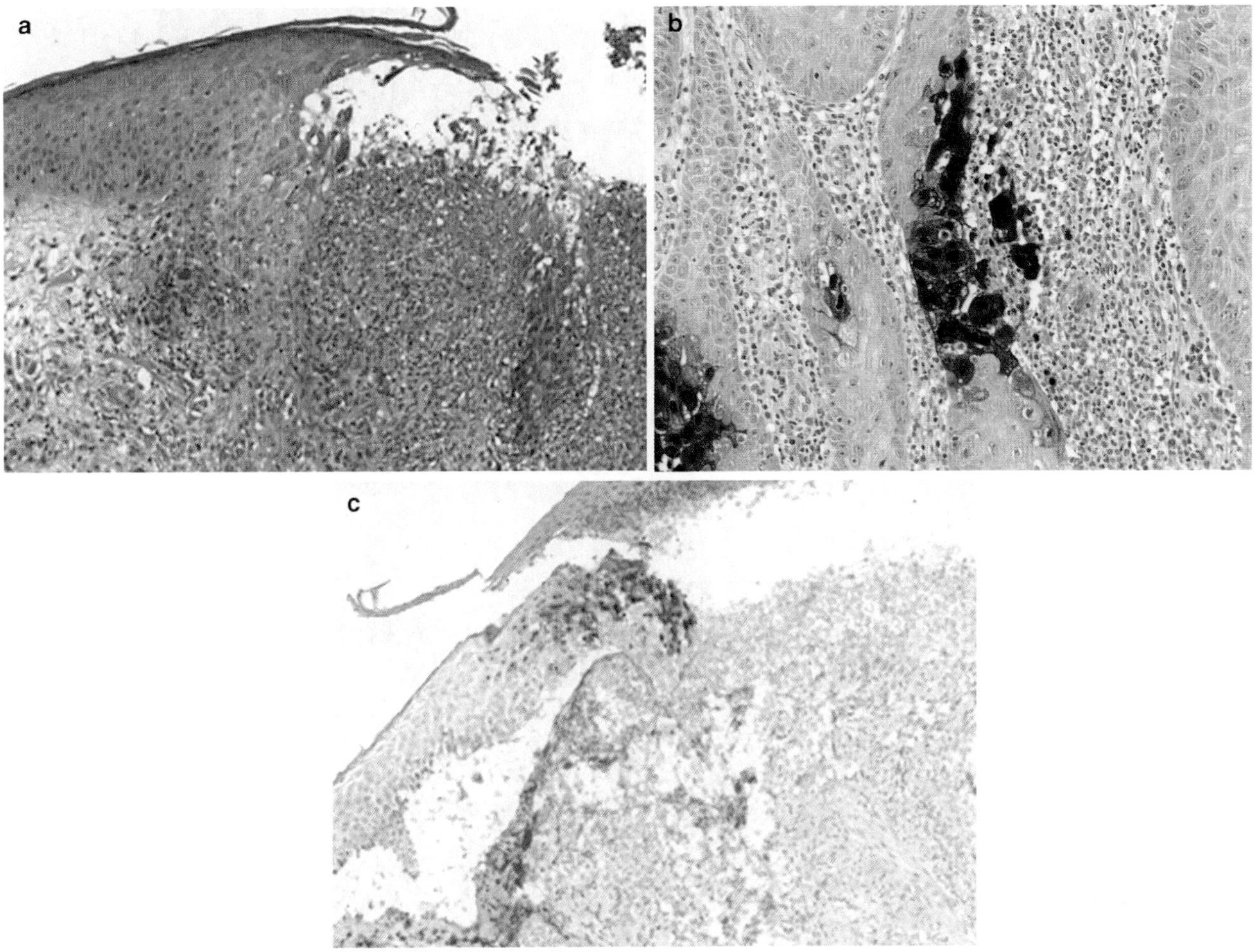

Fig. 29.10 (**a**) Herpes simplex virus (HSV) H&E ×100. (**b**) Herpes simplex virus (HSV) IHC ×200. (**c**) Herpes simplex virus (HSV) ISH ×80

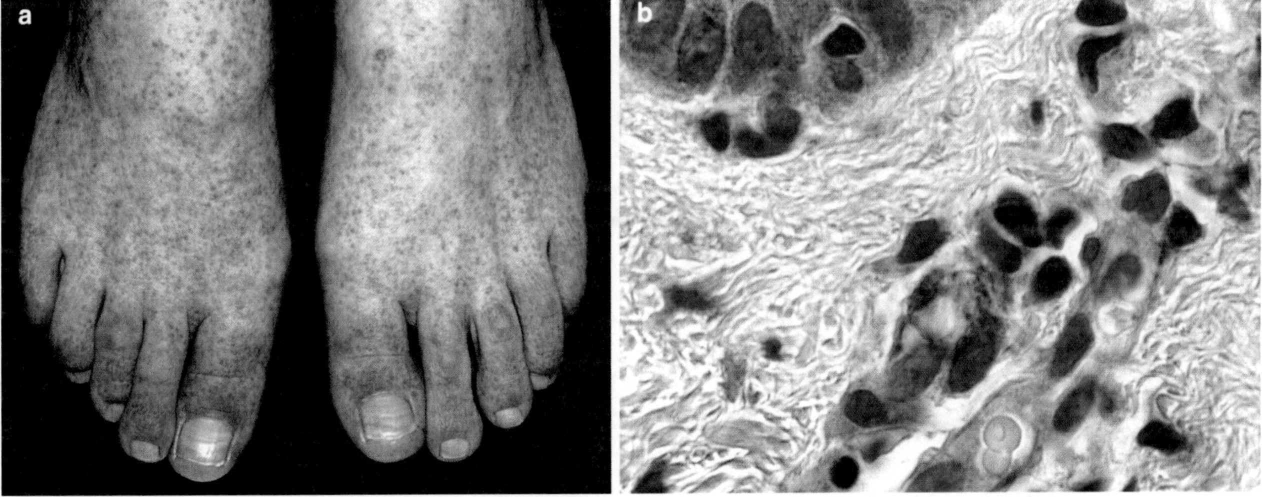

Fig. 29.11 (**a**) Parvovirus B19, purpuric gloves and socks syndrome. (**b**) Parvovirus B19 IHC ×600

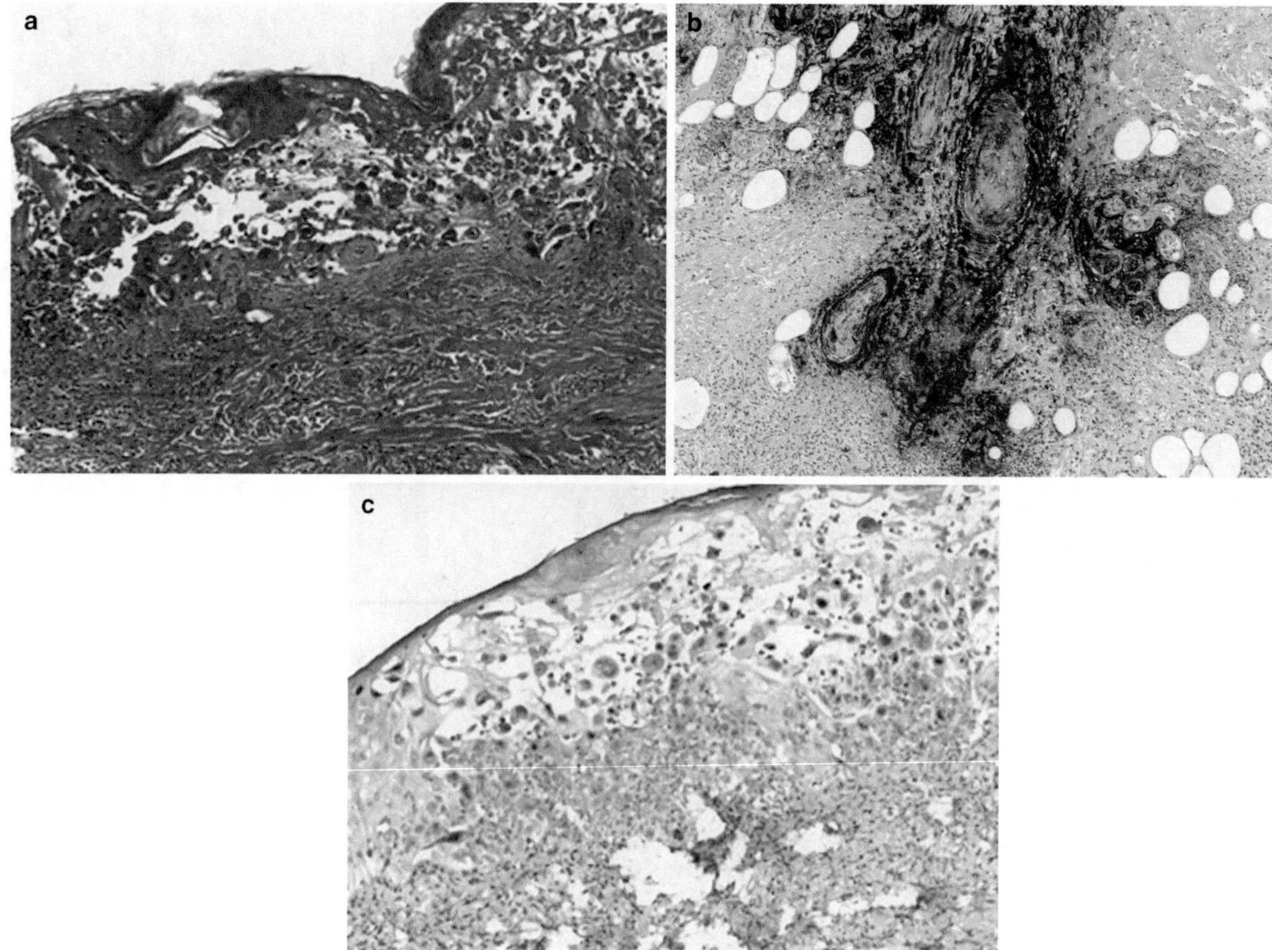

Fig. 29.12 (**a**) Varicella zoster virus (VZV) H&E ×100. (**b**) Varicella zoster virus (VZV) IHC ×200. (**c**) Varicella zoster virus (VZV) ISH ×100

Table 29.3 Commonly used immunohistochemical stains for the detection of viruses

Stain	Comment
CMV	PCR is superior to IHC and ISH if fresh tissue is available
HHV-8	High sensitivity and specificity

29.4 What Tests Are Available to Detect Fungal and Protozoan Pathogens?

29.4.1 Anti-Bacille Calmette-Guerin Antibody Immunostain

Specific IHC tests are being developed, but the BCG antibody immunostain has been the most common stain in use. DAKO recently modified their antibody, and it has lost reactivity with fungal species. PCR and ISH assays are also commonly used and isolation by culture remains the gold standard.

29.4.1.1 How Sensitive Are the Tests?

Results vary by the organism. PCR is more sensitive than IHC using a BCG immunostain for the detection of *Histoplasma capsulatum*. In one study, the 50% quantile to achieve a positive result for each study was determined to be 3 colony-forming units per milligram for PCR, 11 for Grocott stain, 27 for a fluorochrome stain, 190 for immunostaining, and 533 for H&E [57].

29.4.1.2 How Specific Are the Tests?

IHC testing for BCG is quite nonspecific in regard to the identity of the organism, as the antibody reacts with many bacteria, fungi, and protozoa in formalin-fixed paraffin-embedded tissue samples.

29.4.1.3 Does Fixation Affect the Test?

The test works reliably in formalin-fixed tissue.

29.4.2 *Aspergillus Species*

The monoclonal antibody EB-A1 has been used to detect *Aspergillus* species in formalin-fixed, paraffin wax-embedded tissue.

29.4.2.1 How Sensitive Are the Tests?

IHC staining was positive in 89% of cases, including one culture negative case with histological evidence of infection [58]. Polyclonal and monoclonal *Aspergillus* antibodies have shown sensitivities and specificities of 100 and 29%, and 43 and 14%, respectively. Cross reaction with zygomycetes was noted [59].

29.4.2.2 How Specific Are the Tests?

Cross-reactivity was observed with *Pseudallescheria boydii*, but not with *Candida* species, *Apophysomyces elegans*, *Rhizopus oryzae*, or *H. capsulatum*. Polyclonal antibodies have shown a high degree of cross reactivity with other fungi [60].

29.4.2.3 Does Fixation Affect the Test?

Limited data are available.

29.4.3 *Blastomyces dermatitidis, Coccidioides immitis, Cryptococcus neoformans, and Histoplasma capsulatum*

Identification of these yeast-like organisms is of importance particularly in the transplant and immunocompromised patient populations. Most often these organisms can be identified in tissue sections utilizing silver stains (e.g., GMS) or the PAS stain. However, in cases where rapid identification of specific organism is required or in cases where the possibility of more than one infection exists, there is a role for ISH diagnosis. Specific probes designed to detect ribosomal RNA sequences to several fungal organisms including all of the above have been developed.

29.4.3.1 How Sensitive Are the Tests?

Sensitivity for the detection of yeast or hyphal forms is slightly less than traditional silver or PAS stains (83 vs. 95%).

29.4.3.2 How Specific Are the Tests?

Specificity is very high if organisms are present in tissue (100%) vs. 96–100% utilizing traditional silver stains or PAS [61, 62].

29.4.3.3 Does Fixation Affect the Test?

Formalin-fixed, paraffin-embedded tissue may be used. It is recommended, however, that the tissue not be fixed in formalin greater than 24 h before processing and embedding.

29.4.4 *Pneumocystis carinii*

A monoclonal antibody has been developed that recognizes *P. carinii* in tissue, bronchoalveolar lavage fluid, and sputum. The antibody has been adapted to immunoperoxidase staining using an avidin–biotin horseradish peroxidase technique.

29.4.4.1 How Sensitive Are the Tests?

Of the 50 specimens evaluated in one study, there was 94% concordance between conventional Diff-Quik staining and immunoperoxidase staining. The organism is far easier to see with the immunoperoxidase stain [63]. Two Diff-Quik-positive specimens failed to stain with the immunoperoxidase method, and one Diff-Quik-negative specimen was detected by immunoperoxidase staining.

29.4.4.2 How Specific Are the Tests?

In a study of alkaline phosphatase–anti-alkaline phosphatase complex technique for the detection of *P. carinii* in bronchoalveolar lavage fluid from 83 HIV-1 positive patients, 28 samples were positive by immunofluorescence, 26 by Grocott staining, and 29 by IHC [64].

29.4.4.3 Does Fixation Affect the Test?

Limited data are available.

29.4.5 *Leshmaniasis*

29.4.5.1 How Sensitive Are the Tests?

Limited data are available. Some data suggest a sensitivity of 90.9% with PCR vs. 68.8% with IHC [65].

29.4.5.2 How Specific Are the Tests?

Some antibodies cross-react with fungi.

29.4.5.3 Does Fixation Affect the Test?

Limited data are available.

29.4.6 How Should I Incorporate These Tests into My Practice?

Many fungal organisms are quite easily seen in H&E sections, while others such as *H. capsulatum* may be more difficult to find. The BCG antibody is very useful as a screening method to detect a wide variety of pathogens, especially when pathological features suggest an infection, but no microorganism can be cultured or when only formalin-fixed tissue samples are available. Specific IHC testing for is not yet in widespread clinical use but has been developed and tested for a limited number of organisms. These tests are of greatest utility when rapid accurate specific identification is essential for therapeutic purposes (Figs. 29.13–29.19, Table 29.4).

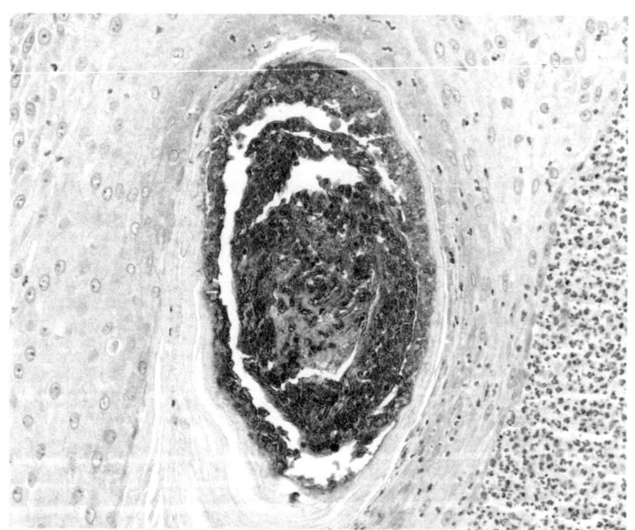

Fig. 29.13 Dermatophytosis anti-BCG IHC ×200

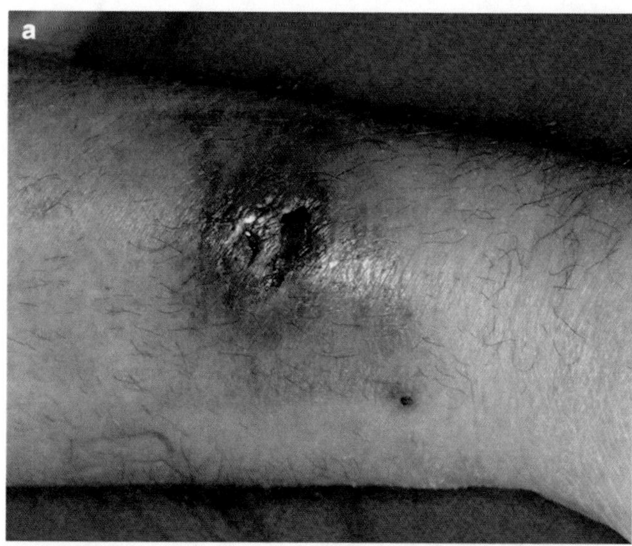

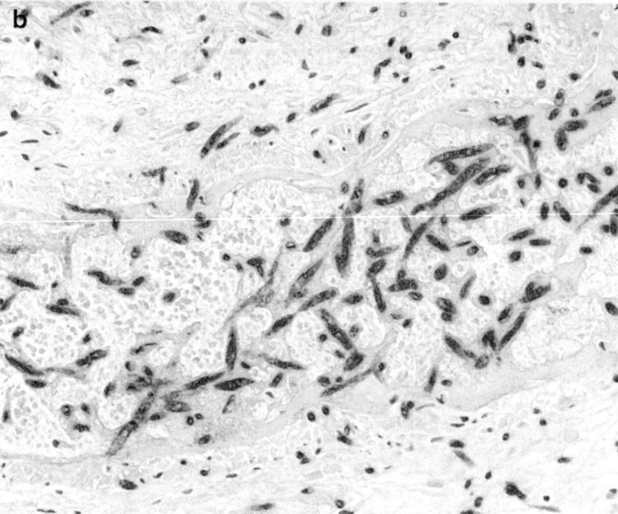

Fig. 29.14 (**a**) *Aspergillus* sepsis. (**b**) *Aspergillus* sepsis anti-BCG IHC ×400

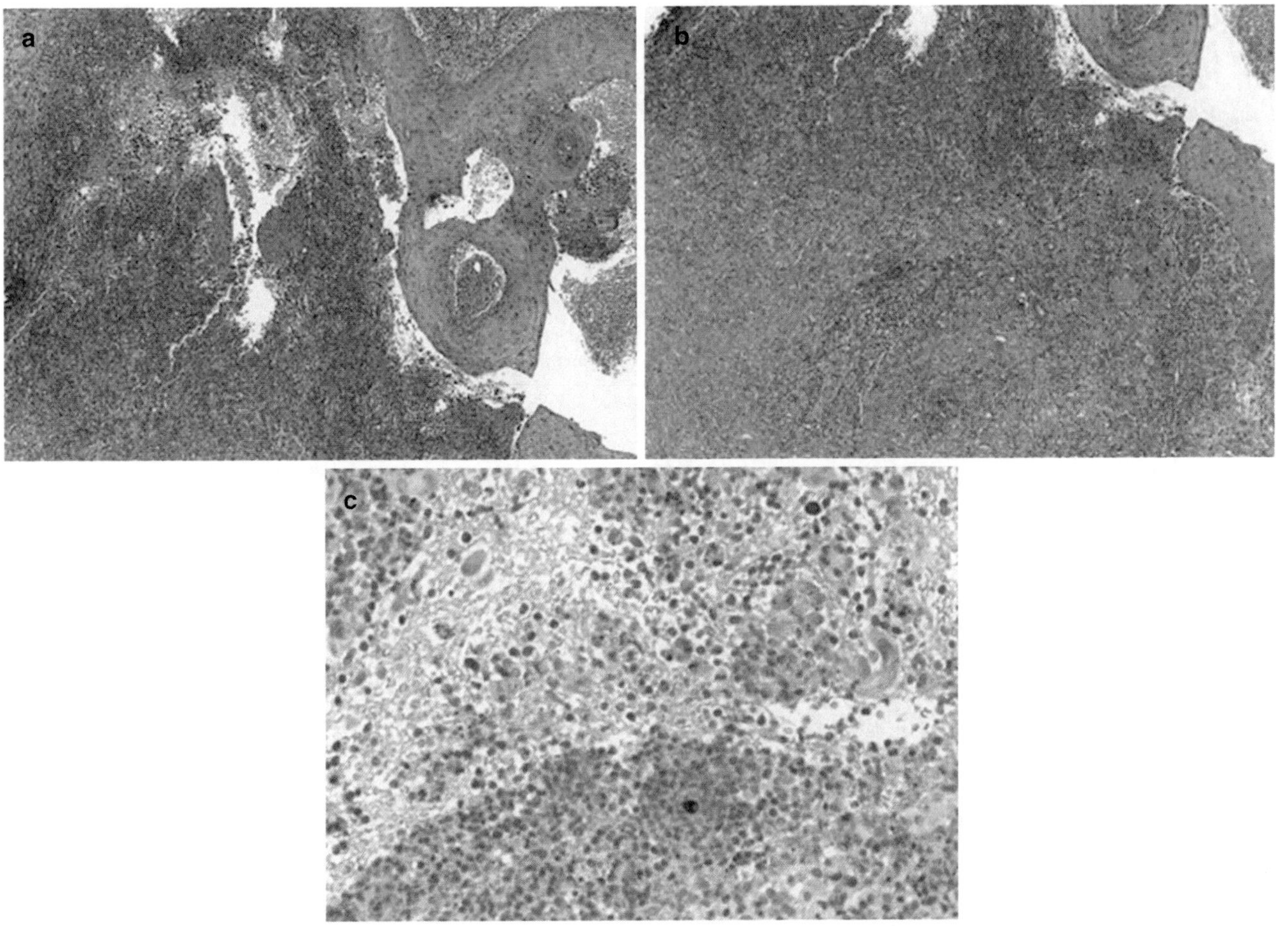

Fig. 29.15 (**a**) *Blastomyces* H&E ×40. (**b**) *Blastomyces* H&E ×60. (**c**) *Blastomyces* ISH ×120

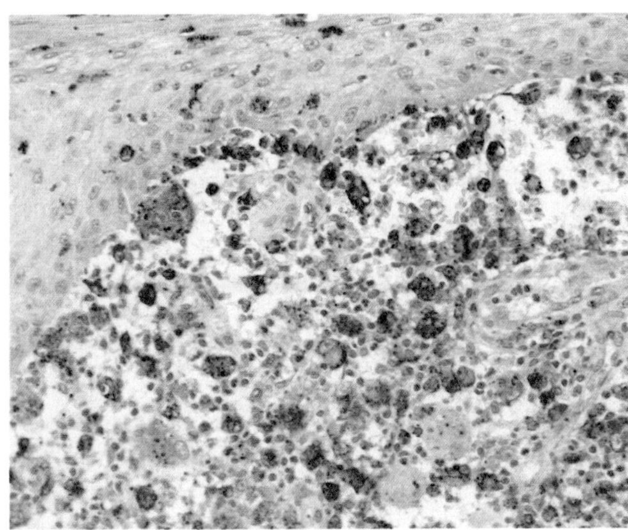

Fig. 29.16 Histoplasmosis ISH ×400

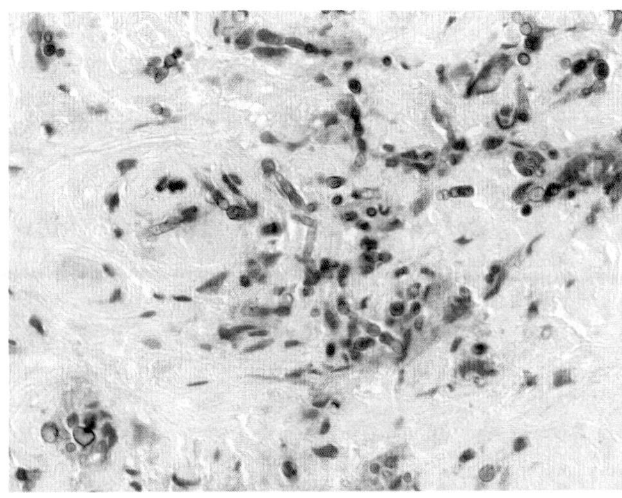

Fig. 29.17 Fungi cross-reacting with leishmanial antibody IHC ×400

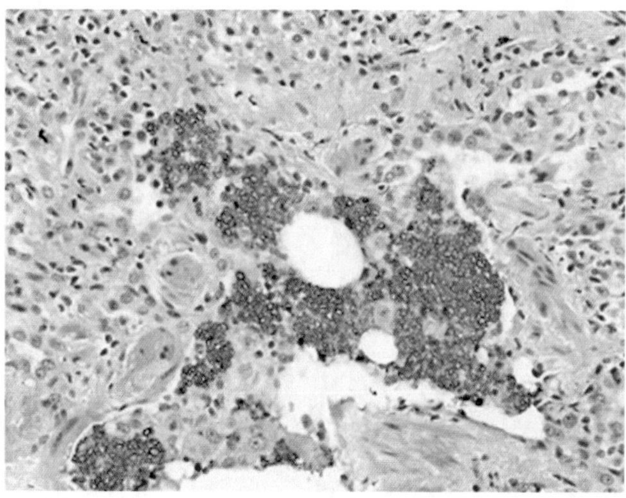

Fig. 29.18 *Pneumocystis carinii* IHC ×200

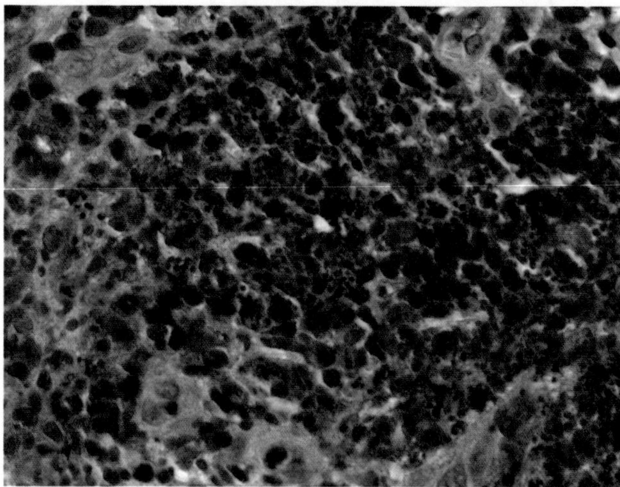

Fig. 29.19 Leishmaniasis (Cristina Riera antibody) IHC ×400

Table 29.4 Commonly used immunohistochemical stains for the detection of fungi

Stain	Comment
Anti-*BCG*	Useful as a screening method to detect a wide variety of pathogens, especially when pathological features suggest an infection, but no microorganism can be cultured or when only formalin-fixed tissue samples are available
Fungal-specific stains	Evolving technology. Cross reactions remain common. ISH is highly specific for a limited number of organisms

References

1. Bacchi CE, Gown AM, Bacchi MM. Detection of infectious disease agents in tissue by immunocytochemistry. Braz J Med Biol Res. 1994;27(12):2803–20.
2. Tatti KM, Greer P, White E, Shieh WJ, Guarner J, Ferebee-Harris T, et al. Morphologic, immunologic, and molecular methods to detect bacillus anthracis in formalin-fixed tissues. Appl Immunohistochem Mol Morphol. 2006;14(2):234–43.
3. Wun-Ju S, Jeannette G, Christopher P, Patricia G, Kathleen T, Marc F, et al. The critical role of pathology in the investigation of bioterrorism-related cutaneous anthrax. Am J Pathol. 2003;163:1901–10.
4. Guarner J, Jernigan J, Shieh W, Tatti K, Flannagan L, Stephens D, et al. Pathology and pathogenesis of bioterrorism-related inhalational anthrax. Am J Pathol. 2003;163:701–9.
5. Caponetti GC, Pantanowitz L, Marconi S, Havens JM, Lamps LW, Otis CN. Evaluation of immunohistochemistry in identifying *Bartonella henselae* in cat-scratch disease. Am J Clin Pathol. 2009;131(2):250–6.
6. Ilhan F, Yener Z. Immunohistochemical detection of *Brucella melitensis* antigens in cases of naturally occurring abortions in sheep. J Vet Diagn Invest. 2008;20(6):803–6.
7. Zeidner NS, Carter LG, Monteneiri JA, Petersen JM, Schriefer M, Gage KL, et al. An outbreak of *Francisella tularensis* in captive prairie dogs: an immunohistochemical analysis. J Vet Diagn Invest. 2004;16(2):150–2.
8. Wabing HR. Comparison of immunohistochemical and modified Giemsa stains for demonstration of *Helicobacter pylori* infection in an African population. Afr Health Sci. 2002;2(2):52–5.
9. Ashton-Key M, Diss TC, Isaacson PG. Detection of *Helicobacter pylori* in gastric biopsy and resection specimens. J Clin Pathol. 1996;49(2):107–11.
10. Ciesielska U, Dziegiel P, Jagoda E, Podhorska-Okołów M, Zabel M. The detection of *Helicobacter pylori* in paraffin sections using the PCR technique and various primers as compared to histological techniques. Folia Morphol (Warsz). 2004;63(2):229–31.
11. Jonkerst D, Stobberingh E, de Bruine A, Arends JW, Stockbrüg R. Evaluation of immunohistochemistry for the detection of *Helicobacter pylori* in gastric mucosal biopsies. J Infect. 1997;35:149–54.
12. Wild CJ, Greenlee JJ, Bolin CA, Barnett JK, Haake DA, Cheville NF. An improved immunohistochemical diagnostic technique for canine leptospirosis using antileptospiral antibodies on renal tissue. J Vet Diagn Invest. 2002;14(1):20–4.
13. Saglam YS, Yener Z, Temur A, Yalcin E. Immunohistochemical detection of leptospiral antigens in cases of naturally occurring abortions in sheep. Small Rumin Res. 2008;74(1–3):119–22.
14. Lebech A, Clemmensen O, Hansen K. Comparison of In Vitro Culture, Immunohistochemical staining, and pcr for detection of *Borrelia burgdorferi* in tissue from experimentally infected animals. J Clin Microbiol. 1995;33(9):2328–33.
15. White WL, Patrick JD, Miller LR. Evaluation of immunoperoxidase techniques to detect *Rickettsia rickettsii* in fixed tissue sections. Am J Clin Pathol. 1994;101(6):747–52.
16. Behrhof W, Springer E, Bräuninger W, Kirkpatrick CJ, Weber A. PCR testing for *Treponema pallidum* in paraffin-embedded skin biopsy specimens: test design and impact on the diagnosis of syphilis. J Clin Pathol. 2008;61(3):390–5.
17. Buffet M, Grange PA, Gerhardt P, et al. Diagnosing *Treponema pallidum* in secondary syphilis by PCR and immunohistochemistry. J Invest Dermatol. 2007;127(10):2345–50.
18. Hoang MP, High WA, Molberg KH. Secondary syphilis: a histologic and immunohistochemical evaluation. J Cutan Pathol. 2004;31(9):595–9.
19. Guarner J, Shieh WJ, Greer PW, Gabastou JM, Chu M, Hayes E, et al. Immunohistochemical detection of *Yersinia pestis* in formalin-fixed, paraffin-embedded tissue. Am J Clin Pathol. 2002;117(2):205–9.
20. Schmengler K, Goldmann T, Brade L, Sánchez Carballo PM, Albrecht S, Brade H, et al. Monoclonal antibody S60-4-14 reveals diagnostic potential in the identification of *Pseudomonas aeruginosa* in lung tissues of cystic fibrosis patients. Eur J Cell Biol. 2010;89(1):25–33.

21. Szeredi L, Glávits R, Tenk M, Jánosi S. Application of anti-BCG antibody for rapid immunohistochemical detection of bacteria, fungi and protozoa in formalin-fixed paraffin-embedded tissue samples. Acta Vet Hung. 2008;56(1):89–99.
22. Prinz BM, Michaelis S, Kettelhack N, Mueller B, Burg G, Kempf W. Subcutaneous infection with *Mycobacterium abscessus* in a renal transplant recipient. Dermatology. 2004;208(3):259–61.
23. Schettini AP, Ferreira LC, Milagros R, Schettini MC, Pennini SN, Rebello PB. Enhancement in the histological diagnosis of leprosy in patients with only sensory loss by demonstration of mycobacterial antigens using anti-BCG polyclonal antibodies. Int J Lepr Other Mycobact Dis. 2001;69(4):335–40.
24. Martinson SA, Hanna PE, Ikede BO, Lewis JP, Miller LM, Keefe GP, et al. Comparison of bacterial culture, histopathology, and immunohistochemistry for the diagnosis of Johne's disease in culled dairy cows. J Vet Diagnos Investig. 2008;20:51–7.
25. Huntley JFJ, Whitlock RH, Bannantine JP, Stabel JR. Comparison of diagnostic detection methods for *Mycobacterium avium* subsp. *paratuberculosis* in North American Bison. Vet Pathol. 2005;42:42–51.
26. Adegboye DS, Rasberry U, Halbur PG, Andrews JJ, Rosenbusch RF. Monoclonal antibody-based immunohistochemical technique for the detection of *Mycoplasma bovis* in formalin-fixed, paraffin-embedded calf lung tissues. J Vet Diagn Invest. 1995;7(2):261–5.
27. Mustafa T, Wiker HG, Mfinanga SG, Mørkve O, Sviland L. Immunohistochemistry using a *Mycobacterium tuberculosis* complex specific antibody for improved diagnosis of tuberculous lymphadenitis. Mod Pathol. 2006;19(12):1606–14.
28. Goel MM, Budhwar P. Immunohistochemical localization of *Mycobacterium tuberculosis* complex antigen with antibody to 38 kDa antigen versus Ziehl Neelsen staining in tissue granulomas of extrapulmonary tuberculosis. Indian J Tuberc. 2007;54:24–9.
29. Wilkens L, Werner M, Nolte M, Wasielewski RV, Verhagen W, Flik J, et al. Influence of formalin fixation on the detection of cytomegalovirus by polymerase chain reaction in immunocompromised patients and correlation to in situ hybridization, immunohistochemistry, and serological data. Diagn Mol Pathol. 1994;3(3):156–62.
30. Strickler J, Manivel J, Copenhaver C, Kubic V. Comparison of in situ hybridization and immunohistochemistry for detection of cytomegalovirus and herpes simplex virus. Hum Pathol. 1990;21:443–8.
31. Bajanowski T, Wiegand P, Brinkmann B. Comparison of different methods for CMV detection. Int J Legal Med. 1994;106:219–22.
32. Lu DY, Qian J, Easley KA, Waldrop SM, Cohen C. Automated in situ hybridization and immunohistochemistry for cytomegalovirus detection in paraffin-embedded tissue sections. Appl Immunohistochem Mol Morphol. 2009;17(2):158–64.
33. Truong CD, Feng W, Li W, Khoury T, Li Q, Alrawi S, et al. Characteristics of Epstein–Barr virus-associated gastric cancer: a study of 235 cases at a comprehensive cancer center in U.S.A. J Exp Clin Cancer Res. 2009;28:14.
34. Fanaian NK, Cohen C, Waldrop S, Wang J, Shehata BM. Epstein–Barr virus (EBV)-encoded RNA: automated in-situ hybridization (ISH) compared with manual ISH and immunohistochemistry for detection of EBV in pediatric lymphoproliferative disorders. Pediatr Dev Pathol. 2009;12(3):195–9.
35. Suh N, Liapis H, Misdraji J, Brunt EM, Wang HL. Epstein–Barr virus hepatitis: diagnostic value of in situ hybridization, polymerase chain reaction, and immunohistochemistry on liver biopsy from immunocompetent patients. Am J Surg Pathol. 2007;31(9):1403–9.
36. Benkoël L, Biagini P, Dodero F, De Lamballerie X, De Micco P, Chamlian A. Immunohistochemical detection of C-100 hepatitis C virus antigen in formaldehyde-fixed paraffin-embedded liver tissue. Correlation with serum, tissue and in situ RT-PCR results. Eur J Histochem. 2004;48(2):185–90.
37. Qian X, Guerrero RB, Plummer TB, Alves VF, Lloyd RV. Detection of hepatitis C virus RNA in formalin-fixed paraffin-embedded sections with digoxigenin-labeled cRNA probes. Diagn Mol Pathol. 2004;13(1):9–14.
38. González-Peralta RP, Fang JW, Davis GL, Gish R, Tsukiyama-Kohara K, Kohara M, et al. Optimization for the detection of hepatitis C virus antigens in the liver. J Hepatol. 1994;20(1):143–7.
39. Pitalia AK, Liu-Yin JA, Freemont AJ, Morris DJ, Fitzmaurice RJ. Immunohistological detection of human herpes virus 6 in formalin-fixed, paraffin-embedded lung tissues. J Med Virol. 1993;41(2):103–7.
40. Patel RM, Goldblum JR, Hsi ED. Immunohistochemical detection of human herpes virus-8 latent nuclear antigen-1 is useful in the diagnosis of Kaposi sarcoma. Mod Pathol. 2004;17(4):456–60.
41. Jeon JH, Shin DM, Cho SY, Song KY, Park NH, Kang HS, et al. Immunocytochemical detection of HPV16 E7 in cervical smear. Exp Mol Med. 2007;39(5):621–8.
42. Mulvany NJ, Allen DG, Wilson SM. Diagnostic utility of p16INK4a: a reappraisal of its use in cervical biopsies. Pathology. 2008;40(4):335–44.
43. Oda Y, Katsuda S, Okada Y, Kawahara EI, Ooi A, Kawashima A, et al. Detection of human cytomegalovirus, Epstein–Barr virus, and herpes simplex virus in diffuse interstitial pneumonia by polymerase chain reaction and immunohistochemistry. Am J Clin Pathol. 1994;102(4):495–502.
44. He F, Du Q, Ho Y, Kwang J. Immunohistochemical detection of influenza virus infection in formalin-fixed tissues with anti-H5 monoclonal antibody recognizing FFWTILKP. J Virol Methods. 2009;155(1):25–33.
45. Samsioe A, Papadogiannakis N, Hultman T, Sjöholm A, Klitz W, Niklasson B. Ljungan virus present in intrauterine fetal death diagnosed by both immunohistochemistry and PCR. Birth Defects Res A Clin Mol Teratol. 2009;85(3):227–9.
46. Escher F, Kuhl U, Sabi T, Suckau L, Lassner D, Poller W, et al. Immunohistological detection of Parvovirus B19 capsid proteins in endomyocardial biopsies from dilated cardiomyopathy patients. Med Sci Monit. 2008;14(6):CR333–8.
47. Ogawa T, Gamoh K, Aoki H, Kobayashi R, Etoh M, Senda M, et al. Validation and standardization of virus neutralizing test using indirect immunoperoxidase technique for the quantification of antibodies to rabies virus. Zoonoses Public Health. 2008;55(6):323–7.
48. Lembo T, Niezgoda M, Velasco-Villa A, Cleaveland S, Ernest E, Rupprecht CE. Evaluation of a direct, rapid immunohistochemical test for rabies diagnosis. Emerg Infect Dis. 2006;12(2):310–3.
49. Inoue S, Sato Y, Hasegawa H, Noguchi A, Yamada A, Kurata T, et al. Cross-reactive antigenicity of nucleoproteins of lyssaviruses recognized by a monospecific antirabies virus nucleoprotein antiserum on paraffin sections of formalin-fixed tissues. Pathol Int. 2003;53(8):525–33.
50. Wacharapluesadee S, Ruangvejvorachai P, Hemachudha T. A simple method for detection of rabies viral sequences in 16-year old archival brain specimens with one-week fixation in formalin. J Virol Methods. 2006;134(1–2):267–71.
51. Donaldson KA, Kramer MF, Lim DV. A rapid detection method for Vaccinia virus, the surrogate for smallpox virus. Biosens Bioelectron. 2004;20(2):322–7.
52. Nikkels AF, Debrus S, Sadzot-Delvaux C, Piette J, Rentier B, Piérard GE. Immunohistochemical identification of varicella-zoster virus gene 63-encoded protein (IE63) and late (gE) protein on smears and cutaneous biopsies: implications for diagnostic use. J Med Virol. 1995;47(4):342–7.
53. Chan EL, Brandt K, Horsman GB. Comparison of Chemicon SimulFluor direct fluorescent antibody staining with cell culture and shell vial direct immunoperoxidase staining for detection of herpes simplex virus and with cytospin direct immunofluorescence staining for detection of varicella-zoster virus. Clin Diagn Lab Immunol. 2001;8(5):909–12.
54. Zaki S, Shieh W, Greer P, Goldsmith C, Ferebee T, Katshitshi J, et al. A novel immunohistochemical assay for the detection of

ebola virus in skin: implications for diagnosis, spread, and surveillance of ebola hemorrhagic fever. J Infect Dis. 1999;179S: 36–47.

55. Smedley RC, Patterson JS, Miller R, Massey JP, Wise AG, Maes RK, et al. Sensitivity and specificity of monoclonal and polyclonal immunohistochemical staining for West Nile virus in various organs from American crows (*Corvus brachyrhynchos*). BMC Infect Dis. 2007;7:49.
56. Bhatnagar J, Guarner J, Paddock CD, Shieh WJ, Lanciotti RS, Marfin AA, et al. Detection of West Nile virus in formalin-fixed, paraffin-embedded human tissues by RT-PCR: a useful adjunct to conventional tissue-based diagnostic methods. J Clin Virol. 2007;38(2):106–11.
57. Bialek R, Ernst F, Dietz K, Najvar LK, Knobloch J, Graybill JR, et al. Comparison of staining methods and a nested PCR assay to detect *Histoplasma capsulatum* in tissue sections. Am J Clin Pathol. 2002;117(4):597–603.
58. Verweij PE, Smedts F, Poot T, Bult P, Hoogkamp-Korstanje JA, Meis JF. Immunoperoxidase staining for identification of *Aspergillus* species in routinely processed tissue sections. J Clin Pathol. 1996;49(10):798–801.
59. Schuetz AN, Cohen C. *Aspergillus* immunohistochemistry of culture-proven fungal tissue isolates shows high cross-reactivity. Appl Immunohistochem Mol Morphol. 2009;17(6):524–9.
60. Fukuzawa M, Inaba H, Hayama M, Sakaguchi N, Sano K, Ito M, et al. Improved detection of medically important fungi by immunoperoxidase staining with polyclonal antibodies. Virchows Arch. 1995;427(4):407–14.
61. Hayden RT, Qian X, Roberts GD, Lloyd RV. In situ hybridization for the identification of yeast-like organisms in tissue sections. Diagn Mol Pathol. 2001;10(1):15–23.
62. Hayden RT, Qian X, Procop GW, et al. In situ hybridization for the identification of filamentous fungi in tissue sections. Diagn Mol Pathol. 2002;11(2):119–26.
63. Blumenfeld W, Kovacs JA. Use of a monoclonal antibody to detect *Pneumocystis carinii* in induced sputum and bronchoalveolar lavage fluid by immunoperoxidase staining. Arch Pathol Lab Med. 1988;112(12):1233–6.
64. Arastéh KN, Simon V, Musch R, Weiss RO, Przytarski K, Futh UM, et al. Sensitivity and specificity of indirect immunofluorescence and Grocott-technique in comparison with immunocytology (alkaline phosphatase anti alkaline phosphatase = APAAP) for the diagnosis of *Pneumocystis carinii* in broncho-alveolar lavage (BAL). Eur J Med Res. 1998;3(12):559–63.
65. Amato VS, Tuon FF, de Andrade HF, Jr BH, Pagliari C, Fernandes ER, et al. Immunohistochemistry and polymerase chain reaction on paraffin-embedded material improve the diagnosis of cutaneous leishmaniasis in the Amazon region. Int J Dermatol. 2009;48(10):1091–5.

Chapter 30
Skin

Tammie Ferringer

Abstract Correlation of the clinical history and histopathology are typically sufficient for accurate diagnosis in dermatopathology. However, in cases where this alone is insufficient, immunohistochemistry can further characterize lesions in the differential diagnosis. As with all immunohistochemical markers, none of those used in dermatopathology are completely sensitive and specific, therefore appropriate selection of a panel of antibodies maximizes the likelihood of making an accurate diagnosis.

The majority of studies evaluating immunohistochemical antibodies are limited to small numbers of cases with variable antibody sources, antigen retrieval methods, and definition of reactivity resulting in inconsistent results. The following chapter summarizes the general trends reported for several of the common conundrums in cutaneous pathology including differentiating spitzoid melanocytic lesions, small blue cell tumors, spindle cell lesions of the skin, sclerosing epithelial neoplasms, and lesions with pagetoid intraepidermal scatter.

Keywords Melanoma • Merkel cell carcinoma • Atypical fibroxanthoma • Cutaneous squamous cell carcinoma • Cellular neurothekeoma • Spitz nevus • Dermatofibroma • Dermatofibrosarcoma protuberans • Cutaneous leiomyosarcoma • Lymphoma • Metastatic small cell lung carcinoma • Paget's disease • Morpheaform basal cell carcinoma • Desmoplastic trichoepithelioma • Microcystic adnexal carcinoma • Sclerosing epithelial neoplasms • Cutaneous adnexal tumors • Metastatic adenocarcinoma to the skin

FREQUENTLY ASKED QUESTIONS

T. Ferringer (✉)
Department of Pathology and Laboratory Medicine, Geisinger Medical Center, 100 N. Academy Ave, Danville, PA 17822, USA

F. Lin and J. Prichard (eds.), *Handbook of Practical Immunohistochemistry: Frequently Asked Questions*,
DOI 10.1007/978-1-4419-8062-5_30,

Table 30.1 Summary of applications and limitations of useful markers

Antibodies	Staining pattern	Function	Key applications and pitfalls
AE1/AE3	C	Epithelial marker; cocktail of high and low molecular weight cytokeratins	Useful in the differential of cutaneous spindle cell neoplasm but does not stain all spindle cell SCCs
CK7	C	Epithelial marker	Positive in Paget's, extramammary Paget's, metastatic breast and lung carcinoma
CK20	C	Marker of gastric and intestinal epithelium, urothelium, and Merkel cells	Positive in metastatic colon carcinoma; positive in Merkel cell carcinoma
EMA	M + C	Epithelial marker; one of human milk fat globule proteins	Marks sebaceous and sweat glands and their neoplasms; positive in sclerosing perineuroma and rudimentary meningocele; labels plasma cells but not a problem distinguishing cytologically
CEA	C	Expressed in various adenocarcinomas and normal glandular epithelium	Marks sweat glands and their neoplasms
Ber-EP4	M + C	Epithelial marker; marks all epithelial cells except the superficial layers of epidermis	Positive in BCC, but negative in SCC
Desmin	C	Skeletal and smooth muscle except vascular smooth muscle	Useful in differential of spindle cell neoplasms of the skin
SMA	C	Labels smooth muscle, including vascular smooth muscle	Stains myofibroblasts, myoepithelial cells, and glomus cells
CD34	M + C	Endothelial and hematopoietic progenitor cell marker; highlights some fibrohistiocytic tumors	Stains vascular tumors and DFSP and also other tumors, including neurofibroma and solitary fibrous tumor
Factor XIIIa	C	Dermal dendrocyte marker	Positive in dermatofibromas
CD31	M+ weak C	Endothelial marker	More specific vascular marker than CD34
D2-40 (podoplanin)	C	Lymphatic endothelial marker	Can help identify lymphatic invasion of tumors
Vimentin	C	Mesenchymal marker, including endothelial cells, all fibroblastic cells, macrophages, melanocytes, vascular smooth muscle, and lymphocytes. Found in all types of sarcoma and lymphoma	In the appropriate panel, positivity excludes most carcinomas
S100	N + C	Neural crest marker: highlights melanocytes, Langerhans cells, sweat glands, nerves, Schwann cells, lipocytes, myoepithelial cells, muscle	Most sensitive melanoma marker, especially for spindle/desmoplastic melanoma, but not specific; for differential identification the use of a panel of antibodies is necessary
HMB-45	C	Recognizes the antigen gp100 expressed on stages 1–3 melanosomes (organelle, rather than lineage-specific marker); indicates active melanosome formation, not present in resting adult melanocytes	Reveals a gradient with decreased staining in the deeper dermal component of benign nevi (Fig. 30.1), with the exception of uniform staining in blue nevi; not reliable in desmoplastic or spindled melanoma; negative or weak in nodal nevi; positive in PEComas
MART-1	C	Melanocytic marker	More specific melanocytic marker than S100 but less sensitive, especially for spindle/desmoplastic melanoma; two antibodies detect the same protein at two different antigenic sites: A-103 (Melan-A) and MART-1; macrophages may aberrantly label with some antigen retrieval techniques, however, the staining is weak and granular
MITF	N	Transcription factor involved in the development of melanocytes and regulation of melanin synthesis; nuclear melanocytic marker	Nuclear staining avoids distraction of cytoplasmic staining of dendritic, overlapping melanocytes when evaluating junctional melanocytic proliferations (Fig. 30.2); positive in most PEComas and can stain histiocytes, lymphocytes, and smooth muscle cells
S100A6 (calcyclin)	N + C	Belongs to family of S100 calcium-binding proteins	Strongly and diffusely positive in Spitz nevi but weak, patchy, or negative in melanoma; stains fibrohistiocytic lesions
NSE	C	Neural and neuroendocrine marker	If neoplastic cells co-express keratin and NSE, neuroendocrine differentiation is probable; positive in Merkel cell carcinoma

(continued)

Table 30.1 (continued)

Antibodies	Staining pattern	Function	Key applications and pitfalls
GLUT-1	C + M	Major glucose transporter at the blood–brain barrier	Reactive in all phases of infantile hemangioma but absent in vascular malformations
Mib-1 (Ki-67)	N	Nuclear proliferation marker; expression in cells in the G1, M, G2, and S phase of the cell cycle (i.e., all phases except the resting G0 phase)	Useful in determining proliferation index in dermal component of melanocytic lesions and other tumors of uncertain malignant potential; not lineage specific so also stains proliferating lymphocytes requiring distinction by cytology or dual staining

Note: *C* cytoplasmic staining, *M* membranous staining, *N* nuclear staining, *SMA* smooth muscle actin, *EMA* epithelial membrane antigen, *CEA* carcinoembryonic antigen, *SCC* squamous cell carcinoma, *BCC* basal cell carcinoma, *DFSP* dermatofibrosarcoma protuberans, *NSE* neuron-specific enolase, *MART-1* melanoma antigen recognized by T-cells, *MITF* microphthalmia transcription factor, *PEComas* perivascular epithelioid cell tumors

References: [1–24, 48–53, 149]

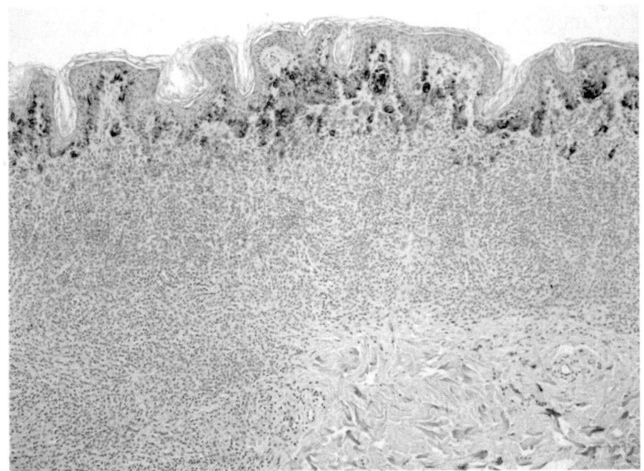

Fig. 30.1 Gradient of decreased expression of HMB-45 with increased depth into the dermis of a benign nevus

Fig. 30.2 Nuclear staining of melanocytes in malignant melanoma in situ with MITF

Table 30.2 Markers for primary cutaneous melanoma

Antibodies	Literature	GML% (*N*)
S100	+[a]	93.4% (91)
HMB-45	+	75% (88)
MART-1	+	88.8% (89)
MITF	+	79.8% (89)
Tyrosinase	+[a]	94.3% (88)
NKI-C3	+[a]	95.5% (88)
PNL2	+	87.1% (85)
SM5-1	+[a]	NA
MUM-1	+[a]	75.6% (86)
SOX-10	+[a]	NA

Note: [a]Greater than 90% of cases are positive

N number studied, *NA* not available

GML% – Geisinger Medical Laboratories data, percentage of melanomas with greater than 25% reactivity

Immunohistochemical markers are virtually never completely specific and sensitive. The published literature on immunohistochemistry of melanoma often is limited to small numbers of cases and the types of melanoma tested (nodular, metastatic, spindle, desmoplastic, etc) varies between studies. The definition of positive reactivity, the antibody source, antigen retrieval methods, and concentrations vary from study to study often resulting in inconsistent results

Table 30.2 (continued)

While the great majority of melanomas are S100 positive, this marker lacks specificity and stains other tissue. Therefore, other antibodies are needed to confirm the melanocytic nature of a S100 positive neoplasm. Tyrosinase has decreased sensitivity with increasing stage and in metastatic lesions. NKI-C3 has poor specificity

Reactivity with melanocytic markers may be less in metastatic melanoma. Spindle/desmoplastic melanomas are often negative for HMB-45 and other specific melanocytic markers. S100 is the most sensitive marker for spindle/desmoplastic melanoma

MITF, MUM-1, and SOX-10 are nuclear markers. This avoids the overlapping cytoplasmic staining of dendritic melanocytes when evaluating junctional melanocytic proliferations (Fig. 30.2)

MUM-1 is primarily used in the workup of hematologic malignancies and is not in routine use for melanoma. Similarly, PNL2 is not yet in widespread use. It superficially stains common nevi and diffusely blue nevi, similar to HMB-45

SM5-1 is a monoclonal antibody developed from mice immunized with melanoma cell lines. There have been limited investigations of its use. It also stains dendritic cells, myofibroblasts, and plasma cells. SOX-10 is a recently described neural crest transcription factor crucial for specification, maturation, and maintenance of Schwann cells and melanocytes. It is also expressed in mast cells, Schwann cells, and myoepithelial cells. None of these newer markers have shown significant advantages over the markers in current use

Mib-1 highlights the nuclei of proliferating cells, including melanocytes. There is increased expression from benign to malignant melanocytic lesions, particularly in the dermal component

Pigmented melanocytes can be difficult to distinguish from pigmented keratinocytes and melanophages. The brown diethylaminobenzidine (DAB) chromogen can be difficult to identify in a background of dense melanin (Fig. 30.3). Alternatives include:

1. Use of aminoethylcarbazole (AEC) resulting in a red product, which is slightly easier to distinguish but can lack the longevity of DAB
2. Melanin bleaching may result in loss of antigenicity, incomplete melanin removal, or loss of cytologic detail
3. Kamino et al. were the first to report replacement of hematoxylin by azure B, which stains the melanin green-blue providing contrast from DAB staining of melanocytes (Fig. 30.4)

Rarely melanomas can exhibit aberrant expression, including smooth muscle actin, CD138, MDM-2, GFAP, CD30, and EMA. CEA reactivity can be seen in melanoma with the polyclonal antibody. Over half of melanomas express CD68. Cytokeratin expression occurs in up to 4% of malignant melanomas with staining tending to be focal and sparse. CAM5.2 is the most frequently positive. There is increased aberrant expression of epithelial-associated markers in metastases. Use of a panel of immunostains, including the previous mentioned melanocytic markers should prevent misdiagnosis

References: [1, 15, 25–64]

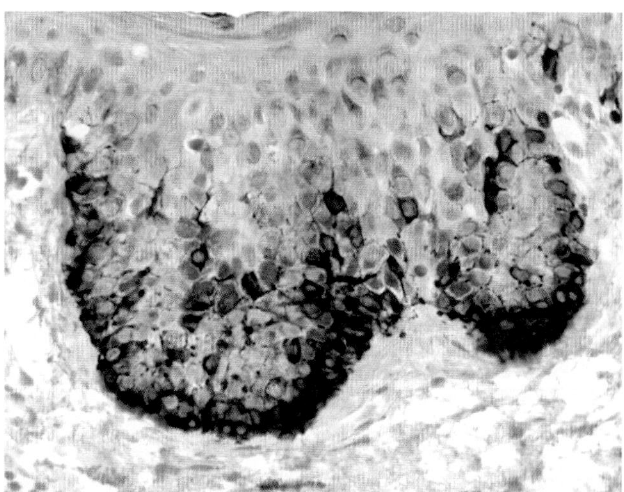

Fig. 30.3 Junctional dysplastic nevus stained with MART-1 using DAB brown chromogen in background of heavy melanin pigmentation of the basal layer keratinocytes

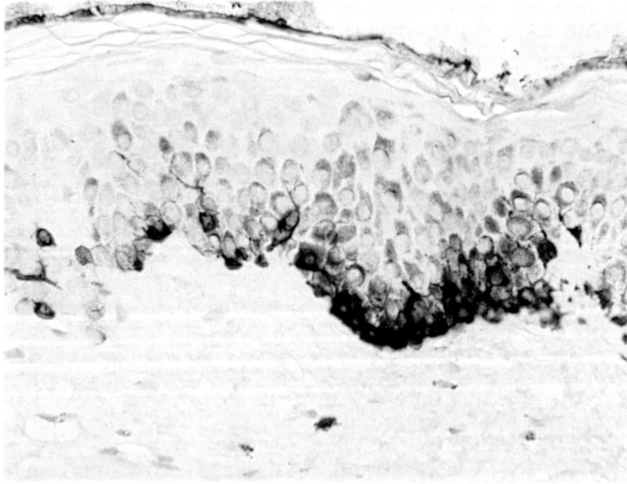

Fig. 30.4 Same heavily pigmented junctional dysplastic nevus as in Fig. 30.3 stained with MART-1 using DAB brown chromogen and azure B counterstain. The melanin is now green-blue and contrasts easily with the DAB brown chromogen

Table 30.3 Markers for Merkel cell carcinoma (MCC)

Antibodies	Literature
NSE	+[a]
Chromogranin	+/–
Synaptophysin	+/–
CK20	+[a]
TTF-1	–
Ber-EP4	+
CD56	+[a]
LCA	–
S100	–/+
CD99	–/+
NFP	+/–
CK7	–/+
Fli-1	–/+
PAX-5	+
Bcl-2	+
TdT	+/–
CD117	+/–

Note: [a]Greater than 90% of cases are positive

TTF-1 thyroid transcription factor, *LCA* leukocyte common antigen (CD45), *NFP* neurofilament protein, CD56 = *NCAM* (neural cell adhesion molecule)

The small blue cell appearance of MCC results in a histologic differential diagnosis including metastatic small cell carcinoma from a primary in the lung or other site, lymphoma, and small cell melanoma. TTF-1 is a nuclear marker expressed in thyroid and pulmonary neoplasms, including small cell carcinoma of the lung and is not identified in MCC. Melanoma can be distinguished by S100 and lymphomas by CD45. The overlapping reactivity of MCC and some hematologic malignancies with CD99, TdT, PAX-5, CD56, Bcl-2, and CD117 can complicate diagnosis of these small blue cell neoplasms. Inclusion of epithelial and neuroendocrine markers in the immunohistochemical panel should avoid confusion

Ewing's sarcoma/primitive neuroectodermal tumor (EWS/PNET) and neuroblastoma are very rare in the skin but have a similar histologic appearance. It is important to recognize that CD99 and Fli-1, markers of EWS/PNET, can be positive in MCC. Ber-EP4 and Bcl-2 reactivity in MCC can be a pitfall if basal cell carcinoma (BCC) is considered in the histologic differential diagnosis, as both are positive in BCC (Fig. 30.5)

CK20 typically highlights aggregates of keratin near the nucleus in a characteristic paranuclear dot pattern (Fig. 30.6). However, in some cases of MCC diffuse cytoplasmic staining predominates. NFP also often has a dot-like pattern in MCC

References: [5, 46, 65–93]

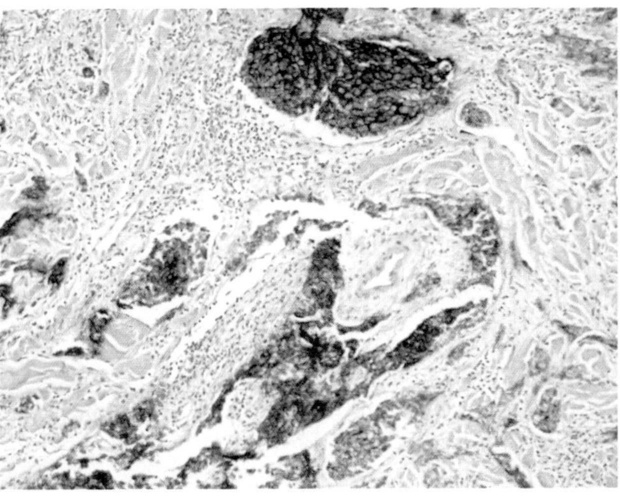

Fig. 30.5 MCC staining with Ber-EP4 can be a potential pitfall if basal cell carcinoma is considered in the differential diagnosis

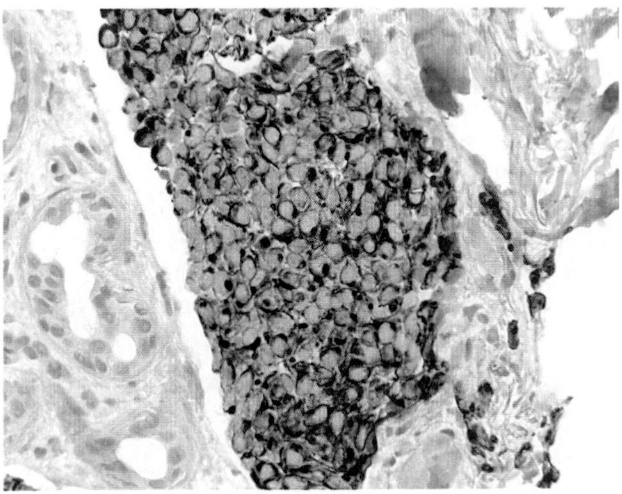

Fig. 30.6 MCC with the typical paranuclear dot pattern with CK20

Table 30.4 Markers for atypical fibroxanthoma (AFX)

Antibodies	Literature
SMA	–/+
Vimentin	+[a]
S100	–
Cytokeratin	–
Desmin	–
S100A6	+
CD10	+[a]
Procollagen (PC-1)	+
CD68	+/–
CD99	+/–
A1AT	+/–
A1ACT	+/–
NKI-C3	+/–
HMB-45	–
EMA	–/+
Factor XIIIa	–/+

Note: [a]Greater than 90% of cases are positive

A1AT alpha-1 antitrypsin, *A1ACT* alpha-1 antichymotrypsin

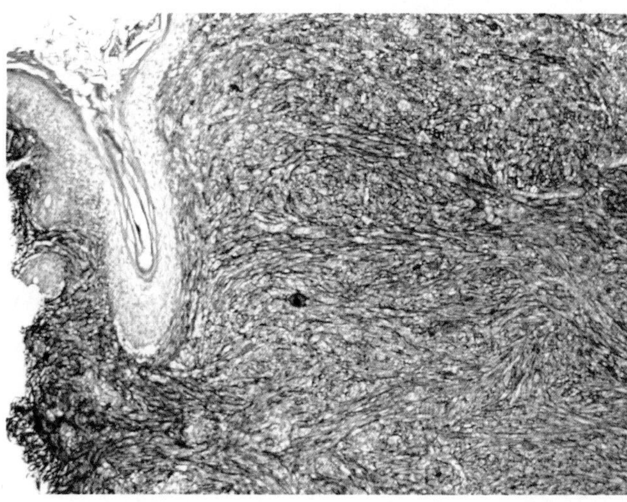

Fig. 30.7 AFX staining with CD10

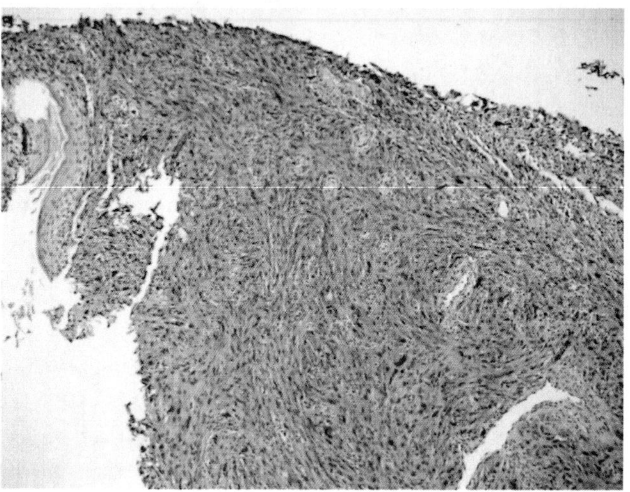

Fig. 30.8 AFX staining with S100A6

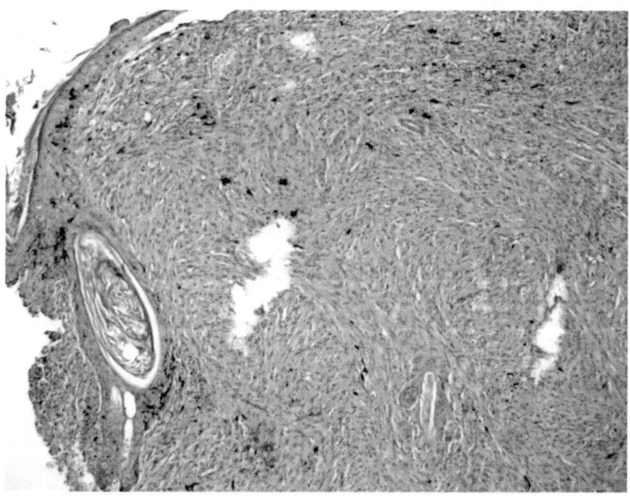

Fig. 30.9 In contrast to the diffuse S100A6 staining in Fig. 30.8, there is an absence of staining with S100 in AFX

AFX is a pleomorphic spindle cell tumor that must be distinguished histologically from spindle or desmoplastic melanoma, spindle cell squamous cell carcinoma, and leiomyosarcoma. While there are immunohistochemical stains that support the later diagnoses, the diagnosis of AFX is generally one of the exclusion. A variety of markers have shown reactivity in AFX, including CD10 (Fig. 30.7) and S100A6 (Fig. 30.8), but these antibodies often stain a variety of other neoplasms and are not specific. For example, CD10, S100A6, and PC-1 also highlight dermatofibromas. Rather than relying on one of these antibodies in isolation, a panel of markers is required to exclude the potential mimics (see Table 30.7). Therefore, AFXs have been defined in the past by the absence of S100 (Fig. 30.9), cytokeratins, and desmin. Occasional atypical spindle cell neoplasms stain with CD10 and/or PC-1, as well as a cytokeratin marker but this is the great minority. The true identity in these cases is uncertain

Focal or weak expression of myogenic markers, indicative of myofibroblastic differentiation, can be seen in AFX. Caution is required in interpreting S100 in atypical spindle cell neoplasms of the skin. There are often scattered S100 positive dendritic cells colonizing AFXs (possibly Langerhans cells) but the neoplastic cells are generally S100 negative (Fig. 30.9)

CD117 reactivity has been reported in AFX, however, it typically highlights a small percentage of dendritic cells that are not highly atypical and many believe represent colonizing cells such as mast cells or Langerhans cells. Therefore, this is not a reliable marker for AFX

References: [19, 87, 94–112, 135]

Table 30.5 Markers for cutaneous spindle cell squamous cell carcinoma (SCSCC)

Antibodies	Literature
AE1/AE3	+
CAM5.2	+/–
CK903	+
CK5/6	+
MNF116	+[a]
p63	+
S100	–
Desmin	–

Note: [a]Greater than 90% of cases are positive

AE1/AE3: Recognizes a mixture of high and low molecular weight cytokeratins 1–6, 8, 10, 14, 15, 16, and 19

CAM5.2: Low molecular weight antibody to cytokeratins 8, 18, and 19

CK903 (34betaE12): High molecular weight antibody to cytokeratins 1, 5, 10, and 14

MNF116: Antibody to cytokeratins 5, 6, 8, 17, and 19

SCSCCs often fail to have an obvious origin from the epidermis or show evidence of keratinization. Due to similarities with AFX, spindle or desmoplastic melanoma, and leiomyosarcoma immunohistochemical confirmation may be required

SCSCCs are often negative or only focally positive with routine cytokeratin stains, including AE1/AE3 (Fig. 30.10) and may express only high molecular weight cytokeratins. The current data suggests that CK5/6, MNF116, and CK903 may be superior to standard cytokeratins in identifying SCSCCs. However, the literature contains studies involving a limited numbers of cases

While vimentin is a mesenchymal marker, co-expression with keratins can be seen in some epithelial tumors, including SCSCCs, possibly due to reduced cell-to-cell contact

p63, a member of the p53 gene family, is a transcription factor involved in the proliferative capacity of epidermal stem cells. It is normally expressed in keratinocytes of the basal and lower spinous layers but is generally not expressed in mesenchymal cells and their neoplasms. This nuclear marker is useful for SCSCC but is not completely specific (Fig. 30.11)

References: [6, 18, 94, 95, 113–115, 135]

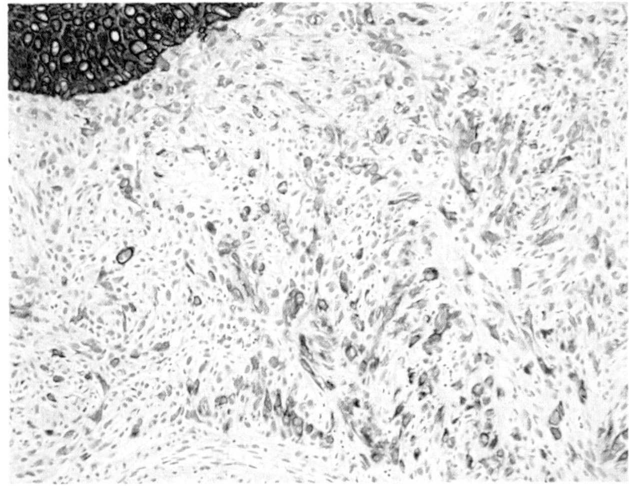

Fig. 30.10 Spindle cell squamous cell carcinoma focally staining with AE1/AE3

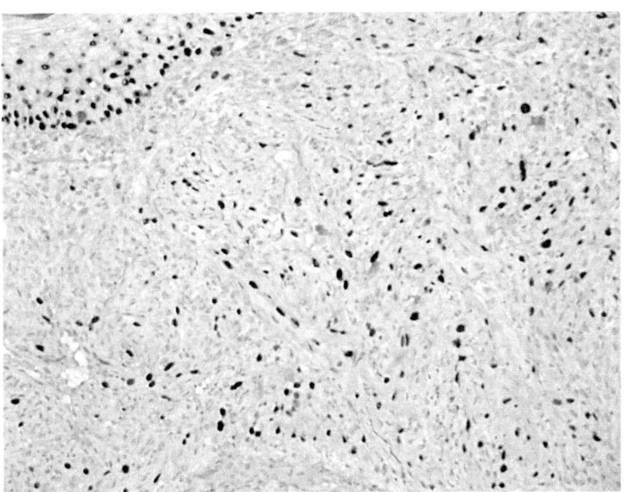

Fig. 30.11 Nuclear staining with p63 in spindle cell squamous cell carcinoma

Table 30.6 Markers for cellular neurothekeoma (CNT)

Antibodies	Literature
S100	–
S100A6	+[a]
SMA	–/+
CD68	+/–
CD10	+[a]
HMB-45	–
NKI-C3 (CD63)	+[a]
MITF	+
PGP9.5	+/–
D2-40 (podoplanin)	+[a]
NSE	+
CD99	+

Note: [a]Greater than 90% of cases are positive

There are three subtypes of neurothekeoma: myxoid, cellular (Fig. 30.12), and mixed. While myxoid neurothekeoma (nerve sheath myxoma) is S100 positive, CNT are negative, suggesting that they are not of peripheral nerve sheath or melanocytic histogenesis, however, the true lineage is uncertain. The absence of S100 is important in differentiating CNT from a melanocytic lesion (Fig. 30.13). Typical melanocytic markers, including S100, HMB-45 and MART-1, are negative in CNT, while other less specific melanocytic markers, such as MITF and NKI-C3 have been identified. In contrast to S100, CNT are S100A6 positive (Fig. 30.14). However, limited numbers of lesions have been studied. Similarly, there is limited data on CD10 and D2-40. While S100A6, CD10, NKI-C3, and D2-40 have been expressed in the great majority of those studied, none of these markers are specific for CNT

References: [116–125]

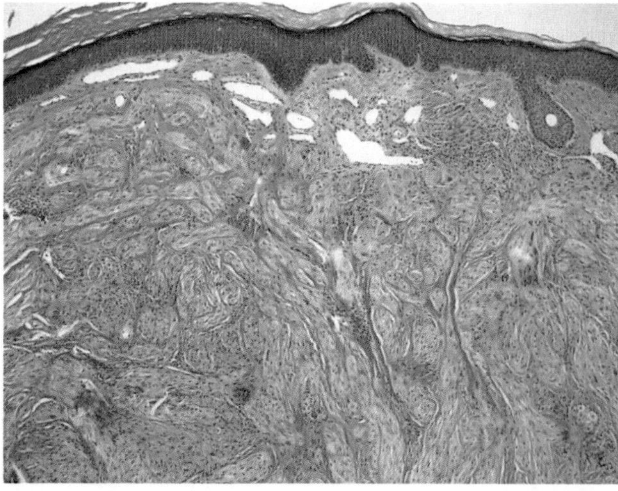

Fig. 30.12 Hematoxylin and eosin-stained sections of a cellular neurothekeoma

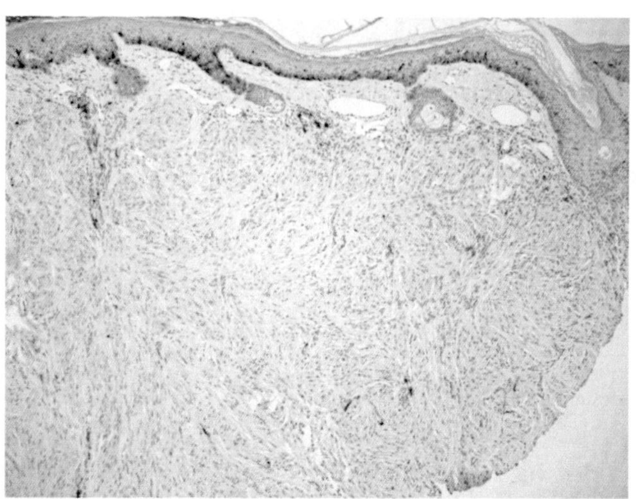

Fig. 30.13 In contrast to the diffuse S100A6 staining in Fig. 30.14, there is an absence of staining with S100 in cellular neurothekeoma

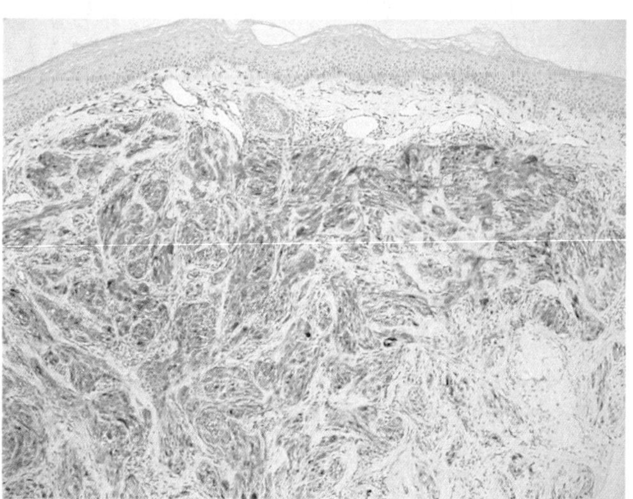

Fig. 30.14 Diffuse S100A6 reactivity in cellular neurothekeoma

Table 30.7 Markers for cutaneous spindle cell neoplasms

Antibodies	AFX	sMM	sSCC	Lms
AE1:AE3	–	–	+	–/+
CK903	–	–	+	–
S100	–	+[a]	–	–/+
Desmin	–	–	–	+
Vimentin	+[a]	+[a]	–/+	+[a]
S100A6	+	+[a]	+[a]	+
PC-1	+	–/+	–/+	+
P75NTR	–	+[a]	–	NA
CD10	+[a]	–/+	–/+	NA
p63	–/+	–/+	+	–/+
CD99	+/–	–/+	–/+	NA
SMA	–/+	–	–	+[a]

Note: [a]Greater than 90% of cases are positive

PC-1 procollagen-1, *AFX* atypical fibroxanthoma, *sMM* spindle cell melanoma, *sSCC* spindle cell squamous cell carcinoma, *Lms* leiomyosarcoma, *NA* not available

The differential diagnosis of atypical spindle cell neoplasms on sun-damaged skin includes AFX, sMM, sSCC, and Lms. Due to potential overlapping reactivity and rare anomalous expression, a panel prevents misdiagnosis

Table 30.7 (continued)

Some melanocytic markers, including HMB-45 and MART-1, are often negative in spindle/desmoplastic melanomas (Figs. 30.15 and 30.16). S100 is the most sensitive marker for spindle/desmoplastic melanoma (Fig. 30.17)

Desmoplastic melanoma may require differentiation from scar tissue, especially in the context of a re-excision specimen or possible recurrence. Based on the high sensitivity, S100 is often used in this context. Care is required in interpretation as scars often contain S100 positive spindle cells but unlike in melanoma, are focal and predominantly in a horizontal pattern (Fig. 30.18). P75 offers the advantage of high sensitivity in desmoplastic melanoma (Fig. 30.19) and lack of expression in scars. P75 expression is strongest in desmoplastic melanomas with less consistent reactivity in other types of melanoma. However, p75 is not specific to desmoplastic melanoma and is seen in other malignant spindle cell tumors

References: [16–19, 50, 59, 94–99, 101–107, 113–115, 126–135]

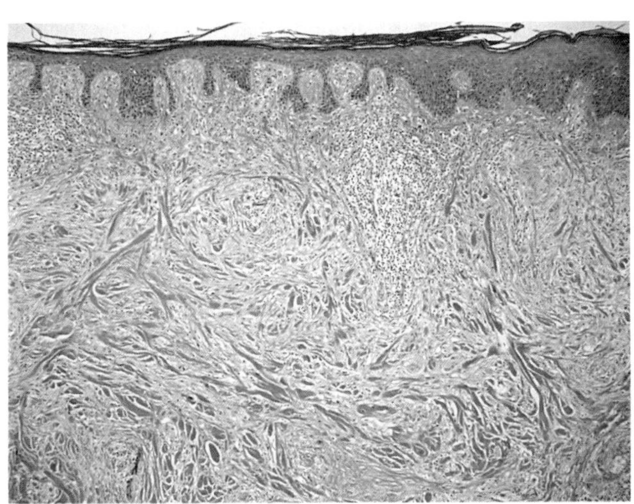

Fig. 30.15 Hematoxylin and eosin-stained sections of desmoplastic melanoma

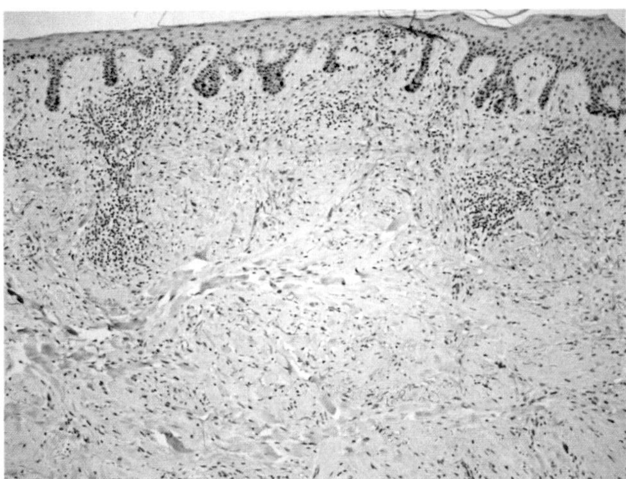

Fig. 30.16 Desmoplastic melanoma is often negative with MART-1

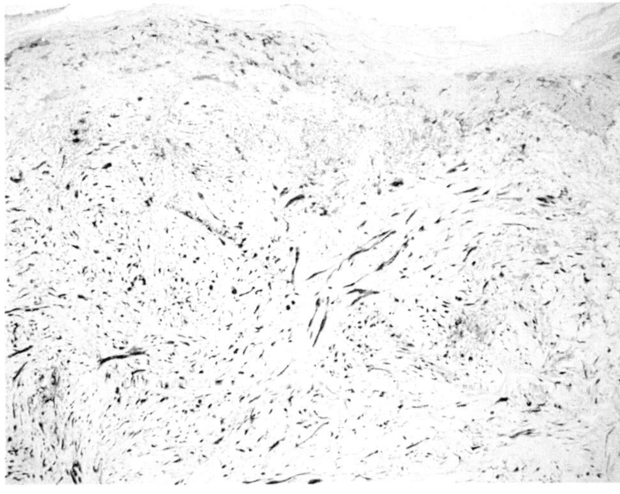

Fig. 30.17 Desmoplastic melanoma staining with S100

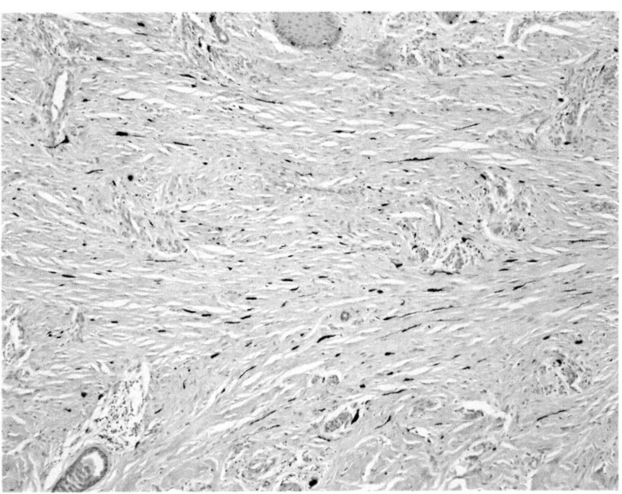

Fig. 30.18 S100 highlighting sparse horizontally oriented spindle cells within a scar. This should not be confused with desmoplastic melanoma

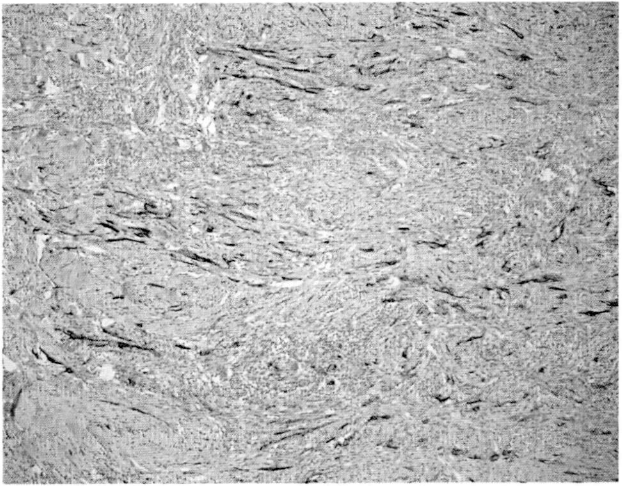

Fig. 30.19 Desmoplastic melanoma staining with p75

Table 30.8 Markers for cutaneous small blue cell tumors

Antibodies	MCC	MM	Mets SCCL
S100	−/+	+[a]	−
NSE	+[a]	+	+/−
CK20	+[a]	−	−
TTF-1	−	−	+[a]
NFP	+/−	NA	−
FLI-1	−/+	−/+	−/+

Note: [a]Greater than 90% of cases are positive

NSE neuron-specific enolase, *NFP* neurofilament protein, *MCC* Merkel cell carcinoma, *MM* malignant melanoma, *Mets SCCL* metastatic small cell carcinoma of the lung, *NA* not available

Small blue cell tumors are composed of round closely packed cells with a high nuclear to cytoplasmic ratio. The histologic differential diagnosis includes neoplasms of vastly different lineages. The most common small blue cell tumor on sun-damaged skin is MCC. Other neoplasms that can have similar cytology include MM, metastatic SCCL, lymphoma, and less commonly involving the skin; Ewing sarcoma/primitive neuroectodermal tumor (EWS/PNET), metastatic neuroblastoma, and rhabdomyosarcoma

Desmin and myogenin identify rhabdomyosarcoma. Lymphoma can be distinguished by lymphoid markers: CD79a, CD3, CD19, and leukocyte common antigen (CD45). EWS/PNET can express S100, NSE, chromogranin, and synaptophysin. CD99 is a marker for EWS/PNET but is not specific and is also seen in lymphoblastic lymphoma, select rhabdomyosarcomas, and small numbers of MCC and MM. FLI-1 antibody is a useful nuclear marker for EWS/PNET, as well as an endothelial marker, but is also expressed in a subset of lymphoma, MCC, SCCL, and MM. Keratin reactivity, particularly CK20, is usually absent in EWS/PNET. Neuroblastoma can express NSE, NFP, synaptophysin, and chromogranin but is usually negative with CD99, CD45, S100, keratins, and skeletal muscle markers

The presence of TTF-1 reactivity is not completely specific to SCCL and can be seen in metastatic small cell carcinoma of extrapulmonary sites, however, it is consistently negative in MCC

Ber-EP4 and bcl-2 reactivity in MCC can be a pitfall if basal cell carcinoma (BCC) is considered in the histologic differential diagnosis (Fig. 30.5). BCCs are negative with S100, CK20, and TTF-1

References: [5, 18, 30, 46, 66, 67, 70, 74, 78–80, 92, 117, 136–141]

Table 30.9 Markers for intra-epidermal or pagetoid scatter

Antibodies	EMPD	SCCIS	MMIS
CEA	+[a]	−	−
S100	−	−	+[a]
CK7	+[a]	−/+	−
EMA	+[a]	+/−	−
CAM5.2	+	−/+	−
Ber-EP4	+	−	−

Note: [a]Greater than 90% of cases are positive

EMPD extramammary Paget's disease, *SCCIS* squamous cell carcinoma in situ, *MMIS* malignant melanoma in situ

EMPD, SCCIS, and MMIS are the most common causes of an atypical intraepidermal pagetoid pattern. Typically, the correct diagnosis can be made on morphology alone. However, in some cases, a panel of immunohistochemical markers is required. The presence of CEA or Ber-EP4 favors EMPD. The percentage of reactivity varies between polyclonal and monoclonal CEA and between EMPD and Paget's disease of the nipple. EMPD is rarely S100 positive but expression has been reported in Paget's disease of the nipple

Positivity with CK7 supports a diagnosis of EMPD (Fig. 30.20), however, CK7 positive SCCIS has been reported. In addition, CK7+ Toker cells and occasionally CK7+ Merkel cells can be seen in the normal epidermis complicating interpretation

Isolated studies have reported CD23 and CD5 reactivity in EMPD, in contrast to absent expression in both MMIS and SCCIS

EMPD is a heterogeneous entity that encompasses case that are limited to the skin and others that are associated with underlying malignancy. This can result in variations in immunohistochemical expression. CK20 is negative in the majority of primary cutaneous EMPD but can be positive in cases with underlying regional malignancy. Similarly, CDX-2 expression suggests an association with underlying rectal carcinoma. On the other hand, GCDFP-15 is more commonly expressed in primary cutaneous EMPD than those associated with underlying malignancy. However, like Paget's disease of the nipple, not all cases of primary cutaneous EMPD are positive with GCDFP-15. Positive expression can help differentiate EMPD or Paget's disease from SCCIS, which has not shown reactivity with GCDFP-15

References: [7, 142–161]

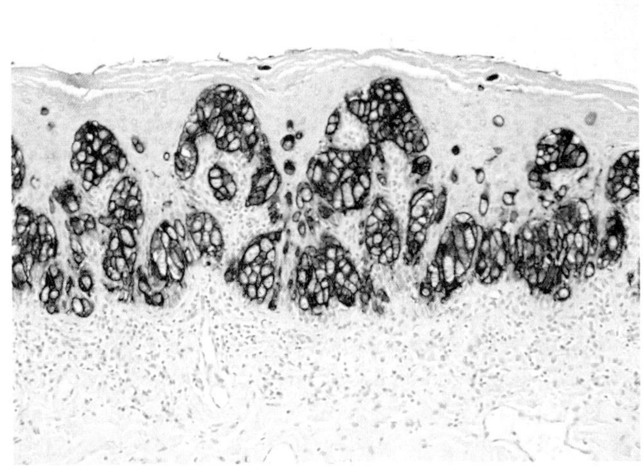

Fig. 30.20 EMPD stained with CK7

Table 30.10 Markers for sclerosing epithelial neoplasms

Antibodies	mBCC	DTE	MAC
CD10	Neoplasm	Stroma	–/+ (neoplasm)
CD34 (stroma)	–/+	+	–
Bcl-2	+[a]	+	–/+
CK20[b]	–	+[a]	–
Mib-1 rate	20–40%	0–13%	<5%
AR	+/–	–	NA
CK15	–	+[a]	+[a]
SMA	+/–	–	+
Stromelysin-3 (stroma)	+	–	NA
Ber-EP4	+[a]	+/–	–/+
CK7	–/+	–	+/–
EMA	–	–/+	+/–
P53	+	–	–/+
CD23	–	–	–/+

mBCC morpheaform basal cell carcinoma, *DTE* desmoplastic trichoepithelioma, *MAC* microcystic adnexal carcinoma, *AR* androgen receptor, *SMA* smooth muscle actin, *EMA* epithelial membrane antigen, *NA* not available

Mib-1, AR, and p53 are nuclear markers

Partial samples of sclerosing epithelial neoplasm can be difficult to classify. Differentiation is not only of academic interest but is also paramount to clinical management. Numerous markers have been evaluated in this context but the great majority evaluated very small numbers of tumors in this differential

When present, CEA positive ductal lumina strongly favor MAC over DTE or mBCC. The pathologist must distinguish expression within the tumor from expression in background sweat ducts

The pattern of reactivity of bcl-2 differs between DTE and mBCC. The tumor islands are diffusely positive in BCC, whereas, typically only the periphery of the basaloid islands is positive in DTE. Focal positivity with bcl-2 has been reported in MAC

Table 30.10 (continued)

Stromelysin 3 is a member of the metalloproteinase family, which is expressed in the stroma of carcinomas. The rate of positivity is highest in the stroma of morpheaform and deeply invasive BCCs. Similarly, SMA reactivity is greatest in the epithelial component of the more aggressive forms of BCC, including morpheaform, micronodular, and infiltrative subtypes

Although there is conflicting data, Pham et al. found that CD10 staining of the basaloid cells favors mBCC over DTE, while expression in the peritumoral stroma favors DTE

References: [7, 13, 159, 162–180]

Note:

[a]Greater than 90% of cases are positive

[b]CK20 highlights sparse Merkel cells colonizing DTE (Fig. 30.21), not the stroma or basaloid neoplastic cells. Merkel cells are not typically identified colonizing morpheaform basal cell carcinomas (Fig. 30.22)

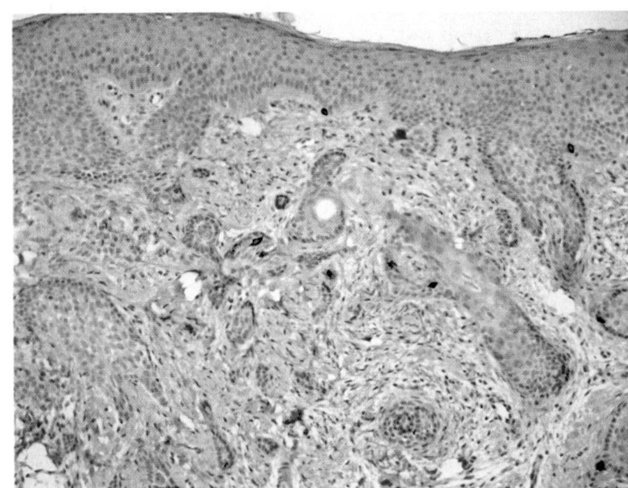

Fig. 30.21 CK20 highlights Merkel cells colonizing DTE

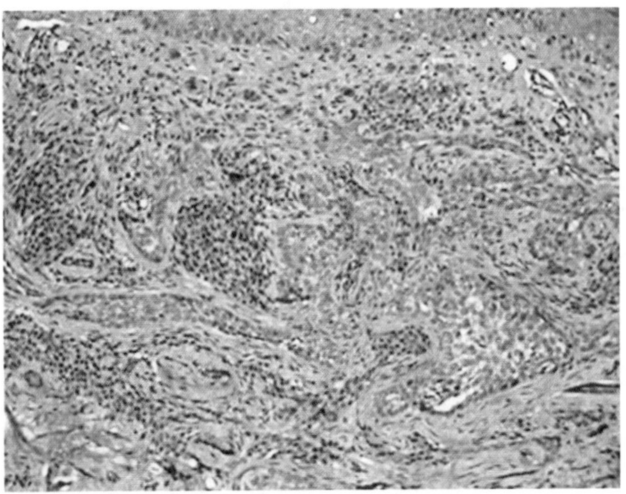

Fig. 30.22 CK20 positive Merkel cells are not identified in mBCC

Table 30.11 Spitz nevus vs. spitzoid melanoma

Antibodies	Spitz	Spitzoid MM
S100A6 (calcyclin)	Strong and diffuse	Weak and patchy
HMB-45	Gradient	No gradient
Mib-1	1.5–5%	13–37%
p16	>40%	<20%
CD99	Variable	Strong and diffuse
p21	>40%	<30%

Note: *MM* malignant melanoma

Differentiating Spitz nevus from spitzoid melanoma can be problematic, even for experts in the field. Misdiagnosis of melanoma as a Spitz nevus is one of the most common causes of malpractice lawsuits in pathology. Many immunohistochemical markers have been investigated to aid in distinguishing Spitz nevus from melanoma without identification of a consistent and reliable method. While overlap exists, general trends have been identified with some markers

S100A6 (calcyclin) is an S100 subtype that stains Spitz nevi in a strong and diffuse pattern (Figs. 30.23 and 30.24) while only one-third of melanomas express S100A6 and usually in a weak and patchy pattern with minimal to no reactivity at the junction. It is important to recognize that nevi other than Spitz react with S100A6 in a weak pattern similar to melanoma and S100A6 also stains fibrohistiocytic lesions

HMB-45 stains melanocytes at the junction and upper dermis but not the deeper melanocytes in Spitz nevi (Fig. 30.25), like most benign nevi (with the exception of blue nevi that are strongly and diffusely positive throughout). This gradient suggests maturation. In contrast, melanomas reveal more heterogeneous, weak and focal staining with HMB-45

A proliferation index, as determined by nuclear Mib-1 staining of melanocytes, over 10% favors melanoma while a proliferation index below 2% favors nevus. However, greater overlap exists between Spitz nevi and melanoma. Mib-1 is not lineage specific and also stains proliferating lymphocytes. When a lesion is heavily inflamed, distinction by cytology or dual staining with a cytoplasmic melanocytic marker is required (Figs. 30.26 and 30.27)

The cell-cycle inhibitor protein p16, is expressed in a greater percentage of Spitz nevi (Fig. 30.28), especially those with increased copy number of chromosome 11p, but is deleted or mutated in a proportion of melanomas resulting in loss of nuclear and sometimes also cytoplasmic staining

One small study found that strong, diffuse CD99 expression favors spitzoid melanoma over Spitz nevus, however, any other staining pattern is not helpful in differentiation. Other types of nevi and melanoma were not studied. In practice, we have found CD99 of minimal assistance in this differential

The tumor suppressor, p21, is the main downstream effector gene mediating p53-induced cell cycle arrest. A high level of p21 nuclear expression suggests Spitz nevus over melanoma, especially when coupled with a low proliferation index

Low levels of cyclin D1, bcl-2, and p53 are seen in Spitz, in contrast to higher expression in melanoma, however, significant overlap exists limiting their usefulness

Differences in the location and frequency of chromosomal aberrations in Spitz nevi and melanomas, as determined by comparative genomic hybridization (CGH) and fluorescence in situ hybridization (FISH), are becoming a more common method to differentiate spitzoid melanocytic neoplasms. The majority of Spitz nevi have no chromosomal abnormalities and those that do, have gains in chromosome 11p, which is rarely present in melanoma; whereas melanoma shows various deletions, including 9p and 10q

References: [12, 16, 33, 181–189]

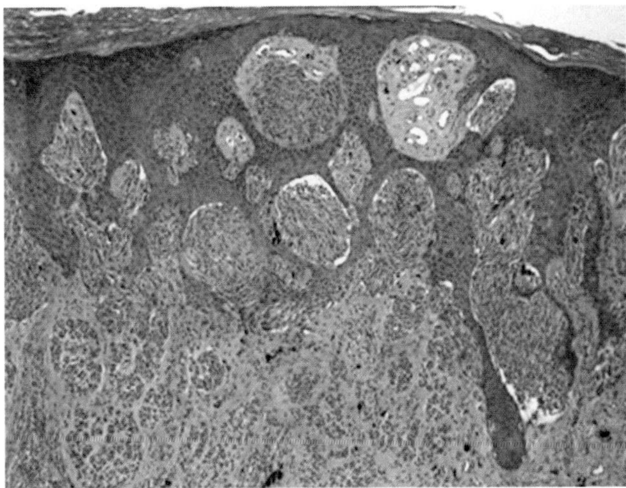

Fig. 30.23 Hematoxylin and eosin-stained sections of Spitz nevus

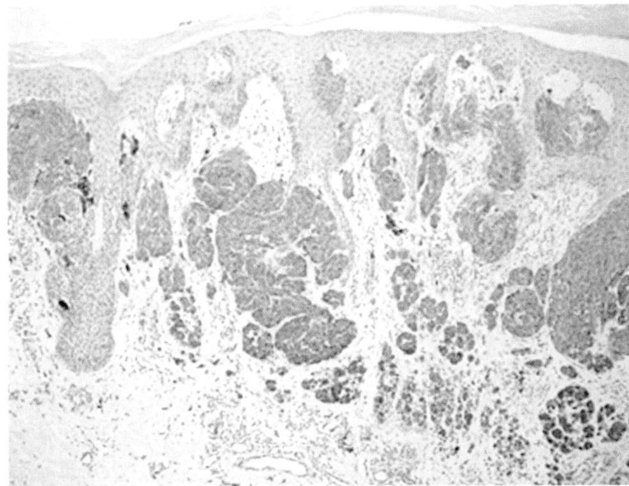

Fig. 30.24 Strong and diffuse staining of Spitz nevus with S100A6

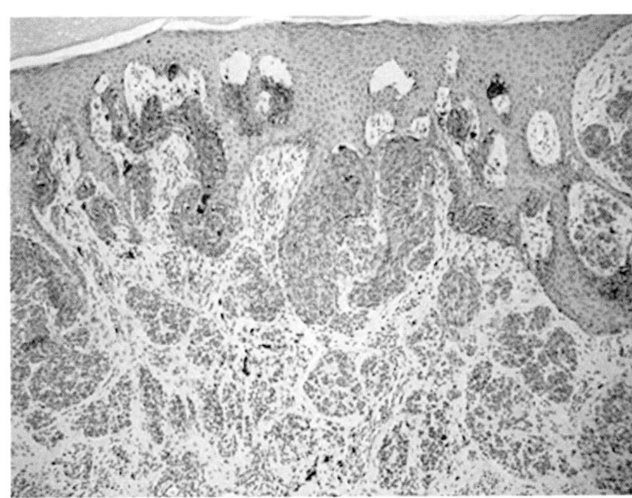

Fig. 30.25 Gradient of decreased expression of HMB-45 with increased depth into the dermis of a Spitz nevus

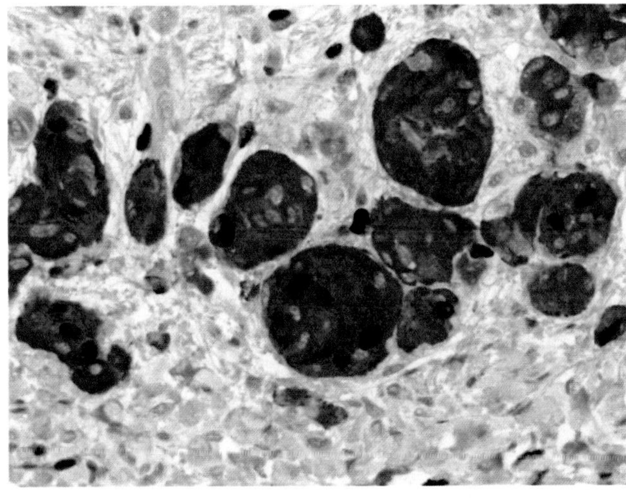

Fig. 30.26 Melanoma with dual MART-1 and Mib-1 staining. MART-1 with Fast Red as the chromogen was used to stain the cytoplasm of the melanocytic cells, while that Mib-1 with DAB was used to highlight the nuclei of proliferating cells. This allows identification of the frequent proliferating melanocytes that have red cytoplasm and brown nuclei in melanoma

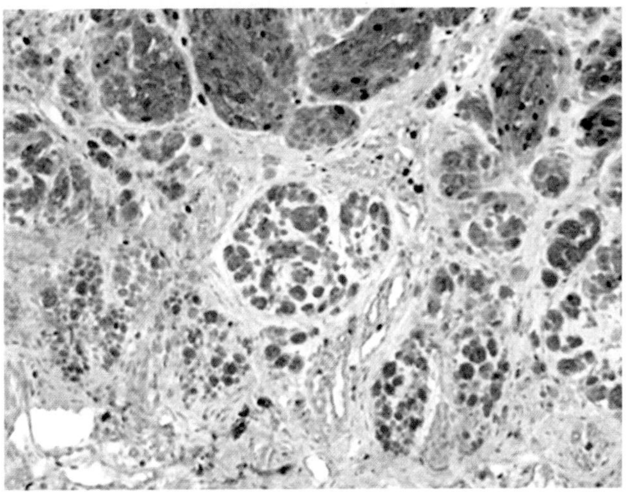

Fig. 30.27 Spitz nevus with MART-1 (Fast Red) and Mib-1 (DAB) revealing a gradient of Mib-1 positive Spitz cells with very few proliferating cells in the deeper dermis

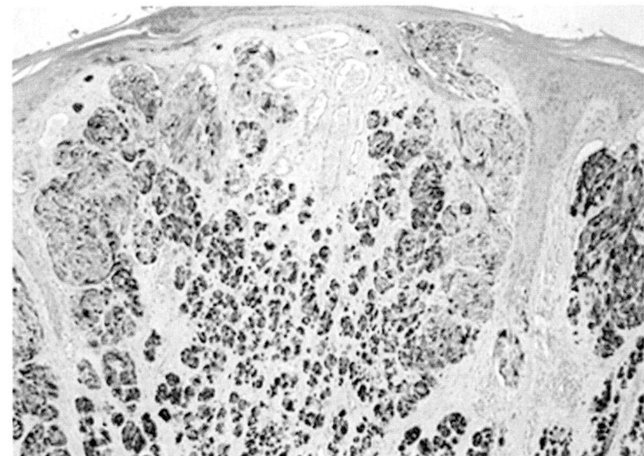

Fig. 30.28 Spitz nevus staining with p16

Table 30.12 Dermatofibroma vs. dermatofibrosarcoma protuberans

Antibodies	DF	DFSP
CD34	–/+	+[a]
Factor XIIIa	+	–/+
Stromelysin-3	+	–
S100A6	+[a]	–
p53	–	+/–
Tenascin (at DEJ)	+[a]	–

Note: [a]Greater than 90% of cases are positive

DF dermatofibroma, *DFSP* dermatofibrosarcoma protuberans, *DEJ* dermal–epidermal junction

Most DFs are easily distinguished from DFSP in adequate samples, however, morphologic differentiation can be difficult in deep or cellular DFs. Classically, the dermal dendritic cell marker, Factor XIIIa has been used with CD34 to differentiate. However, there is overlap and lack of specificity. While CD34 is positive in DFSP (Fig. 30.29), it is not specific and it highlights vascular endothelium, hematopoietic progenitor cells, several other fibrous tumors, and neurofibromas. DFs are often only weakly positive or reactive at the periphery with Factor XIIIa but staining is more diffuse in cellular DFs (Fig. 30.30). Some DFs exhibit focal staining with CD34, especially at the periphery of cellular and deep DF (Fig. 30.31)

Caution is required in the interpretation of DFSP margins with CD34, since CD34 disappears from scars but proliferates in pericicatricial tissue

Stromelysin-3 is a member of the metalloproteinase family that is involved in tissue remodeling, including tumor invasion. Expression is seen in the fibroblastic cells surrounding the epithelial portion of most cancers while most benign tumors, other than DF, are typically negative

Tenascin, an extracellular matrix glycoprotein involved in embryogenesis, carcinogenesis, and wound healing, is noted within the lesion in both DFs and DFSPs and does not assist in differentiation. However, strong tenascin expression is identified at the dermal–epidermal junction overlying DF but not over DFSP

The vast majority of DFs are reactive with S100A6 and CD10, whereas CD10 expression is present in just over half of DFSPs. In contrast, in one small study S100A6 was absent in all DFSPs examined

Expression of p53 in DFSPs ranges from 15 to 92% depending on the study. It has been suggested that the presence of a p53 mutation is associated with tumor progression to fibrosarcoma

References: [10, 19, 102, 170, 190–204]

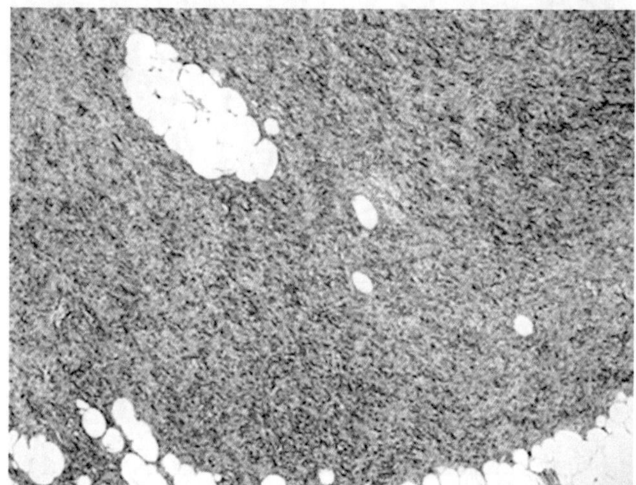

Fig. 30.29 DFSP staining with CD34

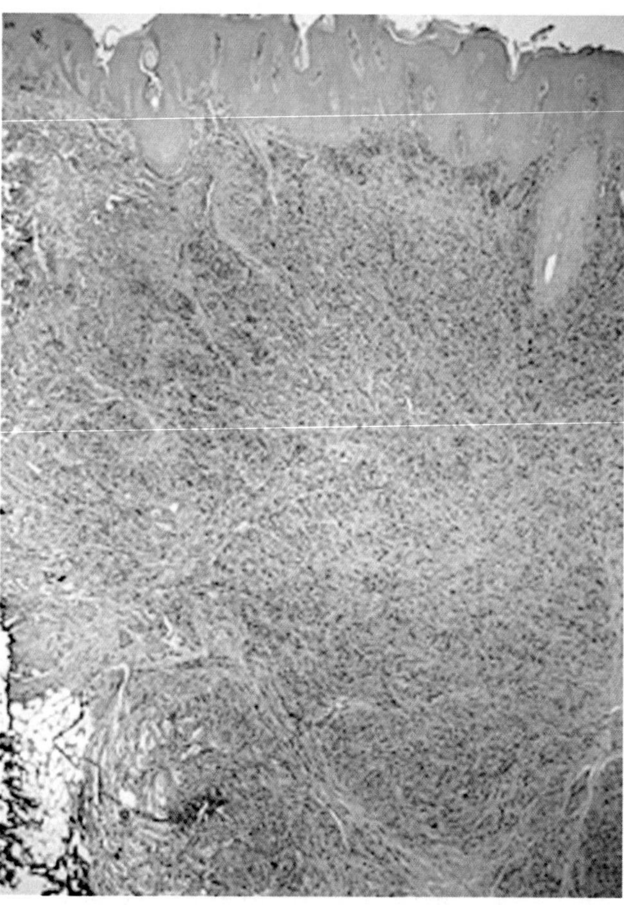

Fig. 30.30 Cellular DF staining with Factor XIIIa

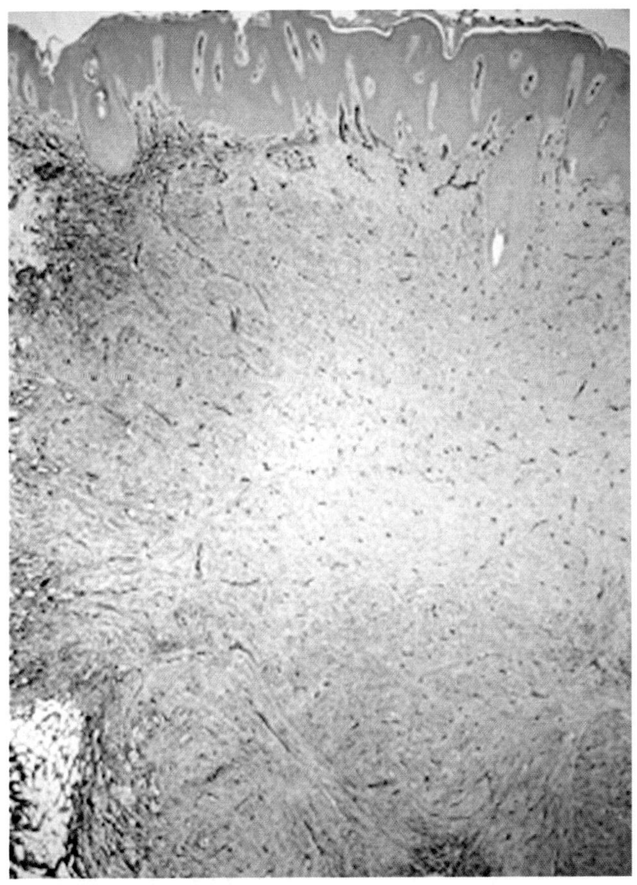

Fig. 30.31 Cellular DF with focal CD34 reactivity at the periphery of the lesion

Table 30.13 Primary cutaneous malignant adnexal tumors vs. metastatic adenocarcinoma to the skin

Antibodies	CAT	Met Adeno
p63	+[a]	–
CK5/6	+[a]	–/+
D2-40 (podoplanin)	+/–	–
CK15	–/+	–

Note: [a]Greater than 90% of cases are positive

CAT cutaneous adnexal tumor, *Met Adeno* metastatic adenocarcinoma

The majority of primary benign and malignant CATs are positive for p63, CK5/6, and D2-40 while expression is rare in metastatic adenocarcinomas (Figs. 30.32 and 30.33). These markers are helpful in distinguishing primary CATs from metastatic adenocarcinoma to the skin but should not preclude systemic evaluation for a primary source. This is not useful in the case of metastatic squamous cell carcinoma or urothelial carcinoma to the skin. In addition, primary cutaneous mucinous carcinoma appears to be an exception and although a primary CAT, does not reliably express p63, D2-40, or CK5/6. Metastases from malignant CATs generally retain p63 and D2-40 expression similar to their associated primary CATs

Table 30.13 (continued)

p63, a homolog of the p53 gene, is mainly expressed in basal cells and myoepithelial cells of the skin. Nuclear expression is known in squamous cell carcinomas. The studies of high molecular weight CK5/6 are small and consist predominantly of benign CATs. In general, metastatic adenocarcinomas express CK5/6 in only one-third of cases, predominantly with weak intensity. However, metastatic breast carcinoma is reactive for CK5/6 in almost half of cases

CK15 is specific in distinguishing CAT from cutaneous metastases but is not sensitive

References: [53, 205–214]

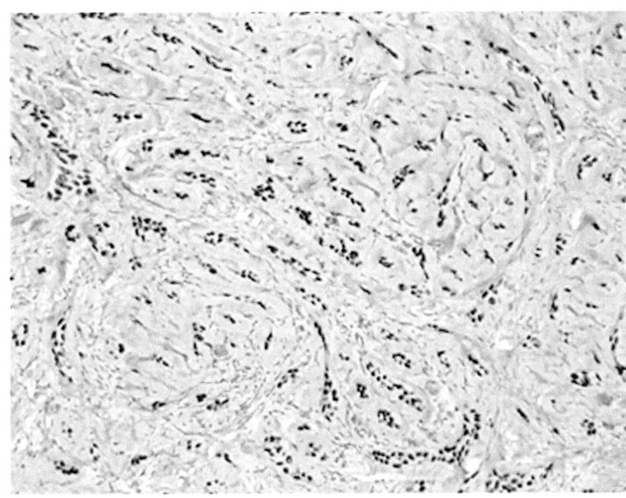

Fig. 30.32 Microcystic adnexal carcinoma with strong p63 expression

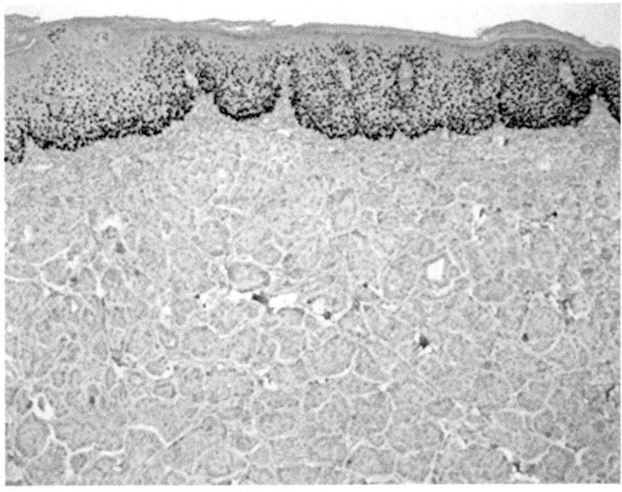

Fig. 30.33 Metastatic breast carcinoma to the skin fails to stain with p63

Note for All Tables

Note: "+" – usually greater than 70% of cases are positive; "–" – less than 5% of cases are positive; "+ or –" – usually more than 50% of cases are positive; "– or +" – less than 50% of cases are positive.

References

1. Nasr MR, El-Zammar O. Comparison of pHH3, Ki-67, and survivin immunoreactivity in benign and malignant melanocytic lesions. Am J Dermatopathol. 2008;30(2):117–22.
2. Liegl B, Hornick JL, Fletcher CD. Primary cutaneous PEComa: distinctive clear cell lesions of skin. Am J Surg Pathol. 2008;32(4):608–14.
3. Kahn HJ, Bailey D, Marks A. Monoclonal antibody D2-40, a new marker of lymphatic endothelium, reacts with Kaposi's sarcoma and a subset of angiosarcomas. Mod Pathol. 2002;15(4):434–40.
4. Ansai S, Hashimoto H, Aoki T, Hozumi Y, Aso K. A histochemical and immunohistochemical study of extra-ocular sebaceous carcinoma. Histopathology. 1993;22(2):127–33.
5. Cheuk W, Kwan MY, Suster S, Chan JK. Immunostaining for thyroid transcription factor 1 and cytokeratin 20 aids the distinction of small cell carcinoma from Merkel cell carcinoma, but not pulmonary from extrapulmonary small cell carcinomas. Arch Pathol Lab Med. 2001;125(2):228–31.
6. Morgan MB, Purohit C, Anglin TR. Immunohistochemical distinction of cutaneous spindle cell carcinoma. Am J Dermatopathol. 2008;30(3):228–32.
7. Smith KJ, Tuur S, Corvette D, Lupton GP, Skelton HG. Cytokeratin 7 staining in mammary and extramammary Paget's disease. Mod Pathol. 1997;10(11):1069–74.
8. Niakosari F, Kahn HJ, Marks A, From L. Detection of lymphatic invasion in primary melanoma with monoclonal antibody D2-40: a new selective immunohistochemical marker of lymphatic endothelium. Arch Dermatol. 2005;141(4):440–4.
9. North PE, Waner M, Mizeracki A, Mihm Jr MC. GLUT1: a newly discovered immunohistochemical marker for juvenile hemangiomas. Hum Pathol. 2000;31(1):11–22.
10. Kahn HJ, Fekete E, From L. Tenascin differentiates dermatofibroma from dermatofibrosarcoma protuberans: comparison with CD34 and factor XIIIa. Hum Pathol. 2001;32(1):50–6.
11. Lohmann CM, Iversen K, Jungbluth AA, Berwick M, Busam KJ. Expression of melanocyte differentiation antigens and ki-67 in nodal nevi and comparison of ki-67 expression with metastatic melanoma. Am J Surg Pathol. 2002;26(10):1351–7.
12. Vollmer RT. Use of Bayes rule and MIB-1 proliferation index to discriminate Spitz nevus from malignant melanoma. Am J Clin Pathol. 2004;122(4):499–505.
13. Beer TW, Shepherd P, Theaker JM. Ber EP4 and epithelial membrane antigen aid distinction of basal cell, squamous cell and basosquamous carcinomas of the skin. Histopathology. 2000;37(3):218–23.
14. Hornick JL, Fletcher CD. Cutaneous myoepithelioma: a clinicopathologic and immunohistochemical study of 14 cases. Hum Pathol. 2004;35(1):14–24.
15. Sun J, Morton Jr TH, Gown AM. Antibody HMB-45 identifies the cells of blue nevi. An immunohistochemical study on paraffin sections. Am J Surg Pathol. 1990;14(8):748–51.
16. Ribe A, McNutt NS. S100A6 protein expression is different in Spitz nevi and melanomas. Mod Pathol. 2003;16(5):505–11.
17. Fullen DR, Garrisi AJ, Sanders D, Thomas D. Expression of S100A6 protein in a broad spectrum of cutaneous tumors using tissue microarrays. J Cutan Pathol. 2008;35 Suppl 2:28–34.
18. Folpe AL, Cooper K. Best practices in diagnostic immunohistochemistry: pleomorphic cutaneous spindle cell tumors. Arch Pathol Lab Med. 2007;131(10):1517–24.
19. Fullen DR, Reed JA, Finnerty B, McNutt NS. S100A6 expression in fibrohistiocytic lesions. J Cutan Pathol. 2001;28(5):229–34.
20. Fukunaga M. Expression of D2-40 in lymphatic endothelium of normal tissues and in vascular tumours. Histopathology. 2005;46(4):396–402.
21. North PE, Waner M, Mizeracki A, et al. A unique microvascular phenotype shared by juvenile hemangiomas and human placenta. Arch Dermatol. 2001;137(5):559–70.
22. Leon-Villapalos J, Wolfe K, Kangesu L. GLUT-1: an extra diagnostic tool to differentiate between haemangiomas and vascular malformations. Br J Plast Surg. 2005;58(3):348–52.
23. Pinkus GS, Kurtin PJ. Epithelial membrane antigen – a diagnostic discriminant in surgical pathology: immunohistochemical profile in epithelial, mesenchymal, and hematopoietic neoplasms using paraffin sections and monoclonal antibodies. Hum Pathol. 1985;16(9):929–40.
24. Miettinen M, Lindenmayer AE, Chaubal A. Endothelial cell markers CD31, CD34, and BNH9 antibody to H- and Y-antigens – evaluation of their specificity and sensitivity in the diagnosis of vascular tumors and comparison with von Willebrand factor. Mod Pathol. 1994;7(1):82–90.
25. Trefzer U, Rietz N, Chen Y, et al. SM5-1: a new monoclonal antibody which is highly sensitive and specific for melanocytic lesions. Arch Dermatol Res. 2000;292(12):583–9.
26. Reinke S, Koniger P, Herberth G, et al. Differential expression of MART-1, tyrosinase, and SM5-1 in primary and metastatic melanoma. Am J Dermatopathol. 2005;27(5):401–6.
27. Trefzer U, Chen Y, Herberth G, et al. The monoclonal antibody SM5-1 recognizes a fibronectin variant which is widely expressed in melanoma. BMC Cancer. 2006;6:8.
28. Banerjee SS, Harris M. Morphological and immunophenotypic variations in malignant melanoma. Histopathology. 2000;36(5):387–402.
29. Pernick NL, DaSilva M, Gangi MD, Crissman J, Adsay V. "Histiocytic markers" in melanoma. Mod Pathol. 1999;12(11):1072–7.
30. Nonaka D, Laser J, Tucker R, Melamed J. Immunohistochemical evaluation of necrotic malignant melanomas. Am J Clin Pathol. 2007;127(5):787–91.
31. Bergman R, Azzam H, Sprecher E, et al. A comparative immunohistochemical study of MART-1 expression in Spitz nevi, ordinary melanocytic nevi, and malignant melanomas. J Am Acad Dermatol. 2000;42(3):496–500.
32. Busam KJ, Chen YT, Old LJ, et al. Expression of melan-A (MART1) in benign melanocytic nevi and primary cutaneous malignant melanoma. Am J Surg Pathol. 1998;22(8):976–82.
33. Skelton 3rd HG, Smith KJ, Barrett TL, Lupton GP, Graham JH. HMB-45 staining in benign and malignant melanocytic lesions. A reflection of cellular activation. Am J Dermatopathol. 1991;13(6):543–50.
34. Ordonez NG, Ji XL, Hickey RC. Comparison of HMB-45 monoclonal antibody and S-100 protein in the immunohistochemical diagnosis of melanoma. Am J Clin Pathol. 1988;90(4):385–90.
35. Rochaix P, Lacroix-Triki M, Lamant L, et al. PNL2, a new monoclonal antibody directed against a fixative-resistant melanocyte antigen. Mod Pathol. 2003;16(5):481–90.
36. Gloghini A, Rizzo A, Zanette I, et al. KP1/CD68 expression in malignant neoplasms including lymphomas, sarcomas, and carcinomas. Am J Clin Pathol. 1995;103(4):425–31.

37. Cassidy M, Loftus B, Whelan A, et al. KP-1: not a specific marker. Staining of 137 sarcomas, 48 lymphomas, 28 carcinomas, 7 malignant melanomas and 8 cystosarcoma phyllodes. Virchows Arch. 1994;424(6):635–40.
38. Polski JM, Janney CG. Ber-H2 (CD30) immunohistochemical staining in malignant melanoma. Mod Pathol. 1999;12(9):903–6.
39. Plaza JA, Suster D, Perez-Montiel D. Expression of immunohistochemical markers in primary and metastatic malignant melanoma: a comparative study in 70 patients using a tissue microarray technique. Appl Immunohistochem Mol Morphol. 2007;15(4):421–5.
40. Kamino H, Tam ST. Immunoperoxidase technique modified by counterstain with azure B as a diagnostic aid in evaluating heavily pigmented melanocytic neoplasms. J Cutan Pathol. 1991;18(6):436–9.
41. Bishop PW, Menasce LP, Yates AJ, Win NA, Banerjee SS. An immunophenotypic survey of malignant melanomas. Histopathology. 1993;23(2):159–66.
42. Selby WL, Nance KV, Park HK. CEA immunoreactivity in metastatic malignant melanoma. Mod Pathol. 1992;5(4):415–9.
43. Ben-Izhak O, Stark P, Levy R, Bergman R, Lichtig C. Epithelial markers in malignant melanoma. A study of primary lesions and their metastases. Am J Dermatopathol. 1994;16(3):241–6.
44. Sanders DS, Evans AT, Allen CA, et al. Classification of CEA-related positivity in primary and metastatic malignant melanoma. J Pathol. 1994;172(4):343–8.
45. Fernando SS, Johnson S, Bate J. Immunohistochemical analysis of cutaneous malignant melanoma: comparison of S-100 protein, HMB-45 monoclonal antibody and NKI/C3 monoclonal antibody. Pathology. 1994;26(1):16–9.
46. Kontochristopoulos GJ, Stavropoulos PG, Krasagakis K, Goerdt S, Zouboulis CC. Differentiation between merkel cell carcinoma and malignant melanoma: an immunohistochemical study. Dermatology. 2000;201(2):123–6.
47. Kocan P, Jurkovic I, Boor A, et al. Immunohistochemical study of melanocytic differentiation antigens in cutaneous malignant melanoma. A comparison of six commercial antibodies and one non-commercial antibody in nodular melanoma, superficially spreading melanoma and lentigo maligna melanoma. Cesk Patol. 2004;40(2):50–6.
48. Mehregan DR, Hamzavi I. Staining of melanocytic neoplasms by melanoma antigen recognized by T cells. Am J Dermatopathol. 2000;22(3):247–50.
49. Prieto VG, Shea CR. Use of immunohistochemistry in melanocytic lesions. J Cutan Pathol. 2008;35 Suppl 2:1–10.
50. Ohsie SJ, Sarantopoulos GP, Cochran AJ, Binder SW. Immunohistochemical characteristics of melanoma. J Cutan Pathol. 2008;35(5):433–44.
51. Mangini J, Li N, Bhawan J. Immunohistochemical markers of melanocytic lesions: a review of their diagnostic usefulness. Am J Dermatopathol. 2002;24(3):270–81.
52. Bahrami A, Truong LD, Ro JY. Undifferentiated tumor: true identity by immunohistochemistry. Arch Pathol Lab Med. 2008;132(3):326–48.
53. Wasserman J, Maddox J, Racz M, Petronic-Rosic V. Update on immunohistochemical methods relevant to dermatopathology. Arch Pathol Lab Med. 2009;133(7):1053–61.
54. Miettinen M, Fernandez M, Franssila K, Gatalica Z, Lasota J, Sarlomo-Rikala M. Microphthalmia transcription factor in the immunohistochemical diagnosis of metastatic melanoma: comparison with four other melanoma markers. Am J Surg Pathol. 2001;25(2):205–11.
55. Nonaka D, Chiriboga L, Rubin BP. Sox10: a pan-schwannian and melanocytic marker. Am J Surg Pathol. 2008;32(9):1291–8.
56. Boyle JL, Haupt HM, Stern JB, Multhaupt HA. Tyrosinase expression in malignant melanoma, desmoplastic melanoma, and peripheral nerve tumors. Arch Pathol Lab Med. 2002;126(7):816–22.
57. Busam KJ, Iversen K, Coplan KC, Jungbluth AA. Analysis of microphthalmia transcription factor expression in normal tissues and tumors, and comparison of its expression with S-100 protein, gp100, and tyrosinase in desmoplastic malignant melanoma. Am J Surg Pathol. 2001;25(2):197–204.
58. Granter SR, Weilbaecher KN, Quigley C, Fletcher CD, Fisher DE. Microphthalmia transcription factor: not a sensitive or specific marker for the diagnosis of desmoplastic melanoma and spindle cell (non-desmoplastic) melanoma. Am J Dermatopathol. 2001;23(3):185–9.
59. Anstey A, Cerio R, Ramnarain N, Orchard G, Smith N, Jones EW. Desmoplastic malignant melanoma. An immunocytochemical study of 25 cases. Am J Dermatopathol. 1994;16(1):14–22.
60. Sundram U, Harvell JD, Rouse RV, Natkunam Y. Expression of the B-cell proliferation marker MUM1 by melanocytic lesions and comparison with S100, gp100 (HMB45), and MelanA. Mod Pathol. 2003;16(8):802–10.
61. Itakura E, Huang RR, Wen DR, Paul E, Wunsch PH, Cochran AJ. RT in situ PCR detection of MART-1 and TRP-2 mRNA in formalin-fixed, paraffin-embedded tissues of melanoma and nevi. Mod Pathol. 2008;21(3):326–33. doi:10.1038/modpathol.3801008.
62. King R, Googe PB, Weilbaecher KN, Mihm Jr MC, Fisher DE. Microphthalmia transcription factor expression in cutaneous benign, malignant melanocytic, and nonmelanocytic tumors. Am J Surg Pathol. 2001;25(1):51–7.
63. Zubovits J, Buzney E, Yu L, Duncan LM. HMB-45, S-100, NK1/C3, and MART-1 in metastatic melanoma. Hum Pathol. 2004;35(2):217–23.
64. Busam KJ, Kucukgöl D, Sato E, Frosina D, Teruya-Feldstein J, Jungbluth AA. Immunohistochemical analysis of novel monoclonal antibody PNL2 and comparison with other melanocyte differentiation markers. Am J Surg Pathol. 2005;29(3):400–6.
65. Buresh CJ, Oliai BR, Miller RT. Reactivity with TdT in Merkel cell carcinoma: a potential diagnostic pitfall. Am J Clin Pathol. 2008;129(6):894–8.
66. Schmidt U, Muller U, Metz KA, Leder LD. Cytokeratin and neurofilament protein staining in Merkel cell carcinoma of the small cell type and small cell carcinoma of the lung. Am J Dermatopathol. 1998;20(4):346–51.
67. Shah IA, Netto D, Schlageter MO, Muth C, Fox I, Manne RK. Neurofilament immunoreactivity in Merkel-cell tumors: a differentiating feature from small-cell carcinoma. Mod Pathol. 1993;6(1):3–9.
68. Leff EL, Brooks JS, Trojanowski JQ. Expression of neurofilament and neuron-specific enolase in small cell tumors of skin using immunohistochemistry. Cancer. 1985;56(3):625–31.
69. Mhawech-Fauceglia P, Herrmann FR, Bshara W, et al. Friend leukaemia integration-1 expression in malignant and benign tumours: a multiple tumour tissue microarray analysis using polyclonal antibody. J Clin Pathol. 2007;60(6):694–700.
70. Mhawech-Fauceglia P, Saxena R, Zhang S, et al. Pax-5 immunoexpression in various types of benign and malignant tumours: a high-throughput tissue microarray analysis. J Clin Pathol. 2007;60(6):709–14.
71. Kennedy MM, Blessing K, King G, Kerr KM. Expression of bcl-2 and p53 in Merkel cell carcinoma. An immunohistochemical study. Am J Dermatopathol. 1996;18(3):273–7.
72. Jensen K, Kohler S, Rouse RV. Cytokeratin staining in Merkel cell carcinoma: an immunohistochemical study of cytokeratins 5/6, 7, 17, and 20. Appl Immunohistochem Mol Morphol. 2000;8(4):310–5.
73. Dong HY, Liu W, Cohen P, Mahle CE, Zhang W. B-cell specific activation protein encoded by the PAX-5 gene is commonly expressed in merkel cell carcinoma and small cell carcinomas. Am J Surg Pathol. 2005;29(5):687–92.

74. Scott MP, Helm KF. Cytokeratin 20: a marker for diagnosing Merkel cell carcinoma. Am J Dermatopathol. 1999;21(1):16–20.
75. Miettinen M. Keratin 20: immunohistochemical marker for gastrointestinal, urothelial, and Merkel cell carcinomas. Mod Pathol. 1995;8(4):384–8.
76. Chan JK, Suster S, Wenig BM, Tsang WY, Chan JB, Lau AL. Cytokeratin 20 immunoreactivity distinguishes Merkel cell (primary cutaneous neuroendocrine) carcinomas and salivary gland small cell carcinomas from small cell carcinomas of various sites. Am J Surg Pathol. 1997;21(2):226–34.
77. Feinmesser M, Halpern M, Fenig E, et al. Expression of the apoptosis-related oncogenes bcl-2, bax, and p53 in Merkel cell carcinoma: can they predict treatment response and clinical outcome? Hum Pathol. 1999;30(11):1367–72.
78. Visscher D, Cooper PH, Zarbo RJ, Crissman JD. Cutaneous neuroendocrine (Merkel cell) carcinoma: an immunophenotypic, clinicopathologic, and flow cytometric study. Mod Pathol. 1989;2(4):331–8.
79. Byrd-Gloster AL, Khoor A, Glass LF, et al. Differential expression of thyroid transcription factor 1 in small cell lung carcinoma and Merkel cell tumor. Hum Pathol. 2000;31(1):58–62.
80. Ordóñez NG. Value of thyroid transcription factor-1 immunostaining in distinguishing small cell lung carcinomas from other small cell carcinomas. Am J Surg Pathol. 2000;24(9):1217–23.
81. Sur M, AlArdati H, Ross C, Alowami S. TdT expression in Merkel cell carcinoma: potential diagnostic pitfall with blastic hematological malignancies and expanded immunohistochemical analysis. Mod Pathol. 2007;20(11):1113–20.
82. Smith KJ, Skelton 3rd HG, Holland TT, Morgan AM, Lupton GP. Neuroendocrine (Merkel cell) carcinoma with an intraepidermal component. Am J Dermatopathol. 1993;15(6):528–33.
83. Su LD, Fullen DR, Lowe L, Uherova P, Schnitzer B, Valdez R. CD117 (KIT receptor) expression in Merkel cell carcinoma. Am J Dermatopathol. 2002;24(4):289–93.
84. Kurokawa M, Nabeshima K, Akiyama Y, et al. CD56: a useful marker for diagnosing Merkel cell carcinoma. J Dermatol Sci. 2003;31(3):219–24.
85. Bobos M, Hytiroglou P, Kostopoulos I, Karkavelas G, Papadimitriou CS. Immunohistochemical distinction between merkel cell carcinoma and small cell carcinoma of the lung. Am J Dermatopathol. 2006;28(2):99–104.
86. Haneke E, Schulze HJ, Mahrle G. Immunohistochemical and immunoelectron microscopic demonstration of chromogranin A in formalin-fixed tissue of Merkel cell carcinoma. J Am Acad Dermatol. 1993;28(2 Pt 1):222–6.
87. Beer TW, Haig D. CD117 is not a useful marker for diagnosing atypical fibroxanthoma. Am J Dermatopathol. 2009;31(7):649–52.
88. Calder KB, Coplowitz S, Schlauder S, Morgan MB. A case series and immunophenotypic analysis of CK20-/CK7+ primary neuroendocrine carcinoma of the skin. J Cutan Pathol. 2007;34(12): 918–23.
89. Acebo E, Vidaurrazaga N, Varas C, Burgos-Bretones JJ, Diaz-Perez JL. Merkel cell carcinoma: a clinicopathological study of 11 cases. J Eur Acad Dermatol Venereol. 2005;19(5):546–51. doi:10.1111/j.1468-3083.2005.01224.x.
90. McNiff JM, Cowper SE, Lazova R, Subtil A, Glusac EJ. CD56 staining in Merkel cell carcinoma and natural killer-cell lymphoma: magic bullet, diagnostic pitfall, or both? J Cutan Pathol. 2005;32(8):541–5.
91. Nicholson SA, McDermott MB, Swanson PE, Wick MR. CD99 and cytokeratin-20 in small-cell and basaloid tumors of the skin. Appl Immunohistochem Mol Morphol. 2000;8(1):37–41.
92. Agoff SN, Lamps LW, Philip AT, et al. Thyroid transcription factor-1 is expressed in extrapulmonary small cell carcinomas but not in other extrapulmonary neuroendocrine tumors. Mod Pathol. 2000;13(3):238–42.
93. Chu P, Wu E, Weiss LM. Cytokeratin 7 and cytokeratin 20 expression in epithelial neoplasms: a survey of 435 cases. Mod Pathol. 2000;13(9):962–72. doi:10.1038/modpathol.3880175.
94. Silvis NG, Swanson PE, Manivel JC, Kaye VN, Wick MR. Spindle-cell and pleomorphic neoplasms of the skin. A clinicopathologic and immunohistochemical study of 30 cases, with emphasis on "atypical fibroxanthomas". Am J Dermatopathol. 1988;10(1):9–19.
95. Monteagudo C, Calduch L, Navarro S, Joan-Figueroa A, Llombart-Bosch A. CD99 immunoreactivity in atypical fibroxanthoma: a common feature of diagnostic value. Am J Clin Pathol. 2002;117(1):126–31.
96. Ma CK, Zarbo RJ, Gown AM. Immunohistochemical characterization of atypical fibroxanthoma and dermatofibrosarcoma protuberans. Am J Clin Pathol. 1992;97(4):478–83.
97. Rudolph P, Schubert B, Wacker HH, Parwaresch R, Schubert C. Immunophenotyping of dermal spindle cell tumors: diagnostic value of monocyte marker Ki-M1p and histogenetic considerations. Am J Surg Pathol. 1997;21(7):791–800.
98. Ricci Jr A, Cartun RW, Zakowski MF. 'Atypical fibroxanthoma. A study of 14 cases emphasizing the presence of Langerhans' histiocytes with implications for differential diagnosis by antibody panels. Am J Surg Pathol. 1988;12(8):591–8.
99. Longacre TA, Smoller BR, Rouse RV. Atypical fibroxanthoma. Multiple immunohistologic profiles. Am J Surg Pathol. 1993;17(12):1199–209.
100. Luzar B, Calonje E. Morphological and immunohistochemical characteristics of atypical fibroxanthoma with a special emphasis on potential diagnostic pitfalls: a review. J Cutan Pathol. 2010;37(3):301–9.
101. Sakamoto A, Oda Y, Yamamoto H, et al. Calponin and h-caldesmon expression in atypical fibroxanthoma and superficial leiomyosarcoma. Virchows Arch. 2002;440(4):404–9.
102. de Feraudy S, Mar N, McCalmont TH. Evaluation of CD10 and procollagen 1 expression in atypical fibroxanthoma and dermatofibroma. Am J Surg Pathol. 2008;32(8):1111–22. doi:10.1097/PAS.0b013e31816b8fce.
103. Patton A, Page R, Googe PB, King R. Myxoid atypical fibroxanthoma: a previously undescribed variant. J Cutan Pathol. 2009;36(11):1177–84.
104. Hultgren TL, DiMaio DJ. Immunohistochemical staining of CD10 in atypical fibroxanthomas. J Cutan Pathol. 2007;34(5):415–9.
105. Weedon D, Williamson R, Mirza B. CD10, a useful marker for atypical fibroxanthomas. Am J Dermatopathol. 2005;27(2):181.
106. Jensen K, Wilkinson B, Wines N, Kossard S. Procollagen 1 expression in atypical fibroxanthoma and other tumors. J Cutan Pathol. 2004;31(1):57–61.
107. Mirza B, Weedon D. Atypical fibroxanthoma: a clinicopathological study of 89 cases. Australas J Dermatol. 2005;46(4):235–8.
108. Hartel PH, Jackson J, Ducatman BS, Zhang P. CD99 immunoreactivity in atypical fibroxanthoma and pleomorphic malignant fibrous histiocytoma: a useful diagnostic marker. J Cutan Pathol. 2006;33 Suppl 2:24–8.
109. Beer TW. CD117 in atypical fibroxanthoma: tumor or stroma? Am J Dermatopathol. 2008;30(4):401–2.
110. Barr KL, Russo JJ, Vincek V. Re: CD117 immunoreactivity in atypical fibroxanthoma. Am J Dermatopathol. 2009;31(1):96–8.
111. Fernandez-Flores A. Mast cell population in atypical fibroxanthoma as a finding with CD117 immunostaining. Am J Dermatopathol. 2008;30(6):640–2.
112. Mathew RA, Schlauder SM, Calder KB, Morgan MB. CD117 immunoreactivity in atypical fibroxanthoma. Am J Dermatopathol. 2008;30(1):34–6.
113. Dotto JE, Glusac EJ. P63 is a useful marker for cutaneous spindle cell squamous cell carcinoma. J Cutan Pathol. 2006;33(6): 413–7.

114. Sigel JE, Skacel M, Bergfeld WF, House NS, Rabkin MS, Goldblum JR. The utility of cytokeratin 5/6 in the recognition of cutaneous spindle cell squamous cell carcinoma. J Cutan Pathol. 2001;28(10):520–4.
115. Gleason BC, Calder KB, Cibull TL, et al. Utility of p63 in the differential diagnosis of atypical fibroxanthoma and spindle cell squamous cell carcinoma. J Cutan Pathol. 2009;36(5):543–7.
116. Laskin WB, Fetsch JF, Miettinen M. The "neurothekeoma": immunohistochemical analysis distinguishes the true nerve sheath myxoma from its mimics. Hum Pathol. 2000;31(10):1230–41.
117. Plaza JA, Torres-Cabala C, Evans H, Diwan AH, Prieto VG. Immunohistochemical expression of S100A6 in cellular neurothekeoma: clinicopathologic and immunohistochemical analysis of 31 cases. Am J Dermatopathol. 2009;31(5):419–22.
118. Page RN, King R, Mihm Jr MC, Googe PB. Microphthalmia transcription factor and NKI/C3 expression in cellular neurothekeoma. Mod Pathol. 2004;17(2):230–4.
119. Calonje E, Wilson-Jones E, Smith NP, Fletcher CD. Cellular 'neurothekeoma': an epithelioid variant of pilar leiomyoma? Morphological and immunohistochemical analysis of a series. Histopathology. 1992;20(5):397–404.
120. Hornick JL, Fletcher CD. Cellular neurothekeoma: detailed characterization in a series of 133 cases. Am J Surg Pathol. 2007;31(3):329–40.
121. Wang AR, May D, Bourne P, Scott G. PGP9.5: a marker for cellular neurothekeoma. Am J Surg Pathol. 1999;23(11):1401–7.
122. Fetsch JF, Laskin WB, Hallman JR, Lupton GP, Miettinen M. Neurothekeoma: an analysis of 178 tumors with detailed immunohistochemical data and long-term patient follow-up information. Am J Surg Pathol. 2007;31(7):1103–14.
123. Fullen DR, Lowe L, Su LD. Antibody to S100a6 protein is a sensitive immunohistochemical marker for neurothekeoma. J Cutan Pathol. 2003;30(2):118–22.
124. Argenyi ZB, LeBoit PE, Santa Cruz D, Swanson PE, Kutzner H. Nerve sheath myxoma (neurothekeoma) of the skin: light microscopic and immunohistochemical reappraisal of the cellular variant. J Cutan Pathol. 1993;20(4):294–303.
125. Kaddu S, Leinweber B. Podoplanin expression in fibrous histiocytomas and cellular neurothekeomas. Am J Dermatopathol. 2009;31(2):137–9.
126. Leinweber B, Hofmann-Wellenhof R, Kaddu S, McCalmont TH. Procollagen 1 and Melan-A expression in desmoplastic melanomas. Am J Dermatopathol. 2009;31(2):173–6.
127. Fernandez-Flores A. Cutaneous squamous cell carcinoma of different grades: variation of the expression of CD10. Cesk Patol. 2008;44(4):100–2.
128. Kanik AB, Yaar M, Bhawan J. P75 nerve growth factor receptor staining helps identify desmoplastic and neurotropic melanoma. J Cutan Pathol. 1996;23(3):205–10.
129. Iwamoto S, Burrows RC, Agoff SN, Piepkorn M, Bothwell M, Schmidt R. The p75 neurotrophin receptor, relative to other Schwann cell and melanoma markers, is abundantly expressed in spindled melanomas. Am J Dermatopathol. 2001;23(4):288–94.
130. Heim-Hall J, Yohe SL. Application of immunohistochemistry to soft tissue neoplasms. Arch Pathol Lab Med. 2008;132(3):476–89.
131. Robson A, Allen P, Hollowood K. S100 expression in cutaneous scars: a potential diagnostic pitfall in the diagnosis of desmoplastic melanoma. Histopathology. 2001;38(2):135–40.
132. Zarbo RJ, Gown AM, Nagle RB, Visscher DW, Crissman JD. Anomalous cytokeratin expression in malignant melanoma: one- and two-dimensional western blot analysis and immunohistochemical survey of 100 melanomas. Mod Pathol. 1990;3(4): 494–501.
133. Chen N, Gong J, Chen X, et al. Cytokeratin expression in malignant melanoma: potential application of in-situ hybridization analysis of mRNA. Melanoma Res. 2009;19(2):87–93.
134. Krustrup D, Rossen K, Thomsen HK. Procollagen 1 – a marker of fibroblastic and fibrohistiocytic skin tumors. J Cutan Pathol. 2006;33(9):614–8.
135. Kanner WA, Brill 2nd LB, Patterson JW, Wick MR. CD10, p63 and CD99 expression in the differential diagnosis of atypical fibroxanthoma, spindle cell squamous cell carcinoma and desmoplastic melanoma. J Cutan Pathol. 2010;37(7):744–50. doi:10.1111/j.1600-0560.2010.01534.x.
136. Battifora H, Silva EG. The use of antikeratin antibodies in the immunohistochemical distinction between neuroendocrine (Merkel cell) carcinoma of the skin, lymphoma, and oat cell carcinoma. Cancer. 1986;58(5):1040–6.
137. Kaufmann O, Dietel M. Expression of thyroid transcription factor-1 in pulmonary and extrapulmonary small cell carcinomas and other neuroendocrine carcinomas of various primary sites. Histopathology. 2000;36(5):415–20.
138. Metz KA, Jacob M, Schmidt U, Steuhl KP, Leder LD. Merkel cell carcinoma of the eyelid: histological and immunohistochemical features with special respect to differential diagnosis. Graefes Arch Clin Exp Ophthalmol. 1998;236(8):561–6.
139. Rode J, Dhillon AP. Neurone specific enolase and S100 protein as possible prognostic indicators in melanoma. Histopathology. 1984;8(6):1041–52.
140. Rossi S, Orvieto E, Furlanetto A, Laurino L, Ninfo V. Dei Tos AP. Utility of the immunohistochemical detection of FLI-1 expression in round cell and vascular neoplasm using a monoclonal antibody. Mod Pathol. 2004;17(5):547–52.
141. Yang DT, Holden JA, Florell SR. CD117, CK20, TTF-1, and DNA topoisomerase II-alpha antigen expression in small cell tumors. J Cutan Pathol. 2004;31(3):254–61.
142. Battles OE, Page DL, Johnson JE. Cytokeratins, CEA, and mucin histochemistry in the diagnosis and characterization of extramammary Paget's disease. Am J Clin Pathol. 1997;108(1):6–12.
143. Helm KF, Goellner JR, Peters MS. Immunohistochemical stains in extramammary Paget's disease. Am J Dermatopathol. 1992; 14(5):402–7.
144. Ramachandra S, Gillett CE, Millis RR. A comparative immunohistochemical study of mammary and extramammary Paget's disease and superficial spreading melanoma, with particular emphasis on melanocytic markers. Virchows Arch. 1996;429(6):371–6.
145. Perrotto J, Abbott JJ, Ceilley RI, Ahmed I. The role of immunohistochemistry in discriminating primary from secondary extramammary Paget disease. Am J Dermatopathol. 2010;32(2):137–43.
146. Olson DJ, Fujimura M, Swanson P, Okagaki T. Immunohistochemical features of Paget's disease of the vulva with and without adenocarcinoma. Int J Gynecol Pathol. 1991;10(3):285–95.
147. Ohnishi T, Watanabe S. The use of cytokeratins 7 and 20 in the diagnosis of primary and secondary extramammary Paget's disease. Br J Dermatol. 2000;142(2):243–7.
148. Nowak MA, Guerriere-Kovach P, Pathan A, Campbell TE, Deppisch LM. Perianal Paget's disease: distinguishing primary and secondary lesions using immunohistochemical studies including gross cystic disease fluid protein-15 and cytokeratin 20 expression. Arch Pathol Lab Med. 1998;122(12):1077–81.
149. Lundquist K, Kohler S, Rouse RV. Intraepidermal cytokeratin 7 expression is not restricted to Paget cells but is also seen in Toker cells and Merkel cells. Am J Surg Pathol. 1999;23(2):212–9.
150. Mai KT, Alhalouly T, Landry D, Stinson WA, Perkins DG, Yazdi HM. Pagetoid variant of actinic keratosis with or without squamous cell carcinoma of sun-exposed skin: a lesion simulating extramammary Paget's disease. Histopathology. 2002;41(4):331–6.
151. Mazoujian G, Pinkus GS, Haagensen Jr DE. Extramammary Paget's disease – evidence for an apocrine origin. An immunoperoxidase study of gross cystic disease fluid protein-15, carcinoembryonic antigen, and keratin proteins. Am J Surg Pathol. 1984;8(1):43–50.

152. Kohler S, Smoller BR. Gross cystic disease fluid protein-15 reactivity in extramammary Paget's disease with and without associated internal malignancy. Am J Dermatopathol. 1996;18(2):118–23.
153. Goldblum JR, Hart WR. Perianal Paget's disease: a histologic and immunohistochemical study of 11 cases with and without associated rectal adenocarcinoma. Am J Surg Pathol. 1998;22(2):170–9.
154. Goldblum JR, Hart WR. Vulvar Paget's disease: a clinicopathologic and immunohistochemical study of 19 cases. Am J Surg Pathol. 1997;21(10):1178–87.
155. Hitchcock A, Topham S, Bell J, Gullick W, Elston CW, Ellis IO. Routine diagnosis of mammary Paget's disease. A modern approach. Am J Surg Pathol. 1992;16(1):58–61.
156. Raju RR, Goldblum JR, Hart WR. Pagetoid squamous cell carcinoma in situ (pagetoid Bowen's disease) of the external genitalia. Int J Gynecol Pathol. 2003;22(2):127–35.
157. Rosen L, Amazon K, Frank B. Bowen's disease, Paget's disease, and malignant melanoma in situ. South Med J. 1986;79(4):410–3.
158. Sellheyer K, Krahl D. Ber-EP4 enhances the differential diagnostic accuracy of cytokeratin 7 in pagetoid cutaneous neoplasms. J Cutan Pathol. 2008;35(4):366–72.
159. Carvalho J, Fullen D, Lowe L, Su L, Ma L. The expression of CD23 in cutaneous non-lymphoid neoplasms. J Cutan Pathol. 2007;34(9):693–8.
160. Bogner PN, Su LD, Fullen DR. Cluster designation 5 staining of normal and non-lymphoid neoplastic skin. J Cutan Pathol. 2005;32(1):50–4.
161. Zeng HA, Cartun R, Ricci Jr A. Potential diagnostic utility of CDX-2 immunophenotyping in extramammary Paget's disease. Appl Immunohistochem Mol Morphol. 2005;13(4):342–6.
162. Poniecka AW, Alexis JB. An immunohistochemical study of basal cell carcinoma and trichoepithelioma. Am J Dermatopathol. 1999;21(4):332–6.
163. LeBoit PE, Sexton M. Microcystic adnexal carcinoma of the skin. A reappraisal of the differentiation and differential diagnosis of an underrecognized neoplasm. J Am Acad Dermatol. 1993;29(4): 609–18.
164. Lum CA, Binder SW. Proliferative characterization of basal-cell carcinoma and trichoepithelioma in small biopsy specimens. J Cutan Pathol. 2004;31(8):550–4.
165. Smith KJ, Williams J, Corbett D, Skelton H. Microcystic adnexal carcinoma: an immunohistochemical study including markers of proliferation and apoptosis. Am J Surg Pathol. 2001;25(4): 464–71.
166. Hoang MP, Dresser KA, Kapur P, High WA, Mahalingam M. Microcystic adnexal carcinoma: an immunohistochemical reappraisal. Mod Pathol. 2008;21(2):178–85.
167. Alessi E, Venegoni L, Fanoni D, Berti E. Cytokeratin profile in basal cell carcinoma. Am J Dermatopathol. 2008;30(3):249–55.
168. Swanson PE, Fitzpatrick MM, Ritter JH, Glusac EJ, Wick MR. Immunohistologic differential diagnosis of basal cell carcinoma, squamous cell carcinoma, and trichoepithelioma in small cutaneous biopsy specimens. J Cutan Pathol. 1998;25(3):153–9.
169. Krahl D, Sellheyer K. Monoclonal antibody Ber-EP4 reliably discriminates between microcystic adnexal carcinoma and basal cell carcinoma. J Cutan Pathol. 2007;34(10):782–7.
170. Thewes M, Worret WI, Engst R, Ring J. Stromelysin-3 (ST-3): immunohistochemical characterization of the matrix metalloproteinase (MMP)-11 in benign and malignant skin tumours and other skin disorders. Clin Exp Dermatol. 1999;24(2):122–6.
171. Cribier B, Noacco G, Peltre B, Grosshans E. Expression of stromelysin 3 in basal cell carcinomas. Eur J Dermatol. 2001; 11(6):530–3.
172. Christian MM, Moy RL, Wagner RF, Yen-Moore A. A correlation of alpha-smooth muscle actin and invasion in micronodular basal cell carcinoma. Dermatol Surg. 2001;27(5):441–5.
173. Law AM, Oliveri CV, Pacheco-Quinto X, Horenstein MG. Actin expression in purely nodular versus nodular-infiltrative basal cell carcinoma. J Cutan Pathol. 2003;30(4):232–6.
174. Izikson L, Bhan A, Zembowicz A. Androgen receptor expression helps to differentiate basal cell carcinoma from benign trichoblastic tumors. Am J Dermatopathol. 2005;27(2):91–5.
175. Katona TM, Perkins SM, Billings SD. Does the panel of cytokeratin 20 and androgen receptor antibodies differentiate desmoplastic trichoepithelioma from morpheaform/infiltrative basal cell carcinoma? J Cutan Pathol. 2008;35(2):174–9.
176. Costache M, Bresch M, Boer A. Desmoplastic trichoepithelioma versus morphoeic basal cell carcinoma: a critical reappraisal of histomorphological and immunohistochemical criteria for differentiation. Histopathology. 2008;52(7):865–76.
177. Abesamis-Cubillan E, El-Shabrawi-Caelen L, LeBoit PE. Merked cells and sclerosing epithelial neoplasms. Am J Dermatopathol. 2000;22(4):311–5.
178. Kirchmann TT, Prieto VG, Smoller BR. Use of CD34 in assessing the relationship between stroma and tumor in desmoplastic keratinocytic neoplasms. J Cutan Pathol. 1995;22(5):422–6.
179. Pham TT, Selim MA, Burchette Jr JL, Madden J, Turner J, Herman C. CD10 expression in trichoepithelioma and basal cell carcinoma. J Cutan Pathol. 2006;33(2):123–8.
180. Yada K, Kashima K, Daa T, Kitano S, Fujiwara S, Yokoyama S. Expression of CD10 in basal cell carcinoma. Am J Dermatopathol. 2004;26(6):463–71.
181. Stefanaki C, Stefanaki K, Antoniou C, et al. Cell cycle and apoptosis regulators in Spitz nevi: comparison with melanomas and common nevi. J Am Acad Dermatol. 2007;56(5):815–24.
182. Chorny JA, Barr RJ, Kyshtoobayeva A, Jakowatz J, Reed RJ. Ki-67 and p53 expression in minimal deviation melanomas as compared with other nevomelanocytic lesions. Mod Pathol. 2003;16(6):525–9.
183. Kanter-Lewensohn L, Hedblad MA, Wejde J, Larsson O. Immunohistochemical markers for distinguishing Spitz nevi from malignant melanomas. Mod Pathol. 1997;10(9):917–20.
184. Bergman R, Malkin L, Sabo E, Kerner H. MIB-1 monoclonal antibody to determine proliferative activity of Ki-67 antigen as an adjunct to the histopathologic differential diagnosis of Spitz nevi. J Am Acad Dermatol. 2001;44(3):500–4.
185. Maldonado JL, Timmerman L, Fridlyand J, Bastian BC. Mechanisms of cell-cycle arrest in Spitz nevi with constitutive activation of the MAP-kinase pathway. Am J Pathol. 2004;164(5): 1783–7.
186. Hilliard NJ, Krahl D, Sellheyer K. p16 expression differentiates between desmoplastic Spitz nevus and desmoplastic melanoma. J Cutan Pathol. 2009;36(7):753–9.
187. King MS, Porchia SJ, Hiatt KM. Differentiating spitzoid melanomas from Spitz nevi through CD99 expression. J Cutan Pathol. 2007;34(7):576–80.
188. Kapur P, Selim MA, Roy LC, Yegappan M, Weinberg AG, Hoang MP. Spitz nevi and atypical Spitz nevi/tumors: a histologic and immunohistochemical analysis. Mod Pathol. 2005;18(2): 197–204.
189. Bastian BC, Wesselmann U, Pinkel D, Leboit PE. Molecular cytogenetic analysis of Spitz nevi shows clear differences to melanoma. J Invest Dermatol. 1999;113(6):1065–9.
190. Calikoglu E, Augsburger E, Chavaz P, Saurat JH, Kaya G. CD44 and hyaluronate in the differential diagnosis of dermatofibroma and dermatofibrosarcoma protuberans. J Cutan Pathol. 2003; 30(3):185–9.
191. Cribier B, Noacco G, Peltre B, Grosshans E. Stromelysin 3 expression: a useful marker for the differential diagnosis dermatofibroma versus dermatofibrosarcoma protuberans. J Am Acad Dermatol. 2002;46(3):408–13.

192. Diaz-Cascajo C, Bastida-Inarrea J, Borrego L, Carretero-Hernandez G. Comparison of p53 expression in dermatofibrosarcoma protuberans and dermatofibroma: lack of correlation with proliferation rate. J Cutan Pathol. 1995;22(4):304–9.
193. Goldblum JR, Tuthill RJ. CD34 and factor-XIIIa immunoreactivity in dermatofibrosarcoma protuberans and dermatofibroma. Am J Dermatopathol. 1997;19(2):147–53.
194. Hanly AJ, Jorda M, Elgart GW, Badiavas E, Nassiri M, Nadji M. High proliferative activity excludes dermatofibroma: report of the utility of MIB-1 in the differential diagnosis of selected fibrohistiocytic tumors. Arch Pathol Lab Med. 2006;130(6):831–4.
195. Kim HJ, Lee JY, Kim SH, et al. Stromelysin-3 expression in the differential diagnosis of dermatofibroma and dermatofibrosarcoma protuberans: comparison with factor XIIIa and CD34. Br J Dermatol. 2007;157(2):319–24.
196. Lee CS, Chou ST. P53 protein immunoreactivity in fibrohistiocytic tumors of the skin. Pathology. 1998;30(3):272–5.
197. Li N, McNiff J, Hui P, Manfioletti G, Tallini G. Differential expression of HMGA1 and HMGA2 in dermatofibroma and dermatofibrosarcoma protuberans: potential diagnostic applications, and comparison with histologic findings, CD34, and factor XIIIa immunoreactivity. Am J Dermatopathol. 2004;26(4): 267–72.
198. Lisovsky M, Hoang MP, Dresser KA, Kapur P, Bhawan J, Mahalingam M. Apolipoprotein D in CD34-positive and CD34-negative cutaneous neoplasms: a useful marker in differentiating superficial acral fibromyxoma from dermatofibrosarcoma protuberans. Mod Pathol. 2008;21(1):31–8.
199. Mori T, Misago N, Yamamoto O, Toda S, Narisawa Y. Expression of nestin in dermatofibrosarcoma protuberans in comparison to dermatofibroma. J Dermatol. 2008;35(7):419–25.
200. Sachdev R, Sundram U. Expression of CD163 in dermatofibroma, cellular fibrous histiocytoma, and dermatofibrosarcoma protuberans: comparison with CD68, CD34, and Factor XIIIa. J Cutan Pathol. 2006;33(5):353–60.
201. Sasaki M, Ishida T, Horiuchi H, MacHinami R. Dermatofibrosarcoma protuberans: an analysis of proliferative activity, DNA flow cytometry and p53 overexpression with emphasis on its progression. Pathol Int. 1999;49(9):799–806.
202. Lee KJ, Yang JM, Lee ES, Lee DY, Jang KT. CD10 is expressed in dermatofibromas. Br J Dermatol. 2006;155(3):632–3. doi:10.1111/j.1365-2133.2006.07375.x.
203. Clarke LE, Frauenhoffer E, Fox E, Neves R, Bruggeman RD, Helm KF. CD10-positive myxofibrosarcomas: a pitfall in the differential diagnosis of atypical fibroxanthoma. J Cutan Pathol. 2010;37(7):737–43. doi:10.1111/j.1600-0560.2010.01532.x.
204. Diwan AH, Skelton 3rd HG, Horenstein MG, et al. Dermatofibrosarcoma protuberans and giant cell fibroblastoma exhibit CD99 positivity. J Cutan Pathol. 2008;35(7):647–50.
205. Cangelosi JJ, Nash JW, Prieto VG, Ivan D. Cutaneous adnexal tumor with an unusual presentation – discussion of a potential diagnostic pitfall. Am J Dermatopathol. 2009;31(3):278–81.
206. Ivan D, Hafeez Diwan A, Prieto VG. Expression of p63 in primary cutaneous adnexal neoplasms and adenocarcinoma metastatic to the skin. Mod Pathol. 2005;18(1):137–42.
207. Ivan D, Nash JW, Prieto VG, et al. Use of p63 expression in distinguishing primary and metastatic cutaneous adnexal neoplasms from metastatic adenocarcinoma to skin. J Cutan Pathol. 2007;34(6):474–80.
208. Liang H, Wu H, Giorgadze TA, et al. Podoplanin is a highly sensitive and specific marker to distinguish primary skin adnexal carcinomas from adenocarcinomas metastatic to skin. Am J Surg Pathol. 2007;31(2):304–10.
209. Plumb SJ, Argenyi ZB, Stone MS, De Young BR. Cytokeratin 5/6 immunostaining in cutaneous adnexal neoplasms and metastatic adenocarcinoma. Am J Dermatopathol. 2004;26(6):447–51.
210. Qureshi HS, Ormsby AH, Lee MW, Zarbo RJ, Ma CK. The diagnostic utility of p63, CK5/6, CK 7, and CK 20 in distinguishing primary cutaneous adnexal neoplasms from metastatic carcinomas. J Cutan Pathol. 2004;31(2):145–52.
211. Sariya D, Ruth K, Adams-McDonnell R, et al. Clinicopathologic correlation of cutaneous metastases: experience from a cancer center. Arch Dermatol. 2007;143(5):613–20.
212. Levy G, Finkelstein A, McNiff JM. Immunohistochemical techniques to compare primary vs. metastatic mucinous carcinoma of the skin. J Cutan Pathol. 2010;37(4):411–5. doi:10.1111/j.1600-0560.2009.01436.x.
213. Mahalingam M, Nguyen LP, Richards JE, Muzikansky A, Hoang MP. The diagnostic utility of immunohistochemistry in distinguishing primary skin adnexal carcinomas from metastatic adenocarcinoma to skin: an immunohistochemical reappraisal using cytokeratin 15, nestin, p63, D2-40, and calretinin. Mod Pathol. 2010;23(5):713–9. doi:10.1038/modpathol.2010.46.
214. Plaza JA, Ortega PF, Stockman DL, Suster S. Value of p63 and podoplanin (D2-40) immunoreactivity in the distinction between primary cutaneous tumors and adenocarcinomas metastatic to the skin: a clinicopathologic and immunohistochemical study of 79 cases. J Cutan Pathol. 2010;37(4):403–10. doi:10.1111/j.1600-0560.2010.01517.x.

Chapter 31
Application of Direct Immunofluorescence for Skin and Mucosal Biopsies: A Practical Review

William B. Tyler

Abstract This is a practical overview of the use of the application of direct immunofluorescence, written in telegraphic style, based on the author's personal experience, and supplemented by a recommended reference reading list, conceptual diagrams, and illustrative examples.

Keywords Anti-epiligrin pemphigoid • Biopsy selection • Bullous pemphigoid • Cicatricial pemphigoid • Combined use of salt split skin and n-serrated/u-serrated patterns • Dermatitis herpetiformis • Dermatomyositis • Discoid lupus • Epidermal proteins diagram • Epidermolysis bullosa acquisita • Henoch Schönlein purpura • IgA pemphigus • Lichen planus • Lichen planus pemphigoides • Linear IgA disease • n-serrated and u-serrated patterns • Nuclear reactions • Other factors • Paraneoplastic pemphigus • Pemphigoid gestationis • Pemphigus erythematosus • Pemphigus foliaceous • Pemphigus vegetans • Pemphigus vulgaris • Porphyria cutanea tarda • Pseudoporphyria • Salt split skin • Shave biopsy or a punch biopsy • Specimen transport • Subacute cutaneous lupus • Systemic lupus • Thin shave biopsies • Vasculitis

Abbreviations

BPAg1	Bullous pemphigoid antigen 1
BPAg2	Bullous pemphigoid antigen 2
DIF	Direct immunofluorescence
EBA	Epidermolysis bullosa acquisita
ELISA	Enzyme-linked immunosorbent serum assay
kDa	kilodaltons
OCT	Optimal cutting temperature

W.B. Tyler (✉)
Dermatopathology Section, Department of Laboratory Medicine, Geisinger Medical Center, 100 North Academy Avenue, Danville, PA 17822, USA
e-mail: wtyler@geisinger.edu

FREQUENTLY ASKED QUESTIONS

1. What is the difference between direct and indirect immunofluorescent testing? (p. 544)
2. Which is better a shave biopsy or a punch biopsy? (p. 544)
3. What is the best biopsy site (Table 31.1)? (p. 544)
4. How should the biopsy specimen be transported (Table 31.2)? (p. 545)
5. How is the specimen processed? (p. 545)
6. What technique is useful for mounting and cutting thin shave biopsies and mucosal biopsies? (p. 545)
7. What antibodies are routinely used? (p. 546)
8. What positive controls are used and how are they prepared? (p. 546)
9. How are immunofluorescent reactions graded? (p. 544)
10. What is salt split skin direct immunofluorescence and how is it useful? (p. 546)
11. What are n-serrated and u-serrated patterns and how are they useful (Figs. 31.4 and 31.5a, b)? (p. 546)
12. What are the characteristic immunofluorescent findings in bullous pemphigoid? (p. 548)
13. What are the characteristic immunofluorescent findings in cicatricial pemphigoid? (p. 550)
14. What are the characteristic immunofluorescent findings in pemphigoid gestationis? (p. 550)
15. What are the characteristic immunofluorescent findings in anti-epiligrin pemphigoid? (p. 550)
16. What are the characteristic immunofluorescent findings in epidermolysis bullosa acquisita? (p. 551)
17. What are the characteristic immunofluorescent findings in dermatitis herpetiformis? (p. 551)
18. What are the characteristic immunofluorescent findings in linear IgA dermatosis? (p. 551)
19. What are the characteristic immunofluorescent findings in discoid lupus erythematosus? (p. 552)
20. What are the characteristic immunofluorescent findings in systemic lupus and bullous systemic lupus erythematosis? (p. 553)
21. What are the characteristic immunofluorescent findings in subacute cutaneous lupus? (p. 554)
22. What are the characteristic immunofluorescent findings in porphyria cutanea tarda (PCT)? (p. 554)

F. Lin and J. Prichard (eds.), *Handbook of Practical Immunohistochemistry: Frequently Asked Questions*, DOI 10.1007/978-1-4419-8062-5_31, © Springer Science+Business Media, LLC 2011

23. What are the characteristic immunofluorescent findings in pseudoporphyria? (p. 555)
24. What are the characteristic immunofluorescent findings in pemphigus vulgaris? (p. 555)
25. What are the characteristic immunofluorescent findings in pemphigus foliaceus? (p. 556)
26. What are the characteristic immunofluorescent findings in pemphigus erythematosus? (p. 556)
27. What are the characteristic immunofluorescent findings in IgA pemphigus? (p. 556)
28. What are the characteristic immunofluorescent findings in paraneoplastic pemphigus? (p. 557)
29. What are the characteristic immunofluorescent findings in pemphigus vegetans? (p. 558)
30. What are the characteristic immunofluorescent findings in lichen planus? (p. 558)
31. What are the characteristic immunofluorescent findings in lichen planus pemphigoides? (p. 558)
32. What are the characteristic immunofluorescent findings in Henoch Schönlein purpura (HSP)? (p. 559)
33. What is the role of direct immunofluorescence in vasculitis? (p. 560)
34. What antibody may be useful in cases of suspected dermatomyositis? (p. 560)
35. What do cytoid bodies mean? (p. 560)
36. How should antinuclear direct immunofluorescent reactions be interpreted? (p. 560)
37. Are immunoperoxidase stains of any use? (p. 561)
38. What other factors should always be considered in any DIF testing? (p. 561)

31.1 What Is the Difference Between Direct and Indirect Immunofluorescent Testing?

Direct immunofluorescent (DIF) examination is performed on tissue biopsies using cryostat sections that are stained with fluorescein conjugated anti-immunoglobulin, anticomplement (C3), and antifibrinogen. The test detects the presence of in vivo deposits of immunoglobulin, complement, and fibrinogen in the tissue sample and displays the distribution pattern of the deposits.

Indirect immunofluorescent examination tests the patient's serum for the presence of circulating antibodies by incubating the serum with a laboratory tissue substrate, such as human skin, monkey esophagus, or rat bladder, and then using a second fluorescein-conjugated anti-immunoglobulin antibody to determine if and where the antibody in the serum is bound to the tissue substrate.

31.2 Which Is Better a Shave Biopsy or a Punch Biopsy?

Either is acceptable. A 3–4-mm punch biopsy provides a good sample and is easy to process for the preparation of frozen sections. Fat attached to the deep edge of the specimen may be trimmed away to make cryostat sectioning of the skin easier.

A shave biopsy provides a larger area for evaluation but the specimen is more tedious to embed with good orientation for cryostat frozen sections.

For routine H&E histology, a deep shave biopsy, i.e., deep enough to get into the upper reticular dermis is preferable for biopsy of a vesicle or bulla because the epidermis may be fragile and easily disrupted by the shearing force of a punch biopsy. The shave biopsy may also allow inclusion of a larger sample of intact skin close to the blister edge.

31.3 What Is the Best Biopsy Site (Table 31.1)?

Table 31.1 Biopsy site selection

Suspected condition	Specimen for DIF	Specimen for routine microscopy
Pemphigus	Perilesional ** intact normal skin or mucosa at lesion edge	Lesion and intact bordering skin and mucosa to show transition zone
Bullous pemphigoid	Perilesional	Lesion and intact bordering skin and mucosa to show transition zone
Pemphigoid gestationis	Perilesional	Lesion and intact bordering skin and mucosa to show transition zone
Linear IgA disease	Perilesional	Lesion and intact bordering skin and mucosa to show transition zone
Epidermolysis bullosa acquisita	Perilesional	Lesion and intact bordering skin and mucosa to show transition zone
Dermatitis herpetiformis	Normal skin close to lesion, i.e., 3 mm from lesion edge	Lesion and intact bordering skin and mucosa to show transition zone
Lichen planus	Perilesional with inclusion of portion of lesion	Lesional
Porphyria cutanea tarda	Perilesional with inclusion of portion of lesion	Lesion and intact bordering skin and mucosa to show transition zone
Pseudoporphyria	Perilesional with inclusion of portion of lesion	Lesion and intact bordering skin and mucosa to show transition zone
Lupus	Lesional	Lesional
Vasculitis	Lesional less than 24–48 h old	Lesional

Modified to table format from Biopsy sites: online at http://beutnerlabs.com/request/biopsy-sites.php

31.4 How Should the Specimen Be Transported (Table 31.2)?

Table 31.2 Specimen transport

Michel's solution	Saline
Tried and true. Standard DIF transport solution in use for many years with consistently good results	Suitable for specimens that will be received in less than 24 h
Preferable to receive within 48–72 h	Fluorescence detection may diminish after 24 h
Stable at room temperature	Stable at room temperature up to 24 h. Use wide mouth screw cap cup like a urine collection cup, tightly closed to avoid dessication
Commercially available in screw cap, glass vials from Zeus Scientific. The vials have a shelf life of several months	Readily available
Not suitable for routine light microscopy. A separate biopsy should be submitted in formalin for routine microscopy. I do not recommend splitting punch biopsies in the clinic. The specimens are small, the tissue is fragile and it is difficult to do without good magnification and a fresh knife blade. It is preferable to have two separate specimens to avoid compromising the quality of one or both samples	Preferable to receive a separate specimen for routine microscopy that has been placed in formalin at the time of the biopsy

References: [1, 2]

31.5 How Is the Specimen Processed?

In lab processing steps	
Buffer wash	Specimens received in Michel's solution are washed in a buffer solution for 30 min at room temperature, after discarding the Michel's solution. The buffer solution is commercially obtained from Zeus Scientific company. It is stored at 4°C once opened and in use
Mounting the specimen	Specimen is oriented and mounted on a cryostat microtome chuck in a button of optimal cutting temperature (OCT) compound. The knife should strike the deep dermal edge of the specimen first and exit through the epidermis last to avoid folded and wrinkled sections
Freezing the specimen	Snap frozen by immersing the mounted specimen in liquid nitrogen
Sectioning the specimen	Cryostat frozen sections are cut at a thickness of 5 mm
Sections are stored at −20°C	Slides are placed in plastic slide boxes and kept at −20°C until they are stained. We also routinely fix an extra slide for each antibody in cold acetone for 3–5 min. Those slides are then air-dried and stained along with the unfixed cryostat sections. The reactions with both sets of slides are typically congruent but sometimes one or the other is superior
Staining the sections	Sections are incubated with fluorescein-conjugated anti-IgA, anti-IgG, anti-IgM, anti-C3, and anti-fibrinogen. We process these specimens with a DAKO robotic stainer that has been programmed with a staining sequence that is an adaptation of a formerly used manual method
Coverslipping the sections	Water-soluble, nonfluorescent mounting medium is used to attach the coverslips
Slide storage	The stained slides are kept refrigerated in a slide folder until the delivery for examination
Reading the slides	The slides are examined in a darkened room using an epiluminescent fluorescence microscope – systematic examination of intercellular space, epidermal BMZ, follicular BMZ, dermal papillae, dermal vessels, epidermal nuclei, and epidermal cytoplasm
Recording the results	For each antibody, the reaction location and intensity of reaction are recorded. Once read, the fluorescent reaction will often remain visible for several days when stored in a slide folder at room temperature but the reaction does not remain visible indefinitely. Permanent record of reactions may be obtained by photomicroscopy

31.6 What Technique Is Useful for Mounting and Cutting Conjunctival Specimens or Large Thin Shave Biopsies?

1. A button of OCT compound is placed on the cryostat chuck and briefly cooled by short immersion in liquid nitrogen to gel the button but not completely solidify it.
2. The thin flimsy fragment of skin, conjunctiva, or other mucosa is then laid flat on the surface of the still liquid OCT compound and it is stretched out flat with the skin or mucosal surface facing up.
3. The chuck is then immersed in liquid nitrogen to freeze the OCT and the specimen solid.
4. Next, the frozen button is pried from the chuck with a scalpel blade after first dribbling a small amount of tap

water around the base of the frozen OCT button to allow it to be easily removed, yet remain frozen.

5. Once removed, the flat piece of frozen tissue and the adherent frozen OCT compound are bisected or trisected and the section fragments including the still frozen OCT compound are turned 90° and immediately reembedded in a fresh button of OCT compound which is then snap frozen in liquid nitrogen.

This method simplifies the embedding process for this type of specimen, and the tissue sections will now be perfectly vertically oriented with the epidermis or mucosa in profile when the tissue is sectioned.

31.7 What Antibodies Are Routinely Used?

Commercially prepared fluorescein-conjugated anti IgA, anti-IgG, anti-IgM, anti-C3, and anti-fibrinogen.

31.8 What Positive Controls Are Used? How Is Positive Control Tissue Prepared and Preserved?

A positive control for each antibody is run with each batch of patient samples. Positive control slides are harvested from positive clinical cases by cutting up to 100 additional slides from the frozen block and storing the slides at −80°C in plastic slide boxes. To store any remaining specimen, the frozen button of OCT compound containing the tissue is removed from the cryostat chuck, wrapped in aluminum foil, and stored at −80°C.

31.9 How Are Immunofluorescent Reactions Graded?

The grading of the intensity of staining is subjective but a general guideline is:

4+ = strong, glaring fluorescence
3+ = strong, bright staining, not glaring
2+ = strong reaction
1+ = dim, but definite
Trace = faint, equivocal

Generally, in positive specimens, staining intensity is in the 2+ to 4+ range.

31.10 How Is a Salt Split Skin Substrate Prepared for Direct Immunofluorescent Study and How Is It Useful?

1. When a biopsy of intact perilesional skin is received in the laboratory, the specimen is placed in a tube of 30–40 ml of 1 M saline that has been previously cooled to 4°C.
2. If the specimen was received in Michel's solution, it should be washed in buffer prior to placing in the saline solution.
3. The specimen is allowed to incubate in the saline solution at 4°C for 48 h.
4. The incubation in cold (4°C) 1 M NaCl causes a cleavage plane in the lamina lucida resulting in portions of the epidermis detaching from the dermis and forming saline induced vesicles of varying size.
5. After the incubation, it is removed from the saline, placed on a paper towel to allow gentle absorption of any surface saline, and then it is mounted in OCT compound and frozen in liquid nitrogen for the preparation of cryostat sections as usual.
6. The undersurface of the epidermis or mucosa forms the roof of the vesicle and the lamina densa regions of the basement membrane zone and the dermis form the floor.

Depending on where the staining reaction now localizes, i.e., along the undersurface of the roof or along the floor provides additional or confirmatory diagnostic information [3] (Figs. 31.1–31.3).

31.11 What Are n-Serrated and u-Serrated Patterns and How Are They Useful (Figs. 31.4 and 31.5a, b)?

1. These are very useful patterns to look for when there is a linear band of immunoglobulin or complement along the epidermal junction because they further define the location of the immunoreactants as either above the lamina densa (n-serrated pattern) as in all forms of pemphigoid and most cases of linear IgA dermatosis or below the lamina densa (u-serrated pattern) as in epidermolysis bullosa acquisita (EBA), bullous lupus erythematosus, and rarely one form of linear IgA dermatosis. The third pattern, true linear, does not aid in defining the location of the immunoreaction.
2. These patterns have been elegantly shown by correlation with immunoelectron microscopy and dual label immunofluorescence mapping to identify the location of the immunoreactants.

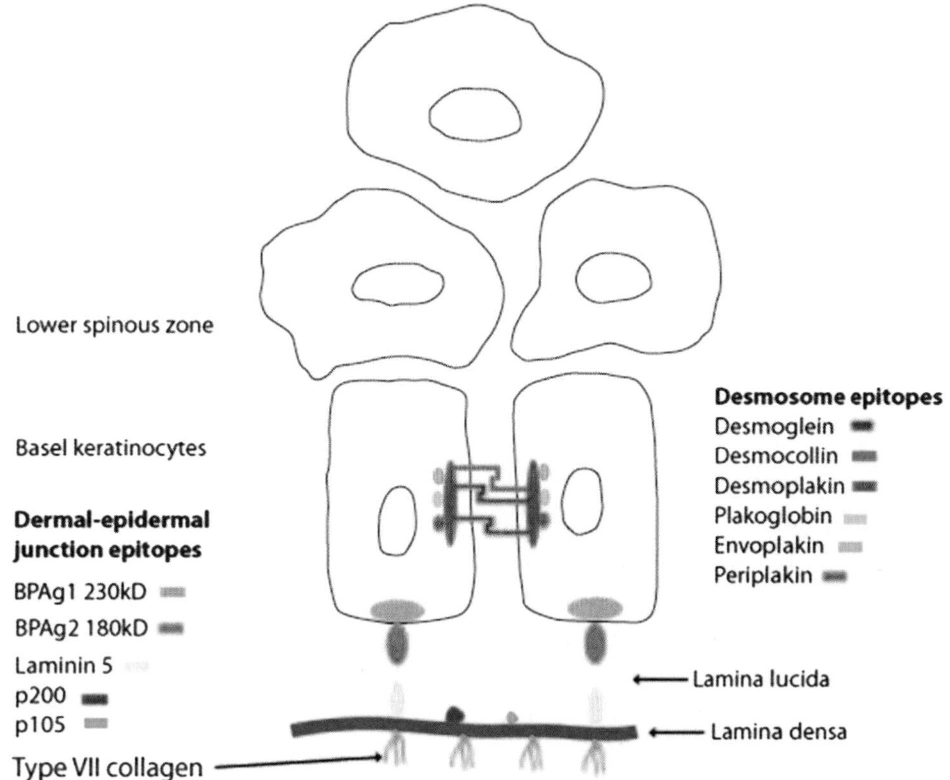

Fig. 31.1 Target epidermal proteins diagram

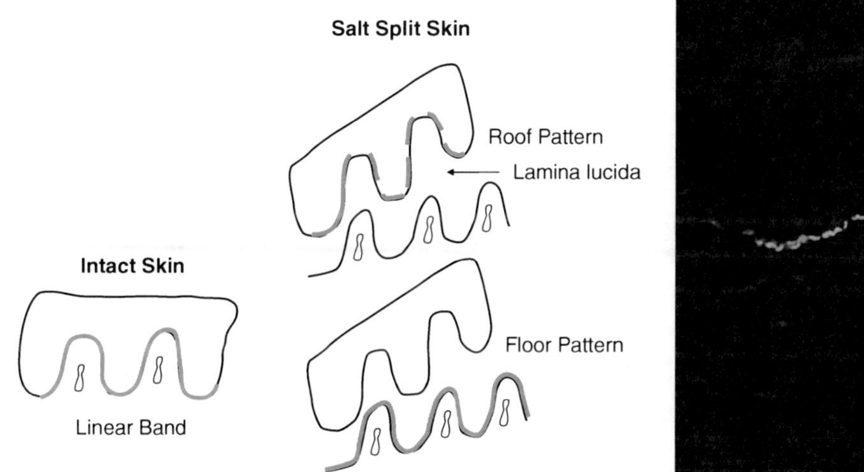

Fig. 31.2 Salt split skin diagram with roof and floor pattern

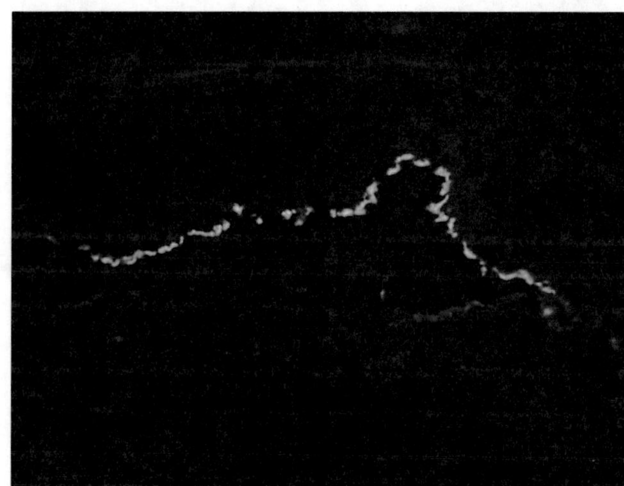

Fig. 31.3 Salt split skin DIF IgG roof pattern

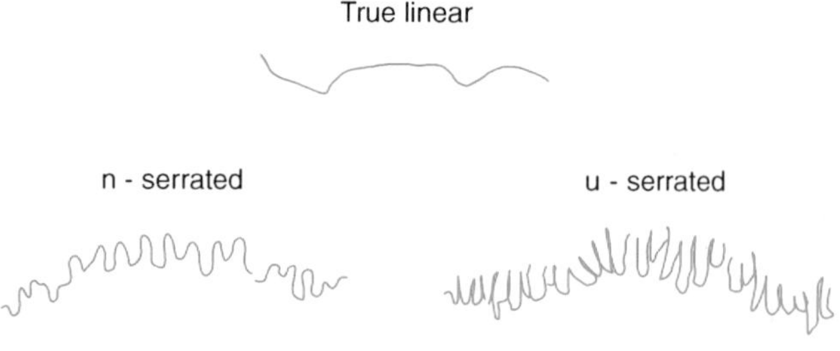

Fig. 31.4 Diagrammatic representation of the fluorescent n-serrated, u-serrated, and true linear basement membrane zone patterns

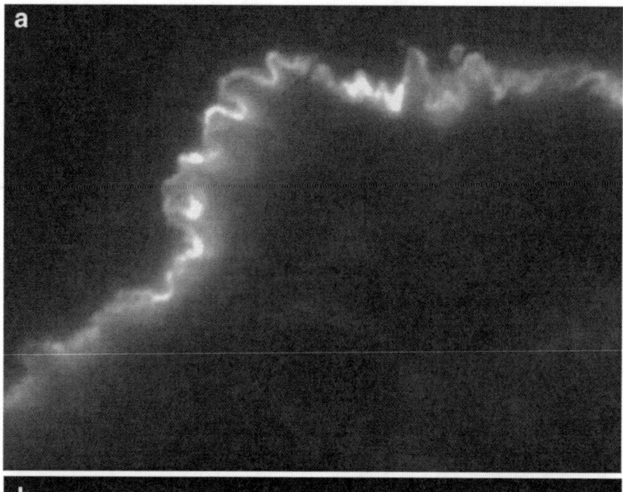

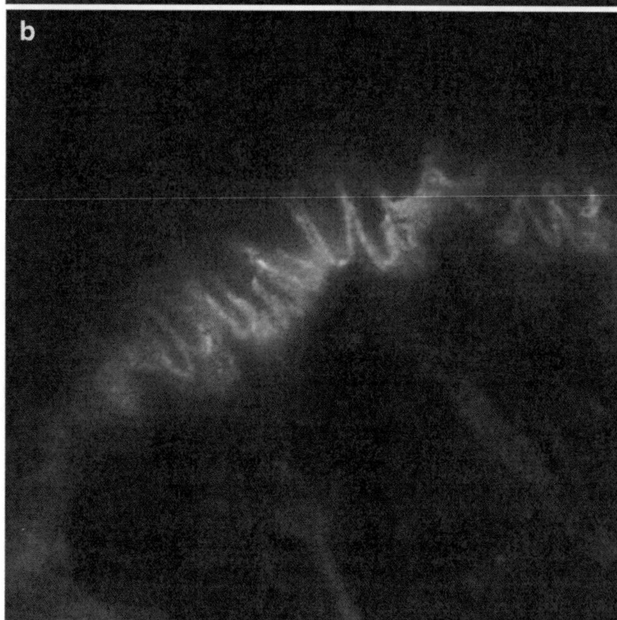

Fig. 31.5 (**a**) n-Serrated, linear, IgG ×1,000 black and white. (**b**) u-Serrated pattern, ×1,000 black and white

3. Once learned, the two patterns are easily distinguished and there is good interobserver agreement.
4. The patterns are visible at 40× magnification but difficult to document photographically without higher magnification, i.e., photograph with digital zoom or use an oil immersion objective.
5. Photography can be performed in black and white if the fluorescence intensity is too great at oil immersion.
6. Identification of either serrated patterns, which in my experience, is nearly always possible, eliminates the need for salt split skin DIF testing (see below) in the most common dilemma of differentiation of bullous pemphigoid and pemphigoid-like forms of EBA, because bullous pemphigoid can be easily distinguished from EBA and bullous lupus by its n-serrated pattern.
7. It may also be useful in combination with salt split skin DIF for recognizing or suspecting unusual often neutrophil rich forms of pemphigoid, such as anti-epiligrin pemphigoid, anti-p200, and anti-p105 pemphigoid, where the target epitopes are at or above the lamina densa but in the floor of salt split skin. In such cases, testing of serum by immunoblot can define the target epitope.
8. In my experience, one of these serrated patterns, most commonly, the n-serrated pattern is visible in variable amounts when there is a linear band of immunoglobulin or complement. The display is often multifocal and quite easily identified, but sometimes it may be limited to a small area and only found on close inspection [4] (Table 31.3).

31.12 What Are the Characteristic Immunofluorescent Findings in Bullous Pemphigoid?

C3 and/or IgG, linear, epidermal basement membrane, usually 2–3+ intensity

May see concurrent weaker identical reactions with IgM and IgA in some cases but IgG and C3 are the dominant immunoreactants

n-serrated pattern

On salt split skin, the roof of the split (undersurface of the detached epidermis) is stained with a continuous or interrupted dash-like (hemi-desmosomal) pattern (Figs. 31.6a–c):

Clinicopathologic correlation.

Histopathology: typically, an eosinophil-rich inflammatory infiltrate with a subepidermal vesicle or bulla. Intact epidermal junction, if urticarial phase. May see eosinophilic spongiosis or eosinophils aligned along the epidermal junction. May be sparsely cellular in some cases. May be neutrophil-rich infiltrate with unusual variants such as anti-p200.

Clinical: The most common immunobullous disorder. Typically elderly, age 70 or greater, tense vesicles and bullae or erythematous patches and plaques or urticarial plaques without blister formation. May occur at any age but uncommon except in older age group. There are occasionally unusual clinical presentations [9, 10].

Table 31.3 Potential for combined use of salt split skin and n-serrated/u-serrated patterns based on known locations of target epitopes

	Salt split skin roof pattern	Target epitope	Salt split skin floor pattern	Target epitope
n-Serrated	Bullous pemphigoid	BPAg1 230 kDa, BPAg2 180 kDa	Anti-epiligrin cicatricial pemphigoid	Laminin 5 serum immunoblot for confirmation
n-Serrated	Pemphigoid gestationis	BPAg2 180 kDa	Unusual neutrophil rich pemphigoid anti-p200	p200 Serum immunoblot for confirmation
n-Serrated	Cicatricial pemphigoid – some forms	BPAg1 230 kDa BPAg2 180 kDa	Unusual pemphigoid anti-p105	p105 Serum immunoblot for confirmation
n-Serrated	Linear IgA disease (most)	Portion of BPAg2 180 kDa		
n-Serrated			Unusual cicatricial pemphigoid other than laminin 5	Need immunoblot to detect other known epitopes laminin 6, uncein, and other incompletely characterized antigens
u-Serrated	Does not occur		Epidermolysis bullosa acquisita	Type 7 collagen
u-Serrated	Does not occur		Bullous systemic lupus	Type 7 collagen Look for other clinical and serologic evidence of lupus
u-Serrated IgA	Does not occur		IgA epidermolysis bullosa acquisita (uncommon)	Type 7 collagen

References: [5–8]

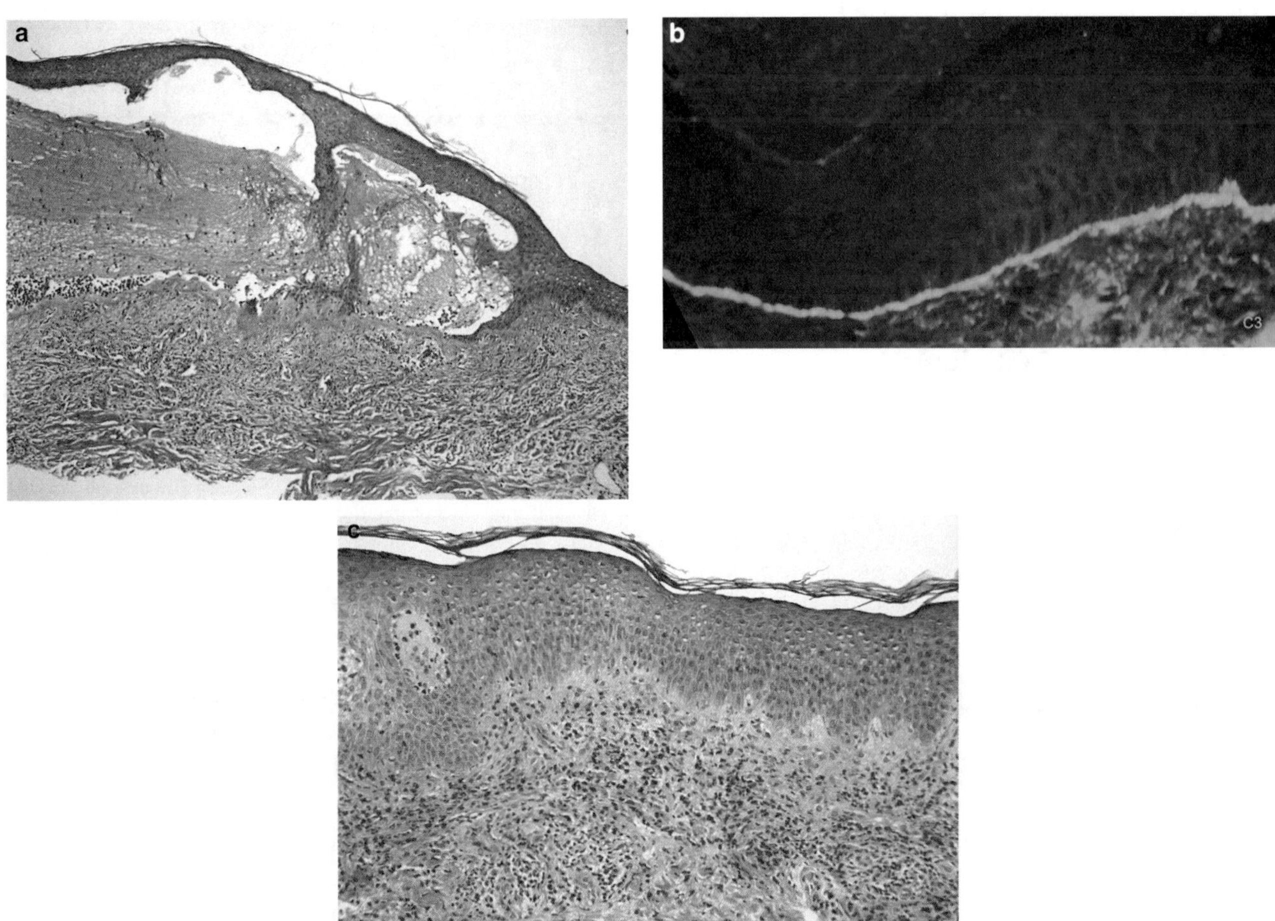

Fig. 31.6 (**a**) Subepidermal vesicle of bullous pemphigoid. (**b**) Linear band of C3 along the epidermal basement membrane zone. (**c**) Urticarial phase bullous pemphigoid. Numerous interstitial eosinophils

31.13 What Are the Characteristic Immunofluorescent Findings in Mucous Membrane Pemphigoid (Cicatricial Pemphigoid)?

2–3+, Linear band with C3, and/or IgG and sometimes IgA. Mucosal involvement: oral and/or conjunctival most commonly. May involve laryngeal, esophageal, and anogenital regions. Skin may also be involved with identical reactions.

n-Serrated as are all forms of pemphigoid.

Salt split skin by direct or indirect methods: roof or floor. If floor pattern, suspect anti-epiligrin pemphigoid. Lack of u-serrated pattern excludes epidermolysis bullosa acquisita.

Clinicopathologic correlation. Mixed inflammatory infiltrate that may include eosinophils, plasma cells, neutrophils, and lymphoid cells. May see fibrosis depending on the duration of the lesion that is biopsied.

Oral ulceration and erosion. Risk of blindness with ocular involvement due to scarring, risk of stricture with laryngeal, esophageal, and anogenital involvement. May have concurrent skin involvement.

Relatively uncommon. Investigate for possible associated malignancy in anti-epiligrin pemphigoid [5, 11].

31.14 What Are the Characteristic Immunofluorescent Findings in Pemphigoid Gestationis (Herpes Gestationis)?

Linear band of C3 with or without IgG. n-serrated pattern. Staining of roof of salt split skin (not usually necessary). Identical to bullous pemphigoid.

Clinicopathologic correlation: Histopathology is essentially identical to bullous pemphigoid. May have a less dense eosinophilic infiltrate. May not be distinguishable histologically from pruritic urticarial papules and plaques, insect bite reaction, or drug-induced inflammatory infiltrate except by immunofluorescent study, which is the gold standard for diagnosis. An ELISA also exists for BPAg2 180 kDa antigen, the target epitope. Onset usually in second or third trimester, urticarial papules and plaques often beginning in the peri-umbilical area and developing tense vesicles and bullae. Usually resolves with delivery. Occasionally, onset is peripartum or postpartum. Distinguished from other pregnancy-related dermatoses by the immunofluorescent findings. Skin involvement in newborn is rare. Onset early in pregnancy and development of blisters reported to be a risk for reduced and low birth weight [12–15] (Fig. 31.7a, b).

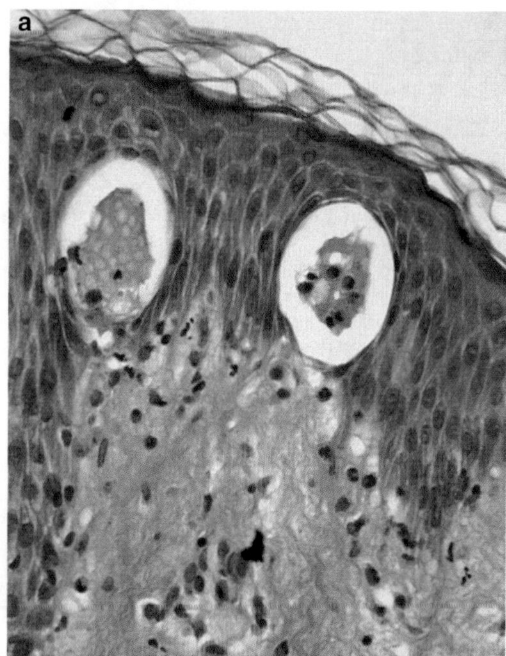

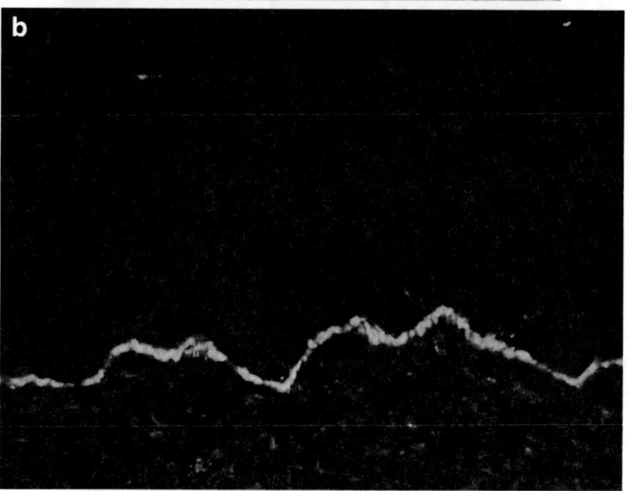

Fig. 31.7 (**a**) Pemphigoid gestationis. Eosinophils, papillary dermal edema and small foci of microvesicle formation. (**b**) Pemphigoid gestationis. Strong linear band of C3 at the epidermal basement membrane zone [11]

31.15 What Are the Characteristic Immunofluorescent Findings in Anti-epiligrin Pemphigoid?

Mucous membrane involvement most commonly oral but may be ocular or other mucosae.

IgG, C3 with or without IgA, linear basement membrane band. n-serrated pattern.

Floor pattern on salt split skin with n-serrated pattern on intact skin is a major clue. Need to send serum for immunoblot or ELISA for immunoblot for confirmation.

Investigate or keep under close surveillance for risk of associated development of carcinoma, typically adenocarcinoma, lung, stomach, uterine [16–19].

31.16 What Are the Characteristic Immunofluorescent Findings in Epidermolysis Bullosa Acquisita?

Strong 2–3+, linear band of IgG and/or C3 at the epidermal basement membrane zone.

Histopathologically, it may be indistinguishable from pemphigoid on H&E or may be cell-poor or neutrophil+rich. The antigenic target is type VII collagen below the lamina densa and a u-serrated pattern distinguishes it from pemphigoid. Distinction from bullous lupus erythematosus is mainly by clinicopathologic correlation with other serologic and clinical features of lupus. Both have type VII collagen as the target epitope.

Clinically, blisters heal with scarring and milia. They tend to occur more prominently in areas of trauma. Mucosal involvement may occur. Serum testing for antibodies to type VII collagen is possible with an ELISA method [20–22].

31.17 What Are the Characteristic Immunofluorescent Findings in Dermatitis Herpetiformis?

Granular deposition of IgA in dermal papillae. Deposition is usually strong 2–3+ and present repetitively in multiple dermal papillae. The deposition may also extend along the epidermal basement membrane zone in some areas. IgA is the dominant immunoreactant. May sometimes see a similar, but weaker, pattern of staining with other conjugates, including fibrinogen, C3 and, IgM (Fig. 31.8a, b).

Clinicopathologic correlation: Classically, neutrophil accumulation with papillary dermal microabscess formation if an early, juicy papule, or early undisturbed small vesicle is biopsied. Many times because of intense pruritus, primary lesions with the classic histology are not found and the H&E morphology may just show erosion and excoriation with a mixed inflammatory infiltrate. Look for clues of neutrophils aligning along the dermal epidermal junction or accumulating in the papillary dermis at the intact skin edge of eroded and ulcerated portions of the epidermis. Characteristic clinical distribution of elbows, knees, upper back and shoulder region, sacral region and buttocks, grouped vesicles on an erythematous base in early onset.

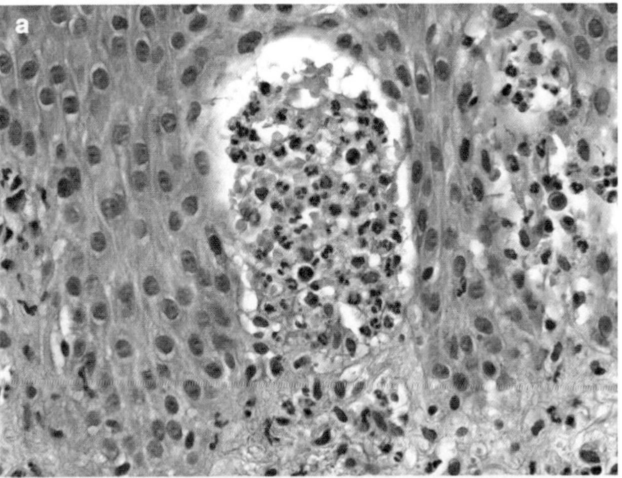

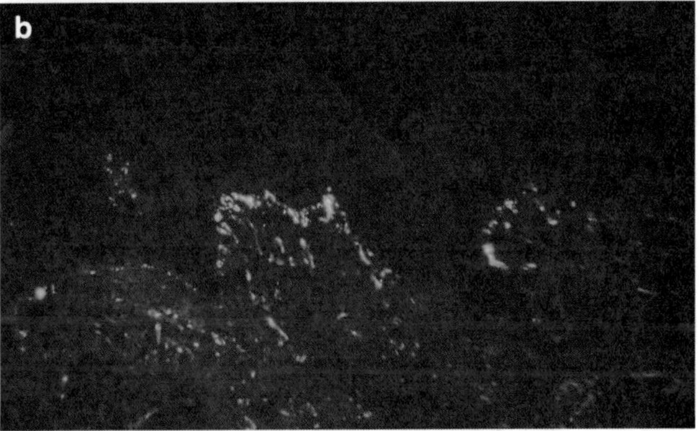

Fig. 31.8 (**a**) Papillary dermal microabscess of dermatitis herpetiformis. (**b**) Granular deposition of IgA in dermal papillae. Dermatitis herpetiformis

H&E morphology with papillary dermal microabscess formation may also be seen with linear IgA dermatosis, bullous systemic lupus, epidermolysis bullosa acquisita, and some forms of bullous pemphigoid. The distinction is made by the direct immunofluorescent study in conjunction with clinicopathologic correlation [9, 20].

31.18 What Are the Characteristic Immunofluorescent Findings in Linear IgA Disease?

Strong, linear band of IgA, 2–3+ along the epidermal basement membrane zone. IgA is the dominant immunoreactant. Most commonly an n-serrated pattern would be anticipated. There is a variant of linear IgA epidermolysis bullosa acquisita that is recognized by a u-serrated pattern (Fig. 31.9a–c).

Clinicopathologic correlation: Neutrophil predominant inflammatory reaction often with papillary dermal microabscess formation mimicking dermatitis herpetiformis,

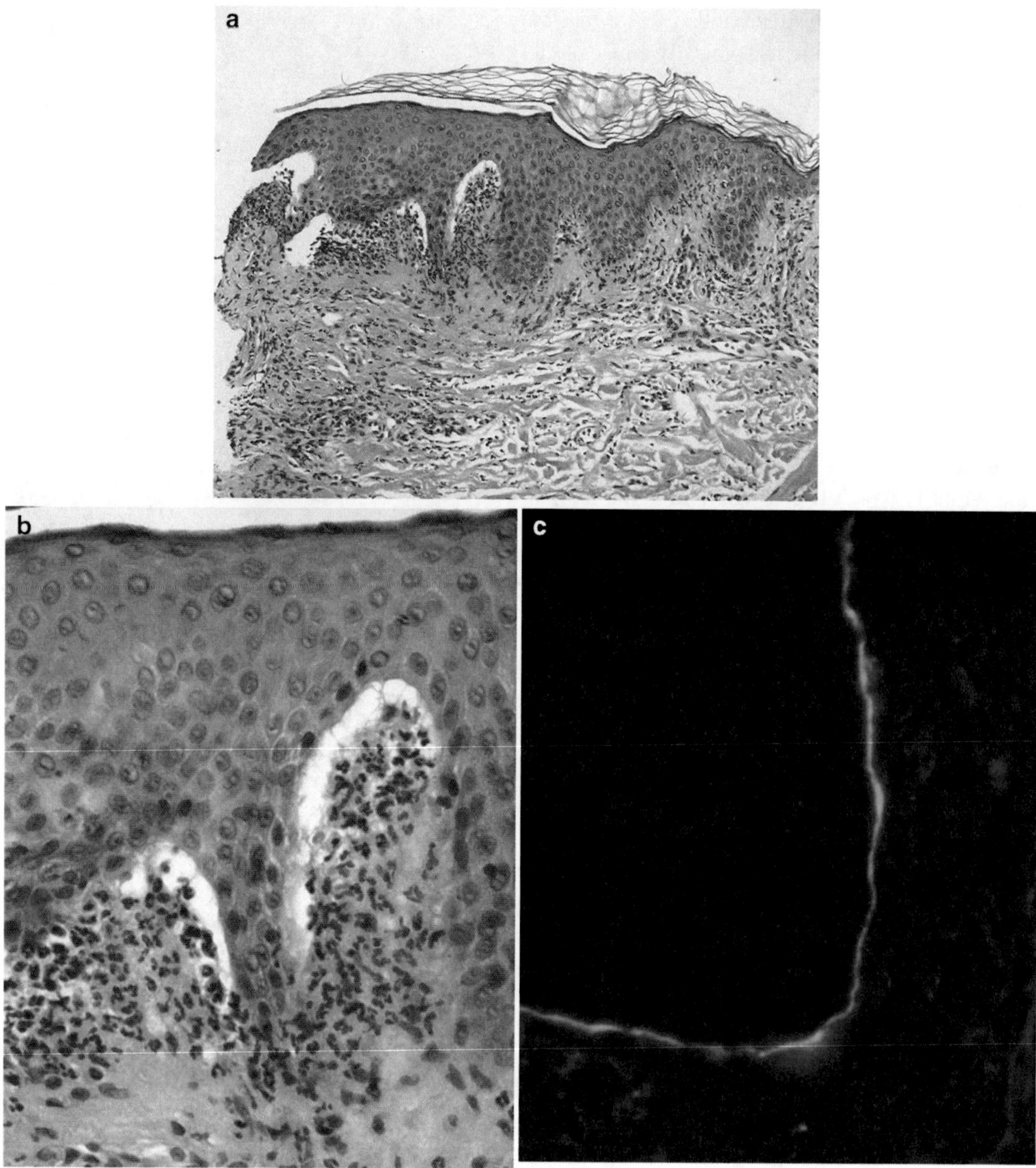

Fig. 31.9 (a) Papillary dermal microabscesses in linear IgA disease. (b) Papillary dermal microabscesses. Linear IgA disease. (c) Linear IgA, epidermal basement membrane zone

histologically. Clinical clues to the diagnosis are the formation of a ring of blisters at the edge of an erythematous plaque. Childhood form is identical, histopathologically, to the adult form. The adult form may be more commonly drug induced. The identification of a drug-induced etiology is made, clinically. It cannot be distinguished from idiopathic forms, histopathologically. The drug-induced form has also been reported to present in some cases with a clinical pattern mimicking toxic epidermal necrolysis. Since the target epitope is usually above the lamina densa, an n-serrated pattern would be expected most commonly. In the event that a u-serrated pattern is found, the possibility of bullous lupus should also be investigated, clinically; however, an IgA form of EBA has been reported [9, 20, 23, 24, 56].

31.19 What Are the Characteristic Immunofluorescent Findings in Discoid Lupus?

A granular deposition of immunoglobulin and complement along the epidermal basement membrane zone with or without an identical deposition along the follicular basement membrane zone. IgM is commonly present but the reaction should be relatively strong, at least 2+, if it is the sole immunoreactant in order to avoid false-positive weak reactions on sun-damaged skin. The specificity of the reaction is increased with the finding of a similar pattern with IgG and/or IgA (Fig. 31.10a, b).

Clinicopathologic correlation: The immunofluorescent findings are reinforced by finding typical H&E morphology of hyperkeratosis, follicular hyperkeratosis, focal epidermal or infundibular epithelial atrophy with epidermal and/or follicular infundibular basement membrane thickening, telangiectasia, and a superficial and deep perivascular and peri-follicular lymphohistiocytic inflammatory reaction that may also focally involve the epidermal interface where there may also be vacuolar change in the basal keratinocyte cytoplasm. There may be increased dermal mucin. Although most commonly it is cutaneous disease only, it cannot be distinguished, histologically, from systemic lupus with discoid lupus lesions. The findings must be integrated, clinically with the clinical morphology, serologic investigation, and other clinical data [25–27].

31.20 What Are the Characteristic Immunofluorescent Findings in Systemic Lupus?

A strong granular band of immunoglobulin often with all three immunoglobulins and usually complement along the epidermal, and often the follicular infundibular, basement membrane zone. There may be staining of epidermal nuclei with immunoglobulin.

The H&E morphology may show an interstitial neutrophilic inflammatory reaction with some leukocytoclasis. Some cases may have associated leukocytoclastic urticarial vasculitis. There may also be relatively sparse lymphocytic inflammation with epidermal atrophy, basal vacuolar change, and increased dermal mucin. Correlation, clinically, with the clinical morphology and serologic tests for lupus are necessary for definitive diagnosis.

In bullous systemic lupus, a linear band of IgG with or without IgA and/or IgM may be seen along the epidermal basement membrane zone. A u-serrated pattern may be

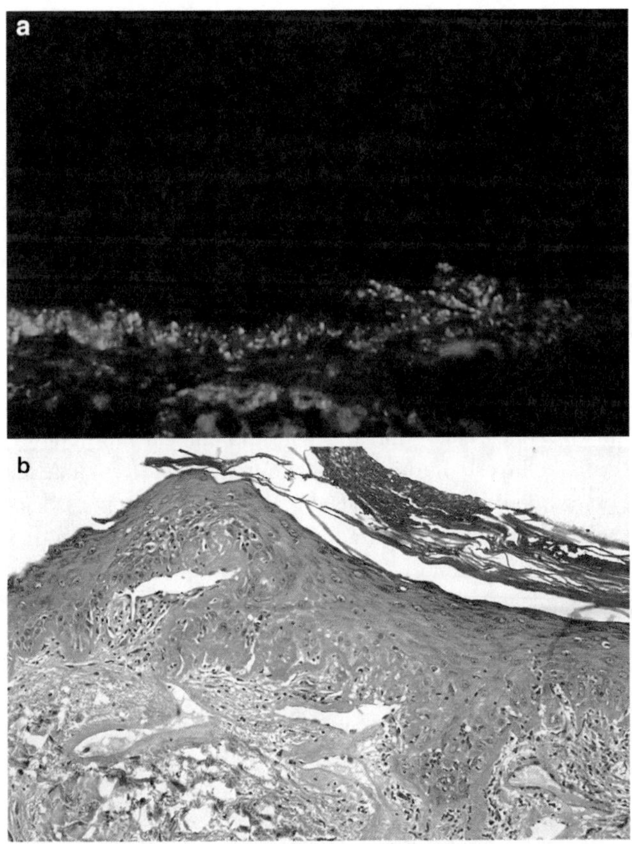

Fig. 31.10 (**a**) Granular, IgG band along the epidermal basement membrane zone in discoid lupus. (**b**) Discoid lupus. Thick, glassy epidermal basement membrane, hypergranulosis, hyperkeratosis, and telangiectasia with thickened vessel basement membranes

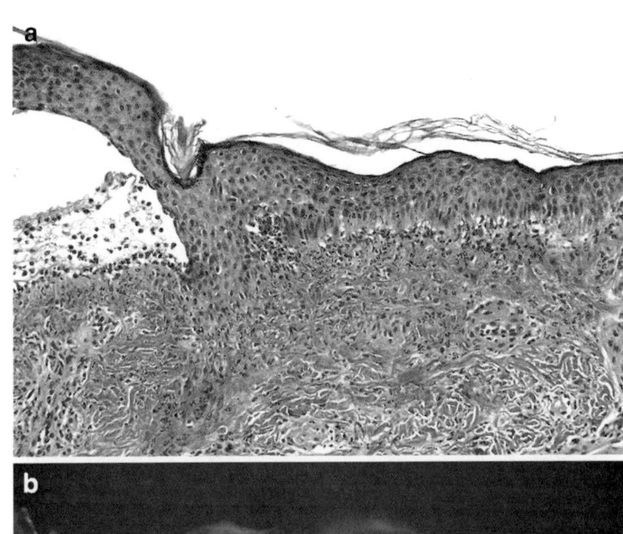

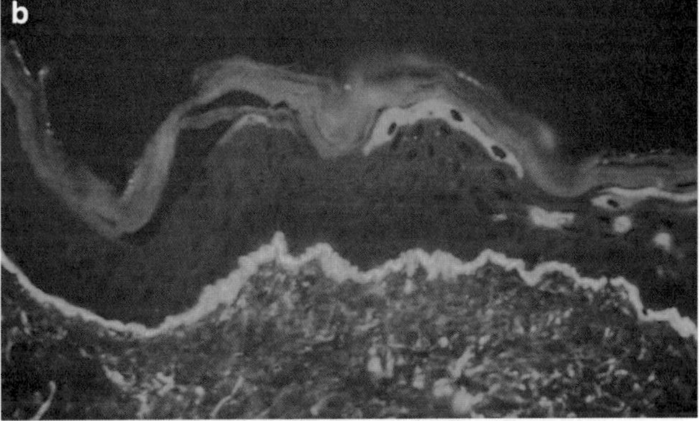

Fig. 31.11 (**a**) Bullous systemic lupus. Interstitial neutrophilic infiltrate and alignment of neutrophils along the epidermal junction at the edge of the bulla. (**b**) Broad linear band of IgG along the epidermal basement membrane zone. (**c**) U-serrated pattern indicative of deposition below the lamina densa

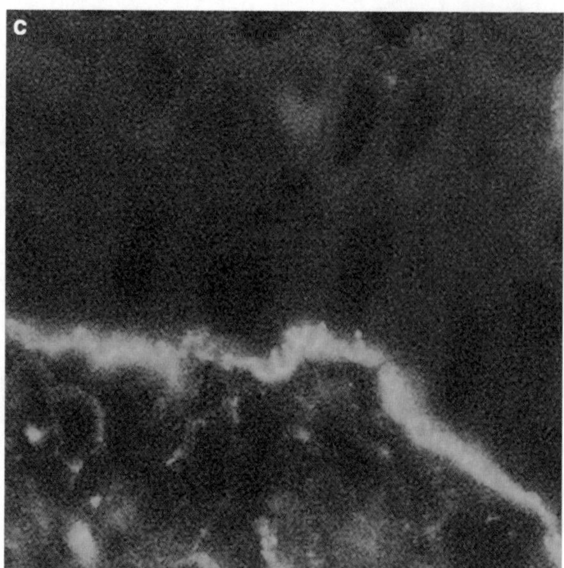

Fig. 31.11 (continued)

evident since the target epitope is type VII collagen (Fig. 31.11a–c).

Clinicopathologic correlation: In bullous systemic lupus, there is a neutrophil-rich inflammatory infiltrate with subepidermal vesicle and bulla formation. Neutrophils may be aligned along the epidermal junction. Papillary dermal microabscess formation may be seen. It must be distinguished from neutrophil-rich EBA and by correlation, clinically, with the clinical morphology and other clinical data, including serologic tests for lupus [27, 28].

31.21 What Are the Characteristic Immunofluorescent Findings in Subacute Cutaneous Lupus?

Deposition of "dust-like" particles in the cytoplasm of lower epidermal keratinocytes with or without speckled staining of epidermal nuclei. This correlates with the antibodies to the Ro cytoplasmic antigen. It is easily distinguished from any nonspecific granular stain precipitate because it is localized to the epidermis in a repetitive, nonrandom, pattern across the width of the specimen and it is not found in the underlying dermis (Fig. 31.12a, b).

Clinicopathologic correlation: H&E morphology is a patchy or widespread lichenoid inflammatory infiltrate without conspicuous basement membrane thickening. There may be hyperkeratosis and focal vacuolar change with occasional apoptotic keratinocytes. There may be increased dermal mucin on colloidal iron stain. The most distinctive finding is the direct immunofluorescent pattern in conjunction

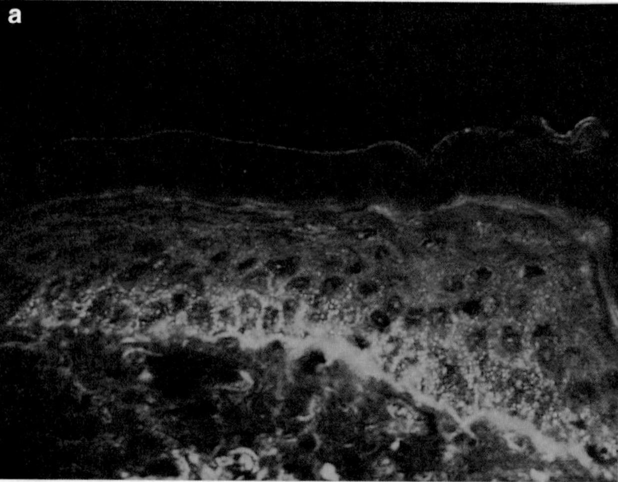

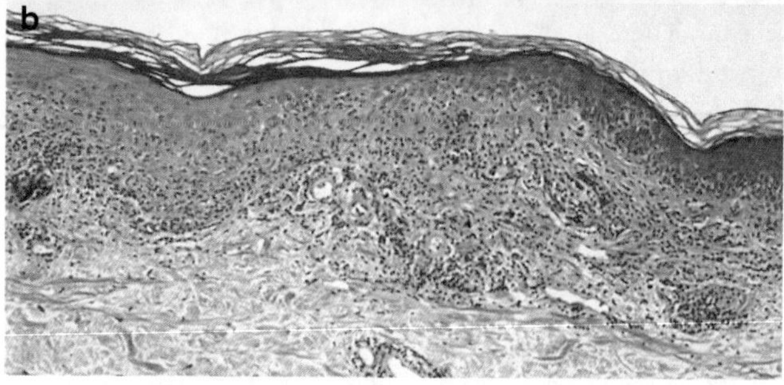

Fig. 31.12 (**a**) "Dusty" granular staining of basal keratinocyte cytoplasm with IgG in subacute cutaneous lupus. (**b**) Perivascular, interstitial, and focal patchy lichenoid interface lymphohistiocytic inflammation with hyperkeratosis. Subacute cutaneous lupus

with the clinical morphology of scaly, annular, polycyclic, or serpiginous plaques usually on the trunk and upper extremities and clinical serologic investigation. Some cases of subacute lupus may be drug induced. These may be suspected histologically, if eosinophils are also evident in the dermal inflammatory infiltrate.

The histopathologic and immunofluorescent findings must be integrated clinically with the clinical morphology, serologic investigation, and other clinical data to exclude the possibility of subacute cutaneous lupus occurring in association with systemic lupus and to aid in the recognition of a drug-induced etiology [29].

31.22 What Are the Characteristic Immunofluorescent Findings in Porphyria Cutanea Tarda?

A thick smudgy band of IgG along the epidermal basement membrane zone and a similar prominent thick, smudgy basement membrane of multiple superficial dermal vessels (Fig. 31.13a, b).

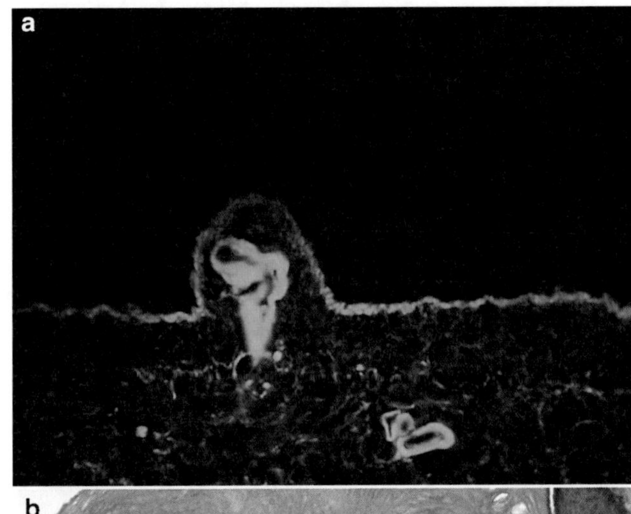

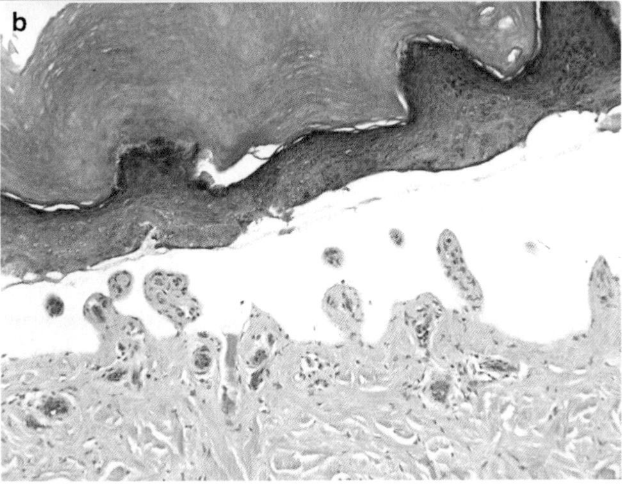

Fig. 31.13 (**a**) Thick band of IgG along epidermal basement membrane zone and smudgy staining of the walls of superficial vessels in porphyria cutanea tarda. (**b**) Noninflammatory subepidermal bulla with festooning of dermal papillae and caterpillar bodies along a portion of the under surface of the detached epidermis in porphyria cutanea tarda

Clinicopathologic correlation: The H&E biopsy is typically from acral skin and shows a noninflammatory or at most pauci-inflammatory subepidermal vesicle or bulla with dermal papillae that protrude from the floor of the vesicle into the blister space, also known as festooning of dermal papillae. The vessels may have visibly thickened basement membranes on H&E and PAS stains. Caterpillar bodies may be seen along the undersurface of the detached epidermis.

Clinically, there is some skin fragility with blisters typically on acral sun-exposed sites that heal with scarring and milia. There may be excess facial hair and sclerodermoid changes may develop in some lesions. There is an elevated level of serum and urine uroporphyrins due to a deficiency of the enzyme uroporphyrinogen decarboxylase. PCT is also associated with hepatic iron overload and there be associated with hemochromatosis, hepatitis C, or alcoholic liver disease [30, 31].

31.23 What Are the Characteristic Immunofluorescent Findings in Pseudoporphyria?

The immunofluorescent findings and the H&E morphology of pseudoporphyria are indistinguishable histologically from porphyria cutanea tarda.

The distinction is made clinically by correlation with the clinical history, drug history, and lack of the abnormal porphyrin level of PCT. Pseudoporphyria occurs in young women who are frequent tanning bed users and it has been causally linked to a variety of drugs, most notably the nonsteroidal anti-inflammatory drug naproxen, and other similar compounds as well as furosemide, chlorothiazide–triamterine and others. It may be seen in children, particularly, in association with nonsteroidal inflammatory drug use in juvenile rheumatoid arthritis. It is not associated with liver disease or iron overload [32].

31.24 What Are the Characteristic Immunofluorescent Findings in Pemphigus Vulgaris?

A delicate smooth staining of the intercellular space in the epidermis with IgG with or without C3. Weaker reactions with IgA and IgM may also be seen but the dominant immunoreactant is IgG. The reaction may be noted throughout the epidermis or it may be concentrated in the lower portions of the epidermis (Fig. 31.14a, b).

Clinicopathologic correlation: There is suprabasal acantholysis in the epidermis and at times in the basal infundibular epithelium of hair follicles. The blisters are fragile and must be handled carefully during gross examination and embedding. Oral mucosal involvement is common and the disease at times may first be found in an oral mucosal biopsy during an investigation of oral mucosal ulcers and erosions. Skin fragility with positive Nikolsky sign and flaccid vesicles and bullae are clinical clues to the diagnosis. Occasionally, limited forms of the disease may occur in areas of prior trauma. Supplemental investigations include indirect immunofluorescent study for the determination of antibody titer and sometimes for further verification of the diagnosis. An ELISA is also available for the main target epitope, desmoglein 3 and it is also available for desmoglein 1 [33, 34].

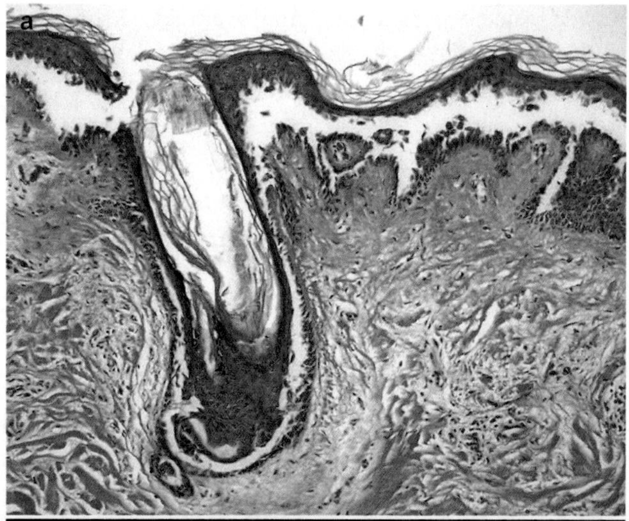

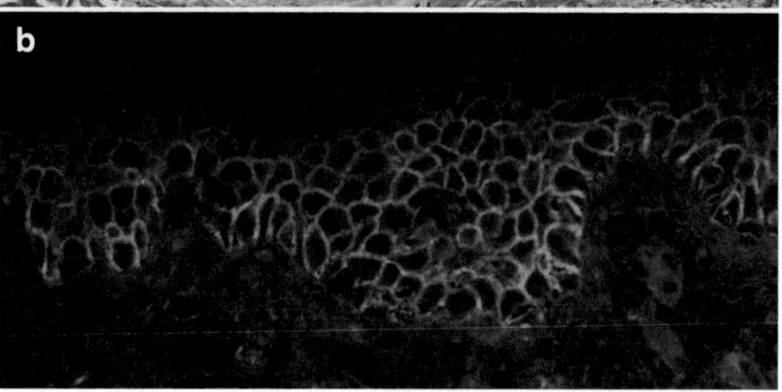

Fig. 31.14 (a) Suprabasal acantholysis of epidermis and follicular infundibular epithelium in pemphigus vulgaris. (b) IgG in the intercellular space of the epidermis in pemphigus vulgaris

31.25 What Are the Characteristic Immunofluorescent Findings in Pemphigus Foliaceus?

Staining of the intercellular space with IgG, particularly in the upper half of the epidermis. There may also be staining with C3 and the staining may extend to involve the entire spinous zone (Fig. 31.15).

Clinicopathologic correlation: The cleavage plane in the H&E sections is in the region of the granular cell layer and upper portion of the spinous zone. The findings may be subtle or obvious. Because the blisters are superficial and fragile, the specimens must be handled carefully during gross examination and embedding to preserve optimal morphology. It may be best to avoid sectioning the specimen, until the time of embedding, if possible. In some cases, a clue to the diagnosis may be the absence of a granular cell layer and stratum corneum due to prior detachment of those structures. An identical cleavage plane occurs with staphylococcal scalded skin syndrome but the immunofluorescent study is negative in that condition. Likewise, a similar pattern of cleavage may be seen in bullous impetigo but in that condition

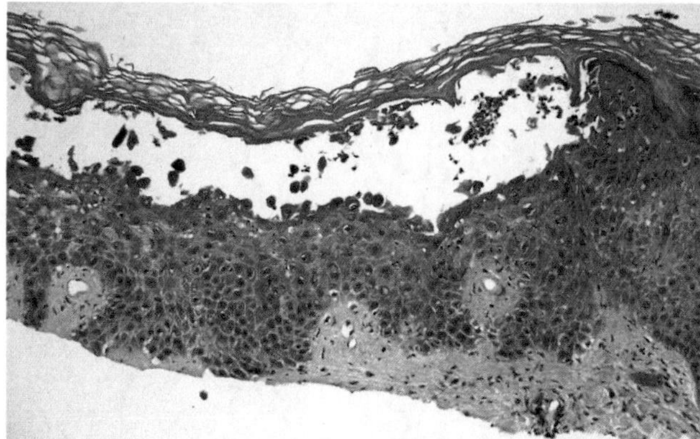

Fig. 31.15 Superficial epidermal acantholytic cleavage plane in pemphigus foliaceous

not only is the direct immunofluorescent study negative but also staphylococci can often be found in abundance in the blister space. Indirect immunofluorescent study may also be used as an adjunctive diagnostic tool and for titer determination. An ELISA is available for desmoglein 1, the target epitope. Clinically, there are scaly crusted plaques with or without visible superficial vesicles and bullae involving the upper trunk but the disease may become widespread. A characteristic corn flake-like scale is sometimes found. The oral mucosa is not involved [35, 36].

31.26 What Are the Characteristic Immunofluorescent Findings in Pemphigus Erythematosus?

Staining of the intercellular space with IgG and granular staining of the epidermal basement membrane zone with IgG.

Clinicopathologic correlation: This is a rare condition with scaly plaques involving the face and upper trunk in a seborrheic distribution. It may be associated with internal malignancy, including thymoma and Castleman's disease. The cleavage plane is also in the region of the granular cell layer and superficial spinous zone of the epidermis. The granular immunoglobulin band at the epidermal junction is lupus-like [37].

31.27 What Are the Characteristic Immunofluorescent Findings in IgA Pemphigus?

Staining of the intercellular space of the epidermis with IgA in the appropriate histopathologic setting (Fig. 31.16a–c).

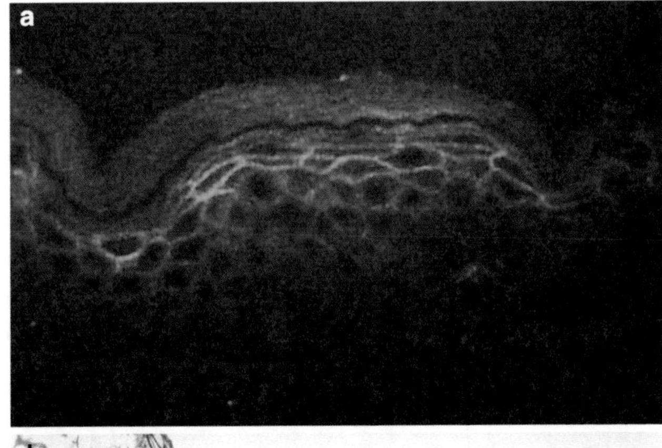

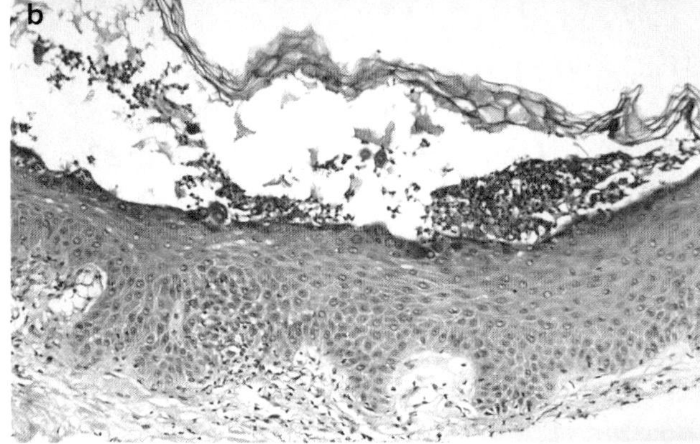

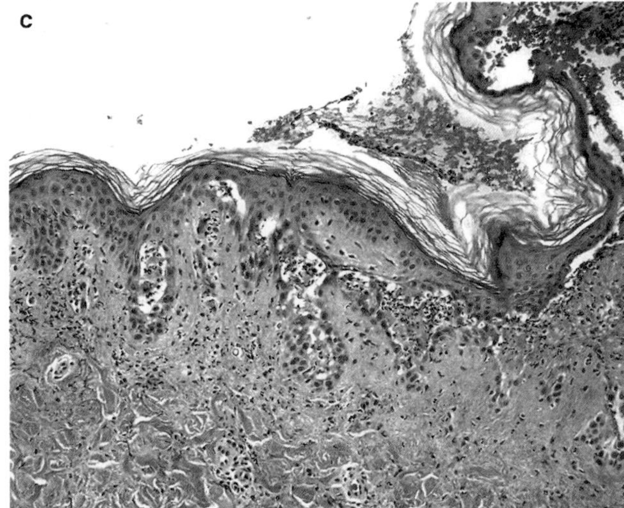

Fig. 31.16 (**a**) Intercellular staining in the superficial epidermis with IgA. (**b**) Subcorneal pustular form of IgA pemphigus. (**c**) Intra-epidermal neutrophilic form of IgA pemphigus

Clinicopathologic correlation: An intra-epidermal neutrophilic and a subcorneal pustular pattern are the two characteristic histopathologic forms of this disease in conjunction with the pemphigus pattern on DIF. Indirect immunofluorescent study may also demonstrate an elevated titer of IgA antibodies with an intercellular reaction pattern. This is an uncommon condition [38–40].

31.28 What Are the Characteristic Immunofluorescent Findings in Paraneoplastic Pemphigus?

Staining of the intercellular space with IgG and also staining of the epidermal basement membrane zone (Fig. 31.17a, b).

Clinicopathologic correlation: The predominant morphology may be an inflammatory reaction along the epidermal interface with focal apoptotic keratinocytes, mimicking erythema multiforme. Acantholysis may be inconspicuous or subtle. Clinically, there is severe oral mucosal, as well as cutaneous, involvement leading to biopsy which reveals the characteristic findings. Indirect immunofluorescent study using rat bladder mucosa is a confirmatory diagnostic test for the detection of desmoplakin antibodies. Immunoblotting using nitrocellulose strips containing separated epidermal proteins may also be performed in a research laboratory with that capability to define the full spectrum of reactivity, which includes BPAg 1–230 kDa,

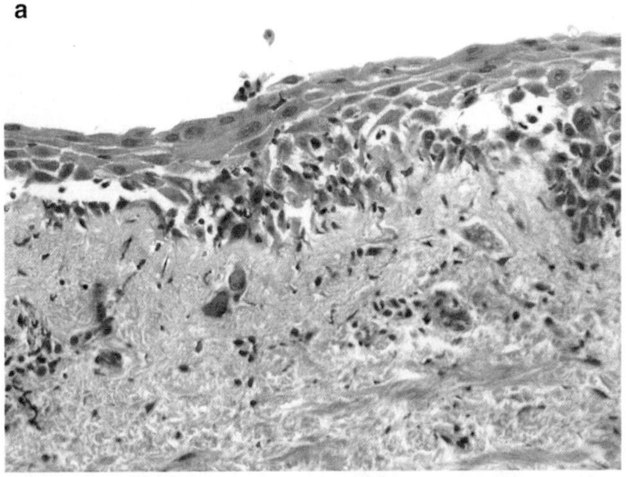

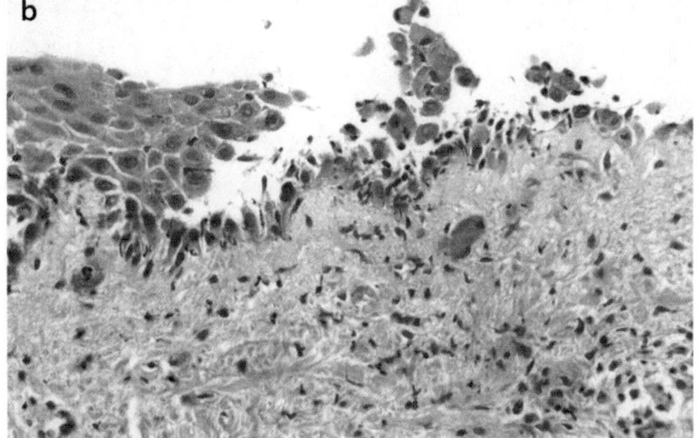

Fig. 31.17 (**a**) Paraneoplastic pemphigus with sparse interface lymphocytic inflammation, occasional apoptotic keratinocytes, and subtle acantholysis. (**b**) The same specimen with a more obvious focus of lower epidermal acantholysis

desmoglein 1 and 3, desmoplakins, and plakoglobin. Clinical investigation for leukemia, lymphoma, or other malignancy should be pursued, if not already evident [41–43].

31.29 What Are the Characteristic Immunofluorescent Findings in Pemphigus Vegetans?

Staining of the intercellular space with IgG (Fig. 31.18a, b).

Clinicopathologic correlation: Histologically, there is prominent prurigo-like epidermal hyperplasia with elongated and thickened rete ridges. A hallmark finding is the presence of intra-epidermal eosinophilic abscesses and foci of supra-basal acantholysis. This is an uncommon condition that is considered as a form of pemphigus vulgaris. It is largely confined to the intertriginous areas as vegetant plaques [44, 45].

31.30 What Are the Characteristic Immunofluorescent Findings in Lichen Planus [46]?

A bright (3–4+), broad, shaggy band of fibrinogen along the basement membrane zone, usually in biopsies from oral mucosa. There may be some focal weak granular staining with C3 (Fig. 31.19a, b).

Clinicopathologic correlation: Biopsies of lichen planus are not usually performed for direct immunofluorescent study except in the investigation of oral mucosal disease. The fibrinogen band is a characteristic, repetitive finding but a definitive diagnosis and distinction from drug-induced lichenoid mucositis requires careful examination of the lichenoid inflammatory infiltrate for the presence of eosinophils or abundant plasma cells. In the presence of either of the latter findings, the possibility of a lichen planus-like drug-induced mucositis should be considered [46, 47].

31.31 What Are the Characteristic Immunofluorescent Findings in Lichen Planus Pemphigoides?

A linear band of C3 at the epidermal or mucosal basement membrane zone with or without IgG and an n-serrated pattern (Fig. 31.20a–d).

Clinicopathologic correlation: This condition is suspected or identified when a patient with an established diagnosis of lichen planus develops vesicles or bullae involving either lesions of lichen planus or previously uninvolved skin. It may also be seen in the oral mucosa of patients with lichen planus. It is an uncommon condition [46, 48, 49].

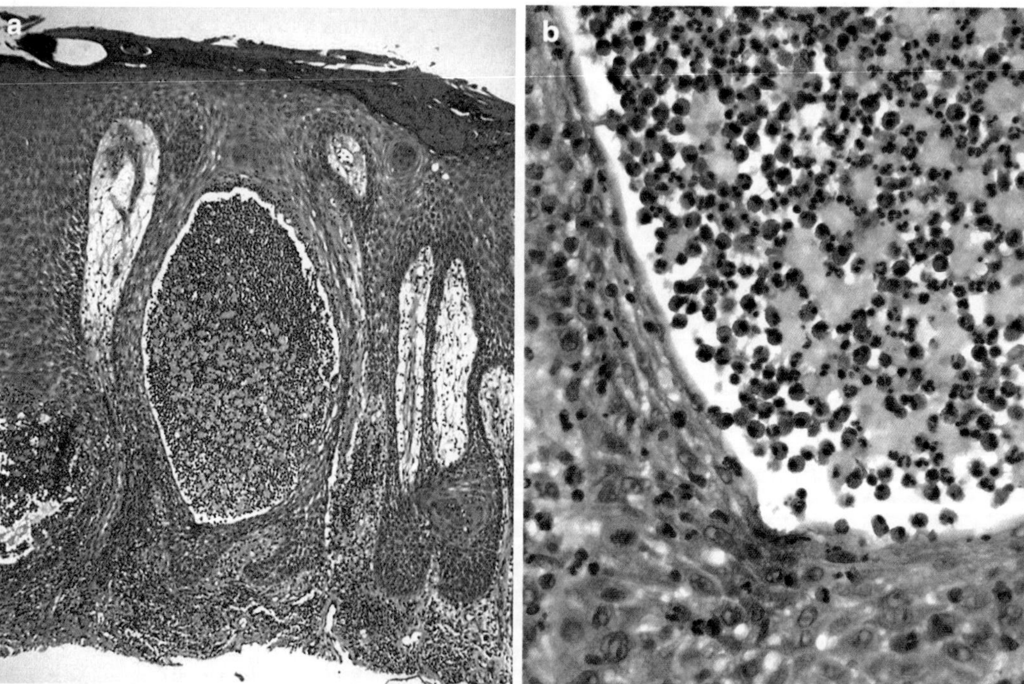

Fig. 31.18 (**a**) Prurigo-like epidermal hyperplasia with a large intra-epidermal abcess that is composed mostly of eosinophils and focal basal epidermal acantholytic change in pemphigus vegetans. (**b**) Portion of the intra-epidermal abscess with numerous eosinophils and some admixed neutrophils

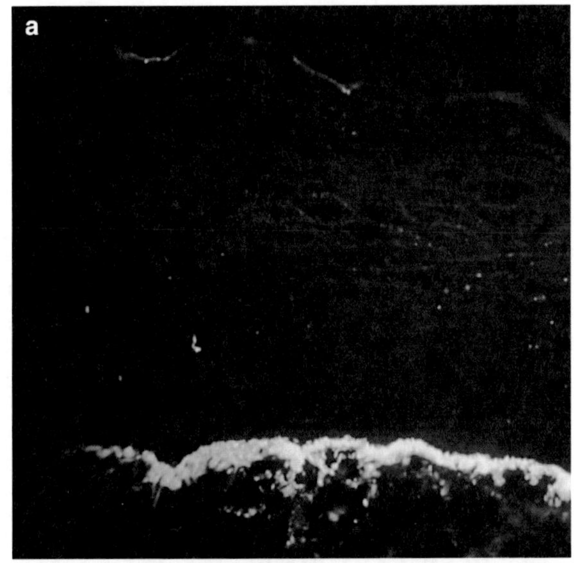

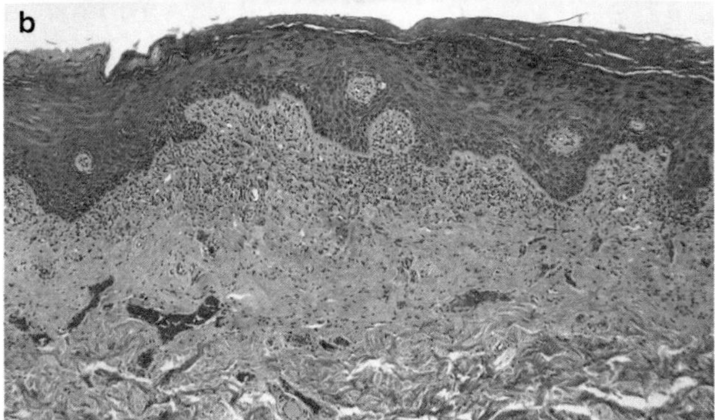

Fig. 31.19 (**a**) Broad, shaggy, strong, fibrinogen band along the basement membrane zone of this oral mucosal biopsy of lichen planus. (**b**) Oral mucosal biopsy of lichen planus with a transition from squamous mucosa to hyperkeratotic mucosa with a granular cell layer and band-like lymphohistiocytic infiltrate in the superficial lamina propria that focally involves the mucosal interface

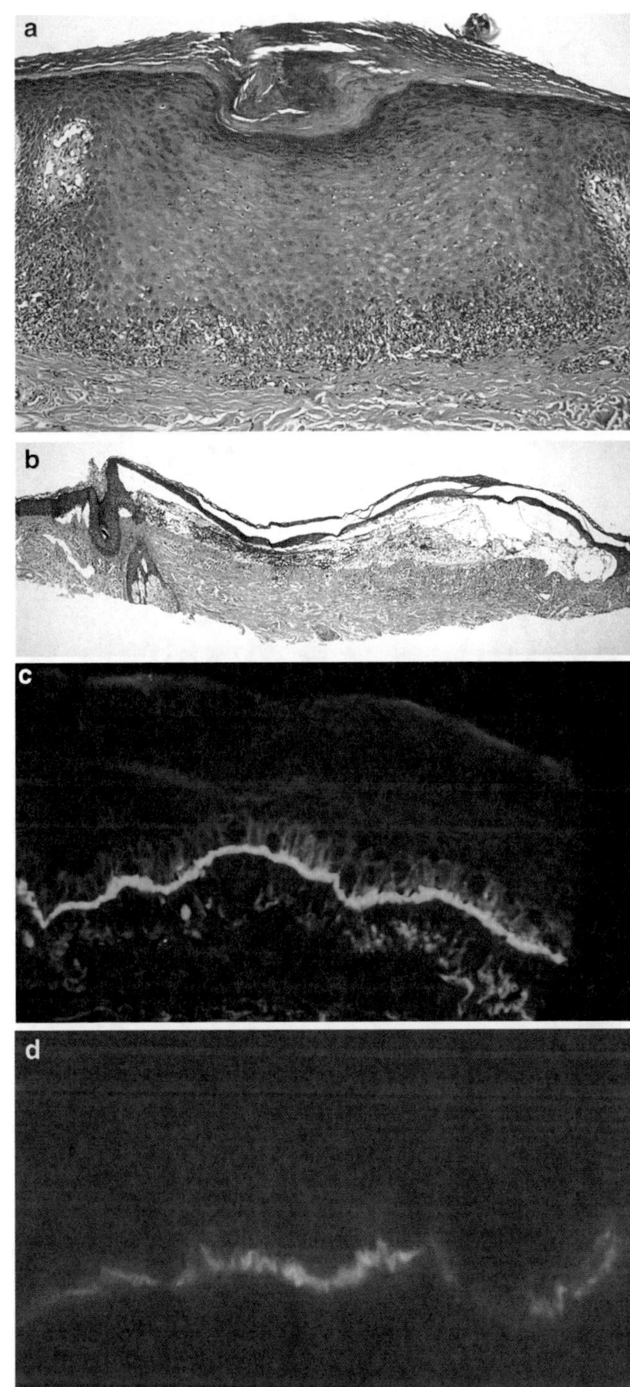

Fig. 31.20 (**a**) Lichen planus. (**b**) Subepidermal vesicle of lichen planus pemphigoides. (**c**) Strong, linear band of C3 along the epidermal basement membrane. Lichen planus pemphigoides p zone. (**d**) Black and white photo of n-serrated pattern visible just to the left of center in this photo. Lichen planus pemphigoides (oil immersion magnification ×1,000)

31.32 What Are the Characteristic Immunofluorescent Findings in Henoch Schönlein Purpura?

A granular deposition of IgA in superficial dermal small vessels. There is also frequently strong staining of dermal vessels with fibrinogen and there may be a granular deposition of C3 and sometimes IgM (Fig. 31.21a, b).

Clinicopathologic correlation: Biopsies are frequently received with a note to "rule out HSP." The presence of IgA in dermal vessels supports a clinical diagnosis of HSP but it is not, by itself, sufficient for the diagnosis of HSP because IgA deposition in dermal vessels may occur in cases of leukocytoclastic vasculitis that are not HSP. A definitive clinical diagnosis should be based on the integration of the biopsy result with the findings of a characteristic clinical

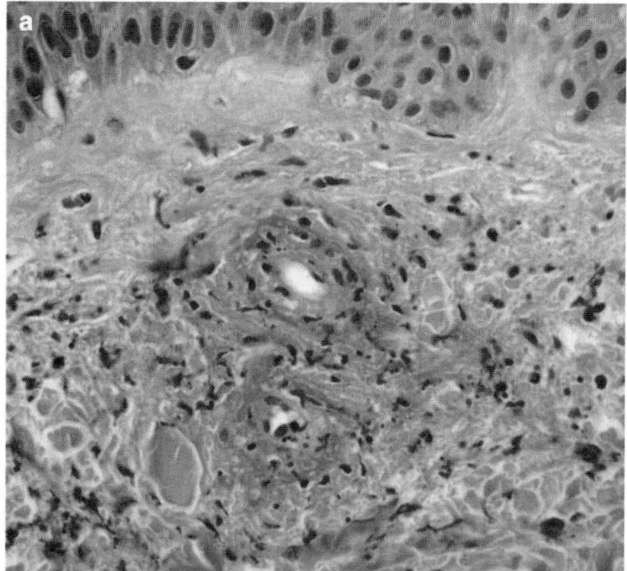

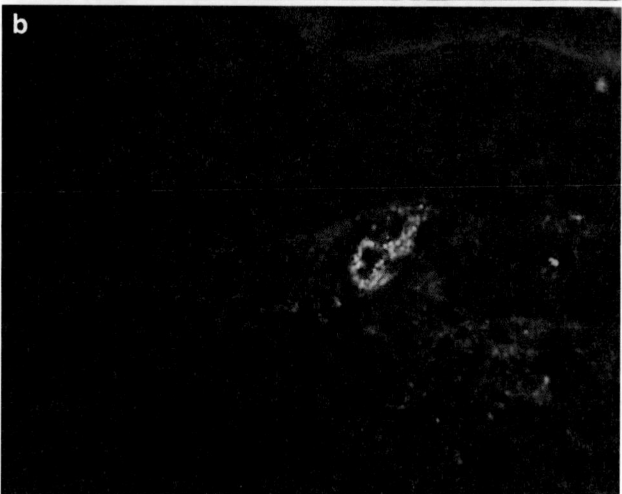

Fig. 31.21 (**a**) Leukocytoclastic vasculitis with prominent fibrin deposition in and around the walls of small vessels and neutrophils and nuclear dust in the surrounding interstitium. (**b**) Granular deposition of IgA in a papillary dermal capillary loop

syndrome of HSP. In summary, the biopsy finding is supportive of a clinical diagnosis of HSP but it is not, by itself, pathognomonic of the disorder [50].

31.33 What Is the Role of Direct Immunofluorescence in Vasculitis?

In my opinion, vasculitis is a diagnosis made by characteristic findings in H&E stained sections. It is not a diagnosis that is made solely by direct immunofluorescent study. It is not uncommon to find staining of some dermal vessels with fibrinogen and sometimes with C3 when there is no clinical and histologic evidence of leukocytoclastic vasculitis. Therefore, a diagnosis of vasculitis should never be based solely on immunofluorescent findings, in my opinion. It may be helpful to look for IgA deposition as support for a clinical diagnosis of HSP. It may be helpful in recognizing urticarial vasculitis, in cases with an urticarial reaction with leukocytoclasis but without overt fibrinoid change in small dermal vessels in the H&E stained sections. In that scenario, I would consider the presence of fibrinogen, and a granular pattern of C3, IgM, or other immunoglobulin in multiple superficial small vessels potentially helpful in supporting a diagnosis of urticarial vasculitis [51].

31.34 What Antibody May Be Useful in Cases of Suspected Dermatomyositis?

Dermatomyositis may mimic lupus histopathologically but it does not show evidence of a granular lupus band. Magro has described a pattern of staining with an antibody to the C5-9 membrane attack complex that may be useful in recognizing dermatomyositis. However, practically speaking, biopsies are seldom submitted for direct immunofluorescent study for dermatomyositis. Consequently, this antibody has not been stocked for routine use [52].

31.35 What Do Cytoid Bodies Mean?

Cytoid bodies are a marker of some prior epidermal injury. They are immunoglobulin-coated dead keratinocytes. They do not have any specific diagnostic value. They are often seen in any condition where there is a component of interface lichenoid inflammatory reaction (Fig. 31.22).

31.36 How Should Antinuclear Reactions Be Interpreted?

Antinuclear staining is sometimes seen in the DIF biopsy specimen. If the staining pattern is moderately strong, i.e., at least 2+ and present throughout the specimen, it will likely correlate well with other clinical data. Weak intensity staining of epidermal nuclei may sometime occur as a spurious finding that I suspect is reagent related. For that reason, in my opinion, the presence or absence of an antinuclear antibody is best determined by conventional serologic testing.

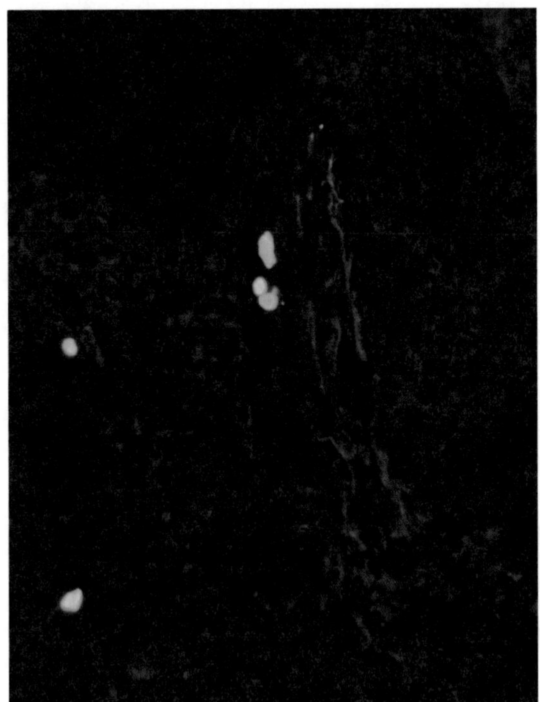

Fig. 31.22 Cytoid bodies in the papillary dermis near the epidermal junction

31.37 Are Immunoperoxidase Stains of Any Use?

An immunoperoxidase stain for type IV collagen on a cryostat section of a biopsy processed for DIF on salt split skin is useful to verify that the separation plane is correct by showing that the basement membrane type IV collagen localized to the floor of the salt split skin. Helm et al. reported the use of immunoperoxidase staining for dermatitis herpetiformis but in general, cryostat sections for DIF are the gold standard for diagnosis, in my opinion. Recently, the use of C3d and C4d immunoperoxidase stains has been described, in formalin-fixed, paraffin-embedded tissue sections. I have no personal experience using either of these antibodies. In general, direct and indirect immunofluorescent testing are the gold standards for the evaluation of these disorders, in my opinion [53–55].

31.38 What Other Factors Should Always Be Considered in Any DIF Testing?

Correlation with the H&E morphology and clinical differential diagnosis are always important. The testing should not be performed blindly in a vacuum without reliable clinical data provided by an experienced clinical dermatologist, in my opinion. Additionally, the findings must be integrated clinically, with all relevant clinical and laboratory data, by an experienced clinician.

References

1. Michel B, Milner Y, David K. Preservation of tissue-fixed immunoglobulins in skin biopsies of patients with lupus erythematosus and bullous diseases – preliminary report. J Invest Dermatol. 1972;59(6):449–52.
2. Vodegel RM, de Jong MC, Meijer HJ, Weytingh MB, Pas HH, Jonkman MF. Enhanced diagnostic immunofluorescence using biopsies transported in saline. BMC Dermatol. 2004;4:10.
3. Lazarova Z, Yancey KB. Reactivity of autoantibodies from patients with defined subepidermal bullous diseases against 1 mol/L salt-split skin. Specificity, sensitivity, and practical considerations. J Am Acad Dermatol. 1996;35(31):398–403.
4. Vodegel RM, Jonkman MF, Pas HH, de Jong MC. U-serrated immunodeposition pattern differentiates type VII collagen targeting bullous diseases from other subepidermal bullous autoimmune diseases. Br J Dermatol. 2004;151(1):112–8.
5. Chan LS, Ahmed AR, Anhalt GJ, et al. The first international consensus on mucous membrane pemphigoid: definition, diagnostic criteria, pathogenic factors, medical treatment, and prognostic indicators. Arch Dermatol. 2002;138(3):370–9.
6. Chan LS. Human skin basement membrane in health and in autoimmune diseases. Front Biosci. 1997;2:d343–52.
7. Zillikens D. Diagnosis of autoimmune bullous skin diseases. Clin Lab. 2008;54(11–12):491–503.
8. Rose C, Weyers W, Denisjuk N, Hillen U, Zillikens D, Shimanovich I. Histopathology of anti-p200 pemphigoid. Am J Dermatopathol. 2007;29(2):119–24.
9. Mutasim DF, Bilic M, Hawayek LH, Pipitone MA, Sluzevich JC. Immunobullous diseases. J Am Acad Dermatol. 2005;52(6):1029–43.
10. Kasperkiewicz M, Zillikens D. The pathophysiology of bullous pemphigoid. Clin Rev Allergy Immunol. 2007;33(1–2):67–77.
11. Fleming TE, Korman NJ. Cicatricial pemphigoid. J Am Acad Dermatol. 2000;43(4):571–91.
12. Castro LA, Lundell RB, Krause PK, Gibson LE. Clinical experience in pemphigoid gestationis: report of 10 cases. J Am Acad Dermatol. 2006;55(5):823–8.
13. Jenkins RE, Hern S, Black MM. Clinical features and management of 87 patients with pemphigoid gestationis. Clin Exp Dermatol. 1999;24(4):255–9.
14. Chi CC, Wang SH, Charles-Holmes R, et al. Pemphigoid gestationis: early onset and blister formation are associated with adverse pregnancy outcomes. Br J Dermatol. 2009;160(6):1222–8.
15. Sitaru C, Dahnrich C, Probst C, et al. Enzyme-linked immunosorbent assay using multimers of the 16th non-collagenous domain of the BP180 antigen for sensitive and specific detection of pemphigoid autoantibodies. Exp Dermatol. 2007;16(9):770–7.
16. Kirtschig G, Marinkovich MP, Burgeson RE, Yancey KB. Anti-basement membrane autoantibodies in patients with anti-epiligrin cicatricial pemphigoid bind the alpha subunit of laminin 5. J Invest Dermatol. 1995;105(4):543–8.
17. Egan CA, Lazarova Z, Darling TN, Yee C, Yancey KB. Anti-epiligrin cicatricial pemphigoid: clinical findings, immunopathogenesis, and significant associations. Medicine (Baltimore). 2003;82(3):177–86.

18. Rose C, Schmidt E, Kerstan A, et al. Histopathology of anti-laminin 5 mucous membrane pemphigoid. J Am Acad Dermatol. 2009;61(3): 433–40.
19. Pas HH. Immunoblot assay in differential diagnosis of autoimmune blistering skin diseases. Clin Dermatol. 2001;19(5):622–30.
20. Mihai S, Sitaru C. Immunopathology and molecular diagnosis of autoimmune bullous diseases. J Cell Mol Med. 2007;11(3):462–81.
21. Remington J, Chen M, Burnett J, Woodley DT. Autoimmunity to type VII collagen: epidermolysis bullosa acquisita. Curr Dir Autoimmun. 2008;10:195–205.
22. Chen M, Chan LS, Cai X, O'Toole EA, Sample JC, Woodley DT. Development of an ELISA for rapid detection of anti-type VII collagen autoantibodies in epidermolysis bullosa acquisita. J Invest Dermatol. 1997;108(1):68–72.
23. Kasperkiewicz M, Meier M, Zillikens D, Schmidt E. Linear IgA disease: successful application of immunoadsorption and review of the literature. Dermatology. 2010;220(3):259–63.
24. Waldman MA, Black DR, Callen JP. Vancomycin-induced linear IgA bullous disease presenting as toxic epidermal necrolysis. Clin Exp Dermatol. 2004;29(6):633–6.
25. Gruschwitz M, Keller J, Hornstein OP. Deposits of immunoglobulins at the dermo-epidermal junction in chronic light-exposed skin: what is the value of the lupus band test? Clin Exp Dermatol. 1988;13(5):303–8.
26. Kontos AP, Jirsari M, Jacobsen G, Fivenson DP. Immunoglobulin M predominance in cutaneous lupus erythematosus. J Cutan Pathol. 2005;32(5):352–5.
27. Crowson AN, Magro C. The cutaneous pathology of lupus erythematosus: a review. J Cutan Pathol. 2001;28(1):1–23.
28. Gammon WR, Woodley DT, Dole KC, Briggaman RA. Evidence that anti-basement membrane zone antibodies in bullous eruption of systemic lupus erythematosus recognize epidermolysis bullosa acquisita autoantigen. J Invest Dermatol. 1985;84(6):472–6.
29. David-Bajar KM, Bennion SD, DeSpain JD, Golitz LE, Lee LA. Clinical, histologic, and immunofluorescent distinctions between subacute cutaneous lupus erythematosus and discoid lupus erythematosus. J Invest Dermatol. 1992;99(3):251–7.
30. Sarkany RP. The management of porphyria cutanea tarda. Clin Exp Dermatol. 2001;26(3):225–32.
31. Egbert BM, LeBoit PE, McCalmont T, Hu CH, Austin C. Caterpillar bodies: distinctive, basement membrane-containing structures in blisters of porphyria. Am J Dermatopathol. 1993;15(3):199–202.
32. Green JJ, Manders SM. Pseudoporphyria. J Am Acad Dermatol. 2001;44(1):100–8.
33. Groves RWH. Pemphigus: a brief review. Clin Med. 2009;9(4): 371–5.
34. Ishii K, Amagai M, Hall RP, et al. Characterization of autoantibodies in pemphigus using antigen-specific enzyme-linked immunosorbent assays with baculovirus-expressed recombinant desmogleins. J Immunol. 1997;159(4):2010–7.
35. Amagai M, Komai A, Hashimoto T, et al. Usefulness of enzyme-linked immunosorbent assay using recombinant desmogleins 1 and 3 for serodiagnosis of pemphigus. Br J Dermatol. 1999;140(2):351–7.
36. Dasher D, Rubenstein D, Diaz LA. Pemphigus foliaceus. Curr Dir Autoimmun. 2008;10:182–94.
37. Amerian ML, Ahmed AR. Pemphigus erythematosus. Presentation of four cases and review of literature. J Am Acad Dermatol. 1984;10(2 Pt 1):215–22.
38. Robinson ND, Hashimoto T, Amagai M, Chan LS. The new pemphigus variants. J Am Acad Dermatol. 1999;40(5 Pt 1):649–71.
39. Duker I, Schaller J, Rose C, Zillikens D, Hashimoto T, Kunze J. Subcorneal pustular dermatosis-type IgA pemphigus with autoantibodies to desmocollins 1, 2, and 3. Arch Dermatol. 2009;145(10): 1159–62.
40. Ishii N, IshidaYamamoto A, Hashimoto T. Immunolocalization of target autoantigens in IgA pemphigus. Clin Exp Dermatol. 2004;29(1):62–6.
41. Anhalt GJ. Paraneoplastic pemphigus. J Investig Dermatol Symp Proc. 2004;9(1):29–33.
42. Kaplan I, Hodak E, Ackerman L, Mimouni D, Anhalt GJ, Calderon S. Neoplasms associated with paraneoplastic pemphigus: a review with emphasis on non-hematologic malignancy and oral mucosal manifestations. Oral Oncol. 2004;40(6):553–62.
43. Probst C, Schlumberger W, Stocker W, et al. Development of ELISA for the specific determination of autoantibodies against envoplakin and periplakin in paraneoplastic pemphigus. Clin Chim Acta. 2009;410(1–2):13–8.
44. Madan V, August PJ. Exophytic plaques, blisters, and mouth ulcers. Pemphigus vegetans (PV), Neumann type. Arch Dermatol. 2009;145(6):715–20.
45. Ma DL, Fang K. Hallopeau type of pemphigus vegetans confined to the right foot: case report. Chin Med J. 2009;122(5):588–90.
46. Helander SD, Rogers 3rd RS. The sensitivity and specificity of direct immunofluorescence testing in disorders of mucous membranes. J Am Acad Dermatol. 1994;30(1):65–75.
47. Raghu AR, Nirmala NR, Sreekumaran N. Direct immunofluorescence in oral lichen planus and oral lichenoid reactions. Quintessence Int. 2002;33(3):234–9.
48. Zillikens D, Caux F, Mascaro JM, et al. Autoantibodies in lichen planus pemphigoides react with a novel epitope within the C-terminal NC16A domain of BP180. J Invest Dermatol. 1999; 113(1):117–21.
49. Cohen DM, Ben-Amitai D, Feinmesser M, Zvulunov A. Childhood lichen planus pemphigoides: a case report and review of the literature. Pediatr Dermatol. 2009;26(5):569–74.
50. Magro CM, Crowson AN. A clinical and histologic study of 37 cases of immunoglobulin A-associated vasculitis. Am J Dermatopathol. 1999;21(3):234–40.
51. Crowson AN, Mihm Jr MC, Magro CM. Cutaneous vasculitis: a review. J Cutan Pathol. 2003;30(3):161–73.
52. Magro CM, Crowson AN. The immunofluorescent profile of dermatomyositis: a comparative study with lupus erythematosus. J Cutan Pathol. 1997;24(9):543–52.
53. Zaenglein AL, Hafer L, Helm KF. Diagnosis of dermatitis herpetiformis by an avidin-biotin-peroxidase method. Arch Dermatol. 1995;131(5):571–3.
54. Chandler W, Zone J, Florell S. C4d immunohistochemical stain is a sensitive method to confirm immunoreactant deposition in formalin-fixed paraffin-embedded tissue in bullous pemphigoid. J Cutan Pathol. 2009;36(6):655–9.
55. Magro CM, Dyrsen ME. The use of C3d and C4d immunohistochemistry on formalin-fixed tissue as a diagnostic adjunct in the assessment of inflammatory skin disease. J Am Acad Dermatol. 2008;59(5):822–33.
56. Vodegel RM, de Jong MC, Pas HH, Jonkman MF. IgA-mediated epidermolysis bullosa acquisita: two cases and review of the literature. J Am Acad Dermatol. 2002 Dec;47(6):919–25. Review.

Chapter 32
In Situ Hybridization in Surgical and Cytologic Specimens

Hong Yin and Barbara Paynton

Abstract Florescence in situ hybridization (FISH) using chromosome-specific probes has become an important cytogenetic tool in the evaluation of many congenital disorders, hematologic malignancies, some solid tumors, and cytologic specimens. Due to its interphase analysis, fast, high sensitivity and specificity, both fresh and fixed specimens, it becomes a very informative and rapid adjunct to standard karyotyping.

Keywords Cytogenetics • Principle of FISH • Dual-fusion probe • Break-apart probe • Aneuploidy probe • 17p deletion/p53 mutation • ATM • High-risk disease • Low-risk disease • 5q- • 7q- • Trisomy 8 • 20q- • t(8;21) • t(15;17) • inv(16) • MLL gene at 11q23 • t(12;21) • Hyperdiploidy • t(9;22) • 11q23 • t(1;19) • t(5;14) • 8q24 • t(9;22)(q34;q11) • ABL/BCR gene • ASS gene • t(11;18) • t(11;14) • t(14;18) • t(8;14) • t(3q27) • t(9;14) • t(2;5) • CECEP7 • CEP17 • LSI9p21 • Polysomy • Tetrasomy • 5p15 • 7p12 (EGFR) • 8q23 (C-MYC) • CEN 6 • EWSR1 • FUS • DDIT3 • SYT • FOXO1A genes • MDM2 gene

FREQUENTLY ASKED QUESTIONS

FISH Overview

H. Yin (✉)
Department of Pathology and Laboratory Medicine, Geisinger Medical Center, 100 N. Academy Avenue, Danville, PA 17822, USA
e-mail: hyin1@geisinger.edu

32.1 Why Do We Need FISH Study, Since We Already Have Cytogenetic Analysis?

Due to the limitations of conventional cytogenetic analysis and interest in more specific genes involved in certain diseases, FISH has become a firmly established technique in the clinical diagnostic area. FISH allows for rapid identification of deletions, translocations, amplifications, duplications, and structural abnormalities of specific genes, loci, or DNA sequences.

32.2 How to Compare Cytogenetic Analysis with FISH Study?

Compare cytogenetic analysis to FISH study as shown in Fig. 32.1.

32.3 What Are the Special Utilities of FISH?

Suboptimal specimen for conventional cytogenetics
Interphase analysis
Clinically suspicious for a specific abnormality but yields normal results (false-negative cytogenetics)
Aids in diagnosis in cases when the abnormality is cryptic (not evident by conventional karyotyping)
Clarifying abnormal or complex conventional karyotype
A surrogate marker for primary genetics

F. Lin and J. Prichard (eds.), *Handbook of Practical Immunohistochemistry: Frequently Asked Questions*,
DOI 10.1007/978-1-4419-8062-5_32, © Springer Science+Business Media, LLC 2011

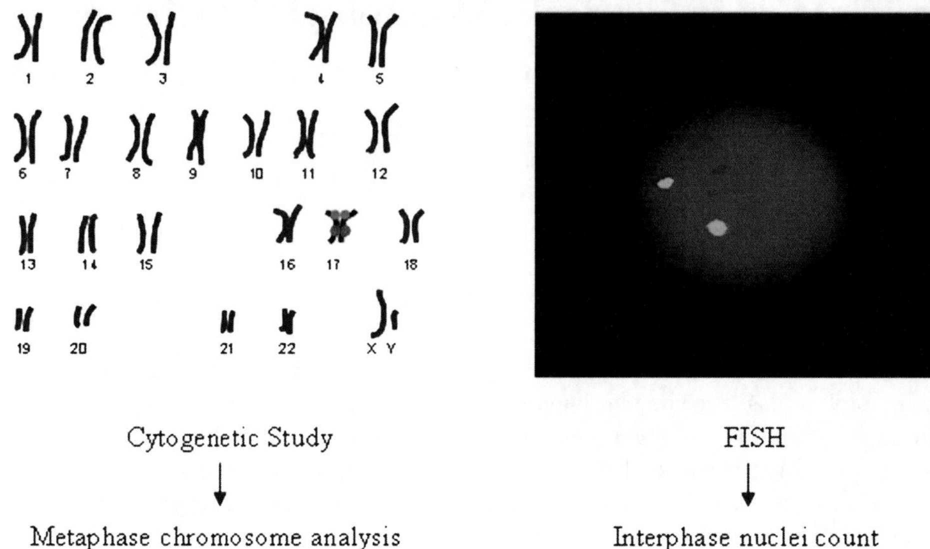

Fig. 32.1 This is an example of Her2/Neu probe. FISH reveals 2 green (CEN17) and 2 red (17q11.2) normal signal pattern

32.4 What Is the Principle of FISH?

A florescent-labeled DNA probe hybridized to targeted genomic sequences of interest.

32.5 What Is the Basic Procedure?

Choose the specific DNA probe to targeted DNA
Prepare the sample (interphase or metaphase)
Denature the targeted DNA and the probe
Hybridize labeled probe to target
Wash
Detect fluorescent signal (manually or automated)

32.6 What Are the Specimen Requirements?

Fresh

Bone marrow, peripheral blood – green or sodium heparin tube

Fine needle aspirate (FNA), solid tumor, or cytology – sterile tube, RPM, or a clean tube

Formalin-fixed, paraffin-embedded tissue

32.7 What Are the Advantages and Limitations?

Advantages

Timing – 24 h
Increased sensitivity
Both interphase nuclei and metaphase cells
Not a large number of cells
Paraffin-embedded tissue and fresh specimen
Automation

Limitations

Limited to a specific abnormality/specific gene

32.8 What Types of Probes Are Used?

There are two types of probes:

1. Locus-specific indicator (LSI) – hybridized to specific loci or genes of interest, to detect translocation/rearrangement or aneuploidy. Under a fluorescence microscope, to determine what abnormal signal patterns (fusion, split) are present in the nucleus of a cell.
2. Centromere enumeration probe (CEP) – hybridized to the pericentromeric region to detect aneuploidy (gain or loss of specific gene region or chromosome). Under a fluorescence

microscope, to determine how many copies of targeted chromosome are present in the nucleus of a cell.

These two basic FISH probes are shown in Fig. 32.2.

Figure 32.3 reveals dual-fusion probes; compares chromosome analysis with FISH study

Figure 32.4 reveals break-apart probes; compares chromosome analysis with FISH study

Figure 32.5 reveals aneuploid probe; compares chromosome analysis with FISH study

32.9 Which Type of Probe Should be Chosen: Break-Apart or Dual-Fusion?

Break-apart

The result is easier to interpret because signals are readily recognized and yield clearly abnormal results, but partner chromosome is unknown.

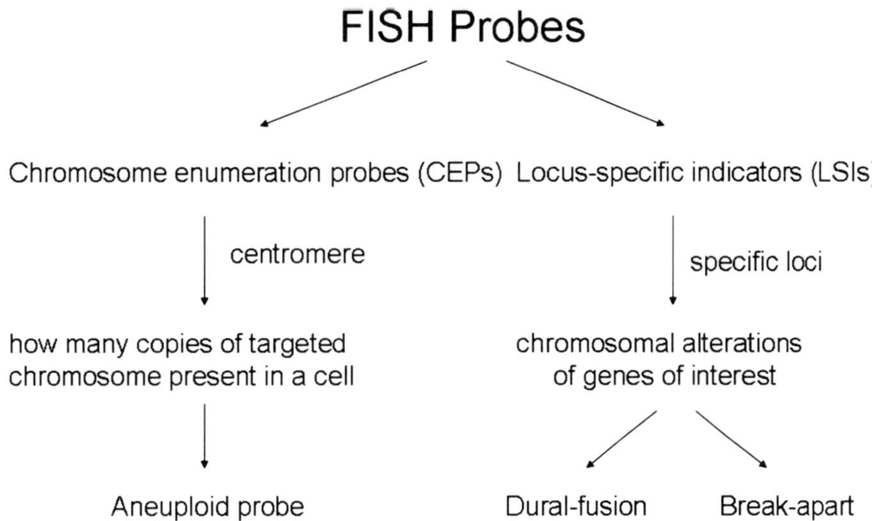

Fig. 32.2 Two basic FISH probes

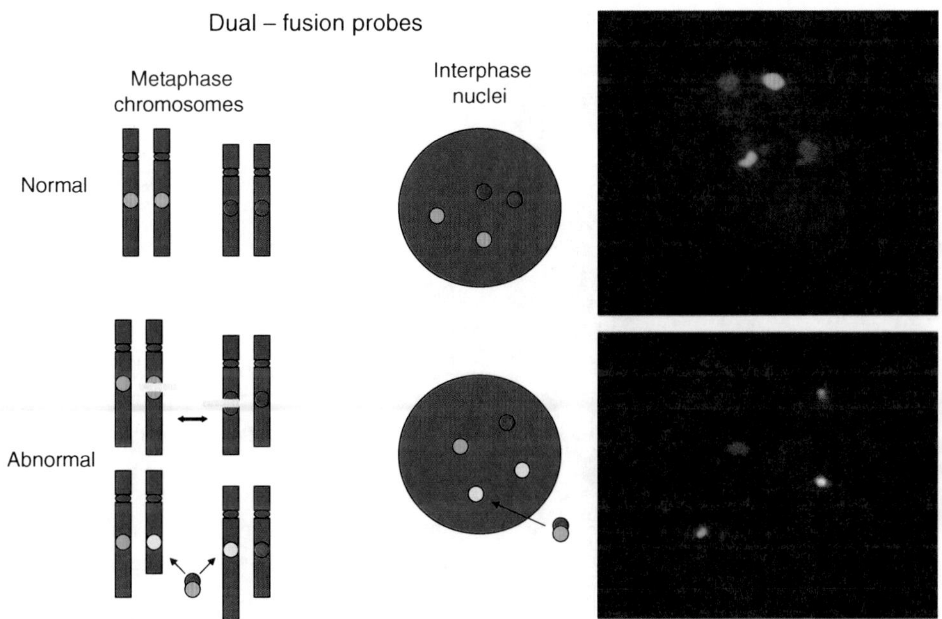

Fig. 32.3 On the left: *Top*: The red and green probes bind to specific loci of chromosomes. Normal FISH yields two red and two green signals. *Bottom*: In the neoplastic cell carrying a translocation, one red and one green signal splits, is rearranged, and yields this new signals - yellow (red/green fusion). The red and green are from normal chromosome. On the right: An example of FISH results: *Top* – normal signal pattern; *bottom* – abnormal signal pattern

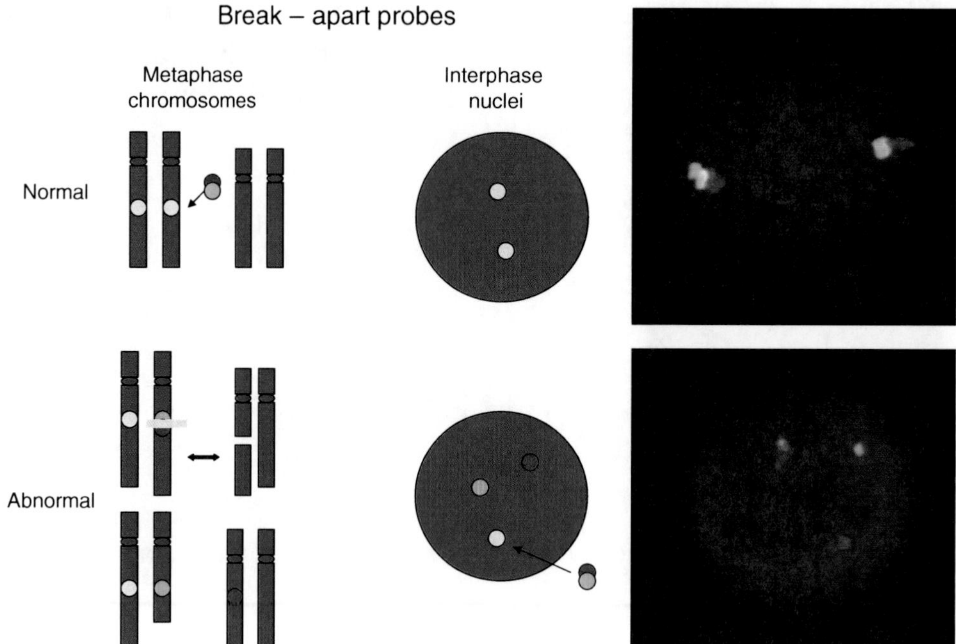

Fig. 32.4 On the left: Top: The red and green probes bind to the loci of interest. FISH analysis yields normal pattern – 2 yellows signals. *Bottom*: In neoplastic cells carrying a translocation, one yellow signal splits and then separated into the red and green signals. The yellow signal is from the normal chromosome. On the right: An example of FISH results: *Top* – normal signal pattern; *bottom* – abnormal signal pattern

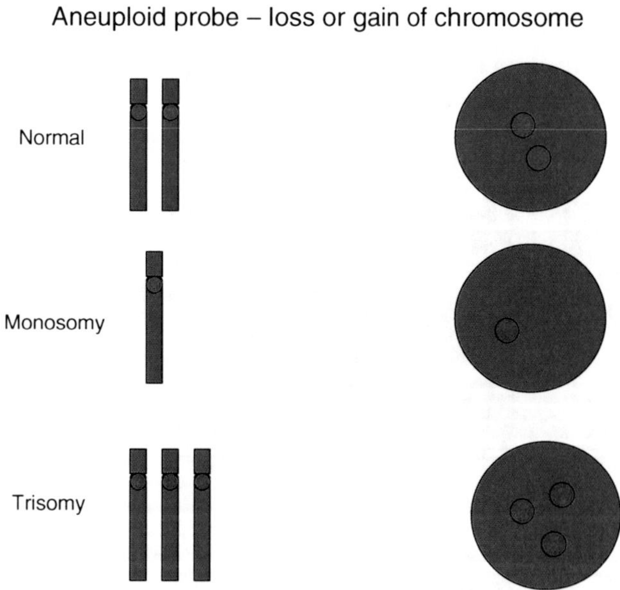

Fig. 32.5 *Top*: Normal cell contains pairs of chromosome. FISH yields two red signals. *Middle* and *bottom*: In neoplastic cells with loss or gain of a particular gene region or chromosome, giving abnormal numbers of chromosomes are observed

Dual-fusion

Superior to break-apart but variant and complex pattern may occur.

32.10 What Are Typical and Atypical Results?

Due to the probe's high specificity, the interpretation is usually straightforward. However, it is not uncommon to have an atypical abnormal interphase. Dual-fusion probes may yield more fusion signals than expected, indicating a possible disease-associated rearrangement. These "unusual" patterns should be considered abnormal and interpreted in conjunction with associated pathology reports and relevant reports in the literature. Complete karyotype analysis may be needed. We will use CML as an example.

Atypical Results: The Most Common Patterns

Aneuploid probe

Monosomy – Two signals overlap; hybridization not 100%
Polysomy – Cells in the S or G2 phase of cell cycle

Dual-fusion probe

Two signals overlap, yield fusion signals

Break-apart probe

Normal signals may appear to be slightly separated, thus the normal pattern needs to be strictly defined
Occasional normal signal can split, yielding an abnormal signal pattern

False Positive

Any disease or situation that causes chromosomal changes, such as autoimmune disease, viral infection, infectious process, or radiation/chemotherapy
Premalignant lesion, for example, tubular adenoma of the colon

False Negative

Low specimen volume
Fewer than expected chromosomal abnormalities in low-grade tumor
Probe sets used to cover the disease chromosomal alterations

References: [1–4]

Hematopoietic Tumor

Chronic Lymphocytic Leukemia (CLL): Modern Diagnostic Workup

1. What is the modern diagnostic workup for CLL? (p. 567)
2. What is an unfavorable prognosis? (p. 567)
3. What are the most frequently used FISH panels and most frequent aberrations? (Table 32.1) (p. 567)

32.11 What Is the Modern Diagnostic Workup for CLL?

Molecular cytogenetic lesions play a major role in the pathogenesis of CLL and they become necessary tools for modern diagnostic workup.

32.12 What Is an Unfavorable Prognosis?

Unmutated IgVh (immunoglobulin heavy chain variable region genes) – early progression
CD38 positive (>30%) – worse prognosis
ZAP70 (>20%) – associated with unmutated IgVh, rapid disease progression
Chromosomal abnormalities

32.13 What Are the Most Frequently Used FISH Panels and Most Frequent Aberrations? (Table 32.1)

Multiple Myeloma (MM)

1. What is the new concept about multiple myeloma? (p. 568)
2. What are the genetic features, abnormalities, genes involved, and clinical features of high-risk disease? (Table 32.2) (p. 568)
3. What are the genetic features, abnormalities, genes involved, and clinical features of low-risk disease? (Table 32.3) (p. 568)
4. What are the recommended tests for all new patients? (Table 32.4) (p. 568)
5. What are the most frequently used FISH panels? (Tables 32.5 and 32.6) (pp. 568–569)

Table 32.1 CLL FISH panels

Abnormality	Gene loci	Gene pattern	Clinical and biological features
13q-	13q14	RB1 deletion	Good prognosis
	13q34	LAMP1 deletion	Most frequent abnormality by FISH
12+	12q13-15	Trisomy	Intermediate to poor prognosis
			Most common by cytogenetics
11q-	11q22.3	ATM gene deletion	Advanced stage; young, extensive lymphadenopathy
			Not detected by routine chromosome analysis
			Third most frequent abnormality by FISH
17p-	17p13.1	P53	Worst prognosis; resistant to therapy
14q32	t(11;14) (q13;32)	CCND/IGH rearrangement	Unfavorable prognosis; atypical CLL
6q	6q21		Intermediate prognosis; atypical CLL

Important factor

17p- and/or p53 mutation is the strongest independent parameter for predicting poor prognosis
Deletion of *TP53* and/or *ATM* identifies a group with poor prognosis, requiring treatment but usually refractory to treatment
References: [5, 6]

32.14 What Is the New Concept About Multiple Myeloma?

Multiple myeloma is not a single disease anymore. Subtypes are:

High-risk myeloma 25%
Low-risk myeloma 75%

32.15 What Are the Genetic Features, Abnormalities, Genes Involved, and Clinical Features of High-Risk Disease? (Table 32.2)

32.16 What Are the Genetic Features, Abnormalities, Genes Involved, and Clinical Features of Low-Risk Disease? (Table 32.3)

32.17 What Are the Recommended Tests for All New Patients? (Table 32.4)

32.18 What Are the Most Frequently Used FISH Panels? (Tables 32.5 and 32.6)

Myelodysplastic Syndrome (MDS)

1. What are the FISH panels for MDS? (p. 568)
2. Why are both FISH and cytogenetics needed for MDS? (p. 569)
3. What is the relationship between gene abnormalities and prognosis? (Table 32.8) (p. 569)

32.19 What Are the FISH Panels for MDS?

Testing for chromosomes 5, 7, 8, 20 (Table 32.7)

Table 32.2 Genetic features of high-risk disease

Abnormalities	Method	Gene	Percentage	Clinical features
t(4;14)(p16.3;q32)	FISH	FGFR3/IgH	13–20%	IgA isotype Usually associated 13- and hypodiploidy
t(14;16)(q32;q23)	FISH	IgH/MAF	2–10%	IgA isotype Usually associated 13-, 17p-, and hypodiploidy
17p-	FISH	P53	5–33% in newly diagnosed 55% in relapsed	Leukemia and central nervous system Usually associated 13-, t(4;14)
13-[a] (monosomy)	Cytogenetics		10–20%	Lambda-light chain Related to t(4;14) and 17p deletion
Plasma cell labeling index >3.0	Serum			

Note: [a]Monosomy 13 by metaphase analysis indicates a very poor prognosis, but interphase FISH analysis has been applied as 13q or monosomy 13, which is one of the most common abnormalities in MM

Table 32.3 Genetic features of low-risk disease

Abnormalities	Method	Gene	Percentage	Clinical features
t(11;14)(q13;q32)	FISH	Cyclin D1	20%	Lymphoplasmacytic Mature morphology CD20 repression
t(6;14)	FISH	Cyclin D3	3–4%	Unknown
Hyperdiploidy			39%	

Table 32.4 Recommend tests for all new patients

Test	Method
t(4;14)(p16.3;q32)	FISH
t(14;16) (q32;q23)	FISH
Deletion of 17p (p53)	FISH
Deletion of chromosome 13	Cytogenetics
Plasma cell labeling index, beta-2-microglobulin, LDH	Serum

Table 32.5 MM FISH panels

Abnormality	Gene loci	Gene pattern	Clinical and biological features
13q- or 13-	13q14.3	RB1 deletion	One of the most frequent abnormalities 30–50% detected by FISH Related to t(4;14) and 17p- Lambda-light chain
14q translocation	14q32	IgH	Mostly cryptic 40–75% detected by FISH Most partner with 11, 4, 16, and 6
17p-	17p13.1	P53	Worst prognosis

Table 32.6 Detailed 14q translocation

14q translocation	Percentage	Clinical features
t(11;14)(q13;q32)	15–20% for MM	Lymphoplasmacytic,maturemorphology
	15–30% for MGUS	Good prognosis
t(4;14)(p16.3;q32)	13–20%	IgA isotype Poor prognosis Correlate 13q-
t(14;16)(q32;q23)	2–10%	Poor prognosis
t(6;14)	3–4%	Unknown

References: [6, 7]

Table 32.7 Most frequent aberrations

Chromosome	Gene	Results	Percentage
5	5q33-q34	5q-; monosomy5	10–20% in newly diagnosed 40% in treated
7	7q31	7q-; monosomy7	16–32%
8	p11.1-q11.1	Trisomy 8	10%
20	20q12	20q-	4–5% in newly diagnosed 7% in treated

Table 32.8 Gene abnormalities and prognosis

Good prognosis group	Normal karyotype 5q- 20q-
Intermediate prognosis group	Trisomy 8 Single or double abnormalities
Poor prognosis group – high risk of progression to AML	Abnormalities of chromosome 7 Complex karyotype (>3)

Reference: [6]

32.20 Why Are Both FISH and Cytogenetics Needed for MDS?

Routine cytogenetic analysis demonstrates aberration in 40–70%

FISH can detect 15–20% of abnormalities in a normal karyotype, which can influence therapy

Combination = cytogenetics + FISH

32.21 What Is the Relationship Between Gene Abnormalities and Prognosis? (Table 32.8)

Acute Myeloid Leukemia (AML)

1. Why is FISH needed in AML? (p. 569)
2. What are the most common chromosome abnormalities associated with AML? (p. 569)
3. What are the recurrent genetic abnormalities? (Table 32.9) (pp. 569–570)
4. What is the relationship between gene abnormalities and prognosis? (Table 32.10) (p. 569–570)
5. What are the FISH panels for AML with recurrent genetic abnormalities? (Table 32.11) (p. 570)

32.22 Why Is FISH Needed in AML?

FISH allows for classification of AML with recurrent cytogenetic abnormalities, provides significant prognostic information, and can also be used to track response to therapy.

FISH is more sensitive than conventional cytogenetics in detecting particular genomic aberrations.

Conventional chromosome analysis remains the gold standard for the identification of common recurrent chromosome abnormalities, but it requires dividing cells (metaphase analysis), and some of the subtle rearrangements can be missed, such as inv[16], *MLL* anomalies, and t(15;17). FISH analysis has a rapid turnaround time, is performed on nondividing cells (interphase analysis), and detects cryptic or subtle rearrangements. Thus, FISH probes used for detecting chromosome abnormalities have widespread use.

32.23 What Are the Most Common Chromosome Abnormalities Associated with AML?

The most common chromosome abnormalities associated with AML include t(8;21), t(15;17), inv(16), 8, inv(3), t(6;9), t(8:16), t(3:21), and abnormalities of the *MLL* gene at 11q23, particularly t(9;11). These recurrent chromosome anomalies are identified in approximately 60% of AML cases.

32.24 What Are the Recurrent Genetic Abnormalities? (Table 32.9)

32.25 What Is the Relationship Between Gene Abnormalities and Prognosis? (Table 32.10)

Table 32.9 Summary of AML with recurrent genetic abnormalities

Genetic abnormalities	Gene	AML type
t(8;21)(q22;q22)	ETO/AML1	M2
t(15;17)(q22;q12)	PML/RARA	Acute promyelocytic leukemia, M3
inv(16)(p13.1q22) or t(16;16)(p13.1;q22)	MYH11/CBFB	M4 Eos
11q23	MLL	M0–M7
t(6;11), t(9;11), t(10;11), t(11;19)		
t(6;9)(p23;q34)	DEK/NUP214	Basophilia and multilineage dysplasia M2, M4
inv(3)(q21q26.2) or t(3;3)(q21;q26.2)	RPN1/EVI1	M1, 2, 4, 6, 7
t(1;22)(p13;q13)	RBM15/MKL1	Infant with Down syndrome

Table 32.10 Summary of prognosis-associated gene abnormalities

Good prognosis	Intermediate prognosis	Poor prognosis
t(8;21)(q22;q22)	– Y	Complex karyotype
inv(16), t(16;16)	+8	3q: inv(3), t(3;3)
t(15;17)	+13	–7
	+21	–5
	+11	5q-
		11q: t(11;19), t(9;11)
		9q-, t(9;9), t(9;22)
		11q23
		t(6;9)
		7q-
		20q-

Table 32.11 Summary of FISH panels for AML

Chromosome abnormalities	Genes involved	Probe type
t(8;21)	ETO/AML1	Dual fusion
t(15;17)	PML/RARA	Dual fusion
Inv(16) ort(16;16)	MYH11/CBFB	Break-apart
11q23	MLL rearrangement	Break-apart

Reference: [6]

32.26 What Are the FISH Panels for AML with Recurrent Genetic Abnormalities? (Table 32.11)

Acute Lymphoblastic Leukemia (ALL)

1. What recurrent genetic abnormalities are associated with a good prognosis? (Table 32.12) (p. 570)
2. What recurrent genetic abnormalities are associated with a poor prognosis? (Table 32.13) (p. 570)
3. What recurrent genetic abnormalities are associated with an uncertain prognosis? (Table 32.14) (pp. 570–571)
4. What recurrent genetic abnormalities are detected by cytogenetics? (Table 32.15) (p. 571)

32.27 What Recurrent Genetic Abnormalities Are Associated with a Good Prognosis? (Table 32.12)

32.28 What Recurrent Genetic Abnormalities Are Associated with a Poor Prognosis? (Table 32.13)

32.29 What Recurrent Genetic Abnormalities Are Associated with an Uncertain Prognosis? (Table 32.14)

Table 32.12 Good prognosis – genetic abnormalities detected by FISH

Chromosomal aberration	Gene/chromosomes involved	Clinical significance
t(12;21) (p13;q22)	TEL-AML1	25% B-ALL Common in children Not seen in infants
Hyperdiploidy	X, 4, 6, 10, 14, 17, 18, 21	25% B-ALL Common in children Not seen in infants

Table 32.13 Poor prognosis – genetic abnormalities detected by FISH

Chromosomal aberration	Gene/chromosomes involved	Clinical significance
t(9;22)(q34;q11.2)	BCR-ABL1	25–30% in adults 3–5% in children
11q23	MLL	10% of ALL Specifically associated with infants (<1 year) Hyperleukocytosis, organomegaly, CNS involvement Variability of partner chromosomal regions
t(1;19)(q23;p13.3)	PBX1/E2A	Both in children and young adults Frequent CNS involvement 5% of ALL, or 20% of pre-B-ALL

Table 32.14 Uncertain prognosis – genetic abnormalities

Chromosomal aberration	Gene/chromosomes involved	Clinical significance
t(5;14)(q31;q32)	IL3/IGH	Both children and adults Hypereosinophilia
8q24	C-MYC	L3 morphology

Table 32.15 Detected by cytogenetics

Hypodiploidy	5% Both children and adults Poor prognosis

References: [8, 9]

32.30 What Recurrent Genetic Abnormalities Are Detected by Cytogenetics? (Table 32.15)

Chronic Myelogenous Leukemia (CML)

1. What is the classical translocation? (p. 571)
2. What are the variant translocation patterns? (p. 571)
3. How to differentiate neoplastic cell vs. normal cell, when FISH yields 1R1G1F signal pattern? (p. 571)
4. How to detect argininosuccinate synthetase (ASS) gene loss? (p. 573)

32.31 What Is the Classical Translocation?

Classical pattern: t(9;22)(q34;q11) ABL/BCR rearrangement

Figure 32.6 shows the classic translocation; compares chromosome analysis with FISH study

32.32 What Are the Variant Translocation Patterns?

Figure 32.7 shows the variant/atypical FISH patterns; compares chromosome analysis with FISH study

32.33 How to Differentiate Neoplastic Cell vs. Normal Cell, When FISH Yields 1R1G1F Signal Pattern?

Figure 32.8 shows the detailed FISH pattern using a tricolor, dual-fusion probe set.

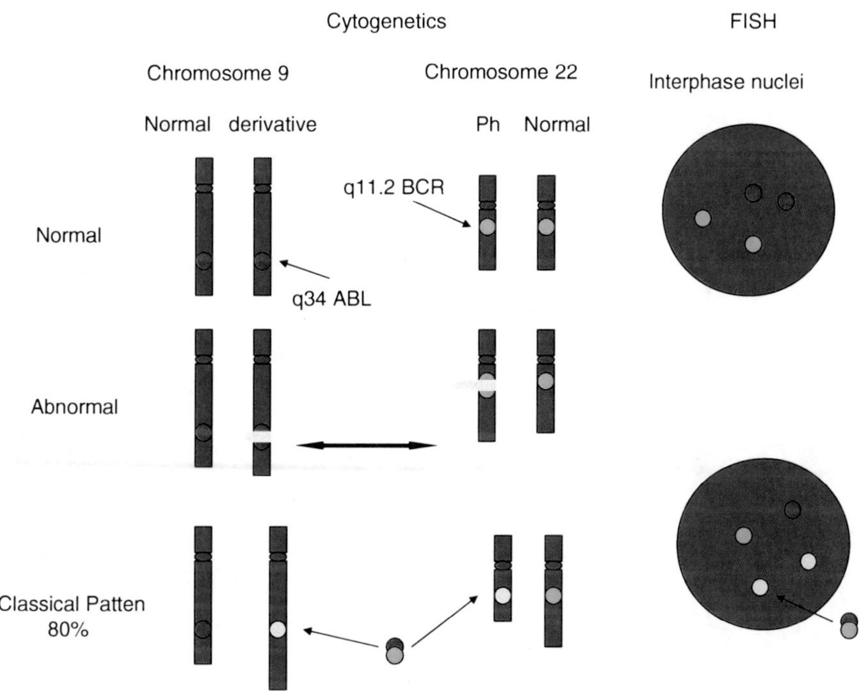

Fig. 32.6 *Top*: The red probe targets ABL on chromosome 9 and green probe targets BCR on chromosome 22. In a normal cell, FISH analysis of interphase nuclei shows two red and two green signals. *Bottom*: In a cell carrying a BCR-ABL fusion gene, derivative chromosome 9 and Ph chromosome 22 have BCR-ABL reciprocal translocations, yielding two fusion signals (yellow); the normal chromosome 9 has a red signal and normal chromosome 22 has a green signal. Thus FISH shows one red, one green and two yellow signals. This is a classic pattern observed in 80% of CML patients

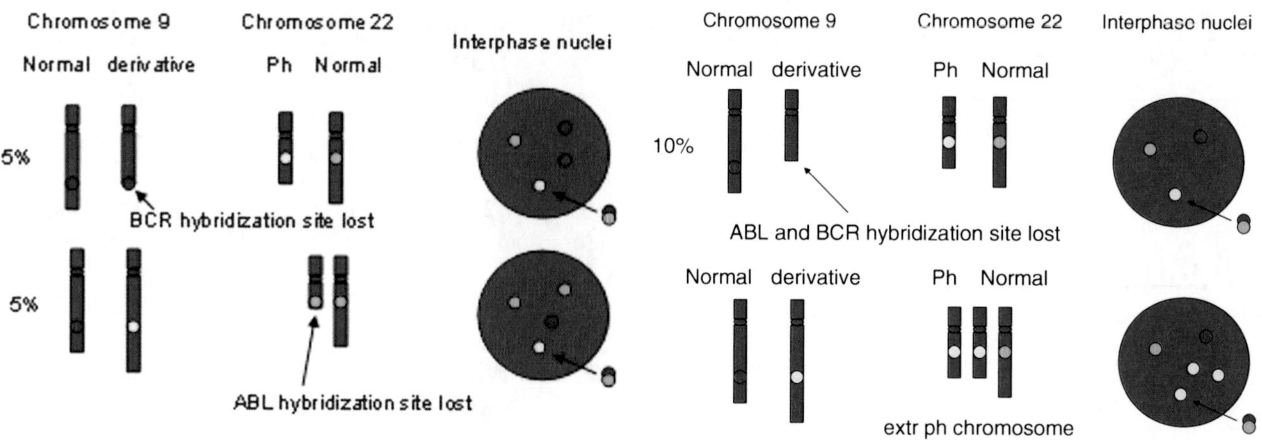

Fig. 32.7-1 *Top*: Loss of the BCR hybridization site that is translocated to the abnormal chromosome 9, yielding two red, one green and one yellow fusion signal. *Bottom*: Loss of the ABL1 hybridization site that normally remains in the abnormal chromosome 9, yielding one red, two green and one fusion signal

Fig. 32.7-2 *Top*: Loss of the ABL1 and BCR hybridization sites that are normally observed on the abnormal chromosome 9, yields one red, one green and one fusion signal. *Bottom*: Having an extra Ph chromosome, then yields one red, one green and three yellow fusion signals. As noted above, when FISH yields 1R1G1F signal pattern due to loss of BCR and ABL hybridization site, the same FISH pattern 1R1G1F seen in normal cells shows coincidental overlap of a red and green signals

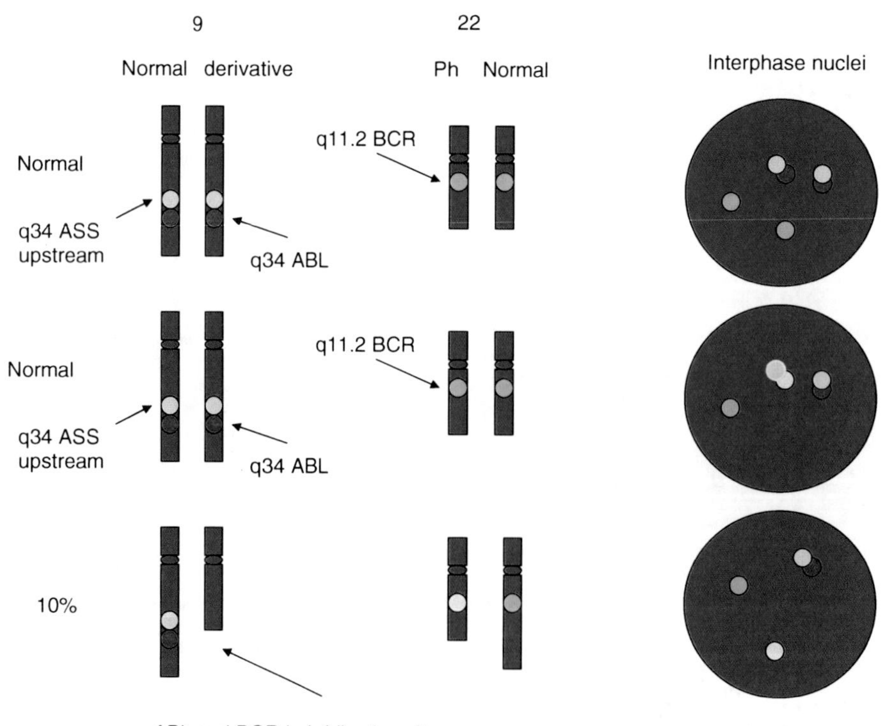

Fig. 32.8 Tricolor, dual-fusion probes were used to distinguish between neoplastic cells with 1R1G1F due to a BCR/ABL translocation and normal cells with 1R1G1F due to the coincidental overlap of a red and green signal. The neoplastic cells lack ASS signal, while normal cells retain ASS signal on derivative chromosome 9. ASS locus is not translocated to Ph chromosome. *Middle*: Normal cells with 1R1G1F due to the coincidental overlap of red and green signals. There are two copies of the ASS signals. *Bottom*: Neoplastic cells with 1R1G1F due to a BCR/ABL translocation. There is only one ASS signal. The fusion yellow signal is not colocalized with the blue signal

32.34 How to Detect Argininosuccinate Synthetase (ASS) Gene Loss?

Triple-probe/three-color system used to detect ASS gene loss – a poor prognosis

Figure 32.9 shows the ASS gene loss; compares chromosome analysis with FISH study

References: [10–13]

Lymphoma

What is the most common chromosomal aberration in B- and T-cell lymphoma? (Tables 32.16 and 32.17) (pp. 571–572)

32.35 What Is the Most Common Chromosomal Aberration in B- and T-Cell Lymphoma? (Tables 32.16 and 32.17)

UroVysion

1. Is UroVysion FDA-approved and what are the criteria for UroVysion testing? (p. 573)
2. What are the types of bladder cancer? (p. 574)
3. What is the basic procedure? (p. 574)
4. What is the principle of UroVysion? (p. 574)
5. What types of probes are used? (p. 574)
6. What are normal results? (p. 575)
7. What are abnormal results? (p. 575)
8. Is FISH a quantitative study? Can it predict cancer recurrence and progression to muscle invasion? (p. 575)
9. What are the normal variant results, or why do normal cells yield abnormal signal patterns? (p. 578)
10. What are the most common false-positive and false-negative results? (p. 578)
11. How to manage positive FISH and negative cystoscopy findings? (p. 578)
12. How to manage positive cytology and negative cystoscopy findings? (p. 578)
13. What are the advantages of UroVysion? (p. 578)
14. How to compare urine cytology with UroVysion? (p. 578)
15. Can UroVysion be used in bladder washing or upper tract urothelial cancer? (p. 578)

32.36 Is UroVysion FDA-Approved, and What Are the Criteria for UroVysion Testing?

UroVysion is FDA approved for testing voided urine.

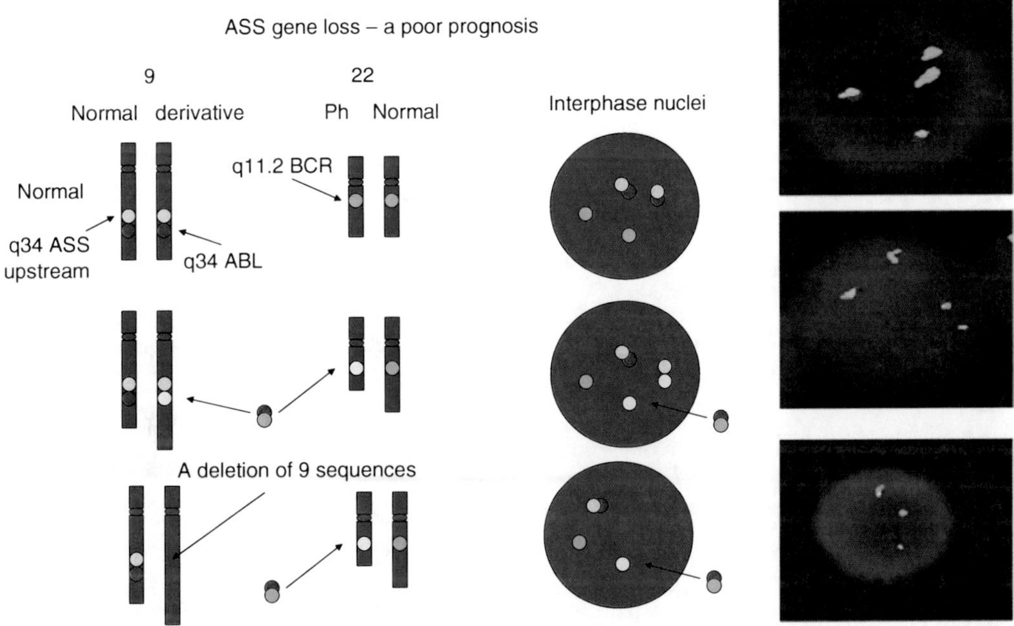

Fig. 32.9 On the left: *Top*: In a normal cell, FISH analysis of interphase nuclei shows colocalization of red and blue signals (ABL and ASS) was seen on the chromosome 9 and green signals on chromosome 22. *Middle*: No ASS gene loss - the classical pattern of CML. Colocalization of red and blue signals was seen on the normal chromosome 9 and a single green signal was seen on the normal chromosome 22. Colocalized red and green signals appeared on both the Ph chromosome and the derivative 9 chromosome. *Bottom*: ASS gene loss - Colocalization of red and blue signals was seen on the normal chromosome 9 and a single green signal was seen on the normal chromosome 22, there is a colocalized red and green signals appeared on the Ph chromosome but not one the derivative 9. On the right: An example of FISH results. *Top* – normal signal pattern; *Middle* – t(9;22) translocation without ASS gene loss; *Bottom* – t(9;22) translocation with ASS gene loss

Table 32.16 B-cell lymphomas

Lymphoid malignancy	Chromosomal aberration	Gene involved	Clinical significance
Marginal zone lymphoma	t(11;18) (q21;q21), 30–50% of MALT cases	API2/MALT1	GI – unfavorable prognosis; *H. pylori* associated, antibiotic resistant
	t(14;18)(q32;q21)	IGH/MALT1	Unknown
	t(1;14)(p22;q32)	BCL10/IGH	Worse prognosis
	Trysomy 3, 50% low-grade MALTomas	3q21-23, 3q25-29, possible BCL6	Unknown
	Trysomy 18, 30% low-grade MALTomas	Unknown	Unknown
Mantle cell lymphoma	t(11;14)(q13;q32) 85%	CCND1/IGH	Detected in ≥90% of cases p16 and p53 related, associated aggressive clinical behavior
Follicular lymphoma	t(14;18)(q32;q21) – 80%	IGH/BCL2	Detected in 90% of cases by FISH, unfavorable prognosis
	3q27 – 15%		
	t(3;14)(q27;q32)	BCL6/IGH	Good prognosis
Burkitt's lymphoma	t(8;14)(q24;q32) 44–100%	MYC/IGH	Detected in nearly 100% of this high-grade lymphoma
	t(2;8)(p11q24)	IGK/MYC	
	t(8;22)(q24;q11)	MYC/IGL	
Diffuse large B-cell lymphoma	t(3q27) 40–50%	BCL6	Good prognosis
	t(14;18)(q32;q21) 20–30%	IGH/BCL2	Unfavorable prognosis
	t(8;14)(q24;q32)	MYC/IGH	
Lymphoplasmacytic lymphoma	t(9;14)(p13;q32) 50%	PAX5/IGH	Usually a low-grade lymphoma

Table 32.17 T-cell lymphoma

Anaplastic large cell lymphoma	t(2;5)(p23;q35)	NPM/ALK	Good prognosis

References: [6, 14, 15]

Two criteria:

1. Monitoring the recurrence of bladder cancer
2. Suspected bladder cancer in patients with hematuria

32.37 What Are the Types of Bladder Cancer?

Two types according to morphology:

- Papillary (75–80%), tend to recur, usually do not progress to invasive cancer
- Flat (20–25%), tend to progress to muscle invasion

Two types according to urologists:

- Nonmuscle invasive
- Muscle invasive

Most bladder cancers grow slowly and are treatable, but recurrence is high (50–75%). Carcinoma in situ (CIS) and tumors with lamina propria invasion are at risk to progress to muscle invasive cancer (54 and 46%). Early detection of cancer recurrence and prevention of muscle invasion is critical.

32.38 What Is the Basic Procedure?

Isolate bladder cells in the voided urine (at least 30 mL), fix cells on a microscopic slide, denature DNA, FISH hybridization, special staining, reading.

32.39 What Is the Principle of UroVysion?

UroVysion is fluorescently labeled DNA probes to detect chromosomal abnormalities, which occur during the development of bladder cancer.

32.40 What Types of Probes Are Used?

Two types of FISH probes are used:

1. Chromosome enumeration probes (CEPs): These hybridize to the centromeres and allow the determination of how many copies of a targeted chromosome are present in a cell, as chromosomes 3, 7, 17.

2. Locus-specific indicators (LSIs): These hybridize to specific loci to detect chromosomal alterations of genes of interest, such as chromosome 9. Four-color, four-DNA probes detect specific regions of chromosomes 3 (red), 7 (green), 17 (aqua), 9 (yellow). Detect aneusomy (polysomy) of chromosomes 3, 7, 9, 17; deletion of 9p21 locus (p16 tumor suppressor gene).

32.41 What Are Normal Results?

Count at least 25 cells or automated/manual scan of the whole slide

Normal: CEP 3 (red), CEP 7 (green), CEP17 (aqua) and LSI 9p21 (gold) – two copies each

Representative sample shown in Fig. 32.10

32.42 What Are Abnormal Results?

1. Polysomy: In at least four cells ≥2 copies of chromosomes – 90% of time with high-grade tumor
   Representative sample shown in Fig. 32.11
2. Homozygous 9p21 deletion: Deletion of 9p21 (chromosome 9) in at least 12 cells – absence of gold signals – low-grade tumor
   Representative sample shown in Fig. 32.12
3. Tetrasomy: Four copies of all four probes – unknown clinical correlation, most often seen in low-grade tumor
   Representative sample shown in Fig. 32.13
4. Trisomy: Three copies of CEP 7, or CEP 3, or CEP 17 and two copies of the other three probes – unknown clinical correlation, most often seen in low-grade tumor
   Representative sample shown in Fig. 32.14.

32.43 Is FISH a Quantitative Study? Can It Predict Cancer Recurrence and Progression to Muscle Invasion?

Yes. The percentage of abnormal cells detected by FISH (polysomy) is associated with bladder cancer recurrence and progression to muscle-invasive cancer. The percent of abnormal cells by FISH is one of the most significant variables for predicting recurrent bladder cancer, with a 2.6% increased chance of recurrence for every 1% increase in the percentage of abnormal cells. Again, the percentage of abnormal cells was one of the most significant variables for identifying disease, with a 1.8% increased risk of muscle-invasive cancer for every 1% increase in the percentage of abnormal cells by FISH; 31% abnormal cells is associated with a high risk of progression to muscle invasion.

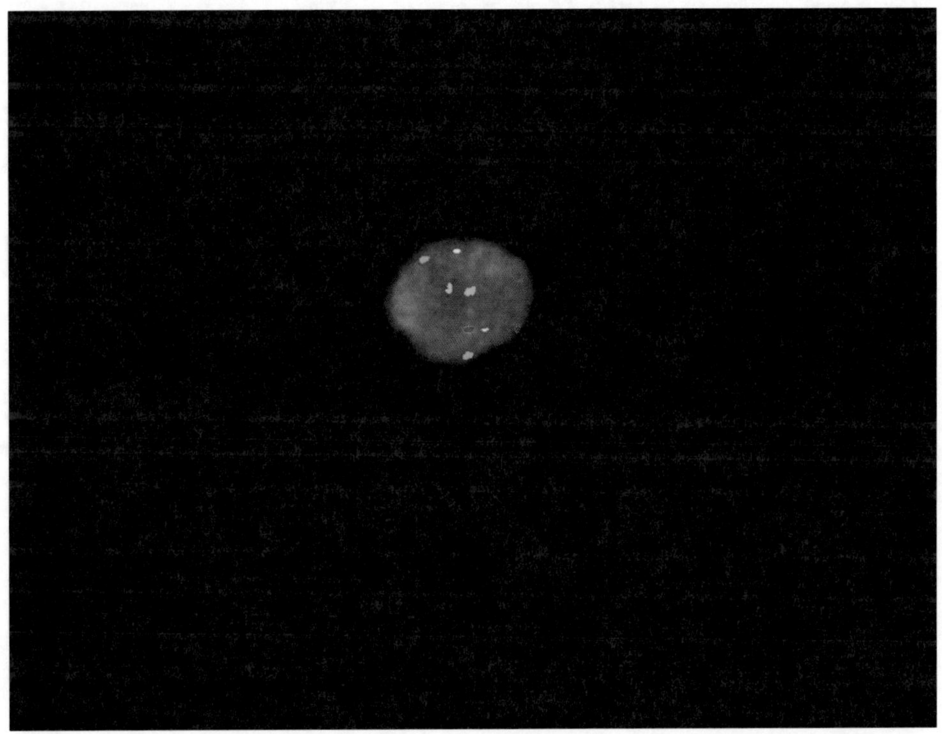

Fig. 32.10 Representative examples of normal cells with UroVysion FISH probe set: 2 signals for all 4 probes. The probe set: CEP 3 (red), CEP 7 (green), CEP 17 (aqua), and 9p21 (gold)

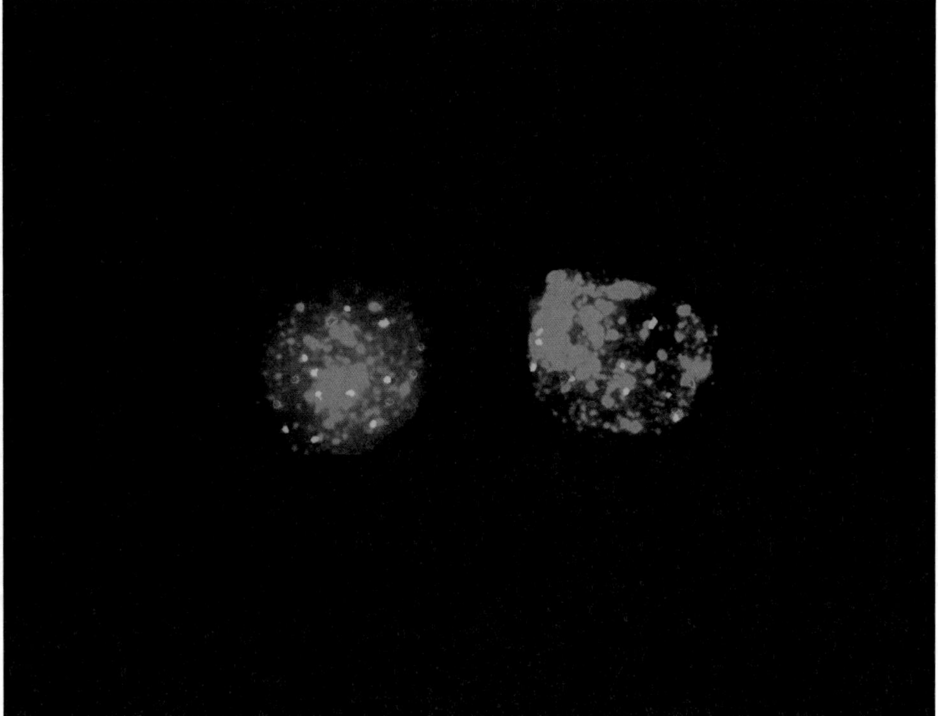

Fig. 32.11 Representative examples of abnormal cells: polysomy, showing gains 3 or more copies for 2 or more of the 4 probes

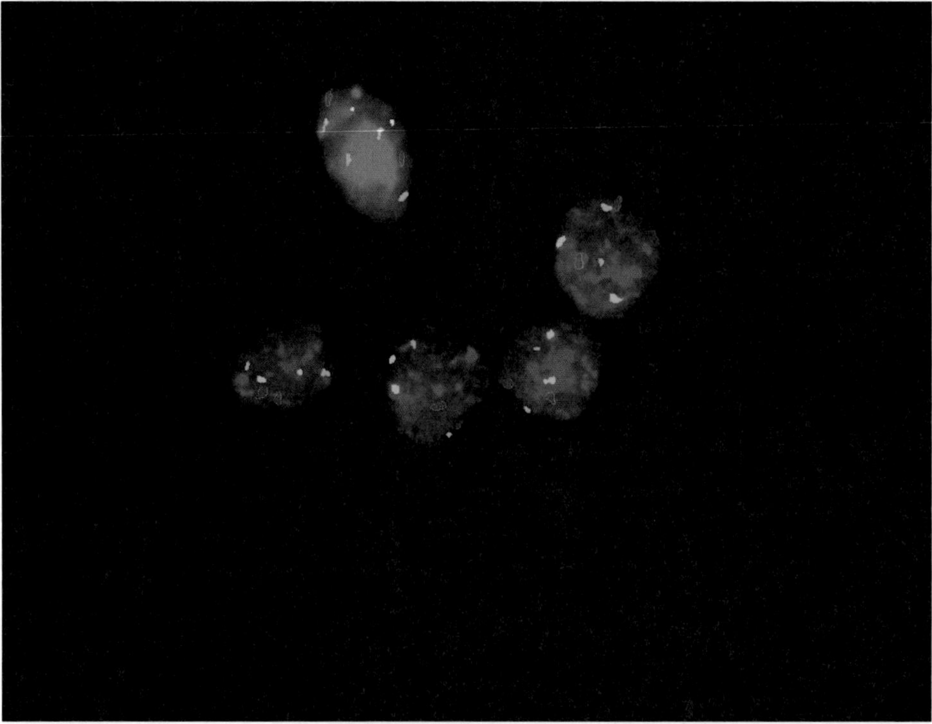

Fig. 32.12 Representative examples of abnormal cells: homozygous deletion (9p21-), showing no yellow signals. The presence of two normal 9p21 copies in normal cell at top left serves as an internal control

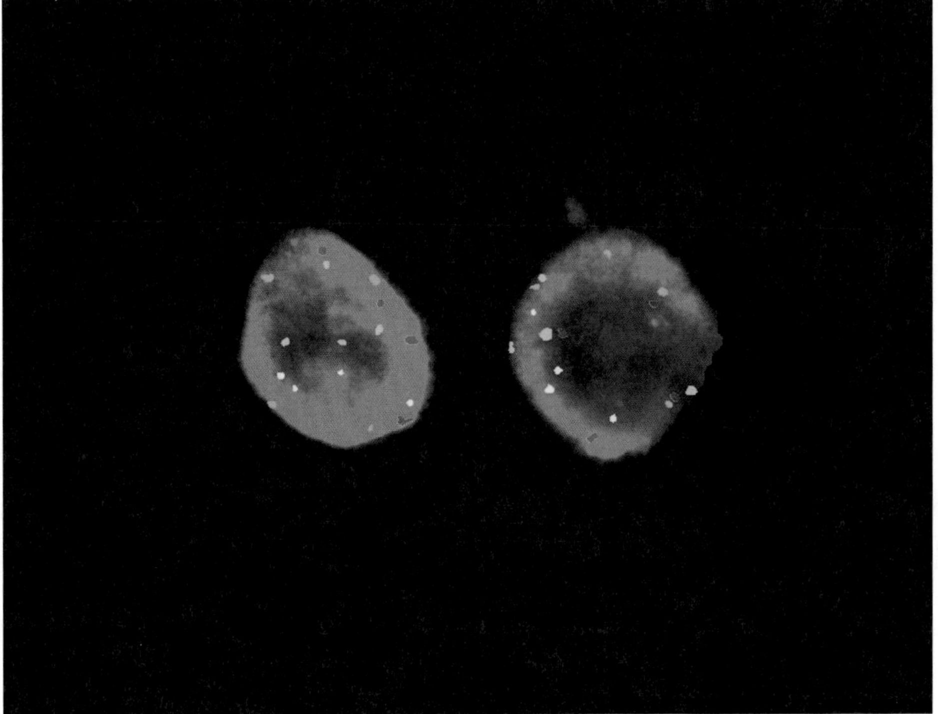

Fig. 32.13 Representative examples of abnormal cells: tetrasomy, showing 4 copies of all 4 probes

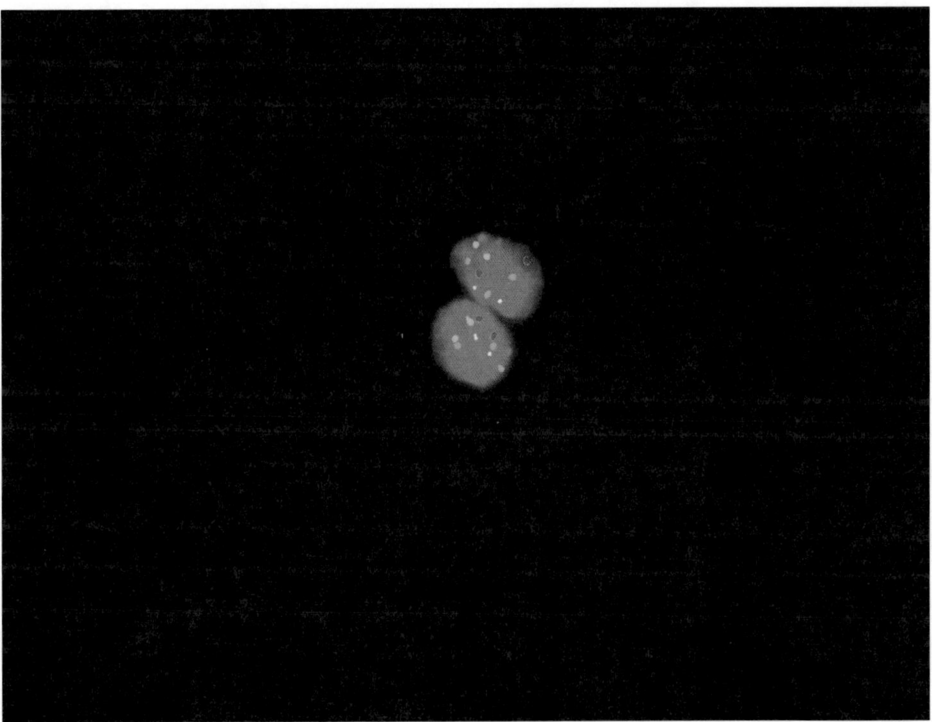

Fig. 32.14 Representative examples of abnormal cells: trisomy 7, showing 3 copies of CEP 7, but 2 copies of the other 3 probes

32.44 What Are the Normal Variant Results, or Why Do Normal Cells Yield Abnormal Signal Patterns?

Technique: Two signals overlap; hybridization not 100%; signal splitting; unrecognized overlapping cells

Cell cycle: Cells in the S or G2 phase give trisomy or tetrasomy

32.45 What Are the Most Common False-Positive and False-Negative Results?

False positive: BK viral infection; radiation/chemotherapy.

False negative: Low-grade noninvasive papillary tumor due to few chromosomal abnormalities; late-stage tumor with deep muscle invasion without mucosal involvement.

32.46 How to Manage Positive FISH and Negative Cystoscopy Findings?

Recommend evaluation for recurrent tumor by random biopsies.

32.47 How to Manage Positive Cytology and Negative Cystoscopy Findings?

Evaluate upper urothelial carcinoma.

32.48 What Are the Advantages of UroVysion?

UroVysion with cystoscopy gives the best result for sensitivity (97%) and specificity (96%).

UroVysion is more sensitive than cytology.

UroVysion can help identify patients with equivocal cytology, who most probably have true malignant cells.

UroVysion frequently detects tumor recurrence before it is detectable by cystoscopy or cytology.

UroVysion is not affected by Bacillus Calmette–Guerin (BCG) treatment; allows assessing for recurrence following BCG treatment.

Interphase nuclear count – chromosomal analysis of all the cells in the urine, including interphase and mitotic phase.

32.49 How to Compare Urine Cytology with UroVysion?

Voided urine cytology is not a very sensitive method to detect abnormal cells, but it is highly specific. The malignant cells can sometimes appear not different from normal cells, while UroVysion detects DNA abnormalities. It is more sensitive than voided urine cytology and detects malignant cells earlier.

32.50 Can UroVysion Can Be Used in Bladder Washing or Upper Tract Urothelial Cancer?

Yes, but it is not FDA-approved for detecting upper tract urothelial carcinoma.

Use bladder washing, obtained by catheterization, and upper tract washing, instead of voided urine. There is little data regarding the appropriate criteria.

References: [4, 16–18]

FISH in Bile Duct Brushing Specimens

32.51 How to Collect the Specimen?

Specimens are collected during endoscopic retrograde cholangiopancreatography (ERCP) as cytology brushing (at least five to-and-fro motions), with sampling stricture area only as possible. Each vial is gently agitated, equally split, and processed for both routine cytology and FISH.

32.52 What Is the Probe Set Used?

Fluorescently labeled probes to the centromeres of chromosomes 3, 7, 17 were used to determine the number of copies of given chromosomes in cells; chromosomal band 9p21 was used to identify abnormalities (UroVysion probe set, Abbott Molecular, Des Plaines, IL).

32.53 What Are the Criteria for Positive FISH Result?

Polysomy: ≥5 cells with ≥3 signals in at least two probes

Trisomy: ≥10 cells with three signals for chromosome 3 or 7; ≤2 signals for the other probes

Tetrasomy: ≥10 cells with four signals for all four probes

32.54 How to Explain Positive FISH?

Polysomy FISH maintains the same high specificity as routine cytology. It plays an important role in clinical practice for identifying additional patients with carcinoma without additional false positives.

Trisomy: It is not specific for carcinoma. It can be seen in both tumor and benign conditions. Recommend following every 6 months for 2 years.

Tetrasomy: It is not specific for carcinoma. It can occasionally be seen in normal cells in the S or G2 phase of cell cycle.

32.55 What Are False-Positive and False-Negative Results?

False Positive: Autoimmune disease, like primary sclerosing cholangitis (PSC)

False negative: Malignant cells may have different chromosomal alterations than were used by UroVysion set

32.56 What Is the Indication?

Evaluate indeterminate pancreatobiliary strictures.

32.57 What Are the Advantages?

FISH has significantly higher sensitivity than routine cytology.

FISH maintains the same high specificity as RC.

FISH detects earlier malignancy than RC.

Combining RC, FISH, age, and PSC status offers valuable data for early intervention.

32.58 How to Analyze the Final Report?

The model generated through multivariable analysis is used to estimate the probability of malignancy for each patient based on their cytologic brushing test result, FISH analysis, age, and PSC status.

32.59 How to Manage If Both RC and FISH Are Negative?

If RC and FISH are both negative and there is high clinical suspicion for malignancy, patient should return within 3–6 months for repeat ERCP, including cytology and FISH study.

Estimate the probability of malignancy based on RC, FISH, age, and PSC status.

32.60 What Is the Recommendation for Bile Duct Brushing?

Recommend performing both RC and FISH as a routine on brushing specimens from all indeterminate pancreatobiliary strictures.

References: [19–21]

FISH in Bronchoscopic Specimens

32.61 What Is the Indication?

Cytology is equivocal, and/or negative, but lung cancer is clinically suspected

32.62 How to Collect the Specimen?

Bronchial brushing specimens are received as ethanol spray-fixed smears. No additional slide preparation is required prior to FISH hybridization.

Bronchial washing specimens are collected in 50 mL conical tubes, then special preparation is required to lyse RBC.

32.63 Is There Any Special Preparation Needed for Prehybridization?

Bronchial brushing specimens – slides are immersed in fresh 3:1 methanol:acetic acid fixative for10 min to help remove debris and prepare for hybridization.

Washing specimens – no special preparation.

32.64 What Is the Probe Set Used?

Use LAVysion multicolor, DNA-based FISH probe (Abbott Molecular, Des Plaines, IL). It contains locus-specific probes – 5p15, 7p12 (EGFR), 8q23 (C-MYC), and a centromeric probe – chromosome 6.

32.65 What Are the Criteria for a Positive FISH Result?

Polysomy: ≥5 cells with ≥2 signals of the four probes

Tetrasomy: ≥10 cells with four signals for all four probes

32.66 How to Obtain Cytology Slides?

Cytology is performed on Papanicolaou-stained bronchial brushing and washing specimens.

32.67 What Are False-Positive and False-Negative Results?

False positive: Radiation or chemotherapy; metastases; premalignant lesions; high-risk patient without cancer

False negative: Malignant cells may have different chromosomal alterations than were used by selected FISH probe set

32.68 What Are the Advantages?

FISH is significantly more sensitive than conventional cytology for detecting lung cancer in bronchial brushing specimens, especially for peripheral tumors.

Combined FISH and conventional cytology improve the detection of early lung cancer.

32.69 How to Manage Negative Cytology and Positive FISH?

Cytology negative, FISH positive – suspicion only, no surgical or chemotherapeutic treatment. Reassess at regular intervals (every 6 months).

Reference: [22]

FISH in the Diagnosis of Soft Tissue Neoplasm

32.70 What Is the Indication for Using FISH in the Diagnosis of Soft Tissue Neoplasm?

Similar histologic appearances with overlapping immunohistochemical profiles

Diagnostic-specific gene involved

Prognostic clinical impact

32.71 What Types of Probe Sets Are Used?

Five break-apart probes, including *EWSR1*, *FUS*, *DDIT3*, *SYT*, and *FOXO1A* genes (Abbott Molecular/Vysis, Des Plaines, IL)

A dual-color MDM2 FISH probe, hybridized to 12q13 to 15, compared CEP 12; a ratio of ≥2 indicates an amplification of MDM2 gene (Cleveland Clinic)

32.72 What Are the Advantages and Limitations?

Advantages
Highly sensitive and specific
Interphase analysis, specific gene abnormalities, and rapid turnaround time
Limitations
Not a screening test
Knowing the possible genetic abnormality prior testing

32.73 What Are the FISH Results for High-Grade Round Cell Sarcoma? (Tables 32.18 and 32.19)

Table 32.18 Genetic abnormalities associated with high-grade round cell sarcoma

Tumor	Genetic abnormality	Genes involved
Ewing sarcoma (ES)/ peripheral neuroecto-dermal tumor (PNET)	t(11;22)(q24;q12)	FLI1-EWS 90%
	t(21;22)(22;q12)	ERG-EWS 5%
	Less common variants	<5%
Poorly differentiated synovial sarcoma	t(X;18)(p11.2;q11.2)	SSX1-SYT 66%
		SSX2-SYT 33%
Alveolar rhabdomyosarcoma	t(1;13)(p36;q14)	PAX7-FKHR 70%
	t(2;13)(q35;q14)	PAX3-FKHR 10%
Desmoplastic small round cell tumor	t(11;22)(p13;q12)	WT1-EWS >90%
Extraskeletal myxoid chondrosarcoma	t(9;22)(q22;q12)	NOR1-EWS 70%
	t(9;17)(q22;q11)	NOR1-RBP56 20%

Note: Alveolar rhabdomyosarcoma: t(1;13)(p36;q14) – better prognosis, t(2;13)(q35;q14) – poorer prognosis

Table 32.19 Summary of genes involved and clinical features

Tumor	Gene test percentage	Clinical significance
Ewing sarcoma (ES)/peripheral neuroectodermal tumor (PNET)	EWSR1 gene (22q12) 96%	Distinguish from other SRCN
Poorly differentiated synovial sarcoma	SYT 100%	Diagnostic
Alveolar rhabdomyosarcoma	FOXO1A 80%	Diagnostic and prognostic
Desmoplastic small round cell tumor	EWSR1 100%	Poor prognosis
Extraskeletal myxoid chondrosarcoma	NOR1 >90% EWSR1 70%	Diagnostic

32.74 What Is the Most Common Use of FISH in Spindle Cell Sarcoma?

Monophasic synovial sarcoma

Malignant peripheral nerve sheath tumor (MPNST)

Both have similar histologic appearance and overlapping immunophenotypes. Thus molecular studies play an important role in the differential diagnosis. Malignant peripheral nerve sheath tumors do not harbor the t(X;18). The absence of rearrangement of the STY gene can be helpful in supporting the diagnosis. In addition, 25–50% of MPNSTs are associated with neurofibromatosis. Loss of p53 is involved in the progression from neurofibroma to MPNST.

Leiomyosarcoma

Histology and immunohistochemical panels for diagnosis

Dermatofibrosarcoma protuberans

FISH does not play a role in the diagnosis; immunohistochemistry (loss of CD34 expression) aids the diagnosis.

Table 32.20 Genetic abnormalities associated with low-grade myxoid neoplasm

Tumor	Genetic abnormality	Gene involved
Low-grade fibromyxoid sarcoma	t(7;16)(q33;p11)	CREB3L2-FUS 96%
	t(11;16)(p11;p11)	CREB3L1-FUS
Myxoid/round cell liposarcoma	t(12;16)(q13;p11)	DDIT3[a]-FUS 90–95%
	t(12;22)(q13;q11-12)	DDIT3-EWS

Note: [a]DDIT3 was formerly known as CHOP

32.75 What Are the FISH Results for Low-Grade Myxoid Neoplasm? (Tables 32.20 and 32.21)

Myxofibrosarcoma is characterized by a highly complex karyotype. No consistent cytogenetic findings. Usually does not require FISH study. FISH can play a role in ruling out neoplasms. No rearrangement of FUS or DDIT3 was observed.

Table 32.21 Summary of genes involved and clinical features

Tumor	Gene test percentage	Clinical significance
Low-grade fibromyxoid sarcoma	FUS 91%	Both LGFMS and myxoid liposarcoma harbor FUS
Myxoid/round cell liposarcoma	DDIT3 100%	Diagnostic

Note: Myxoid/round cell liposarcoma: Morphology as small round blue cell and occasional rearrangement of EWSR1, but negative CD99 is useful to differentiate in this situation

Table 32.22 Genetic abnormalities associated with adipocytic neoplasms

Tumor	Genetic abnormality	Gene involved
Well-differentiated liposarcoma[a]	12q rings and giant markers 12q13 to 15	MDM2 (amplified), 100%
Dedifferentiated liposarcoma	12q13 to 15	MDM2 (amplified), 100%
Pleomorphic liposarcoma	12q13 to 15	MDM2 (amplified), 40%

Note: [a]The same region of gene rearrangement, not amplification, can be seen in lipoma

Myxoma may be considered as a differential diagnosis of the sarcoma. The role of FISH in the diagnosis is restricted to exclusion.

32.76 What Are the FISH Results for Adipocytic Neoplasms? (Table 32.22)

It is important to differentiate dedifferentiated liposarcoma from pleomorphic liposarcoma due to a better prognosis of dedifferentiated liposarcoma. If MDM2 is negative, it strongly argues against the diagnostic possibility of dedifferentiated liposarcoma.

32.77 What Are the FISH Results for Melanocytic Neoplasm? (Table 32.23)

32.78 Which Type of Soft Tissue Tumor Is Associated with the EWSR1 Gene?

Ewing sarcoma/PNET
- Desmoplastic small round cell tumor
- Clear cell sarcoma

Table 32.23 Summary of FISH results

Tumor	Genetic abnormality	Percentage	Gene involved
Clear cell sarcoma	t(12;22)(q13;q12)	EWSR1 88%	ATF1-EWS 100%
Melanoma	No consistent translocations	EWSR1 0%	

32.79 Which Type of Soft Tissue Tumor Is Associated with the SYT Gene?

SYT – most common soft tissue neoplasm
- Poorly differentiated synovial sarcoma
- Monomorphic synovial sarcoma

32.80 Which Type of Soft Tissue Tumor Is Associated with the FOXO1A Gene?

Alveolar rhabdomyosarcoma

32.81 Which Type of Soft Tissue Tumor Is Associated with the DDIT3 Gene?

Myxoid/round cell liposarcoma

32.82 Which Type of Soft Tissue Tumor Is Associated with the FUS Gene?

Low-grade fibromyxoid sarcoma
- Myxoid liposarcoma

32.83 Which Type of Soft Tissue Tumor Is Associated with the MDM2 Gene?

Well-differentiated liposarcoma
- Dedifferentiated liposarcoma

References: [23–25]

Acknowledgment Special thanks for Jenny Pettengill, CT (ASCP), Cytotechnologist at Mayo Clinic, providing UroVysion pictures and Neogenomics providing the rest of FISH pictures.

References

1. Levsky JM, Singer RH. Fluorescence in situ hybridization: past, present and future. J Cell Sci. 2003;116(Pt 14):2833–8.
2. Liehr T, Claussen U. Current developments in human molecular cytogenetics techniques. Curr Mol Med. 2002;2(3):283–97.
3. Ventura RA, Martin-Subero JI, Jones M, et al. FISH analysis for the detection of lymphoma-associated chromosomal abnormalities in routine-paraffin-embedded tissue. J Mol Diagn. 2006;8(2):141–51.
4. Kalling KC, Kipp BR. Bladder cancer detection using FISH (UroVysion assay). Adv Anat Pathol. 2008;15(5):279–86.
5. Cavazzini F, Ciccone M, Negrini M, et al. Clinicobiologic importance of cytogenetic lesions in chronic lymphocytic leukemia. Expert Rev Hematol. 2009;2(3):305–14.
6. Sreekantaiah C. FISH panels for hematologic malignancies. Cytogenet Genome Res. 2007;118(2):284–96.
7. Stewart AK, Bergsagel PL, Greipp PR, et al. A practical guide to defining high-risk myeloma for clinical trials, patient counseling and choice of therapy. Leukemia. 2007;21(3):529–34.
8. Avet-Loiseau H. FISH analysis at diagnosis in acute lymphoblastic leukemia. Leuk Lymphoma. 1999;33(5–6):441–9.
9. Harrison CJ. The detection and significance of chromosomal abnormalities in childhood acute lymphoblastic leukaemia. Blood Rev. 2001;15(1):49–59.
10. Dewald GW, Wyatt WA, Juneau AL, et al. Highly sensitive fluorescence in situ hybridization method to detect double BCR/ABL fusion and monitor response to therapy in chronic myeloid leukemia. Blood. 1998;91(9):3357–65.
11. Wolff DJ, Bagg A, Cooley LD, et al. Guidance for fluorescence in situ hybridization testing in hematologic disorders. J Mol Diagn. 2007;9(2):134–43.
12. Smoley SA, Brockman SR, Paternoster SF, Meyer RG, Dewald GW. A novel tricolor, dual-fusion fluorescence in situ hybridization method to detect BCR/ABL fusion in cells with t(9;22)(q34;q11.2) associated with deletion of DNA on the derivative chromosome 9 in chronic myelocytic leukemia. Cancer Genet Cytogenet. 2004;148(1): 1–6.
13. Sinclair PB, Nacheva EP, Leversha M, et al. Large deletions at the t(9;22) breakpoint are common and may identify a poor-prognosis subgroup of patients with chronic myeloid leukemia. Blood. 2000;95(3):738–43.
14. Niitsu N, Okamoto M, Nakamura N, et al. Prognostic impact of chromosomal alteration of 3q27 on nodal B-cell lymphoma: correlation with histology, immunophenotype, karyotype, and clinical outcome in 329 consecutive patients. Leuk Res. 2007;31(9): 1191–7.
15. Espinet B, Bellosillo B, Gregori E, et al. Fish is the best method to detect BCL2/IgH translocation in follicular lymphoma at diagnosis. A comparative study with conventional cytogenetics, Fish and PCR (Biomed-2 Primers) techniques [American Society of Hematology abstract #1377]. Blood. 2004;104(11):1377.
16. Kipp BR, Tanasescu M, Else TA, et al. Quantitative fluorescence in situ hybridization and its ability to predict bladder cancer recurrence and progression to muscle-invasive bladder cancer. J Mol Diagn. 2009;11(2):148–54.
17. Halling KC, King W, Sokolova IA, et al. A comparison of cytology and fluorescence in situ hybridization for the detection of urothelial carcinoma. J Urol. 2000;164(5):1768–75.
18. Halling KC. Vysis UroVysion for the detection of urothelial carcinoma. Expert Rev Mol Diagn. 2003;3(4):507–19.
19. Levy MJ, Clain JE, Clayton A, et al. Preliminary experience comparing routine cytology results with the composite results of digital image analysis and fluorescence in situ hybridization in patients undergoing EUS-guided FNA. Gastrointest Endosc. 2007;66(3): 483–90.
20. Barr Fritcher EG, Kipp BR, Slezak JM, et al. Correlating routine cytology, quantitative nuclear morphometry by digital image analysis, and genetic alterations by fluorescence in situ hybridization to assess the sensitivity of cytology for detecting pancreatobiliary tract malignancy. Am J Clin Pathol. 2007;128(2):272–9.
21. Fritcher EG, Kipp BR, Halling KC, et al. A multivariable model using advanced cytologic methods for the evaluation of indeterminate pancreatobiliary strictures. Gastroenterology. 2009;136(7): 2180–6.
22. Halling KC, Rickman OB, Kipp BR, Harwood AR, Doerr CH, Jett JR. A comparison of cytology and fluorescence in situ hybridization for the detection of lung cancer in bronchoscopic specimens. Chest. 2006;130(3):694–701.
23. Anderson J, Gordon T, McManus A, et al. Detection of the PAX3-FKHR fusion gene in paediatric rhabdomyosarcoma: a reproducible predictor of outcome? Br J Cancer. 2001;85(6):831–5.
24. Mehra S, de la Roza G, Tull J, Shrimpton A, Valente A, Zhang S. Detection of FOXO1 (FKHR) gene break-apart by fluorescence in situ hybridization in formalin-fixed, paraffin-embedded alveolar rhabdomyosarcomas and its clinicopathologic correlation. Diagn Mol Pathol. 2008;17(1):14–20.
25. Tanas MR, Goldblum JR. Fluorescence in situ hybridization in the diagnosis of soft tissue neoplasms: a review. Adv Anat Pathol. 2009;16(6):383–91.

Appendix A

F. Lin and J. Prichard (eds.), *Handbook of Practical Immunohistochemistry: Frequently Asked Questions*,
DOI 10.1007/978-1-4419-8062-5,

Antibody name and synonyms	Vendor	Catalog no.	Approved use	Clonality	Host animal	Dilution	Inc. time (min)	AR method/time/ temp./pH	Localization	Control tissue
Actin, smooth muscle (SMA, smooth muscle actin)	DAKO	M0851	IVD	1A4	Mouse	1:50	40	EDTA/15/100/8	C	Leiomyosarcoma
Adrenocorticotropic hormone (ACTH)	CellMq	206A	IVD	Polyclonal	Rabbit	1:100	40	EDTA/15/100/8	C	Normal pituitary
Alpha-1-antichymotrypsin (A-ACT, A1ACT)	DAKO	A0012	IVD	Polyclonal	Rabbit	1:500	30	None	C	Liver
Alpha-1-antitrypsin (A1AT)	DAKO	N1533	IVD	Polyclonal	Rabbit	1:700	30	ProtK/9/Ambient/7.5	C	Tonsil
Alpha-fetoprotein, (AFP)	DAKO	N1501	IVD	Polyclonal	Rabbit	1:2	40	None	C	Germ cell tumor
Alpha-methylacyl-CoA racemase (AMACR, P504S)	ZETA	Z2001	RUO	13H4	Rabbit	1:80	30	Hi pH/20/99/9.9	C	Prostate
Anaplastic lymphoma kinase-1 (ALK-1, ALK1)	DAKO	M7195	IVD	ALK1	Mouse	1:30	30	AR/15/100/6	N, C	ALK+ tissue
Androgen receptor protein (ARP)	CellMq	200M-15	IVD	AR441	Mouse	1:10	40	EDTA/15/100/8	N	Prostate
Annexin A1 (ANXA-1)	CellMq	221M	IVD	MRQ-3	Mouse	1:100	40	EDTA/15/100/8	M, C	Hairy cell leukemia
B cell Oct binding protein 1 (BOB.1)	Leica	NCL-L-BOB-1	ASR	TG14	Mouse	1:20	60	EDTA/15/100/8	N, C	B-cell lymphoma
B72.3, (TAG 72, BRST-3, BRST3)	CellMq	337M-85	IVD	B72.3	Mouse	1:200	30	EDTA/15/100/8	C	Block #1
B-cell CLL/lymphoma 1 (Bcl-1, Cyclin D1, Bcl1)	DAKO	M7155	IVD	DSC-6	Mouse	1:75	30	Hi pH/20/99/9.9	N	Mantle cell lymphoma
B-cell CLL/lymphoma 2 (Bcl-2, Bcl2)	CellMq	226M-95	IVD	124	Mouse	1:100	40	EDTA/15/100/8	C	Tonsil
B-cell CLL/lymphoma 6 (Bcl-6, Bcl6)	DAKO	M7211	IVD	PG-B6p	Mouse	1:10	60	Hi pH/20/99/9.9	N	Tonsil
Beta-catenin	CellMq	224M-16	IVD	14	Mouse	1:50	40	EDTA/15/100/8	N, M, C	Block #1
Breast cancer-1 (BRCA-1)	BioM	345 A	IVD	MS110	Mouse	1:50	60	EDTA/15/100/8	C	Breast CA
C4d	Alpco	BI-RC4D	RUO	Polyclonal	Rabbit	1:50	30	AR/15/100/6	M, C	Transplanted kidney
Calcitonin	DAKO	A0576	IVD	Polyclonal	Rabbit	1:600	60	TRS/20/99/6.1	C	Medullary thyroid CA
Caldesmon	CellMq	230R-15	IVD	E89	Rabbit	1:25	40	Hi pH/20/99/9.9	C	Smooth muscle
Calponin (CALP)	CellMq	231M-16	IVD	Calp	Mouse	1:100	40	TRS/20/99/6.1	C	Breast, uterus
Calponin-1 (CALP-1)	CellMq	231R-15	IVD	EP798Y	Rabbit	1:50	40	TRS/20/99/6.1	C	Uterus
Calretinin (CALRET)	Zymed	18-0211	IVD	Polyclonal	Rabbit	1:500	40	TRS/20/99/6.1	N, C	Mesothelial cells
Cancer antigen 15-3 (CA15-3)	CellMq	353M-15	IVD	DF3	Mouse	Pre-diluted	40	EDTA/15/100/8	C	Normal breast, pancreas CA
Cancer antigen 19-9 (CA19-9, CA 19-9)	CellMq	399M-15	IVD	121SLE	Mouse	1:50	30	EDTA/15/100/8	C	Block #1
Cancer antigen-125 (CA-125, CA 125)	Covance	SIG-3617	IVD	OC125	Mouse	1:20	40	TUF/10/99/8	C	Ovarian CA
Carbonic anhydrase IX (CA IX, CAIX, CA-IX)	SantaC	Sc-25599	ASR	Polyclonal	Rabbit	1:50	60	EDTA/15/100/8	C	RCC
Carcinoembryonic antigen (CEA)	Biogx	MU009-UC	IVD	B01-94-11M-P	Mouse	1:350	30	ProtK/9/100/7.5	C	Colon
CD10	CellMq	110M-15	IVD	56C6	Mouse	1:10	40	EDTA/15/100/8	M, C	Tonsil
CD105 (endoglin)	DAKO	M3527	IVD	SN6h	Mouse	1:50	40	EDTA/15/100/8	C	Tonsil

CD117 (c-kit)	Ventana	790-2951	IVD	9.7	Rabbit	Pre-diluted	30	EDTA/15/100/8	M, C	GIST
CD13	SantaC	Sc-53970	RUO	BR2	Mouse	1:25	40	EDTA/15/100/8	M	Duodenum
CD138 (syndecan 1)	AbD	MCA681A647	RUO	B-B4	Mouse	1:300	30	AR/15/100/6.0	M, C	Tonsil
CD15 (Leu-M1)	Ventana	760-2504	IVD	MMA	Mouse	Pre-diluted	40	EDTA/15/100/8	M, C	Tonsil
CD163	CellMq	163M-15	IVD	MRQ-26	Mouse	Pre-diluted	40	EDTA/15/100/8	M, C	Tonsil
CD19	DAKO	M7296	IVD	LE-CD19	Mouse	1:50	40	EDTA/15/100/8	M	Tonsil
CD1a	DAKO	M3571	IVD	10	Mouse	1:50	60	TRS/20/99/6.1	C	Skin
CD2	Vector	VP-C313	ASR	AB75	Mouse	1:50	30	EDTA/15/100/8	M, C	Tonsil
CD20	DAKO	M0755	IVD	L26	Mouse	1:700	30	None	M	Tonsil
CD21	DAKO	M0784	IVD	1F8	Mouse	1:30	60	TRS/20/99/6.1	M	Tonsil
CD23	DAKO	M0763	IVD	MHM6	Mouse	Pre-diluted	30	TRS/20/99/6.1	M	Tonsil
CD25	CellMq	125M-15	IVD	4C9	Mouse	Pre-diluted	40	EDTA/15/100/8	M, C	Tonsil
CD3	DAKO	M7254	IVD	F7.2.38	Mouse	1:100	30	TRS/20/99/6.1	M	Tonsil
CD30 (Ber H-1, Ber-H1)	DAKO	M0751	IVD	BerH2	Mouse	1:30	40	TRS/20/99/6.1	C	Tonsil
CD31	CellMq	131M-15	IVD	1A10	Mouse	1:30	40	TRS/20/99/6.1	M, C	Tonsil
CD34	CellMq	134M-15	IVD	QBEnd/10	Mouse	1:50	40	EDTA/15/100/8	C	Tonsil
CD35 (follicular dendritic cell)	DAKO	M0846	IVD	Ber-MAC-DRC	Mouse	1:15	30	None	M, C	Tonsil
CD4	NOVO	NCL-CD4-1F6	IVD	IF6	Mouse	1:20	30	EDTA/15/100/8	M, C	Tonsil
CD43	DAKO	M0786	IVD	DF-T1	Mouse	1:80	30	TRS/20/99/6.1	M	Tonsil
CD44	DAKO	M7082	IVD	DF1485	Mouse	1:160	40	TRS/20/99/6.1	M	Tonsil
CD45 (LCA)	DAKO	M0701	IVD	2B11 + PD7/26	Mouse	1:1600	30	None	M	Tonsil
CD45RO	DAKO	M0742	IVD	UCHL1	Mouse	1:100	30	None	M	Tonsil
CD5	Vector	VP-C322	IVD	4C7	Mouse	1:30	30	AR/15/100/6	M	Tonsil
CD56 (NCAM)	CellMq	156M-85	IVD	123C3.D5	Mouse	1:100	40	EDTA/15/100/8	C	Appendix
CD57	CellMq	157M-94	IVD	NK1	Mouse	1:100	30	EDTA/15/100/8	C	Tonsil
CD61	DAKO	M0753	IVD	Y2/51	Mouse	1:50	40	TRS/20/99/6.1	C	Bone marrow
CD68	DAKO	M0814	IVD	KP1	Mouse	1:100	30	None	C	Tonsil
CD7	NOVO	NCL-CD7-580	IVD	LP15	Mouse	1:50	60	AR/15/100/6	M	Tonsil
CD74	Ventana	760-2628	IVD	LN2	Mouse	Pre-diluted	40	EDTA/15/100/8	M, C	Tonsil
CD79a	DAKO	M7051	IVD	HM57	Mouse	1:100	30	None	C	Tonsil
CD8	DAKO	M7103	IVD	C8/144B	Mouse	1:40	30	AR/15/100/6	M	Tonsil
CD99 (MIC-2, MIC2)	CellMq	199R-15	IVD	EPR3097Y	Rabbit	1:100	40	EDTA/15/100/8	M, C	Ewing's sarcoma
CDX-2 (CDX2)	CellMq	235R-15	IVD	EPR2764Y	Rabbit	1:100	40	EDTA/15/100/8	N	Colon
Chromogranin A (chrom)	BioM	CM010 B	IVD	LK2H10+PHE5	Mouse	1:120	30	EDTA/15/100/8.0	C	Pancreas
Claudin 1 (claudin-1, CLDN1, CLDN-1)	CellMq	359A-15	IVD	Polyclonal	Rabbit	1:25	40	EDTA/15/100/8	M	Colon, small intestine
Claudin 18 (claudin-18, CLDN18, CLDN-18)	Invitro	38-8100	ASR	Polyclonal	Rabbit	1:100	50	AR/15/100/6.0	C	Lung, stomach
Claudin 4 (claudin-4, CLDN4, CLDN-4)	Invitro	32-9400	ASR	3E2C1	Mouse	1:100	60	EDTA/15/100/8.0	C	Colon ADC
Claudin 8 (claudin-8, CLDN8, CLDN-8)	Invitro	40-2600	RUO	Polyclonal	Rabbit	1:100	40	EDTA/15/100/8.0	C	Colon ADC
Collagen type IV	DAKO	M0785	IVD	CIV 22	Mouse	1:75	60	TRS/20/99/6.1	C, E	Basement membranes
COX-2 (COX2)	CellMq	240R-16	IVD	SP21	Rabbit	1:10	40	EDTA/15/100/8.0	C	Colon ADC
Cyclin-dependent kinase 4 (CDK4, CDK-4)	Thermo	MS-469P	RUO	DCS-31	Mouse	1:300	40	EDTA/15/100/8.0	M, C	Liposarcoma
Cytokeratin 14 (CK14)	CellMq	314M-16	IVD	LL002	Mouse	1:100	40	EDTA/15/100/8.0	C	Skin
Cytokeratin 15 (CK15)	Vector	VP-C411	RUO	LHK15	Mouse	1:40	60	EDTA/15/100/8.0	C	Skin, hair follicles

(continued)

(continued)

Antibody name and synonyms	Vendor	Catalog no.	Approved use	Clonality	Host animal	Dilution	Inc. time (min)	AR method/time/temp./pH	Localization	Control tissue
Cytokeratin 17 (CK17)	DAKO	M7046	IVD	E3 (1)	Mouse	1:80	30	EDTA/15/100/8.0	C	Block #1
Cytokeratin 19 (CK19)	Ventana	760-4281	IVD	(A53-B/A2.26)	Mouse	1:100	30	EDTA/15/100/8.0	C	Block #1
Cytokeratin 20 (CK20)	CellMq	320M-15	IVD	Ks20.8	Mouse	1:500	30	EDTA/15/100/8.0	C	Block #1
Cytokeratin 5 (CK5)	CellMq	305R-15	IVD	EP1601Y	Rabbit	1:50	40	EDTA/15/100/8.0	C	Mesothelioma
Cytokeratin 5 and 6 (CK5/6, CK 5 and 6)	CellMq	356M-16	IVD	D5 and 16B4	Mouse	1:25	60	EDTA/15/100//8.0	C	Tonsil, prostate
Cytokeratin 7 (CK7)	CellMq	307M-95	IVD	OV-TL12/30	Mouse	1:200	30	ProtK/9/Ambient/7.5	C	Breast
Cytokeratin 8 (CK8, 35betaH11)	DAKO	M7010	IVD	DC 10	Mouse	1:25	30	EDTA/15/100/8.0	C	Prostate
Cytokeratin 8 and 18 (CK8/18, CK 8 and 18)	CellMq	818M-95	IVD	B22.1 and B23.1	Mouse	1:100	40	EDTA/15/100/8.0	C	Pancreas, prostate, salivary gland
Cytokeratin AE1 (CK AE1, AE1/AE3)	Biogx	MU-075-UC	IVD	AE1	Mouse	1:150	30	ProtK/9/Ambient/7.5	M, C	Skin
Cytokeratin AE1/AE3 (AE1/AE3)	DAKO	M3515	IVD	AE1/AE3	Mouse	1:75	40	ProtK/9/Ambient/7.5	C	Appendix
Cytokeratin, CAM 5.2 (CAM 5.2, LMW cytokeratin, low molecular weight cytokeratin, LMWCK)	BD	349205	IVD	CAM5.2	Mouse	1:4	30	None	C	Appendix
Cytokeratin, HMW/CK903 (CK903, 34betaE12, HMWCK, high molecular weight cytokeratin)	CellMq	334M-85	IVD	34betaE12	Mouse	1:100	30	EDTA/15/100/8.0	C	Prostate
Cytomegalovirus (CMV)	DAKO	M0767	ASR	CCH2	Mouse	1:30	30	ProtK/9/Ambient/7.5	N	CMV
D2-40 (podoplanin, D240)	CellMq	322M	IVD	D2-40	Mouse	1:40	60	EDTA/15/100/8.0	C	Tonsil
Desmin	DAKO	M0760	IVD	D33	Mouse	1:200	30	TUF/10/99/8.0	C	Appendix
Desmoglein3 (desmoglein-3)	Abcam	Ab14416	RUO	3G133	Mouse	1:25	60	TRS/20/99/6.1	C	Lung SQCC
DOG1	CellMq	244R-15	IVD	SP31	Rabbit	1:25	40	EDTA/15/100/8.0	M, C	GIST
E-cadherin	DAKO	M3612	IVD	NCH-384	Mouse	1:200	30	EDTA/15/100/8.0	M	Breast
Epithelial cell adhesion molecule antibody (Ber-EP4, EPCAM, ESA, epithelial specific antigen)	DAKO	M0804	IVD	Ber-EP4	Mouse	1:100	30	TRS/20/99/6.1	M, C	Block #1
Epithelial membrane antigen (EMA)	DAKO	M0613	IVD	Monoclonal	Mouse	1:200	30	None	M	Colon
Estrogen receptor (ER)	DAKO	M7047	IVD	1D5	Mouse	1:300	60	AR/15/100/6.0	N	Breast
Factor VIII (FVIII)	CellMq	250A-15	IVD	Polyclonal	Rabbit	1:100	30	ProtK/9/Ambient/7.5	C	Tonsil
Factor XIIIa (FXIIIa)	CellMq	251R-15	IVD	EP3372	Rabbit	1:60	30	EDTA/15/100/8.0	C	Tonsil
Fascin	DAKO	M3567	RUO	55K-2	Mouse	1:200	30	EDTA/15/100/8.0	C	Tonsil
Follicle-stimulating hormone (FSH)	CellMq	207A	IVD	Polyclonal	Rabbit	1:50	60	EDTA/15/100/8.0	C	Pituitary gland
Friend leukemia virus integration-1 (FLI-1, FLI1)	CellMq	254M-15	IVD	MRQ-1	Mouse	1:25	40	EDTA/15/100/8.0	N	Angiosarcoma, Ewing's sarcoma
Galectin-3 (galectin 3, GAL3, GAL-3)	SantaC	Sc-20157	ASR	Polyclonal	Rabbit	1:200	45	EDTA/15/100/8.0	N, C	Pancreas or thyroid CA
Gastrin	Ventana	760-2643	IVD	Polyclonal	Rabbit	Pre-diluted	40	EDTA/15/100/8.0	C	Stomach

Glial fibrillary acidic protein (GFAP)	CellMq	258M-15	IVD	GA5	Mouse	1:50	40	Hi pH/20/99/9.9	C	Brain
Glucagon	DAKO	A0565	IVD	Polyclonal	Rabbit	1:900	30	None	C	Pancreas
Glucose transporter 1 (GLUT1, GLUT-1)	DBS	RP128-05	RUO	Polyclonal	Rabbit	1:25	40	EDTA/15/100/8.0	M	Malignant mesothelioma, or block #1
Glycophorin A	CellMq	260M-15	IVD	GA-R2 and HIR2	Mouse	Pre-diluted	40	EDTA/15/100/8.0	M	Bone marrow
Glypican-3, (GPC3)	CellMq	261M-95	IVD	1G12	Mouse	1:100	40	EDTA/15/100/8.0	C	HCC
Granzyme B	NOVO	NCL-GRAN-B	IVD	11F1	Mouse	1:40	60	AR/15/100/6.0	C	Tonsil
Gross cystic disease fluid protein 15 (GCDFP-15, BRST-2)	CellMq	257M-15	IVD	23A3	Mouse	1:50	40	EDTA/15/100/8.0	C	Breast carcinoma
Growth hormone (GH)	CellMq	208A	IVD	Polyclonal	Rabbit	1:50	40	EDTA/15/100/8.0	C	Pituitary gland
HBME-1 (HBME1, mesothelial cell)	CellMq	CXA128	IVD	HBME-1	Mouse	Pre-diluted	40	TRS/20/99/6.1	M, C	Mesothelioma, thyroid carcinoma
Helicobacter pylori (*H. pylori*, HP)	DAKO	B0471	ASR	Polyclonal	Rabbit	1:20	30	ProtK/9/Ambient/7.5	E	*H. Pylori*
Hep Par1 (Hep-Par1, Hep Par-1, hepatocyte specific antigen)	DAKO	M7158	IVD	OCH1E5	Mouse	1:600	40	EDTA/15/100/8.0	C	Liver
Hepatitis B virus core antigen (HBVCA)	Biogx	PU082-UP	ASR	Polyclonal	Rabbit	1:20	30	None	N	HEP B.C.
Hepatitis B virus surface antigen (HBVSA)	Biogx	Mu-364-UC	ASR	A34060259P	Mouse	Pre-diluted	30	None	C	HEP B.S
Her-2/neu (c-erbB-2, Her-2)	Zymed	28-8003	ASR	TAB250	Mouse	1:800	30	ProtK/9/Ambient/7.5	M	Herpes
Herpes simplex virus I and II (HSV I and II, HSV1&2)	DAKO	B 0114	IVD	Polyclonal	Rabbit	1:100	60	ProtK/9/Ambient/7.5	N	Herpes
Human chorionic gonadotropin (hCG)	DAKO	A0231	IVD	Polyclonal	Rabbit	1:2000	30	ProtK/9/Ambient/7.5	C	Placenta
Human herpes virus 8 (HHV-8, HHV8)	Ventana	760-4260	IVD	13B10	Mouse	Pre-diluted	40	EDTA/15/100/8.0	N	Kaposi's sarcoma
Human melanoma black-45 (HMB-45, HMB45)	DAKO	M0634	IVD	HMB45	Mouse	1:75	30	TUF/10/99/8.0	C	Skin
Human placental lactogen (hPL)	Ventana	7604443	IVD	Polyclonal	Rabbit	Pre-diluted	40	EDTA/15/100/8.0	C	Placenta
Immunoglobulin A (IgA)	DAKO	A0262	IVD	Polyclonal	Rabbit	1:1200	60	ProtK/9/Ambient/7.5	C	Tonsil
Immunoglobulin D (IgD)	DAKO	A0093	IVD	Polyclonal	Rabbit	1:300	30	ProtK/9/Ambient/7.5	C	Tonsil
Immunoglobulin G (IgG)	DAKO	A0423	IVD	Polyclonal	Rabbit	1:1600	60	ProtK/9/Ambient/7.5	C	Tonsil
Immunoglobulin M (IgM)	DAKO	A0425	IVD	Polyclonal	Rabbit	1:2000	60	ProtK/9/Ambient/7.5	C	Tonsil
Inhibin alpha (INH-A, inhibin-α, inhibin-alpha)	DAKO	M3609	IVD	R1	Mouse	1:25	30	AR/15/100/6.0	C	Adrenal gland
INI-1 (hSNF5, INI 1, SMARCB)	CellMq	272M-16	IVD	MRQ-27	Mouse	1:50	40	EDTA/15/100/8.0	N	Tonsil
Insulin	DAKO	A0564	IVD	Polyclonal	Guinea pig	1:400	30	None	C	Pancreas
Insulin-like growth factor 2 mRNA binding protein 3 (IGF-2, KOC, IMP-3, IGF2, IGF2BP3)	DAKO	M3626	IVD	69.1	Mouse	1:50	40	EDTA/15/100/8.0	C	Pancreatic ADC or Block #1
Kappa light chains (kappa)	DAKO	A0192	IVD	Polyclonal	Rabbit	1:2000	30	ProtK/9/Ambient/7.5	C	Tonsil
Ki-67 (MIB-1)	DAKO	M7240	IVD	MIB-1	Mouse	1:75	40	EDTA/15/100/8.0	N	Tonsil
Kidney-specific cadherin (ksp-cad, cadherin 16)	CellMq	276M-98	IVD	MRQ-33	Mouse	Pre-diluted	30	EDTA/15/100/8.0	M, C	Kidney

(continued)

(continued)

Antibody name and synonyms	Vendor	Catalog no.	Approved use	Clonality	Host animal	Dilution	Inc. time (min)	AR method/time/ temp./pH	Localization	Control tissue
Lambda light chains (lambda)	DAKO	A0193	IVD	Polyclonal	Rabbit	1:1200	30	ProtK/9/Ambient/7.5	C	Tonsil
Leutenizing hormone (LH)	CellMq	209A	IVD	Polyclonal	Rabbit	1:100	40	EDTA/15/100/8.0	C	Pituitary gland
Lysozyme (LYZ)	DAKO	A0099	IVD	Polyclonal	Rabbit	1:600	30	AR/15/100/6.0	C	Tonsil
Mammaglobin (MGB)	DAKO	M3625	IVD	304-1A5	Mouse	1:100	40	EDTA/15/100/8.0	C	Breast carcinoma (ductal)
MART-1	BioM	CM077C	IVD	M2-7c10+M2-9E3	Mouse	1:80	40	Borg/20/99/9.5	C	Melanoma
Maspin	BD	554292	RUO	G167-70	Mouse	1:200	40	EDTA/15/100/8.0	N, C	Pancreatic ADC
Melan-A	DAKO	M7196	IVD	A103	Mouse	1:30	30	AR/15/100/6.0	C	Skin
Melanoma (NL-2, PNL2)	DAKO	N1601	RUO	PNL-2	Mouse	Pre-diluted	30	EDTA/15/100/8.0	C	Melanoma
Melanoma-associated antigen (NKI-C3, MAA)	Biogx	MU077-UC	IVD	NKI-C3	Mouse	1:40	30	None	M, C	Skin
Microphthalmia transcription factor (MiTF)	DAKO	M3621	IVD	D5	Mouse	1:100	40	EDTA/15/100/8.0	N	Melanoma
Mini chromosome maintenance protein-2, (MCM-2, MCM2)	Vector	VP-M651	RUO	CRCT2.1	Mouse	1:25	60	EDTA/15/100/8.0	N	Tonsil
MLH1	BD	550838	RUO	G168-15	Mouse	1:5	60	AR/15/100/6.0	N	Colon ADC
MOC-31 (MOC31)	DAKO	M3525	IVD	MOC-31	Mouse	1:100	30	TRS/20/99/6.1	M, C	Colon
MSH2 (MSH-2)	CellMq	286M-16	IVD	G219-1129	Mouse	1:25	60	EDTA/15/100/8.0	N	Colon ADC
MSH6 (MSH-6)	Invitro	18-0443	IVD	2D4B5	Mouse	1:25	60	EDTA/15/100/8.0	N	Colon ADC
MUC (MUC-1)	Vector	VP-M654	RUO	Ma 552	Mouse	1:100	60	TRS/20/99/6.1	M, C	Breast CA
MUC2 (MUC-2)	Vector	VP-M656	RUO	Ccp 58	Mouse	1:100	60	EDTA/15/100/8.0	C	Small bowel
MUC4 (MUC-4)	Sigma	HPA005895	RUO	Polyclonal	Rabbit	1:150	30	AR/15/100/6.0	M, C	Block #1
MUC5AC (MUC-5AC)	Vector	VEC.VP-M657	RUO	CLH2	Mouse	1:50	60	Hi pH/20/99/9.9	C	Stomach
MUC6, MUC-6	Vector	VP-M658	RUO	CLH5	Mouse	1:50	60	Hi pH/20/99/9.9	C	Stomach
MUM1, MUM-1	DAKO	M7259	IVD	MUM1p(1)	Mouse	1:30	60	EDTA/15/100/8.0	N	Skin
Muscle specific actin (MSA)	DAKO	M0635	IVD	HHF35	Mouse	1:300	30	TUF/10/99/8	C	Soft tissue tumors with muscle
Myelin basic protein (MBP)	CellMq	295A-15	IVD	Polyclonal	Rabbit	1:200	40	EDTA/15/100/8.0	C	Brain
Myeloperoxidase (MPO)	DAKO	A0398	IVD	Polyclonal	Rabbit	1:2400	30	None	C	Myeloid leukemia
MyoD1	DAKO	M3512	IVD	5.8A	Mouse	1:25	40	TRS/20/99/6.1	N	Rhabdomyosarcoma
Myogenin	CellMq	296M-15	IVD	F5D	Mouse	1:25	40	TRS/20/99/6.1	N	Rhabdomyosarcoma
Myoglobin	CellMq	297A-75	IVD	Polyclonal	Rabbit	1:200	40	EDTA/15100/8.0	C	Skeletal muscle
Myosin, smooth muscle (SMMH1, smooth muscle myosin, heavy chain)	CellMq	298M-15	IVD	SMMS-1	Mouse	1:25	40	EDTA/15/100/8.0	C	Smooth muscle
Napsin A	CellMq	352A-76	IVD	Polyclonal	Rabbit	1:100	40	EDTA/15/100/8.0	C	Lung ADC
NB84a (neuroblastoma antibody)	Abcam	Ab49504	RUO	NB84a	Mouse	1:100	40	Trypsin/15/Ambient/ NA	C	Neuroblastoma
Nerve growth factor receptor (NGFR)	DBS	Mob 495-05	IVD	ME20.4	Mouse	1:50	40	TRS/20/99/6.1	C	Melanoma
Neurofilament (NF)	DAKO	M0762	IVD	2F11	Mouse	1:250	30	TRS/20/99/6.1	C	GFAP positive tissue
Neuron-specific anolase (NSE)	CellMq	306M-15	IVD	E27	Mouse	1:400	30	TRS/20/99/6.1	C	Appendix
OCT3/4	BioM	PM 313 A	IVD	SEMGC	Mouse	Pre-diluted	30	EDTA/15/100/8.0	N	Seminoma
OCT4	CellMq	CXA122	IVD	MRQ-10	Mouse	Pre-diluted	40	EDTA/15/100/8.0	N	Seminoma
p120 catenin, (p120ctn)	BD	610134	RUO	98/pp120	Mouse	1:400	30	TRS/20/99/6.1	M, C	Epithelial carcinoma
p53	Biogx	MU195-UC	IVD	BP53-12	Mouse	1:100	30	AR/15/100/6.0	N	Block #1

p57Kip2	CellMq	457M-95	IVD	Kp10	Mouse	1:600	40	TRS/20/100/6.1	N	Placenta
p63	CellMq	463M-15	RUO	4A4	Mouse	1:50	40	TRS/20/100/6.1	N	Breast/prostate
Paired box gene 2 (PAX2, PAX-2)	CellMq	311A-15	IVD	Polyclonal	Rabbit	1:10	40	AR/15/100/6.0	N	Renal carcinoma
Pancrease/duodenum homeobox 1 (PDX1, IPF1)	R&D	MAB2419	RUO	267712	Mouse	1:25	40	EDTA/15/100/8.0	N	Pancreatic carcinoma
Pancytokeratin (pan-CK, MNF116)	DAKO	M0821	IVD	MNF116	Mouse	1:100	40	ProtK/9/100/7.5	C	Epithelial tumors
Pancytokeratin (pan-CK, MNF116)	DBS	MOB 052-05	IVD	MNF116	Mouse	1:25	40	EDTA/15/100/8.0	M, C	Skin
Parafibromin (HRPT2)	SantaC	Sc-33638	RUO	2H1	Mouse	1:100	40	EDTA/15/100/8.0	N, C	Parathyroid adenoma
Parathyroid hormone (PTH)	CellMq	310M-25	IVD	MRQ31	Mouse	1:100	40	EDTA/15/100/8.0	C	Parathyroid adenoma
Parvalbumin	Vector	VP-P963	RUO	2E11	Mouse	1:100	60	EDTA/15/100/8.0	N, C	Oncocytoma/ chromophobe RCC
PAX5 (BSAP, PAX-5)	CellMq	312M	IVD	24	Mouse	Pre-diluted	40	EDTA/15/100/8	N	Tonsil
PAX-8 (PAX8)	BioM	PP379AA	IVD	Polyclonal	Rabbit	Pre-diluted	60	EDTA/15/100/8.0	N	Renal tissue
P-cadherin (p-cad)	Vector	VP-P965	IVD	56C1	Mouse	1:50	60	TRS/20/100/6.1	M	Placenta, skin
Phosphatase and tensin homology (PTEN)	DAKO	M3627	IVD	6H2.1	Mouse	1:100	40	EDTA/15/100/8.0	N, C	Endometrium
Phospho-histone (H3, PHH3)	Cell Sig	9714	RUO	Polyclonal	Rabbit	1:50	40	EDTA/15/100/8.0	N	Tonsil
Placental alkaline phosphatase (PLAP)	DAKO	M7191	IVD	8A9	Mouse	1:75	60	TRS/20/100/6.1	C	Placenta
PMS2 (PMS-2)	SantaC	Sc-11440	RUO	Polyclonal	Rabbit	1:25	60	EDTA/15/100/8.0	N	Colon carcinoma
Pneumocystis jiroveci (*carinii*)	Ventana	760-2665	ASR	3F6	Mouse	Pre-diluted	40	EDTA/15/100/8.0	M	Lung
ProExC (Pro-ExC)	BD	005-11000-40	IVD	MCM2 26H6.19, MCM2 27C5.6, Top2A SWT3D1	Mouse	Pre-diluted	40	EDTA/15/100/8.0	N	Cervical SQCC
Progesterone receptor (PR)	CellMq	323R-16	ASR	Y85	Rabbit	1:25	40	EDTA/15/100/8.0	N	Breast carcinoma
Prolactin (PRL)	CellMq	210A-15	IVD	Polyclonal	Rabbit	1:100	40	EDTA/15/100/8.0	C	Pituitary gland
Proliferating nuclear cell antigen (PCNA)	DAKO	M0879	IVD	PC10(5)	Mouse	1:200	30	EDTA/15/100/8.0	N	Block #1
Prostate stem cell antigen (PSCA)	NeoMK	RB9098-P1	IVD	IG8	Rabbit	1:25	30	AR/15/100/6.0	C	Bladder/prostate carcinoma
Prostate-specific acid phosphatase (PSAP)	CellMq	326M-15	IVD	PASE/4LJ	Mouse	1:25	60	EDTA/15/100/8.0	C	Prostate
Prostate-specific antigen (PSA)	DAKO	M0750	IVD	ER-PR8	Mouse	1:75	30	TUF/10/99/8.0	C	Prostate
Protein gene product 9.5 (PGP 9.5, PGP9.5)	BioM	CM329 BK	IVD	31A3	Mouse	1:250	60	EDTA/15/100/8.0	C	Kidney
Renal cell carcinoma marker (RCCMa)	Vector	Vp-R150	RUO	66.4.C2	Mouse	1:25	60	TRS/20/99/6.1	M, C	Kidney, RCC
Ron oncogene	BD	610745	RUO	29	Mouse	1:750	60	EDTA/15/100/8.0	C	Renal oncocytoma
S100	DAKO	Z0311	IVD	Polyclonal	Rabbit	1:800	30	TRS/20/99/6.1	N, C	Melanoma
S100A1	NeoMK	MS-1801-S	RUO	DAK-S100A1/1	Mouse	1:40	30	EDTA/15/100/8.0	N, C	Kidney, RCC
S100A6 (anti-calcyclin)	Sigma	S5049	RUO	CACY-100	Mouse	1:1000	30	ProtK/9/Ambient/7.5	N, C	Block #1
S100P	BD	610307	RUO	Clone 16	Mouse	1:100	30	ProtK/12/Ambient/7.5	N, C	Urothelial CA
Sal-like protein 4 (SALL4, SALL-4)	BioM	CM384 C	IVD	6E3	Mouse	1:100	30	EDTA/15/100/8.0	N	Seminoma

(continued)

(continued)

Antibody name and synonyms	Vendor	Catalog no.	Approved use	Clonality	Host animal	Dilution	Inc. time (min)	AR method/time/temp./pH	Localization	Control tissue
Serotonin	DAKO	M0758	IVD	5HT-H209	Mouse	1:25	40	ProtK/9/Ambient/7.5	C	EC cells in colon
Smoothelin	BioM	CM372 C	IVD	R4A	Mouse	1:50	40	EDTA/15/100/8.0	C	Bladder or colon CA
SOX10	Abcam	Ab25978	RUO	Polyclonal	Rabbit	1:200	40	TRS/20/99/6.1	N	Block #1
SV40 (BK virus)	EMO	DP02	RUO	PAb416	Mouse	1:100	40	AR/15/100/6.0	N	BK Virus (trans-planted kidney)
Synaptophysin (synap)	BioM	CM371 CK	IVD	27G12	Mouse	1:150	30	EDTA/15/100/8.0	C	Pancreas
Tartrate resistant acid phos-phatase (TRAP, TRAcP)	CellMq	341M-95	IVD	9C5	Mouse	1:100	40	EDTA/15/100/8.0	C	Hairy cell leukemia
Terminal deoxynucleotidyl transferase (TdT)	DAKO	A3524	IVD	Polyclonal	Rabbit	1:40	60	Hi pH/20/99/9.9	N	Lymphoblastic lymphoma
Thrombomodulin (TM)	DAKO	M0617	IVD	1009	Mouse	1:100	40	None	C	Block #1
Thyroglobulin (TGB)	DAKO	M0781	IVD	DAK-Tg6	Mouse	1:2000	30	None	C	Thyroid
Thyroid transcription factor I (TF1, TTF-1)	CellMq	343M-95	IVD	8G7G3/1	Mouse	1:100	40	EDTA/15/100/8.0	N	Lung ADC
Thyroid-stimulating hormone (TSH)	CellMq	211A-15	IVD	Polyclonal	Rabbit	1:50	60	EDTA/15/100/8.0	C	Pituitary gland
Topo II-alpha (top II-α, topoIIa, topo-IIa, topo IIalpha)	Vector	VP-T484	RUO	3F6	Mouse	1:20	30	EDTA/15/100/8.0	N	Tonsil
Transcription factor E3 (TFE3)	Sigma	HPA023881	RUO	Polyclonal	Rabbit	1:450	40	EDTA/15/100/8.0	N	Translocation RCC
Triple stain (CK5/CK14/p63+/P504S, PIN-4 cocktail)	BioM	PPM 225 DS AA, H, L	RUO	XM26 + LL002 + BC4A4 + N/A	Mouse, rabbit	Pre-diluted	40	EDTA/15/100/8.0	N, M, C	Prostate carcinoma
Tyrosinase	CellMq	344M-95	IVD	T311	Mouse	1:100	40	EDTA/15/100/8.0	C	Skin
Ulex Europaeus agglutinin-1 (UEA-1, UEA1)	Sigma	U4754	RUO	Polyclonal	Rabbit	1:200	40	EDTA/15/100/8.0	C	Prostate
Uroplakin III (UPIII, UP-III)	CellMq	345M-15	IVD	AU-11	Mouse	1:25	40	EDTA/15/100/8.0	M, C	Urothelial CA
Vascular endothelial growth factor (VEGF)	DAKO	M7273	RUO	VG1(1)	Mouse	1:50	30	EDTA/15/100/8.0	C	Block #1
Vasoactive intestinal peptide (VIP)	SantaC	Sc-25347	RUO	H6	Mouse	1:150	60	TRS/20/100/6.1	C	Colon
Villin	CellMq	346M-15	IVD	CWWB1	Mouse	1:100	40	EDTA/15/100/8.0	M, C	Block #1
Vimentin (Vim)	Biogx	MU074-UC	IVD	V9	Mouse	1:300	30	None	C	Block #1
Von Hippel-Lindau tumor suppressor gene protein (VHL, pVHL)	SantaC	Sc-5575	RUO	Polyclonal	Rabbit	1:50	30	ProtK/9/Ambient/7.5	M, C	Kidney
Von Willebrand factor (VWF)	DAKO	M0616	IVD	F8/86	Mouse	1:25	60	EDTA/15/100/8.0	M	Tonsil
Wilms tumor gene 1 (WT1, WT-1, WTG1, WTG-1)	NeoMK	RB-9267P	IVD	Polyclonal	Rabbit	1:200	30	EDTA/15/100/8.0	N	Wilms' tumor, mesothelial cells

Localization (N, M, C, E: nuclear, membranous, cytoplasmic, extracellular)

IVD in vitro diagnostic use, *ASR* analyte-specific reagent, *RUO* for research use only

Block #1 contains: endometrial ADC, kidney, tonsil, breast, melanoma, colon ADC, renal cell carcinoma, lung ADC

ADC adenocarcinoma, *SQCC* squamous cell carcinoma, *CA* carcinoma, *RCC* renal cell carcinoma, *HCC* hepatocellular carcinoma, *Inc* incubation, *AR* antigen retrieval, *NA* not applicable

Vendor Information

AbD: AbD Serotec(USA). 3200 Atlantic Avenue, Ste 125, Raleigh, NC 27604. Tel.: 919-878-7978; Fax: 919-878-3751.

Abcam: Abcam Inc. 1 Kendall Square, Ste 341, Cambridge, MA 02139-01517. Tel.: 617-225-2272; Fax: 866-739-9884.

Alpco: American Laboratory Products Company. 26-G Keewaydin Drive, Salem, NH 03079. Tel.: 603-893-8914; Fax: 603-898-6854.

BD: Becton Dickinson Immunocytometry Systems (BD Biosciences). 2350 Qume Drive, San Jose, CA 95131. Tel.: 877-232-8995; Fax: 800-325-9637.

Biogx: BioGenex Laboratories Inc. 4600 Norris Canyon Road, San Ramon, CA 94583. Tel.: 925-275-0550; Fax: 925-275-1999.

BioM: Biocare Medical. 4040 Pike Lane, Concord, CA 94520. Tel.: 800-799-9499; Fax: 925-603-8080.

CellMq: Cell Marque Corporation. 6600 Sierra College Blvd, Rocklin, CA 95677. Tel.: 916-746-8900; Fax: 916-746-8989.

Cell Sig: Cell Signaling Technology, Inc. 3 Trask Lane, Danvers, MA 01923. Tel.: 877-616-2355; Fax: 978-867-2488.

Covance: Covance. 5858 Horton Street, Suite 500, Emeryville, CA 94608. Tel.: 800-922-2226; Fax: 888-320-4837.

DAKO: Dako North America, Inc. 6392 Via Real, Carpinteria, CA 93013. Tel.: 800-235-5763; Fax: 800-566-3256.

DBS: Diagnostic Biosystems Inc. Diagnostic BioSystems, 1020 Serpentine Ln. Suite #114, Pleasanton, CA 94566. Tel.: 888-896-3350; Fax: 925-484-3390.

EMD: EMD Chemicals, Inc. (Calbiochem). 480 S. Democrat Road, Gibbstown, NJ 08027. Tel.: 800-854-3417; Fax: 800-776-0999.

GeneTex: GeneTex, Inc. 2456 Alton Pkwy, Irvine, CA 92606. Tel.: 877-436-3839; Fax: 949-309-2888.

Invitro: Invitrogen Corporation. 1600 Faraday Ave, Carlsbad, CA 92008. Tel.: 800-955-6288; Fax: 800-331-2286.

Leica: Leica Biosystems Newcastle Ltd. 2345 Waukegan Road, Bannockburn, IL 60015. Tel.: 800-248-0123; Fax: 847-405-0164.

Millipo: Millipore Corporate Headquarters. 290 Concord Road, Billerica, MA 01821. Tel.: 800-645-5476; Fax: 800-645-5439.

NeoMK: Neo Markers, Inc. 47790 Westinghouse Drive, Fremont, CA 94539. Tel.: 510-991-2800; Fax: 510-991-2826.

NOVO: Novocastra Laboratories Ltd. Balliol Business Park West, Benton Lane, Newcastle upon Tyne NE12 8EW, UK. Tel.: 44 (0) 191-215-0567; Fax: 44 (0) 191-215-1152.

R&D: R&D systems, Inc. 614 McKinley Place N.E, Minneapolis, MN 55413. Tel.: 800-343-7475; Fax: 612-656-4400.

SantaC: Santa Cruz Biotechnology, Inc. 2145 Delaware Avenue, Santa Cruz, CA 95060. Tel.: 800-457-3800; Fax: 831-457-3801.

Sigma: Sigma Aldrich Corporation. 3050 Spruce Street, Saint Louis, MO 63103. Tel.: 314-771-5765; Fax: 314-286-7828.

Thermo: Thermo Fisher Scientific. 46360 Fremont Blvd, Fremont, CA 94538. Tel.: 510-771-1560; Fax: 510-771-1570.

Vector: Vector Laboratories, Inc. 30 Ingold Road, Burlingame, CA 94010. Tel.: 650-697-3600; Fax: 650-697-0339.

Ventana: North American Corporate Headquarters. 1910 Innovation Park Drive, Tucson, AZ 85755. Tel.: 520-887-2155; Fax: 520-229-6855.

ZETA: Zeta Corporation. PO Box 282, Sierra Madre, CA 91205. Tel.: 626-355-2053; Fax: 626-836-9149.

Zymed: Zymed. 458 Carlton Court, San Francisco, CA 94080. Tel.: 800-874-4494; Fax: 415-871-4499.

Appendix B

Antibody name and synonyms	Vendor ID	Catalog no.	Approved use	Clonality	Host animal	Dilution	Inc. time (mins)	AR method/time/temp./pH	Localization	Control tissue
Actin, smooth muscle (SMA, smooth muscle actin)	DAKO	M0851	IVD	1A4	Mouse	1:150	8	CC1 short/8/95/8	C	Leiomyosarcoma
Adrenocorticotropic hormone (ACTH)	CellMq	206A	IVD	Polyclonal	Rabbit	1:100	48	CC1 mild/32/95/8	C	Normal pituitary
Alpha-1-antichymotrypsin (A-ACT, A1ACT)	Ventana	760-2604	IVD	Polyclonal	Rabbit	Pre-diluted	32	CC1 mild/32/95/8	C	Liver
Alpha-1-antitrypsin (A1AT)	Ventana	760-2605	IVD	Polyclonal	Rabbit	Pre-diluted	32	CC1 mild/32/95/8	C	Tonsil
Alpha-fetoprotein (AFP)	DAKO	N1501	IVD	Polyclonal	Rabbit	1:2	40	CC1 standard/64/95/8	C	Germ cell tumor
Alpha-methylacyl-CoA racemase (AMACR, P504S)	BioM	PP365JJ	ASR	Polyclonal	Rabbit	Pre-diluted	16	CC1 mild/32/95/8	C	Prostate
Anaplastic lymphoma kinase-1 (ALK-1, ALK1)	Ventana	790-2918	IVD	ALK01	Mouse	Pre-diluted	16	CC1 standard/64/95/8	N	ALK+ tissue
Androgen receptor protein (ARP)	CellMq	200M-18	IVD	AR441	Mouse	Pre-diluted	36	CC1 standard/64/95/8	N	Prostate
Annexin A1 (ANXA-1)	Ventana	760-4435	IVD	MRQ-3	Mouse	Pre-diluted	40	CC1 mild/32/95/8	M, C	Hairy cell leukemia
B cell Oct binding protein 1 (BOB.1)	NOVO	NCL-L-BOB-1	ASR	TG14	Mouse	1:20	40	CC1 standard/64/95/8	N	B-cell lymphoma
B72.3 (TAG 72, BRST-3,BRST3)	Ventana	760-2669	IVD	B72.3	Mouse	Pre-diluted	24	CC1 mild/32/95/8	C	Block #1
B-cell CLL/lymphoma 1 (Bcl-1, Cyclin D1, Bcl1)	Ventana	760-4282	IVD	SP4	Rabbit	Pre-diluted	32	CC1 standard/64/95/8	N	Mantle cell lymphoma
B-cell CLL/lymphoma 2 (Bcl-2, Bcl2)	Ventana	760-4240	IVD	124	Mouse	Pre-diluted	16	CC1 standard/64/95/8	C	Tonsil
B-cell CLL/lymphoma 6 (Bcl-6, Bcl6)	Ventana	760-4241	IVD	GI191E/A8	Mouse	Pre-diluted	32	CC1 standard/64/95/8	N	Tonsil
Beta-catenin (B-catenin)	Ventana	760-4242	IVD	14	Mouse	Pre-diluted	16	CC1 mild/32/95/8	N, M, C	Block #1
C4d	Ventana	760-4436	IVD	Polyclonal	Rabbit	1:50	32	CC1 standard/64/95/8	M, C	Transplanted kidney
Calcitonin	Ventana	760-2611	IVD	Polyclonal	Rabbit	Pre-diluted	32	CC1 mild/32/95/8	C	Medullary thyroid CA
Caldesmon	Ventana	760-4375	IVD	E89	Rabbit	Pre-diluted	32	CC1 standard/64/95/8	C	Smooth muscle
Calponin 1 (CALP-1)	Ventana	760-4376	IVD	EP798Y	Rabbit	Pre-diluted	32	CC1 standard/64/95/8	C	Uterus
Calretinin (CALRET)	Ventana	760-2700	IVD	Polyclonal	Rabbit	Pre-diluted	32	CC1 mild/32/95/8	N, C	Mesothelial cells
Cancer antigen 15-3 (CA15-3, CA 15-3)	Ventana	760-2608	IVD	DF3	Mouse	Pre-diluted	32	CC1 standard/64/95/8	C	Normal breast pancreas CA
Cancer antigen 19-9 (CA19-9, CA 19-9)	Ventana	760-2609	IVD	121SLE	Mouse	Pre-diluted	16	CC1 mild/32/95/8	C	Block #1
Cancer antigen-125 (CA-125, CA 125)	Ventana	760-2610	IVD	OC125	Mouse	Pre-diluted	12	CC1 mild/32/95/8	C	Ovarian CA
Carcinoembryonic antigen (CEA)	Biogx	MU009-UC	IVD	B01-94-11M-P	Mouse	1:250	40	CC1 short/8/95/8	C	Block #1
CD10	Ventana	760-2705	IVD	56C6	Mouse	Pre-diluted	56	CC1 mild/32/95/8	M, C	Tonsil
CD105 (endoglin)	DAKO	M3527	IVD	SN6h	Mouse	1:5	32	Protease 1/8/37/NA	C	RCC
CD117 (c-kit)	Ventana	790-2951	IVD	9.7	Rabbit	Pre-diluted	20	CC1 mild/32/95/8	M, C	CD117 (GIST)
CD138 (syndecan 1)	Ventana	760-4248	IVD	B-A38	Mouse	Pre-diluted	28	CC1 mild/32/95/8	M, C	Tonsil
CD15 (Leu-M1)	Ventana	760-2504	IVD	MMA	Mouse	Pre-diluted	40	CC1 mild/32/95/8	M, C	Tonsil
CD163	Ventana	760-4437	IVD	MRQ-26	Mouse	Pre-diluted	40	CC1 standard/64/95/8	M, C	Tonsil
CD19	DAKO	M7296	IVD	LE-CD19	Mouse	1:50	40	CC1 standard/64/95/8	M	Tonsil

CD1a	Ventana	760-4244	IVD	MTB1	Mouse	Pre-diluted	40	CC1 mild/32/95/8	C	Skin
CD2	Biogx	MU438UC	ASR	AB75	Mouse	1:30	32	CC1 mild/32/95/8	M, C	Tonsil
CD20	Ventana	760-2531	IVD	L26	Mouse	Pre-diluted	16	CC1 short/8/95/8	M	Tonsil
CD21	Ventana	760-4245	IVD	2G9	Mouse	Pre-diluted	32	CC1 mild/32/95/8	M	Tonsil
CD23	Ventana	760-2616	IVD	1B12	Mouse	Pre-diluted	28	CC1 mild/32/95/8	M	Tonsil
CD25	Ventana	760-4439	IVD	4C9	Mouse	Pre-diluted	40	CC1 mild/32/95/8	M, C	Tonsil
CD3	Ventana	760-4341	IVD	2GV6	Rabbit	Pre-diluted	32	CC1 standard/64/95/8	M	Tonsil
CD30 (Ber H-1, Ber-H1)	Ventana	790-2926	IVD	BerH2	Mouse	Pre-diluted	20	CC1 standard/64/95/8	C	Embryonal CA, or block #1
CD31	DAKO	M0823	IVD	JC7OA	Mouse	1:30	32	Protease 1/8/37/NA	M, C	Tonsil
CD34	Ventana	790-2927	IVD	QBEnd/10	Mouse	Pre-diluted	8	None	C	Tonsil
CD35 (follicular dendritic cell)	Ventana	760-4255	IVD	CNA.42	Mouse	Pre-diluted	16	CC1 mild/32/95/8	M, C	Tonsil
CD4	Ventana	790-4423	IVD	SP35	Rabbit	Pre-diluted	24	CC1 standard/64/95/8	M, C	Tonsil
CD43	Ventana	7600-2511	IVD	L60	Mouse	Pre-diluted	20	CC1 mild/32/95/8	M	Tonsil
CD44	DAKO	M7082	IVD	DF1485	Mouse	1:80	40	CC1 standard/64/95/8	M	Tonsil
CD45 (LCA)	DAKO	M0701	IVD	2B11 + PD7/26	Mouse	1:80	28	CC1 mild/32/95/8	M	Tonsil
CD45RO	DAKO	M0742	IVD	UCHL1	Mouse	1:1600	20	None	M	Tonsil
CD5	CellMq	205R-18	IVD	SP19	Rabbit	Pre-diluted	40	CC1 standard/64/95/8	M	Tonsil
CD56 (NCAM)	Ventana	760-2625	IVD	123C3.D5	Mouse	Pre-diluted	40	CC1 mild/32/95/8	C, M	Neuroendocrine tumors
CD57	Ventana	760-2626	IVD	NK1	Mouse	Pre-diluted	20	CC1 standard/64/95/8	C	Tonsil
CD61	DAKO	M0753	IVD	Y2/51	Mouse	1:50	32	CC1 mild/32/95/8	C	Bone marrow, megakaryocytes
CD68	DAKO	N1576	IVD	PGM1	Mouse	Pre-diluted	28	CC1 mild/32/95/8	C	Tonsil
CD7	CellMq	107M-18	IVD	MRQ-12	Mouse	Pre-diluted	20	CC1 mild/32/95/8	M	Tonsil
CD74	Ventana	760-2628	IVD	LN2	Mouse	Pre-diluted	32	CC1 standard/64/95/8	M, C	Tonsil
CD79a	Ventana	790-2932	IVD	1.10E + 04	Mouse	Pre-diluted	12	CC1 standard/64/95/8	C	Tonsil
CD8	Ventana	760-4250	IVD	C8/144B	Mouse	Pre-diluted	8	CC1 standard/64/95/8	M	Tonsil
CD99 (MIC-2, MIC2)	Ventana	760-2631	IVD	H036-1.1	Mouse	Pre-diluted	16	CC1 mild/32/95/8	M, C	Ewing's sarcoma
CDX-2 (CDX2)	Biogx	MU392A-UC	IVD	CDX2-88	Mouse	1:30	32	CC1 mild/32/95/8	N	Colon CA
Chromogranin A (chrom)	BioM	PM010-AA	IVD	LK2H10 + PHE5	Mouse	Pre-diluted	32	CC1 standard/64/95/8	C	Pancreas
Claudin 1 (claudin-1, CLDN1, CLDN-1)	CellMq	359A-15	IVD	Polyclonal	Rabbit	1:25	40	CC1 standard/64/95/8	M	Colon, small intestine
Collagen type IV	Ventana	760-2632	IVD	CIV22	Mouse	Pre-diluted	32	Protease 1/4/37/NA	C, E	Basement membranes
COX-2 (COX2)	Ventana	760-4254	IVD	SP21	Rabbit	Pre-diluted	16	CC1 mild/32/95/8	C	Colon carcinoma
Cyclin-dependent kinase 4 (CDK4, CDK-4)	Thermo	MS-469P	RUO	DCS-31	Mouse	1:200	32	CC1 standard/64/95/8	M, C	Liposarcoma
Cytokeratin 14 (CK14)	CellMq	314M-16	IVD	LL002	Mouse	1:200	32	CC1 mild/32/95/8	C	Block #1
Cytokeratin 17 (CK17)	DAKO	M7046	IVD	E3 (1)	Mouse	1:80	32	CC1 standard/64/95/8	C	Block #1
Cytokeratin 19 (CK19)	Ventana	760-4281	IVD	(A53-B/A2.26)	Mouse	Pre-diluted	20	CC1 short/8/95/8	C	Block #1
Cytokeratin 20 (CK20)	Ventana	760-2635	IVD	Ks20.8	Mouse	Pre-diluted	28	CC1 mild/32/95/8	C	Block #1
Cytokeratin 5 (CK5)	CellMq	305R15	IVD	EP1601Y	Rabbit	1:50	32	CC1 standard/64/95/8	C	Mesothelioma
Cytokeratin 5 and 6 (CK5/6, CK 5 and 6)	Ventana	760-4253	IVD	D5 and 16B4	Mouse	Pre-diluted	32	CC1 mild/32/95/8	C	Tonsil, prostate
Cytokeratin 7 (CK7)	CellMq	307M-95	IVD	OV-TL12/30	Mouse	1:200	32	CC1 mild/32/95/8	C	Block #1
Cytokeratin 8 (CK8, 35betaH11)	CellMq	335M-96	IVD	35betaH11	Mouse	1:100	32	CC1 mild/32/95/8	C	prostate
Cytokeratin 8 and 18 (CK8/18, CK 8 and 18)	CellMq	818M	IVD	B22.1 and B23.1	Mouse	Pre-diluted	32	CC1 standard/64/95/8	C	Pancreas, prostate, salivary gland

(continued)

(continued)

Antibody name and synonyms	Vendor ID	Catalog no.	Approved use	Clonality	Host animal	Dilution	Inc. time (mins)	AR method/time/temp./pH	Localization	Control tissue
Cytokeratin AE1/AE3 (AE1/AE3)	DAKO	M3515	IVD	AE1/AE3	Mouse	1:100	32	Protease 1/4/37/NA	C	Block #1
Cytokeratin, CAM 5.2 (CAM 5.2, LMW cytokeratin, low molecular weight cytokeratin, LMWCK)	BD	349205	IVD	CAM5.2	Mouse	1:4	20	CC1 mild/32/95/8	C	Block #1
Cytokeratin, HMW/CK903 (CK903, 34betaE12, HMWCK, high molecular weight cytokeratin)	Ventana	790-4373	IVD	34betaE12	Mouse	Pre-diluted	24	Protease 1/4/37/NA	C	Prostate
Cytomegalovirus (CMV)	CellMq	213M-18	ASR	DDG9/CCH2	Mouse	Pre-diluted	32	CC1 standard/64/95/8	N	CMV infected tissue
D2-40 (podoplanin, D240)	DAKO	M3619	IVD	D2-40	Mouse	1:50	32	CC1 short/8/95/8	C	Tonsil
Desmin	Leica	ORG-8889	IVD	DE-R-11	Mouse	Pre-diluted	28	CC1 standard/64/95/8	C	Block #1
DOG1	CellMq	244R-15	IVD	SP31	Rabbit	1:50	32	CC1 standard/64/95/8	M, C	GIST
E-cadherin	DAKO	M3612	IVD	NCH-384	Mouse	1:200	48	CC1 mild/32/95/8	M	Block #1
Epithelial cell adhesion molecule antibody (Ber-EP4, EPCAM, ESA, epithelial specific antigen)	DAKO	M0804	IVD	Ber-EP4	Mouse	1:100	32	Protease 1/4/37/NA	M, C	Block #1
Epithelial membrane antigen (EMA)	Ventana	760-4259	IVD	E29	Mouse	Pre-diluted	16	CC1 mild/32/95/8	M	Block #1
Estrogen receptor (ER)	Ventana	790-4324	IVD	SP1	Rabbit	Pre-diluted	40	CC1 mild/32/95/8	N	ER
Factor VIII (FVIII)	Ventana	760-2642	IVD	Polyclonal	Rabbit	Pre-diluted	32	CC1 mild/32/95/8	C	Tonsil
Factor XIIIa (FXIIIa)	CellMq	251R-15	IVD	EP3372	Rabbit	1:60	44	CC1 mild/32/95/8	C	Tonsil
Fascin	Ventana	760-2702	IVD	55K-2	Mouse	Pre-diluted	32	CC1 mild/32/95/8	C	Tonsil
Follicle stimulating hormone (FSH)	CellMq	207A	IVD	Polyclonal	Rabbit	1:100	32	CC1 standard/64/95/8	C	Normal pituitary
FOXP1	CellMq	350A-18	IVD	Polyclonal	Rabbit	Pre-diluted	16	CC1 mild/32/95/8	N	Tonsil
Friend leukemia virus integration-1 (FLI-1, FLI1)	CellMq	254M-15	IVD	MRQ-1	Mouse	1:50	32	CC1 standard/64/95/8	N	Angiosarcoma, Ewing's sarcoma
Galectin-3 (galectin 3, GAL3, GAL-3)	Ventana	760-4256	IVD	9C4	Mouse	Pre-diluted	24	CC1 mild/32/95/8	N, C	Pancreas CA
Gastrin	Ventana	760-2643	IVD	Polyclonal	Rabbit	Pre-diluted	40	CC1 mild/32/95/8	C	Stomach
Glial fibrillary acidic protein (GFAP)	DAKO	M0761	IVD	6F2	Mouse	1:150	32	CC1 mild/32/95/8	C	Brain
Glucose transporter 1 (GLUT1, GLUT-1)	CellMq	355A-15	IVD	Polyclonal	Rabbit	1:100	32	CC1 mild/32/95/8	M	Malignant mesothelioma, colorectal carcinoma
Glycophorin A	CellMq	260M-18	IVD	GA-R2 and HIR2	Mouse	Pre-diluted	32	CC1 mild/32/95/8	M	Bone marrow
Glypican-3 (GPC3)	CellMq	261M-98	IVD	1G12	Mouse	Pre-diluted	32	CC1 mild/32/95/8	C	HCC
Granzyme B	Ventana	760-4283	IVD	Polyclonal	Rabbit	Pre-diluted	32	CC1 standard/64/95/8	C	Tonsil
Gross cystic disease fluid protein 15 (GCDFP-15, BRST-2)	CellMq	257M-18	IVD	23A3	Mouse	Pre-diluted	32	CC1 standard/64/95/8	C	Breast CA
Growth hormone (GH)	CellMq	208A	IVD	Polyclonal	Rabbit	1:100	48	CC1 mild/32/95/8	C	Normal pituitary
HAM-56	Ventana	760-2657	IVD	HAM-56	Mouse	Pre-diluted	32	CC1 mild/32/95/8	C	Tonsil

HBME-1 (HBME1, mesothelial cell)	CellMq	283M-18	IVD	HBME-1	Mouse	Pre-diluted	32	CC1 mild/32/95/8	M, C	Mesothelioma
Helicobacter pylori (*H. pylori*, HP)	Ventana	760-2645	IVD	Polyclonal	Rabbit	Pre-diluted	32	CC1 standard/64/95/8	E	*H. pylori* infected tissue
Hep Par1 (Hep Par 1, Hep-Par1, Hep Par-1, Hepatocyte specific antigen)	DAKO	M7158	IVD	OCH1E5	Mouse	1:80	20	CC1 mild/32/95/8	C	Liver
Hepatitis B virus core antigen (HBVCA)	CellMq	216A-18	ASR	Polyclonal	Rabbit	Pre-diluted	32	CC1 standard/64/95/8	N	Hepatitis B infected tissue
Hepatitis B virus surface antigen (HBVSA)	CellMq	217M-18	ASR	S1-210	Mouse	Pre-diluted	32	CC1 standard/64/95/8	C	Hepatitis B infected tissue
Her-2/neu (c-erbB-2, Her-2)	Ventana	790-100	IVD	4B5	Rabbit	Pre-diluted	16	CC1 mild/32/95/8	M	Breast carcinoma
Herpes simplex virus I (HSV I, HSV1)	CellMq	361A-18	ASR	Polyclonal	Rabbit	Pre-diluted	32	Protease 1/4/37/NA	N, C	Herpes I infected tissue
Herpes simplex virus II (HSV II, HSV2)	CellMq	362A-18	ASR	Polyclonal	Rabbit	Pre-diluted	32	Protease 1/4/37/NA	N, C	Herpes II infected tissue
Human chorionic gonadotropin (hCG)	DAKO	A0231	IVD	Polyclonal	Rabbit	1:2000	32	CC1 mild/32/95/8	C	Placenta
Human herpes virus 8 (HHV-8, HHV8)	Ventana	760-4260	IVD	13B10	Mouse	Pre-diluted	32	CC1 mild/32/95/8	N	Kaposi's sarcoma
Human melanoma black-45 (HMB-45, HMB45)	CellMq	282M-98	IVD	HMB45	Mouse	Pre-diluted	24	CC1 standard/64/95/8	C	Melanoma
Human placental lactogen (hPL)	Ventana	760-4443	IVD	Polyclonal	Rabbit	Pre-diluted	40	CC1 mild/32/95/8	C	Placenta
Immunoglobulin A (IgA)	Ventana	760-2652	IVD	Polyclonal	Rabbit	Pre-diluted	16	CC1 mild/32/95/8	C	Tonsil
Immunoglobulin D (IgD)	Ventana	760-4444	IVD	Polyclonal	Rabbit	Pre-diluted	16	CC1 mild/32/95/8	C	Tonsil
Immunoglobulin G (IgG)	Ventana	760-2653	IVD	Polyclonal	Rabbit	Pre-diluted	16	CC1 mild/32/95/8	C	Tonsil
Immunoglobulin M (IgM)	Ventana	760-2654	IVD	Polyclonal	Rabbit	Pre-diluted	16	CC1 mild/32/95/8	C	Tonsil
Inhibin alpha (INH-A, inhibin-a, inhibin-alpha)	Ventana	760-2634	IVD	R1	Mouse	Pre-diluted	24	CC1 mild/32/95/8	C	Adrenal gland
INI-1 (hSNF5, INI 1, SMARCB)	CellMq	272M-16	IVD	MRQ-27	Mouse	1:30	24	CC1 standard/64/95/8	N	Tonsil
Insulin	DAKO	A0564	IVD	Polyclonal	Guinea pig	1:400	32	CC1 short/8/95/8	C	Pancreas
Insulin-like growth factor 2 mRNA binding protein 3 (IGF-2, KOC, IMP-3, IGF2, IGF2BP3)	DAKO	M3626	IVD	69.1	Mouse	1:100	32	CC1 extended/92/95/8	C	Pancreatic ADC, or block #1
Kappa light chains (Kappa)	Ventana	760-2514	IVD	L1C1	Mouse	Pre-diluted	32	Protease 1/4/37/NA	C	Tonsil
Ki-67 (MIB-1)	Ventana	790-4286	IVD	K2	Mouse	Pre-diluted	16	CC1 mild/32/95/8	N	Tonsil
Kidney-specific cadherin (ksp-cad, cadherin 16)	Ventana	760-4387	IVD	MRQ-33	Mouse	Pre-diluted	16	CC1 mild/32/95/8	M, C	Kidney
Lambda light chains (lambda)	Ventana	760-2515	IVD	Polyclonal	Rabbit	Pre-diluted	8	CC1 standard/64/95/8	C	Tonsil
Leutenizing hormone (LH)	CellMq	209A	IVD	Polyclonal	Rabbit	1:100	48	CC1 mild/32/95/8	C	Pituitary
Lysozyme (LYZ)	Ventana	760-2656	IVD	Polyclonal	Rabbit	Pre-diluted	20	CC1 mild/32/95/8	C	Tonsil
Mammaglobin (MGB)	Ventana	760-4263	IVD	31-A5	Mouse	Pre-diluted	40	CC1 standard/64/95/8	C	Breast CA (ductal)
MART-1	Ventana	790-2990	IVD	A103	Mouse	Pre-diluted	16	CC1 mild/32/95/8	C	Melanoma
Maspin	BD	554292	RUO	G167-70	Mouse	1:200	40	CC1 mild/32/95/8	N, C	Pancreatic ADC
Melan-A, (melanA)	DAKO	M7196	IVD	A103	Mouse	1:30	32	CC1 mild/32/95/8	C	Skin

(continued)

(continued)

Antibody name and synonyms	Vendor ID	Catalog no.	Approved use	Clonality	Host animal	Dilution	Inc. time (mins)	AR method/time/temp./pH	Localization	Control tissue
Microphthalmia transcription factor (MiTF)	DAKO	M3621	IVD	D5	Mouse	1:80	32	CC1 mild/32/95/8	N	Melanoma
MLH1	Ventana	760-4264	IVD	G168/728	Mouse	Pre-diluted	32	CC1 standard/64/95/8	N	Block #1
MOC-31 (MOC-31)	DAKO	M3525	IVD	MOC-31	Mouse	1:50	32	CC1 mild/32/95/8	M, C	Block #1
MSH2 (MSH-2)	Ventana	760-4265	IVD	G219-1129	Mouse	Pre-diluted	32	CC1 mild/32/95/8	N	Block #1
MSH6 (MSH-6)	Zymed	610918	RUO	44/MSH6	Mouse	1:50	48	CC1 standard/64/95/8	N	Block #1
MUC1, MUC-1	Vector	VP-M654	RUO	Ma 552	Mouse	1:200	40	CC1 standard/64/95/8	M, C	Breast CA
MUC2 (MUC-2)	Vector	VP-M656	RUO	Ccp 58	Mouse	1:100	40	CC1 standard/64/95/8	C	Small bowel
MUC4 (MUC-4)	BioM	CM326	IVD	8G-7	Mouse	1:200	40	CC1 mild/32/95/8	M, C	Block #1
MUC5AC (MUC-5AC)	Vector	VP-M657	RUO	CLH2	Mouse	1:50	40	CC1 standard/64/95/8	C	Stomach
MUC6 (MUC-6)	Vector	VP-M658	RUO	CLH5	Mouse	1:50	40	CC1 standard/64/95/8	C	Stomach
MUM1 (MUM-1)	BioM	CRM352	IVD	BC5	Mouse	1:50	40	CC1 standard/64/95/8	N, C	Skin
Muscle specific actin (MSA)	Ventana	760-2601	IVD	HHF35	Mouse	Pre-diluted	16	None	C	Soft tissue tumors with muscle
Myelin basic protein (MBP)	CellMq	295A-15	IVD	Polyclonal	Rabbit	1:100	32	CC1 short/8/95/8	C	Brain
Myeloperoxidase (MPO)	DAKO	A0398	IVD	Polyclonal	Rabbit	1:2400	32	CC1 mild/32/95/8	C	Myeloid leukemia
Myosin, smooth muscle (SMMH1, smooth muscle myosin, heavy chain)	DAKO	M3558	IVD	SMMS-1	Mouse	1:500	40	CC1 standard/64/95/8	C	Smooth muscle
Napsin A	Ventana	760-4446	IVD	Polyclonal	Rabbit	Pre-diluted	40	CC1 mild/32/95/8	C	Lung adenocarcinoma, PRCC
NB84a (neuroblastoma antibody)	Abcam	Ab49504	RUO	NB84a	Mouse	1:100	32	Protease 2/8/37/NA	C	Neuroblastoma
Nerve growth factor receptor (NGFR)	GeneTex	GTX23125	RUO	NGFR5	Mouse	1:100	40	CC1 mild/32/95/8	C	Melanoma
Neurofilament (NF)	Ventana	760-2661	IVD	2F11	Mouse	Pre-diluted	36	CC1 mild/32/95/8	C	GFAP positive tissue
Neuron-specific enolase (NSE)	Ventana	760-2662	IVD	E27	Mouse	Pre-diluted	12	CC1 mild/32/95/8	C	Appendix
OCT4	CellMq	CXA122	IVD	MRQ-10	Mouse	Pre-diluted	32	CC1 mild/32/95/8	N	Seminoma
p120 catenin (p120ctn)	BD	610134	RUO	98/pp120	Mouse	1:50	32	CC1 standard/64/95/8	M, C	Epithelial CA
p53	Ventana	790-2912	IVD	D0-7	Mouse	Pre-diluted	20	CC1 mild/32/95/8	N	Block #1
p63	DAKO	M7247	RUO	4A4	Mouse	1:150	32	CC1 standard/64/95/8	N	Breast/prostate
Paired box gene 2 (PAX2, PAX-2)	CellMq	311A-18	IVD	Polyclonal	Rabbit	Pre-diluted	24	CC1 standard/64/95/8	N	Renal CA
Pancytokeratin (pan-CK, MNF116, panCK)	DAKO	M0821	IVD	MNF116	Mouse	1:100	20	CC1 mild/32/95/8	C	Epithelial tumors
Parafibromin (HRPT2)	SantaC	Sc-33638	RUO	2H1	Mouse	1:50	60	CC1 mild/32/95/8		Parathyroid adenoma
Parathyroid hormone (PTH)	CellMq	310M-26	IVD	MRQ-31	Mouse	1:100	32	CC1 mild/32/95/8	M, C	Parathyroid adenoma
Parvalbumin	Vector	VP-P963	RUO	2E11	Mouse	1:100	40	CC1 mild//32/95/8	N, C	Oncocytoma/chromophobe RCC
Parvovirus B19	CellMq	218M-18	ASR	R92F6	Mouse	Pre-diluted	32	[a]CC2 mild/36/95/6	N, C	Parvovirus B19 infected tissue
PAX5 (BSAP, PAX-5)	Ventana	760-4270	IVD	24	Mouse	Pre-diluted	32	CC1 standard/64/95/8	N	Tonsil
PAX-8 (PAX8)	BioM	CP379AK	IVD	Polyclonal	Rabbit	1:20	32	CC1 standard/64/95/8	N	Renal tissue
Phospho-histone H3 (PHH3)	CellSig	9714	RUO	Polyclonal	Rabbit	1:50	40	CC1 standard/64/95/8	N	Tonsil

Placental alkaline phosphatase (PLAP)	Ventana	760-2664	IVD	NB10	Mouse	Pre-diluted	32	CC1 mild/32/95/8	C	Placenta
PMS2 (PMS-2)	BD	Parmingen 556415	RUO	A16-4	Mouse	1:30	48	CC1 standard/64/95/8	N	Colon CA
Progesterone receptor (PR)	Ventana	790-2223	IVD	1.00E+02	Rabbit	Pre-diluted	24	CC1 mild//32/95/8	N	Breast CA
Programmed death-1 (PD-1, PD1, CD28, NAT)	CellMq	315M-96	IVD	MRQ-22	Mouse	1:100	40	CC1 standard/64/95/8	C	Tonsil, lymph node
Prolactin (PRL)	CellMq	210A-15	IVD	Polyclonal	Rabbit	1:100	48	CC1 mild/32/95/8	C	Pituitary
Prostate stem cell antigen (PSCA)	CellMq	326M	IVD	PASE/4LJ	Mouse	1:120	24	None	C	Prostate
Prostate-specific antigen (PSA)	Ventana	760-2506	IVD	Polyclonal	Rabbit	Pre-diluted	16	CC1 short/8/95/8	C	Prostate
Protein gene product 9.5 (PGP 9.5, PGP9.5)	Ventana	760-4434	IVD	Polyclonal	Rabbit	Pre-diluted	40	CC1 mild/32/95/8	C	Kidney
Renal cell carcinoma marker (RCCMa)	Ventana	760-4273	IVD	PN-15	Mouse	Pre-diluted	40	Protease 1/8/37/NA	M, C	RCC
S100	Ventana	790-2914	IVD	4C4.9	Mouse	Pre-diluted	8	CC1 mild/32/95/8	N, C	Melanoma
S100A1	NeoMK	MS-1801-S	RUO	DAK-S100A1/1	Mouse	1:40	40	CC1 standard/64/5/8	N, C	Normal kidney, RCC
S100A6 (anti-calcyclin)	Sigma	S5049	RUO	CACY-100	Mouse	1:1000	32	Protease 1/4/37/NA	N, C	Block #1
S100P	BD	610307	RUO	Clone 16	Mouse	1:200	48	CC1 mild/32/95/8	N, C	Urothelial CA
Sal-like protein 4 (SALL4, SALL-4)	BioM	CM 384 C	IVD	6E3	Mouse	1:100	40	CC1 standard/64/95/8	N	Seoma
Serotonin	DAKO	M0758	IVD	5HT-H209	Mouse	1:25	32	Protease 1/8/37/NA	C	EC cells in colon
Smoothelin	BioM	CM372C	IVD	R4A	Mouse	1:50	32	CC1 standard/64/95/8	C	Bladder or colon carcinomas
Somatostatin	CellMq	332A-18	IVD	Polyclonal	Rabbit	1:200	40	CC1 standard/64/95/8	C	Pancreas
SV40 (BK virus)	EMD	DP02	RUO	Pab416	Mouse	1:100	32	CC1 standard/64/95/8	N	BK virus (transplanted kidney)
Synaptophysin (synap)	BioM	PM371	IVD	27G12	Mouse	Pre-diluted	52	CC1 standard/64/95/8	C	Pancreas
Terminal deoxynucleotidyl transferase (TdT)	Ventana	760-2670	IVD	Polyclonal	Rabbit	Pre-diluted	32	CC1 mild/32/95/8	N	Lymphoblastic lymphoma
Thrombomodulin (TM)	DAKO	M0617	IVD	1009	Mouse	1:60	32	None	C	Block #1
Thyroglobulin (TGB)	DAKO	M0781	IVD	DAK-Tg6	Mouse	1:200	32	None	C	Thyroid
Thyroid transcription factor 1 (TTF1, TTF-1)	Ventana	790-4398	IVD	8G7G3/1	Mouse	Pre-diluted	32	CC1 mild/32/95/8	N	Thyroid
Thyroid-stimulating hormone (TSH)	CellMq	211A-14	IVD	Polyclonal	Rabbit	1:100	48	CC1 mild/32/95/8	C	Pituitary
Topo II-alpha (top II-a, topoIIa, topo-IIa, topo IIalpha)	Vector	VP-T484	RUO	3F6	Mouse	1:20	40	CC1 standard/64/95/8	N	Tonsil
Toxoplasma gondii	CellMq	220A-18	ASR	Polyclonal	Rabbit	Pre-diluted	24	[a]CC1 standard/64/95/8	M, C	*Toxoplasma Gondii* infected tissue
Transcription factor E3 (TFE3)	Sigma	HPA023881	RUO	Polyclonal	Rabbit	1:400	40	CC2 standard/68/95/6	N	Translocation RCC
Triple stain (CK5/CK14/p63+/P504S, PIN-4 Cocktail)	BioM	PM364AAK, PP365AA	RUO	XM26+LL002 +BC4A4, Polyclonal	Mouse, rabbit	Pre-diluted	(1) 32 (2) 32	CC1 standard/64/5/8	N, M, C	Prostate
Tryptase	Ventana	760-4276	IVD	G3	Mouse	Pre-diluted	32	CC1 short/8/95/8	C	Mast cells
Tyrosinase	CellMq	344M-98	IVD	T311	Mouse	Pre-diluted	32	CC1 standard/64/95/8	C	Skin
Vascular endothelial growth factor (VEGF)	SantaC	Sc-7269	RUO	C-1	Mouse	1:80	32	CC1 mild/32/95/8	C	Block #1

(continued)

(continued)

Antibody name and synonyms	Vendor ID	Catalog no.	Approved use	Clonality	Host animal	Dilution	Inc. time (mins)	AR method/time/temp./pH	Localization	Control tissue
Villin	Ventana	760-4277	IVD	CWWB1	Mouse	Pre-diluted	32	CC1 mild/32/95/8	M, C	Block #1
Vimentin (Vim)	Ventana	790-2917	IVD	V9	Mouse	Pre-diluted	32	CC1 mild/32/95/8	C	Block #1
Von Hippel-Lindau tumor suppressor gene protein (VHL, pVHL)	SantaC	Sc-5575	RUO	Polycolonal	Rabbit	1:150	40	Protease 1/8/37/NA	M, C	Normal kidney
Von Willebrand factor (VWF)	DAKO	M0616	IVD	F8/86	Mouse	1:25	32	Protease 1/8/37/NA	M	Tonsil
Wilms tumor gene 1 (WT1, WT-1, WTG1, WTG-1)	NeoMK	RB-9267P	IVD	Polyclonal	Rabbit	1:200	20	CC1 mild/32/95/8	N	Mesothelial cells, Wilms tumor
ZAP-70 (ZAP70)	Ventana	760-4278	IVD	2F3.2	Mouse	Pre-diluted	32	CC1 mild/32/95/8	C	Chronic lymphocytic leukemia

Localization (N, M, C, E: nuclear, membranous, cytoplasmic, extracellular)

IVD in vitro diagnostic use, *ASR* analyte-specific reagent, *RUO* for research use only

Block #1 contains: endometrial ADC, kidney, tonsil, breast, melanoma, colon ADC, renal cell carcinoma, lung ADC

ADC adenocarcinoma, *SQCC* squamous cell carcinoma, *CA* carcinoma, *RCC* renal cell carcinoma, *HCC* hepatocellular carcinoma, *Inc* incubation, *AR* antigen retrieval, *NA* not applicable

[a]Manufacturer's suggested protocol

Vendor Information

AbD: AbD Serotec(USA). 3200 Atlantic Avenue, Ste 125, Raleigh, NC 27604. Tel.: 919-878-7978; Fax: 919-878-3751.

Abcam: Abcam Inc. 1 Kendall Square, Ste 341, Cambridge, MA 02139-1517. Tel.: 617-225-2272; Fax: 866-739-9884.

Alpco: American Laboratory Products Company. 26-G Keewaydin Drive, Salem, NH 03079. Tel.: 603-893-8914; Fax: 603-898-6854.

BD: Becton Dickinson Immunocytometry Systems (BD Biosciences). 2350 Qume Drive, San Jose, CA 95131. Tel.: 877-232-8995; Fax: 800-325-9637.

Biogx: BioGenex Laboratories Inc. 4600 Norris Canyon Road, San Ramon, CA 94583. Tel.: 925-275-0550; Fax: 925-275-1999.

BioM: Biocare Medical. 4040 Pike Lane, Concord, CA 94520. Tel.: 800-799-9499; Fax: 925-603-8080.

CellMq: Cell Marque Corporation. 6600 Sierra College Blvd, Rocklin, CA 95677. Tel.: 916-746-8900; Fax: 916-746-8989.

Cell Sig: Cell Signaling Technology, Inc. 3 Trask Lane, Danvers, MA 01923. Tel.: 877-616-2355; Fax: 978-867-2488.

Covance: Covance. 5858 Horton Street, Suite 500 Emeryville, CA 94608. Tel.: 800-922-2226; Fax: 888-320-4837.

DAKO: Dako North America, Inc. 6392 Via Real, Carpinteria, CA 93013. Tel.: 800-235-5763; Fax: 800-566-3256.

DBS: Diagnostic Biosystems Inc. Diagnostic BioSystems, 1020 Serpentine Ln. Suite # 114, Pleasanton, CA 94566. Tel.: 888-896-3350; Fax: 925-484-3390.

EMD: EMD Chemicals, Inc (Calbiochem). 480 S. Democrat Road, Gibbstown, NJ 08027. Tel.: 800-854-3417; Fax: 800-776-0999.

GeneTex: GeneTex, Inc. 2456 Alton Pkwy, Irvine, CA 92606. Tel.: 877-436-3839; Fax: 949-309-2888.

Invitro: Invitrogen Corporation. 1600 Faraday Ave, Carlsbad, CA 92008. Tel.: 800-955-6288; Fax: 800-331-2286.

Leica: Leica Biosystems Newcastle Ltd. 2345 Waukegan Road, Bannockburn, IL 60015. Tel.: 800-248-0123; Fax: 847-405-0164.

Millipo: Millipore Corporate Headquarters. 290 Concord Road, Billerica, MA 01821. Tel.: 800-645-5476; Fax: 800-645-5439.

NeoMK: Neo Markers, Inc. 47790 Westinghouse Drive, Fremont, CA 94539. Tel.: 510-991-2800; Fax: 510-991-2826.

NOVO: Novocastra Laboratories Ltd. Balliol Business Park West, Benton Lane, Newcastle upon Tyne NE12 8EW, UK. Tel.: 44 (0) 191-215-0567; Fax: 44 (0) 191-215-1152.

R&D: R&D systems, Inc. 614 McKinley Place N.E, Minneapolis, MN 55413. Tel.: 800-343-7475; Fax: 612-656-4400.

SantaC: Santa Cruz Biotechnology, Inc. 2145 Delaware Avenue, Santa Cruz, CA 95060. Tel.: 800-457-3800; Fax: 831-457-3801.

Sigma: Sigma Aldrich Corporation. 3050 Spruce Street, Saint Louis, MO 63103. Tel.: 314-771-5765; Fax: 314-286-7828.

Thermo: Thermo Fisher Scientific. 46360 Fremont Blvd, Fremont, CA 94538. Tel.: 510-771-1560; Fax: 510-771-1570.

Vector: Vector Laboratories, Inc. 30 Ingold Road, Burlingame, CA 94010. Tel.: 650-697-3600; Fax: 650-697-0339.

Ventana: North American Corporate Headquarters. 1910 Innovation Park Drive, Tucson, AZ 85755. Tel.: 520-887-2155; Fax: 520-229-6855.

ZETA: Zeta Corporation. PO Box 282, Sierra Madre, CA 91205. Tel.: 626-355-2053; Fax: 626-836-9149.

Zymed: Zymed. 458 Carlton Court, San Francisco, CA 94080. Tel.: 800-874-4494; Fax: 415-871-4499.

Index

Q

R

S